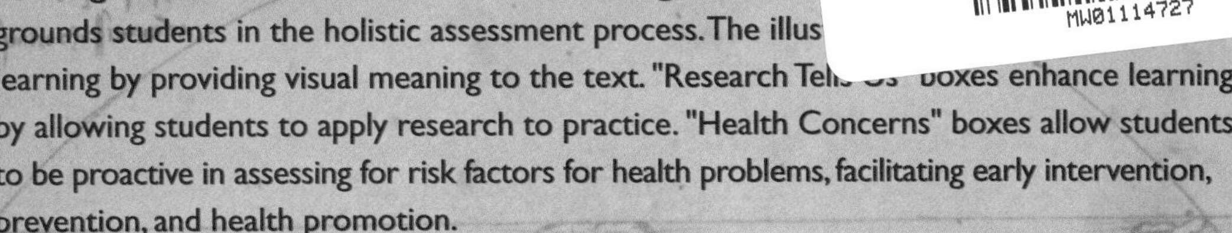

Nursing Health Assessment: A Critical Thinking, Case Stu grounds students in the holistic assessment process. The illus learning by providing visual meaning to the text. "Research Tel boxes enhance learning by allowing students to apply research to practice. "Health Concerns" boxes allow students to be proactive in assessing for risk factors for health problems, facilitating early intervention, prevention, and health promotion.

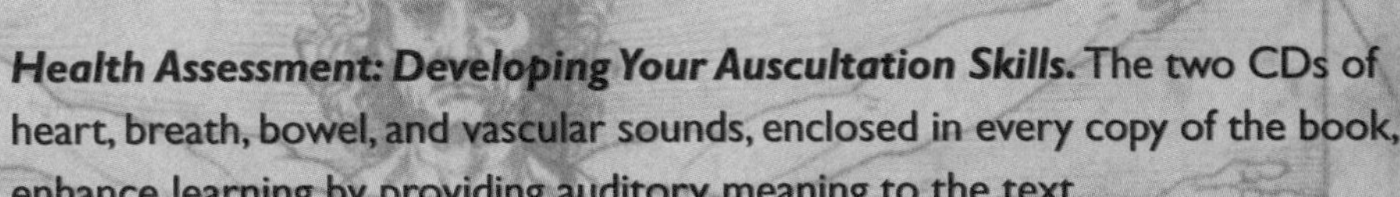

Health Assessment: Developing Your Auscultation Skills. The two CDs of heart, breath, bowel, and vascular sounds, enclosed in every copy of the book, enhance learning by providing auditory meaning to the text.

Nursing Health Assessment: An Interactive, Case Study Approach. The case studies CD-ROM enhances learning by allowing students to apply the assessment process in various situations through an interactive approach, asking them to cluster the data in support of the nursing diagnoses they have selected and giving them practice in documenting their findings.

Nursing Health Assessment: Student Applications. The applications exercises enhance learning by allowing students to review anatomy and physiology, apply the assessment process, and identify learning needs through self-evaluation in an engaging, fun way.

Nursing Health Assessment: Clinical Pocket Guide. The clinical pocket guide enhances learning by providing students with a resource in the clinical area to validate and perfect their skills.

Web Support. Access to the F.A. Davis website enhances learning by providing additional resources, such as symptom analysis tables, and encourages students to use and develop their technological skills. Go to "Explore this Product" at *http://www.fadavis.com/detail.cfm?id=0882-9.*

THE TOOLS OF NURSING HEALTH ASSESSMENT

The Dillon Difference

...any medications, prescri...

Case Study Evaluation

Before you proceed with the physical examination of the skin, hair, and nails, document the key information you have learned from Mrs. Green's health history and the integumentary history related to her.

CRITICAL THINKING ACTIVITY #1

What history findings put Mrs. Green at risk for skin problems?

CRITICAL THINKING ACTIVITY #2

What strengths can you identify that will help Mrs. Green adapt to or prevent skin disorders?

Physical Assessment

...ou have taken the history, proce... ...through your phy...

- **Assessment is a thinking, doing, and feeling process.** Rather than discuss critical thinking and clinical decision-making at the end of the text, we address these issues in the very first chapter and thereafter throughout the text. We ask students to think as they learn the assessment process. Students are not only doing and feeling, but are also thinking every step of the way.

- **Assessment is about connections.** Instead of presenting content as a series of systems, never making explicit the interaction between the systems, never fully demonstrating that a problem in one system eventually affects every other system, we show students this connection in both the anatomy and physiology review and the assessment process itself. In each system's chapter, we demonstrate the relationship of that particular system to all other systems graphically as well as in the text. Prior to the specific physical assessment of each system, we tell students to perform a general head-to-toe scan, looking for the relationships among systems. This provides a truly holistic picture of the client; not only will students assess the physical, psychosocial, cultural, developmental, and spiritual status of their clients, but they will do so in relation to the whole being.

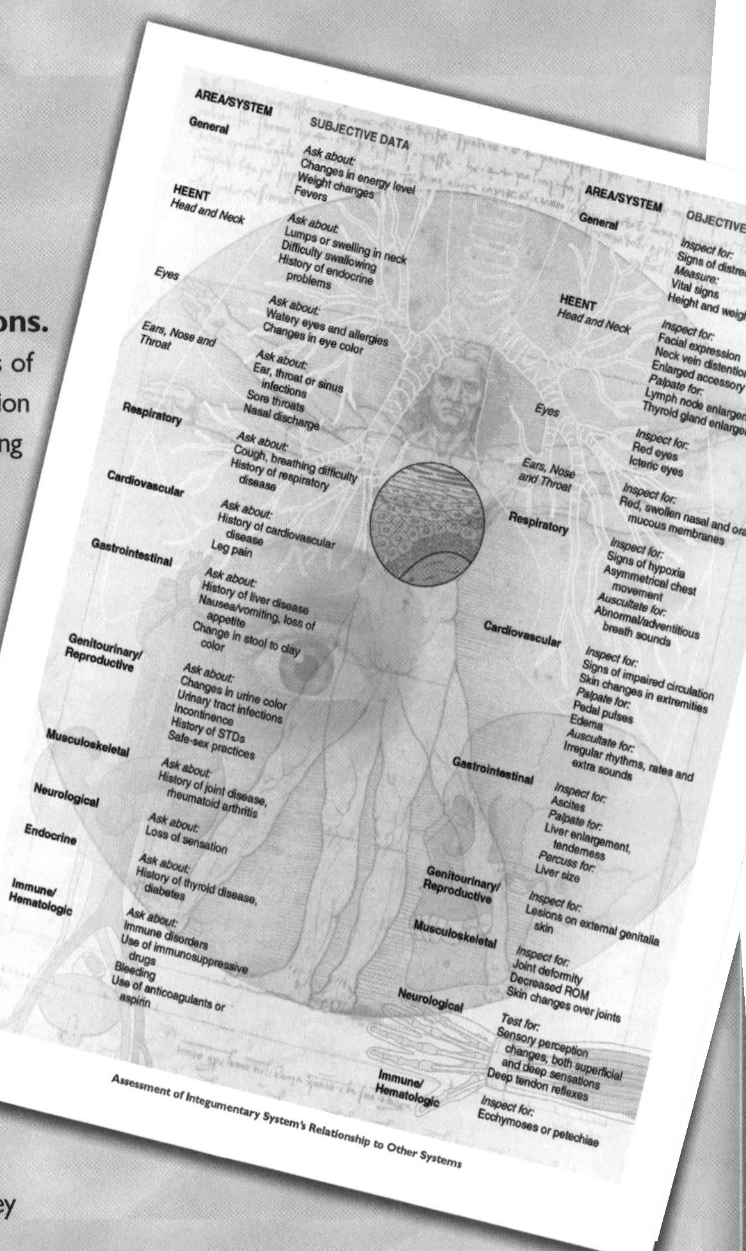

Assessment of Integumentary System's Relationship to Other Systems

is founded on the beliefs that...

- ***Assessment is about people.*** Without clinical experence, many students have difficulty understanding and applying assessment techniques. The case study approach gives students a context in which to apply assessment. The case study gives meaning to the assessment. The case study engages students in the assessment process and allows them to experience assessment.

Introducing the Case Study

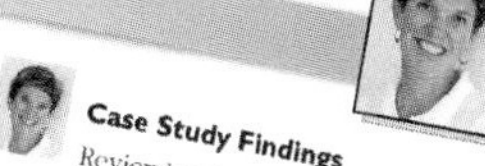

As a nurse in a community health setting, you have volunteered to participate as an examiner in a community skin cancer screening program. Eva Green, a 48-year-old woman with fair, freckled skin, presents for a total skin assessment. She states that several of her relatives have been diagnosed with skin cancer and she is very much afraid that she might have it. She goes on to say that because she has always had very freckled skin that "easily blemishes," she has difficulty determining what is normal and what should be a concern. As part of the screening program, you will complete a health history and physical examination that focuses on the integumentary system.

Case Study Findings

Reviewing Mrs. Green's biographical data:

- 48-year-old woman, married, with two adult children (27 and 22 years old)
- Works part-time in retail sales
- Born in the United States, of English-Scottish descent
- Protestant religion
- Husband is accountant and provides insurance through his employer

Current Health Status

Performing the Integumentary Assessment

- ***Unique pedagogical features enhance learning.***

Research Tells Us

Skin cancer is the most common form of malignancy in the United States. A projected one-third of Caucasians born in the U.S. after 1994 will develop at least one skin cancer. In the past, there was limited empirical evidence showing that ultraviolet light exposure actually caused skin cancers, rather than simply stimulating existing cancers. However, a recent study by the National Institute of Arthritis and Musculoskeletal and Skin Diseases of clients receiving ultraviolet treatments for psoriasis showed that those who received initial high doses of ultraviolet light, even when later treatments were at lower doses, continued to develop new skin cancers, both squamous and basal cell types. The investigators interpreted their findings as supporting the theory that ultraviolet light was capable of actually starting the cancers. Based on these findings, the institute finds strong support for using sun protection, including using a sunscreen (SPF $\geq$ 15); wearing long sleeves, pants, and wide-brimmed hats; avoiding sunlight during peak hours (10 AM to 3 PM); and seeking protection under shaded areas.

Some day there may be added measures to prevent skin cancer. Recent studies revealed that mice fed a COX-2 inhibitor (celecoxib) developed squamous cell cancers at only half the rate of mice that did not receive the drug. Further studies might find that COX-2 inhibitors or other drugs help prevent skin cancer. But for the time being, avoiding sun exposure is very important (NIH, 2000).

Health Concerns

Facts about Melanoma

- The incidence of malignant melanoma has greatly increased over the past several decades. In 1997, the overall incidence of melanoma in the United States was 14.3/100,000, up from 7.6/100,000 in 1977.
- The exact cause of the increase is not known, but sun exposure is a major contributing factor.
- The rate is higher in whites (19.3/100,000) than in blacks (0.9/100,000) and increases with age. For instance, the incidence is 10.1/100,000 for all people under age 65 and 45.5/100,000 for those aged 65 and older.
- The 5-year survival rate for persons from 1989 to 1996 averaged 88.3 percent. However, when melanoma is diagnosed at an early stage when it presents as a local site, the 5-year survival rate is 98.3/100,00. It drops to 12.5/100,000 when it has spread distally.

Common Abnormalities

ABNORMALITY	ASSESSMENT FINDINGS
Acne vulgaris Caused by sebaceous gland overactivity with plugging of hair follicles and retention of sebum, resulting in comedones, papules and pustules. Onset is typically at puberty, but acne may last into advanced age. Greater incidence in males.	• Pimples present as papules or pustules. • Cysts may develop and leave extensive scarring. • Most common on face, back, and shoulders. • Bacillus is cause. • Lesions may be sore and painful. • Aggravated by emotional distress, greasy topical applications (cosmetics) and certain medications (oral contraceptives, isoniazide,rifampin, lithium, phenobarbital) 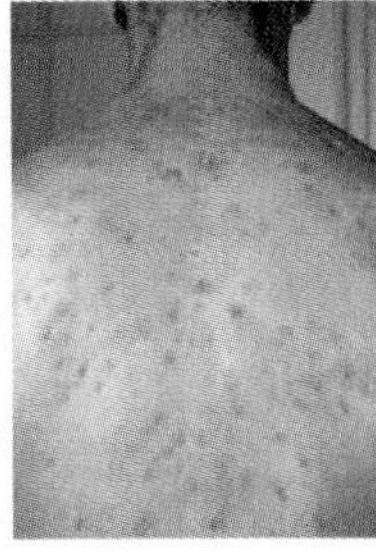

Meeting Your Resource Needs Too!

Finally, we haven't forgotten you, the educator. To enhance and augment your teaching, we have created the **Instructor's Resource Disk**, a CD containing

- ***Instructor's Guide.*** Outlines; expected outcomes; teaching strategies; student assignments; lab practicum with point values assigned for preparation, assessment process, and documentation; "Jeopardy"-style game; and "Name that…" identification exercise for each systems chapter.
- ***PowerPoint Presentation.*** Almost 300 slides covering all of health assessment which you can change to suit you and to which you can add your own slides.
- ***Electronic Test Bank and Test Constructor.*** More than 800 multiple choice questions and answers, organized by chapter, and coded with nursing process step, patient care area, and learning level. You can alter the questions and answers as necessary, you can add your own questions to the bank, you can sort questions by any number of key words, and you can create individual tests and answer sheets for every student in each class if you choose.
- ***Image Bank.*** Electronic files of every illustration used in the text—over 1300—that you can print out or import into other applications such as Word and PowerPoint, and from which you can create transparencies.

Our goal was to create a complete set of tools to help your students learn and experience assessment. Select those that best meet the learning needs of your students. If you think of other tools that we should consider for the future, don't hesitate to let us know!

Patricia M. Dillon

Patricia M. Dillon, RN, MSN, DNSc

Nursing Health Assessment

A CRITICAL THINKING, CASE STUDIES APPROACH

PATRICIA M. DILLON, DNSc, RN
Adjunct Faculty
Temple University
College of Allied Health Professions
Department of Nursing
Philadelphia, Pennsylvania

Illustrated by Dimitri Karenitkov
Photography by B. Proud

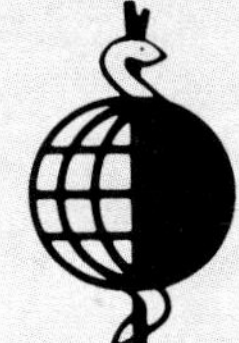

F. A. DAVIS COMPANY / PUBLISHERS • PHILADELPHIA

F. A. Davis Company
1915 Arch Street
Philadelphia, PA 19103
www.fadavis.com

Printed in the United States of America

Last digit indicates print number: 10 9 8 7 6 5 4 3 2

Acquisitions Editor: Lisa B. Deitch
Developmental Editors: Marylou Ambrose, Melanie Freely
Production Editor: Jessica Howie Martin
Cover Designer: Louis J. Forgione

As new scientific information becomes available through basic and clinical research, recommended treatments and drug therapies undergo changes. The author and publisher have done everything possible to make this book accurate, up to date, and in accord with accepted standards at the time of publication. The author, editors, and publisher are not responsible for errors or omissions or for consequences from application of the book, and make no warranty, expressed or implied, in regard to the contents of the book. Any practice described in this book should be applied by the reader in accordance with professional standards of care used in regard to the unique circumstances that may apply in each situation. The reader is advised always to check product information (package inserts) for changes and new information regarding dose and contraindications before administering any drug. Caution is especially urged when using new or infrequently ordered drugs.

Library of Congress Cataloging-in-Publication Data

Dillon, Patricia M.
Nursing health assessment : a critical thinking, case studies approach / Patricia M. Dillon.
p. ; cm.
Includes bibliographical references and index.
ISBN 0-8036-0882-9 (hard cover)
1. Nursing assessment. 2. Nursing assessment—Case studies. I. Title.
[DNLM: 1. Nursing Assessment—Case Report. 2. Medical History Taking—methods—Case Report. 3. Physical Examination—methods—Case Report. WY 100.4 D579n 2003]
RT48 .D54 2003
616.07′5—dc21

2002041005

To my patients and students, who have taught me so much.

Dear Students:

Welcome to F. A. Davis's *Nursing Health Assessment: A Critical Thinking, Case Study Approach*. Assessment is the **first step** of the nursing process and probably the **most important** because your assessment **directs the rest of the process.** It does not matter what your outcomes and goals are if you "missed it" on the assessment!

Assessment is a **thinking, doing, and feeling process.** You need to think as you act and interact with your patients. **Think critically** as you proceed through the assessment process and make clinical decisions.

Assessment is a skill, and as with any skill, the more you **practice,** the better you become. This book will walk you through the assessment process, but it is up to you to develop the skill. As a beginning practitioner, focus on learning the normal. Once you are able to identify the normal, if something abnormal occurs, you will know! Initially, you may not be able to identify the abnormal, but you will know that it does not belong. Don't worry; with practice you will be able not only to identify the normal, but also to differentiate it from the abnormal.

You will use assessment in every area of nursing. As you perfect your assessment skills, you will find that you can apply them in all levels of health care, in acute care, in the home, and in long-term care.

F. A. Davis has a variety of resources available to meet your learning needs and develop your assessment skills. Here is a brief guide on how to use them.

- **Interact** with the case study in the text. This is your patient.
- **Review** your anatomy and physiology, apply the assessment process, and identify your learning needs through the self-evaluation exercises in the applications text.
- **Listen** to the auscultatory CD of heart, breath and bowel sounds again and again until you can clearly hear each sound.
- **Practice** your assessment skills using the case studies CD-ROM.
- **Visit** the F. A. Davis Web site for additional resources, such as the symptom analysis tables for every major system chief complaint.
- **Validate** your assessment findings and perfect your skills by using your pocket guide in the clinical area.

Consider this text your guide to assessment. Take ownership of it as you learn to assess. Consider the case studies as your patients. As you interact with them, you will learn assessment. Every patient encounter provides you with an opportunity to assess, so seize the opportunity. You can learn so much from your patients. Make each encounter with your patient a learning experience as you develop the skill--and art--of assessment. So practice, practice, practice! And have fun as you develop your assessment skills!

Patricia M. Dillon

PATRICIA M. DILLON, MSN, DNSC

I would like to tell my colleagues, the contributors, and the reviewers how much I appreciate their excellent contributions to this project, particularly Dr. Daniel Mason, who so generously made available his outstanding collection of heart, lung, and abdominal sounds. And to those who provided the photos that will enhance students' understanding of the assessment findings, thank you.

For believing in my vision and for their unending support throughout this project I, would like to acknowledge the staff at F. A. Davis, especially Lisa Deitch and Melanie Freely. I would also like to thank Marylou Ambrose for her editorial expertise.

Finally, and most importantly, a special thank-you to my family—Joe, Joey, Katie, and Patty—for their understanding and unending support.

Noreen Chikotas, MSN, CRNP
Assistant Professor
Department of Nursing
Bloomsburg University
Bloomsburg, Pennsylvania

Linda C. Curry, RN, PhD
Professor of Nursing
Harris School of Nursing
Texas Christian University
Fort Worth, Texas

Denise Demers, RN, MS
Assistant Professor of Nursing
St. Joseph's College
Standish, Maine

Patricia M. Dillon, DNSc, RN
Adjunct Faculty
Temple University
College of Allied Health Professions
Department of Nursing
Philadelphia, Pennsylvania

Pamela Jean Frable, RN, ND
Assistant Professor
Harris School of Nursing
Texas Christian University
Fort Worth, Texas

Mary Jo Goolsby, MSN, EdD, ANP-C, FAANP
Director of Research and Education
American Academy of Nurse Practitioners
Austin, Texas
Patient Care Research Specialist
University Health Care System
Augusta, Georgia

Diane Greslick, RNc, MSN
Assistant Professor of Nursing
St. Joseph's College
Standish, Maine

Annette Gunderman, RN, DEd
Associate Professor
Department of Nursing
Bloomsburg University
Bloomsburg, Pennsylvania

Shelton M. Hisley, RNC, PhD, WHNP, ACCE
Assistant Professor
Graduate Clinical Coordinator
School of Nursing
The University of North Carolina at Wilmington
Wilmington, North Carolina

Mildred O. Hogstel, RNC, PhD
Professor Emeritus
Harris School of Nursing
Texas Christian University
Fort Worth, Texas

Barbara Jones, RN, MSN, DNSc
Associate Professor
Gwynedd-Mercy College
Gwynedd Valley, Pennsylvania

Kathleen Kellinger, MSN, PhD, CRNP
Chairperson of Department of Nursing
Slippery Rick University
Slippery Rock, Pennsylvania

Judith Ann Kilpatrick, RN, MSN, DNSc
Assistant Professor of Nursing
Widener University
Chester, Pennsylvania

Maryanne Lachat, RNC, PhD
Associate Professor
Georgetown University
Washington, DC

Daniel Mason, MD, FACC
Professor of Medicine (Cardiology)
Hahnemann University School of Medicine
Philadelphia. Pennsylvania

Carol Meadows, RNP, MNSc, APN
Instructor
University of Arkansas
Eleanor Mann School of Nursing
Fayetteville, Arkansas

Donna Molyneaux, RN, MSN, DNSc
Associate Professor
Gwynedd-Mercy College
Gwynedd Valley, Pennsylvania

Louise Niemer, RN, BSN, MSN, PhD, CPNP, ARNP
Associate Professor, Nursing
Northern Kentucky University
Highland Heights, Kentucky

Sandra G. Raymer Raff, RN, MS, FNP
Perinatal Educator
Natividad Medical Center
Salinas, California

Barbara Resnick, PhD, CRNP, FAAN, FAANP
Associate Professor, University of Maryland
School of Nursing
Baltimore, Maryland

S. Anne Stewart, ARNP, PhD, CS
Associate Professor
California State University
Sacramento, California

Joanne L. Thanavaro, RN, MSN, ARNP, BC
Assistant Professor of Nursing
Jewish Hospital College of Nursing and Allied Health at Washington University
St. Louis, Missouri
Private Practice: Clayton Medical Consultants, Inc.
St. Louis, Missouri

Rose Utley, RN, PhD
Assistant Professor
Department of Nursing
Southwest Missouri State University
Springfield, Missouri

Case studies used in the companion *Nursing Health Assessment: Student Applications* were provided by N. Chitokas and A. Gunderman (Musculoskeletal), P. Frable (Teaching), M.J. Goolsby (Integumentary and Head, Face, and Neck), D. Greslick and D. Demers (Abdomen), J. Kilpatrick (Spirituality), C. Meadows (Male Genitourinary and Adolescent), L. Niemer (Nutrition and Toddler), J. Thanavero (Peripheral-Vascular and Lymphatic), and S. Raff (Putting It All Together).

Lisa M. Abdallah, RN, PhD
College of Nursing and Health Sciences
University of Massachusetts-Boston
Boston, Massachusetts

Carol B. Allen, RN, BSN, MSN
Instructor
Intercollegiate College of Nursing
Washington State University College of Nursing
Spokane, Washington

Rachel R. Boersma
Professor
College of Nursing
Fitchburg State College
Fitchburg, Massachusetts

Simone Bollaerts, BN
Professor of Nursing; Coordinator of Assessment Program and Wound Management
Mohawk College, Health Sciences Division
Hamilton, Ontario, Canada

Barbara Scott Cammuso, PhD, EdD, APRN, BC
Professor
Chairperson of the Graduate Program in Forensic Nursing
Fitchburg State College
Fitchburg, Massachusetts

Patricia Carroll, RN, BC, CEN, RRT, MS
Owner, Educational Medical Consultants
Founder, *www.nursesnotebook.com*
Meridien, Connecticut

Lynn Chilton, DSN, GNP/FNP, BC
Professor of Graduate Nursing
Nurse Practitioner Program
Mississippi University for Women
Columbus, Mississippi

Alice E. Davis, RN, PhD
Assistant Professor
University of Michigan, Ann Arbor
School of Nursing
Canton, Michigan

Jean E. DeMartinis, PhD, FNPc
Nurse Practitioner, Cardiology and Prevention
Physicians' Clinic, Inc.
Methodist Health Systems
Omaha, Nebraska

Virginia B. Dory, RN, MSN, ARNP
Clinical Instructor
Florida Southern College
6035 S. Rio Grande Avenue
Orlando, Florida

Mary Jo Goolsby, MSN, ARNP, EdD
Practicing Adult Nurse Practitioner
Florida State University, School of Nursing
Tallahassee, Florida

Kelly A. Goudreau, MSN, DSNc
Associate Professor
University of Maine at Fort Kent
Fort Kent, Maine

Lee Ann Grogan, ADN
Home Health Nurse
Bayley Place, Ohio

Deborah J. Gutshall, NP, MSN
Harrisburg Area Community College
Harrisburg, Pennsylvania

Mary B. Haq, FNP, PhD
Associate Professor
Felician College
Lodi, New Jersey

Janice Hausauer, RN, MS, FNP
Adjunct Assistant Professor
Montana State University, College of Nursing
Bozeman, Montana

Mary E. Hazzard, PhD
National University
Nursing Program
La Jolla, California

Jeanna M. Hicks, ASN, BSN
Assistant Professor of Nursing
Jackson State Community College
Jackson, Tennessee

Helen F. Hodges, RN-BSN, PhD
Coordinator, Professor
George Baptist College of Nursing of Mercer University
Atlanta, Georgia

Judy Johnson-Russell, RN, EdD
Associate Professor
Texas Woman's University
College of Nursing
Dallas, Texas

David C. Keller, APRN, MS
Assistant Teaching Professor
College of Nursing
Brigham Young University
College of Nursing
Provo, Utah

Darrice E. Kelley, MSN
Faculty
Excelsior College
School of Nursing
Albany, New York

Ramona M. Leslie, RN, MS
Nurse Educator
Excelsior College
Albany, New York

Robyn Levy, RN, MSN, CS, ANP
Assistant Professor
Jewish Hospital College of Nursing and Allied Health
St. Louis, Missouri

Mary Delia Linthacum, RN, MS, MSN
Associate Professor
Department of Registered Nurse Education
Del Mar College
Corpus Christi, Texas

Janet A. Lohan, PhD, MS, BS
Assistant Professor
Intercollegiate College of Nursing
Washington State University
Spokane, Washington

Katharina Loock, RN, MD, BSN
Education Coordinator
Wadley Regional Medical Center
Texarkana, Texas

Sally K. Miller, BSN, MS
Assistant Professor
MCP Hahnemann University
School of Nursing
Philadelphia, Pennsylvania

Patricia Ann O'Leary, RN, DSN, MSN, BSN
Associate Professor
Middle Tennessee State University
School of Nursing
Murfreesboro, Tennessee

Karen J. Pagnotta, MSN
Family Nurse Practitioner/ Nursing Instructor
Alamance Community College
Graham, North Carolina

Judith Pollachek, RNBC, CANP, CGNP, PhD
Certified Adult and Geriatric Nurse Practitioner, Assistant Professor
Rutgers University
School of Nursing
Newark, New Jersey

Donna I. Rae, BScN, Med, ENC(c)
Professor, College of Nursing
University of Saskatchewan
Saskatoon, Saskatchewan, Canada

Clare E. Safran-Norton, MS, BS
Assistant Professor
Simmons College
Physical Therapy Department
Boston, Massachusetts

Sheila A. Sarver, RN, MEd, BS
Program Director of Nursing Eduction
Lee County School of Practical Nursing
Fort Myers, Florida

Linda Scott, BSN, MS, EdD
Assistant Professor
Winona State University
Rochester, Minnesota

Rita A. Seeger Jablonski, RN, MSN, CS, ANP
Clinical Associate Professor
Virginia Commonwealth University
Richmond, Virginia

Diane R. Smith, MSN, FNP, APNP
Clinical Assistant Professor
School of Nursing
University of Wisconsin
Wisconsin

Craig R. Telesz, BSN (Student at time of review)
University of Akron
School of Nursing
Akron, Ohio

Donna M Thompson, MSN, BSN, APRN, FNE
Department of Nursing
Salt Lake Community College
Salt Lake City, Utah

Lindsay A. Thompson, BSN (Junior-level student at time of review)
University of North Carolina at Greensboro
School of Nursing
Greensboro, North Carolina

Saundra L. Turner, RN, EdD
Associate Professor and Interim Chair
Family Nurse Practitioner
Medical College of Georgia
School of Nursing
Augusta, Georgia

Susan Urbanski, RN, MN, CCDN
President/Executive Director
CIGNA Behavioral Health of California
Glendale, California

Vickie Valenziano, RN, MSN
Adjunct Nursing Faculty
College of the Canyons
Valencia, California

Mark van Viegen, RN, MS, FNP, PNP
Family Nurse Practitioner
Duke University
Myrtle Beach, South Carolina

Julee B. Waldrop, MSN, BSN
Clinical Assistant Professor
School of Nursing
University of North Carolina at Chapel Hill
Pediatric Nurse Practitioner
North Carolina Children's Hopsital
Chapel Hill, North Carolina

Mariann B. Ward, MSN, BSN, CFNP
St. Frances Hospital
Wilmington, Delaware

Getting Started

Health Assessment and the Nurse

Before You Begin

INTRODUCTION TO THE HEALTH ASSESSMENT

You are doing blood pressure screening at a health fair. You take the blood pressure of a middle-aged man. Your reading is 170/100.

You are working in the Emergency Department (ED) when a father comes in with his 9-year-old daughter. He states that she fell off her bike and hit her head but did not lose consciousness. But she has a terrible headache and feels sick.

You are making a postpartum follow-up visit to the home of a young mother who had her first baby 2 days ago.

You are making an initial hospice visit to a 74-year-old woman with pancreatic cancer.

What do you do? Where do you begin? You begin with assessment. How well you perform your assessment will affect everything else that follows. You will ask questions, and you will use four of your senses to collect data.

The Nursing Process

Nursing is the diagnosis and treatment of human responses to actual or potential health problems. Diagnosis and treatment are achieved through a process that guides nursing practice, called the nursing process. The nursing process is a systematic problem-solving method that has five steps: assessment, nursing diagnoses, planning, implementation, and evaluation.

The nursing process (Fig. 1–1) is used to identify, prevent, and treat actual or potential health problems and promote wellness. It provides a framework in which to practice nursing. Think of it as a continuous, circular process that revolves around your client. You begin with assessment, collect data, cluster the data, and then formulate nursing diagnoses. Once you have identified the nursing diagnosis, you will develop a plan of care, determine the goals and expected outcomes, implement your plan, and then evaluate it. Then you will begin the nursing process again.

Step 1: Assessment

Assessment involves collecting, validating, and clustering data. It is the first and most important step in the nursing process. The assessment phase sets the tone for the rest of the process, and the rest of the process flows from it. If your assessment is off the mark, then the rest of the process will be too. Assessment identifies your client's strengths and limitations and is performed continuously throughout the nursing process. After performing your initial assessment, you establish your baseline, identify nursing diagnoses and develop a plan. Then, as you implement your plan, you also assess your client's response. Finally, you assess the effectiveness of your plan of care for your client.

Step 2: Nursing Diagnoses

Formulating nursing diagnoses involves identifying and prioritizing. Once you collect your data, you need to analyze it and then identify actual and potential health problems or responses to life processes and state them as nursing diagnoses. Nursing diagnoses can be actual, potential, possible, or collaborative problems as well as wellness issues. An actual nursing diagnosis identifies an occurring health problem for your client. A potential nursing diagnosis identifies a high-risk health problem that most likely will occur unless preventive measures are taken. A possible nursing diagnosis is one that needs further data to support it. A collaborative problem is a potential medical complication that warrants both medical and nursing interventions. Because nursing's focus is not limited to illness, wellness diagnoses focus on promoting or enhancing a client's level of wellness. Once the diagnoses have been identified, you need to prioritize them in order to develop a plan of care.

Step 3: Planning

The planning phase involves setting goals and outcomes. Once you have prioritized your diagnoses, you are ready to develop an individualized plan of care for your client. First, you establish goals and determine measurable outcomes. Next, you identify nursing interventions needed to meet the outcome. Then you communicate your plan to maintain continuity of care and ensure success.

Step 4: Implementation

Implementation (also called intervention) involves carrying out your plan to achieve goals and outcomes. This is the "doing" phase of the nursing process, in which you

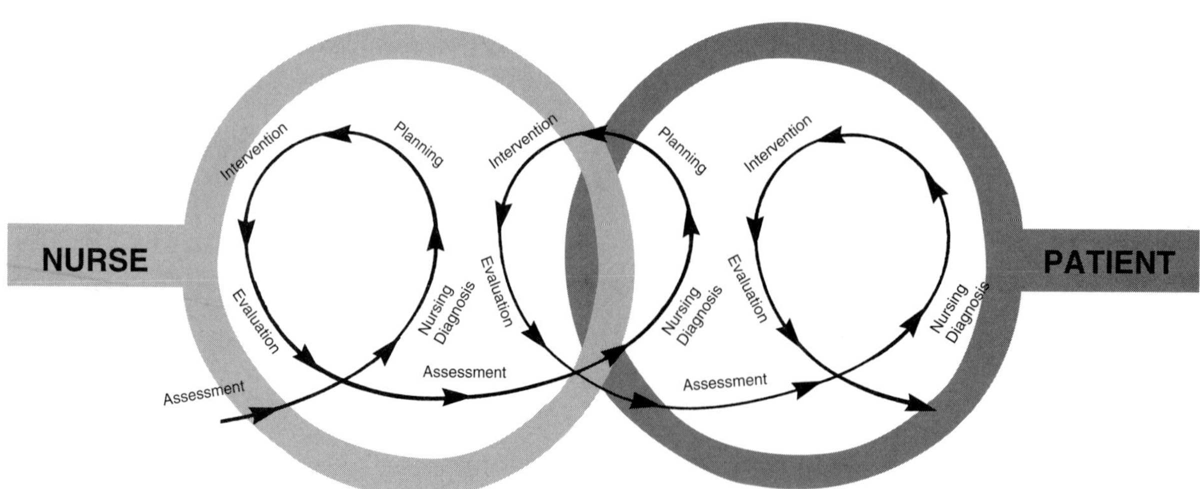

FIGURE 1–1. The nursing process.

NANDA nursing diagnoses

The following list of nursing diagnoses was endorsed by the North American Nursing Diagnosis Association in 2001.

- Activity Intolerance
- Activity Intolerance, Risk for
- Adjustment, Impaired
- Airway Clearance, Ineffective
- Allergy Response, Latex
- Allergy Response, Risk for Latex
- Anxiety
- Anxiety, Death
- Aspiration, Risk for
- Attachment, Risk for Impaired Parent/Infant/Child
- Autonomic Dysreflexia
- Autonomic Dysreflexia, Risk for
- Body Image, Disturbed
- Body Temperature, Risk for Imbalanced
- Bowel Incontinence
- Breastfeeding, Effective
- Breastfeeding, Ineffective
- Breastfeeding, Interrupted
- Breathing Pattern, Ineffective
- Cardiac Output, Decreased
- Caregiver Role Strain
- Caregiver Role Strain, Risk for
- Communication, Impaired Verbal
- Conflict, Decisional
- Conflict, Parental Role
- Confusion, Acute
- Confusion, Chronic
- Constipation
- Constipation, Perceived
- Constipation, Risk for
- Coping, Ineffective
- Coping, Ineffective Community
- Coping, Readiness for Enhanced Community Coping
- Coping, Defensive
- Coping, Compromised Family
- Coping, Disabled Family
- Coping, Readiness for Enhanced Family
- Denial, Ineffective
- Dentition, Impaired
- Development, Risk for Delayed
- Diarrhea
- Disuse Syndrome, Risk for
- Diversional Activity, Deficient
- Energy Field, Disturbed
- Environmental Interpretation Syndrome, Impaired
- Failure to Thrive, Adult
- *Falls, Risk for
- Family Processes, Dysfunctional: Alcoholism
- Family Processes, Interrupted
- Fatigue
- Fear
- Fluid Volume, Deficient
- Fluid Volume, Excess
- Fluid Volume, Risk for Deficient
- Fluid Volume, Imbalanced, Risk for
- Gas Exchange, Impaired
- Grieving, Anticipatory
- Grieving, Dysfunctional
- Growth and Development, Delayed
- Growth, Risk for Disproportionate
- Health Maintenance, Ineffective
- Health-Seeking Behaviors (Specify)
- Home Maintenance, Impaired
- Hopelessness
- Hyperthermia
- Hypothermia
- Identity, Disturbed Personal
- Incontinence, Functional Urinary
- Incontinence, Reflex Urinary
- Incontinence, Stress Urinary
- Incontinence, Total Urinary
- Incontinence, Urge Urinary
- Incontinence, Risk for Urge Urinary
- Infant Behavior, Disorganized
- Infant Behavior, Risk for Disorganized
- Infant Behavior, Readiness for Enhanced Organized
- Infant Feeding Pattern, Ineffective
- Infection, Risk for
- Injury, Risk for
- Injury, Risk for Perioperative-Positioning
- Intracranial Adaptive Capacity, Decreased
- Knowledge, Deficient (Specify)
- Loneliness, Risk for
- Memory, Impaired
- Mobility, Impaired Bed
- Mobility, Impaired Physical
- Mobility, Impaired Wheelchair
- Nausea
- Neglect, Unilateral
- Noncompliance

Nutrition, Imbalanced, Less Than Body Requirements
Nutrition, Imbalanced, More Than Body Requirements
Nutrition, Imbalanced, Risk for More Than Body Requirements
Oral Mucous Membrane, Impaired
Pain, Acute
Pain, Chronic
Parenting, Impaired
Parenting, Risk for Impaired
Peripheral Neurovascular Dysfunction, Risk for
Poisoning, Risk for
Post-Trauma Syndrome
Post-Trauma Syndrome, Risk for
Powerlessness
*Powerlessness, Risk for
Protection, Ineffective
Rape-Trauma Syndrome
Rape-Trauma Syndrome: Compound Reaction
Rape-Trauma Syndrome: Silent Reaction
Relocation Stress Syndrome
*Relocation Stress Syndrome, Risk for
Role Performance, Ineffective
Self-Care Deficit, Bathing/Hygiene
Self-Care Deficit, Dressing/Grooming
Self-Care Deficit, Feeding
Self-Care Deficit, Toileting
Self-Esteem, Chronic Low
Self-Esteem, Situational Low
*Self-Esteem, Risk for Situational Low
*Self-Mutilation
Self-Mutilation, Risk for
Sensory Perception, Disturbed (Specify: Visual, Auditory, Kinesthetic, Gustatory, Tactile, Olfactory)
Sexual Dysfunction
Sexuality Patterns, Ineffective
Skin Integrity, Impaired
Skin Integrity, Risk for Impaired
Sleep Deprivation
Sleep Pattern, Disturbed
Social Interaction, Impaired
Social Isolation
Sorrow, Chronic
Spiritual Distress
Spiritual Distress, Risk for
Spiritual Well-Being, Readiness for Enhanced
Suffocation, Risk for
*Suicide, Risk for
Surgical Recovery, Delayed
Swallowing, Impaired
Therapeutic Regimen: Effective Management
Therapeutic Regimen: Ineffective Management
Therapeutic Regimen: Community, Ineffective Management
Therapeutic Regimen: Family, Ineffective Management
Thermoregulation, Ineffective
Thought Process, Disturbed
Tissue Integrity, Impaired
Tissue Perfusion, Ineffective (Specify Type: Renal, Cerebral, Cardiopulmonary, Gastrointestinal, Peripheral)
Transfer Ability, Impaired
Trauma, Risk for
Urinary Elimination, Impaired
Urinary Retention
Ventilation, Impaired Spontaneous
Ventilatory Weaning Response, Dysfunctional
Violence, Risk for Other-Directed
Violence, Risk for Self-Directed
Walking, Impaired
*Wandering

*New to the 14th Conference

actually carry out your plan. As you implement your plan, you continue to assess your client's responses and modify the plan as needed. Be sure to document your care.

CHARACTERISTICS OF THE NURSING PROCESS

- Dynamic and cyclic
- Client centered
- Goal directed
- Flexible
- Problem oriented
- Cognitive
- Action oriented
- Interpersonal
- Holistic
- Systematic

Step 5: Evaluation

Evaluation involves determining the effectiveness of your plan. Did you meet your goals and outcomes? Once again, assess your client's response based on the criteria you set for the outcome. If the goals and outcomes have not been met, you'll need to rethink the plan and work through the process again to develop a more effective plan of care for your client.

The Assessment Process

The American Nurses Association (ANA) has identified assessment as the first Standard of Nursing Practice. The Standard describes assessment as the systematic, continuous collection of data about the health status of clients. Nurses are responsible not only for data collection, but for making sure that the data are accessible, communicated, and recorded. Assessment is an ongoing process. Every client encounter provides you with an opportunity for assessment.

Purpose of Assessment

The purpose of assessment is to collect data pertinent to the client's health status, to identify deviations from normal, to discover the client's strengths and coping resources, to pinpoint actual problems and to spot factors that place the client at risk for health problems.

Skills of Assessment

Assessment requires cognitive, problem-solving, psychomotor, affective/interpersonal, and ethical skills.

Cognitive Skills

Assessment is a "thinking" process. Cognitive skills are needed for critical thinking, creative thinking, and clinical decision making. Your theoretical knowledge base enables you to assess your client holistically. The knowledge base includes not only biophysical knowledge, but also developmental, cultural, psychosocial, and spiritual knowledge. This knowledge base enables you to differentiate normal from abnormal findings and to identify and prioritize actual and potential problems.

You will use both deductive and inductive reasoning to assess your client and interpret the data. For example, suppose your client is admitted to the hospital with the diagnosis of congestive heart failure (CHF). Knowing this enables you to look for specific signs and symptoms as you perform the assessment and determine your client's response to this illness. In this case, you will use deductive reasoning, looking for specific clues that support the diagnosis of decreased cardiac output.

Inductive reasoning would be appropriate when assessing a postoperative client who states, "It hurts too much to take deep breaths" and who has decreased breath sounds and crackles at the bases, pulse oximetry of 90 percent on room air, temperature of 101°, pulse of 106 BPM, and respirations 26 and shallow. When you piece together all of the pertinent assessment data, you formulate a diagnosis of Gas Exchange, Impaired and Airway Clearance, Ineffective.

Assessment requires sharp observation skills and the ability to distinguish relevant from irrelevant and important from unimportant data. Once the data are collected, they need to be organized, categorized, and validated.

Assessment also requires clinical decision making. As you collect data, you will make clinical decisions as to its relevance. You will look for cues and make inferences. With experience, you will be able to identify patterns and recognize what differs from the norm. Use your knowledge, experience, and what the client says to validate the data. Then use the data to formulate nursing diagnoses.

Problem-Solving Skills

Various problem-solving methods can be used as you assess your client and work through the nursing process. With experience, you will develop your problem-solving skills. Do not limit yourself to one method; instead, select the method that best suits your client's needs.

Reflexive thinking is automatic, without conscious deliberation and comes with experience. For example, if you are working in the ED and a 45-year-old man is admitted with "crushing chest pain," you will automatically take his vital signs and do an electrocardiogram to assess his cardiac status as you ask him questions.

The trial-and-error approach is hit-or-miss thinking—random, not systematic and inefficient. This would never be your primary problem-solving approach, but it may prove helpful at times because it allows you to "think outside of the box." Trial-and-error thinking fosters creativity and allows you to formulate new ideas. Use it for situations that don't quite fit the picture, look beyond the obvious, and keep looking until you find an answer.

The scientific method is a systematic, critical-thinking approach to problem solving. It involves identifying a problem and collecting supporting data, formulating a hypothesis, planning a solution, implementing the plan, and then evaluating its effectiveness. Assessment corresponds with the "collection of supporting data phase" of the scientific method. The nursing process is similar to the scientific method, but the nursing process offers nurses the flexibility to practice both the art and science of nursing.

Intuition is a problem-solving method that develops through experience, in which theory and practice are intertwined. This is how the "expert" nurse solves problems. Through experience, she has a well-established experiential base of pattern recognition, an intuitive grasp of the situation and the ability to zero in on problem areas. For example, suppose a client says "I just don't feel right," even though his or her vital signs are stable and everything seems fine on the chart. The objective data may not support it, but the expert nurse senses that something is not quite right and returns to further assess her client, only to find him or her in distress. She intervenes swiftly and saves the client's life.

Psychomotor Skills

Assessment is "doing." Psychomotor skills are needed to perform the four techniques of physical assessment: inspection, palpation, percussion, and auscultation. As a beginning practitioner, you may feel unsure of your technique and your findings, but practice will hone your skills. Input from your colleagues will help you perfect your skills and interpret your findings. Through experience, you will become competent at performing the physical assessment and confident in interpreting your findings.

Affective/Interpersonal Skills

Assessment is a "feeling" process. Affective skills are needed to practice the "art" of nursing. Affective skills are essential in developing caring, therapeutic nurse-client relationships. Interpersonal skills include both verbal and nonverbal communication skills. The quality of your assessment depends on your communication skills and the relationship that you develop with your client. Establishing trust and mutual respect is essential before you begin the assessment. Seeing your client as an individual and being sensitive to his or her feelings conveys a message of caring and promotes human dignity. Illness often makes a client very vulnerable, but the power of a caring relationship can have a major impact on the client's sense of worth and well-being. Such a relationship can be mutually rewarding, affecting both your client and you both personally and professionally.

Your interpersonal skills are also needed to communicate with family members and members of the healthcare team. Communicating effectively with the healthcare team is essential in order to successfully meet your client's goals.

Ethical Skills

Assessment is being responsible and accountable. You are responsible and accountable for your practice. You are also an advocate for your client. Your client has rights that need to be respected and confidentiality assured. The ANA describes the ethical standards that guide nursing practice in its Code for Nurses.

Role of the Nurse and Assessment

The role of the nurse has changed drastically over the years. So have the nurse's responsibilities. The importance of assessment can be traced to the beginning of modern nursing. Florence Nightingale (1859) stressed the importance of observation and experience as essential in maintaining or restoring one's state of health. The scope of assessment has also expanded from simple observation to a holistic view of the client that includes the biophysical, psychosocial, developmental, and cultural assessment. The skills of assessments have also expanded as the scope of practice has expanded from simple observations to detailed use of physical assessment skills.

Nursing Assessment vs. Medical Assessment

Assessment is not unique to nursing. It is also an integral part of medical practice. Although the assessment process may be the same for nursing and medical practice, the outcome differs. The goal of medical practice is to diagnose and treat disease. The goal of nursing practice is to diagnose and treat human responses to actual or potential health problems. Nursing assessment focuses not only on physiological and psychological responses, but also on psychosocial, cultural, developmental, and spiritual dimensions. It identifies clients' responses to health problems as well as their strengths. Nursing's aim is to help the client reach his or her optimal level of wellness.

The Code for Nurses

1 The nurse, in all professional relationships, practices with compassion and respect for the inherent dignity, worth and uniqueness of every individual, unrestricted by considerations of social or economic status, personal attributes, or the nature of health problems.

2 The nurse's primary commitment is to the patient, whether an individual, family, group, or community.

3 The nurse promotes, advocates for, and strives to protect the health, safety, and rights of the patient.

4 The nurse is responsible and accountable for individual nursing practice and determines the appropriate delegation of tasks consistent with the nurse's obligation to provide optimum patient care.

5 The nurse owes the same duties to self as to others, including the responsibility to preserve integrity and safety, to maintain competence, and to continue personal and professional growth.

6 The nurse participates in establishing, maintaining, and improving healthcare environments and conditions of employment conducive to the provision of quality health care and consistent with the values of the profession through individual and collective action.

7 The nurse participates in the advancement of the profession through contributions to practice, education, administration, and knowledge development.

8 The nurse collaborates with other health professionals and the public in promoting community, national, and international efforts to meet health needs.

9 The profession of nursing, as represented by associations and their members, is responsible for articulating nursing values, for maintaining the integrity of the profession and its practice, and for shaping social policy.

Source: American Nurses Association, Code for nurses with interpretive statements (Kansas City, Mo.: American Nurses Association, 2004), Reprinted with permission.

Medical and nursing assessments should complement, not contradict each other in promoting the client's health and wellness. Often data obtained through the nursing assessment contributes to the identification of medical problems. By working together in a collaborative relationship, nursing and medicine ensure the best possible care for clients.

The nurse-physician relationship has changed through the years. In the late 1800s nurses were subservient to physicians; their primary duty was to serve physicians. By 1936, the nurse-physician relationship was that of coworkers with the primary goal of restoring the client to health. This relationship was further refined with the formation of the National Joint Practice Commission (NJPC) in 1972. Established by the American Medical Association (AMA) and the ANA, this interprofessional organization recognized the importance of a collaborative nurse-physician relationship in improving client care. The NJPC identified five components that promote collaboration: primary nursing, integrated client records, individual decision making by nurses, a joint practice committee, and joint care reviews. Today nurses practice both independently and collaboratively.

Levels of Preventive Health Care

Preventive health care can be classified as primary, secondary, and tertiary. Nurses have a vital role in all three

The nurse's changing role

In the past 60 years, the nurse's role has changed dramatically, and so has the scope of nursing practice. A mirror of the times, the nurse's role has grown from that of a skilled observer in the 1930s to that of a health care professional who performs holistic assessment. The following excerpts from actual nursing notes reflect this change in the nurse's role.

1930s

"Patient admitted to ward in a wheelchair. Stated that he is unable to walk due to pinched nerves of right foot. Patient is crying, says he is homesick. Condition of skin good. Made as comfortable as possible."

This note includes observations only. The nurse's role is limited to that of a skilled observer.

1950s

"25-year-old female admitted ambulatory. Past history of ulcerative colitis. Now in because of abdominal cramps and vomiting X 4 days. Is 8 months pregnant. TPR 99.4, 80, 20. Ht 5'4". Wt 116½. Urine to lab."

This note traces the past and present history of illness as well as observations. The nurse's role has expanded to include interviewing skills that assess the client's past and current heaith status.

1970s

"12-year-old white female admitted to Room 203 via stretcher from E.R. with leukemia. Parents don't seem to know of diagnosis. TPR 102.8°, 120,24. Ht 62¼". Wt 100 lb. No known allergies. Has not been eating much for last few days. Appears extremely pale. BP 150/70. No urine obtained. I.V. started. Blood started. Vital signs relatively stable. T 103° when blood started."

This note records intravenous and blood therapy and includes observations as well as information about past illnesses and diet. The nurse's role now includes observation, interviewing, performing procedures (venipuncture), and monitoring.

1990s to present

"Young, obese Caucasian female states she came here to 'get the sugar out of her blood.' States she found out about her sugar 3 months ago by glucose tolerance test results (in Jan. 1990 miscarried 2-month pregnancy and GTT was part of workup); states she has seen her husband test his blood (fingerstick method) and give himself insulin but has done neither herself; has tried to prepare both 1,800 and 2,200 calorie American Diabetic Association diets as ordered for husband but 'he doesn't stick to it'; has noted increased hunger, increased thirst, increased urination for several months and occasional blurred vision.

"Lives with husband and daughter next door to sister-in-law; husband makes playground equipment; states they are able to 'get by' on his salary, sometimes borrow money and have difficulty paying it back; have Blue Cross/Blue Shield which should pay for this hospitalization; husband has diabetes mellitus (takes insulin), is losing weight but refuses to see doctor—she is concerned about him; states husband will not be able to visit her because of work."

This note records observation and assessment of the client as well as the biophysical, psychosocial, and cultural factors that influence the client's health problem. The nurse's role has grown to include holistic health assessment.

levels of health care, and assessment skills are needed at all levels.

Primary preventive care focuses on health promotion and prevention. Examples are health fairs, immunizations, and providing breast self-examination instructions. Nurses use assessment skills to screen, identify, and educate clients about the risk factors for health problems.

Secondary preventive care focuses on early detection, prompt intervention and health maintenance for

The NJPC's elements of collaboration

According to the National Joint Practice Commission (NJPC) study, five elements foster nurse-physician collaboration and provide the following benefits.

ELEMENT AND DESCRIPTION	BENEFITS
Primary nursing	
Nursing with little or no delegation of nursing tasks to others. One nurse is responsible for a client's comprehensive care	• Direct communication between the primary nurse and physician • Client care coordination by one person • Nursing autonomy • Shared accountability with the physician • Fewer errors in client care • Increased client satisfaction
Integrated client records	
Interdisciplinary client progress notes that combine nurse and physician observations, judgments, and actions and provide a formal means of nurse-physician communication about client care	• Substantive and concise nursing notes • Opportunity for health care professionals to read each others' notes • Less duplication of charted information • Validation of observations and judgments by cosigning of nurse's and physician's notes
Individual decision-making by nurses	
Ability to exercise independent judgment and initiate care based on the judgment. Decisions must lie within the scope of nursing practice	• Greater nursing control of the environment • Greater job satisfaction for nurses
Joint practice committee	
A committee of nurses and physicians that monitors nurse-physician relationships and recommends actions that support collaboration	• Opportunity for nurses and physicians to discuss collaborative practice and work out problems • Improved understanding between nurses and physicians
Joint care reviews	
Monthly review of client charts by a review committee of nurses and physicians to evaluate collaborative care	• Identification of ways to improve client care and collaborative practice

clients with health problems. It addresses acute health problems seen with inpatient hospitalization. Accurate assessment is crucial to establish the client's baseline and to continually monitor his or her condition and response to treatment.

Tertiary preventive care deals with rehabilitative or extended care. Although the client's health status is usually more stable than in secondary care, clients usually have a chronic illness. Skilled nursing care facilities, rehabilitative hospitals, long-term care facilities, home care, and hospice are examples of tertiary-level care. Assessment skills are needed to continually monitor health status.

Remember: At every level of preventive care, you have opportunities to practice assessment. You are often the one who decides when the client's condition warrants medical intervention.

Collecting Data

Data can be classified as subjective and objective. Subjective data are covert and not measurable. They reflect what the client is experiencing and include thoughts, beliefs, feelings, sensations, and perceptions. Subjective findings are referred to as symptoms. The health history is an example of subjective data.

Objective data are overt and measurable. Objective data are referred to as signs. The physical examination and diagnostic studies are examples of objective data. Data sources are either primary or secondary. The client is a primary data source. Secondary data sources are anyone or anything aside from the client, including family members, friends, other healthcare providers and old medical records. Both primary and secondary data can also be subjective or objective.

CRITICAL THINKING ACTIVITY # 1

Identify the following data as subjective or objective:

Headache
BP 170/110
Nausea
Diaphoresis
Equal pupillary reaction
Tingling sensation
Dizziness
Decreased muscle strength
Slurred speech
Numbness, left arm

CRITICAL THINKING ACTIVITY #2

Elaine Ploransky is a 29-year-old married woman, gravida 1, para 0. She is having contractions 5 minutes apart, which she describes as "severe cramps." Her husband states, "I think her water broke on the way to the hospital."

Physical examination reveals that Mrs. Ploransky is 6 cm dilated. Fetal monitor reveals a fetal heart rate of 120 BPM. The client's vital signs include BP 140/80, pulse 90 BPM, respirations 22/minute. Prenatal records reveal hemoglobin 12.0, hematocrit 45 and blood type AB+.

Identify:

Primary data source
Secondary data source
Subjective data
Objective data

Types of Assessment

Assessments can be comprehensive or focused. A comprehensive assessment is usually the initial assessment. It is very thorough and includes a detailed health history and physical examination. A comprehensive assessment examines the client's overall health status. A focused assessment is problem oriented and may be the initial assessment or an ongoing assessment. If a client's condition does not warrant a comprehensive assessment, a focused assessment of the client's present health problem is done. Once the client's condition improves and stabilizes, the comprehensive assessment can be completed. A focused assessment is frequently performed on an ongoing basis to monitor and evaluate the client's progress, interventions, and response to treatments.

No matter what type of assessment you are performing, realize that even though you may be looking at one specific area or system, you also need to look at the entire picture. A problem in one system will affect or be affected by every other system. So scan your client from head to toe and note any changes in other systems. Look for clues or pertinent data that will help you formulate your diagnosis.

Communication

To assess, you must be able to communicate and communicate well! Communication is a process of sharing information and meaning, of sending and receiving messages. The messages we communicate are both verbal and nonverbal. The sections below describe the many factors that influence communication. You need to consider all of them when communicating with your client to be sure that the message you want to send is the one your client actually receives.

Nonverbal Messages

Nonverbal behavior is an important source of data. Often the nonverbal message being sent is more accurate than the verbal one. So examine both your nonverbal behavior and your client's. Be conscious of your beliefs and values and do not let them influence your verbal or nonverbal communication. Nonverbal behavior includes vocal cues or paralinguistics, action cues or kinetics, object cues, personal space, and touch.

Vocal Cues and Paralinguistics

Vocal cues describe the quality of your voice and its inflections, tone, intensity, and speed when speaking. These voice characteristics usually reflect underlying feelings. If your client is in pain, moaning or the inflections in his or her speech may alert you to the pain's severity. Someone who is afraid may speak softly, with trepidation. Anger, doubt, disbelief, or disapproval can all be conveyed by the tone of your voice.

Vocal characteristics may also reflect underlying physiological or psychological problems. For example, older clients may speak loudly because of hearing loss. Clients with hyperthyroidism may have rapid speech. Rapid speech is also associated with manic depression.

Be aware of the characteristics of your own speech. What message are you sending to your client? Your speech should be calm, reassuring, and without inflections that convey judgment or disapproval. Speak slowly enough and loudly enough so that your client can hear you and respond appropriately.

Action Cues and Kinetics

Action cues or kinetics are body movements that convey messages. Posture, arm position, hand gestures, body movements, facial expressions, and eye contact all convey a message. The message may reflect a feeling, a mood or an underlying physiological or psychological problem. A relaxed posture with arms at the sides conveys openness; whereas a tense posture with arms crossed may reflect anger or mistrust. A tense, guarded posture may also indicate pain. A tripod position is assumed to ease breathing.

Hand gestures can convey approval, but they may signal anxiety when overused. Abnormal movements may indicate an underlying neurological problem. Facial expressions reflect a variety of emotions, including happiness, sadness, fear, anger, approval, and disapproval.

Facial expressions may also signal an underlying problem, such as anguish from excruciating pain or fear and anxiety from shortness of breath. Eye contact usually conveys interest, caring, and trust. Lack of eye contact may reflect shyness, depression, disinterest, or mistrust.

Your body language is as important as your client's. During history taking, keep your body posture relaxed to convey a calm, reassuring attitude. Work at the same level as your client. Standing over him or her conveys a sense of dominance and authority, enhancing his or her sense of dependence. Give reaffirming gestures such as nodding. Your facial expression should convey care and concern. Maintain eye contact to show the client you are interested in what he or she has to say.

Object Cues

Your client's dress and grooming reflect his or her identity and how he or she feels about himself or herself. Poor grooming or disheveled clothing may indicate a psychological problem such as depression. A depressed client may not take much interest in how he or she looks. Poor grooming may also signal an underlying physical problem that has affected the client's ability to care for himself or herself.

Your appearance is equally important. Your grooming and dress should be neat and appropriate for the situation and reflect your professionalism. Be sure to wear a tag with your name and title. Object cues can also be furnishings or possessions—for example, your jewelry or the seating arrangement for a meeting. These cues are usually selected on a conscious level to convey a specific message, so they are not as revealing as nonverbal communications.

Personal Space

Personal space is the territory surrounding a person that he or she perceives as private or the physical distance that needs to be maintained for the person to feel comfortable. When our personal space is invaded, we feel uncomfortable and anxious, often backing away to regain control of our territory. Personal space is often defined by culture and is also influenced by the situation. Public space is about 12 feet or more, such as in a classroom or when giving a speech. Social-consultative space is about 4 to 12 feet, such as in impersonal conversations or interviews. Personal distance is about 18 inches to 4 feet, such as in personal conversation. Intimate distance is 0 to 18 inches, such as in intimate conversations and maximum sensory stimulation. A person who is withdrawn or mistrusting may widen his or her personal space. An aggressive, angry person may invade your personal space.

Be aware of your position in relation to your client. Assessment entails working in close proximity to your client—about 3 to 4 feet when taking the health history and much closer, within your client's personal or intimate space, when performing the physical assessment. Be sure to explain what you are doing, and look for clues that your client is becoming uncomfortable. If so, you may need to back off and try another approach.

Touch

Touch is a means of communication. An array of feelings can be conveyed through touch, including anger, caring, and protectiveness. The interpretation of touch is often culturally prescribed. Touch can be easily misconstrued. It may be seen as an invasion of one's personal space or a threat. How a person responds to touch often depends on the trust established within a relationship.

Nursing involves touch. We often use touch to convey a sense of caring to our clients. Assessment involves touch. We must touch clients in order to collect data. Gaining your client's trust can help you obtain an accurate, comprehensive health history. It can also make the physical assessment quicker and easier for both of you.

Cultural Considerations

Cultural communication patterns need to be considered when obtaining a health history.

Obviously, if you and your client do not speak the same language, you will need an interpreter to communicate. Even if your client speaks English, he or she still might misinterpret some words or expressions. They may convey a totally different meaning to him or her.

TIPS FOR USING INTERPRETERS

- Use an interpreter rather than a translator. A translator only restates the words; an interpreter translates the words with meaning.
- Use dialect-specific interpreters when possible.
- Allow time for the interpreter and client to become acquainted.
- Allow extra time for the health history.
- Be aware that some of the data may be lost through interpretation.
- Avoid using relatives—they may distort the interpretation.
- Avoid using children, especially for sensitive topics.
- Match interpreter with client by age and gender when possible.
- Maintain eye contact with both the client and the interpreter and read nonverbal cues.
- Be aware of your body language. The client may understand more than he or she can express verbally.
- Speak clearly and slowly, but do not exaggerate or speak loudly.

- Use active rather than passive tense and wait for feedback.
- Use a reference book with common phrases such as *Taber's Cyclopedic Medical Dictionary*.
- Use as many words as possible in the client's language to convey your message.
- Use nonverbal communication when you are unable to understand the language.

Source: Data from Purnell and Paulanka.

Also consider the context in which the language is spoken. For example, German, English, and French are not very contextual because so many words are needed to express a thought. However, Chinese and Native-American languages are very contextual because they use fewer words with more emphasis on what is unspoken.

Vocal characteristics also vary with different cultures. For example, European-Americans and African-Americans talk loudly compared to people of Chinese and Hindu backgrounds, who might misinterpret relative loudness as anger. Arabs often speak excitedly or passionately, another vocal characteristic that can easily be misinterpreted as anger.

European-Americans tend to be open and willing to communicate their feelings and thoughts. Japanese often appear shy and withdrawn to strangers, whereas Jews and Italians are often seen as assertive. Appalachians and Mexican-Americans are not willing to share information with a healthcare provider until a relationship is established.

Use of touch as a means of communication varies with culture. For example, Egyptian-Americans do not usually accept touch except between spouses and family. Even though Mexican-Americans often use touch in communicating; they may be modest during a physical examination performed by someone of the opposite sex.

Personal space also varies with culture. European-Americans keep a much greater distance between each other (about 18 inches) than people of Arabian or Turkish descent, who are comfortable with a much shorter personal space.

Direct eye contact is usually acceptable for European-Americans, but not for Asian-Americans when speaking with someone they consider a superior. Sustained eye contact is considered rude in Bolivia. Sustained eye contact between a child and an adult is considered an "evil eye" or "bad eye" in many cultures.

Facial expression is also influenced by culture. Smiling conveys a warm, friendly message for most cultures, but for the Cofer Indians of Ecuador, smiling is seen as a sign of aggression.

Acceptable greetings vary from culture to culture. The handshake is accepted in most cultures as a friendly sign. Finns consider it rude to speak with your hands in your pockets. A relaxed posture usually conveys confidence and competence in America, but a tense posture conveys the same meaning in Japan and Korea.

Communication Techniques

Because there is a purpose to your interaction with your client, your interview will be focused. You will direct the conversation in order to obtain the data needed to complete the assessment. Even though you want your client to be as open as possible, you may still need to redirect his or her conversation so that you can complete the task at hand. Follow cues that he or she gives you that may lead you to a better understanding of his or her health status.

The following communication techniques will help you direct the interview:

Affirmation/Facilitation: Acknowledge your client's responses through both verbal and nonverbal communication to reassure him or her that you are paying attention to what he or she is saying. Nonverbal gestures, such as nodding or sitting up and leaning forward, encourage your client to continue. Verbal cues, such as saying "ah ha," "go on," or "tell me more" send the same message.

Silence: Although silence is difficult to maintain at times, it can be very effective at facilitating communication. Periods of silence allow your client to collect his or her thoughts before responding and help prevent hasty responses that may be inaccurate. Silence is usually more uncomfortable for you than for your client. You may feel compelled to fill the silence by asking more questions or even by trying to answer the question for your client. Resist the urge! You may end up losing valuable data and sending the wrong message to your client. Silence also gives *you* more time to think and plan your responses. Use this "quiet time" to focus on your client's nonverbal behavior.

Clarifying: If you are unsure or confused about what your client is saying, rephrase what he or she said and then ask the client to clarify. Use phrases like "Let me see if I have this right," or "I want to make sure I'm clear on this," or "I'm not sure what you mean."

Restating: Restating the client's main idea shows him or her that you are listening, allows you to acknowledge your client's feelings, and encourages further discussion. It also helps clarify and validate what your client has said and may help identify teaching needs. For example, if the client states, "I take a water pill every day for my blood pressure," your response might be, "I see—you take Lasix every morning for your blood pressure." If the client replies, "No, I take a water pill every morning," this identifies a teaching need.

Active Listening: Pay attention, maintain eye contact, and really listen to what your client tells you both verbally and nonverbally. As you listen, keep in mind what you are telling your client nonverbally. Active listening conveys interest and acceptance.

Broad or General Openings: This technique is effective when you want to elicit what is important to your client. Use open-ended questions such as, "What would you like to talk about?"

Reflection: Reflection allows you to acknowledge your client's feelings, encouraging further discussion. When your client expresses a thought or feeling, you echo it back, usually in the form of a question. For example, if the client states, "I am so afraid of having surgery," your response would be "You're afraid of having surgery?"

Humor: Humor can be very therapeutic when used in the right context. It can reduce anxiety, help clients cope more effectively, put things into perspective, and decrease social distance.

Informing: Giving information allows your client to be involved in his or her healthcare decisions. An example would be explaining the postoperative course and the importance of coughing and deep breathing to your client preoperatively.

Redirecting: Redirecting your client helps keep the communication goal-directed. It is especially useful if your client goes off on a tangent. To get your client on track again you might say, "Getting back to what brought you to the hospital. . ."

Focusing: Focusing allows you to hone in on a specific area, encouraging further discussion. Examples include: "You said your mother and sister had breast cancer?" or "Do you do BSE, and have you ever had a mammogram?" In this case, you have identified a risk factor and a potential area for health education.

Sharing Perceptions: With this technique, you give your interpretation of what has been said in order to clarify things and prevent misunderstandings. You may need to question your client if there is a discrepancy in the message sent. For example, you might say, "You said you weren't upset, but you're crying."

Identifying Themes: Identifying recurrent themes may help your client make a connection and focus on the major theme. For example, you might say, "From what you've told me, it sounds that every time you were discharged from the hospital to home you had a problem."

Sequencing Events: If your client is having trouble sequencing events, you may need to help him or her place the events in proper order. Start at the beginning and work through the event until the conclusion. You might say, "What happened before the problem started?" "Then what happened?" "How did it end?"

Suggesting: Presenting alternative ideas gives your client options. This is particularly helpful if the client is having difficulty verbalizing his or her feelings. Suggesting is also a good teaching tool. For example, if the client says, "I've tried so hard to lose weight, but I can't," you might say, "Have you tried combining diet and exercise?"

Presenting Reality: If your client seems to be exaggerating or contradicting the facts, help him or her re-examine what has already been said and be more realistic. For example, if he or she says, "I waited all day for someone to answer my call light," you might respond, "All day?"

Summarizing: Summarizing is useful at the conclusion of a major section of the interview. It allows the client to clarify any misconseptions you may have. For example, you might say, "Let me see if I have this correct: You came to the hospital with chest pain, which started an hour ago, after eating lunch."

How You Communicate

Always be aware of the messages you are sending your client, both verbally and nonverbally. How you respond is crucial in establishing the nurse-client relationship. Qualities that help establish and maintain this relationship include genuineness, respect, and empathy.

Genuineness: Be open, honest, and sincere with your client. Your client can detect a less-than-honest response or inconsistencies between your verbal and nonverbal behavior.

Respect: Everyone should be respected as a person of worth and value. You need to be nonjudgmental in your approach. You may not always agree with your client's decisions or like or approve of his or her behavior, but everyone needs to feel accepted as a unique individual.

Empathy: Empathy is knowing what your client means and understanding how he or she feels. Showing empathy acknowledges your client's feelings; shows acceptance, care, and concern; and fosters open communication. Phrases that recognize your client's feelings help build a trusting relationship—for example, "That must have been very difficult for you."

Methods of Data Collection

Data collection can occur through interviews, observation, and physical assessment.

Interviews

The interview is usually structured communication with the purpose of obtaining subjective data. It is most useful when taking the health history. For an interview to be successful, you need good interpersonal communication skills. Many factors can impair effective communication with your client, including cultural or developmental differences or life experiences. You need to examine your values and beliefs to minimize any bias that may interfere with the interview.

When you use your interpersonal skills in a healing way to help your client, this is known as "therapeutic use of self." Showing empathy, demonstrating acceptance, and giving recognition are three techniques that enhance therapeutic use of self. Being empathetic is the ability to understand another's feelings. Maintaining a neutral, nonjudgmental position and demonstrating acceptance of your client's verbal and nonverbal communication is essential in developing a trusting relationship. Acknowledging the client's verbal and nonverbal communication conveys true interest and encourages further communication.

Types of Interviews

Interviews can be either directive or nondirective. Directive interviews are structured with specific questions and are controlled by the nurse. These interviews require less time and are very effective for obtaining factual data. Nondirective interviews are controlled by the client, although the nurse often needs to summarize and clarify the data. These interviews require more time than directive interviews but are very effective at eliciting the client's perceptions and feelings. Nondirective interviews help you to identify what is important to the client.

Types of Questions

Questions are classified as closed or open. Closed questions are often those that elicit a yes or no response. This type of question takes little time and is very effective for factual data. Directive interviews frequently use many closed questions. Open questions elicit the client's perceptions. More time is needed for this type of question. They are frequently used in nondirective interviews.

Interviewing Techniques

Begin the interview by establishing trust and conveying a caring attitude. Make sure that the environment is comfortable and that privacy is ensured with minimal distractions. The following tips will help you get the most from your interviews:

- Introduce yourself.
- Don't rush! Allow enough time for the interview.
- Avoid interruptions.
- Explain that information from the interview is confidential.
- Actively listen to what your client is saying.
- Maintain eye contact.
- Work at the same level as your client. Pull up a chair and sit next to him or her.
- Don't invade your client's personal space. Two to four feet away is a comfortable distance for most clients.
- Explain what you are doing and why.
- If the client presents with a problem, begin by asking questions about that.
- Begin with nonsensitive issues. Leave more sensitive topics until the end.
- Consider your client's cultural background. How does it affect the interview and your interpretation of the data?
- Consider your client's developmental level. How does it affect the interview and your interpretation of the data?
- Don't become preoccupied with writing. You may convey to the client that the forms you are completing are more important than he or she is.
- Be nonjudgmental.
- Avoid "why" questions; they tend to put clients on the defensive.
- Nonverbal behavior is more accurate than verbal. Take a look at yours—what is it telling your client?
- Take a good look at your client's nonverbal behavior. Is it consistent with what he or she is telling you?
- Now look at your client's nonverbal behavior another way. Does it indicate health problems?
- Never pass up an opportunity to teach.
- Present reality.
- Be honest!
- Provide reassurance and encouragement.
- Be respectful.

Interviewing Pitfalls

Try not to fall into the following traps when interviewing a client:

Leading the client: People will tell you what you want to hear. So don't lead the client. Having him or her describe what is happening in his or her own words is much more helpful.

Biasing yourself: You can bias yourself because of the client, a particular disease, or a particular physician. But if you fail to check your biases, you limit your objectivity during assessment.

Letting family members answer for client: You will learn a lot more by having the client describe things in his or her own words.

Asking more than one question at a time: If you do, the client may not know which one to answer. Or, you may not be sure which question is being answered.

Not allowing enough response time: Give the client time to think through his or her answer. This is especially important with older clients.

Using medical jargon: Express your questions in lay terms to make sure your client understands you.

Assuming rather than clarifying and validating: Assuming can lead to inaccurate interpretations and incorrect conclusions.

Taking the client's responses personally: An angry or frustrated client may verbally attack you or the healthcare facility. Realize that the client is displacing his or her feelings on you and using you as a sounding board.

Feeling personally uncomfortable: This often happens with beginning students. Stay focused. It will get easier with experience.

Using clichés: Interviewers often resort to clichés when they feel uncomfortable or unsure of an answer. No one expects you to have all the answers. If you do not have an answer, tell the client that you will try to find one and get back to him or her. Clichés show a disregard for your client's feelings. Examples are "Where there's life there's hope," or "You'll feel better in the morning."

Offering false reassurance: Telling the client that everything will be fine is condescending. It may not be.

Asking persistent or probing questions: Persistent or probing questions make your client uncomfortable. Remember: The client has a right not to answer a question.

Changing the subject: Some nurses change the subject when the interview is making them uncomfortable. This is not very helpful for the client. Remember: You are attending to the client's needs, not your own.

Taking things literally: Literal responses may lead to misunderstanding. Clients who have difficulty expressing feelings directly may use figurative language. So always consider the context in which the statement is made, and clarify if you are still unsure. For example, an extremely frustrated client might say, "If I don't get out of here soon, I'll go crazy!" Don't rush to have a psychiatric consultation—recognize the client's feelings of frustration and focus on them.

Giving advice: The client needs to be informed, but can make his or her own decisions.

Jumping to conclusions: Make sure you have all the facts before drawing conclusions.

Phases of the Interview

The interview is divided into three phases: the introductory phase, the working phase, and the termination phase. Each phase has a specific purpose and different communication patterns.

Introductory Phase

The introductory phase is the time to introduce yourself to your client, put him or her at ease, and explain the purpose of the interview and the time frame needed to complete it. Questions should be nonprobing and client centered. Explain that you will be taking notes, but keep your writing to a minimum.

The Working Phase

The working phase is often where data collection occurs. It is usually very structured; it is also the longest phase. Make sure you allot enough time for the working phase. Although you will need to take notes, stay focused on your client. Listen to what he or she is saying both verbally and nonverbally. With experience, you will become skilled at taking minimal notes and then documenting your data *after* the interview rather than during it.

The Termination Phase

The end of the interview is the termination phase. During this phase, you need to summarize and restate your findings. This provides an opportunity to clarify the data and share your findings with the client. Based on this information, both you and the client can discuss follow-up plans.

Observation

The second method of data collection is observation. Observation entails deliberate use of your senses of sight, smell, and hearing to collect data. Look at both your client and his or her environment to detect anything out of the ordinary. Your initial observations may provide

clues to underlying problems. These clues can be further investigated during the physical examination.
Ask yourself:

- Does the client show signs of physical or psychological stress?
- Does the client seem comfortable?
- What is the client doing?
- What position is he or she assuming?
- Are there any abnormal movements?
- What is the client's body language telling you?
- Is the client's verbal language consistent with his or her nonverbal language?
- Do you notice any unusual odors?
- Do you hear any unusual sounds?
- Is there anything unusual, unsafe, or risky in the client's environment?

Look for:

- Facial expression, color changes, breathing problems
- Grimacing, guarding, diaphoresis
- Eye contact
- Tone of voice and flow of speech
- Position, orthopnea
- Grooming and dress
- Nervousness, restlessness, voluntary/involuntary movements
- Unusual odors, such as fruity smell associated with diabetic ketoacidosis, or foul odor
- Drainage associated with infection
- Unusual sounds, such as grunting, wheezing, rhonchi, or stridor associated with respiratory problems; swishing sounds associated with murmurs

Physical Assessment

Physical assessment provides the objective database. It helps you assess your client's health status and identify actual or potential problems. During physical assessment, you use your senses to collect data through the techniques of inspection, palpation, percussion, and auscultation.

During inspection, look at your client and compare his or her appearance to what you know as normal. Use your sense of smell to detect any unusual odor that may warrant further investigation into a possible health problem. During palpation, use light touch to assess surface characteristics, to put your client at ease, and to convey concern and caring. Use deep palpation to assess organs and masses. During percussion, you use direct, indirect, and fist percussion to assess organ size and areas of tenderness. During auscultation you listen to your client directly and indirectly to hear sounds produced by the body.

The extent of physical assessment depends on the client's condition and your expertise. Physical assessment skills can be used with clients at all levels of health care. Your skills will develop over time with practice and provide invaluable, objective data essential in planning your client's care. (For more information, see Chapter 3, *Approach to the Physical Assessment.*)

COMMON DATA COLLECTION PITFALLS

Because assessment affects every step of the nursing process, the accuracy of your information is critical. To help ensure accurate data collection, avoid the following common pitfalls:

Omitting data: You are not thorough enough, are in a hurry, fail to follow clues that your client gives you or simply lack experience. If you do not know what to look for, you will never see it!

Misinterpreting data: You fail to validate the data and then misinterpret them, or you lose your objectivity and allow your biases to enter into your interpretation of the data.

Hasty interpretation: You make hasty interpretations before you have completed a thorough assessment.

Irrelevant data: You have difficulty deciding which data are important. Experience and knowledge will help you distinguish what is relevant and what is not.

Failure to follow up: You fail to continually assess for changes in your client's responses. Assessment is not a one-shot deal; it is an ongoing process.

Poor communication: You fail to communicate effectively with your client verbally, nonverbally, or both. Your communication skills directly affect the quality of your assessment.

Avoid these problems by listening carefully to what your client is telling you, both verbally and nonverbally. Be thorough and systematic in your approach, be objective, use your knowledge, and develop a strong experiential base for assessment.

▶ Validating Data

Once you have collected the data, you need to validate it to ensure its accuracy. Validation can occur simultaneously with the assessment process. Validating every piece of data is unrealistic, but you do need to validate any time you notice an inconsistency or are unsure of your findings. There are numerous ways to validate data. You can use the same sources that you used to collect data to validate it. For example, as your perform the health history, validate the subjective findings as you perform the physical examination by comparing them with the objective findings. The subjective and objective findings should support each other.

You can also call on your client to validate the assessment data. Often the client can be very helpful. Other sources for validation include family members, other healthcare providers, past health records, and diagnostic tests.

As a beginning practitioner, you may initially feel unsure of your findings. Take advantage of the expertise of your colleagues to validate them. For example, maybe you think you hear an abnormal heart sound, but you are not sure. Ask a colleague to double-check. With experience, you will develop confidence in the accuracy of your assessment. When assessment findings are way out of line from the normal, even experienced nurses will rely on colleagues to validate findings.

Organizing Data

After you have validated the assessment data, you need to organize it. Begin by identifying pertinent data—any findings that are out of the norm and any findings that identify client strengths. The pertinent data provides cues that will help you identify any actual or potential problems. Once you have identified these cues, "cluster" the data, grouping all cues that support a problem. Clustering relevant data gives meaning to the data. These clustered data will be the basis for formulating nursing diagnoses for your client.

Several frameworks can be used for organizing data. A framework provides a way of looking at your client and the data. All frameworks have a common thread—they address the physical, psychosocial, and spiritual needs of a client in a holistic approach.

Common frameworks include the following:

Maslow's Hierarchy of Human Needs: Organizes data according to the client's basic human needs: physiological, safety and security, love and belonging, self-esteem, and self-actualization (Fig. 1–2).

Roy's Adaptation Theory: Organizes data according to the client's adaptation to physiological, self-concept, social role, and interdependence demands.

Gordon's Functional Health Patterns: Organizes data into 11 functional groups that contribute to a person's overall health and well-being, quality of life, and attainment of human potential. These groups include health perception/health management pattern, nutritional-metabolic pattern, elimination pattern, activity-exercise pattern, sleep-rest pattern, cognitive-perceptual pattern, self-perception/self-concept pattern, role-relationship pattern, sexuality-reproductive pattern, coping/stress pattern, and value belief pattern.

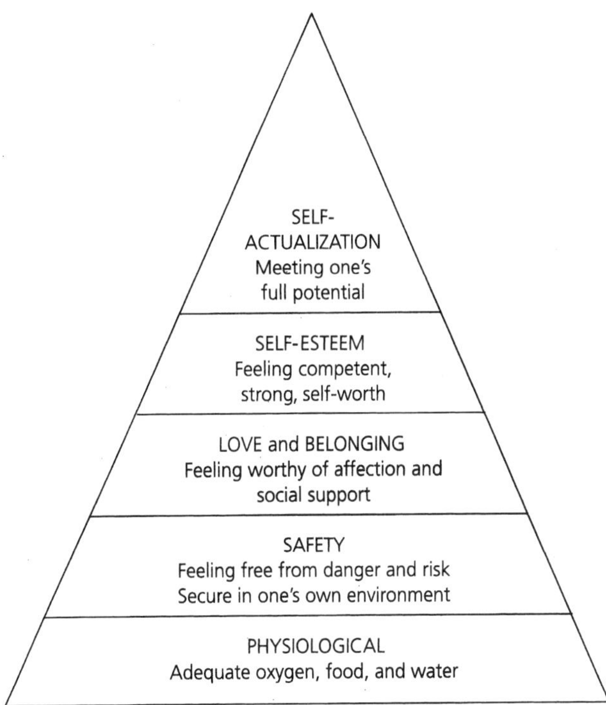

FIGURE 1–2. Maslow's Hierarchy of Human Needs.

NANDA-Unitary Person Framework: Organizes data based on the concept that a person is an open system in constant interaction with the environment. Nine human responses result from this interaction: exchanging, communicating, relating, valuing, choosing, moving, perceiving, knowing, and feeling.

No matter what framework you choose to organize your data, be consistent. The framework allows you to view your client in a particular way and makes your data meaningful.

Prioritizing Data

You need to prioritize the client's problems. When prioritizing, consider the acuity of the problem, the client's perception of the problem, and the situation at hand. Put life-threatening problems that require immediate attention at the top of the list, then problems affecting basic needs that require prompt attention, and finally problems affecting psychosocial needs.

Top-priority or primary problems—such as airway problems—are life-threatening. Secondary problems—such as pain—require prompt attention to prevent further progression or deterioration in your client's condition. Although important, third-level problems—such as teaching needs—do not require immediate attention and can be addressed once your client's condition has stabilized.

CRITICAL THINKING ACTIVITY #3

Give an example of a nursing diagnosis that would correspond to Maslow's Hierarchy of Human Needs.
Physiological needs
Safety needs
Love and belonging
Self-esteem needs
Self-actualization

CRITICAL THINKING ACTIVITY # 4

Prioritize the problems below, assigning primary, secondary, and tertiary levels of priority.
Bleeding
Fatigue, pallor, hemoglobin 7.0
Nausea and vomiting
Grieving
Sleep disturbance, fever, night sweats
Knowledge deficit on self-administration of insulin
Impaired mobility, fractured hip
Irregular heart rate > 140 BPM
BP 70/40
New parent role

Although actual problems usually take precedence over potential ones, potentially serious problems may also have high priority. Also consider the nature and context of the problem. For example, if a new mother is being discharged with her baby, providing instruction regarding care for her and the newborn would be a priority.

HELPFUL HINT

A person's basic needs must be met before addressing higher-level needs that address self-esteem or self-actualization.

Identifying what is important to your client must be considered when prioritizing problems. If your client does not believe that he or she has a problem that you have identified, it will be difficult to develop and implement an effective plan to resolve the problem. Working together with your client to identify actual or potential problems is the best way to develop an effective plan, ensure compliance, and resolve the problem.

ASSESSMENT TIPS

- Involve your client in planning care.
- Common problems occur commonly, rare problems, rarely. So concentrate on common problems.
- On the other hand, be open and expect the unexpected.
- Determine if the onset is acute or chronic.
- Determine if the problems are life threatening and need immediate attention.
- Know what is normal before you try to identify abnormal. Experience will help you refine your ability to differentiate the two.
- Look at your client holistically and identify relevant health risk factors. For example, a middle-aged, African-American male is at risk for hypertension because of this biographical data.
- Validate any inconsistencies.
- Realize that multiple problems will lead to varied human responses.
- Identify problems, but also look for strengths.
- Remember that every system is related. So if you identify a problem in one area, realize that this problem can affect every other system.

Documenting Your Findings

Once you have completed your assessment, document your findings. Your client's initial assessment may require documenting a detailed health admission record that contains both the history and physical assessment data. Every assessment that follows also needs to be documented. To ensure continuity of care, your client's assessment needs to be communicated to all members of the healthcare team involved in his or her care.

Documentation Methods

The approach to documentation is usually source-oriented or problem-oriented. Source-oriented documentation is done by department, so each healthcare group has a section to document findings. This method easily identifies each discipline, but it tends to fragment the data, making it difficult to follow the sequencing of events. With problem-oriented medical records (POMR), everyone involved in the care of the client charts on the same form. This allows for better communication of data to collaboratively resolve the client's problems.

No matter which approach you use, a variety of methods and forms is available for documentation. Many healthcare facilities use standardized nursing assessment forms in a checklist format, which is efficient and time-saving. Computerized documentation is also available in a standardized checklist format. The narrative format may also be used, but this is very time consuming.

Two popular methods of problem-oriented documentation are SOAPIE and PIE. A third popular method, DAR, is used with FOCUS® charting, which focuses more holistically on the client, identifying both strengths and problems that can be incorporated into his or her care. These methods are explained in subsequent text. Another method—charting by exception—is a shorthand documentation method frequently used to save time. It includes only significant data, that is, findings that deviate from well-defined standards.

DOCUMENTATION METHODS

Case Study:
Mary Rutherford, age 43, is one day postoperative after a cholecystectomy. Her assessment data includes the following:
"It hurts to take a deep breath."
Pain rated 8/10
Guarding abdomen
Vital signs: BP 144/90; Pulse 108; Respirations 24 and shallow; Temperature 100.8 °F
Pulse oximeter 92% on room air
Decreased breath sounds at bases due to poor ventilatory effort, also few crackles noted at bases
Receiving PCA morphine
Dressings dry and intact

Here is how you would document Mrs. Rutherford's findings using each method:

SOAPIE Method:

S = subjective data
O = objective data
A = assessment/clinical judgment
P = plan
I = implementation
E = evaluation

Documentation:

S = "It hurts to take a deep breath": Pain increases with activity and breathing, PCA helps; Pain is sharp; Pain located in right upper quadrant (RUQ) and epigastric region; Pain rated 8/10; Pain only when moving.
O = First-day postop cholecystectomy; Vital signs: BP 144/90, pulse 108, Respirations 24 and shallow, Temperature 100.8°F; pulse oximeter 92% on room air; client guarding abdomen; Decreased breath sounds at bases because of poor ventilatory effort, also few crackles noted at bases; Receiving PCA morphine.
A = Ineffective breathing pattern related to incisional pain.
P = Client will establish effective breathing pattern; client will experience no signs of respiratory complications.
I = Enourage coughing and deep breathing; teach client to splint incision; control pain with PCA; encourage ambulation; provide instruction on use of incentive spirometer; maintain adequate hydration.
E = Client coughing and deep breathing, splinting incision; using incentive spirometer; ambulating; using PCA morphine as needed; lungs clear; Vital signs: BP 130/86, temperature 99°F, pulse 80, respirations 20, pulse oximeter 96% on room air.

DAR Method:

D = data
A = action
R = response

Documentation:

D = "It hurts to take a deep breath"; Pain increases with activity and breathing, PCA helps; Pain is sharp; Pain located in RUQ and epigastric region; Pain rated 8/10; Pain only when moving; First-day postop cholecystectomy; Vital signs: BP 144/90; pulse 108; respirations 24 and shallow; temperature 100.8°F; pulse oximeter 92% on room air; client guarding abdomen; Decreased breath sounds at bases because of poor ventilatory effort, also few crackles noted at bases; Receiving PCA morphine.
A = Encourage coughing and deep breathing; teach client to splint incision; control pain with PCA; encourage ambulation; provide instruction on use of incentive spirometer; maintain adequate hydration.
R = Client coughing and deep breathing, splinting incision; using incentive spirometer; ambulating; using PCA morphine as needed; lungs clear; VS: BP = 130/86, t = 99°F, p = 80, r = 20, pulse ox = 96% on room air.

PIE Method:

P = problem
I = implementation
E = evaluation

Documentation:

P = Ineffective breathing pattern related to incisional pain
I = Encourage coughing and deep breathing; teach client to splint incision; control pain with PCA; encourage ambulation; provide instruction on use of incentive spirometer; maintain adequate hydration.
E = Client coughing and deep-breathing, splinting incision; using incentive spirometer; ambulating; using PCA morphine as needed; lungs clear; Vital signs: BP 130/86, temperature 99°F, pulse 80, respirations 20, pulse oximeter 96% on room air.

DOCUMENTATION TIPS

- Be brief and to the point.
- Use acceptable abbreviations.
- If documentation is handwritten, make sure writing is legible.
- No need to write in complete sentences.
- State the facts! Avoid interpretations.
- Avoid terms such as "normal," "good," "usual," and "average."
- Avoid generalizations.
- Document sequentially, in chronological order.
- Do not leave blanks or skip lines.
- Use correct spelling and grammar.
- No erasures or whiting out.
- Record date and time and sign your full signature.

Whatever format or method is used, you need to document accurately and concisely. Documentation is a part of your client's permanent record, and the information is confidential. Because the data should be available to all healthcare members involved in your client's care, it should be readily accessible and easy to read. Other members of the healthcare team should be able to quickly peruse the data and identify pertinent findings. Remember, if your plan of care is to be successful, everyone involved in your client's care needs to have access to the data.

Summary

- The nursing process is a systematic, problem-solving method that guides nursing practice. Assessment is the first step of the nursing process. From your assessment of your client, the rest of the process flows.
- Assessment is a process of continuous data collection; a thinking, doing, feeling process with ethical and legal ramifications.
  - As a thinking process, it requires cognitive skills needed for critical thinking, creative thinking, and clinical decision making.
  - As a doing process, assessment requires psychomotor skills to perform a physical assessment.
  - As a feeling process, assessment requires affective and interpersonal skills to develop caring, therapeutic nurse-client relationships.
- Assessment is responsibility and accountability for your practice and to your client.
- Assessment has always been a part of nursing practice, but the nurse's role, particularly in physical assessment, has expanded through the years. Assessment is now an expected part of every nurse's practice.
- Even though the assessment process may be the same for nursing and medical practice, the outcome differs.
  - The goal of medical practice is to diagnose and treat disease.
  - The goal of nursing practice is to diagnose and treat human responses to actual or potential health problems. Nursing assessment focuses not only on the client's physiological and psychological responses, but also on his or her psychosocial, cultural, developmental, and spiritual dimensions. It identifies the client's responses to health problems as well as his or her strengths. Nursing's aim is to assist the client to his or her optimal level of wellness.
- You will use interviewing, observation, and physical assessment to collect data. Once the data have been collected, you will need to validate them. The data are then organized into clusters and prioritized. From this you will formulate your nursing diagnosis and develop a plan of care.
- Document your findings to communicate the plan of care to all members involved in your client's care.
- Initially, as you begin to develop your assessment and clinical decision-making skills, your focus is limited. You have difficulty looking at your client as a whole; instead, you tend to focus on the parts while you strive to develop skills. With experience, as you develop your assessment and clinical decision-making skills, you will begin to recognize patterns and to see the entire picture while zooming in on the acute problems.
- With practice, you will develop competence in your skills and confidence in your findings. So practice and learn from your clients, for they can teach you so much!

CHAPTER 2

The Health History

Before You Begin

INTRODUCTION TO THE HEALTH HISTORY

The health history provides the subjective database for your assessment. Often the health history is your first major interaction with your client—so make it count! You have only one chance to make a good first impression, and it is often the first impression that your client will remember. This first encounter provides the foundation and sets the tone for your nurse-client relationship.

The health history is subjective, allowing you to see your client through his or her "eyes." It consists of what the client tells you, what the client perceives, and what the client thinks is important. It provides a holistic, qualitative picture of your client. Clues that you obtain from the health history will direct your physical assessment and are essential in developing a successful plan of care for your client.

Purpose of the Health History

The purpose of the health history is to identify not only actual or potential health problems, but also your client's strengths. It should also identify discharge needs. In fact, a successful discharge plan begins on admission with the health history. To create a successful discharge plan, you must take a holistic view of your client and all that affects him or her. Remember: The plan you develop will be successful only if your client is able to follow through with it after discharge.

The purpose of the health history is to:

- Provide the subjective database
- Identify client strengths
- Identify client health problems, both actual and potential
- Identify supports
- Identify teaching needs
- Identify discharge needs
- Identify referral needs

Types of Health Histories

A health history may be either complete or focused. A complete health history includes biographical data, reason for seeking care, current health status, past health status, family history, a detailed review of systems, and a psychosocial profile. A focused health history focuses on the acute problem, so all of your questions will relate to that problem.

Complete Health History

The complete health history begins with biographical data, including the client's name, age, gender, birthdate, birthplace, marital status, race, religion, address, education, occupation, contact person, and health insurance/social security number. It should also include the source of the health history and his or her reliability, who referred the client, and whether or not the client has an advance directive. Once you have obtained this information, you should then identify the reason for seeking health care, followed by a description of current health status.

The past health history includes childhood illnesses, surgeries, injuries, hospitalizations, adult medical problems, medications, allergies, immunizations, travel, and military service. The family history will identify familial or genetically linked disorders. The review of systems provides a comprehensive assessment to determine your client's physiologic status. Past or current problems may be identified and warrant further investigation. The psychosocial profile gives you a picture of your client's health promotion and preventative patterns. It includes a description of health practices and health beliefs, a typical day, nutritional patterns, activity/exercise patterns, recreational patterns, sleep/rest patterns, personal habits, occupational and environmental risk factors, socioeconomic status, developmental level, roles and relationships, self-concept, religious and cultural influences, supports, sexuality patterns and, finally, the emotional health status of your client. Once you have completed the health history, summarize any pertinent data.

A complete health history provides a comprehensive, holistic picture of your client. It screens for actual or potential problems and identifies your client's strengths and health-promotion patterns. A complete health history may be obtained in a primary setting as a screening tool, in a secondary setting once your client's condition stabilizes, or in a tertiary setting to establish a baseline from which to develop your plan of care.

Focused Health History

A focused health history contains necessary biographical data, including the client's name, age, birth date, birthplace, gender, marital status, dependents, race, religion, address, education, occupation, contact person, and health insurance/social security number. It also includes the source of the health history and his or her reliability, who referred the client, and whether or not the client has an advance directive. You should then identify the reason for seeking care, followed by a complete symptom analysis.

In your past health history, address any areas that relate to the reason for seeking care, including diseases of high incidence in the United States, such as heart disease, hypertension, cancer, diabetes, and alcoholism. In your review of systems, ask questions about every system and how it relates to the presenting health problem. The questions in the psychosocial profile identify the impact of the presenting health problem on your client's life.

A focused health history may be indicated when your client's condition is unstable or when time constraints are an issue. Focused health histories may also be used for episodic follow-up visits for your client. In this case, you have already obtained a detailed health history at an earlier point and have established the subjective database. During the follow-up visits, you need to obtain further subjective data to monitor and evaluate your client's progress. Once you have completed the focused health history, remember to document any pertinent findings (Table 2–1).

Table 2–1 Components of Health Histories

COMPLETE HEALTH HISTORY	FOCUSED HEALTH HISTORY
Biographical data	Biographical data
Reason for seeking care	Reason for seeking care
Current health status and symptom analysis if indicated	Current health status and symptom analysis
Past health history	Past health history only as it relates to specific reason for seeking care Check for history of the most prevalent diseases in the United States: heart disease, hypertension, cancer, diabetes, and alcoholism
Family history	Family history only as it relates to specific reason for seeking care
Review of systems	Review of systems only as it relates to specific reason for seeking care
Psychosocial profile	Psychosocial profile only as it relates to specific reason for seeking care
Developmental considerations	Developmental considerations only as they would affect the acute problem
Ethnic considerations	Ethnic considerations only as they would affect the acute problem

Which Type to Do?

Deciding which type of health history to do depends on two factors: your client's condition and the amount of time you have.

Client's Condition

First, determine the condition of your client. It may prohibit a detailed health history upon admission. For example, if you are working in the emergency department and John Harrison, a 49-year-old man, presents with acute chest pain, a detailed health history is not indicated. Instead, you should obtain a focused history while you perform a physical assessment, draw laboratory studies, obtain an electrocardiogram, and connect your client to a cardiac monitor. When a client is in acute distress, trying to obtain a complete health history is not only detrimental, but also provides little valuable or accurate information. So ask key questions that focus on the acute problem; then once your client's condition stabilizes, obtain a more detailed health history.

CRITICAL THINKING ACTIVITY #1

Suppose you were caring for Mr. Harrison. What questions would you ask him to assess his chest pain?

CRITICAL THINKING ACTIVITY #2

What question(s) would you ask Mr. Harrison related to his past health history, family history, review of systems, and psychosocial profile?

Amount of Time

Allot at least 30 minutes to an hour to obtain a complete health history. Be sure to let your client know why you are asking these questions and that it will take time. If you do not have enough time to complete the history, do not rush. Instead, perform a focused history first, and then complete the history at later sessions.

HELPFUL HINT

To save time: Ask the client to fill out a standard history form; then review it with him or her. If necessary, use secondary sources, such as family members, to obtain data. Ask questions while you're bathing the client or performing other care.

Some information may already have been provided; for example, biographical data from the admission sheet. Do not repeat questions unless you need your client's perspective. If the client is asked the same questions several times by different members of the healthcare team, he or she may become frustrated. So, if you need to repeat questions, be sure to tell him or her the reason why.

Medical History vs. Nursing History

The areas addressed and the questions asked during a medical health history are very similar to those in a nursing health history. However, some important differences exist. These differences are defined by the focus and scope of medical vs. nursing practice. Although the history questions are similar, the underlying rationale differs. Remember: Physicians diagnose and treat illness. Nurses diagnose and treat the client's response to a health problem.

For example, Mary Johnson, an 81-year-old woman, is admitted to the hospital with a fractured right hip. The focus of the medical history would be to identify what caused the fracture in order to determine the extent of injury. The history would also try to identify any preexisiting medical problems that might make her a poor surgical risk. The physician will use the data that he or she obtains to develop a treatment plan for the fracture.

Although the nursing health history also focuses on the cause of the injury, the purpose is to determine Mary Johnson's *response* to the injury, or what effect it has on her. You will look at much more than the fractured hip. You will consider how the injury affects every aspect of your client's health and life. Your history will provide clues about the impact of the injury on her ability to perform her everyday activities and help you identify strengths she has that can be incorporated into her plan of care. You will also identify supports and begin your discharge plan. Then you will use the data to develop a care plan with Mary Johnson that includes not only her perioperative phase, but also her discharge rehabilitative planning.

Setting the Scene

Before you begin your assessment, look at your surroundings. Do you have a quiet environment that is free of interruptions? A private room is preferred, but if one is not available, provide privacy by using curtains or screens. Prevent interruptions and distractions so that both you and your client can stay focused on the history. Also make sure that the client is comfortable and that the room is warm and well lit.

Before you begin asking questions, tell your client what you will be doing and why. Inform him or her if you will be taking notes, and reassure the client that what he or she says will be confidential. However, avoid excessive note taking—it sends the message to your client that the health history form is more important than he or she is. Also, if you are too preoccupied with writing and continually break eye contact, you may miss valuable nonverbal messages. Excessive note taking may also inhibit your client's responses, especially when discussing personal and sensitive issues such as sexuality or drug or alcohol use.

Be sure to work at the same level as your client. Sit across or next to him or her. Avoid anything that may break the flow of the interview. If the interview is being recorded or videotaped, be sure to get your client's permission before starting. Position the equipment as unobtrusively as possible so that it does not distract you or your client.

Your approach to your client depends on his or her cultural background, age, and developmental level. Ask yourself, "Are there any cultural considerations that might influence our interaction?" "What approach is best, considering my client's age?"

KEY POINTS TO REMEMBER WHEN OBTAINING A HEALTH HISTORY

- Listen to what your client is telling you both verbally and nonverbally.
- Don't rush! Allow enough time to obtain the data.
- Ensure confidentiality.
- Provide a private, quiet, comfortable environment.
- Avoid interruptions.
- Tell your client how long the interview will take and why you need to ask these questions.
- Do not be so concerned about completing forms that you neglect the client.
- Start with what the client perceives as the problem.
- Use open-ended questions to elicit the client's perspective.
- Attend to any acute problems, such as pain, before obtaining a detailed history.
- Remember that quality is more important than the quantity of information obtained.

Components of the Health History

The components of a complete health history address health and illness patterns, health promotion and protective patterns, and roles and relationships. The parts of the health history that focus on health and illness patterns include the biographical data, reason for seeking health care, current health status, past health history, family history, and review of systems. You identify not only current health problems, but also past health problems and any familial factors that place your client at risk for health problems. Your client's health promotions, protective patterns, and role and relationship patterns are assessed through the psychosocial component of the health history. Here, you assess for risk factors that pose a threat to your client's health in every aspect of his or her life. Also, you need to consider your client's cultural and developmental status as it affects his or her health status.

Biographical Data

The biographical data provide you with direct information related to a current health problem, alert you to risk factors for health problems, and point out the need for referrals. Your client's ability to accurately provide biographical data reflects his or her mental status.

Biographical data include the client's name, address, phone number, contact person, age/birth date, place of birth, gender, race, religion, marital status, educational level, occupation, and social security number/health insurance. They also include the person who provided the history and his or her reliability and the person who referred the client. Information on advance directives may also be obtained for hospital admissions. Also note any special considerations, such as the use of an interpreter (Table 2–2).

Table 2–2 Biographical Data

DATA	SIGNIFICANCE/CONSIDERATIONS
Name (full name and maiden name)	Prevents confusion when clients have similar names. Formats of names may differ culturally (e.g., Cambodians put last name first; married Hispanic women take husband's surname while retaining both parents' last names).
Address and Phone Number	May provide socioeconomic information and identify environmental health risks (e.g., urban vs. suburban or rural neighborhoods).
Contact Person	May be a source for further data and support for client. Essential in case of medical emergency.
Age/Birthdate/Place of Birth	Allows you to compare stated age to apparent age (e.g., chronic illness can make a person appear older). Identifies age-related risk factors for health problems (e.g., children more at risk for accidents; incidence of cardiovascular disease and cancer increases with age). Age helps identify client's developmental stage. Place of birth may correlate with environmental risks.
Gender	Identifies risk for gender-related health problems (e.g., women have a much higher incidence of breast cancer than men).
Race/Ethnicity/Nationality	Identifies risk for health problems associated with a particular race or ethnic group (e.g., African-American males have high incidence of hypertension, Native-Americans have high incidence of diabetes). Identifies possible ethnic influences on healthcare practices.
Religion	Alerts you to religious beliefs that may influence health practices (e.g., Judaism and diet, Jehovah's Witnesses and blood products). May identify sources of support for your client.
Marital Status (never married, married, widowed, separated, divorced)	Identifies possible support people. Present health status may affect family relationships, client's economic status, and ability to support family. Referral may be necessary.
Number of Dependents	Do not assume that unmarried clients live alone. Ask if they live with someone.
Educational Level	Helps determine teaching approaches. Do not assume that educational level correlates with knowledge and understanding (e.g., newly diagnosed diabetic may have a PhD but be totally unfamilar with disease and its management). Do not talk down to client who has had little formal education. **HELPFUL HINT** Ask your client what teaching method he or she prefers (e.g., videos, pamphlets, group, one on one).
Occupation	Identifies possible occupational risk factors. Provides clues about socioeconomic status. Current health status also may affect client's occupational status. Referral may be necessary.

(Continued)

Table 2–2 Biographical Data *(Continued)*

DATA	SIGNIFICANCE/CONSIDERATIONS
Social Security Number/Health Insurance	Social Security number may help in retrieving records. Insurance type may influence length of stay. Referrals may be needed depending on type of health insurance.
Source of History/Reliablity	Ideally, client is source of history. Secondary source is necessary with children or clients unable to provide history—usually a family member or friend. Establish reliability of person providing history by noting consistency in responses and willingness to communicate.
Referral	Identifies primary care physician/practitioner. If no referral source identified, may need to make referral for follow-up.
Advance Directives	Allows you to comply with client's healthcare wishes if advance directives exist.

Reason for Seeking Health Care

Ask your client why he or she is seeking health care; then document his or her direct quote. The client's reason for seeking care is usually related to the healthcare setting—primary, secondary, or tertiary. If the setting is a primary level of health care, there is usually no acute problem. The reason usually relates to health maintenance or promotion. For example, the client states, "I am here for my annual physical examination."

If there is an acute problem, ask the client to state what the problem is and how long it has been going on. For example, "I have had chest pain for the last hour." If your client identifies more than one problem, he or she may be confusing associated symptoms with the primary problem. Help him or her clarify and prioritize the problems by asking questions such as, "Which problems are giving you the most difficulty?"

Usually clients identify problems that affect their ability to do what they usually do. In an acute-care setting, the reason for seeking care is called the chief complaint. The chief complaint gives you the client's perspective on the problem, a view of the problem through his or her eyes.

At the tertiary level, the problem may be well defined, a chronic problem, or an acute problem that is resolving. In this case, the problem does not have the acuity or life-threatening urgency of an acute problem.

Current Health Status

Once you have identified the client's reason for seeking health care, assess his or her current health status. At a primary level of health care (no acute problem), the current health status should include the following:

- Usual state of health
- Any major health problems
- Usual patterns of health care
- Any health concerns

For example: Client is Maryanne Weller, age 42, married, mother of three, full-time teacher. Usual state of health good. Has yearly physical with pelvic examination and dental examination. Last eye examination 1 year ago. Expresses concern regarding family history of hypertension and ovarian cancer.

Clients in secondary or tertiary healthcare settings have an existing problem. So you will need to perform a symptom analysis to thoroughly assess your client's presenting symptoms. Although many questions come to mind, your client's condition and time constraints may preclude you from going into too much detail. If so, you'll need to zero in on several key areas to evaluate your client's symptoms.

As you perform the symptom analysis, try to determine how disabling this problem is for your client. Also ask if he or she has any medical problems related to the current problems and if he or she is taking any medications for this current problem.

HELPFUL HINT

Perform a symptom analysis for any positive symptom that your client reports.

The helpful mnemonic PQRST provides key questions that will give you a good overview of any symptom. Although you can ask additional questions, the following ones provide a thorough analysis of any presenting symptom:

P = Precipitating/Palliative Factors

Ask: What were you doing when the problem started? Does anything make it better, such as medications or certain positions? Does anything make it worse, such as movement or breathing?

Q = Quality/Quantity

Ask: Can you describe the symptom? What does it feel like, look like, or sound like? How often are you experiencing it? To what degree does this problem affect your ability to perform your usual daily activities?

R = Region/Radiation/Related Symptoms

Ask: Can you point to where the problem is? Does it occur or spread anywhere else? (Take care not to lead your client.) Do you have any other symptoms? (Depending on the chief complaint, ask about related symptoms. For example, if the client has chest pain, ask if he or she has breathing problems or nausea.)

S = Severity

Ask: Is the symptom mild, moderate, or severe? Grade it on a scale of 0 to 10, with 0 being no symptom and 10 being the most severe. (Grading on a scale helps objectify the symptom.)

T = Timing

Ask: When did the symptom start? How often does it occur? How long did it last?

PAIN SCALES

Several scales are used for assessing pain, but they can be adapted to assess any symptom. Besides the numeric (0 to 10) scale, you may use scales that rate pain/symptoms with words like "little pain" or "worst pain possible." For children, scales are available with drawings of happy to sad faces or photographs of children's faces representing "no hurt" to "worst hurt ever." Crayons may also be used, with different colors representing different degrees of symptoms or pain.

Past Health History

The past health history assesses childhood illnesses, hospitalizations, surgeries, serious injuries, adult medical problems (including serious or chronic illnesses), immunizations, allergies, medications, recent travel, and military service. The purpose is to identify any health factors from the past that may have a direct relationship to your client's current health status. For example, a history of rheumatic fever as a child may explain mitral valve disease as an adult.

The past health history also identifies any chronic pre-existing health problems, such as diabetes or hypertension, which may directly affect the current health problem. For example, clients with diabetes often have poor wound healing. Also, even though the chronic disease may be well controlled, the current health problem may cause an exacerbation. For instance, a client with well-controlled diabetes may need to adjust his or her medication when scheduled for surgery, because the stress of surgery can elevate blood glucose. In addition, the past health history can identify additional health risks cause by pre-existing conditions.

Finally, the past health history may explain your client's response to illness, health care, and healthcare workers. If he or she has a history of multiple medical problems requiring frequent hospitalizations, these experiences may affect his or her perception of health care either positively or negatively.

When obtaining the past health history, be sure to ask for dates, physicians' names, names of hospitals, and reasons for hospitalizations or surgeries. This information is important if past records are needed. Also avoid using terms such as usual, general, or routine. For example, "usual" childhood illnesses vary depending on the age of your client and available immunizations. (Table 2–3).

Table 2–3 Past Health History

DATA	SIGNIFICANCE/CONSIDERATIONS
Childhood Illnesses	Positive history of mumps, chickenpox, rubella, frequent ear infections, frequent streptococcal infections or sore throats, rheumatic fever, scarlet fever, pertussis, or asthma may have a direct link to current health problem (e.g., history of chickenpox explains current shingles).
Hospitalizations	Previous hospitalizations may have a direct link to current problem or provide clues to pre-existing problems. Knowing name of hospital and dates facilitates record retrieval. Ask about hospitalizations for both physical and psychological problems.
Surgeries	Knowing past surgical procedures may rule out certain problems or explain others. For example, a client with right lower quadrant pain cannot have appendicitis if his or her appendix has been removed, but pain may be caused by adhesions.

(Continued)

Table 2–3 Past Health History *(Continued)*

DATA	SIGNIFICANCE/CONSIDERATIONS
Serious Injuries	History of serious injuries (fractures, head injuries with loss of consciousness, motor vehicle accidents, burns, or lacerations) may relate to current problem or explain findings during physical examination. For example, past motor vehicle accident (MVA) may cause lingering musculoskeletal problems or scars.
Serious/Chronic Illness	Encourages clients with well-controlled chronic illnesses (e.g., heart disease, hypertension, diabetes, cancer, seizures) to identify these illnesses. Otherwise, they may fail to mention them if they are not currently causing problems. Consider client's age and ask about most prevalent diseases for his or her age group.
Immunizations	Lack of immunization may explain current problem. Consider client's age: In the United States today, children receive many more immunizations than they did 20 years ago. Also, the need for some immunizations (e.g., smallpox) no longer exists. Ask if children have had the following immunizations: measles, mumps, rubella, chickenpox, hepatitis B, diphtheria, tetanus, polio, and *Haemophilus influenzae B* (HIB). Ask older adults if they have had a pneumococcal vaccine (pneumovax) and influenza (flu shot). If not vaccinated against tuberculosis (TB), ask about last purified protein derivative (PPD) test. Consider where client lives: In the United States, people are not routinely immunized against TB, but in other countries where incidence of TB is high, Bacille Calmette-Guerin (BCG) vaccine may be used.
Allergies	Allergy may explain current problem. **HELPFUL HINTS** ■ A client vaccinated against TB with BCG will have a positive PPD. ■ Clients often confuse drug side effects with allergic reactions. If client has an allergy, note type of reaction. Allergic reactions include hives, pruritus, and respiratory problems. Side effects include GI upset, nausea, and diarrhea. Remember that immune systems change, so client may become sensitive to something he or she was not allergic to before, or vice versa. Ask if he or she has ever received penicillin, and if there was a reaction.
Medications	Medications may be causing current problem. For example, over-the-counter medication may be interacting with a prescribed medication, causing adverse effects or negating desired effects. Allows you to assess client's understanding of his or her medications, which may identify teaching needs. Ask about prescribed and over-the-counter medications, including vitamins, supplements, and herbs. Obtain name of medication, dose, frequency, and last time taken.
Recent Travel	May identify exposure to health hazards and explain presenting symptoms (e.g., traveler's diarrhea or "Montezuma's revenge").
Military Service	Recent or past military service may identify exposure to health hazards. For example, exposure to Agent Orange during Vietnam War is risk factor for cancer, and exposure to chemical toxins during Operation Desert Storm is risk factor for later health problems.

Family History

The family history provides clues to genetically linked or familial diseases that may be risk factors for your client. Ask about the health status and ages of your client's family members. Family members include the client, spouse, children, parents, siblings, aunts and uncles, and grandparents. Ask about genetically linked or common diseases, such as heart disease, high blood pressure, stroke, diabetes, cancer, obesity, bleeding disorders, tuberculosis, renal disease, seizures. or mental disease. If the client's family members are deceased, record the age and cause of death.

The family history may be recorded in one of two ways. You can list family members along with their age and health status, or you can use a genogram (family tree). A genogram allows you to identify familial risk factors at a glance. When developing a genogram, use symbols to represent family members, and include a key to explain the symbols and abbreviations.

FAMILY HISTORY BY LISTING FAMILY MEMBERS

The following history is for a 37-year-old female client.

- Client: Age 37, alive and well
- Spouse: Age 40, divorced, alcoholism
- Daughter: Age 12, alive and well
- Son: Age 8, alive and well
- Brother: Age 32, alive and well
- Sister: Age 30, alive and well
- Father: Age 66, hypertension (HTN)
- Mother: Age 60, mitral valve prolapse (MVP)
- Paternal aunt: Age 65, breast cancer
- Maternal uncle: Age 62, HTN
- Maternal uncle: Deceased age 28, tuberculosis (TB)
- Maternal aunt: Age 64, MVP
- Maternal aunt: Age 58, HTN
- Maternal aunt: Deceased age 9, ruptured appendix
- Paternal grandfather: Deceased age 68, cancer
- Paternal grandmother: Age 80, HTN
- Maternal grandmother: Age 77, HTN, breast cancer
- Maternal grandfather: Deceased age 70, cardiovascular disease (CVD)

Family History by Genogram

Here is the same 37-year-old female client's family history recorded as a genogram.

Family History by Genogram

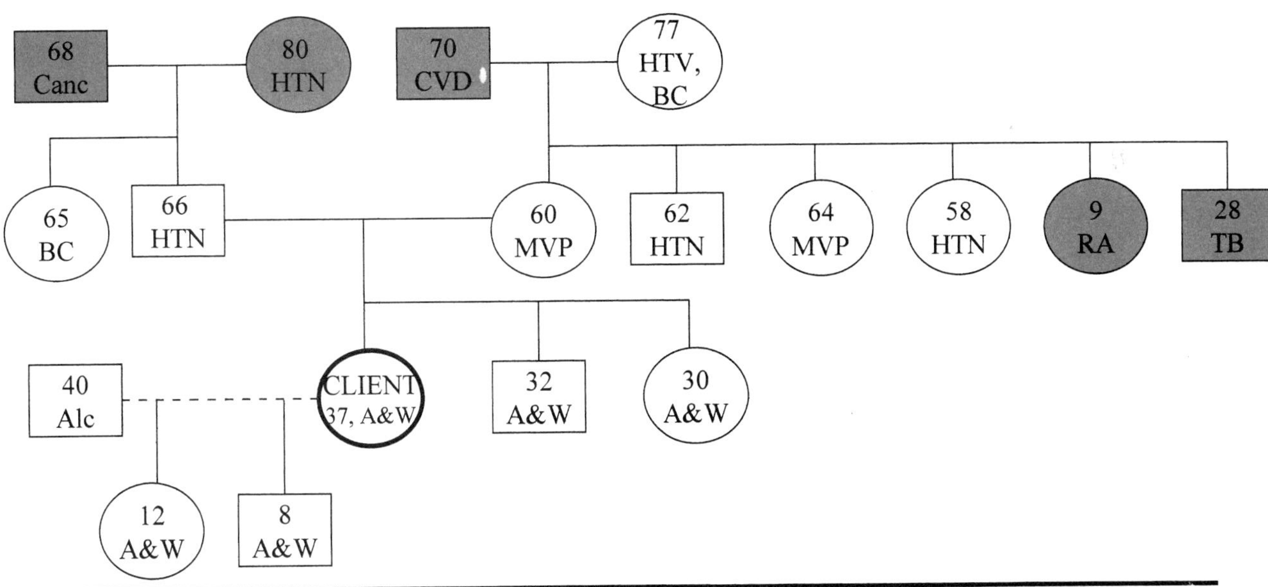

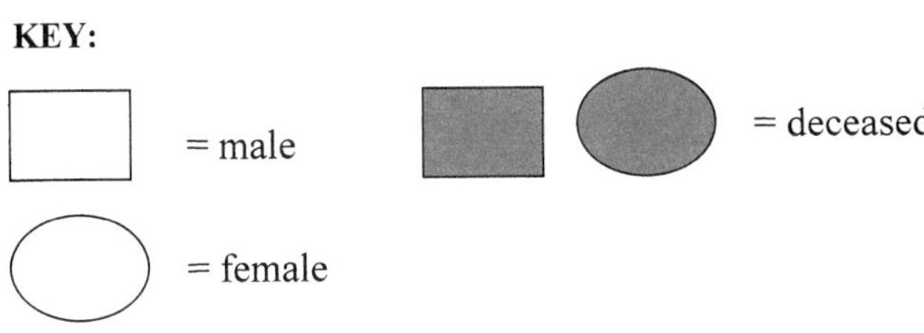

A&W = alive and well
Canc = cancer
HTN = hypertension
BC = breast cancer
RA = ruptured appendicitis
TB = tuberculosis
CVD = cardiovascular disease
MVP = mitral valve prolapse
Alc = alcoholic
- - - = divorced

FIGURE. 2–1. Family history by genogram.

 CRITICAL THINKING ACTIVITY #3

After studying the above family history, what familial health risks would you identify for this client?

Review of Systems

The review of systems (ROS) is a litany of questions specific to each body system. The questions are usually about the most frequently occurring symptoms related to a specific system. The ROS is used to obtain the current and past health status of each system and to identify health problems that your client may have failed to mention previously. Remember: If your client has an acute problem in one area, every other body system will be affected, so look for correlations as you proceed with the ROS. Then perform a symptom analysis for every positive finding and determine the effect of and the client's response to this symptom. The ROS also provides clues to health promotion activities for each particular system. Identify health promotion activities and provide instruction as needed (Table 2–4).

Table 2–4 Review of Systems

AREA/SYSTEM	ASK ABOUT
General Health Survey	Unusual problems or symptoms, fatigue, exercise intolerance, unexplained fevers, night sweats, weakness, difficulty doing activities of daily living (ADLs), number of colds or illnesses per year.
Integumentary	Skin diseases, such as psoriasis, itching, rashes, scars, sores, ulcers, warts, and moles; changes in skin lesions; skin reaction to hot and cold. Changes in hair texture, baldness, usual patterns of hair care (e.g., shampooing, coloring, permanents). Changes in nails (e.g., color, texture, splitting, cracking, breaking); usual patterns of nail care (e.g., use of polish, acrylic nails). **HELPFUL HINT** Recommend an annual skin examination for all adults.
HEENT *Head and Neck*	Headaches, lumps, scars, recent head trauma, injury or surgery, history of concussion or loss of consciousness, dizzy spells, fainting, stiff neck, pain with movement of head and neck, swollen glands, nodes, or masses.
Eyes	Wearing glasses or contact lenses, visual deficit, last eye examination, last glaucoma check, eye injury, itching, tearing, drainage, pain, floaters, halos, loss of vision or parts of fields, blurred vision, double vision, colored lights, flashing lights, light sensitivity, twitching, cataracts or glaucoma, eye surgery, retinal detachment, strabismus, or amblyopia. **HELPFUL HINT** Recommend a routine eye examination and glaucoma check for adults every 2 years.
Ears	Last hearing test, difficulty hearing, sensitivity to sounds, ear pain, drainage, vertigo, ear infections, ringing, fullness in ears, ear wax problems, use of hearing aids, ear-care habits, such as use of cotton-tipped swabs. **HELPFUL HINT** Test your client's hearing during the physical examination and screen for hearing losses routinely in elderly clients.

Table 2–4 Review of Systems

AREA/SYSTEM	ASK ABOUT
Nose and Sinuses	Nosebleeds, broken nose, deviated septum, snoring, postnasal drip, runny nose, sneezing, allergies, use of recreational drugs, difficulty breathing through nose, problem with ability to smell, pain over sinuses, sinus infections.
Mouth and Throat	Sore throats, streptococcal infections, mouth sores, oral herpes, bleeding gums, hoarseness, changes in voice quality, difficulty chewing or swallowing, changes in sense of taste, dentures and bridges, description of dental health, dental surgery, last dental examination, dental hygiene patterns.
	HELPFUL HINT Recommend an annual dental examination.
Respiratory	Breathing problems, cough, sputum (color and amount), bloody sputum, shortness of breath (SOB) with activity, noisy respirations such as wheezing, pneumonia, bronchitis, TB, last chest x ray and results, PPD and results, history of smoking.
Cardiovascular	Chest pain, palpitations, murmurs, skipped beats, HTN, awakening at night with SOB, dizzy spells, cold or numb hands and feet, color changes in hands and feet, pain in legs while walking, swelling of extremities, hair loss on legs, sores that do not heal, results of electrocardiogram if ever done.
	HELPFUL HINT Recommend a blood pressure reading every 1 to 2 years.
Breasts	Breast masses, lumps, pain, discharge, swelling, changes in breast or nipples, cystic breast disease, breast cancer, breast surgery, reduction, enhancements, breast self-examination (BSE) (when and how), date of last clinical breast examination, date of last mammogram, if ever done.
	HELPFUL HINT Recommend BSE monthly, clinical breast examination yearly and mammogram yearly for clients over age 40, unless indicated earlier.
Gastrointestinal	Loss of appetite, indigestion, heartburn, GERD, nausea, vomiting, vomiting blood, liver or gallbladder disease, jaundice, abdominal swelling, regular bowel patterns, changes in bowel patterns, color of stool, diarrhea, constipation, hemorrhoids, weight changes, use of laxatives and antacids, date and results of last fecal occult blood test, if ever done.
	HELPFUL HINT Recommend annual fecal occult blood test and sigmoidoscopy/colonoscopy every 5–10 years for clients over age 50.
Genitourinary	Pain on urination, burning, frequency, urgency, dribbling, incontinence, hesitancy, changes in urine stream, color of urine, history of urinary tract infections, kidney infections, kidney disease, kidney stones, frequent nighttime urination.

(Continued)

Table 2–4 Review of Systems *(Continued)*

AREA/SYSTEM	ASK ABOUT
Female Reproductive	Menarche, description of cycle, last menstrual period, painful menstruation, excessive bleeding, irregular menses, bleeding between periods, last Pap test and results, satisfaction with sexual performance, painful intercourse, use of contraceptives, history of sexually transmitted disease (STD), knowledge of prevention of STDs including HIV, infertility problems, obstetrical history including pregnancies, live births, miscarriages, abortions. **HELPFUL HINT** Recommend a yearly pelvic examination with Pap test for all sexually active women.
Male Reproductive	Lesions, discharge, pain on urination, painful intercourse, prostate or scrotal problems, history of STDs, infertility problems, impotence or sterility, satisfaction with sexual performance, knowledge of prevention of STDs including HIV, use of contraceptives, frequency and technique for testicular self-examination, if ever done, date and results of last prostate examination, if ever done. **HELPFUL HINT** Recommend monthly testicular self-examination and annual digital rectal examination of prostate for men age 50 and over.
Musculoskeletal	Fractures, sprains, muscle cramps, pain, weakness, joint swelling, redness, limited range of motion, joint deformity, noise with movement, spinal deformities, low back pain, loss of height, osteoporosis, degenerative joint disease or rheumatoid arthritis, use of calcium supplements, impact on ability to do activities of daily living (ADLs). **HELPFUL HINT** Recommend a dexascan for bone density for high-risk postmenopausal women.
Neurological	Loss of consciousness, fainting, seizures, head injury, changes in cognition or memory, hallucinations, disorientation, speech problems, sensory disturbances such as numbness, tingling or loss of sensations, motor problems, problems with gait, balance or coordination, and impact on ability to do activities of daily living.
Endocrine	Endocrine disorders such as thyroid disease or diabetes, unexplained changes in weight or height, increased thirst, hunger or urination, heat and cold intolerance, goiter, weakness, hormone therapy, changes in hair or skin.
Immune/Hematologic	Anemia, bleeding disorders, recurrent infections, cancers, HIV, fatigue, blood transfusion, bruising, allergies, unexplained swollen glands.

HELPFUL HINT

As you proceed with the ROS, consider any prescribed or over-the-counter medications your client is taking and how they affect every system. This may help explain some of your findings.

Developmental Considerations

The last part of your health history is taking a psychosocial profile, but before you do this, consider the developmental stage of your client. A person's development crosses the life span. Developmental assessments are often performed on children because the developmental changes that occur at this age are very observable and measurable. Yet adults also go through developmental changes that you need to consider during the assessment. Illness and hospitalization can have a major impact on a child's growth and development, by either halting its progression or regressing it to an earlier stage. For example, when Johnny, age 4, is admitted to the hospital for a hernia repair, he begins wetting the bed during the night, even though his mother assures you that he has been "potty trained" since age 3.

Several developmental theories exist and will provide a framework for your psychosocial profile. These theories focus on specific areas of development, such as physical, psychosocial, cognitive, and behavioral. Identifying your client's developmental stage will help you determine the relationship between the client's health status and his or her growth and development. Because many of these theories do not cross the life span, do not limit yourself to one developmental model. Each theorist views development from a different perspective. So be open and choose the theory or theories that will best help you assess your client's development (Boxes 2–1 and 2–2).

Box 2–1 Developmental Stages and Theories

Stage	Freud	Erikson	Piaget	Kolberg
Infancy (birth to one year)	Oral-sensory	Trust vs. mistrust	Sensorimotor	
Toddler (1 to 3 years)	Anal	Autonomy vs. shame	Preoperational thought—Preconceptual phase	Preconventional level Punishment and obedience
Preschool (3 to 6 years)	Phallic	Initiative vs. guilt	Preoperational–intuitive phase	Preconventional level
School age (6 to 12 years)	Latency	Industry vs. inferiority	Concrete operations—inductive reasoning and beginning to think logically	Conventional level—conformity and loyalty, responds to authority
Adolescence (12 to 18 years)	Genital	Identity vs. role diffusion	Formal operation—deductive and abstract reasoning	Postconventional—behavior corresponds with society
Young adult (18 to 40 years)		Intimacy vs. isolation		
Middle adult (40 to 64 years)		Generativity vs. stagnation		
Older adult (64 to death)		Integrity vs. despair		

Box 2–2 Developmental Tasks

Stage	Freud	Erikson	Piaget	Kolberg	Havighurst
Infancy	Receives pleasure (oral gratification) through sucking.	Begins to trust caregiver. Develops drive and hope.	Understanding of the world is through overt physical actions. Moves from simple reflexes to organized set of schemes of permanent objects.		*Between infancy & school age:* Learns to walk, talk, eat, control elimination. Learns sex differences and modesty. Attains psychological stability. Learns to relate emotionally. Learns right from wrong.

(Continued)

Box 2–2 Developmental Tasks *(Continued)*

Stage	Freud	Erikson	Piaget	Kolberg	Havighurst
					Develops a conscience.
Toddler	Delays gratification through bowel and bladder control.	Becomes independent and learns to cooperate with others. Achieves self-control and willpower.	Develops symbolic play, graphic imagery, mental imagery and language. Egocentric thinking, inflexible, semilogical reasoning and limited social cognition.	Stage 1: Punishment/ obedience. Decisions based on avoiding punishment.	
Pre-schooler	Curious about gender differences and genitals.	Achieving confidence in own abilities. Has direction and purpose.		Naïve instrumental orientation—actions are directed to meet his or her own needs. Very concrete sense of justice/fairness.	
School age	Transition period, develops peer relationships, identifies with parent or caregiver of same sex.	Accomplishments are source of pleasure. Develops methods and competence.	Develops the understanding of conservation of quantity.	Stage 2: Instrumental/ relativist. More self-reliant. Behavior directed to satisfy needs. Negotiate and trade off to meet needs. Stage 3: Approval seeking. Behavior is directed to gain approval by significant others.	Develops physical skills; positive self-image; personal independence, relationships with peers, appropriate gender roles, cognitive skills of reading, writing, and calculations; concepts for everyday living (conscience, values, and morality) and opinions of social and institutional groups.
Adolescent	Attains sexual maturity and becomes interested in sex.	Realizes a stable sense of identity. Develops devotion and fidelity.	Able to combine systems. Develops hypothetical-deductive thinking.	Stage 4: Law and order. Behavior guided by law and order, the rules of society.	Acceptance and development of gender role. Develops more mature relationships. Attains emotional, financial independence from parents.

(Continued)

Box 2–2 Developmental Tasks

Stage	Freud	Erikson	Piaget	Kolberg	Havighurst
					Begins to think of choosing a career and partner for marriage. Intellectual skills and socially acceptable behavior develop further.
Young adult		Develops personal and professional relationships. Attains affiliation and love.		Stage 5: Social contract. Respects individual differences. Realizes that social laws may contradict moral principles. Tries to better the social condition.	Selects mate. Learns to live together with partner. Starts career and family. Rears family. Manages career, family, and home. Assumes civic responsibility. Has social group of friends.
Middle adult		Productive and creative in both work and relationships. Develops productivity and caring for family, friends, and community.		Stage 6: Universal-ethical. Universal-ethical principles guide moral judgment with underlying good of humanity as driving force even at expense of the individual. (This stage is rarely met by most individuals over the course of a lifetime.)	Assumes more civic and social responsibility. Maintains career and family. Develops leisure activities. Strengthens spousal relationship. Accepts mid-life changes. Cares for aging parents.
Older adult		Has had purpose in life and fulfillment. Achieves sense of fulfillment and wisdom.	Adjusts to physical changes, retirement, reduced income, loss of spouse, family members, and friends.		Develops explicit identity with own age group. Modifies living arrangements. Meets social and civic obligations.

Source: Data from Craven and Hirnle, 2000.

Summary of cognitive developmental theories

Knowledge of the various developmental theories provides the nurse with a framework for cultural and psychosocial assessment. The chart below lists selected developmental theorists and summarizes the focus of their theories.

THEORIST	THEORY FOCUS
Sigmund Freud	Psychosexual. Biological drives influence a person's psychological and personality development.
Erik Erikson	Psychosocial. The human life cycle is composed of eight developmental stages, each containing a developmental crisis to be resolved. Psychosocial strengths emerge with resolution of the crisis.
Abraham Maslow	Self-actualization. People are innately motivated toward psychological growth, self-awareness, and personal freedom. Basic needs must be met before a person can advance to higher needs.
Jean Piaget	Cognitive development. An individual's knowledge comes from the interaction between genetic potential and culturally influenced environmental experiences.
Lawrence Kohlberg	Moral development. Cognitive development and emotional growth affect the individual's ability to make autonomous decisions.
Carol Gilligan	Moral development from a female perspective. Women have moral concern for others based on their innate nurturing instincts. They maintain social rules and the expectations of families, social groups, or culture.
Robert Butler	Life review. Elderly clients spend time reviewing past events and concentrating on past conflicts. This life review correlates with the elderly client's good long-term memory.
Robert Peck	Psychosocial. This theory emphasizes aspects of development from middle age through old age by dividing Erikson's last stage into two parts. There is a developmental crisis to be resolved in each part.
Robert Havighurst	Activity during aging. Elderly clients who stay active and maintain or find substitutes for activities of middle age are more satisfied with life than elderly clients who do not. Diminished activity is equated with increased social isolation and accelerated physical decline.
Elaine Cumming and **William Henry**	Disengagement during aging. A person naturally gives up roles (a career, for example) and undergoes losses (through death) as aging occurs. As losses occur, a person withdraws from the high activity level of middle age. At the same time, society withdraws from the elderly client to avoid assigning crucial roles to a group with a high death rate. This mutual disengagement helps society and the elderly client prepare for death.
Evelyn Duvall	Family development. Family goes through identifiable stages with tasks to be mastered.

Psychosocial Profile

The last section of the health history is the psychosocial profile. This section focuses on health promotion, protective patterns, and roles and relationships. It includes questions about healthcare practices and beliefs, a description of a typical day, a nutritional assessment, activity and exercise patterns, recreational activities, sleep/rest patterns, personal habits, occupational risks, environmental risks, roles and relationships, and stress and coping mechanisms.

In a primary healthcare setting, the psychosocial assessment enables you to identify how your client incorporates health practices into every aspect of his or her life. You can then teach and reinforce health promotion activities that your client can incorporate into his or her everyday life. If he or she has an acute problem, the psychosocial assessment helps you determine the impact of this illness on every facet of the client's life and assists you in determining discharge planning needs. For your plan of care to be successful, the client must be able to follow through with it after discharge. Help ensure success by identifying clues as you perform the assessment and then making appropriate referrals (Table 2–5).

Table 2–5 Psychosocial Profile

DATA	SIGNIFICANCE/CONSIDERATIONS
Health Practices and Beliefs	Your client's overall health is affected by his or her values, beliefs, financial status, expectations of health care, and other factors. How does the client perceive his or her role in maintaining health? Does he or she get a yearly physical examination or seek health care only when ill? Does he or she perform self-examinations and other self-care measures? Health is a component of every aspect of life. Determine whether your client's life positively or negatively affects his or her health.
Typical Day	Describing a typical day may identify health risk factors. Or, if the client has a health problem, it helps determine what effect this problem has on his or her everyday life.
Nutritional Patterns	Eating habits can positively or negatively affect your client's health. Religious beliefs or culture may influence eating habits. Financial problems, such as being on a fixed income, may limit food purchases. Ask about special diets, food preferances, food allergies, weight changes, happiness with weight, and history of eating disorders. Ask who does the cooking, who does the shopping, and who dines with the client. All of these factors have an effect on nutrition. Screen for nutritional deficits by doing a 24-hour recall. Ask the client, "What did you eat yesterday?" Do the recall on a weekday rather than a weekend because it is more reflective of the usual diet. After you complete the 24-hour recall, compare the diet to the food groups (meat, poultry and fish, grains, dairy, vegetables and fruits), and note any deficits. Take note of number and size of servings. Also note if your client is taking vitamin or mineral supplements. Make nutritional referrals as indicated. (See Chapter 8, Nutritional Assessment.)
Activity and Exercise Patterns	Activity and routine exercise can help maintain both physical and mental health. Ask about type and amount of activity or exercise. If your client participates in contact sports, assess use of protective equipment and provide instruction as needed. If he or she has a health problem, determine its effect on his or her ability to maintain usual activity and exercise patterns.
Recreation, Pets, Hobbies	Recreational activities, hobbies, and pets usually enhance health by reducing stress. But they can also pose health risks. For example, stained glass work exposes one to lead, and pets may trigger allergies or carry diseases such as toxoplasmosis.
Sleep/Rest Patterns	Many physical and psychological problems can affect sleep or are affected by lack of sleep. Ask your client how many hours of sleep he or she gets, if sleep is interrupted, how many hours he or she needs to feel rested, any medication taken to aid sleep, or if client has any sleeping disorders such as narcolepsy or sleep apnea.
Personal Habits	Unhealthy personal habits, such as use of tobacco, alcohol, caffeine, and drugs, can adversely affect health. **HELPFUL HINT** Ask for specific information about the amount and length of use. *Tobacco:* Ask about cigarettes (filtered/unfiltered), pipe, cigars, or chewing tobacco.

(Continued)

Table 2–5 Psychosocial Profile *(Continued)*

DATA	SIGNIFICANCE/CONSIDERATIONS
	Alcohol: Ask what kinds (wine, beer, mixed drinks), when client drinks, if he or she drinks to help deal with stress, and whether client notices a change in his or her drinking patterns (more or less). The CAGE questionnaire can be used to screen for alcohol abuse (see Chapter 25.) *Caffeine:* Ask what kinds (coffee, tea, chocolate) and if client has trouble sleeping, nervousness, or palpitations. *Drugs:* Ask what kinds (prescription, over-the-counter, recreational, or street drugs), when client last took drug, and method of use (e.g., inhalation, intravenous, oral). **ALERT** *IV drug users are at risk for hepatitis B and HIV.*
Occupational Health Patterns	Certain occupations pose health risks. Ask your client if his or her job requires exposure to toxins such as asbestos, PCPs, pesticides, plastics, anesthetics, radiation, or solvents; if it requires protective gear (e.g., construction workers, welders, landscapers, and tree trimmers), or requires heavy physical activity, such as nursing. Job satisfaction can also affect health. Ask your client if he or she is satisfied with the job, what he or she likes best and least, how many hours a week he or she works, how far he or she travels to and from work, if there are occupational health programs, if he or she gets work breaks, how much vacation he or she gets, if he or she considers the job stressful, and if he or she is satisfied with the salary received.
Socioeconomic Status	Socioeconomic status can have a major impact on your client's health and health care. Ask your client if he or she has health insurance, dental insurance, or a prescription plan. Limited financial resources may limit available healthcare services or prevent your client from following through with a treatment plan. You may need to make referrals to social service agencies for assistance.
Environmental Health Patterns	The client's home and type of community can have an impact on his or her health. Ask if the client's community is urban, suburban, or rural. Urban dwellers are exposed to more noise and air pollution, whereas rural dwellers are exposed to more polluted water sources and septic systems. Determine type of neighborhood. Ask the client if he or she feels safe, are there adequate sidewalks and lighting, with police and fire departments and ambulance nearby, public transportation, accessibility to food and drug stores, easy access to churches, schools, healthcare facilities and community supports, such as senior citizen centers. Determine type of home client lives in. Ask if it is a single home or apartment; if he or she rents or owns it; if living space, heating, water, and plumbing are adequate; if it is one story, two stories, or more; if there are smoke detectors, fire extinguishers, carbon monoxide detectors, and a burglar alarm system; and what type of heating is used. Also ask if medications and cleaning supplies are kept out of the reach of children and if the family uses seat belts, car seats, and bike helmets. Identify teaching needs or areas that warrant referrals or further follow-up.

Table 2–5 Psychosocial Profile

DATA	SIGNIFICANCE/CONSIDERATIONS
Roles, Relationships, Self-Concept	Your client's feelings, attitudes, past experiences, and relationships contribute to his or her sense of value and worth and affect his or her overall health. A person with a positive self-concept and an internal locus of control takes charge and assumes responsibility for his or her life and for achieving health goals. Find out if your client has a positive or negative self-image by asking what he or she feels are his or her strengths and weaknesses, what he or she likes best and least about himself or herself, and if he or she considers himself or herself outgoing or shy. Find out if his or her locus of control is internal or external by asking if he or she feels in control of what happens to him or her or believes that "whatever will be will be." Does he or she assume responsibility or place the responsibility on others? Illness or changes in body image can pose a threat to self-concept. Be alert for risk factors such as serious illness, loss of function, or surgery that threaten your client's self-image. Use the supports and resources necessary to help him or her maintain the integrity of his or her self-concept.
Cultural Influences	Culture can influence communication patterns, health beliefs and practices, dietary habits, family roles, and life-and-death issues. Ask yourself: "Is there a language barrier? Cultural practices that conflict with the prescribed treatment plan? Dietary preferences that need to be considered? Cultural practices that can be included in the client's plan of care?" As long as cultural beliefs will not harm the client's health, accepting them and incorporating them into the plan of care can only help ensure compliance. Individualizing the plan of care gives the client a feeling of ownership and makes him or her more likely to follow through.
Religious/Spiritual Influences	Religion and spirituality influence health beliefs and practices, dietary preferences, family roles, and life-and-death issues. Ask about religious beliefs that conflict with prescribed treatment plan. For example, a Jehovah's Witness may refuse a blood transfusion even in a life-threatening situation. Ask about dietary preferences, such as kosher food for Jewish clients. Ask about religious rites that should be incorporated into the plan of care, such as receiving the sacrament of the sick for Catholic clients. As long as religious beliefs will not harm the client's health, accepting them and incorporating them into the plan of care will only help ensure its success.
Family Roles and Relationships	The family is an important support system for most ill people. Also, when people become ill, their role in the family changes and the family unit may need to reorganize to sustain itself. Determine what effect this change has on your client and his or her family; then plan how to meet their needs. You may need to rely on outside supports. Ask your client about his or her role within the family and other social groups. Is he or she head of the household, responsible for parenting and housekeeping, or are the roles shared? Today's family structure varies greatly, from traditional nuclear family, to single-parent family, to restructured family through divorce or remarriage, to alternative families, to the extended family of the past. But all families share common functions. (See box, Assessing the Family.)

(Continued)

Table 2–5 Psychosocial Profile *(Continued)*

DATA	SIGNIFICANCE/CONSIDERATIONS
Sexuality Patterns	Illness can have both physical and psychological effects on your client's sexuality. Changes in body image or self-concept, changes in ability to perform sexually, prescribed medications and depression can all have adverse affects on sexuality. Developmental, cultural, and religious factors influence your client's perspective and expression of sexuality and his or her willingness to discuss sexuality with you. Sexuality concerns also vary according to your client's age and developmental stage. Sexuality is a sensitive topic that both you and your client may feel uncomfortable discussing. Pick up on clues from your client and address sexuality issues when most appropriate, either during the ROS or the psychosocial history. Be open and nonjudgmental. Ask if your client is sexually active and, if so, whether he or she is satisfied with his or her sexual role, performance and relationship. Find out the source of his or her knowledge of sexuality, reproduction, birth control, and safe sex practices.
Social Supports	Support systems outside the family are important during illness. Ask your client if there is anyone aside from family that he or she can call on for help—for example, friends, coworkers, community agencies, or clergy. Ask if he or she belongs to a church or to community organizations or clubs and if he or she attends on a regular basis. If your client's social supports are limited, tell him or her about resources available within the community and church, and help him or her access those that meet his or her needs.
Stress and Coping Patterns	The amount of stress in your client's life and how he or she copes with it can impact on his or her health. Illness only adds stress and anxiety. Ask your client how he or she deals with everyday stress, what he or she does when feeling upset, if he or she has ever felt sad or depressed, and whom he or she talks to when upset. Keep in mind that normal developmental changes and changes associated with illness can threaten a person's ability to cope. If you determine that your client's coping skills are ineffective, develop a plan of care to help him or her deal with stress more effectively, including sources of support.

Documenting Your Findings

Once you have completed the health history, summarize pertinent findings and share them with your client to confirm their accuracy. Then document your findings and begin to formulate a plan of care.

Documentation of history findings varies from one healthcare facility to another. Many acute-care facilities use computerized programs that enable you to enter the history directly into the computer. Standardized nursing admission assessment forms that combine both history and physical assessments are also commonly used. Regardless of the system, here are some helpful hints for documenting a health history:

- Be accurate and objective. Avoid stating opinions that might bias the reader.
- Do not write in complete sentences. Be brief and to the point!
- Use standard medical abbreviations.
- Don't use the word "normal." It leaves too much room for interpretation.
- Record pertinent negatives.
- Be sure to date and sign your documentation.

Assessing the family

Assessment of how and to what extent the client's family fulfills its functions is an important part of the health history. The nurse should assess the family into which the client was born (family of origin) and, if different, the current family.

Use this guide to assess how the client perceives family functions. Because the questions target a nuclear family—that is, mother, father, and children—they may need modification for single-parent families, families that include grandparents, clients who live alone, or unrelated individuals who live as a family.

Affective function

Assessing how family members feel about, and get along with, each other provides important information. In some families, one person performs the "sick role," and the other family members support the illness and keep the member sick. For example, a child whose parents have marital problems may be sick to get attention. The parents may allow the child to be sick so they can focus their attention on the child and avoid dealing with their problems. To assess affective function, ask the following questions:

- How do the members of your family treat each other?
- How do family members regard each other?
- How do the members of your family regard each other's needs and wants?
- How are feelings expressed in your family?
- Can family members safely express both positive and negative feelings?
- What happens in the family when members disagree?
- How do family members deal with conflict?

Socialization and social placement

These questions provide information about the flexibility of family responsibilities, which is helpful for planning a client's discharge. For example, a mother of small children who has just had major surgery may need household help when she goes home, if the husband is not expected to help or does not want to. To assess socialization and social placement, ask the following questions:

- How satisfied are you with your role and your partner's role as a couple?
- How did you decide to have (or not to have) children?
- Do you and your partner agree about how to bring up the children? If not, how do you work out differences?
- Who is responsible for taking care of the children? Is this mutually satisfactory?
- How well do you feel your children are growing up?
- Are family roles negotiable within the limits of age and ability?
- Do you share cultural values and beliefs with the children?

Healthcare function

This assesssment will uncover many cultural beliefs. Identify the family caregiver and then use that information when planning care. For example, if the client is the caregiver, then the client may need household help when discharged. To assess healthcare function, ask the following questions:

- Who takes care of family members when they are sick? Who makes doctor appointments?
- Are your children learning skills, such as personal hygiene, healthful eating habits, and the importance of sleep and rest?
- How does your family adjust when a member is ill and unable to fulfill expected roles?

Family and social structures

The client's view of the family and of other social structures affects health care. For example, if the client needing home health care belongs to an ethnic group with a strong sense of family responsibility, then the family probably will care for the client. To assess the importance of family and social structures, ask the following questions:

- How important is your family to you?
- Do you have any friends that you consider family?
- Does anyone other than your immediate family (for example, grandparents) live with you?
- Are you involved in community affairs? Do you enjoy these activities?

Economic function

Financial problems frequently cause family conflict. Ask these questions to explore money issues and how they relate to power roles within the family:

- Does your family income meet the family's basic needs?
- Does money allocation consider family needs in relation to individual needs?
- Who makes decisions about family money allocation?

Sample Documentation of Health History

You are now familiar with each step in the history-taking process. If you were interviewing Janet Perry, here is how you would document your findings:

Biographical Data:

- Name: Janet Perry
- Address: 1234 Happy Valley Road, Abington, Pennsylvania 19001
- Home Phone: 215-884-1234
- Work Phone: 215-675-2468
- Sex: Female
- Age: 37
- Birth Date: 4/5/64
- Social Security Number: 123-45-6789
- Place of Birth: Philadelphia, Pennsylvania
- Race: Caucasian
- Nationality: American
- Culture: German-American
- Marital Status: Divorced
- Dependents: 2: Kate, age 15; Joe, age 12
- Contact Person: Sister, Marge Jones: 215-885-2345
- Religion: Episcopalian
- Education: B.S. Chemistry
- Occupation: Lab Assistant, Acme Chemical Corp.
- Health Insurance: BC/BS
- Source and Reliability: Client, seems reliable
- Referral: Self, currently has no primary care provider
- Advance Directives: None

Reason for Seeking Health Care

"I've been feeling tired lately, so I wanted a health exam to make sure nothing is wrong."

Current Health Status

Says she's been feeling tired for about a month. Denies any other symptoms. Denies loss of appetite or history of anemia or blood loss. States that she has been busier at work than usual and hasn't had enough time to spend with her children because she's going to night school for her master's degree. Thinks fatigue may be related to a busy schedule rather than a physical problem. Last had a complete physical 4 years ago, including a Pap smear.

Past Health History

- Childhood illnesses: Positive for measles, rubella, mumps, chickenpox, frequent sore throats.
- Hospitalizations and surgeries: Hospitalized at age 6 for tonsillectomy and adenoidectomy, St. Mary's Hospital, Philadelphia, Dr. Smith. Hospitalized 1986 and 1989 for childbirth, St. Mary's Hospital, Dr. Ballay.
- Serious Injuries: Fractured left arm and concussion from bicycle accident age 10; resolved with no complications.
- Serious/Chronic Illness: No history of cardiovascular disease, hypertension, diabetes, cancer, seizures.
- Immunizations: Up to date, had diphtheria-pertussis-tetanus (DPT), oral polio, smallpox vaccine, last tetanus shot 4 years ago.
- Allergies: No known drug, food, or environmental allergies; has had penicillin without reaction.
- Medications: Takes Tylenol occasionally for headaches and multivitamin daily.
- Travel: No recent travel outside U. S.
- Military Service: Never served in military.

Family History

Documented by listing family members and health status:

- Client—age 37, alive and well
- Spouse—age 40, divorced, alcoholism
- Daughter—age 12, alive and well
- Son—age 8, alive and well
- Brother—age 32, alive and well
- Sister—age 30, alive and well
- Father—age 66, HTN
- Mother—age 60, MVP
- Paternal aunt—age 65, breast cancer
- Maternal uncle—age 62, HTN
- Maternal uncle—deceased age 28, tuberculosis
- Maternal aunt—age 64, MVP
- Maternal aunt—age 58, HTN
- Maternal aunt—deceased age 9, ruptured appendix
- Paternal grandfather—deceased age 68, colon cancer
- Paternal grandmother—age 80, HTN
- Maternal grandmother—age 77, HTN, breast cancer
- Maternal grandfather—deceased age 70, CVD

Figure 2–2 is the same information documented as a genogram.

Pertinent findings: Positive family history for CVD, HTN, MVP, TB and breast and colon cancer. No family history of stroke, diabetes, obesity, bleeding disorders, renal disease, seizures, or mental disease.

Review of Systems

- **General Health Survey:** Complains of fatigue. Had two head colds in past year. No other illnesses. Good exercise tolerance.

Family History by Genogram

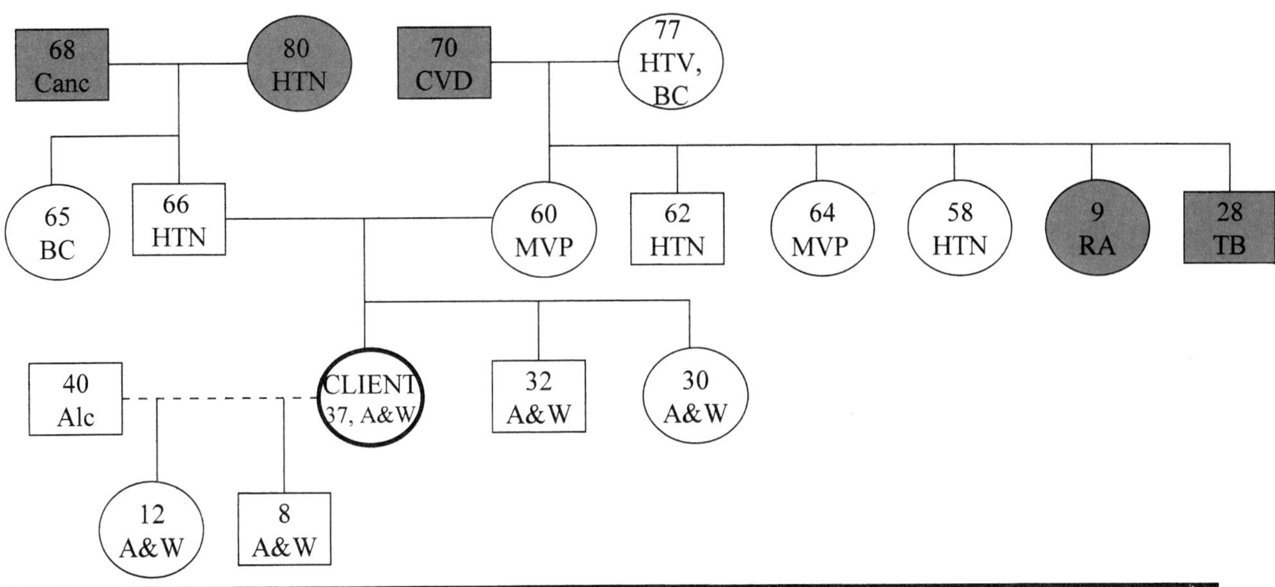

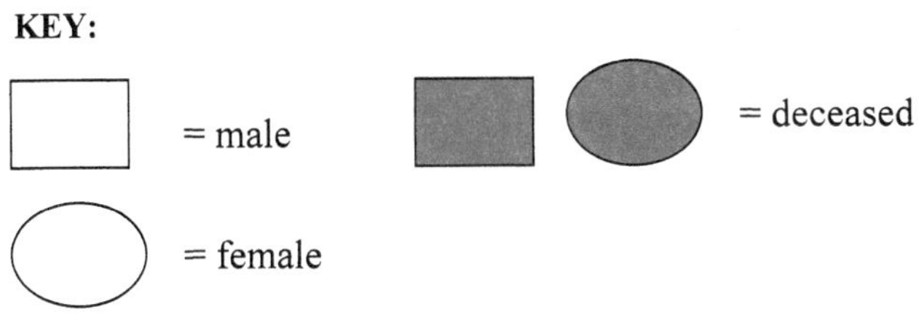

A&W = alive and well
Canc = cancer
HTN = hypertension
BC = breast cancer
RA = ruptured appendicitis
TB = tuberculosis
CVD = cardiovascular disease
MVP = mitral valve prolapse
Alc = alcoholic
- - - = divorced

FIGURE 2–2. Family history by genogram.

- **Skin, Hair, and Nails:** No suspicious lesions, no changes in hair or nails.
- **Head and Neck:** Positive headaches, once a month caused by tension, 6/10 pain scale, relieved with Tylenol. Had concussion as a child, no seizures. No neck pain, masses, has full ROM of neck.
- **Nose and Sinuses:** No history of nosebleeds, rhinorrhea, or sinus infections.
- **Mouth and Throat:** Last dental exam 1 year ago, few fillings, brushes twice a day and flosses. Had T and A as child, no further sore throats.
- **Eyes:** Last eye exam 2 years ago. Wears contact lenses for myopia, wears protective goggles in the lab.
- **Ears:** Reports no hearing problems or ear infections. Last hearing exam 5 years ago.
- **Respiratory:** No breathing difficulties, no history of pneumonia, bronchitis or asthma; exposed to second-hand smoke while married.
- **Cardiovascular:** No chest pain, palpitations, murmurs, HTN, coldness/numbness/color changes in hands or feet, varicose veins, or swelling. Never had an ECG.
- **Breasts:** Reports left breast slightly larger than right, no pain, masses or discharge. BSE about 3–4 times/year. Never had a mammogram.
- **Gastrointestinal:** No history of weight changes, appetite change, indigestion, ulcers, liver or gallbladder disease. Had hemorrhoids during last pregnancy, but resolved after delivery. Regular daily bowel movement, formed and brown in color.
- **Genitourinary:** No history of kidney stones. Had bladder infections 4 years ago, treated with Macrodantin. No problems with urination or incontinence; voids clear yellow urine several times a day.
- **Reproductive:** Menarche at age 12, menses every 30 days, lasts 3–4 days, moderate flow, no discomfort. Obstetrical history: Para 3, gravida 2, 1 miscarriage before oldest child, no complications. No problems with subsequent pregnancies, vaginal deliveries, full term. No history of sexually

transmitted diseases (STDs). Used contraceptive pills in past with no adverse reaction. Sexual relations during marriage described as "fine." Currently not sexually active.

- **Neurological:** History of concussion (see Past Health History), occasional headache (see Review of Systems, Head and Neck), no history of loss of cognition or memory, no balance or coordination problems, no loss of sensation.
- **Musculoskeletal:** No muscle or joint pain/stiffness. History of fractured arm (see Past Health History).
- **Immune/Hematological:** Anemic during last pregnancy even when taking iron. No history of blood loss, anemia, or blood transfusion. Blood type A+. No reported swollen lymph nodes or glands.
- **Endocrine:** No history of thyroid disease or diabetes. No hot/cold intolerance, no increased thirst, urination, or appetite.

Developmental Considerations

In "young adult" stage of development. Divorced for 2 years but has a good relationship with ex-husband, a recovering alcoholic. Feels she is emotionally stable, but feels down and lonely now and then because she hasn't had much time to socialize since divorce.

Psychosocial Profile

- **Health Practices and Beliefs:** Believes each person is responsible for leading a lifestyle conducive to health. Realizes she's overdue for physical exam, in search of new primary care provider. Satisfied with past experiences with healthcare providers.
- **Typical Day:** Wakes at 6:30 AM, gets children up and ready for school, has breakfast, takes children to school, arrives at work at 8:30 AM and works till 5:00 PM, picks children up at after-school program, makes dinner, helps children with homework, gets children ready for bed by 9:00–10:00 PM, studies after children are in bed, retires between 11:30 PM and 12 midnight. Goes to night school 2 nights a week from 6:00 to 9:00 PM.
- **Nutritional Patterns:** 24-hour recall indicates deficits in iron, protein, and calcium. Takes vitamin and mineral supplement. Frequently skips lunch. Happy with weight, no recent changes.
- **Activity and Exercise Patterns:** Jogs 2 miles three times a week during lunch, would like to do more but can't find time.
- **Recreation, Pets, Hobbies:** Enjoys swimming, hiking, and camping; goes camping with children in summer. Would like to do more, but has no time. No pets.
- **Sleep/Rest Patterns:** Says she is a morning person. Awakens at 6:30 AM, goes to bed around 12 midnight. Has no trouble falling asleep, rarely awakens during the night. Would like 8 hours of sleep but rarely gets it.
- **Personal Habits:** Never smoked or used recreational drugs, has two cups of caffeinated coffee a day, drinks one to two glasses of wine a week. Takes vitamin and mineral supplement daily and occasional Tylenol for headache.
- **Occupational Health Patterns:** Works 7 1/2 hours/day with 1-hour lunch. Works well with co-workers. Has had job for 3 years; before divorce was homemaker. Feels under a lot of pressure at work. Is not very satisfied with job and is trying to improve credentials to get better job. Is exposed to toxic chemicals at work but uses proper safety precautions (mask, gloves, goggles).
- **Socioeconomic Status:** States she makes enough to make ends meet—around $25,000 plus child support of $800 a month. Has health insurance and retirement plan through work, children's insurance covered by husband.
- **Environmental Health Patterns:** Lives in three-bedroom single home in suburbs. Considers neighborhood safe. Police and fire departments within 5 miles; schools, stores and church within 10 minutes driving distance from home. Has smoke and carbon monoxide detectors in home, has a burglar alarm system. Drives 20 minutes to work every day. Family uses seat belts and bicycle helmets.
- **Roles, Relationships, Self-Concept:** Describes self as fairly attractive with good sense of humor. Divorce was very difficult, received counseling for 6 months, but is doing OK now.
- **Cultural Influences:** No specific cultural influences that would affect healthcare practices.
- **Religious/Spiritual Influences:** Practicing Episcopalian, but doesn't consider self very religious. Feels it is important for children to attend Sunday services and Sunday school weekly. No religious influences that would affect healthcare practices.
- **Family Roles and Relationships:** Single parent, lab assistant, student with never enough time to do all she wants. Communicates with ex-husband on child-care issues. He is cooperative and provides some financial support. Children get along well for the most part with occasional arguments over her time with them. They help with light chores around the house. Her sister and brother-in-law are major source of support and help with child care. Relationship with parents is distant both geographically and emotionally.

- **Sexuality Patterns:** Currently not sexually active. Says dating again is difficult and she doesn't really have the time.
- **Social Supports:** Aside from sister and brother-in-law, has three close friends in the neighborhood. Doesn't belong to any organized groups, but is aware of such community resources as Parents without Partners.
- **Stress and Coping Patterns:** Says she usually deals with stress by avoiding problem until it is staring her in the face and she has to deal with it. Job is stressful, but she manages on a day-to-day basis, uses co-workers as support. Feels she is easygoing, but when she hasn't had a break in a while, occasionally "blows up" at the kids.

Summary of Pertinent Findings

Client, 37-year-old divorced woman experiencing much stress from work, single parenting, and school. No significant physical problems noted. Positive family history of CVD, HTN, MVP, and breast cancer. Needs physical exam and lab studies to rule out iron deficiency anemia or other physical problems. Needs health promotion instruction re: diet, time and stress management, expanded use of community resources. Positive findings include self-motivated to seek health care; exercises routinely; has family, friends, and coworkers who are source of support; self-motivated to further education to expand career options.

Summary

- The health history provides the subjective database for your client's assessment. It is usually your first major interaction with your client and often provides the foundation of your nurse-client relationship.
- As you proceed with the history, listen to both your client's verbal and nonverbal messages.
- Phrase your questions with your client's developmental stage and cultural background in mind.
- After you complete the history, document your findings and summarize pertinent data.
- Sharing your findings with your client allows you to validate your assessment. You will begin to identify not only actual and potential health problems, but also your client's strengths. Use these strengths in planning his or her care.
- The health history provides clues that will direct your physical assessment as you complete your database and develop a plan of care for your client.

CHAPTER 3

Approach to the Physical Assessment

Before You Begin

INTRODUCTION TO THE PHYSICAL ASSESSMENT

The physical examination is a process during which you use your senses to collect objective data. You will need all of the skills of assessment—cognitive, psychomotor, interpersonal, affective, and ethical/legal—to perform an accurate, thorough physical assessment. You also need to know normal findings before you can begin to distinguish abnormal ones. The best way to perfect your physical assessment skills is through practice. Effective communication skills are essential in establishing the trust needed to proceed with the examination. Finally, you need to remember your ethical and professional responsibility to your client in respecting his or her right to privacy and confidentiality.

Physical assessment provides another perspective. Whereas the health history allows you to see your client *subjectively* through *his* or *her* eyes, the physical examination now allows you to see your client *objectively* through *your* senses. The objective data complete the client's health picture.

PURPOSE OF THE PHYSICAL ASSESSMENT

Like the health history, the goal of physical assessment is not only to identify actual or potential health problems, but also to discover your client's strengths. Data from the physical assessment can be used to validate the health history. For example, you can use the physical examination to further assess clues you obtained from the history. Combined with the history data, your physical assessment findings are essential in formulating nursing diagnoses and developing a plan of care for your client.

Types of Physical Assessment

Physical assessment may be either complete or focused. A **complete physical assessment** includes a general survey; vital sign measurements; assessment of height and weight; and physical examination of *all* structures, organs, and body systems. Perform it when you are examining a client for the first time and need to establish a baseline.

On the other hand, a **focused physical assessment** zeros in on the acute problem, and so you assess only the parts of the body that relate to that problem. It is usually performed when your client's condition is unstable or you are pressed for time.

Complete Physical Assessment

The complete physical examination begins with a general survey. This includes your initial observations of the client's general appearance and behavior, vital signs, and **anthropometric measurements.** Vital signs include temperature, pulse, respirations, blood pressure, and pulse oximetry, if available. Anthropometric measurements include height and weight.

Next, perform a head-to-toe systematic physical assessment. As you proceed from one area to another, remember that all systems are related, so a problem in one area eventually will affect or be affected by every other system. Therefore look for the relationships between the systems as you proceed. For example, a skin lesion or a sore that is not healing may be the first sign of an underlying vascular problem or endocrine problem such as diabetes.

This assessment can be performed at any level of health care prevention—primary, secondary, or tertiary. In a primary setting, a complete physical examination is often performed to establish or monitor health status (for example, it may be required for school, camp, or a job). In an acute-care setting, a complete physical examination is often performed shortly after admission to establish a baseline and detect any other actual or potential problems. In a long-term-care setting, a complete physical examination is also helpful in establishing a baseline from which the client's condition can then be monitored and evaluated.

Because a complete physical assessment takes from 30 minutes to an hour, save time by asking some of the history questions (especially the review of systems) as you perform parts of the physical examination. Perform the assessment as soon as possible because the findings help to establish a baseline.

Focused Physical Assessment

The focused physical assessment consists of a general survey, vital sign measurements, and assessment of the specific area or system of concern. It also includes a quick head-to-toe scan of the client, checking for changes in every system as they relate to the problem at hand. This scan may reveal associated problems and help you determine the severity of the problem. For example, if your client is having breathing problems, do not limit your assessment to the respiratory system alone, because detecting confusion or cyanotic skin color changes may reflect severe hypoxia. The extent of the head-to-toe and focused examinations will depend on your client's condition and your findings.

A focused physical examination is indicated when your client's condition is unstable, when time constraints exist, or for episodic follow-up visits. In the last case, you have already performed a complete physical examination, and so now you perform focused physical assessments to monitor or evaluate your client's health status.

Focused physical assessments can be performed at any level of health-care prevention. In a primary setting, they may be used to monitor your client's health status; for example, to perform a breast examination and teach breast self-examination. In a secondary setting, after you have performed the initial physical assessment, focused assessments are often used to monitor and evaluate your client's health problem. For example, you might take vital signs or auscultate the lungs of a client who was admitted with pneumonia. In a long-term-care setting, a focused assessment is often used to monitor and evaluate your client's progress. For instance, if your client is recovering from a total hip replacement, you will probably assess his or her musculoskeletal system, including gait, muscle strength, and prescribed ROM of joints (Table 3–1).

WHICH TYPE TO DO?

Which type of physical assessment you do depends on:

- The reason for performing the examination
- The condition of your client
- The amount of time you have

Medical Physical Assessment vs. Nursing Physical Assessment

The physical assessment techniques used by physicians and nurses are essentially the same. However, as with the health history, some critical differences exist. These differences are defined by the focus and scope of nursing and medical practice. The techniques are similar, but the underlying rationale differs. Remember: Physicians diagnose and treat illness, but nurses diagnose and treat the client's response to a health problem in an effort to promote his or her health and well-being.

For example, remember the patient in Chapter 2—81-year-old Mary Johnson, who was admitted to the hospital

Table 3–1 Components of Physical Assessments

COMPLETE PHYSICAL ASSESSMENT	FOCUSED PHYSICAL ASSESSMENT
General Survey	**General Survey**
General observations of appearance and behavior	General observations of appearance and behavior as they relate to area of concern
Measurements	**Measurements**
Vital Signs: Temperature, pulse, respirations, blood pressure (BP), and pulse oximetery, if available	Vital Signs: Temperature, pulse, respirations, BP, and pulse oximetry, if available
	Height and weight if client's condition permits
Height and weight	If client's condition does not permit, may need to make estimate
Complete head-to-toe physical assessment of every system or area	Head-to-toe scan as it relates to area of concern
	Focused physical assessment of area or system of concern

with a fractured right hip? The physician would perform a physical assessment to confirm the extent of Mrs. Johnson's injury and ensure that she was medically stable for surgery. The nurse would also perform a physical examination, but his or her focus would be to identify the extent to which this injury affects Mrs. Johnson's physical, psychological, and social well-being. The nurse would also use physical assessment to work collaboratively with the physician to identify any potential complications that might pose a threat to Mrs. Johnson.

The sharper your assessment skills, the better you will be able to detect subtle changes in your client. Alerting the physician to these changes may prevent a more serious complication. You will also use your physical assessment skills to monitor Mrs. Johnson's progress through the perioperative phase to rehabilitation and discharge. Along with the history findings, the data you obtain through physical assessment will be used to develop and evaluate a nursing plan of care for Mrs. Johnson.

Tools of Physical Assessment

The most important tools that you have for physical assessment are your senses. You will use your *eyes* to inspect, looking for both physical changes and nonverbal clues from your client. You will use your *ears* to listen, hearing both sounds produced by various body structures and also what your client is saying. You will use your *nose* to detect any unusual odors that may indicate an underlying problem. You will use your *hands* to feel for physical changes and also to convey a sense of caring to your client.

You will also use a variety of equipment to perform the physical assessment and enhance your assessment abilities. As with any piece of equipment, assessment equipment needs to be periodically checked and calibrated for accuracy, especially equipment that is used for measurement (Table 3–2).

Table 3–2 Physical Assessment Equipment

EQUIPMENT	PURPOSE	TYPES, HINTS, AND CAUTIONS
Thermometer	The thermometer measures body temperature. Measurements may be oral, rectal, tympanic, axillary, or skin. A rectal measurement is most reflective of core temperature, whereas skin or surface measurements are the least reflective. Thermometers measure temperature in either degrees Fahrenheit (°F) or centigrade/Celsius (°C). Types of thermometers include: *Glass mercury:* Used for oral, rectal, or axillary temperature measurements *Electronic digital:* Used for oral, rectal, or axillary temperature measurements	Because mercury is very toxic, many healthcare agencies have stopped using glass mercury thermometers. Electronic thermometers are much faster than mercury thermometers. Disposable probe covers for electronic and tympanic thermometers minimize the risk of cross-contamination. When using a tympanic thermometer, pull the helix up and back for the adult client. Although tympanic thermometers are frequently used in children, studies show conflicting results, especially in infants and children under age 6.

(Continued)

Table 3–2 Physical Assessment Equipment *(Continued)*

EQUIPMENT	PURPOSE	TYPES, HINTS, AND CAUTIONS
	Tympanic: Uses infrared sensors to sense temperature measurements of the tympanic membrane *Disposable paper strips with temperature sensitive dots:* Used for oral or skin/surface temperature measurements	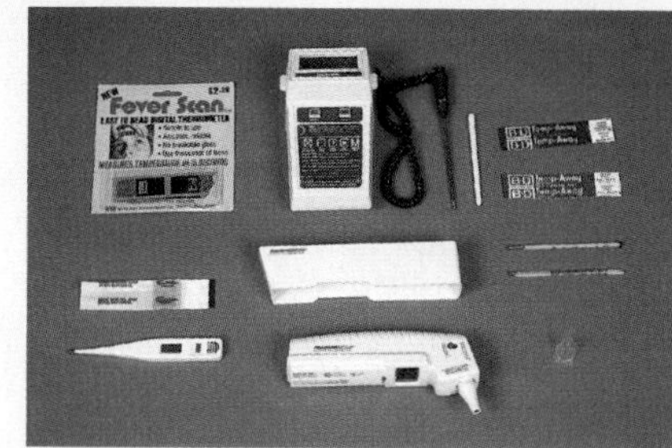 **Types of thermometers**
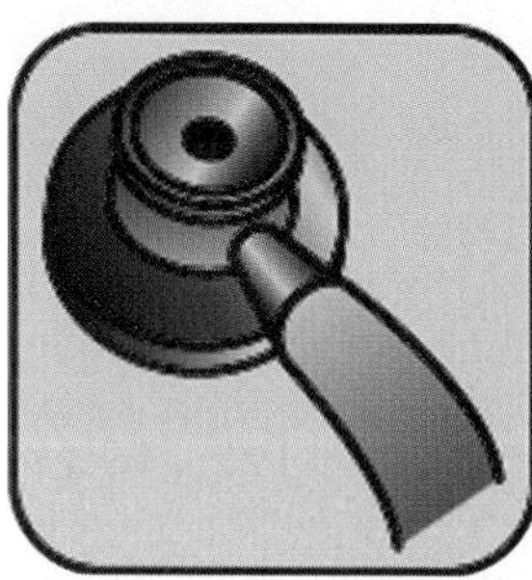 **Stethoscope**	The stethoscope is used to auscultate sounds produced by various body structures (e.g., breath sounds, bowel sounds, heart sounds, BP, and vascular sounds). It should have the ability to detect both high- and low-pitched sounds and may have a single tube, a double tube, or a double tube sealed as one. The average length of a stethoscope is 22 to 27 inches. The diameter of the chestpiece is approximately 1¾ inches. Types of stethoscopes include: *Combination stethoscope with bell and diaphragm:* The bell is the cupped part of the stethoscope. It is best for detecting low-pitched sounds, such as the third and fourth heart sounds, some murmurs, bruits, and Korotkoff sounds. The deeper the cup, the better its ability to detect low-pitched sounds. The diaphragm is the flat part of the stethoscope. It is best for detecting high-pitched sounds, such as breath sounds and some heart and bowel sounds. *Pressure-sensitive single-head stethoscope:* This scope also has the ability to detect high- and low-pitched sounds by the amount of pressure applied. For high-pitched sounds, apply firm pressure. For low-pitched sounds, use light pressure. *Electronic stethoscope:* This scope also has the ability to detect high- and low-pitched sounds. It also allows you to adjust the volume of the sound. This scope is ideal for anyone with a hearing impairment. *Fetoscope:* This scope is used to auscultate fetal heart sounds. It is designed to transmit sound through your ears (air	Your ability to auscultate is only as good as the instrument you use! Always have earpieces pointing forward. Double tubing is better for transmitting sound. The longer or lighter the scope, the less effective it is at transmitting sound. When using the bell portion of the stethoscope, apply light pressure. When using the diaphragm portion of the stethoscope, apply firm pressure. Use a smaller chest piece on infants and small children. 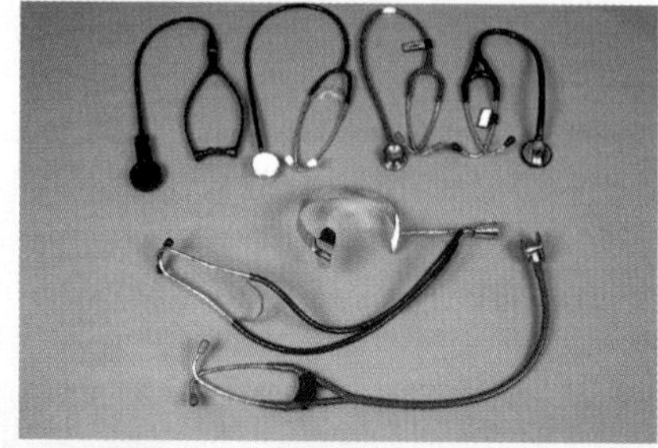 **Types of stethoscopes**

Table 3–2 Physical Assessment Equipment

EQUIPMENT	PURPOSE	TYPES, HINTS, AND CAUTIONS
	conduction) and through your skull (bone conduction), thus increasing your ability to hear the sounds.	
Doppler	The Doppler is used to detect fetal heart sounds. It is also used to locate pulses that may be difficult to palpate, such as the pedal pulses.	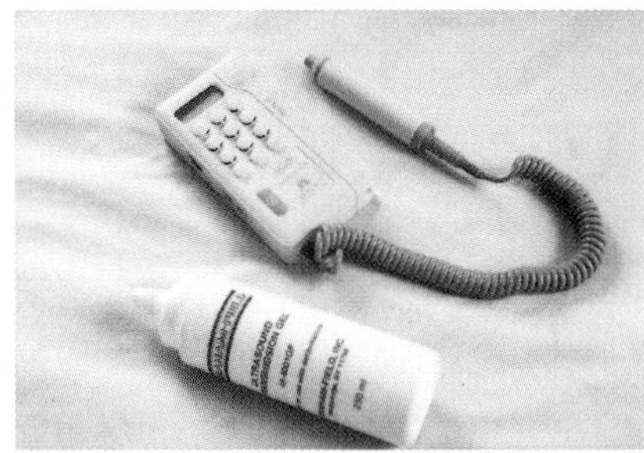 **Doppler**
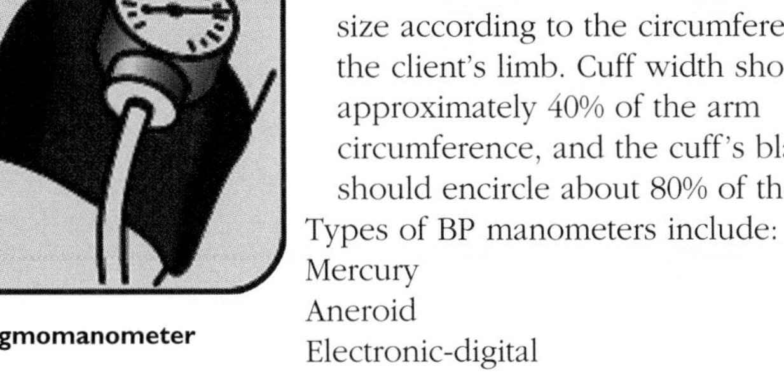 **Sphygmomanometer**	The sphygmomanometer or BP manometer is used to measure BP. Choose a cuff size according to the circumference of the client's limb. Cuff width should be approximately 40% of the arm circumference, and the cuff's bladder should encircle about 80% of the arm. Types of BP manometers include: Mercury Aneroid Electronic-digital This equipment may be wall-mounted or portable.	Incorrect cuff size can lead to inaccurate readings. Mercury manometers are more accurate than aneroid types and require less maintenance. But many healthcare facilities are replacing the mercury type with aneroid types because of the toxicity of mercury. 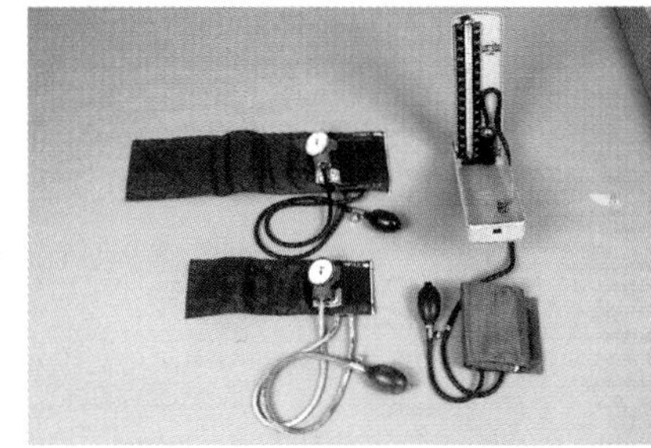 **Types of blood pressure manometers**
Visual Acuity Charts 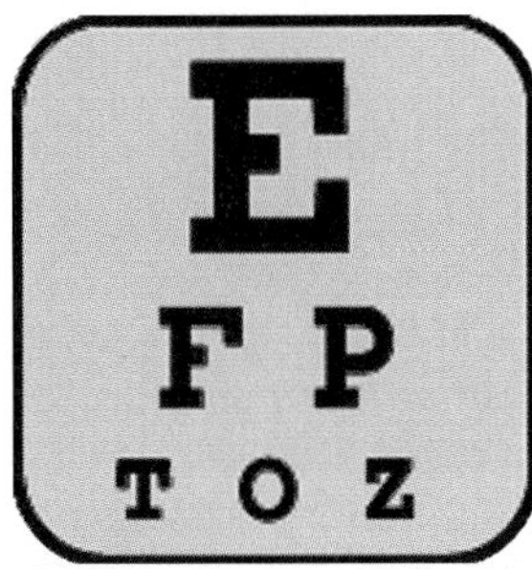 **Snellen eye chart**	Visual acuity charts are used to assess far and near vision. Far vision testing for adults is 20 feet from chart. Far vision for children is 10 feet from chart. Near vision testing is at a distance of about 14 inches. The red and green color bars on the Snellen eye chart can be used to screen for color blindness. Types of visual acuity charts include: *Snellen eye chart:* The "E" chart is used to test children under age 6 or illiterate or non–English-speaking clients. The letter chart can be used for school-age children and literate adults. *Stycar chart:* Uses commonly recognizable letters such as X and O to test vision. Used for children over age 2½ and illiterate adults.	Test each eye separately, then both eyes together. If your client wears glasses or contact lenses, test him or her both with and without them. No more than two mistakes are allowed when using the Snellen chart. 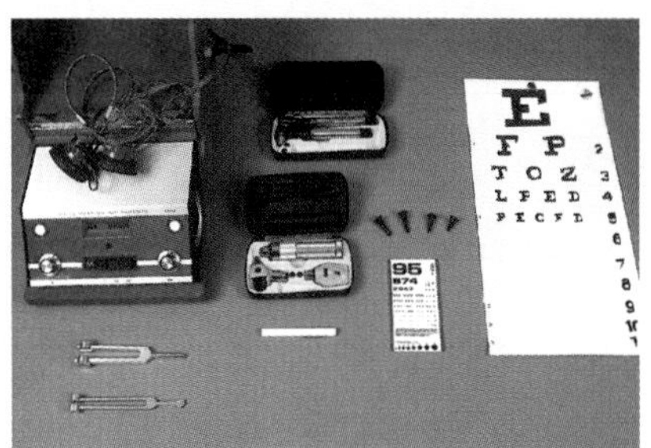 **Types of visual acuity charts**

(Continued)

Table 3–2 Physical Assessment Equipment *(Continued)*

EQUIPMENT	PURPOSE	TYPES, HINTS, AND CAUTIONS
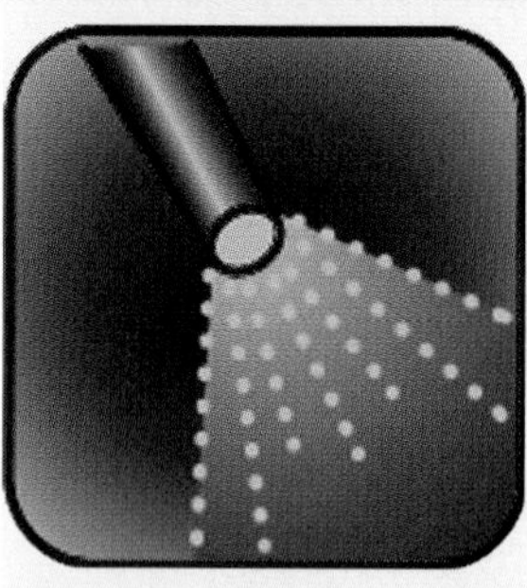 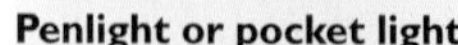 **Penlight or pocket light**	*Allen cards:* Pictures of familiar objects, such as a car, house, or horse are used to test vision of children as young as 24 months. *Pocket vision screener or printed material:* Can be used to test near vision. The penlight is used to assess eyes and hard-to-see places, such as the mouth, throat, and nose.	Check your batteries!
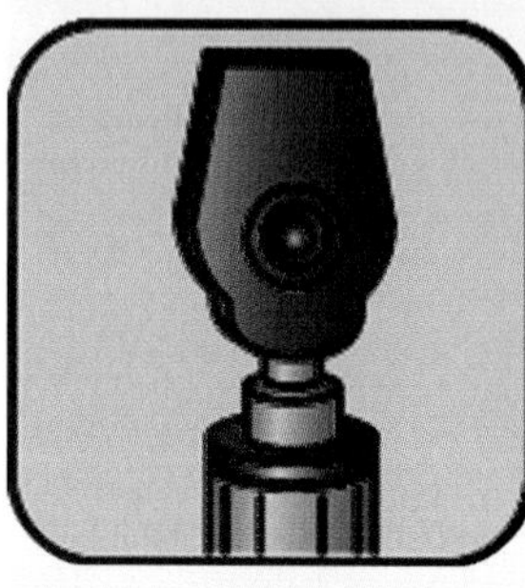 **Ophthalmoscope**	The ophthalmoscope is used to assess the internal structures of the eye. It contains two wheels, the light wheel and the lens wheel. The light wheel includes: Small white light used for undilated pupil Large white light used for dilated pupil Green light to filter out the color red Blue light used to detect lesions when fluorocine dye is used Grid used to locate structures and lesions Slit of light used to determine shape of lesions The lens wheel contains: Red or negative numbers that are concave lenses, which focus far Black or positive numbers that are convex lenses, which focus near Types of ophthalmoscopes include: Battery-operated (some with rechargeable batteries) Penlight type or a combination oto/ophthalmoscope with interchangeable heads Portable or wall-mounted (For more information, see Chapter 10.)	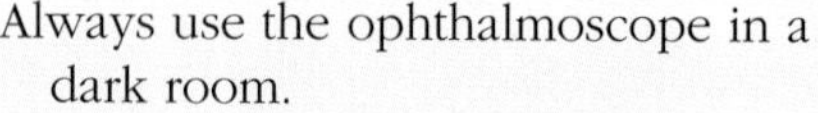 Always use the ophthalmoscope in a dark room. When assessing the client's right eye, use your right eye. When assessing the client's left eye, use your left eye.
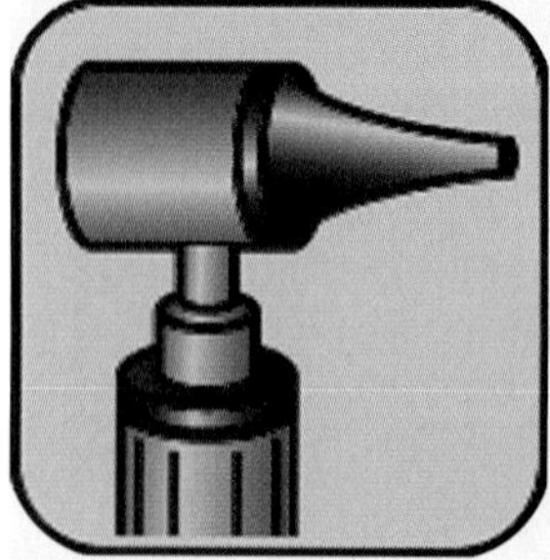 **Otoscope**	The otoscope is used to illuminate and magnify the external ear canal and tympanic membrane. Disposable specula of 3, 4, or 5 mm and about ½ inch in length are used. When choosing a speculum, use the largest one the client's ear can accommodate in order to seal the canal. Also use the shortest speculum possible to prevent trauma or discomfort because the inner two-thirds of the ear canal is over the temporal bone and is very sensitive. For an adult, insert the scope about ½ inch; for a child, about ¼ inch. Many otoscopes also have a	Always palpate the tragus, helix, and mastoid process for tenderness before inserting an otoscope. If they are tender, proceed carefully. For an adult, pull the helix up and back to straighten the canal. For a preschool child, pull the ear lobe down and back to straighten the canal.

Table 3–2 Physical Assessment Equipment

EQUIPMENT	PURPOSE	TYPES, HINTS, AND CAUTIONS
	pneumatic tube attachment to assess the mobility of the tympanic membrane. This is especially valuable when assessing children's ears. Types of otoscopes include: Battery-operated (some with rechargeable batteries) Penlight type or a combination oto/ophthalmoscope with interchangeable heads Portable or wall-mounted (For more information, see Chapter 10.)	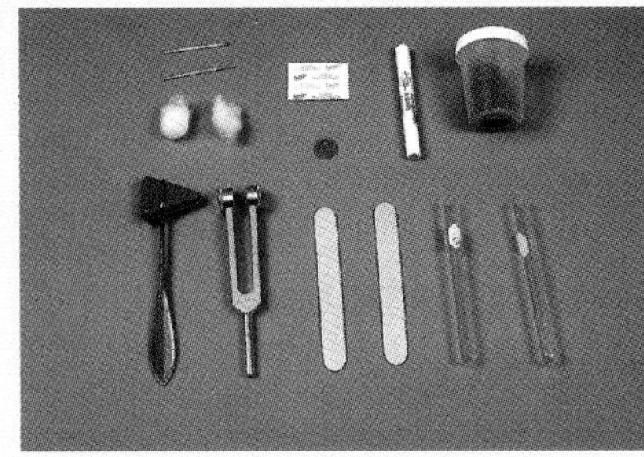 **Equipment used to test hearing**
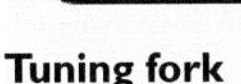 **Tuning fork**	The tuning fork is used to assess hearing and vibratory sensations. Types of tuning forks include: *Low-frequency (256-Hz)*: Best for testing vibratory sensation during the neurological examination *High-frequency (512-Hz)*: Best for assessing hearing	Strike the tuning fork firmly against a hard surface, being careful not to touch the tines—this dampens the vibrations.
Nasoscope	A nasoscope is used to illuminate the nostrils. Types of nasoscopes include: A metal nasal speculum attached to a penlight that illuminates and opens the nostrils to allow visualization An oto/ophthalmoscope with a special nasal tip to illuminate and open the nostrils, allowing better visualization	
 Transilluminator	A transilluminator is used to assess for fluid in the sinuses, the fontanels of the newborn, and the male scrotum. When pressed against a body surface, the light produces a red glow. You can then detect whether the underlying surface contains air, fluid, or tissue.	Transillumination should be performed in a dark room.
	The transilluminator is an attachment that fits on the combination oto/ophthalmoscope with interchangeable heads.	If you do not have a transilluminator, use a penlight instead.
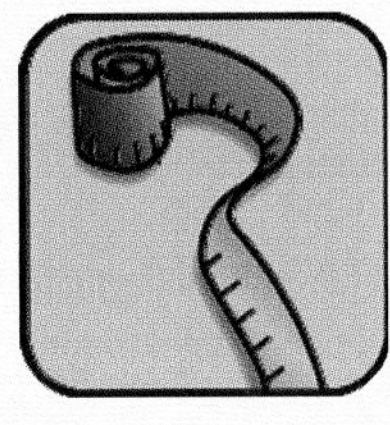 **Tape measure**	A tape measure is used to measure lengths and circumferences of extremities and abdominal girth. In pregnant clients, it isused to measure fundal heights. In newborns, it is used to measure head, chest, and abdominal circumference and length. A stationary wall-mounted tape measure is more accurate for measuring height in children.	Tape measures and rulers are usually calibrated in both centimeters and inches. Centimeters are used more often than inches.

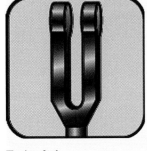

(Continued)

Table 3–2 Physical Assessment Equipment *(Continued)*

EQUIPMENT	PURPOSE	TYPES, HINTS, AND CAUTIONS
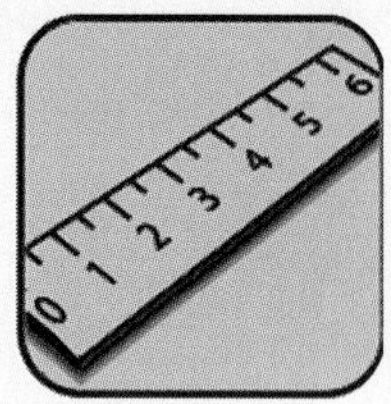 **Pocket ruler**	A pocket ruler is used to measure liver size, respiratory excursion, jugular venous pressure, and any lesion found during the examination.	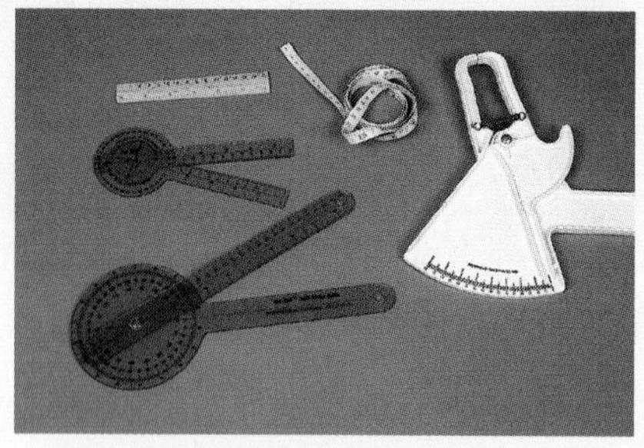 **Types of measuring equipment**
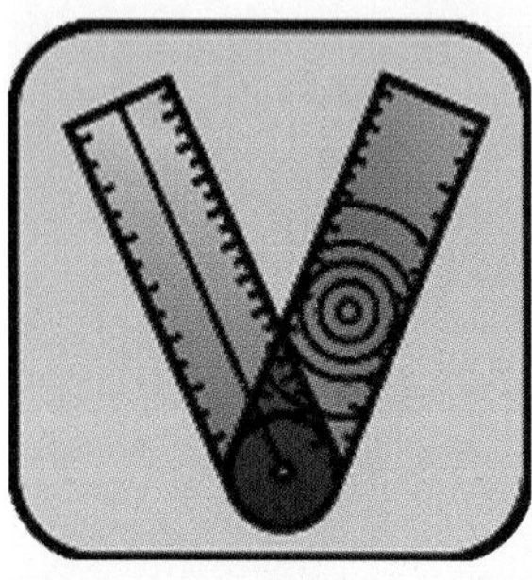 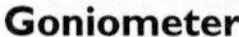 **Goniometer**	A goniometer is used during a musculoskeletal examination to assess the ROM of a joint. It is a protractor with a movable arm and a fixed arm (axis).The center (zero point) is placed at the joint with the fixed arm perpendicular to the joint. As the joint moves, the movable arm is moved to measure the joint's ROM in degrees.	
 **Triceps skinfold calipers**	Triceps skinfold calipers are used to measure body fat. They measure the thickness of the subcutaneous tissue in millimeters.	
 **Marking pen**	Marking the skin with a marking pen helps ensure accuracy. A marker is commonly used for liver sizes and diaphragmatic excursion measurements. Pulses that are difficult to find may also be marked for subsequent assessments.	Markers should be washable and nontoxic.
	A scale is used to measure weight in pounds and kilograms. Be sure the scale is calibrated and balanced. Types of scales include: *Platform scale with height attachment:* Appropriate for weighing a child or	If obtaining daily weights, weigh client at the same time with the same scale. Weights should be taken with the client wearing as little clothing as possible.

Table 3–2 Physical Assessment Equipment

EQUIPMENT	PURPOSE	TYPES, HINTS, AND CAUTIONS
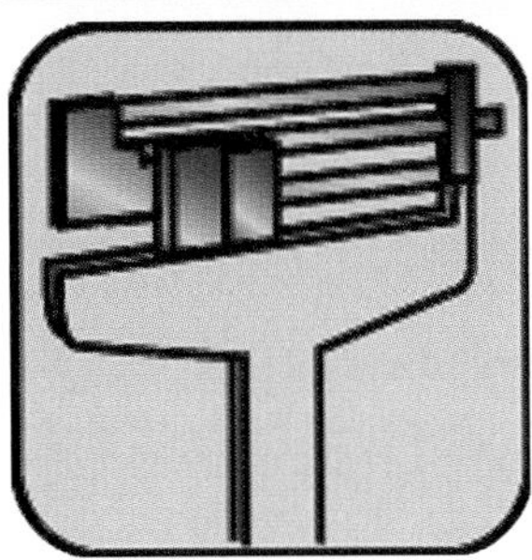 **Scale**	adult. Height attachment appropriate for adults; measure children with a wall-mounted measure. *Portable floor scale:* Appropriate for a child or adult. *Bed scale:* Appropriate for bedridden clients. *Smaller platform "baby" scale:* Appropriate for infants. Has curved sides to prevent infant from rolling off.	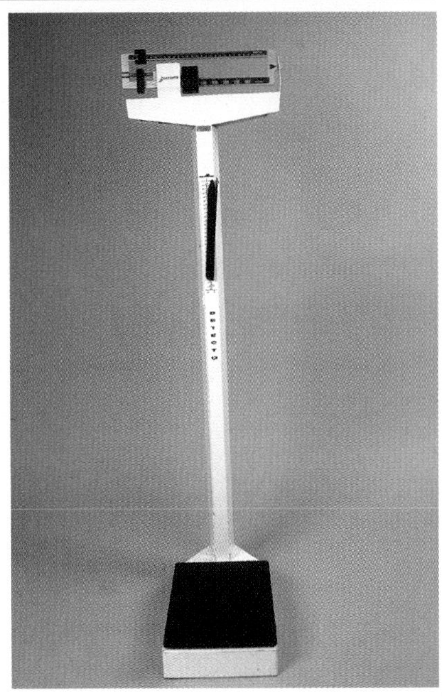 **Platform scale with height attachment**
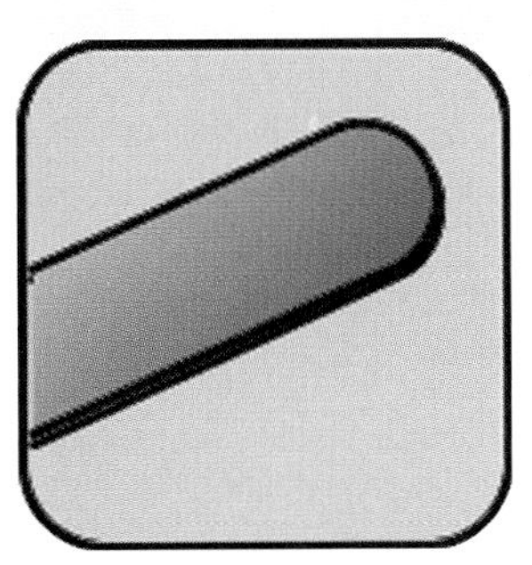 **Wooden tongue depressor**	A wooden tongue depressor allows better visualization of the pharynx. It is also useful in assessing the gag reflex, CN V (trigeminal cranial nerve), and the strength of the muscles of mastication.	Break tongue depressors after use.
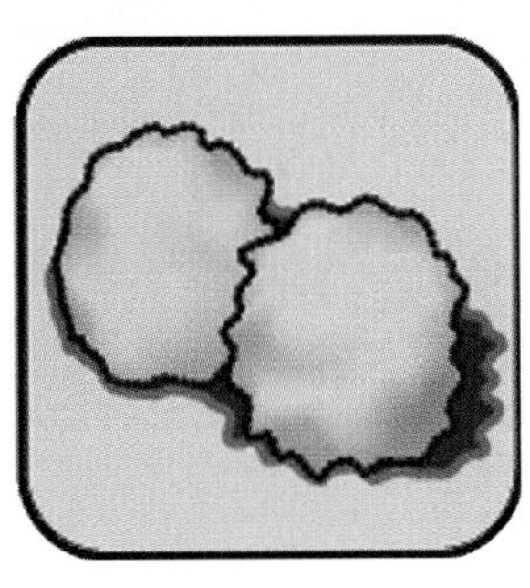 **Cotton balls**	Cotton balls are used during the neurological examination to assess light touch. A wisp of cotton may also be used to assess the corneal reflex.	
Test tubes	Test tubes are used during the neurological examination to assess hot and cold sensation.	If test tubes are not readily available, use the cold metal portion of your stethoscope to assess cold sensation.

(Continued)

Table 3–2 Physical Assessment Equipment *(Continued)*

EQUIPMENT	PURPOSE	TYPES, HINTS, AND CAUTIONS
 **Coffee**	A substance with a strong scent, such as coffee or vanilla, is needed to assess the sense of smell.	
Sugar and lemon	Sugar and lemon are needed to assess the sense of taste.	
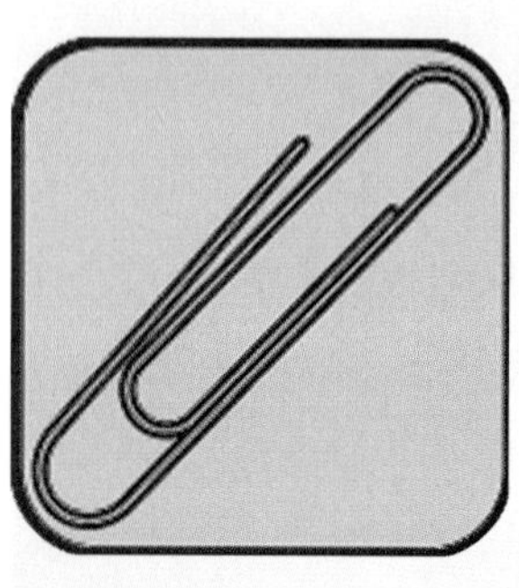 **Cup of water**	A cup of water is needed to assess your client's swallowing ability and thyroid.	
Paper clip	A familiar object, such as a paper clip or coin, is needed to assess for stereognosis during the neurological examination. Stereognosis is the ability to identify a familiar object through the sense of touch.	
Safety pin	A safety pin or other sharp object is used during the neurological examination to assess light touch and pain.	Discard safety pins or straight pins after use. Be careful not to break the skin! A toothpick can be used in place of a safety pin, minimizing the risk of breaking the skin.
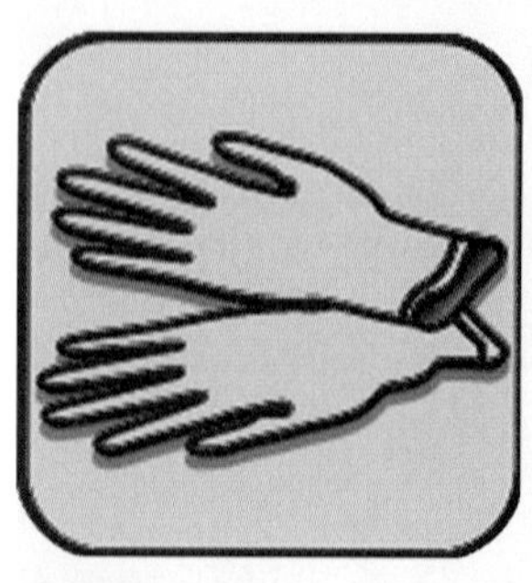 **Gloves**	Wear gloves at any point during the assessment when there is a risk of exposure to blood or body fluids, such as examination of the mouth, pelvic structures of a female client, male reproductive structures, or rectum.	Wear nonlatex gloves. Change gloves as needed.

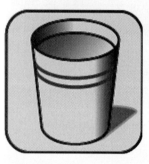

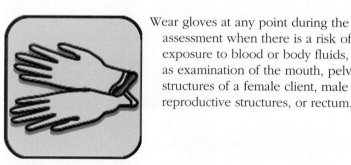

Table 3–2 Physical Assessment Equipment

EQUIPMENT	PURPOSE	TYPES, HINTS, AND CAUTIONS
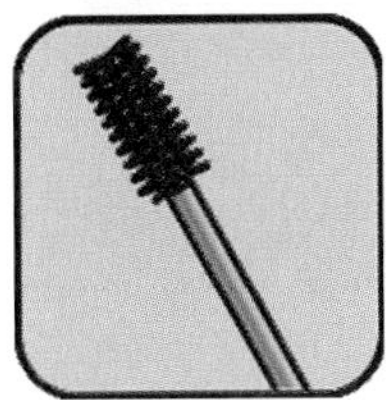 **Cytology brush** 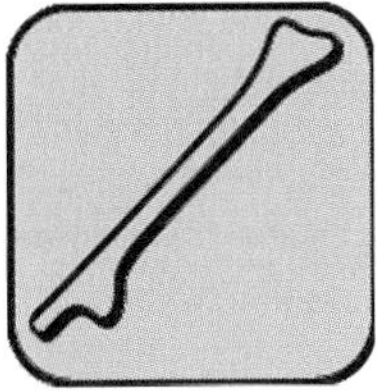 **Scraper**  **Thin Pap test slides** 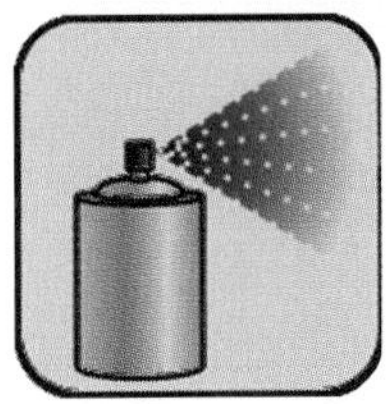 **Fixative**	A cytology brush and scraper and thin Pap test slides are used for specimens obtained during a pelvic examination. If a thin Pap test is not available, use a slide and fixative.	Make sure specimens are labeled and sent to the lab promptly. 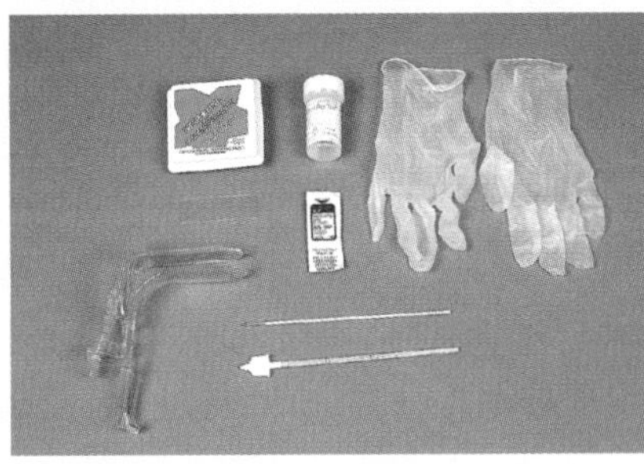 **Equipment used for pelvic exam**
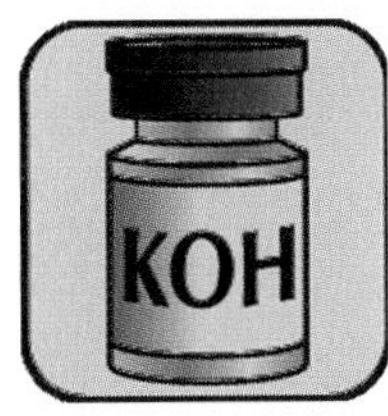 **KOH**	Slides and potassium hydroxide may also be needed for specimen examination.	
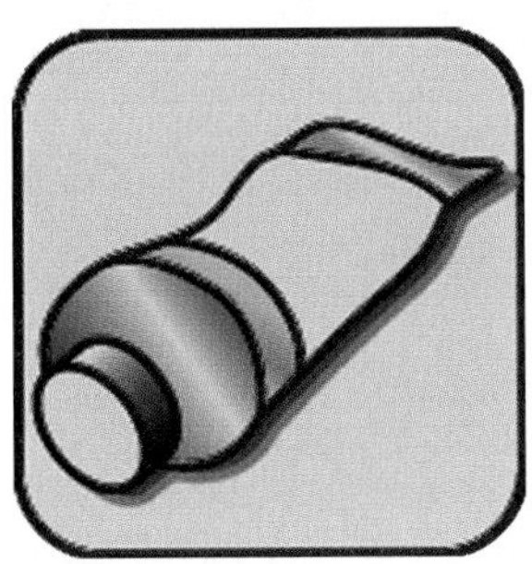 **Lubricant**	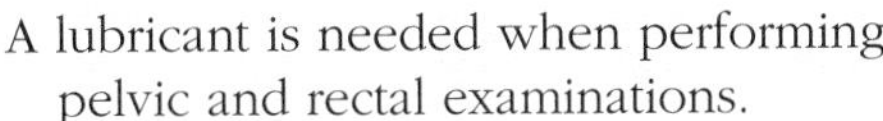 A lubricant is needed when performing pelvic and rectal examinations.	Use a water-soluble lubricant.

(Continued)

Table 3–2 Physical Assessment Equipment *(Continued)*

EQUIPMENT	PURPOSE	TYPES, HINTS, AND CAUTIONS
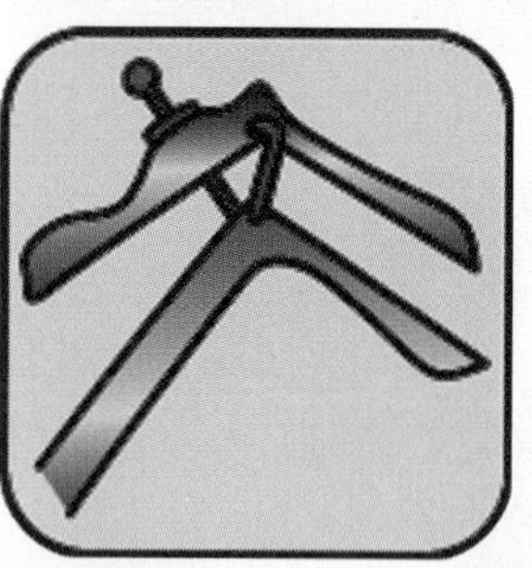 **Speculum**	A vaginal speculum is used to assess the female reproductive system. Specula come in various sizes. After the speculum is inserted into the vaginal canal, it is opened to allow for better visualization of the canal and cervix. Some specula are equipped with a light to illuminate the canal and cervix.	
Hemoccult test	A hemoccult test is used during a rectal examination to test the stool for blood.	

Techniques of Physical Assessment

The four techniques of physical assessment are **inspection, palpation, percussion,** and **auscultation.** They are performed in this order, with the exception of the abdominal assessment. In this case, auscultation precedes palpation and percussion so as not to alter the bowel sounds.

Inspection

Always begin with inspection (Fig. 3–1. Inspection is the most frequently used assessment technique, but its value is often overlooked. With inspection, you not only use your sense of sight, but also your senses of hearing and smell to critically inspect your client. Do not rush the process; take your time and really look at your client. Perform inspection at every encounter with your client.

Be sure you have adequate lighting, and sufficiently expose that area being assessed. Be systematic in your approach, working from head to toe and noting key landmarks and normal findings. Use your client as a comparative when possible. Ask yourself, "Does it look the same on the left side as the right?" Look for surface characteristics such as color, size, and shape. Ask yourself, "Are there color changes? Is the client symmetrical?" Look for gross abnormalities or signs of distress. Do you notice any unusual odors or hear any unusual sounds that warrant further investigation? Always view your findings in light of the client's growth and developmental stage and cultural background, which may influence your interpretation.

Inspection may be direct or indirect. **Direct inspection** involves directly looking at your client. **Indirect inspection** involves using equipment to enhance visualization. For example, the oto/ophthalmoscope allows better visualization of the ears and eyes, and specula, such as the nasal speculum and vaginal speculum, open and illuminate allowing for better visualization.

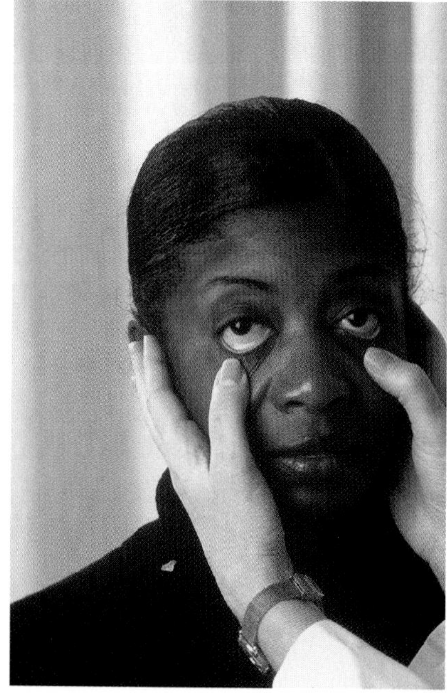

FIGURE 3–1. Inspection.

Palpation

During palpation (Fig. 3–2), you are using your sense of touch to collect data. Palpation is used to assess every system. It usually follows inspection, but both techniques are often performed simultaneously. Palpation al-

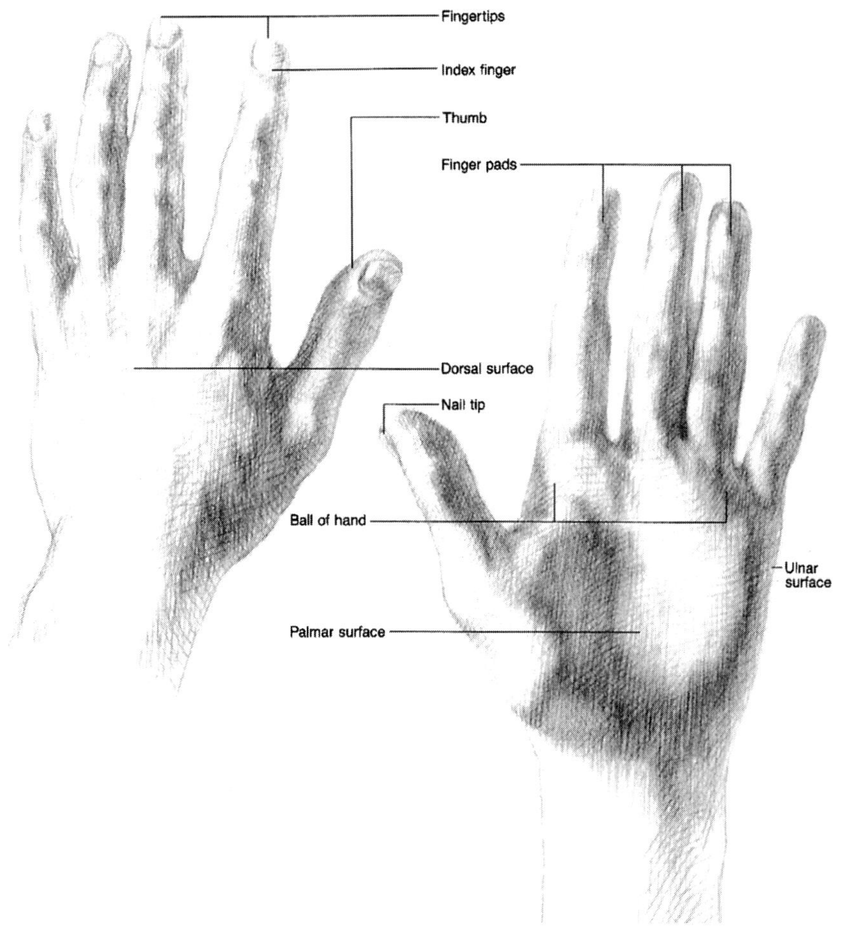

FIGURE 3–2. Parts of hands used in palpation.

lows you to assess surface characteristics, such as texture, consistency, and temperature, and allows you to assess for masses, organs, pulsations, muscle rigidity, and chest excursion. It also lets you differentiate areas of tenderness from areas of pain.

HELPFUL HINT

Tenderness is elicited on palpation; pain is present even without palpation.

Different parts of the hand are best suited for specific purposes. For example, the dorsal aspect of the hand is best for assessing temperature changes (Fig. 3–3); the ball of the hand on the palm and ulnar surface is best for detecting vibration <Fig. 3–4), and the fingertips are the most discriminatory for detecting fine sensations such as pulsations (Fig. 3–5).

Types of Palpation

Two types of palpation may be performed—light and deep. Always begin with light palpation (Fig. 3–6), if for no other reason than to put your client at ease and convey a message of caring. Light palpation is applying very gentle pressure with the tips and pads of your fingers to a body area and then gently moving them over the area, pressing about ½ inch. Light palpation is best for assessing surface characteristics, such as temperature, texture, mobility, shape, and size. It is also useful in assessing pulses, areas of edema, and areas of tenderness. Closing your eyes while palpating will help you concentrate better on what you are feeling.

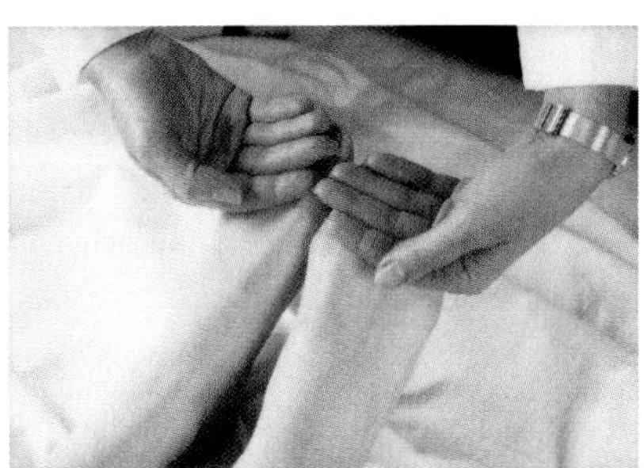

FIGURE 3–3. Palpating temperature changes with dorsal part of hand.

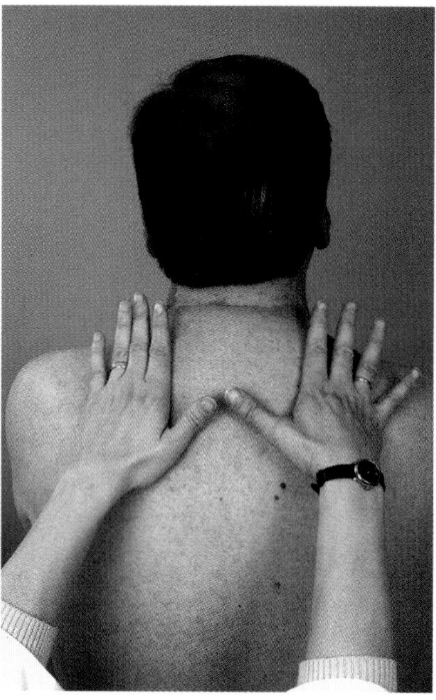

FIGURE 3–4. Palpating vibratory sensations and tactile fremitus with balls of hands.

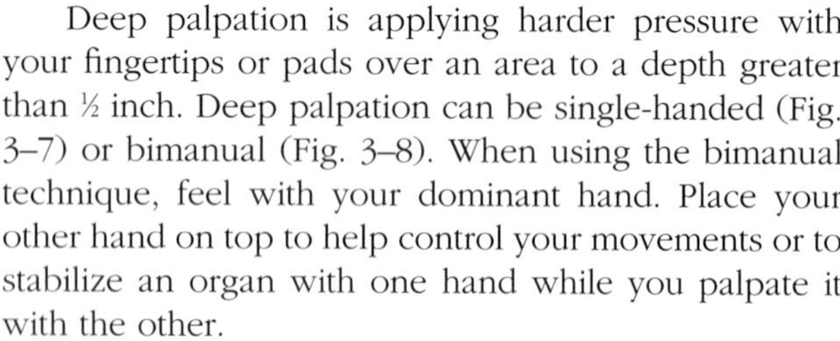

Deep palpation is applying harder pressure with your fingertips or pads over an area to a depth greater than ½ inch. Deep palpation can be single-handed (Fig. 3–7) or bimanual (Fig. 3–8). When using the bimanual technique, feel with your dominant hand. Place your other hand on top to help control your movements or to stabilize an organ with one hand while you palpate it with the other.

Deep palpation is used to assess organ size, detect masses, and further assess areas of tenderness. To assess for rebound tenderness, press down firmly with your dominant hand and then lift it up quickly. An increase in the client's pain when you release the pressure signals rebound tenderness. If your client's muscles tense on palpation (voluntary guarding), have the client take a few slow, deep breaths or place his or her hands over yours during palpation (Fig. 3–9).

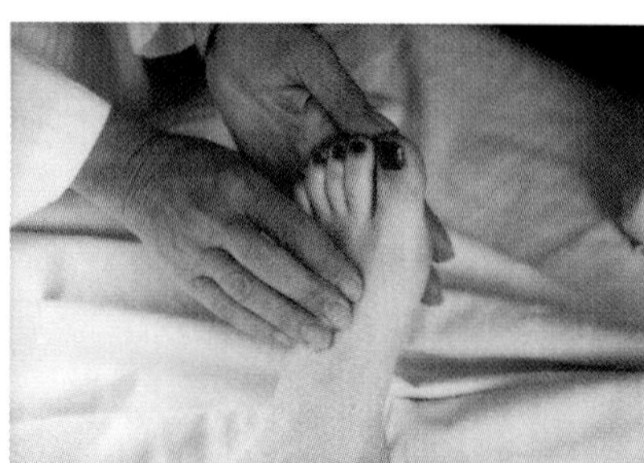

FIGURE 3–5. Palpating with fingertips to assess pulsations.

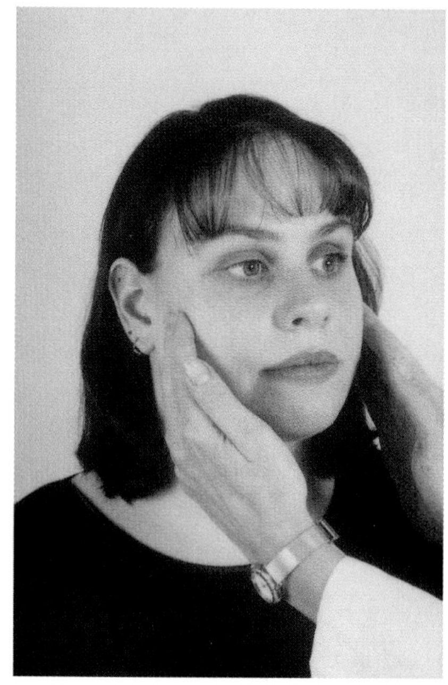

FIGURE 3–6. Light palpation.

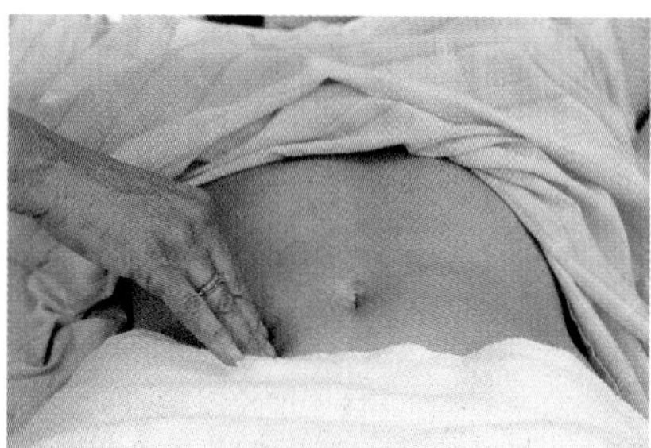

FIGURE 3–7. Deep palpation, single hand.

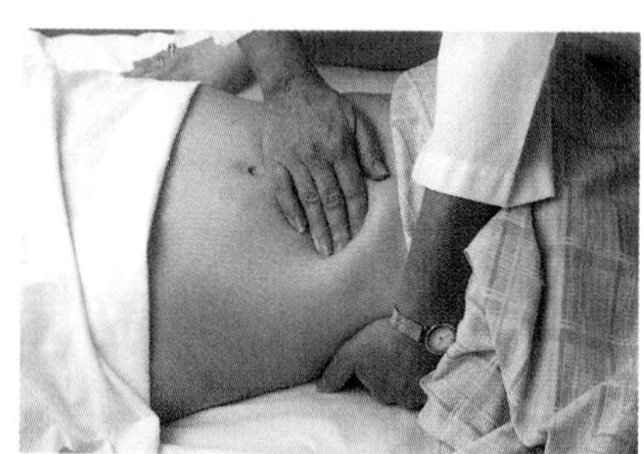

FIGURE 3–8. Deep palpation, bimanual.

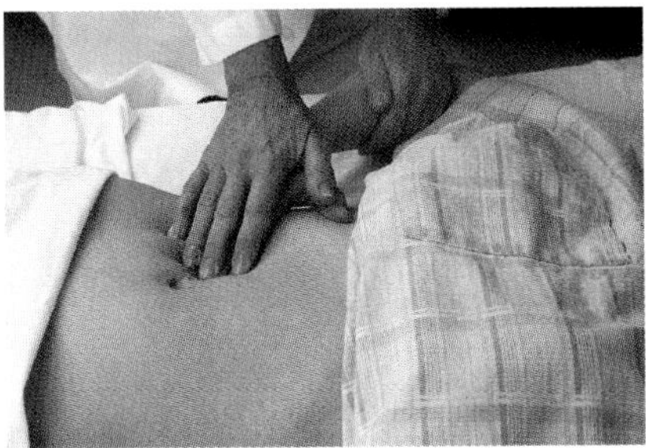

FIGURE 3–9. Palpation using client's hands.

HELPFUL HINT

Wash and warm your hands before palpating.

Ballottement

Ballottement <Fig. 3–10) is a palpation technique used to assess a partially free-floating object. Deep palpation is applied in one area, causing the partially attached object to become palpable in another area. It is frequently used to assess the fetus during pregnancy. It is also used to assess for fluid in the suprapatellar pouch, which, if present, results in a floating kneecap that bounces back on your finger when tapped.

HELPFUL HINT

If you identify an area of tenderness, palpate that area last.

Percussion

Percussion is used to further assess areas of tenderness and to assess deep tendon reflexes (DTRs). It entails striking a body surface with quick, light blows and eliciting vibrations and sounds. The sound determines the density of the underlying tissue and whether it is solid tissue or filled with air or fluid. By determining the density, you can also "outline" the underlying structure. The value of such a finding is that, besides density, you can also determine the size and shape of the underlying structure.

Two factors influence the sound produced during percussion—the thickness of the surface being percussed and your technique. The more tissue you have to percuss through, the duller the sound. Percussion is a skill that usually requires practice to perfect. You also need to develop skill at identifying and differentiating the percussion sounds.

Types of Percussion

Direct or immediate percussion (Fig. 3–11) is directly tapping your hand or fingertip over a body surface to elicit a sound or to assess for an area of tenderness. Direct percussion may be used on an infant's chest instead of indirect percussion. It is also used to assess for sinus tenderness. To perform indirect or mediate percussion (Fig. 3–12), place your nondominant hand over a body surface, pressing firmly with your middle finger. Then place your dominant hand over it. Flexing the wrist of your dominant hand, tap the middle finger of your nondominant hand with the middle finger of your dominant hand. Do not rest your entire hand on the body surface because this dampens the sound. Keep only your middle finger on the body surface, and hyperextend it as you percuss. Tap lightly and quickly, removing your top finger after each tap.

HELPFUL HINT

Trim your nails! Percussing with long fingernails may injure your finger or the area being percussed. An alternative technique is to flex the fingers of the striking hand and use your proximal interphalangeal joint as the hammer.

Using a percussion hammer (Fig. 3–13) to test reflexes is also a type of indirect percussion. Instead of your finger, you use the hammer to tap a body surface. The purpose of this type of percussion is to elicit DTR responses.

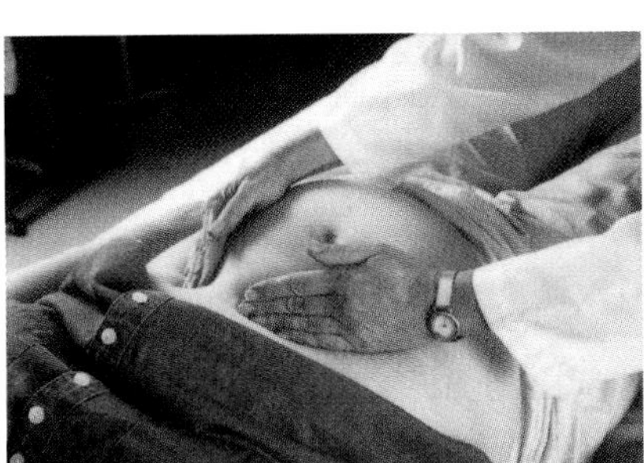

FIGURE 3–10. Ballottement.

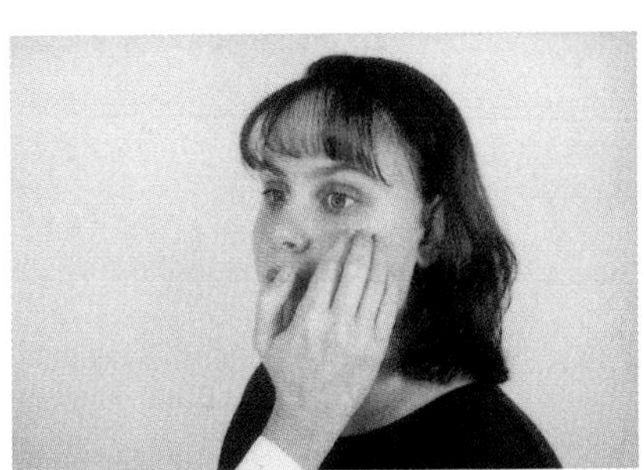

FIGURE 3–11. Direct percussion.

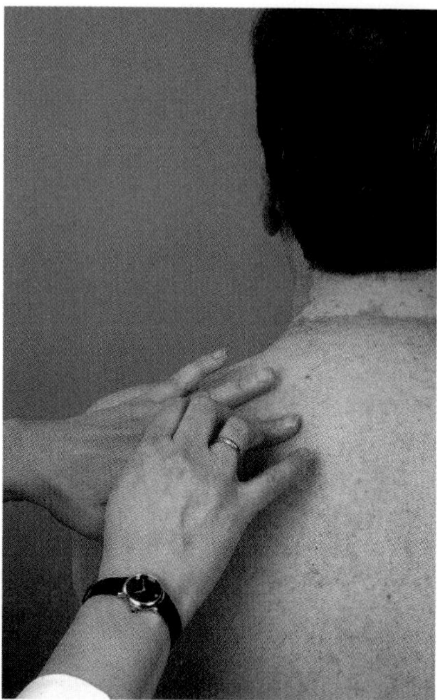

FIGURE 3–12. Indirect percussion.

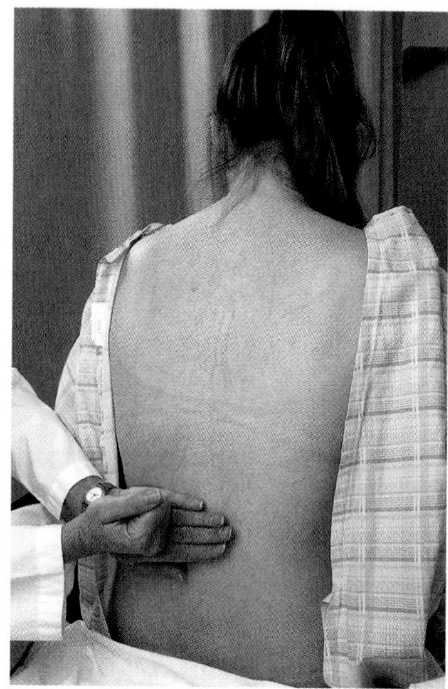

FIGURE 3–14. Percussing for costovertebral angle tenderness.

Fist or blunt percussion is used to assess for organ tenderness (Fig. 3–14. It may be direct or indirect. Direct fist percussion involves striking a body surface with the ulnar surface of your fist. Indirect percussion involves placing your nondominant hand over the body surface and then striking that hand with the ulnar surface of your other fist.

See Percussion Sounds, p. 65.

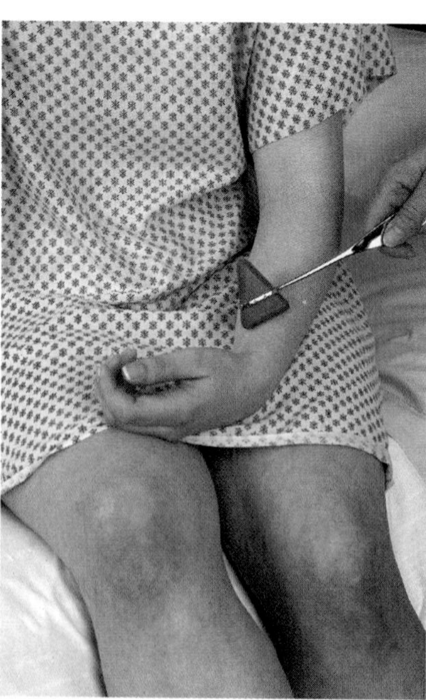

FIGURE 3–13. Using a percussion hammer.

HELPFUL HINT

When performing indirect percussion, be careful not to slap your stationary finger; striking your stationary finger like a hammer will get you the best sound.

Auscultation

Auscultation involves using your sense of hearing to collect data. You will listen to sounds produced by the body, such as heart sounds, lung sounds, bowel sounds, and vascular sounds. Auscultation can be both direct and indirect. Direct auscultation is listening for sounds without a stethoscope, but only a few sounds can be heard this way. Two examples are respiratory congestion in a client who requires suctioning and the loud audible murmur of mitral valve replacement. For most of the sounds produced by the body, you will need to perform indirect auscultation with a stethoscope (Figs. 3–15 and 3–16). Your ability to hear is affected by the quality of the stethoscope. The stethoscope should have the ability to detect both high- and low-pitched sounds.

HELPFUL HINT

Do not percuss over bone—this produces a dull sound and may be misleading. For example, when percussing the chest, percuss in the intercostal spaces rather than across the ribs.

Percussion sounds

Percussion produces sounds that vary according to the tissue being percussed. This chart shows important percussion sounds along with their characteristics and typical locations.

SOUND	INTENSITY	PITCH	DURATION	QUALITY	SOURCE
Resonance	Moderate to loud	Low	Long	Hollow	Normal lung
Tympany	Loud	High	Moderate	Drumlike	Gastric air bubble; intestinal air
Dullness	Soft to moderate	High	Moderate	Thudlike	Liver; full bladder; pregnant uterus
Hyperresonance	Very loud	Very low	Long	Booming	Hyperinflated lung (as in emphysema)
Flatness	Soft	High	Short	Flat	Muscle

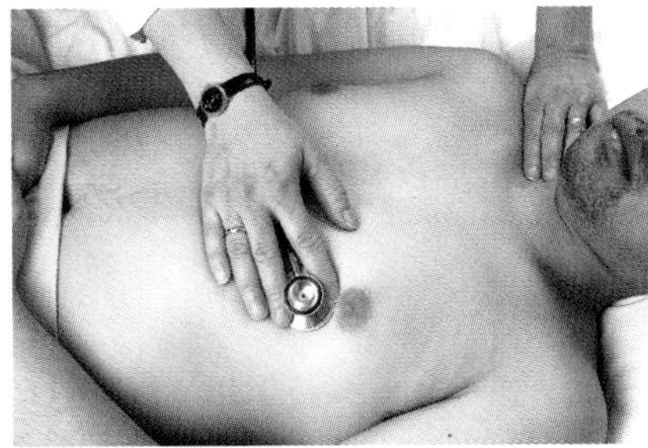

FIGURE 3–15. Listening with diaphragm of stethoscope.

Auscultation is also a skill that requires practice. You need to know what constitutes normal sounds before you can begin to identify abnormal sounds. Listen for the characteristics of sound—the pitch, intensity, duration, and quality. Pitch may be high, medium, or low. Ask yourself, "Which part of the stethoscope was I using when I heard the sound best?" Intensity can range from soft to loud or can be graded on a scale. Ask yourself, "Could I hear the sound easily, or did I have to listen closely?" Duration may be short or long. Ask yourself, "How long was the sound?" Quality describes the sound. Ask yourself, "What did it sound like? Was it harsh, blowing, etc.?"

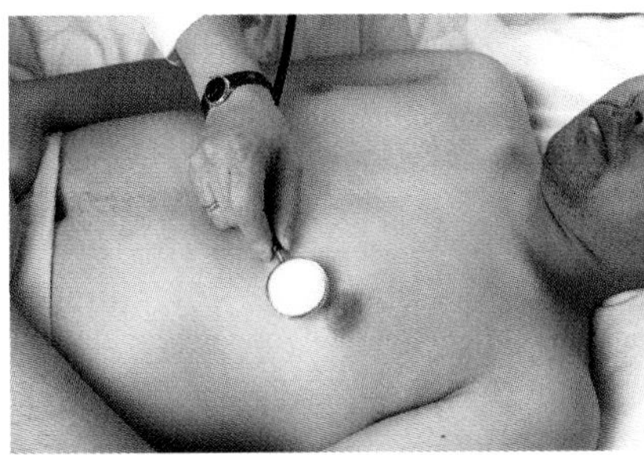

FIGURE 3–16. Listening with bell of stethoscope.

Practice listening to normal sounds. Be a selective listener and focus only on the sounds that you are auscultating, filtering out other sounds. For example, when auscultating heart sounds, close your eyes and block out background breath sounds so that you can concentrate on heart sounds. Once you become skilled at identifying normal sounds, you will then be able to identify anything that sounds different. You may have difficulty identifying abnormal sounds at first, but with practice you will be able to differentiate them. If you are not sure of what you are hearing, ask a more experienced nurse to validate your findings. Also, do not rely on just one assessment technique to assess your client. If you hear something abnormal, look for other data to support or negate that finding.

Besides comparing the sounds you hear to what you know is normal, be sure also to consider your client's size.

AUSCULTATION TIPS

- Always have earpieces pointing forward to seal the ear canal. Warm your stethoscope.
- Work on the client's right side. This stretches your stethoscope across the client's chest and minimizes interference.
- Never listen through clothes.
- Make sure that the environment is quiet.
- If hair is a problem, wet it to minimize artifact.
- Use light pressure to detect low-pitched sounds
- Use firm pressure to detect high-pitched sounds.
- Close your eyes to help you focus.
- Learn to become a selective listener.
- Most of all—practice!

It may affect the sounds you hear. The thicker the chest wall, the softer the sound and the more difficult it is to hear. Use your client as his or her own comparative. For example, it may be easier to hear breath sounds in a client who weighs 110 pounds than in one who weighs 220 pounds. But both clients' breath sounds may be normal.

Approach to the Physical Assessment

Whether you are doing a complete physical assessment or a focused physical assessment, you need to be systematic in your approach. You can approach the physical examination either by systems or by region. With a systems approach, you perform all assessments related to one system before proceeding to the next system. With a regional approach, you perform a thorough assessment of one region, thus encompassing many systems, before proceeding from head to toe. Each approach is systematic and comprehensive and elicits the same data.

Which approach should you use? That depends on the client's health status, the purpose of the assessment, and your own preference. The systems approach is best suited for a focused physical assessment and corresponds with the documentation of findings. The regional approach is best suited for a complete physical assessment because it minimizes client position changes and requires less time. No matter which approach you use, be consistent. You may find it helpful to develop a written checklist so that you do not miss any areas. If you use the same approach consistently and adjust it to meet your clients' needs, it will eventually become second nature to you.

As you proceed, remember that every system is related, and every system has an effect on every other. Be systematic: Work from head to toe, and whenever possible, from side to side so that you can use your client as his or her own comparative. Always consider the developmental stage of your client, and adjust your approach to meet his or her needs. Also be aware of cultural influences that may affect the assessment and your findings. For example, Hindu and Mexican women are very modest and may request a nurse of the same gender to perform the physical examination.

Begin by introducing yourself and telling your client what you are going to do and why. The examination itself may be stressful for your client, especially if he or she is concerned over health problems that may be validated by the examination. Because clients often equate the length of the examination with the severity of a problem, let your client know that the examination normally takes time. Also be conscious of your nonverbal behavior, maintain a professional demeanor and caring attitude, and be sensitive to your client's needs. Explain what you are doing every step of the way, and encourage the client to ask questions.

Make sure that the examination room is quiet and private and that you will not be interrupted. The room also needs to be warm and well lit. Ask the client if he or she needs to void before the examination. While he or she is changing into a gown, assemble all your equipment and make sure that everything is in working order. Designate one area as clean for the unused equipment and one area as dirty for the used equipment. If your client is uncomfortable removing all of his or her clothing, allow him or her to leave undergarments on and remove them only during the parts of the examination when it is necessary. Wash your hands before you begin, and wear gloves if the possibility of exposure to blood or body fluids exists. Drape your client. Work from the right side when possible, and expose only the area being assessed.

During the examination, you will use all four techniques of physical assessment: inspection, palpation, percussion, and auscultation. If your client has identified an area of concern, begin there; otherwise, proceed from head to toe. Usually, the more private areas of the examination, such as the pelvic and rectal examination, are performed last. Do not rush! Pay attention to your client's responses, both verbal and nonverbal, and respond accordingly. For example, if you see that your client is tiring, you may need to provide a short rest period. If you have identified any health teaching needs, the physical examination is an ideal opportunity for health teaching.

Clients with Special Needs

Children and pregnant, elderly, or disabled clients need special consideration during physical assessment. The following paragraphs contain some tips for assessing these clients. In each case, remember to incorporate teaching into your assessment.

Children

- *Infants:* Allow parents to be present and help, if appropriate.
- *Children 1 to 2 years old:* May be fearful, so use games or toys during examination. Leave eye, ear, and mouth assessment until last.
- *Children 2 to 3 years old:* Most difficult to examine. May cling to parents, so let parents help. Allow child to see and touch equipment. Demonstrate use of equipment on doll or parent.
- *Children 4 to 5 years old:* More cooperative, respond well when play is incorporated into examination.
- *School-age children:* Usually cooperative; can converse and follow instructions.

- *Adolescents:* May be sensitive and modest. May not want parent present during examination. Let client know that it is okay to ask questions.
- *All ages:* Look for normal growth and developmental changes. (For more information, see Chapters 23 and 24.)

Pregnant Clients

- Assess both the mother-to-be and the fetus.
- Include fundal heights and future heart tones in the examination.
- Assess for normal changes that occur during pregnancy.
- Pay special attention to nutritional assessment.
- Remember that client may have difficulty changing or assuming positions during last trimester.
- Be aware that hormonal swings may exaggerate client's responses. (For more information, see Chapter 21.)

Elderly Clients

- Do not rush.
- Look for developmental changes.
- Do not assume! For example, your client may be elderly, but that does not mean he or she is hard of hearing.
- Conserve your client's energy by minimizing position changes and helping him or her change positions as needed.
- Allow enough time for client to respond to questions or instructions. (For more information, see Chapter 25.)

Disabled Clients

- Identify the disability.
- Focus on the client's functional ability and mental capacity.
- Modify your assessment based on the client's assets and needs. For example, if he or she is deaf, you may need to write instructions or have someone available who can sign.
- Be alert and sensitive to your client's needs, especially if he or she is unable to communicate verbally.

CRITICAL THINKING ACTIVITY #1:

How might you adjust your assessment if your client were blind?

Positions for Physical Assessment

In order to perform a thorough physical assessment, you must ask the client to assume various positions. Table 3–3 describes the positions needed to assess each area.

Table 3–3 Examination Positions

POSITION	AREAS ASSESSED	ADVANTAGES/DISADVANTAGES
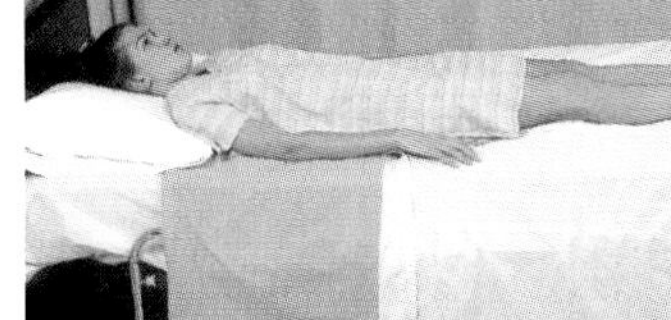 Supine	Anterior chest for respiratory, cardiac, and breast exams (should be supine for breast exam) Pulses and extremities	If client has trouble breathing in supine position, use semi-Fowler's position (semisitting with knees flexed and supported by pillows).
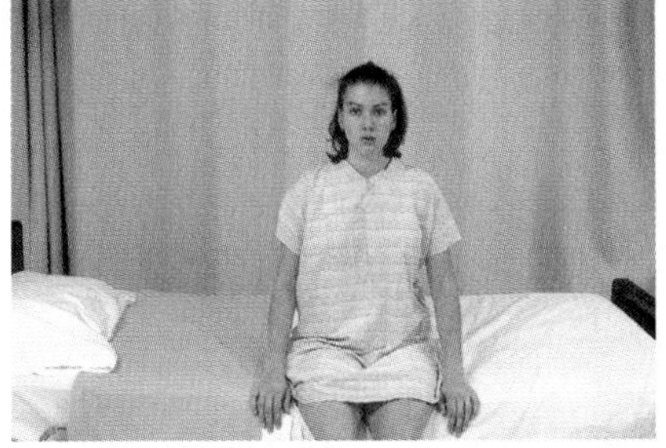 Sitting	Head and neck Anterior and posterior chest for respiratory, cardiac and breast exams Vital signs and upper extremities	Provides good visualization. Allows full lung expansion for respiratory assessment. Clients with weakness or paralysis may have difficulty assuming position and need assistance.

(Continued)

Table 3–3 Examination Positions *(Continued)*

POSITION	AREAS ASSESSED	ADVANTAGES/DISADVANTAGES
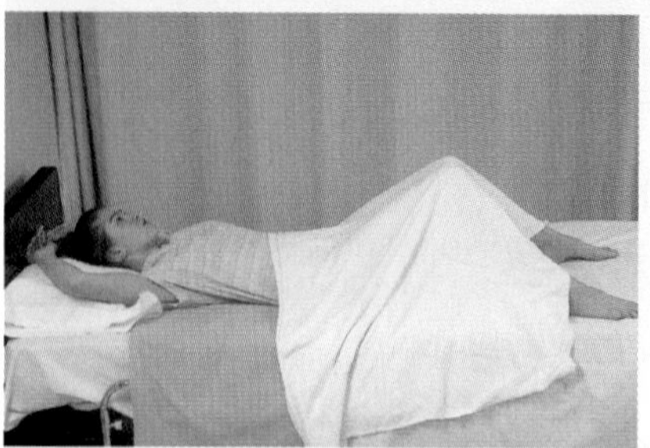 **Dorsal recumbent**	Abdomen: Basically supine position with knees slightly flexed to relax abdominal muscles Female pelvic area if client is unable to assume lithotomy or Sims' position Lithotomy position for female pelvic and rectal areas essentially same as dorsal recumbent but legs and feet in stirrups	If client has abdominal pain, flexing knees is usually more comfortable. Older clients may have difficulty assuming lithotomy position.
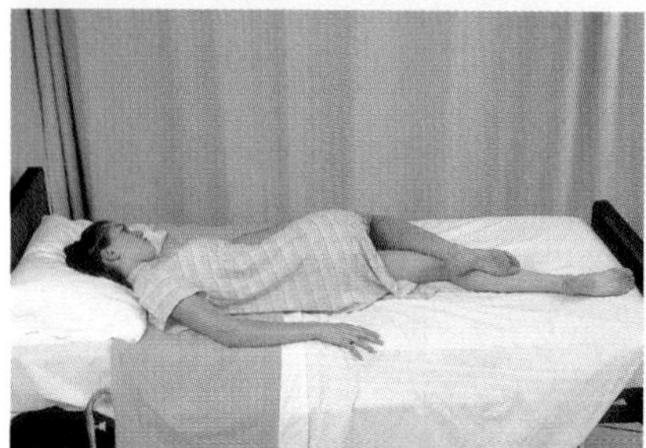 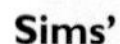 **Sims'**	Female pelvic and rectal areas: Best alternative if client is unable to assume lithotomy position	May be difficult to assume if client has arthritis. Contraindicated if client has had total hip replacement.
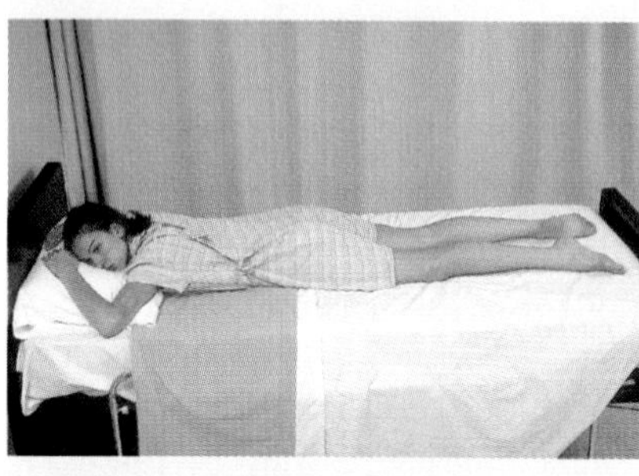 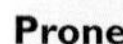 **Prone**	Musculoskeletal system	Difficult position for many clients, especially those with respiratory disease.
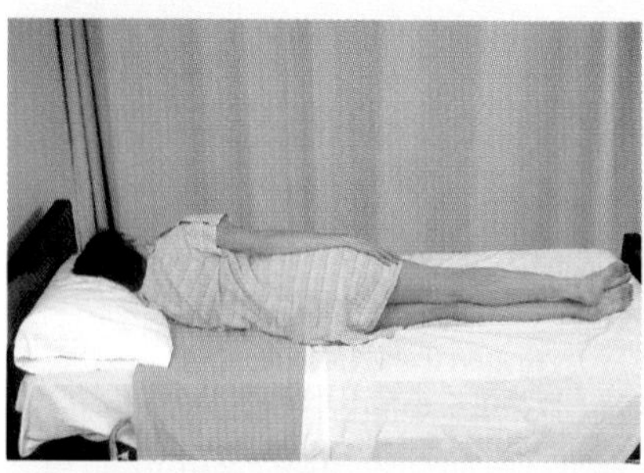 **Left lateral recumbent**	Chest: Best for cardiac auscultation, particularly of S_3, S_4, and some murmurs	Clients with respiratory problems may have trouble assuming this position.

Table 3–3 Examination Positions

POSITION	AREAS ASSESSED	ADVANTAGES/DISADVANTAGES
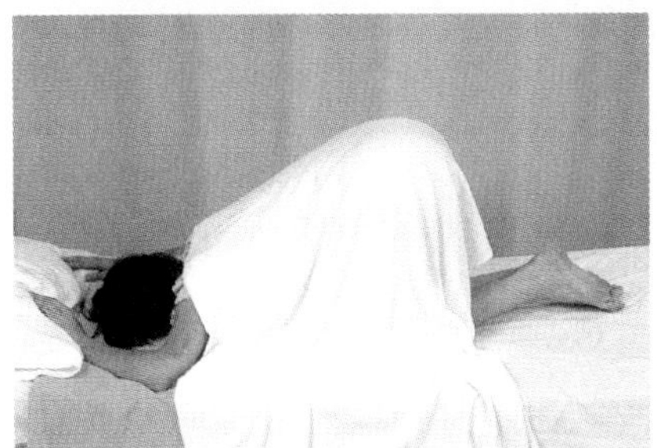 Knee-chest	Male rectal and prostate areas: Best position for these exams	This position and its alternative (bending over a table) are very difficult and embarrassing for most clients.
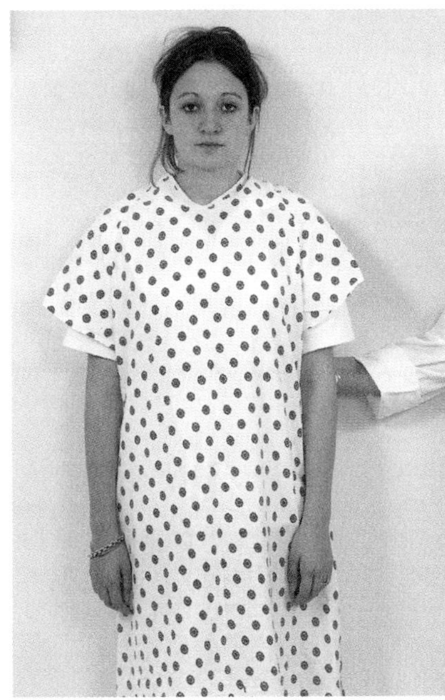 Standing	Spine and joints (ROM): Best musculoskeletal for these areas; used for both and neurological exam and to assess gait and cerebellar function	Clients who are weak, disabled, or paralyzed may need assistance or may not be able to assume this position.

Components of the Physical Assessment

Before you focus on a particular system or area, perform a general survey and measure vital signs, height, and weight. During the health history, you performed a review of systems to detect possible problems in other systems. This provided you with a subjective look at the relationship of these systems. Now take an objective look at each system as it affects each other system before you focus on a specific system or area.

General Survey

Always begin the physical assessment with the general survey. This "first impression" of your client begins as soon as you meet him or her. Use your senses and your observational skills to look, listen, and take note of any unusual odors. First, look for the obvious: Apparent age, gender, and race. Then look closer for clues that might signal a problem. Also consider your client's developmental stage and cultural background; these may influence your findings and interpretation. Make a mental note of any clues detected on the general survey that you may need to follow up during the physical examination.

When looking for clues, watch for signs of distress and check facial characteristics, body size and type, posture, movements, speech, grooming, dress, and hygiene.

Signs of Distress

Ask yourself, "Are there any obvious signs of distress (for example, breathing problems)?" If signs of acute distress are apparent, do a focused physical assessment and address the acute problem.

CRITICAL THINKING ACTIVITY #2:

What other signs would indicate acute distress?

Facial Characteristics

Ask yourself, "What is the client's face telling me?" Do you see pain, fear or anxiety? Does the client maintain eye contact? Is his or her facial expression happy or sad? Facial expression may signal an underlying problem, such as masklike expression in Parkinson's disease. Look at the client's facial features. Are they symmetrical? Ptosis of the eyelid may indicate a neurological problem; drooping on one side of the face may indicate a transient ischemic attack (TIA) or cerebrovascular accident (CVA); and exophthalmos suggests hyperthyroidism. Also look at the condition of your client's skin. It may reflect your client's age, but excessive wrinkling from excessive sun exposure or illness may make the client appear older than his or her stated age.

Body Type and Posture

View your client's body size and build in respect to his or her age and gender. Is he or she stocky, slender, or of average build? Obese or cachectic? Proportional? Does your client have abnormal fat distribution, such as the truncal obesity and buffalo hump seen with Cushing's syndrome? Greet your client with a handshake. The handshake will convey that you care, but also allow you to assess muscle strength, hydration, skin temperature, and texture. Then take a close look at your client's hands. Do you see clubbing, edema, or deformities? Clubbing and edema may reflect a cardiopulmonary problem; deformities may reflect arthritic changes.

Watch how your client enters the room. Are his or her movements smooth and coordinated, or does he or she have an obvious gait problem? Does he or she walk with an assistive device such as a cane or walker? Do you see a wide base of support with short stride length? Gait problems may suggest a musculoskeletal or neurological problem. Spastic movements or unsteady gaits may be seen in clients with cerebral palsy or multiple sclerosis. A shuffling gait is seen with Parkinson's disease. Clients with a wide base of support and short stride length may have a balance or cerebellar problem.

If your client is bedridden, observe his or her ability to move from side to side, sit up in bed, and change positions. Determine how much assistance he or she needs with moving. Any problem detected during the general survey should be further evaluated during the physical examination.

The client's posture may also reveal clues about his or her overall health status. Is he or she sitting upright or slumped? Can he or she assume a supine position? Is there a position that he or she prefers? A slumped position may indicate fatigue or depression. Clients with cardiopulmonary disease often cannot assume a supine position. They prefer a sitting or tripod position because it eases breathing. Clients with abdominal pain also may find it difficult to assume a supine position. Sitting hunched over or in a side-lying position with legs flexed often eases the pain.

Speech

Listen to your client's speech pattern and pace. Speech reflects the mental state, thought process, and affect. Are your client's responses appropriate? Speech patterns and appropriateness of responses reflect his or her thought process. Pressured speech, inappropriate responses, and illogical or incoherent speech may be associated with psychiatric disorders. Pressured, hurried speech may also be seen in clients with hyperthyroidism. Note the tone and quality of his or her voice. Do you hear anger? Sadness? Changes in voice quality may indicate a neurological problem; specifically, a problem with CN IX (glossopharyngeal) or CN X (vagus). Note whether his or her speech is clear or garbled. Aphasia can be expressive (motor/Broca's), receptive (sensory/ Wernicke's), or global, a combination of both. Aphasia of any type is often associated with a TIA or CVA.

The client's vocabulary and sentence structure offer clues to his or her educational level, which you will need to consider when developing teaching plans. Also be alert for foreign accents. You need to determine if there is a language barrier and solicit an interpreter, if needed.

Dress, Grooming, and Hygiene

The way your client is dressed and groomed tells a great deal about his or her physical and psychological well-being. Is he or she neatly dressed and well groomed or disheveled? Disinterest in appearance may reflect depression or low self-esteem. Poor hygiene and a disheveled appearance may also reflect the client's inabilty to care for himself or herself.

Also take note of the appropriateness of dress for the season and situation. Inapproriate dress may be a sign of hyperthyroidism, which causes heat intolerance. Worn clothing may indicate financial problems. Be sure to take note of any unusual odors, such as alcohol or urine, that may indicate a problem and warrant further investigation.

Mental State

Determine if your client is awake, alert, and oriented to time, place, and person. Are his or her repsonses appropriate? Bizarre responses suggest a psychiatric problem. Is your client lethargic? Many conditions can affect the level of consciousness. Determine if this is a change in your client's mental status. If so, investigate further. Also take note of your client's medications, because they may be contributing to the change in mental status.

Cultural Considerations

Note any cultural influences that may affect your client's physical characteristics, response to pain, dress, grooming, and hygiene. Patterns of verbal and nonverbal communication may also be culturally influenced. Keeping these factors in mind will help you avoid making hasty, inaccurate interpretations.

Here are a few examples of cultural differences:

- Chinese-Americans are usually shorter than Westerners.
- European-Americans and African-Americans tend to speak loudly; whereas Chinese-Americans speak softly.
- Asians may avoid eye contact with anyone considered a superior.
- Japanese and Koreans maintain a tense posture to convey confidence and competence, whereas Americans assume a relaxed posture to convey the same message. (For more information on cultural influences, see Chapter 1.)

Developmental Considerations

Consider the developmental stage of your client. Here are some points to keep in mind when performing the general survey:

Children

- Behavior should correspond with the child's developmental level.
- Children tend to regress when ill.
- Take note of the relationship between child and parent.

Pregnant Clients

- General appearance should reflect gestational age.
- Look for normal changes that occur with pregnancy, such as wide base of support and lordosis.
- Look for swelling.
- Note client's affect and response to pregnancy.

Older Adults

- Look for normal changes that occur with aging.
- Look for clues of decreasing ability to function, especially dress and grooming problems.
- Pay attention to your client's affect, especially signs of depression.
- Note changes in mental status such as confusion, and then consider medications, hydration, and nutritional status or an underlying infection as a possible cause.

Documenting the General Survey

Documentation of the general survey records your first overall impression of your client. It should include age (actual and apparent), gender, race, level of consciousness, dress, posture, speech, affect, and any obvious abnormalities or signs of distress.

Here is an example of documentation:

Joe Dunleavy, 50-year-old white male, looks younger than stated age; alert and oriented to time, place, and person. Neatly dressed, well groomed. Well developed. Speech clear, responds appropriately, affect pleasant. No signs of acute distress.

▶ Vital Signs

Vital signs include measurements of temperature, pulse, respirations, and blood pressure. They are the most frequent assessments performed, reflecting cardiopulmonary function and the overall functioning of the body.

The purpose of taking vital signs is to:

- Establish a baseline
- Monitor the client's condition
- Evaluate the client's response to treatments
- Identify problems

The initial set of vital signs serves as the baseline. How often you will need to take vital signs depends on the client's condition. Serial measurements are more reflective of health than one-time measurements. For example, a blood pressure of 150/98 in a client who was hurrying to be on time for his appointment and was upset because he was late may not be a reflection of his usual blood pressure. Stress can cause abnormal elevations. Also check your equipment periodically to make sure that it is reliable and accurate. Last, do not rely on one assessment finding—look for other data to support or negate your finding. For example, if your client's temperature is 102°F, his or her skin should be warm and flushed.

Temperature

Body temperature is the difference between heat produced and heat lost. The hypothalamus acts as the body's thermostat to maintain a constant body temperature. The balance is maintained between the body's

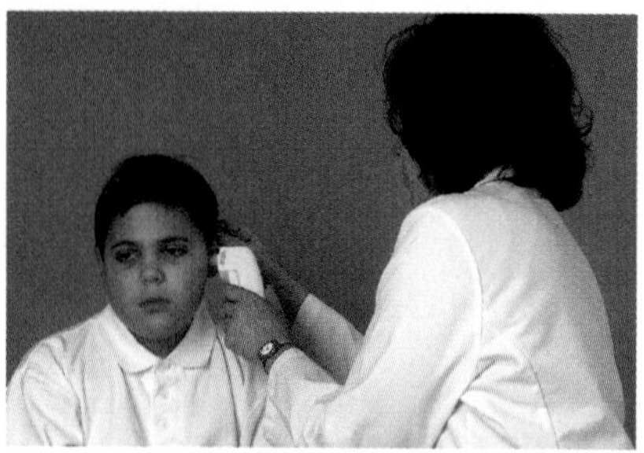

FIGURE 3–17. Taking a tympanic temperature.

heat-producing functions (metabolism, shivering, muscle contraction, exercise, and thyroid activity) and heat-losing functions (radiation, convection, conduction, and evaporation). When one becomes greater than the other, temperature changes are seen; therefore heat-producing functions result in temperature elevations (fever/**hyperthermia**), and greater heat-losing functions result in temperatures decreases (**hypothermia**).

Keep in mind that a fever can be a part of the inflammatory response that helps the body fight diseases. Diseases that affect metabolism, such as thyroid disease, can also affect body temperature. Because the hypothalamus is the body's thermostat, disorders that affect the hypothalamus, such as a CVA, will affect the temperature.

Temperature is measured in either degrees Fahrenheit (°F) or degrees centigrade, or Celsius (°C). The average normal oral temperature is 98.6°F (37°C). Rectal and tympanic temperatures (Fig. 3–17) are more reflective of the body's core temperature, with the average temperature being one degree higher than oral temperature. Axillary temperature measures skin temperature and is on average one degree lower than the oral temperature (Table 3–4).

Various factors can influence the normal temperature reading. They include the following:

Age: Newborns are **homeothermic,** stabilizing temperature within a small range, which makes them easily susceptible to temperature variations, especially hypothermia. Children have slightly higher normal temperatures than adults—99°F until age 3. Elderly people have decreased thermoregulation, also making them vulnerable to temperature changes. They tend to have lower-than-normal temperatures—97°F.

Gender: Women have greater fluctuations in body temperature than men because of hormonal changes. For example, increases in progesterone during ovulation can cause a woman's body temperature to increase by 0.5°F to 1°F.

Circadian rhythms *(diurnal, sleep/wake cycle)*: Body temperature changes at different times of the day. It is usually lowest in the morning and highest in the evening. Temperature fluctuations can range from 1°F to 2°F.

HELPFUL HINT

The conversion from °F to °C is (°F − 32) × 5/9 = °C,
The conversion from °C to °F is (°C × 9/5) + 32 = °F

Table 3–4 Advantages and Disadvantages of Temperature Routes

ROUTE	ADVANTAGES	DISADVANTAGES
Oral (Normal: 98.6°F, 37°C)	Easy, fast, accurate	Cannot be used for clients who are unconscious, confused, prone to seizures, recovering from oral surgery, or under age 6 Need to wait 15–20 minutes after eating
Rectal (Normal: 99.5°F, 37.5°C)	More reflective of core temperature	Cannot be used for clients who have rectal bleeding, hemorrhoids, or diarrhea or who are recovering from rectal surgery
	Fast	Contraindicated for cardiac clients because it may stimulate the vagus nerve and decrease heart rate Not recommended for newborns because of risk of perforating anus
Tympanic (Normal: 99.5°F, 37.5°C)	More reflective of core temperature Safe, good for children	Reports of accuracy are conflicting.
Axillary (Normal: 97.6°F, 36.5°C)	Safe, good for children and newborns	Measures skin surface temperature, which can be variable.
Forehead (Normal: 94°F, 34.4°C)	Safe and easy	Measures skin surface temperature Least accurate method

Exercise/stress: Stress and exercise cause an increase in epinephrine and norepinephrine, increasing the metabolic rate and in turn increasing temperature.

Environmental factors: Exposure to temperature extremes can lead to hypothermia (low temperature from exposure to excessive cold) and hyperthermia (high temperature from exposure to excessive heat).

Pulse

The pulse reflects the force of the heart contracting. This force creates a wave of pressure as blood circulates throughout the systemic circulation. The pulse reflects stroke volume, the amount of blood ejected with each contraction.

Assess the client's pulse for rate and rhythm. The radial pulse (Fig. 3–18) is usually used when assessing vital signs. Normal pulse rate varies with age (see The Effect of Age on Vital Signs, below). The average rate for a newborn is 125 beats per minute (BPM). By age 4, it decreases to about 100 BPM, and by adolescence, the rate is in the normal adult range of 60 to 100 BPM.

Cardiac output is equivalent to stroke volume times heart rate (CO = SV × HR). The fastest way to increase cardiac output is to increase the heart rate. Heart rates above 100 BPM are called tachycardia; below 60 BPM, bradycardia. Athletes' hearts work more efficiently, so they often have heart rates lower than 60 BPM. To meet the increased oxygen demands associated with exercise, stroke volume increases over time.

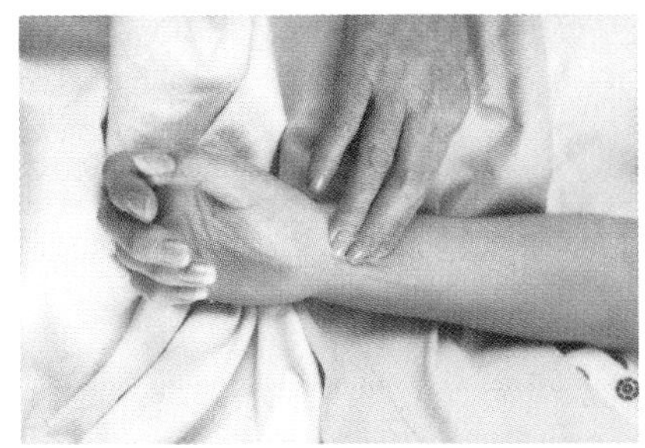

FIGURE 3–18. Taking a radial pulse.

If you have trouble finding your client's radial pulse, use a larger, more central pulse, such as the carotid or femoral. Whenever you obtain an irregular rhythm, auscultate an apical heart rate (Fig. 3–19) for one full minute. Children often have a rhythm that varies with

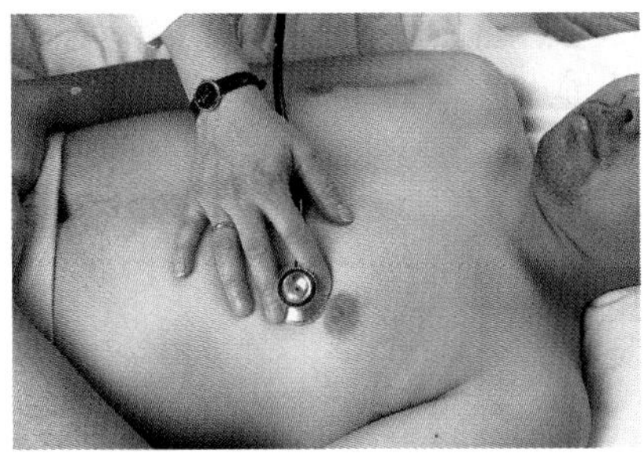

FIGURE 3–19. Taking an apical pulse.

The effect of age on vital signs

Normal vital sign ranges vary with age, as this chart shows.

AGE	TEMPERATURE ° Fahrenheit	TEMPERATURE ° Celsius	PULSE RATE	RESPIRATORY RATE	BLOOD PRESSURE
Newborn	98.6 to 99.8	37 to 37.7	120 to 160	30 to 80	systolic: 50 to 52 diastolic: 25 to 30 mean: 35 to 40
3 years	98.5 to 99.5	36.9 to 37.5	80 to 125	20 to 30	systolic: 78 to 114 diastolic: 46 to 78
10 years	97.5 to 98.6	36.3 to 37	70 to 110	16 to 22	systolic: 90 to 132 diastolic: 56 to 86
16 years	97.6 to 98.8	36.4 to 37.1	55 to 100	15 to 20	systolic: 104 to 108 diastolic: 60 to 92
Adult	96.8 to 99.5	36 to 37.5	60 to 100	12 to 20	systolic: 95 to 140 diastolic: 60 to 90
Older adult	96.5 to 97.5	35.9 to 36.3	60 to 100	15 to 25	systolic: 140 to 160 diastolic: 70 to 90

respirations, causing a sinus arrythmia. During inspiration, there is an increased venous return to the right side of the heart, causing a slight increase in rate to handle the increased load. The apical pulse is also used in infants and small children. (See Chapter 13 for a more detailed assessment of the pulses.)

Respirations

Assessing respirations includes checking rate, rhythm, and depth. It includes assessing inspiration (taking oxygen into the lungs) and expiration (removing carbon dioxide from the lungs). Many factors influence respirations, including the client's metabolism and whether the cardiovascular, musculoskeletal, and neurological systems are intact. The respiratory rate is a count of one full inspiration/expiration cycle for one full minute.

The normal respiratory rate varies with age. The newborn's respiratory rate is quite rapid, averaging about 40 breaths per minute. The respiratory rate gradually decreases with age until it reaches the adult rate of 12 to 20 breaths per minute. Respiratory rates that are within normal range are termed **eupnea;** those above normal range are termed **tachypnea;** and those below normal range are called **bradypnea.** Absent breathing is **apnea** and difficult breathing is **dyspnea.**

The rhythm of respirations for adults and children is usually regular, with an occasional "sigh," or deeper breath. Infants normally have irregular respiratory rhythms, but be alert for prolonged periods of apnea. Apnea lasting for more than 15 seconds is cause for alarm and warrants further assessment. Irregular breathing patterns may also indicate an underlying problem such as a neurological problem.

The depth of respirations reflects the tidal volume—the amount of air inhaled with each breath. In adults, the normal tidal volume is about 300 to 500 mL. Ask yourself, "Are the client's respirations deep or shallow?" Deep and rapid respirations may indicate that your client is hyperventilating. Conditions such as metabolic acidosis can cause hyperventilation. Shallow respirations may indicate hypoventilation, which may be caused by conditions such as sedation and guarding from pain.

As you are counting the respirations, take note of signs of distress, such as cyanotic color changes and retraction or use of accessory muscles to breathe. Also listen for audible sounds such as wheezing or congestion that may signal distress and warrant further assessment. (See Chapter 11 for further assessment of the respiratory system.)

Blood Pressure

Blood pressure (BP) is a measurement of the pressure within the vascular system as the heart contracts (systole) and relaxes (diastole). Blood pressure indirectly reflects your client's overall cardiovascular functioning. It is equal to cardiac output times peripheral vascular resistance (BP = CO × PVR). Normal BP varies with age. Other factors that can affect BP include stress, genetics, medications, heavy meals, diurnal variations, exercise, and weight.

Box 3–1 explains the procedure for measuring a client's blood pressure.

Normal BP for an adult ranges from 100 to 140 mm Hg (systolic) and from 60 to 90 mm Hg (diastolic). Normal BP for children and infants is much lower. Because BP reflects the pressure within the vascular system, a person cannot maintain a high BP without serious effects. A systolic reading of greater than 140 mm Hg and a diastolic reading greater than 90 mm Hg are considered hypertensive, whereas a systolic reading less than 90 mm Hg and a diastolic reading less than 60 mm Hg is considered hypotensive. An elevated BP reading should be followed up with a serial reading to see if the BP is consistently elevated. Keep in mind that the systolic pressure changes more readily in response to external stimuli, whereas the diastolic is more constant. Consequently, an elevated diastolic pressure may be more worrisome than an isolated elevation of the systolic pressure.

The pulse pressure—the difference between the systolic and the diastolic reading—is normally about 40 mm Hg. A widened pulse pressure is often seen in elderly people because of a decreased elasticity of the arterial walls, but it may also be a sign of increased intracranial pressure. A narrow pulse pressure can be seen when the client is hypovolemic or going into shock and heart failure.

Blood pressure measurements are often taken with the client in several positions—supine, sitting, and standing. Measuring BP in several positions allows you to check for orthostatic hypotension or postural hypotension (a drop in BP with position change). If the client has orthostatic hypotension, the systolic reading will drop 20 mm Hg, and the pulse rate will increase by about 20 BPM, causing dizziness or lightheadedness. Certain medications and hypovolemia can cause orthostatic hypotension.

HELPFUL HINT

If you are unsure about a BP reading, double-check or have another nurse retake it.

If you are having difficulty hearing the BP, try using an electronic BP device. Or, if electronic equipment is not available, do a palpable BP. Inflate the cuff and palpate the brachial artery. As you deflate the cuff, note at what point the brachial pulse becomes palpable. This number represents the systolic reading. A diastolic reading cannot be obtained using the palpation method. An example of documentation of a palpable BP is "90/palpated."

BOX 3–1 Measuring Blood Pressure

To assess a client's blood pressure accurately, the nurse should follow this procedure.

Preparing the Client

Before beginning, make sure the client is relaxed and has not eaten or exercised in the past 30 minutes. The client can sit, stand, or lie down during blood pressure measurement.

Applying the Cuff and Stethoscope

To obtain a reading in an arm (the most common measurement site), wrap the sphygmomanometer cuff snugly around the arm 1 inch (2.5 cm) above the antecubital area (the inner aspect of the elbow), with the cuff bladder centered over the brachial artery (Fig.3-20). Most cuffs have arrows that should be placed over the brachial artery. Make sure to use the proper-size cuff for the client.

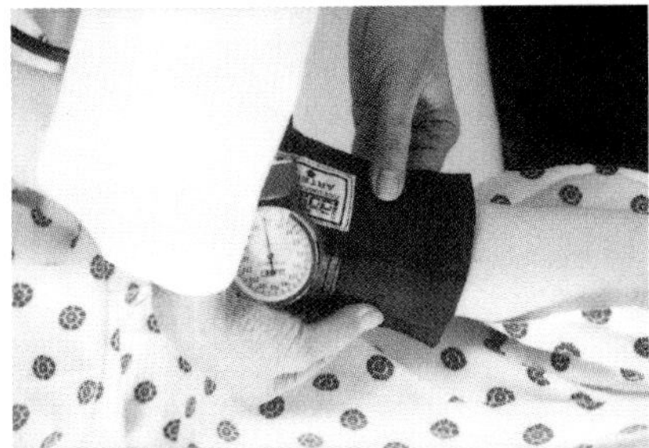

FIGURE 3–20. Measuring cuff size.

Keep the mercury manometer at eye level; if using an aneroid gauge, place it level with the client's arm. Keep the client's arm level with the heart. *Do not* use the client's muscle strength to hold up the arm; tension from muscle contraction can elevate systolic pressure. Have a recumbent client rest the arm at the side.

Then, palpate the brachial pulse just below and slightly medial to the antecubital area. Rapidly inflate the cuff to about 30 mm Hg above the level at which the pulsations disappear. Deflate the cuff slowly until you feel the pulse again. Then, deflate the cuff completely. Place the earpieces of the stethoscope in your ears and position the stethoscope head over the brachial atery, just distal to the cuff or slightly beneath it (Fig. 3-21). Although the diaphragm is more frequently used, the bell is best for detecting the low-pitched Korotkoff sounds.

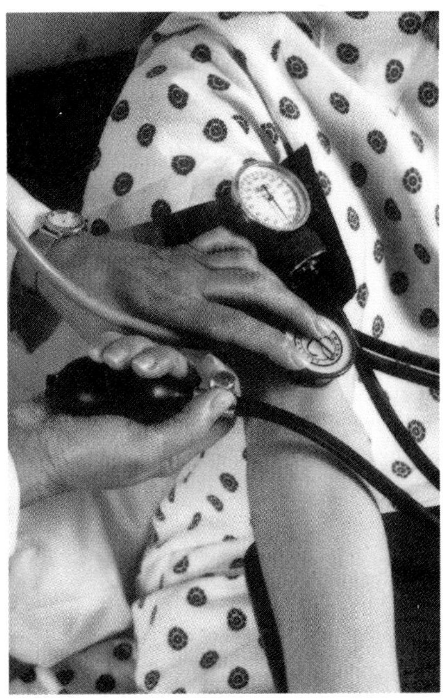

FIGURE 3–21. Taking blood pressure with bell of stethoscope.

Obtaining the Blood Pressure Reading

Watching the manometer, pump the bulb until the mercury column or aneroid gauge reaches about 30 mm Hg above the point at which the pulse disappeared. Then, slowly open the air valve and watch the mercury drop or the gauge needle descend. Release the pressure at a rate of about 3 mm Hg per second and listen for pulse sounds (Korotkoff sounds).

These sounds, which determine the blood pressure measurement, are classified as follows:

Phase I
Onset of clear, faint tapping, with intensity that increases to a thud or louder tap

Phase II
Tapping that changes to a soft, swishing sound

Phase III
Return of clear, crisp tapping sound

Phase IV (first diastolic sound)
Sound becomes muffled and takes on a blowing quality

Phase V (second diastolic sound)
Sound disappears.

As soon as you hear blood begin to pulse through the brachial artery, note the reading on the aneroid dial or mercury column. Reflecting phase I (the first Korotkoff sound), this sound coincides with the client's systolic pressure. Continue deflating the cuff, noting the point at which pulsations diminish or become muffled—phase IV (the fourth Korotkoff sound)—and then disappear—phase V (the fifth Korotkoff sound). For children and highly active adults, many authorities consider phase IV the most accurate reflection of blood pressure.

The American Heart Association and the World Health Organization recommend documenting phases I, IV, and V. However, phase IV is often not indicated in practice. To avoid confusion and make your measurements more useful, follow this format for recording blood pressure: systolic/muffling/disappearance (for example, 120/80/76).

BP may also be difficult to hear in infants. If so, use the flush method. As you inflate the cuff and occlude the artery, the extremity will become pale; as you release the pressure, blood flow returns and the extremity will flush. The point at which the extremity flushes coincides approximately with the mean arterial pressure (MAP). (MAP = diastolic pressure + 1/3 of the pulse pressure).

BLOOD PRESSURE TIPS

- Too-narrow cuff: False high reading.
- Too-wide cuff: False low reading.
- Cuff wrapped too loosely: False high reading.
- Arm above heart level during reading: False low reading.
- Muscle contracted on arm during BP reading: False high reading.
- Arm pressures should not differ more than 10 mm Hg.
- Leg pressures should be the same or slightly higher than arm pressures.

WHICH ARM TO USE?

You can usually use either arm for BP measurement. However, there are a few restrictions. They are:

- Arm with injury or cast
- Arm with IV site
- Arm of client who has had a mastectomy
- Arm that has a vascular access for dialysis

Documenting Vital Signs

Vital signs are often documented on graphic charts, which allow you to monitor or plot the patterns of the vital signs. This is very helpful in evaluating the effectiveness of treatment. Vital signs may also be documented in narrative form. For example: T 98.8°F, P 88, regular, R 16 unlabored, regular and deep, BP 120/80 lying, 118/80 sitting, and 118/80 standing.

Height and Weight

Anthropometric measurements provide valuable data about your client's growth and development, nutritional status and overall general health. Accurate assessment of height (Fig. 3–22) and weight (Fig. 3–23)is also a vital assessment used to determine medication dosages. This is particularly true with children because medication dosages are calculated based on the child's weight. For adults, weight is used to determine chemotherapy dosages and anesthesia administration. Weight can also be used to evaluate the effectiveness of a treatment, such as IV fluids, drugs, or nutritional therapy.

Weight and height for adults who can stand can be obtained using a platform scale with a sliding ruler to measure height. Be sure your scale is balanced. Weigh the client while he or she is wearing minimal clothing (gown) and no shoes. If the client cannot stand, use a bed scale. Children may also be weighed on a platform scale, but they should be measured with a wall-mounted measure to ensure accuracy. Weigh infants with a small table platform scale. To measure an infant's length, use

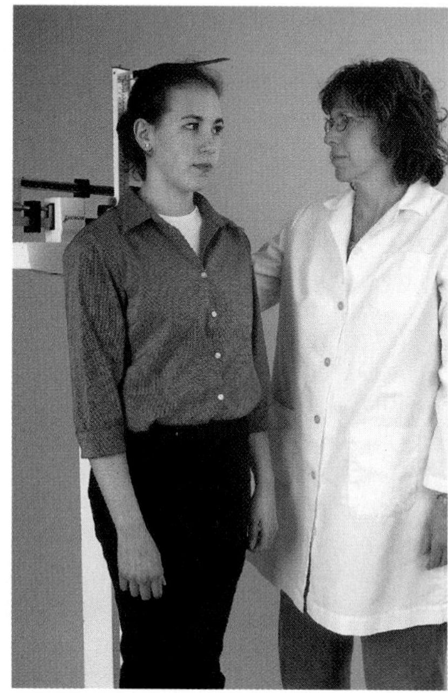

FIGURE 3–22. Measuring height.

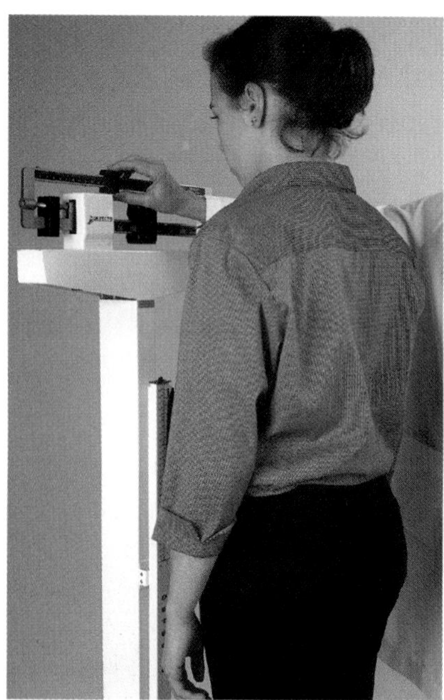

FIGURE 3–23. Measuring weight.

a stationary measure or mark disposable examination paper at the top of the head and the heel of the extended foot and then measure the distance between the two. If serial weights are being done, weigh the client on the same scale at the same time of day. Be sure to document the measurements in centimeters or inches. Because children have frequent changes in growth and development, their measurements are often documented on growth charts for easy monitoring. (See Appendix B).

Head-to-Toe Scan

Whether you are doing a complete or focused physical assessment, remember that all body systems are interrelated. A problem in one system will eventually affect or be affected by every other system. When performing a complete physical assessment, perform a thorough assessment of each system, looking for relationships. When you perform a focused physical assessment—an in-depth assessment of one system—begin by scanning the other systems, looking for changes as they relate to the system being assessed.

For example, suppose you were performing a focused assessment of the cardiovascular system. Here are some of the effects you should look for:

- **Integumentary:** Look for color changes, pallor, edema, and changes in skin and hair texture and growth. Clients with cardiovascular problems may have edema and thin, shiny, hairless skin.
- **HEENT:** Look for periorbital edema. Funduscopic examination may reveal vascular changes.
- **Respiratory:** Look for cyanosis and breathing difficulty. Auscultate for adventitious sounds such as crackles that are associated with CHF.
- **Breast:** Assess for male breast enlargement that may occur with cardiac medications such as digoxin.
- **Abdominal:** Assess for ascites and hepatomegaly, which may be associated with CHF.
- **Musculoskeletal:** Assess for muscle weakness and atrophy associated with disuse.
- **Neurological:** Assess level of consciousness. Confusion, fatigue, and lethargy may be associated with decreased cardiac output and hypoxia.

After you look for the relationships between the systems, you are ready to perform the focused physical assessment. This text is structured to emphasize the relationship of one system to another. The relationship between the systems is presented for every system assessed.

Documenting Your Physical Assessment Findings

Once you have completed the physical assessment, document your findings. Because writing should be kept to a minimum during the examination, document your findings as soon as possible, while they are uppermost in your mind. Document accurately, objectively, and concisely. Avoid general terms such as "normal." Record your findings system by system, being sure to chart pertinent negative findings. Once you have completed your objective database, combine it with your subjective database, cluster your data, identify pertinent nursing diagnoses, and develop a plan of care for your client. (For more information on documentation, see Chapter 1.)

Summary

- The physical assessment provides objective data for the database. It involves using your senses to collect data. You look, listen, smell, and feel!
- Specific equipment may be used to enhance the data collection process.
- The four techniques of physical assessment include inspection, palpation, percussion, and **auscultation.**
- The physical examination may be complete (an entire, thorough assessment) or focused (an assessment of one system or area).
- The physical assessment also helps you validate subjective data found in the history, identify any health problems, and evaluate the client's response to treatment.
- The physical examination should always begin with a general survey and a measurement of vital signs, height, and weight.
- For a focused physical examination, a head-to-toe scan identifies the system's effects on every other system.
- Physical assessment requires the use of cognitive, psychomotor, interpersonal, affective, and ethical skills.
- As with any skills—practice! The more you practice, the more competent and confident you will be in performing an accurate physical assessment and in interpreting your findings—findings that are essential to the plan of care for your client.

UNIT II

Promoting Health

4

Teaching the Client

Before You Begin

Introducing the Case Study

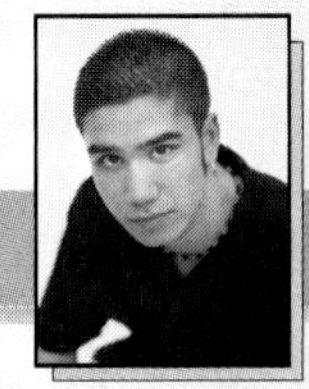

Lucas Hernandez, a 21-year-old college junior, arrives for his annual checkup. He has no health complaints, but he is concerned about juggling school and work responsibilities. Lucas is studying to become a teacher and also moonlights as a bartender 4 nights a week, from 7 pm to 3 am. He usually sleeps from 6 am to noon on workdays, but he is about to start student teaching and must be at school from 7 am to 4 pm. He says he plans to sleep in two shifts.

Lucas's past health history, family history, and review of systems are negative. His psychosocial profile reveals that he is gay and has been living with a partner for 2 years. He drinks only occasionally and is a vegetarian who includes eggs and milk in his diet. His physical assessment findings are also negative. His immunizations are current, but he has not been immunized against hepatitis B, and he declines HIV testing, stating that he is in a monogamous relationship.

What kind of teaching plan would you develop for Lucas? Before you can begin to develop this plan, you need to consider how his assessment findings will affect his learning needs.

Introduction to Teaching the Client

As a nurse, you have a primary role in educating clients that is essential in preventing, promoting, and restoring health. This chapter will help you to:

- Assess the learner and yourself in preparation for teaching
- Understand how to use information from your assessment to develop effective teaching plans
- Recognize opportunities for teaching during the assessment

Purpose and Goals of Teaching

Teaching is a key nursing intervention at all levels of health care. As a nurse, you teach individuals, families, groups, and communities. At the primary level, you teach healthy people to reinforce desired behaviors, promote continued wellness, and anticipate and prevent potential health problems. At the secondary level, you teach ill people to help them cope with their immediate illness, restore and promote optimal wellness, and work most effectively with their healthcare team. At the tertiary level, you teach people how to manage chronic illnesses and maintain an optimal level of health.

The goals of teaching are to:

- Promote health and wellness
- Prevent disease and illness
- Restore and maintain health and wellness
- Promote coping

Tips for Effective Teaching

- Polish your verbal and nonverbal communication skills.
- Establish a relationship that is focused on the individual, holistic, and interactive.
- Identify factors that will affect learning needs and compensate for them.
- Involve the individual in identifying his or her learning needs and planning your teaching strategy.
- Be sure that the individual values learning and that you both agree on his or her learning needs.
- Engage as many of the person's senses as possible—he or she will be more likely to learn.
- Build on what the person already knows.
- Consider the person's lifestyle and resources available to him or her to develop a practical plan.
- Be realistic in your expectations.
- Remember: No matter how well you teach, you cannot make someone learn!

Developmental, Cultural, and Ethnic Variations

Developmental Level

To develop an effective teaching plan, you must identify the individual's developmental level and understand normal growth and developmental tasks. Determine the person's developmental readiness to learn. Be aware of how he or she compares with developmental standards physically, cognitively, emotionally, and socially. Anticipate teaching content related to current and future growth and development issues.

Provide opportunities for learners of all ages to ask questions or voice concerns. For example, if the person is a young adolescent, you might say, "People's bodies and feelings go through many changes from ages 9 to 20. Are there any particular changes that you would like to discuss?" Or if he or she is a parent introducing a new baby to an older sibling, you might say, "Older siblings have conflicting feelings about a new baby. How have you prepared your older child for the baby's homecoming?"

Also consider the cognitive and physical development of the individual. For example, teaching a newly diagnosed diabetic who is 5 years old about diabetes would be very simplistic compared to teaching a newly diagnosed 25-year-old. If you are teaching skills, remember to consider the person's motor development level. Fine motor skill development is needed to give self-injections, and young and older clients may have difficulty mastering this.

Culture and Ethnicity

Culture refers to characteristics that create common patterns of living or belief among people. Working at the same company or having similar incomes creates common patterns of living just as much as ethnic origin does. Identifying a person's cultural and religious background will help you approach him or her in a respectful manner, more accurately interpret body language and oral communication, be aware of taboos or practices that could affect learning or teaching, and be aware of the priority that wellness has in his or her life.

Performing the Assessment

Before you can develop a teaching plan for an individual, you need to assess him or her. Collect both subjective and objective data. Identify the person's learning needs, factors that could affect learning, and his or her stressors, strengths, and deficits. Then plan your teaching around them.

Health History

Reflect carefully on everything you learn during the health history. It provides you with the background data needed to develop an effective teaching plan and tells you who the learner is! As you gather information in the following categories, keep asking yourself, "How will this affect my teaching?"

Biographical Data

Asking for biographical information is a good place to start when developing a teaching plan. Age and gender allows comparison to standards for demographic cohorts. Age also helps identify developmental stage and appropriate teaching level. Occupation and address identify environmental concerns that may affect learning and community learning resources near the person's home or job. Knowledge of religion and culture identifies beliefs that may influence your teaching plan.

HELPFUL HINT

Do not assume that the person's educational level corresponds with knowledge or understanding.

Current Health Status

Knowing the person's current state of health and reason for seeking care will help you identify whether significant or unexpected changes are occurring in his or her health status, whether he or she has a preventative or crisis focus, and whether he or she understands the health problem and perceives it as serious. If he or she has an acute problem, you may need to address it before you begin teaching. If the person has major teaching needs but does not consider his or her problem serious, you need to help him or her understand the severity of the illness and the necessity of a teaching plan. Otherwise, learning will be difficult if not impossible.

Having the person describe the problem in his or her own words gives you his or her perception of it and may reveal teaching needs. For example, an older woman with congestive heart failure may say that her problem is "swollen ankles" and make no association with the heart.

Other factors that affect learning include fear, anxiety, and medications. For example, a person who is depressed or anxious will have trouble concentrating. Or the person may be taking medications that make him or her drowsy and limit the amount of time you can teach per session.

Ask the person: "Is there anything going on in your life now that makes it particularly easy or difficult for you to manage your health or practice good health habits?" This question alerts you to current stressors, strengths, and deficits that could affect learning. It allows you to:

- Plan teaching to accommodate for current issues.
- Be sensitive to learners' priorities in planning.
- More effectively assist learners to prioritize learning needs for short- and long-term time periods.

Past Health History

Questions about the person's past health history shed light on his or her learning abilities, new learning needs, or misconceptions that need clarification. Ask him or her: "Do you have any medical problems?" If the answer is yes, ask: "Did you receive instructions from heathcare providers? What were they?" Multiple health problems may affect the person's ability to learn. Negative experiences with healthcare providers may make him or her less receptive to learning.

Family History

The family history helps identify health risks that in turn identify teaching needs. Ask your client: "Are there any major medical problems in your family?" This question identifies genetic or familial risk for health problems and points out the need for further education. Past experience with specific illnesses also may influence the person's perception of the disease.

Review of Systems

The review of systems (ROS) helps you recognize changes in one body system that may influence other body systems. As you perform the ROS, identify any areas that may affect learning.

Review of Systems

AREA/QUESTIONS TO ASK	RATIONALE/SIGNIFICANCE
General Health Survey	
How have you been feeling?	Identifies problems that may interfere with learning and alerts you to adjust your teaching plan. For example, depression or anxiety may interfere with learning. Fatigue may limit the person's tolerance, so short teaching sessions may be more effective.

(Continued)

Review of Systems *(Continued)*

AREA/QUESTIONS TO ASK	RATIONALE/SIGNIFICANCE
Integumentary	
Do you have any problems with your skin, hair, or nails?	Helps identify problems that can affect learning. Helps identify teaching needs.
Head, Eyes, Ears, Nose, and Throat (HEENT)	
Do you have headaches?	Headaches can interfere with learning. Vision or hearing problems need to be addressed when developing an effective teaching approach. Vision problems may affect ability to perform tasks requiring psychomotor skills, such as self-administration of insulin.
Do you have hearing problems? Do you wear a hearing aid? When was your last hearing test? Do you have vision problems? Do you wear glasses or contact lenses? When was your last eye examination?	
Respiratory	
Do you have a history of lung disease or breathing problems such as shortness of breath (SOB)?	SOB may limit tolerance, so short teaching sessions may be more effective.
Cardiovascular	
Do you have any history of cardiovascular disease?	Fatigue associated with chronic cardiac problems such as CHF limits tolerance, so short teaching sessions may be more effective.
Gastrointestinal/Genitourinary	
Do you have any gastrointestinal (GI) or genitourinary (GU) problems?	GI complaints, such as nausea or diarrhea, and GU complaints, such as urinary urgency and frequency, may affect learning.
Neurological	
Do you have any memory problems, numbness, or tingling?	Forgetfulness or difficulty concentrating affect ability to learn. Numbness and tingling may affect ability to learn psychomotor skills, such as self-administration of insulin.
Musculoskeletal	
Do you have a history of arthritis, joint pain, or weakness?	Joint pain, deformity, stiffness, or weakness may affect ability to perform tasks requiring psychomotor skills.
Endocrine	
Do you have thyroid disease or diabetes?	You may need to adjust the climate of the teaching environment if the person has heat or cold intolerance.
Immune/Hematologic	
Do you have cancer, HIV, or a bleeding disorder?	History of immunosuppression may prohibit group teaching programs. Anemias can cause fatigue.

Psychosocial Profile

The psychosocial profile can provide clues that are vital to planning a successful teaching plan, including areas in which health education is needed.

Psychosocial Profile

AREA/QUESTIONS TO ASK	RATIONALE/SIGNIFICANCE
Health Practices and Beliefs/ Self-care Activities	
What are you doing now to stay healthy?	Identifies client's focus (preventive or crisis). Identifies current level of self-care activities.

Psychosocial Profile

AREA/QUESTIONS TO ASK	RATIONALE/SIGNIFICANCE
Why? How did you learn to do it?	Identifies why learner practices and adheres to existing health behaviors.
How do you usually learn about health matters (e.g., nurse, physician, pharmacist, newspaper, radio, TV, friends, family member, Internet)?	Identifies usual sources of health information.
Typical Day	
How do you usually spend your day? How does a typical week go for you?	Identifies times of day or week when learners are most rested and comfortable, and when they prefer to learn.
Nutritional Patterns	
Are you on a special diet? What times do you usually eat?	Consider special diets or special eating times when scheduling teaching sessions. Hunger can affect learning.
Activity and Exercise Patterns	
What activities do you do involving your body (e.g., hobbies, playing instruments, tasks at home or work)?	If possible, incorporate client's activities into your teaching plan.
Sleep/Rest Patterns	
When do you have the most energy? Feel most relaxed? When are you most tired or uncomfortable?	Helps identify best times for teaching/learning.
Personal Habits	
Do you use tobacco, drugs, or alcohol?	Use of drugs and alcohol can be a barrier to learning and identify additional learning needs.
Occupational Health Patterns	
Does your place of employment offer health and wellness programs?	Identifies resources within the workplace.
Socioeconomic Status	
Does your health insurance program offer or cover health programs? Are you on a fixed income?	Makes you aware of time, responsibility, and economic barriers or assets. Identifies resources so that you can make appropriate referrals. Health programs or coverage may be available through health insurance programs.
Environmental Health Patterns	
What is your usual means of transportation?	Lack of transportation may be a barrier to learning. May need to identify alternative means, such as public transportation.
Roles and Relationships	
How do you balance your role responsibilities?	Learning must fit into your client's current role responsibilities.
Social Supports	
Will other people be coming to class with you? Are there family members or friends who need to know what you are learning?	Prepares you for other family members or supporters who may attend teaching session. Alerts you to people who may reinforce or impede the client's learning/behavior change.
Are there relationships in your life that will make it easier or harder for you to make changes?	Anticipates and addresses logistical barriers to learning, such as having unreliable transportation or being responsible for dependent care.
Stress and Coping	
Do you have any stress in your life currently? How do you usually deal with stress?	Be aware of current stressors, strengths, and deficits that could affect learning.

The Physical Assessment

Once you have completed the health history, identify physical assessment findings that could affect learning. Further investigate areas identified in the health history that might affect learning. As you perform the head-to-toe assessment, ask open-ended questions to determine the learner's baseline knowledge of your teaching content.

Physical Assessment

AREA/ASSESSMENT	ABNORMAL FINDINGS/RATIONALE
General Health Survey	
Inspect level of consciousness, posture, signs of acute distress. Measure vital signs.	If person is in acute distress or has altered level of consciousness, postpone teaching until his or her condition improves.
Integumentary	
Inspect for color changes such as cyanosis, pallor, jaundice.	Cyanosis may indicate hypoxia, and jaundice may indicate liver disease. Both conditions may alter mental status. Pallor is associated with anemia, which causes fatigue.
HEENT	
Test visual acuity and hearing.	Identify impaired vision or peripheral field and hearing deficits and adjust teaching plan to meet person's needs. Type and severity of deficit influence teaching strategies and tools.
Respiratory	
Measure respiratory rate. Auscultate lungs.	Hypoxia can cause confusion and decrease ability to concentrate.
Cardiovascular	
Measure blood pressure and pulse rate.	Cardiovascular problems such as CHF are often associated with fatigue.
Abdominal	
Palpate for tenderness and organomegaly.	Liver disease can result in a confused mental state and weakness.
Musculoskeletal	
Inspect joints. Test muscle strength, ROM.	Muscle weakness, joint deformity, and pain may affect ability to learn motor skills.
Neurological	
Test balance and coordination, fine motor skills, and senses.	Problems in these areas may make learning motor skills difficult.

HELPFUL HINT

To assess motor skills, observe the learner dressing, undressing, moving around the room, or performing a task such as writing.

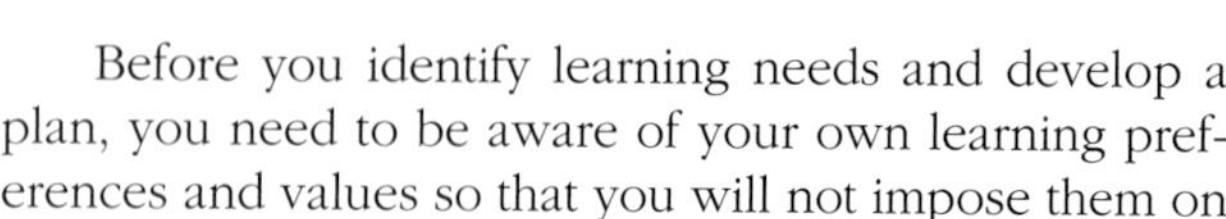

Case Study Analysis and Plan

Before you identify learning needs and develop a plan, you need to be aware of your own learning preferences and values so that you will not impose them on your client. For example, if your are an independent learner and your client is a dependent learner, a self-study approach is not likely to work.

HELPFUL HINT

As a nurse, you may feel that you never have enough time to teach, but remember that teaching can be informal as well as formal. Every time you interact with your client presents a potential for teaching.

Now that you know what factors to consider when devising a teaching plan, write a plan for Lucas based on his learning needs related to sleep.

CRITICAL THINKING ACTIVITY

Can you identify any additional learning needs for Lucas?

Summary

- Like the nursing process, the teaching process begins with assessment.
- During the health history, consider cultural, developmental, and psychosocial factors.
- During the physical examination, assess the person for factors that could affect learning, and identify both deficits and strengths.
- After you complete your assessment, identify the person's learning needs, readiness to learn, learning preferences, and learning styles. Then identify methods and strategies needed to develop and implement a successful teaching plan.
- Implement your plan, evaluating and revising as needed. Be sure to document every step of the teaching process.

5

Assessing Wellness

Before You Begin

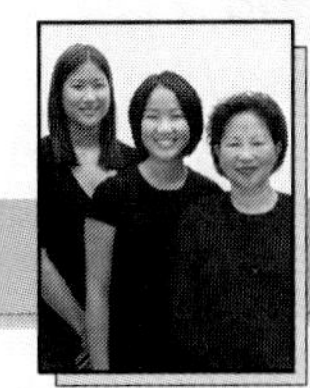

Introducing the Case Study

Mrs. Evelyn Chen (age 40); her daughter, Jan (age 15); and Mrs. Chen's mother, Mrs. Emily Wong (age 60) are attending a women's health fair sponsored by several large hospital systems and pharmaceutical companies. Health screenings and educational materials are available for women of all ages. If these three women asked you which screenings to have, what would you tell them? Before you can offer advice, you need to have an understanding of what health is and what factors influence a person's decision to live a healthy lifestyle.

Introduction to Assessing Wellness

Health is a broad concept that is difficult to define. Older definitions viewed health as the absence of disease. But today health is seen as a goal, a dynamic process that involves the self and self-care ability; optimal functioning of body, mind, and spirit; the ability to adapt; feelings of well-being and wholeness; and growing and becoming. People also have their own definitions of health, which are affected by gender, sociocultural factors, previous experience, age, and personal goals. These personal definitions influence their health promotion goals.

The three basic levels of prevention are primary, secondary, and tertiary. Primary prevention is essential to maintaining a state of wellness. At this level, the assessment process should include screening procedures, immunizations, and, especially, prevention education.

How do you teach people to stay well? Follow these steps:

- Set an example with a healthy lifestyle.
- Motivate them to change unhealthy behaviors.
- Propose strategies for behavior change.
- Show them how to care for themselves more effectively.
- Build on their strengths.
- Help them find and use available resources.
- Provide support through telephone, individual, and group counseling and continuing education.

This chapter focuses on four key areas fundamental to maintaining wellness—rest and sleep, exercise, stress management, and injury prevention—and suggests questions to ask at each developmental stage.

HELPFUL HINT

Do not assume that people know how to stay well. We may be bombarded with health information in the media and on the Internet, but what seems simple and obvious to the healthcare professional may still seem complex to the layperson.

Factors Affecting Health Behaviors

Support Systems

The encouragement of friends and family can mean the difference between achieving personal health goals or falling short of them. Ask the person about his or her support systems, and then use these systems in the assessment process when needed. Other types of supports include organized religious groups, nurses and other caregiving professionals, and self-help groups such as Weight Watchers.

Psychological State

A person's psychological state affects his or her physical state. For example, if a person knows that he or she needs to stop smoking, start eating more healthfully, and start exercising more, then why doesn't he or she do it? Part of the assessment process is determining these reasons and working with people to change harmful behaviors.

Access to Health Care

People may be motivated to maintain or improve their state of wellness but be prevented from doing so because they lack access to health care. Causes include lack of finances or insurance coverage, rural location, lack of transportation, crowding at available healthcare resources, age, gender, ethnicity and/or religion (possibly because of prejudice), and healthcare rationing based on these factors).

Motivational Level

Because people tend to resist change, convincing them to trade unhealthy behaviors for healthy ones can be dif-

ASSESSING PEOPLE'S STRENGTHS

Knowing your client's strengths and weaknesses will help both of you set realistic goals and help you plan appropriate interventions. Ask some or all of the following questions:

- What abilities do you possess to take care of your health?
- What activities help you to maintain or improve your health?
- What changes have you made in your lifestyle to improve your health in the past 2 years?
- What goals have you set to improve your health? Do you have a plan for reaching them?
- What changes in your life do you see in the future?
- What people currently give you the most support?
- What current activities make you feel happy?
- When you were younger, what activities gave you strength, comfort, and support?
- What helps you cope in a crisis?
- What gives you direction in your life?
- How do you spend a typical day?
- What do you feel motivated to do in terms of a lifestyle change?
- What barriers do you think will inhibit your lifestyle change?
- What health problems have you successfully dealt with in the past?

ficult. Teaching them the importance of primary prevention does not ensure that they will practice what you preach. For example, people know that smoking, obesity, and lack of exercise are dangerous to their health, but they still have trouble changing long-standing behaviors unless they are truly motivated.

HELPFUL HINT

Individualize your client's health promotion plan—it increases the chance of success.

HEALTH PROMOTION PLAN OF ACTION

- Identify the person's healthcare goals.
- Identify behavioral or health outcomes.
- Develop a behavior change plan.
- Reiterate benefits of change.
- Address environmental and interpersonal facilitators and barriers to change.
- Determine a time frame for implementation.
- Ask the person to make a commitment to healthcare goals.

Performing the Wellness Assessment

The wellness assessment consists of asking the person and/or caregiver general questions about health promotion behaviors and then specific questions about sleep and rest, exercise, stress management, and injury prevention. Health promotion behaviors and needs differ according to the person's developmental stage. (For a description of developmental stages see Chapter 2, The Health History.)

General Questions to Ask at Each Developmental Stage

Tailor your assessment questions to the person's developmental level—infant, toddler/preschool/school age, adolescent, young adult, middle age, or older adult. Include younger children in the interview as maturational level permits, and definitely include them by late school age. For young children, also assess health promotion behaviors for the family and the ability of the family to meet the child's needs.

Infants/Toddlers/Preschoolers

Ask the parent(s) or caregiver(s): Has your child's blood pressure been checked? Does the child brush his or her own teeth? How often? Are his or her immunizations up to date (polio, diphtheria-tetanus-pertussis, measles-mumps-rubella, *Haemophilus influenzae* type b, hepatitis A and B, chickenpox, pneumococcal disease)? Has he or she had a vision and hearing assessment? If so, when? If the assessment was abnormal, what follow-up has occurred? What are your child's nutritional habits? (For more information, see Chapter 6, *Nutritional Assessment*.) Has he or she been tested for anemia or tuberculosis? What are your childcare arrangements? Have you ever harmed your child or wanted to? Do you know what community resources are available related to child abuse?

School-Age Children

Adapt the questions in the previous paragraph and also ask the following: Has your child been part of home, school, or community education programs related to alcohol, drugs, sexuality, AIDS, birth control, or sexually transmitted diseases (STDs)? Does the child brush his or her teeth and practice other health promotion behaviors without being reminded? How is he or she doing in school?

Adolescents

Ask the adolescent the same questions as you asked about the school-age child, and also ask the following: Who are your community role models?

Young Adults

Primary physical growth is completed during the 20s, and body systems usually reach peak functioning. Although most young adults are healthy, some major threats include accidental injury, cancer, heart disease, suicide, AIDS, and homicide. Men are more likely to die than women, especially as a result of homicide involving handguns. Ask the following questions: Are your immunizations up to date? Do you visit a family doctor? Do you perform self-screening (e.g., breast or testicular self-examination)? How often? What do you eat in a 24-hour period? Are there behaviors affecting your health that you would like to change?

Middle-Aged Adults

At this stage, people are likely to be knowledgeable and assertive about their health and health care. However, they may not know what specific screening tests they should have. Middle-aged men are less likely to seek routine preventive care than women, which may be one reason why women's life expectancy is approximately 7 years longer than men's. Ask the following questions: How do you care for your teeth? What screening tests have you had and when (e.g., mammograms and prostate-specific antigen blood tests). What were the results? Do you keep a written record of your physician visits, immunizations, and screenings? Do you get a yearly flu shot? How about pneumonia vaccinations, tetanus-diphtheria, and hepatitis B injections?

Older Adults

Many older people begin to develop health problems, but they need to know that it is never too late to begin living more healthfully. Social support is the key in maintaining wellness in the later years. Research shows that older people who attend religious services regularly are less likely to require hospitalization and, if they do, have shorter hospital stays. Ask the same questions you asked the middle-aged person, but stress the importance of getting immunized, limiting medication use, eating nutritious foods, drinking enough fluids, interacting with family and friends, and keeping active in the church or community.

Questions to Ask All Adults

What is your or your family's definition of health? Do you believe you are healthy? Do other family members believe they are healthy? What health practices are included in your and your family's lifestyle? How is the family affected when someone is ill? Do you and your family have access to health care? Do you all have health insurance? Do you all receive regular physical and dental examinations? What religious or cultural beliefs do you all have that guide your purpose in life and your health practices?

Assessing Areas of Wellness

The following four areas are critical to maintaining wellness: rest and sleep, exercise, stress management, and injury prevention.

Rest and Sleep

Sleep restores, rejuvenates, and sometimes heals the body. Lack of sleep causes fatigue, stress, depression, and a decrease in lymphatic system functioning, increasing the risk of infection and disease. The following factors can directly affect how well and how long we sleep:

- *Circadian rhythms:* Also called the "**biological clock,**" these rhythms help regulate the sleep/wake cycle, body temperature, and hormonal levels within a 24-hour period. Disruption affects muscle strength and coordination, attention, memory, and concentration.
- *Age:* Infants sleep 16 to 20 hours a day; preschoolers, 10 to 12 hours a day; school-age children, 9 to 10 hours a day; adolescents 7 1/2 hours a day; and adults and older adults, 6 to 8 hours a day. Babies spend more time in **rapid eye movement (REM) sleep** than adults. Young children may experience sleep problems such as **nocturnal enuresis** (bedwetting), **nightmares** (bad dreams), **night terrors** (nightmare from which child awakens screaming), and **somnambulism** (sleepwalking). Older adults may take more time to fall asleep (**sleep latency**), have a fragmented sleep pattern with less deep sleep, and may awaken early. (For more information on sleep problems in children, see Chapter 24. Assessing the Preschool/School-Age Child.)
- *Exercise:* Moderate exercise has little or no effect on sleep; however, vigorous exercise before retiring may inhibit sleep.
- *Nicotine, caffeine, alcohol:* Smoking increases the time needed to fall asleep and causes lighter sleeping and more frequent awakening. Caffeine near bedtime can increase sleep latency and reduce total sleep time, especially in older adults. Alcohol affects REM sleep, causing a fragmented sleep pattern, and also exacerbates sleep apnea.
- *Diet and weight:* Sleep apnea is more common in obese people. High-protein foods increase alertness; carbohydrates promote relaxation. People who are gaining weight usually sleep more; those who are losing weight sleep less.
- *Medical problems:* COPD, CHF, and pain can affect sleep patterns.
- *Stress:* Stress often increases arousal and inhibits sleep.
- *Medications:* Some prescription and OTC drugs can affect the number of hours a person sleeps as well as the sleep process.

Questions to Ask at Each Developmental Stage

Infants: Ask the parent(s) or caregiver(s): Where does the infant sleep? In what position do you place him or her? Does the infant sleep through the night? Does he or she go to sleep with a bottle? If so, do you remove it once he or she is asleep? (Having a nipple drip milk into

Medications That Affect Sleep

Medication	Effect on Sleep
Amphetamines	Difficulty falling asleep
Antidepressants	Difficulty falling asleep
Barbiturates	Shallow, fragmented sleep; "hangover"
Phenylpropanolamine (found in OTC decongestants and cold and diet remedies)	Difficulty falling asleep
Diuretics before sleep	Frequent awakening
Beta blockers (e g , Inderal)	Nightmares

the mouth once the child is asleep can cause tooth decay and ear infections, in addition to the danger of choking.)

Toddlers/Preschoolers/School-Age Children: Ask the parent(s) or caregiver(s): Where does the child sleep? How many hours does he or she sleep? Does the child take naps? Does he or she sleep through the night? If not, how do you console the child when he or she awakens? What bedtime rituals do you practice? Does the child act tired during the day?

Adolescents: Ask the adolescent: How many hours do you sleep? Are you tired during the day? Do you have trouble paying attention at school or at work because of fatigue? Do you have a regular time you go to bed, and do you stick to it? Do you usually sleep through the night? If not, what causes you to wake up? How do you get back to sleep?

Young Adults: Ask the young adult: How many hours of sleep do you need to feel rested? How many hours of uninterrupted sleep do you get each night? Do you usually sleep through the night? If not, what causes you to wake up? How do you promote sleep or get back to sleep? Do you have a bedtime routine? Do you take medications that interrupt a normal sleep cycle? Do you take medications to help you sleep? Do you maintain a physical fitness program? Do you have problems concentrating because of fatigue? What are your usual work hours?

Middle-Aged Adults: Ask the same questions as you asked the young adult, as well as the following: How would you describe your quality of sleep? What time do you usually go to bed? How long does it take you to go to sleep? What time do you usually wake up and get up? What do you do for relaxation and how often do you do it?

Older Adults: Adapt the questions you asked the young and middle-aged adults, as well as the following: What activities do you engage in during late afternoon or early evening? If you have trouble falling asleep, have you tried a light, warm snack at bedtime?

Exercise

Today, with so many people working at sedentary jobs, exercise needs to be planned for. Research shows that women are less active than men; people with lower incomes and less education are less active than those with higher incomes and education; people with disabilities are less active than people without disabilities; African-Americans and Hispanics are less physically active than Caucasians; and many children and youth are overweight and exercising less, except for those active in organized sports. Major barriers to increasing physical activity are lack of time, access to convenient facilities, and safe environments in which to be active.

Questions to Ask at Each Developmental Stage

Infants: Keep in mind what gross and fine motor skills are normal at this age. Ask the parent(s) or caregiver(s): Does the infant play with his or her hands and feet and make noises? What kinds of toys do you give him or her? Which toys does the infant prefer? How often do you change his or her toys and play environment? Do you check toys regularly for loose parts and other safety hazards?

Toddlers/Preschoolers: Keep in mind what gross and fine motor skills are normal at this age. Ask the parents(s) or caregiver(s): Does the child have any physical limitations? Does he or she tire easily? What activities does he or she like? Does the child have a safe environment to explore and play? Whom does he or she play with? How many hours does your child watch TV or participate in other sedentary activities? What do you do to encourage physical activity during bad weather?

School-Age Children: Ask the same questions as you asked about the toddler/preschool child, as well as the following: *To the child:* Do you play organized sports? What precautions do you take, and what protective equipment do you wear? *To the parent(s) or caregiver(s):* Do you encourage physical activity? Do you engage in physical activities with your children?

Adolescents: Ask the adolescent: What competitive sports or other physical activities do you like? Do you schedule exercise during your week? How often and for how long? Do you exercise with friends? Do you have any physical limitations? Have you ever been injured during exercise? Does your school encourage participation in physical activities? What precautions do you take and what protective equipment do you wear? Do you gain satisfaction from exercising?

Young Adults: Ask the young adult: What physical activities do you include during an average week? How often and for how long? Do you have any physical limitations? Do you have any health conditions that should be evaluated before beginning an exercise program? Where do you exercise? Do you participate in activities that raise your heart rate? Do you include a warm-up and cool-down period? Do you participate in organized sports? What precautions do you take and what protective equipment do you wear? Have you had any exercise-related injuries? With whom do you exercise? Do you engage in physical activities as a family? Do you enjoy your exercise program?

Middle-Aged Adults: Ask the middle-aged adult: What kinds of exercise do you do? How often and for how long? Where do you exercise? With whom do you exercise? Describe them. Do you warm up before and cool down after each exercise period? Have you had any unusual or uncomfortable feelings before, during, or after exercising? (If so, refer back to the person's cardiovascular, respiratory, and musculoskeletal history data.)

Older Adults: Ask the same questions as you asked the middle-aged client, but emphasize that the older adult should check with his or her doctor before starting a new exercise program.

HELPFUL HINT

Teach older people to take their pulses when exercising. The recommended formula for maximum heart rate at this age group is: 220 minus age, multiplied by 60–80%. For example, in an 80-year-old, the range would be 84–112, with 84 being the minimum heart rate and 112 the maximum heart rate for cardiovascular functioning.

Stress Management

Multiple stressors can occur at any age, even infancy, although different age groups are subject to different stressors. Over time, stress can cause hypertension, cardiac arrhythmias, cardiovascular disease, gastrointestinal problems, headaches, and decreased immunological functioning, which can contribute to cancer and other diseases.

Questions to Ask at Each Developmental Stage

Infants: Keep in mind what social developmental milestones are normal for this age. Ask the parent(s) or caregiver(s) the following: What emotions have you seen the infant express? How does the infant calm himself or herself when crying? How do you calm the infant when he or she is unable to become calm? How would you describe his or her temperament? Does the infant entertain himself or herself when alone? How do you set limits for him or her? Does your home environment provide cognitive, physical, and psychosocial stimulation for the infant? Who provides child care when needed? Does the caregiver stick to the infant's usual routines?

Toddlers/Preschoolers: Adapt the questions above, and also ask the following: How does your child calm himself or herself after an emotional outburst? Children tend to regress when ill, so what do you do to support the child's developmental level when he or she is ill? How do you show affection to your child, and how does he or she respond? How well does your child play with other children? What kinds of conflicts occur with other children? How do you set disciplinary guidelines for your child? How do you encourage his or her development of autonomy and initiative? How does he or she interact with siblings? How does he or she express positive emotions (love, affection, happiness, joy) and negative emotions (hate, jealousy, anger, fear)? Do you actively model healthy expression of emotions in the home? Does your child enjoy childcare experiences?

School-Age Children: To the child: Do you usually feel happy and contented? Do you like yourself? What do you do when you feel bored or sick? Do you like to compete with others in organized or informal activities? Do you enjoy learning new things? Do you feel confident as you begin new projects? Do you enjoy the challenge of solving new problems? Do you feel like your parents or caregivers support your activities and enjoy your successes? Do they support you even when you do not meet their expectations? Do you think of the consequences of your behavior before acting? Who are your friends? Do you feel included in most peer-group activities? If you have conflicts with friends, what is the source of the conflict, and how do you resolve it? Do you receive an allowance or have an opportunity to earn money? How do you manage your money? Do you feel good about your progress at school? What do you like most and least about school? How often do you miss school or other activities because you do not feel well? What types of physical activities do you do? How often and for how long? *To the parent(s) or caregiver(s):* Do you give your child an allowance and provide general guidelines for money management? How do you display your interest in your child's school work/progress? How do you support your child when he or she does not feel well? How would you describe your child's friends? What stress-management techniques do you model or actively teach your child? How does your child act when he or she is tired or stressed out? How does he or she cope with emotional stress? What types of changes have affected your family and the child during the last year?

Adolescents: Adapt the questions for the school-age child, and also ask the following: Do you feel comfortable with the physical changes accompanying puberty? What accomplishments are most important to you? What stressors do you experience weekly? How do you reduce stress or the effects of stress? Are you able to be assertive when you need to be? Can you give an example? What risks have you taken in the last year? Do you use tobacco, alcohol, or street drugs? What about OTC and prescription drugs? If so, what kinds, how often, and how much? How would you describe your peer group and your relationship with the group? How would you describe your relationships with the same sex, the opposite sex, and adults? How do you usually make decisions? What plans do you have once you leave or complete high school? Who are your role models for stress management? How do your parents support your efforts to be an independent person? What are the most common sources of conflict with your family and your peers? How do you resolve conflicts when they occur? Whom do you go to for support when you have a problem? What steps would you take if you were depressed or had thoughts of suicide or if you saw these characteristics in a friend? Have you ever been the victim of violence? Have you ever abused an animal or another person?

Young Adults: What stressors do you experience weekly? How do you reduce stress or the effects of stress? What risks have you taken in the last year? How do you make decisions? How would you describe your relationships with the same sex and the opposite sex? What are the most common sources of conflict with your family, friends, and coworkers? How do you resolve conflicts when they occur? Do you use tobacco, alcohol, or street drugs? What about OTC and prescription drugs?

If so, what kinds, how often, and how much? Have you ever been the victim of violence? Have you ever wanted to hurt or abuse another person? Are you satisfied with your career choice? If not, what are your plans for a change? Do you have problems with time management? If you have children, what parenting rewards and challenges do you encounter? Do you feel confident and satisfied with your parenting skills?

Middle-Aged Adults: Ask the same questions that you asked the young adult.

Older Adults: Adapt the questions you asked the young adult and middle-aged adult, and also ask the following: When do you plan to retire from a full-time position? Are your financial resources adequate? Do you plan to work part-time after retirement? What activities are you interested in (e.g., travel, hobbies, volunteer work in the community)?

Injury Prevention

Injuries can occur at any age, and most people have a significant injury at some time in their lives. Although most accidents are predictable and preventable, accidental injuries are the leading cause of death in the 1-to-34 age group. Additional millions are incapacitated by accidental injuries.

Questions to Ask at Each Developmental Stage

Infants: Ask the parent(s) or caregiver(s): What have you done to make your home safe for the infant? Do you use an infant car seat? Is the infant regularly exposed to tobacco smoke? Has he or she been injured as a result of an accident in the home, in another's home, or while riding in a motor vehicle? How often do you check equipment and toys for possible hazards? Are there guns in your home or in your caretaker's home? If so, are they securely stored?

Toddlers/Preschoolers/School-Age Children: Adapt the questions above, and also ask the parent(s) or caregiver(s) the following: Have you taught your child personal safety guidelines? Does he or she use protective equipment when participating in physical activities like skating or bicycling? Who supervises your child when he or she is playing? Can he or she swim and does he or she know water safety guidelines?

Adolescents: Ask the adolescent: Do you like to take risks? Have you completed a driver education course? What safe-driving behaviors do you practice? Do you talk on a cell phone while driving? Do you consider yourself well informed regarding the transmission, signs, symptoms, and treatment of STDs? Are you sexually active, and if so, do you practice safe sex? Do you know where to get confidential medical attention if you believe you have an STD or may be pregnant? Do you use alcohol, tobacco, or street drugs? What about OTC and prescription drugs? If so, what kinds, how often, and how much? Do you ever drive while under the influence of alcohol or drugs? Do you have guns in your home, and if so, are they securely stored? Have you ever been injured as a result of participation in physical activities? What protective measures do you take? Would you recognize signs and symptoms of depression in yourself or a peer? What would you do if you or a peer were depressed or had thoughts of suicide?

Young Adults: Adapt the questions above, and also ask: Have you evaluated your occupational health risks? What resources are available to you at work related to health maintenance or injury prevention? Do you have smoke and carbon monoxide detectors in your home, and do you check them frequently?

Middle-Aged Adults: Adapt the questions above, and also ask: Are you aware of environmental hazards in the home (e.g., loose rugs, electrical cords, stairways, steps)?

Older Adults: Adapt the questions for young and middle-aged adults, but focus on the prevention of falls. Ask: Can you describe any hazards in your home, especially in the bathroom, kitchen, or outside steps and sidewalks? Do you use an assistive device, such as a cane, walker, or wheelchair? Do you keep them in good repair? Have you made any modifications to your home, such as a wheelchair ramp or grab bars in the tub and by the toilet?

Case Study Analysis and Plan

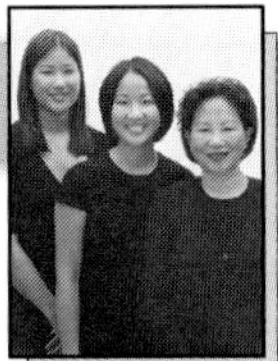

Now that you know what factors to consider when assessing health and wellness, what screening would you recommend for Jan, Mrs. Chen, and Mrs. Wong?

Summary

- There is no uniform definition of health as it applies to individuals, families, and communities. Yet a definition forms the foundation for personal perceptions and is crucial in determining individual health promotion behaviors.
- Other factors that affect health behaviors are the person's motivation, support system, psychological state, and access to health care.
- The key is to identify the person's perspective of health and any factors that affect health behaviors, and then work with him or her to develop a plan that promotes healthy living.

CHAPTER 6

Assessing Nutrition

Before You Begin

INTRODUCTION TO ASSESSING NUTRITION

Nutrition is the relative state of balance between nutrient intake and physiologic requirements for growth and physical activity. Optimal nutrition helps protect against disease, facilitates recovery, and decreases complications during illness. Good nutrition helps people stay healthy!

Malnutrition has traditionally been defined as a deficit of appropriate nutrients. However, malnutrition literally means "bad nutrition" and can encompass any situation that contributes to an imbalance in nutrient intake relative to actual needs. Therefore, malnutrition can mean a nutrient deficit or excess. Although nutritional deficits remain a significant health problem in Third-World countries, the major problem in the United States is nutritional excess.

As a nurse, you are in a unique position to assess people's nutritional status and provide information on proper nutrition. You can reinforce positive nutritional patterns, identify people at risk for malnutrition, and encourage more healthful eating habits.

Assessing nutritional status achieves the following:

- Identifies actual nutritional deficiencies.
- Illuminates dietary patterns that may contribute to health problems.
- Provides a basis for planning for more optimal nutrition.
- Establishes baseline data for evaluation.

This chapter covers basic screening considerations and the procedures for conducting a complete nutritional assessment.

Review of Nutrients

The goal of eating is to supply body cells with necessary nutrients. Ingestion, digestion, absorption, and metabolism are the processes that normally accomplish this goal. Interference with any of these functions can contribute to nutritional problems. (For more information on these functions, see Chapter 15, Assessing the Abdomen.)

Primary Nutrients

Nutrients are substances contained in food that are essential for optimal body functioning. The **primary nutrients** are carbohydrates, proteins, fats, vitamins, minerals, and water. Carbohydrates, protein, and fat are the body's major energy sources. Carbohydrates and protein each supply 4 calories per gram, and fat provides 9 calories per gram. Vitamins are essential to specific functions in the body. Minerals are inorganic elements that are essential to cell structure and physiologic functions in the body. Water comprises 50 to 60 percent of the adult weight. It is required for many functions, and humans cannot survive for more than a few days without it.

Carbohydrates

Carbohydrates are the body's major energy source. Foods that contain the most carbohydrates are grains, legumes, potatoes, corn, fruits, and vegetables. Adult carbohydrate intake should range from 50 to 100 g daily, depending on level of activity. In a normal diet, this means that 50 to 60 percent of the daily caloric intake should be derived from carbohydrates.

Protein

Protein is the primary building block of all tissues and organs and serves an important function in cell structure and tissue maintenance. Integrity of the skin, internal organs, and muscles depends on adequate protein intake and metabolism. The body can synthesize most of the necessary amino acids from nonprotein dietary sources. However, there are nine essential amino acids that the body cannot synthesize and that must be obtained through dietary sources. For this reason, adults require 0.8 grams/kilogram (g/kg) per day of protein (about 10 to 20 percent of the daily caloric intake). Primary sources of protein include meat, milk and milk products (e,g., cheese and yogurt), nuts, and legumes.

More protein is needed during tissue building; for example, in pregnancy and lactation, childhood, adolescence, postoperative recovery, tissue damage, and long-term illness. Athletes also require additional protein to build and maintain muscle. Animal products are the most common source of protein in industrialized countries. However, well-planned vegetarian diets can also provide ample dietary protein.

VEGETARIAN DIETS

Vegetarian diets consist primarily of plant foods. ***Vegans*** *avoid all animal products in the diet,* ***lactovegetarians*** *eat dairy products, and* ***lacto-ovovegetarians*** *also eat eggs. Although these diets provide less protein than nonvegetarian diets, they meet or exceed the recommended dietary allowances. Whole grains, legumes, vegetables, seeds, and nuts contain all the essential and nonessential amino acids. As long as food intake is varied and calories are sufficient, protein deficiencies will not occur. Furthermore, soy protein provides all essential and nonessential amino acids and is nutritionally equivalent to animal sources of protein. It can serve as the sole source of protein if desired. However, because considerable variation exists, evaluate the adequacy of vegetarian diets on an individual basis.*

Fats

Lipids or fats are insoluble in water and soluble in alcohol, ether, and chloroform. They include true fats, lipids, and sterols, such as cholesterol. Fat supplies twice as much energy as carbohydrates or proteins. It provides essential fatty acids (linoleic and linolenic acids) and promotes the absorption of the fat-soluble vitamins A, D, E, and K. The typical American diet usually contains adequate fat, and recommended daily allowances in grams do not exist. However, because triglycerides and cholesterol are major contributors to heart disease, diabetes mellitus, and obesity, the U. S. Department of Agriculture (USDA) and the American Heart Association recommend that fat intake not exceed 20 to 30 percent of a person's total daily calories.

Highly **saturated fat** (solid at room temperature) significantly contributes to elevated serum triglyceride and cholesterol levels. So USDA/United States Department of Health and Human Services (USDHHS) guidelines recommend that no more than 10 percent of daily calories be derived from saturated fats. Unsaturated and polyunsaturated fats are recommended because of their inverse relationship with heart disease.

Cholesterol occurs naturally and exclusively in all animal food products. The body needs cholesterol for cell structure, as a precursor for certain hormones and vitamins, and to aid in the digestive process. But even if no cholesterol were consumed in the diet, the body would synthesize the needed supply.

Lipoproteins

Serum cholesterol and lipids attach to proteins and are transported throughout the body as **lipoproteins.** The relative ratio of lipid to protein determines the density of the molecule. A low lipid-to-protein ratio results in a high-density lipoprotein (HDL). HDLs are produced during cellular metabolism. They lower serum cholesterol by transporting it from the cell to the liver for metabolism and excretion. Conversely, a high lipid-to-protein ratio produces a larger and low-density lipoprotein (LDL). LDLs are produced in the gastrointestinal wall after eating and transport dietary cholesterol and triglycerides to the cells. Thus, HDLs guard against heart disease by lowering cholesterol, and LDLs contribute to heart disease by raising cholesterol. The risk for heart disease is particularly high when total serum cholesterol exceeds 200 mg/dL. The risk also increases as the HDL level decreases. An HDL less than 35 mg/dL is considered a major risk factor for heart disease, and an HDL above or equal to 60 mg/dL is a negative risk factor.

Vitamins and Minerals

Vitamins are organic compounds that play a major role in enzyme reactions associated with the metabolism of carbohydrate, protein, and fat. Although vitamins are required in small amounts, the body does not synthesize them, so they must be present in the diet. Vitamins are classified as water soluble or fat soluble. The body does not store water-soluble vitamins (B complex and C vitamins), so any surplus in daily intake is excreted in the urine. Fat-soluble vitamins (A, D, E, and K) are obtained through dietary fat and are stored in adipose tissue, where they can accumulate and become toxic. Toxicity generally results from self-administered large doses of a vitamin or excessive intake of foods that contain the vitamin.

Minerals are inorganic compounds found in nature. They play a wide variety of roles in human nutrition. Minerals are required in varying amounts and are divided into major and trace elements. Major minerals are required in excess of 100 mg per day and include calcium, chloride, magnesium, phosphorus, potassium, sodium, and sulfur. The remaining minerals are known as trace elements.

Water

We usually do not think of water as being related to nutrition. But without it, humans cannot survive more than a few days. Water helps regulate body temperature, serves as a solvent for vitamins, minerals, and other nutrients, acts as a medium for chemical reactions, serves as a lubricant, and transports nutrients to and wastes from the cells. Adults consume about 6 cups of water per day through beverages; another 4 cups are obtained through food; and about 1 cup is produced as a by-product of metabolism. **Sensible water loss** occurs through perspiration, urine, and gastrointestinal secretions. Evaporative or **insensible water loss** occurs via the lungs and skin.

More than half of the body's weight is comprised of water, and therefore rapid weight changes are usually a reflection of fluid balance. This is especially true for infants who have a greater proportion of water weight and proportionately more extracellular fluid. Thirst is not an accurate indicator of hydration status because it does not occur until about 10 percent of the intravascular volume is lost, or 1 to 2 percent of the intracellular volume is depleted. Assessment of hydration and signs and symptoms of dehydration are discussed later in this chapter.

Nutritional Guidelines and Standards

Early guidelines addressed the nutritional needs of the entire population, so they exceed the needs of most normal, healthy people. A diet that meets roughly two-thirds of the Recommended Daily Allowances (RDAs) for each nutrient is considered adequate.

Dietary Guidelines and the Food Guide Pyramid

The RDAs provide guidelines for specific nutrient quantities for clinical applications. The six-group Food Guide Pyramid (Fig. 6–1) was developed to make these recommendations easier for the public to understand and follow. The pyramid can be used to evaluate individual nutritional status and to educate people about nutrition.

SERVING EQUIVALENTS FOR FOOD GUIDE PYRAMID GROUPS

1. Bread, cereal, rice, pasta:
1 cup ready-to-eat cereal
1/2 cup cereal nuggets or granola
1 1/2 cups puffed cereal
1/2 cup cooked cereal, rice, or pasta

2. Vegetables:
1 cup raw leafy vegetables
1/2 cup other vegetables, cooked or chopped raw
3/4 cup vegetable juice

3. Fruit:
1 medium apple, banana, or orange
1/2 cup chopped, cooked, or canned fruit
3/4 cup fruit juice

4. Milk, yogurt, cheese:
1 cup milk or yogurt
1 1/2 oz natural cheese
2 oz processed cheese

5. Meat, poultry, fish, dry beans, eggs, nuts:
2–3 oz cooked lean meat, poultry, or fish
1/2 cup cooked dry beans or one egg = 1 oz lean meat
2 tablespoons peanut butter or 1/3 cup nuts = 1 oz meat

6. Fats, oils, sweets:
Use sparingly

(Adapted from USDA Center for Nutrition Policy and Promotion)

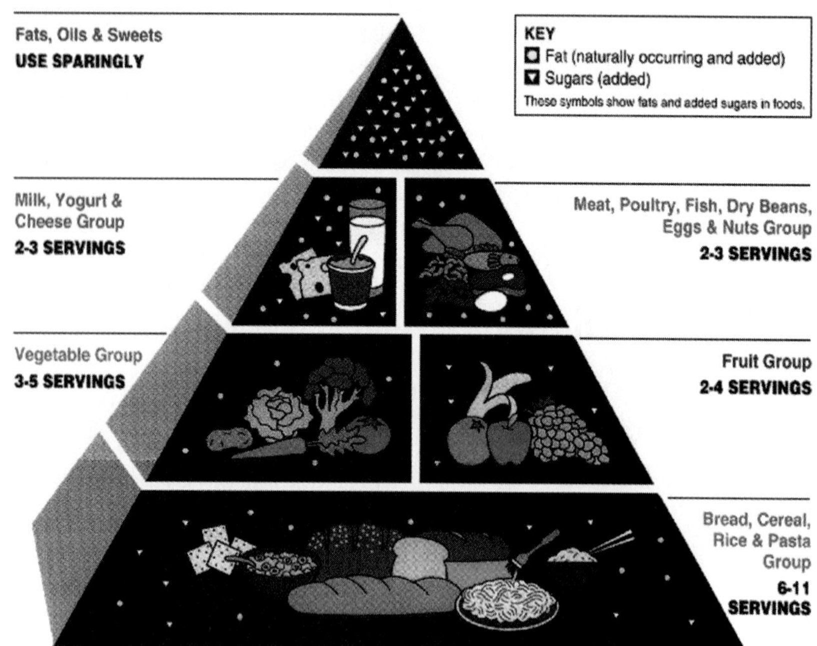

FIGURE 6–1. Food Guide Pyramid (Courtesy of United States Department of Agriculture and Department of Health and Human Services).

How a Nutritional Deficiency Develops

Nutritional deficiencies have characteristics that are relatively unique to the specific nutrient that is lacking in the diet. For example, diminished night vision is a classic symptom of vitamin A deficiency, and fetal deformities are associated with folic acid deficiencies in pregnancy. A thorough nutritional assessment can identify deficiencies long before actual clinical symptoms occur. The section below describes the four stages of nutritional deficiency.

Stage 1: Nutritional Deficiency Occurs

Malnutrition occurs when the nutrient in question is not available for digestion, absorption, and metabolism. **Primary malnutrition** results when a specific nutrient is lacking in the diet. Iron-deficient diets that result in anemia in infants and young children and calcium-deficient diets that cause osteoporosis in postmenopausal women are examples. **Secondary malnutrition** results from impaired bioavailablity of nutrients to the body. Intake of nutrients may be adequate, but physiologic processes prevent them from being digested, absorbed, or metabolized. Primary and secondary malnutrition can occur together.

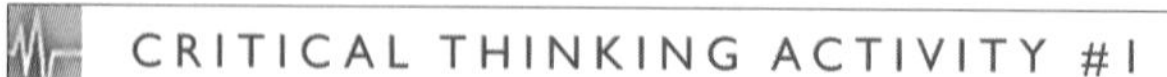
CRITICAL THINKING ACTIVITY #1

Identify some other causes of primary malnutrition.

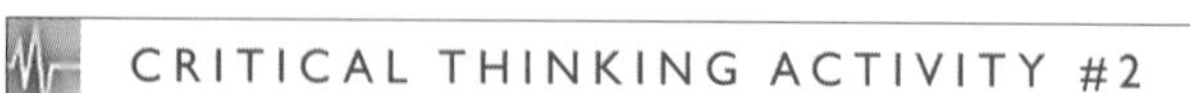
CRITICAL THINKING ACTIVITY #2

Identify some causes of secondary malnutrition.

Stage 2: Tissue Reserves Decrease

When a nutritional deficiency occurs, the body mobilizes tissue reserves to sustain metabolic processes. Nutrient levels in the blood generally will remain within normal limits as long as there are tissue reserves that the body can depend on. However, if the intake deficiency persists, tissue reserves become depleted and blood levels of nutrients drop, causing biochemical abnormalities.

Stage 3: Biochemical Lesions Occur

Biochemical lesions are changes in serum values that signal depletion of tissue reserves. Biochemical testing is a valuable adjunct to nutritional assessment and may reveal nutrient deficiencies well before clinical signs and symptoms occur.

Stage 4: Clinical Lesions Occur

Clinical lesions are physical changes that result from an inadequate supply of one or more nutrients necessary for tissue growth and maintenance.

Developmental, Cultural, and Ethnic Variations

As people grow and develop, their nutritional needs change. Developmental groups especially at risk for nutritional problems include pregnant and lactating women, infants and children, adolescents, and older adults.

Infants, Children, and Adolescents

The growth and development that occur in infancy, childhood, and adolescence determine nutritional needs. For example, brain development is at its peak from birth through the second year of life, but after this, improved nutrition will not enhance brain growth. Growth charts are the standard against which infant and child growth is evaluated (see Appendix B). Table 6–1 lists indications of good nutrition in school-age children, and Table 6–2 summarizes pertinent growth and developmental factors and corresponding nutritional needs of infants, children, and adolescents.

Table 6–1 Indications of Good Nutrition in the School-Age Child

General Appearance	Alert, energetic Normal height and weight
Skin and Mucous membranes	Skin smooth, slightly moist; Mucous membranes pink, no bleeding
Hair	Shiny, evenly distributed
Scalp	No sores
Eyes	Bright, clear, no fatigue circles
Teeth	Straight, clean, no discoloration or caries
Tongue	Pink, papillae present, no sores
Gastrointestinal system	Good appetite, regular elimination
Musculoskeletal system	Well-developed, firm muscles; erect posture, bones straight without deformities
Neurological system	Good attention span for age; not restless, irritable, or weepy

Source: Lutz & Przytulski (2001).

Table 6–2 Nutritional Needs of Infants, Children, and Adolescents

AGE	DEVELOPMENTAL AND GROWTH FACTORS	CORRESPONDING NUTRITIONAL NEEDS
Infants: Birth–12 months	Energy needs largely a result of high metabolic rate, increased skin-to-body-size ratio (facilitates heat loss and requires more thermal energy), and sucking and crying activities.	100–200 kcal/day at birth, decreases to 80–100 kcal/day by 12 months.
	Increased protein needs result from rampant growth in first year	2.5–3.5 g protein at birth, decreases to 2 g by 12 months.
	Fat is critical to developing nervous system and is also an important energy source at this age.	30–55% of daily caloric intake should be derived from fat.
	Fetal iron stores depleted around 4–6 months.	Solids usually introduced around 4–6 months. Cereal is important source of iron. Provide iron supplements if solids not introduced. Do not give eggs and cheese

(Continued)

Table 6–2 Nutritional Needs of Infants, Children, and Adolescents *(Continued)*

AGE	DEVELOPMENTAL AND GROWTH FACTORS	CORRESPONDING NUTRITIONAL NEEDS
		until immune system has matured, around 12 months of age.
Toddlers: 1–3 years	Growth rate slows drastically and appetite decreases. Wish for autonomy also contributes to selective appetite or refusal to eat. Parents usually become concerned about decreased/erratic appetite.	Require all essential nutrients. Intake should adhere to Food Pyramid guidelines. Serving size roughly 1 tablespoon per year of child's age (e.g., 2–1/2 tablespoons of rice for a 2-1/2-year-old).
	Fat remains an essential nutrient for energy and neurological development.	Whole milk is necessary through the second year.
	Risk of iron deficiency anemia related to decreased intake of iron-rich foods.	Milk contains no iron, so limit it to 1 quart daily because more will diminish food intake.
	Children usually dislike vegetables, so fiber intake throughout childhood tends to be low.	Beginning at age 2, daily fiber intake should be equal to child's age + 5 grams of fiber.
Preschoolers: 3–6 years	Continue to be very active. Growth continues at approximately 4–5 lb and 1–2 inches a year.	Needs average of 1800 calories/day. Requires same nutrients as adults but in lesser amounts. 1 tablespoon per age in years remains appropriate serving size.
	At risk for iron-deficiency anemia, especially those from low-income families, who are also at risk for vitamin A and C deficiency.	Monitor for iron-deficiency anemia.
	Children are trying to master behaviors that emulate the social norm and are internalizing nutritional patterns and habits.	Children should be learning optimal dietary practices.
School Age: 6–12 years	Doubles first year's weight by age 6. Energy needs and requirements correspond to age and activity.	RDA for caloric intake is 2000 calories/day.
	Breakfast is important for optimal school performance	Breakfast should include 25–30% of daily nutrient intake.
	Calcium and phosphorus are critical to prepubertal skeletal development.	RDA for calcium is 800 mg/day. Calcium and phosphorus retention is greatest just preceding puberty, so encourage milk intake.
Adolescence: 12–20 years	Growth is erratic and occurs in spurts.	60 to 80 calories/kg needed to support dramatic growth and intense physical and cognitive activity.
	Sex hormones influence growth differences between boys and girls: Boys' needs related to increased size, muscle mass, and sexual maturation.	Boys have greater calorie, iron, and zinc needs for sexual maturation. Girls' needs related to menstrual function. Girls require even more iron for menstrual function. Both sexes (especially athletes) need vitamins B and C for protein synthesis.
	Continued skeletal growth with enhanced needs for calcium and phosphorus Development characterized by identity-seeking behaviors and need to fit in with peers. Consumption of soft drinks and fast food increases. White female adolescents are at greatest risk for anorexia nervosa and bulimia.	Need four servings of milk or dairy products/day. At risk for developing obesity or calcium deficiency if soft drinks are substituted for milk.

Pregnant Women

Good nutrition is critical to the developing fetus. Women who fail to receive adequate nutrition before and during pregnancy are at risk for premature birth, low-birth-weight (LBW) infants, or infants who are small for gestational age (SGA). These infants are at higher risk for mental and physical disabilities and other congenital anomalies. In addition, pregnant women who are poorly nourished endanger their own health because maternal nutrients are sacrificed to compensate for the increasing demands of the growing fetus.

Pregnant women need an additional 300 calories a day, and lactating women an additional 500 calories a day. Development of the placenta, amniotic fluid, and fetal tissues, and increases in maternal blood volume during pregnancy require 10 g of protein a day. This requirement can be met simply by adding one additional serving each of milk and meat to the daily diet. Prenatal vitamins and mineral supplements during pregnancy and lactation are also critically important. Table 6–3 summarizes the vitamin and mineral needs of pregnant and lactating women.

Older Adults

Older adulthood begins at age 65. The senses become less acute, and diminished taste of sweet and salty foods may cause people to compensate by increasing sugar and salt. Decreased gastric acidity can impede vitamin B_{12} absorption. Antacid use impedes it further. Skin changes associated with aging impair vitamin D synthesis; so does spending less time outdoors. Diminished physical strength and decreased activity predispose older adults to bone demineralization and loss. This problem is especially common in women who do not consume adequate calcium and in postmenopausal women who have lost the protective advantage of estrogen. In addition, loss of urinary sphincter muscle tone in women and urination difficulty associated with prostate changes in men may discourage fluid intake. Confusion, a common consequence of dehydration, may impair mental status. Decreased income, loss of the social context for eating (e.g., death of spouse), and lack of accessibility to food markets are social and economic aspects of aging that may adversely affect nutrition.

The RDA amounts beginning in early adulthood change only moderately through the middle adult years. The most significant changes beginning in midlife and extending into older adulthood are related to the physical changes associated with aging. Energy requirements are thought to decrease by about 5 percent per decade after age 40. However, without dietary modifications, weight gain will occur, with the risk for obesity-related diseases. The RDA reflect a 200-mg increase in calcium and a twofold increase for vitamin D to 10 μg after age 50. Unless fluid intake is restricted for medical reasons, older adults still need 6 to 8 glasses of water daily.

People of Different Cultural/Ethnic Groups

Sociocultural patterns of food intake also influence nutritional status. Cultural patterns of eating are learned and reinforced early in life and are difficult to change without conscious efforts and external support. Many cultures have healthy eating habits. For example, the traditional Asian diet provides adequate nourishment and is associ-

Table 6–3 Vitamin and Mineral Needs During Pregnancy and Lactation

VITAMIN/MINERAL	FUNCTION
Vitamin C	Activates folic acid (folate), facilitates iron absorption, and helps build connective tissue.
Folic acid (400 μg)	Needed for fetal brain development. Deficiencies have been correlated with mental retardation and neural tube defects.
Iron (30 mg)	Important for development of red blood cells. Is supplied to fetus regardless of mother's iron status, increasing risk of maternal anemia.
Calcium (1200 mg)	Necessary for fetal skeletal tissue. Derived from mother's circulating supply, and unless calcium reserves are replenished, pregnant women will experience compensatory bone demineralization.
Fluoride (1 mg)	Fetal tooth bud development begins near end of first trimester. No recommendations exist for fluoride supplementation during pregnancy, but children whose mothers took fluoride daily during pregnancy have fewer cavities.
Zinc	A structural element of cells and an important mineral for a growing, developing fetus. Not mobilized from maternal tissues and must be supplied to fetus through mother's diet. Deficiencies associated with small, malformed infants and difficult labor.

Source: Data from Glenn et al, 1982, and Lutz et al, 1997.

ated with lower rates of the chronic diseases that plague Western populations. However, now that Asians are beginning to adopt Western food preferences, chronic diseases are on the rise in these countries. In contrast, diets in Western industrialized cultures are high in meat, sugar, and fat (Table 6–4).

Table 6–4 Cultural Dietary Preferences

CULTURE	DIETARY HABITS
African-American	High-fat, high-sodium foods, fried foods, large amounts of animal fat, little fruit and vegetables.
Amish	High in fats and carbohydrates.
Appalachian	Believe that plenty of food is associated with wealth. Use large amounts of lard and preserve meats and other foods with salt.
Arab-American	Cook with spices and herbs, eat lamb and chicken, but no pork, believe it is unhealthy to drink and eat at same time or mix hot and cold foods. Main meal is at mid-day.
Chinese-American	Food at meals is eaten in specific order. Food often used as medicine to cure disease and increase strength. Peanuts and soybeans popular.
Cuban-American	Staples include root crops, plantains, and grains. Meat is usually chicken and pork. Typical diet is high in calories, starch, and saturated fats. Leisurely noontime meal, late dinner.
Egyptian-American	Food is well done and well seasoned. Rice is main staple. Usually do not eat pork. Do not mix hot and cold, sweet and sour foods. Main meal is at mid-day.
Fillipino-American	Meals are a time for socialization. Sharing food is important. Salt and vinegar used as preservatives, leading to high sodium intake. Plants and herbs also used for medicinal purposes.
Mexican-American	Celebrate with food. Food rich in color, flavor, and spice. Rice, beans, and tortillas are staples. Hot and cold theory applies to food.
Navajo Native American	Food used to celebrate life events. Corn is a staple. Many have lactose intolerance and do not drink milk, leading to Vitamin D deficiency.
Vietnamese-American	Because of people's smaller size, normal caloric intake 2/3 less than that of other Americans. Rice is main staple. Hot and cold theory applies to food. High incidence of lactose intolerance.

Source: Adapted from Purnell and Paulanka, 1998.

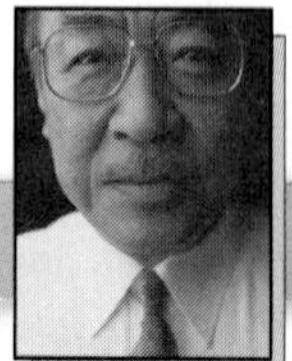

Introducing the Case Study

James Thomas, a 76-year-old African-American man, lives alone in a two-story urban row home. His wife passed away 6 months ago. He has a history of hypertension (HTN), which is controlled with Lasix 40 mg od and Vasotec 5 mg bid. He has come for a routine blood pressure (BP) check but complains that he doesn't feel well and has lost 10 lb since his wife's death. He states, "I have no energy, and I'm always tired."

Performing the Nutritional Assessment

One of the first steps in assessing nutrition is screening the client for possible nutritional risks. At the very least, you should evaluate the health history for symptoms and situations related to nutritional problems, perform a basic physical examination, and obtain laboratory data associated with malnutrition. A comprehensive nutritional assessment involves a detailed dietary history, focused **anthropometry,** and evaluation of laboratory values. It is recommended for people with any of the following nutritional risks:

- Weight less than 80 percent or more than 120 percent of ideal body weight (IBW)
- History of unintentional weight loss (greater than 10 lb or 10 percent of usual weight)
- Serum albumin concentration lower than 3.5 g/dL
- Total lymphocyte count lower than 1500 cells/mm^3
- History of illness, surgery, trauma, or stress
- Symptoms associated with nutritional deficiency or depletion
- Factors associated with inadequate nutritional intake or absorption

Health History

Nutritional health risks and problems are not always obvious to the client or the nurse. So during the health history, stay alert for clues. The following sections summarize health history data that may signal nutritional problems that warrant further investigation.

Biographical Data

Scan the biographical data for clues that may affect the client's nutritional status. Note age to determine normal dietary requirements. Nutritional needs also vary according to gender. Religion and cultural background may influence dietary preferences. Financial status may also affect the person's ability to maintain a healthy diet.

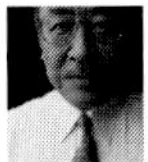

Case Study Findings

Reviewing Mr. Thomas' biographical data:

- 78-year-old African-American male
- Wife died 6 months ago
- Lives alone in urban area
- Retired postal worker
- Baptist religion
- Medicare/Medicaid health insurance
- Daughter is primary contact

Current Health Status

Inadequate nutrition is often discovered indirectly during a routine health history and physical examination. For instance, diminished growth and delayed development related to inadequate nutrition may be identified during a routine well-child checkup. Client concerns that result from malnutrition usually present as a specific symptom or functional problem rather than a focused nutritional problem. For example, a person with iron-deficiency anemia may complain of a lack of energy and an inability to concentrate.

Ask your client if his or her health status has changed. If so, consider the potential influence of the health change on nutrition. Acute and chronic illnesses, debilitating conditions, medications, surgery, and trauma all affect nutrition. Illness and trauma stimulate the stress response and increase nutritional requirements. Vomiting and diarrhea can cause fluid and electrolyte loss. Febrile illnesses accelerate metabolic processes and insensible fluid loss. Energy and fluid requirements are also greater during infections and febrile illnesses. Certain diseases, such as diabetes mellitus, cystic fibrosis, and celiac disease, are linked to specific nutritional deficits.

Ask about changes in diet or weight. Diet changes may be a result of physical, economic, or other factors that could contribute to malnutrition. Weight gains can occur with certain endocrine problems, and weight loss may accompany cancer, diabetes mellitus, and hyperthyroidism. Sudden weight changes are more likely to be related to fluctuations in hydration status caused by such conditions as congestive heart failure (CHF) or severe diarrhea.

Ask about prescription and over-the-counter (OTC) medications. Many of these drugs adversely affect nutrition (Box 6–1). Note the client's use of diuretics because they can cause non-nutritional weight changes.

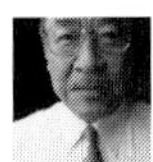

Case Study Findings

Mr. Thomas' current health status includes:

- Vague complaints of not feeling well, being very tired, and having no energy; 10-lb weight loss since wife's death.
- Current medications are Lasix 40 mg od and Vasotec 5 mg bid. No over-the-counter (OTC) medications except occasional milk of magnesia (MOM) for constipation. No illegal drug use.

Past Health History

Ask the person if he or she has experienced a major illness, surgery, or trauma. These are usually associated with increased nutritional needs and, depending on how recently they occurred and the person's recovery status, they may continue to pose a nutritional risk. Also ask if he or she has any chronic conditions such as cancer that could affect utilization of nutrients. In addition, inquire about dental or oral problems. Loss of teeth or pain and discomfort associated with eating can significantly impair ingestion. Last, ask about recent camping trips or foreign travel because of the risk of food- and waterborne pathogens.

Box 6–1 Drugs That Adversely Affect Nutritional Status

Drug Class	Drug	Possible Adverse Reactions
Antacids	calcium carbonate	Hypercalcemia, milk-alkali syndrome
	magnesium hydroxide	Fluid and electrolyte imbalances
	sodium bicarbonate	Metabolic alkalosis
Anti-infectives	amphotericin B	Hypokalemia, hypomagnesemia, reversible normochromic, normocytic anemia
	aminoglycosides	Sprue-like syndrome with steatorrhea, malabsorption, and electrolyte imbalance
	tetracyclines	Impaired absorption of calcium, magnesium, and iron
	sulfasalazine	Inhibition of folic acid absorption
Antilipemics	cholestyramine resin	Impaired folic acid or phosphorus absorption, steatorrhea, fat-soluble vitamin absorption with long-term use of high doses
	niacin	Hyperglycemia and abnormal glucose tolerance with long-term use of high doses
	colestipol hydrochloride	Impaired absorption of vitamins A, D, E, and K
Antineoplastics	cisplatin	Severe electrolyte disturbances
	cyclophosphamide	Hyperkalemia, hyponatremia
Diuretics	thiazides	Hypokalemia, hypochloremic alkalosis, hypercalcemia, hypophosphatemia, hypomagnesemia
	bumetanide, furosemide	Hypokalemia, hypomagnesemia, hypochloremia, hyponatremia, hypocalcemia, metabolic alkalosis
	mannitol	Fluid and electrolyte imbalances
	amiloride hydrochloride, spironolactone, triamterene	Hyperkalemia
Steroids	prednisone, methylprednisolone, dexamethasone	Sodium retention, hypokalemic alkalosis, hypocalcemia
Miscellaneous agents	alcohol	Decreased vitamin B_{12} absorption; thiamine, magnesium, or folic acid deficiencies
	chlorpropamide, tolbutamide	Hyponatremia
	oral contraceptives	Decreased glucose tolerance, altered carbohydrate and lipid metabolism, folic acid or B_6 deficiency
	orlistat	Impaired absorption of vitamins A, D, E, and K

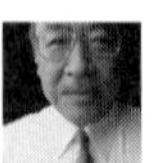

Case Study Findings

Mr. Thomas' past health history reveals:

- Positive history of HTN for 10 years
- Hospitalized last year for uncontrolled HTN
- Appendectomy at age 12
- No allergies to food, drugs, or environmental factors
- Medications listed previously

Family History

Certain genetic and hereditary conditions affect digestion, absorption, and metabolism. Ask the person if he or she has a history of food intolerance or allergies, such as lactose intolerance. Ask about hereditary or familial health problems, such as Crohn's disease, diabetes mellitus, or cystic fibrosis; or anemias, such as thalassemia. Inquire about a family history of cardiovascular disease, atherosclerotic disease, or obesity.

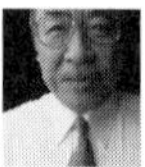

Case Study Findings

Mr. Thomas' family history reveals:

- Daughter, age 50, alive and well
- Wife deceased age 74, breast cancer
- Mother, deceased age 75, HTN, CVA
- Father, deceased age 80, HTN, MI
- Sister, age 70, HTN
- Sister, age 73, alive and well
- Brother, age 75, DM, HTN, CAD
- Maternal aunt, deceased age 80, CAD, MI
- Maternal uncle, deceased age 78, CVA
- Paternal aunt, deceased age 82, colon cancer
- Paternal uncle, deceased age 81, CVA

Review of Systems

The review of systems (ROS) provides a focused screening for past and present problems related to or affecting each of the physical systems. It may also identify problems or symptoms that indicate a nutritional risk (Table 6–5).

Table 6–5 Review of Systems

SYSTEM/QUESTIONS TO ASK	RATIONALE/SIGNIFICANCE
General Health Survey	
Have you had unexplained weight loss, fatigue, activity intolerance, or inability to concentrate?	May indicate metabolic problems (e.g., diabetes mellitus, hyperthyroidism, or malignancy), iron-deficiency anemia, or dehydration.
Integumentary	
Have you noticed changes in skin texture, skin discolorations, poor wound healing, or bruising?	May signal vitamin and mineral deficiencies, protein malnutrition, or metabolic disorders.
HEENT/*Eyes*	
Do you have poor night vision or eye dryness?	May indicate vitamin A deficiency or dehydration.
HEENT/*Nose, Mouth, Throat*	
Do you have nosebleeds or bleeding gums?	Possible vitamin, mineral, or protein deficiencies.
Cavities or lost teeth?	May indicate excess sugar intake.
Cardiovascular	
Do you have chest pain or pressure?	*Cardiac disease:* May be caused by high cholesterol, elevated triglycerides, or high-calorie diet.
Gastrointestinal	
Are you constipated?	*Constipation:* Low-fiber diet, poor fluid intake.
Do you have diarrhea?	*Diarrhea:* High-fiber diet, food allergies, hereditary and genetic disorders (e.g., cystic fibrosis).
Reproductive	
Women: Have you had frequent miscarriages or irregular menses?	Maternal malnutrition can lead to fetal growth restriction.
How much caffeine do you consume a day?	Consumption of 300 mg of caffeine/day increases risk for spontaneous abortion. Eating disorders can result in irregular menses.
Men: Do you suffer from impotence?	Alcohol intake increases risk for impotence.
Musculoskeletal	
Do you have muscle weakness?	May be caused by potassium deficiency or dehydration.
Neurological	
Are you nervous or irritable? Do you have headaches, numbness or tingling, or muscle tics?	Possible vitamin B deficiencies or hypocalcemia.
Lymphatic	
Do you have frequent infections?	*Frequent infections:* Protein malnutrition.
Allergies?	*Allergies:* Food sensitivity (e.g., lactose).

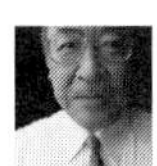

Case Study Findings

Mr. Thomas' ROS reveals:

- **General Health Survey**: 10-lb weight loss, fatigue.
- **Integumentary**: Dry, flaky skin.
- **HEENT**: Wears dentures.
- **Respiratory**: No changes.
- **Cardiovascular**: No chest pain; positive history of HTN.
- **Gastrointestinal**: Bowel movement every 2–3 days, brown and formed. Takes MOM as needed.
- **Genitourinary/Reproductive**: On Lasix; no problems

with urination; voids about 8 times/day. Not sexually active since wife died.

- **Musculoskeletal**: Weakness and occasional cramping in legs.
- **Neurological**: No sensory changes. States that he is very lonely since wife's death.
- **Lymphatic**: No allergies or recent infections.

Psychosocial Profile

Because physical problems are frequently assumed to have a physical origin, nurses may underestimate the relationship of everyday life to health. Taking a psychosocial profile can yield valuable clues about a person's nutritional status. Helping the person change unhealthy lifestyle behaviors may also be the most viable avenue of intervention (Table 6–6).

Table 6–6 Psychosocial Profile

CATEGORY/QUESTIONS TO ASK	RATIONALE/SIGNIFICANCE
Health Practices and Beliefs/Self-Care Activities	
Who shops and prepares meals in your family?	Dependent people may not eat properly if caregivers are lax or uninformed about good nutrition.
Are you able to plan and cook meals yourself, or do you depend on others to do this?	Diminished mental capacity or physical limitations from aging or debilitation may impair ability to buy, prepare, or eat food.
When was your last dental exam?	Good dentition is required for proper mastication and digestion of food.
Do you go for routine physical exams?	Identifies teaching needs.
Typical Day	
How do you usually spend your days? Do you go to restaurants frequently, and if so, where do you go and what types of foods do you eat? How much time do you spend shopping, preparing, and eating food?	Shows importance of food and good nutrition in person's life, what types of food person normally eats, and how often and where he or she eats out.
Nutritional Patterns	
What is your typical daily diet? How much water do you drink daily?	Can immediately point to malnutrition and/or poor hydration.
Do you actively try to maintain good nutrition and healthy weight? How?	Indicates conscious modifications of diet, although not necessarily correct information or awareness of health risks.
Have your eating habits and appetite changed recently?	Appetite changes can accompany depression, medication therapy, and some physical illnesses.
Activity and Exercise Patterns	
What is your usual activity and exercise level?	Validates that the person has a normal, active lifestyle.
Do you feel that you have adequate energy? What activities do you not pursue because of lack of energy?	Some changes may be a normal part of aging. Loss of energy or inability to pursue simple functional activities can accompany iron and protein/calorie deficiencies.
Sleep/Rest Patterns	
How many hours of sleep do you get a night? Do you wake up during the night? Are you taking more naps than usual? Do you feel rested? Do you use sleep aids? If so, what kinds?	Hunger or mild dehydration can interrupt sleep. Lack of energy or excessive sleep can be caused by iron or protein/calorie deficiency.

Table 6–6 Psychosocial Profile

CATEGORY/QUESTIONS TO ASK	RATIONALE/SIGNIFICANCE
Personal Habits	
Do you smoke?	Smoking interferes with absorption of vitamin C.
Do you drink alcohol? If so, how much/day? Do you drink coffee, tea, or soft drinks every day? If so, how much?	Alcohol and soft drinks are non-nutritive food sources. Excessive amounts impede adequate nutrition. Caffeine is mildly addictive. Withdrawal can cause nervousness and irritability. Excessive intake can contribute to calcium deficiency.
Do you use OTC drugs?	Some OTC drugs impair nutrient absorption and metabolism. Artificial sweeteners help avert obesity but have potential cancer risks
Do you use illegal drugs?	Purchase of food may be sacrificed to support an addictive drug habit.
Occupational Health Patterns	
What do you do for a living?	Exposure to chemical substances (e.g., lead) can interfere with absorption/ metabolism of nutrients.
How does your job affect daily meal routines?	Rotating or night shifts can interfere with meal routines and planning. People may substitute fast or convenience foods for more appropriate food sources.
Socioeconomic Status	
Is your income adequate to meet your food needs?	Good-quality food and food variety are expensive. Poverty and homelessness put people at serious risk for malnutrition. A significant number of the poor and homeless are women, children, and adolescents. Alcoholics and the chronically mentally ill are another large component of the homeless population. (See *USDA Nutrition-Assistance Programs.)*
Environmental Health Patterns	
Where do you buy your food? How do you store it? How do you prepare it?	Contamination and spoilage may be a concern. Poor hygiene and inadequate cooking increase risk of foodborne pathogens.
Roles and Relationships	
Do you have regular social interaction? Do you usually eat with other people or alone?	Eating and preparing food have a strong basis in culture and serve important social functions. Changes in this structure (for example, the death of a spouse) can affect nutrition.
Cultural Influences	
Do you have any cultural influences that may affect your dietary practices? If so, what are they?	Different cultures have different dietary preferences that can affect overall nutrition.
Religious/Spiritual Influences	
Do you have any religious influences that may affect your dietary practices? If so, what are they?	Some religions restrict certain foods, which can affect overall nutrition.
Stress and Coping	
Are your social relationships satisfying or stressful? How much stress do you have in your life? How do you cope with it?	Food can become a substitute for satisfying relationships. Emotional or psychological stress can weaken the immune system. Loss of appetite can occur with stress.

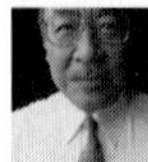

Case Study Findings

Mr. Thomas' psychosocial profile includes:

- Finds it hard to cook for one person; wife used to prepare meals.
- Says that his dentures are a little loose since he lost weight.
- Visits doctor every 6 months for BP check.
- Typical day: Awakens at 7 AM, has breakfast, walks to corner for newspaper, takes midmorning nap, usually skips lunch, watches TV, has dinner around 5 PM., watches TV after dinner, usually falls asleep while watching TV, goes to bed after the 10 PM news.
- Has three 8-oz glasses of water a day, not trying to lose weight. Eats out about once a week, likes fried foods. Not much appetite since wife died. Usually eats alone.
- Daily walk to corner for paper, no other scheduled exercise.
- Sleeps 7–8 hours a night. Awakens at least once to go to bathroom. Takes two 20 to 30–minute naps during day.
- Never smoked or used drugs. Occasional alcoholic drink about 2 times a month.
- Retired postal worker on fixed income with government pension; able to meet financial needs.
- Most close friends have passed away.
- No cultural or religious influence on dietary habits.
- Says life is "pretty routine without much stress."
- Daughter is main source of support; lives 1 hour away, visits once a week, takes him shopping.

Focused Nutritional History

If the situation or time prohibits a detailed nutritional history, focus on the person's weight, symptoms of malnutrition, and identification of nutritional risk factors. The person's response will help you appropriately focus your assessment. Key questions include the following:

- Have you lost or gained weight unintentionally in the past 6 months?
- What is the most you have ever weighed?
- How much did you weigh 6 months ago, and how much do you weigh now?
- What do you normally eat every day? Has your diet changed significantly? If so, how?
- Do you have any stomach or bowel symptoms (e.g., nausea, vomiting, diarrhea, or anorexia) that have lasted more than 2 weeks?
- Has anything happened in your life that has affected your ability to obtain or prepare food? If so, what?

Comprehensive Nutritional History

If the person has one or more known nutritional risks, perform a comprehensive nutritional history. Although nutritional patterns are learned early in life and are hard to break, weight and nutrition are major health issues in Western cultures. Information on dieting, exercise, and nutrition pervades the news media, along with the message that people should take responsibility for making healthy changes. Consequently, many people worry that they will be scolded for poor nutritional practices, so they withhold or embellish information. So remember to convey an attitude of acceptance and caring, and never be authoritarian or paternalistic.

Two dietary analysis techniques are discussed below—24-hour recall and food intake records. You can use either technique as part of your comprehensive history.

24-Hour Recall

Ask the person to write down what he or she ate and drank during the previous 24 hours. Then use the Food Guide Pyramid to sort and categorize the foods and determine the general quality of his or her diet. People often have trouble accurately recalling what they ate, so prompt them by saying, "Start with the first thing you had when you got out of bed." Also ask them to record between-meal drinks and snacks, desserts, bedtime snacks, condiments (e.g., mayonnaise, butter, sugar, or cream), and food preparation items (e.g., cooking oil or lard). Water is critical to nutritional metabolic processes, so ask them to record water intake, too. Last, be sure to have them record the amount of each food or liquid they consumed, and translate these into standard servings according to the Food Pyramid. A person's typical serving may actually equal several servings.

The 24-hour recall is a valuable screening and assessment tool only if it represents the person's typical daily intake. If a person is ill or has a change in routine, his or her intake will vary from normal. So be sure to ask if what he or she recorded represents a typical day. If he or she says no, ask him or her to substitute foods typically eaten.

Use the Food Pyramid to categorize 24-hour-recall data. Then tabulate food items alongside each corresponding Pyramid group, and document them in the person's health record.

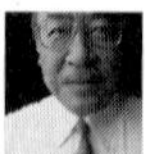

Case Study Findings

Mr. Thomas' 24-hour recall includes:

- Breakfast: 8 ounces black coffee, 8 ounces water, bowl of Cheerios with whole milk
- No lunch
- Afternoon snack: 4 pretzels

- Dinner: Frozen prepared dinner of Salisbury steak, potatoes, and corn, piece of apple pie, 8 ounces water, 8 ounces black coffee.

Food Intake Records

Food intake records are typically done on people who are debilitated, have severe burns, or are on chemotherapy. A Food Intake Record is a quantitative listing of all food and fluid consumed within a designated time frame—usually 3 to 5 days. Because food intake patterns often change on weekends and holidays, records kept during outpatient or home-care situations should reflect one atypical day for a 3-day period and one weekend for a 5-day period. Again, be sure to clarify serving sizes.

To analyze the data, reduce the recorded food items into their constituent nutrients, using USDA food composition tables. To get a daily average intake for each nutrient, add up the total nutrients and divide by the number of days the record was kept. Evaluate the averages against the RDA. Two-thirds of the RDA is considered adequate for the general healthy population. However, acceptable levels may vary in disease, risk, or deficiency situations and will be reflected in therapeutic treatment decisions.

A less specific but more practical approach involves analyzing the client's Food Intake Record using food labels on packages. USDA food composition tables for foods that do not have package labels can be found at *http://www.rahul.net/cgi-bin/fatfree/usda/usda.cgi*. Once you have determined the total number of calories consumed, calculate the total grams of carbohydrate, protein, and fat and the percentage of caloric intake contributed by each of these. Protein should comprise 10 percent of the diet; fat, 20 to 30 percent, and carbohydrates, the remaining calories.

Case Study Evaluation

Before you conduct an objective health assessment on Mr. Thomas, review his health history information from the comprehensive nutritional assessment.

CRITICAL THINKING ACTIVITY #3

What information from the health history indicates that Mr. Thomas is at risk for or has a nutritional deficiency?

Physical Assessment

Now proceed to the objective part of the assessment. Findings from the health history will determine the depth and scope of your physical examination. As you perform the examination, be alert to findings in various body systems that might signal malnutrition. Remember, determination of malnutrition cannot be made on physical findings alone. Many diseases and disorders mimic nutritional deficiencies. Always corroborate your physical findings with the health history and the results of laboratory assessments. The assessment includes performing a head-to-toe scan and taking various anthropometric measurements.

Approach

You will mainly use the techniques of inspection and palpation. Examining the skin and mucous membranes is crucial, but additional data are derived from assessment of other body systems.

Optimal nutrition cannot occur without adequate hydration. Therefore evaluate the person's hydration status simultaneously. Red flags include reports of minimal fluid intake, excessive thirst or excessive fluid intake, increased urination, diarrhea, or diuretic use. Very young infants, very frail older adults, and chronically ill and debilitated people are less tolerant of fluid loss and are at particular risk for dehydration from vomiting and/or diarrhea.

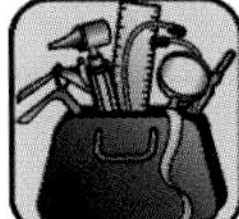

Toolbox

The tools for a comprehensive nutritional assessment include a weight scale, flexible measuring tape, calipers, and stethoscope. You should also have access to growth charts, weight and height tables, anthropometric tables, and laboratory values. To help the person accurately estimate quantities of food, have a variety of containers on hand.

Performing a Head-to-Toe Physical Assessment

Look for changes in every system that might signal a nutritional problem. Table 6–7 summarizes physical examination findings that are commonly associated with nutritional deficiencies and excesses.

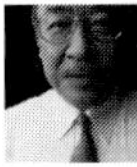

Case Study Findings

Mr. Thomas' physical assessment findings include:

- **General Health Survey:** AAO × 3; cooperative, neatly dressed 76-year-old black male who appears stated age. Affect sad, poor eye contact, responds appropriately.
- **Vital Signs:** BP 130/70; pulse 100 and regular; respirations 20; temperature 97.5°F; height 5'11"; weight 175; 10-lb weight loss since last visit 6 months ago.
- **Integumentary:** Skin dry and flaky, hair evenly distributed, no alopecia.

Table 6–7 Performing a Head-to-Toe Physical Assessment

SYSTEM/NORMAL VARIATIONS	ABNORMAL FINDINGS/RATIONALE
General Health Survey	
No unexplained weight changes	Weight changes within a short period of time usually reflect fluid loss or gain (1 mL = 1 g).
Vital signs within normal limits for person's age	Elevated BP may reflect fluid overload, high sodium intake, and obesity. Low BP may reflect dehydration.
INSPECT/PALPATE	
Integumentary/*Skin*	
Skin intact, warm, and dry	*Scaling:* Low or high vitamin A, zinc, essential fatty acids.
Texture smooth, no lesions	*Transparent, cellophane appearance:* Protein deficit.
Color consistent with ethnicity	*Cracking (flaky paint, cracked-pavement appearance):* Protein deficit. *Follicular hyperkeratosis:* Vitamins A, C deficits. *Petechiae (especially perifollicular):* Vitamin C deficit. *Purpura:* Vitamins C, K deficits. *Pigmentation/desquamation of sun-exposed areas:* Niacin deficit. *Edema:* Protein and thiamine deficits. *Skin lesions, ulcers, wounds that do not heal:* Protein, vitamin C, zinc deficits. *Yellow pigmentation (except sclerae):* Excess carotene (benign). *Poor skin turgor:*Dehydration.
Integumentary/*Hair*	
Even hair distribution; no alopecia	*Transverse pigmentation of hair shaft:* Protein deficit. *Hair easy to pluck, breaks easily:* Protein deficit. *Sparse hair distribution:* Protein, biotin, zinc deficits, excess vitamin A. *Corkscrew hairs, unemerged hair coils:* Vitamin C deficit.
Integumentary/*Nails*	
Nails smooth and pink	*Transverse ridges in nails:* Protein deficit. *Concave "spoon" nails:* Iron deficit.
Head, Eyes, Ears, Nose, Throat (HEENT)/*Eyes*	
Eyes clear and bright, vision intact	*Papilledema:* Vitamin A excess. *Night blindness:* Vitamin A deficit. *Sunken eyeballs, dark circles, decreased tears:* Dehydration. *Sunken fontanels:* Dehydration.
HEENT/*Nose*	
Sense of smell intact	Anosmia can affect taste.
HEENT/*Mouth*	
Oral mucosa pink, moist, and intact without lesions. Tonsils pink; gums pink and intact with no bleeding.	*Angular stomatitis:* Riboflavin, niacin, pyridoxine deficits. *Cheilosis (dry, cracked, ulcerated lips):* Riboflavin, niacin, pyridoxine deficits. *Atrophic lingual papillae (coated tongue):* Riboflavin, niacin, folic acid, vitamin B_{12}, protein, iron deficits. *Glossitis (raw, red tongue):* Riboflavin, niacin, pyridoxine, folic acid, vitamin B_{12} deficits.
Taste sensation intact	*Hypogeusia (blunting of sense of taste):* Zinc deficit.
Swallow and gag reflex intact Full mobility of tongue	Absent swallow and gag reflexes may make eating difficult. Impaired tongue mobility may cause dysphagia.
HEENT/*Nose*	
Sense of smell intact.	*Hyposmia (defect in sense of smell):* Zinc deficit.
Nasal mucosa pink, moist, and intact without lesions.	*Swollen, retracted, bleeding gums (if teeth present):* Vitamin C deficit.

Table 6–7 Performing a Head-to-Toe Physical Assessment

SYSTEM/NORMAL VARIATIONS	ABNORMAL FINDINGS/RATIONALE
	Dry mucous membranes: Dehydration. *Parotid gland enlargement:* Protein deficit (consider bulimia).
Respiratory Lungs clear, respirations within normal limits	*Increased respiratory rate:* Iron-deficiency anemia.
Cardiovascular Regular heart rate/rhythm. PMI 1 cm at apex. No extra sounds.	*Heart failure, S_3:* Thiamin, phosphorus, iron deficits. *Sudden heart failure, death:* Vitamin C deficit. *Tachycardia and systolic murmur:* Iron-deficiency anemia.
Gastrointestinal Abdomen soft, nontender, no organomegaly	*Hepatomegaly, ascites:* Protein deficits, vitamin A excess. *Hyperactive bowel sounds:* May indicate hyperperistalsis associated with an absorption problem.
Musculoskeletal No deformities, tenderness, or swelling	*Beading of ribs, epiphyseal swelling, bowlegs:* Vitamin D deficit. *Tenderness, superperiosteal bleeding:* Vitamin C deficit.
Neurological No headache AAO × 3 DTR + 2/4 Senses intact	*Headache:* Vitamin A excess. *Drowsiness, lethargy, vomiting:* Vitamin A, D excess. *Dementia:* Niacin, vitamin B_{12} deficit. *Confusion, irritability:* Dehydration. *Disorientation:* Thiamin (Korsakoff's psychosis) deficit. *Ophthalmoplegia:* Thiamin, phosphorus deficit. *Peripheral neuropathy (weakness, paresthesia, ataxia, and decreased deep tendon reflexes, and diminished tactile, vibratory, and position sensation:* Niacin, pyridoxine, vitamin B_{12} deficits. *Tetany, increased deep tendon reflexes (DTRs):* Calcium, magnesium deficits.

- **HEENT:** Dry, pink mucous membranes, dentures poorly fitted.
- **Respiratory:** Breath sounds equal bilaterally, clear to auscultation but decreased at bases because of poor inspiratory effort.
- **Cardiovascular:** Normal heart rate and rhythm, $+S_4$, PMI 2 cm at apex.
- **Gastrointestinal:** Bowel sounds present, regular, slightly diminished; abdomen soft, nontender, with no masses or organomegaly.
- **Musculoskeletal:** +4 muscle strength on upper and lower extremities.
- **Neurological:** Cranial nerves intact; deep tendon reflexes +2, senses intact.

Anthropometry

Anthropometry literally means "human measurement." It includes measuring overall body mass (particularly growth, fat reserves, and somatic protein stores) and evaluation of related laboratory values. Growth charts that plot height, weight, and head growth are used for children up to age 18. By adulthood, growth has stabilized and ratio measurements of body mass are used. The following sections describe common anthropometric techniques for assessing nutrition in children and adults.

Growth Charts

Children

Growth charts for height, weight, and head circumference (Appendix B) are excellent indicators of nutrition in children because they allow you to visualize the child's growth progress. Two sets of charts are commonly used: one for birth to 36 months includes head circumference) and one for age 2 to 18 (does not include head circumference because cerebral growth is complete by age 2). New charts have also been developed to track the unique growth patterns of premature infants.

Until age 2, take growth measurements with the child nude or wearing only a diaper and lying supine.

For children age 2 to 18, take a standing height without shoes, with the client dressed in usual examination clothing. Record measurements on the corresponding axes of the chart at the point that intersects with the child's current age. To visualize a growth pattern, take serial measurements. The important factor is the relative consistency of the child's growth within the norms of the curve.

As long as a child receives adequate nutrition, his or her growth largely reflects genetic heritage. If a child shows a consistent decline into a lower percentile or falls below the fifth percentile, suspect undernutrition. Suspect overnutrition in children who begin to deviate into higher percentiles or who fall above the 95th percentile. Growth chart abnormalities can also signify problems of a non-nutritional nature, such as endocrine disorders. If your history does not support a nutritionally related growth problem, a medical referral is warranted.

Adults

By age 18, growth is largely complete and weight-for-height tables replace growth charts. The Metropolitan Life Insurance Company's height and weight tables, revised in 1983 (Appendix B), are the standard, although they do not reflect ideal weights. Instead, they represent the weights of people with the most longevity in each height category and recommend weight ranges based on height and skeletal frame size. Figures 6–2 and 6–3 illustrate height and weight measurement.

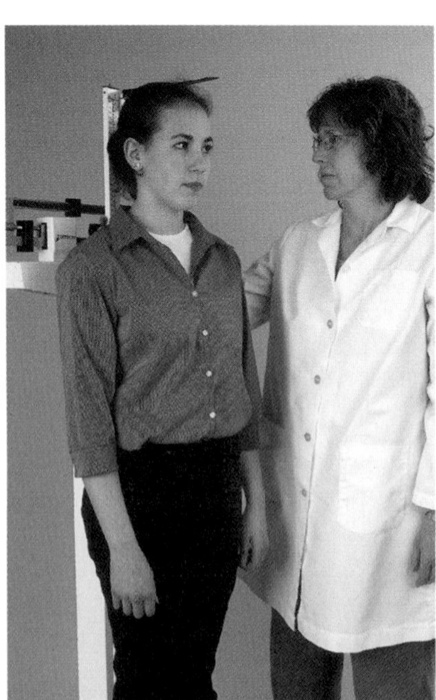

FIGURE 6–2. Measuring height.

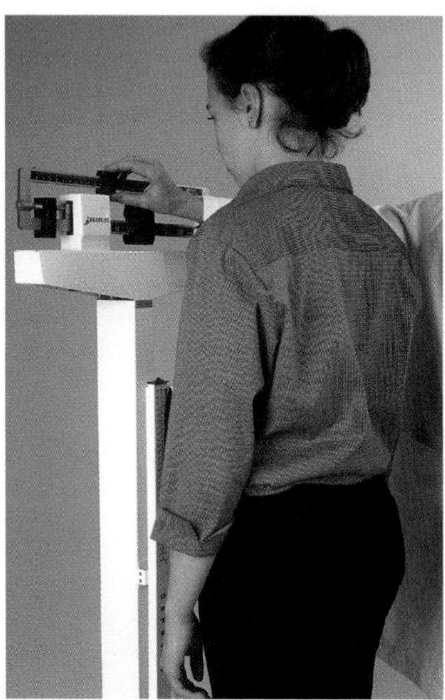

FIGURE 6–3. Measuring weight.

HELPFUL HINT

To estimate frame size, have the person wrap the thumb and middle finger of one hand around his or her opposite wrist. If the fingers overlap by 1 cm or more, he or she has a small frame; if the fingertips meet, a medium frame; and if the fingertips do not meet by 1 cm or more, a large frame.

Body Mass Index

Body mass index (BMI) is an accurate indicator of fat in adults. The most commonly used BMI is Quetelet's Index, which is obtained by dividing weight in kilograms by height in meters squared. BMIs between 20 and 25 kg/m^2 are associated with the least mortality; BMIs under 16 kg/m^2 are associated with eating disorders. The relatively larger proportion of muscle in athletes and body builders and the greater blood and tissue volume in pregnant and lactating women make BMI measurements inappropriate for these groups. It is also not recommend for growing children or frail and sedentary older adults. You can determine BMI by consulting the table in Box 6–2.

Arm Measurements

Triceps Skin Fatfold

Triceps skin fatfold (TSF) estimates body fat using a double fold of skin and subcutaneous adipose tissue from the client's dominant arm. With the client's arm at his or her side and elbow flexed at 90 degrees, measure and

Box 6–2 Body Mass Index

BMI	19	20	21	22	23	24	25	26	27	28	29	30	31	32	33	34	35
Height								*Weight in pounds*									
4'10" (58")	91	96	100	105	110	115	119	124	129	134	138	143	148	153	158	162	167
4'11" (59")	94	99	104	109	114	119	124	128	133	138	143	148	153	158	163	168	173
5' (60")	97	102	107	112	118	123	128	133	138	143	148	153	158	163	168	174	179
5'1" (61")	100	106	111	116	122	127	132	137	143	148	153	158	164	169	174	180	185
5'2" (62")	104	109	115	120	126	131	136	142	147	153	158	164	169	175	180	186	191
5'3" (63")	107	113	118	124	130	135	141	146	152	158	163	169	175	180	186	191	197
5'4" (64")	110	116	122	128	134	140	145	151	157	163	169	174	180	186	192	197	204
5'5" (65")	114	120	126	132	138	144	150	156	162	168	174	180	186	192	198	204	210
5'6" (66")	118	124	130	136	142	148	155	161	167	173	179	186	192	198	204	210	216
5'7" (67")	121	127	134	140	146	153	159	166	172	178	185	191	198	204	211	217	223
5'8" (68")	125	131	138	144	151	158	164	171	177	184	190	197	203	210	216	223	230
5'9" (69")	128	135	142	149	155	162	169	176	182	189	196	203	209	216	223	230	236
5'10" (70")	132	139	146	153	160	167	174	181	188	195	202	209	216	222	229	236	243
5'11" (71")	136	143	150	157	165	172	179	186	193	200	208	215	222	229	236	243	250
6' (72")	140	147	154	162	169	177	184	191	199	206	213	221	228	235	242	250	258
6'1" (73")	144	151	159	166	174	182	189	197	204	212	219	227	235	242	250	257	265
6'2" (74")	148	155	163	171	179	186	194	202	210	218	225	233	241	249	256	264	272
6'3" (75")	152	160	168	176	184	192	200	208	216	224	232	240	248	256	264	272	279

The National Institutes of Health (NIH) interpret BMI values for adults with one fixed number, regardless of age or sex, using the following guidelines: Underweight: <18.5 Overweight: 25.0–29.9 Obese: 30.0 or more

Source: Evidence Report of Clinical Guidelines on the Identification, Evaluation, and Treatment of Overweight and Obesity in Adults, 1998. NIH/National Heart, Lung, and Blood Institute (NHLBI). Centers for Disease Control and Prevention, United States Department of Health and Human Services.

mark the midpoint overlying the triceps muscle between the elbow and shoulder. Tell the client to relax the arm. Then use your thumb and index finger to compress a symmetrical fold of skin and adipose tissue 1/2 inch above the marked site. Use calipers to measure in the middle of the skin fold at the marked site, about 1/2 inch below your fingers. Release the calipers, and wait 4 seconds before reading the measurement. To ensure reliability, take two to three additional measurements at least 15 seconds apart. They should not vary by more than 1 mm.

Compare fatfold measurements with equivalent age and gender-specific percentiles (Appendix B). Values below the 10th percentile or above the 90th percentile indicate diminished or extensive fat reserves, respectively. Figure 6–4 illustrates triceps skin fatfold measurement.

Midarm Circumference

Mid-arm circumference (MAC) provides a crude estimate of muscle mass and is most useful when combined with TSF. Measure the circumference of the client's dominant arm at the same site where you obtained the TSF. Wrap the measuring tape firmly around the client's arm without compressing the skin. Take two or three more measurements to ensure reliability. They should not vary by more than 1 mm. Compare midarm measurements with equivalent age and gender-specific percentiles (Appendix B). Figure 6–5 illustrates midarm circumference measurement.

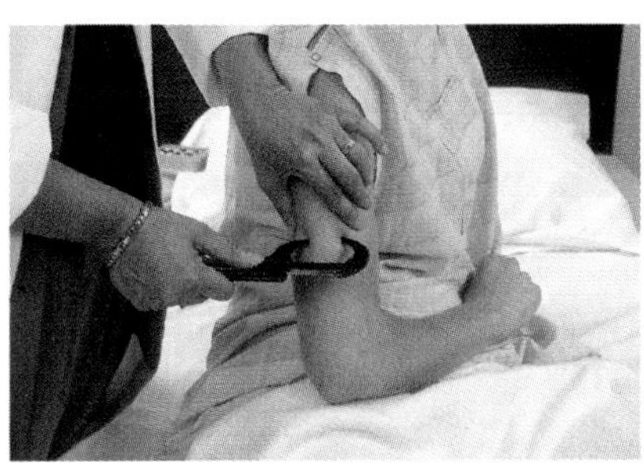

FIGURE 6–4. Measuring triceps skin fatfold.

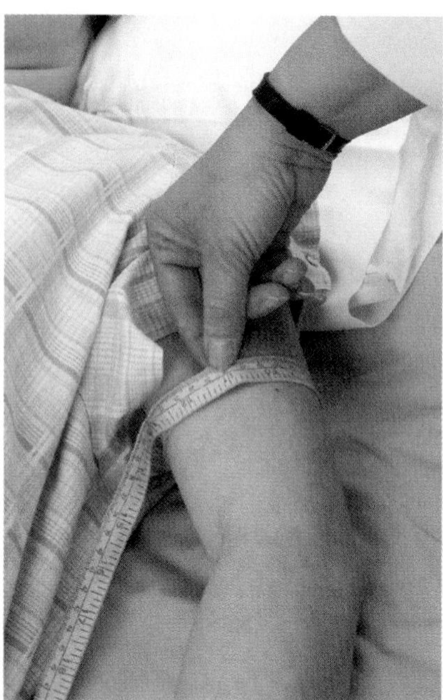

FIGURE 6–5. Measuring midarm circumference.

Midarm Muscle Circumference

Midarm muscle circumference (MAMC) is mathematically derived using TSF and MAC values. As an indirect measurement of muscle mass, it provides an index of protein stores. To calculate MAMC, multiply the TSF (in centimeters) by 3.143 and subtract the result from the MAC. Because MAMC estimates skeletal muscle reserves, it should generally fall within 90 percent of standard. Values falling between 60 and 90 percent suggest moderate protein deficiency and those less than 60 percent indicate severe malnutrition. Compare midarm muscle circumference measurements with equivalent age- and gender-specific percentiles (Appendix B).

Waist-to-Hip Ratio

The **waist-to-hip ratio** (WHR) estimates obesity by evaluating the amount of abdominal fat. People with a greater proportion of upper body fat are at greater risk for hypertension, diabetes, elevated triglycerides, and other atherosclerotic risk factors. WHR is calculated simply by dividing the waist circumference by the hip circumference. A WHR of 1.0 or greater in men and 0.8 or greater in women indicates upper body obesity.

Case Study Analysis and Plan

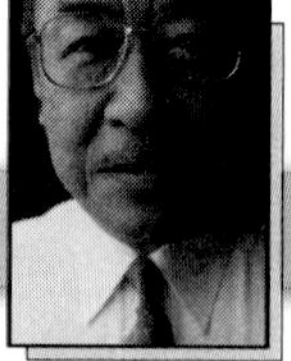

Now that you have completed your comprehensive nutritional assessment of Mr. Thomas, list key history and physical examination findings that will help you formulate your nursing diagnoses.

Nursing Diagnoses

Consider all of the data you have collected during your assessment of Mr. Thomas, and then use this information to develop a list of nursing diagnoses. Some possible ones are listed below. Cluster the supporting data.

1. Nutrition: imbalanced, less than body requirements, related to inadequate iron intake
2. Fluid Volume, deficient, related to medications and poor intake
3. Knowledge, deficient, related to nutrition

Identify any additional nursing diagnoses and any collaborative nursing diagnoses.

CRITICAL THINKING ACTIVITY #4

Now that you have identified some nursing diagnoses for Mr. Thomas, select one from above and develop a brief teaching plan for him. Include learning outcomes and teaching strategies.

Research Tells Us

Iron deficiency is the most common nutritional deficiency in children and adults. Blood loss and chronic disease states are the most common causes of iron deficiency anemia among adults. However, among infants, young children, adolescent girls, and women of childbearing age, iron-deficiency anemia is predominantly the result of nutritional deficiency and is most prevalent among minority and low-income groups. (Looker, Dallman, Carroll, Gunter, & Johnson, 1997). Iron deficiency without anemia can cause developmental and behavioral deviations; with anemia, it can result in irreversible effects on brain function (Ritchey, 1987).

For unknown reasons, pica (the persistent eating of non-nutritive substances) is associated with iron-deficiency anemia and occurs most commonly in pregnant women and children in lower socioeconomic groups (Rose, Porcerelli, & Neale, 2000). In homes with lead paint where hygiene is lacking, pica can contribute to lead poisoning and helminthic infestations. In addition to serious neurological damage, severe or long-term lead poisoning also inhibits heme production, which further compounds the initial effects of iron deficiency. Helminthic infections can result in subtle but significant blood loss that further contributes to anemia.

Health Concerns

Facts about obesity and disease

- Obesity affects roughly 35 percent of women and 31 percent of men in the United States. This is an increase of 1/3 over the past decade, and the rate continues to rise.
- Genetics account for only 33 percent of variations in body weight and have a greater overall influence on fat distribution than on total body fat.
- Moderate obesity, particularly abdominal obesity, can increase the risk of non–insulin-dependent diabetes mellitus (adult onset) by tenfold.
- The risk of cardiovascular disease increases with increasing levels of obesity, independent of other risk factors.
- Overweight men have a significantly higher mortality rate for colorectal and prostate cancer.
- Overweight women are three times as likely to have breast, uterine, cervical, and ovarian cancer, and are seven times more likely to have endometrial cancer.
- Obese girls begin to menstruate at a younger age than normal-weight girls.
- Obese women have more irregular menstrual cycles and a greater frequency of other menstrual abnormalities than normal-weight women.
- Overweight women have more problems during pregnancy, including toxemia and hypertension.
- Overweight people have an increased risk of developing gallbladder disease.
- Increased weight causes more wear and tear on the joints, leading to osteoarthritis.
- As weight increases, breathing at night becomes progressively more difficult, leading to sleep apnea or Pickwickian syndrome (obesity hypoventilation syndrome).
- In the United States, obesity-related illness is second only to smoking-related illness as a leading cause of death.

Common Abnormalities

ABNORMALITY	AREA	ASSESSMENT FINDINGS
Anorexia Nervosa A preoccupation with being thin and dieting, leading to excessive weight loss.	General Health Survey Behavioral	• Continued dieting despite weight loss • Feeling fat despite weight loss • Intense fear of weight gain • Preoccupation with food, especially calories and fat content • Eating in isolation, lying about food • Exercising compulsively
	Integumentary	• Cold intolerance, cold hands and feet • Weakness and exhaustion • Dry, brittle skin and hair; hair loss • Growth of fine body hair on extremities • Blotchy or yellow skin
	Respiratory	• Shortness of breath

(Continued)

Common Abnormalities *(Continued)*

ABNORMALITY	AREA	ASSESSMENT FINDINGS
	Cardiovascular	• Low blood pressure • Dysrhythmias
	Gastrointestinal	• Constipation
	Musculoskeletal	• Skeletal muscle atrophy • Loss of fatty tissue
	Neurological	• Depression, anxiety
	Genitourinary	• Amenorrhea
Bulimia Nervosa Uncontrolled binge eating (excessive quantities of food consumed in one sitting) alternated with purging (ridding the body of food) in an attempt to lose weight. It is characterized by intense feelings of guilt and shame.	Behavioral	• Preoccupation with body weight • Uncontrolled eating alternating with periods of strict dieting and exercise • Inducing vomiting or taking laxatives to lose weight • Frequent use of bathroom after a meal
	HEENT	• Swollen glands in neck and face • Deterioration of dental enamel from related to gastric acidity of vomitus • Sore throat
	Integumentary	• Poor skin turgor; dehydration
	Cardiovascular	• Arrythmias related to electrolyte imbalances; cardiac arrest possible
	Gastrointestinal	• Hemoptysis from damage to throat when inducing vomiting • Heartburn, bloating, indigestion
	Neurological	• Depression, mood swings, feeling out of control
	Genitourinary	• Amenorrhea or irregular menses
Diabetes Mellitus A disorder in the metabolism of carbohydrates caused by decreased production of insulin or decreased ability to use insulin.	General Health Survey	• Increased thirst
	Integumentary	• Fatigue • Poor skin turgor • Frequent skin infections
	HEENT	• Blurred vision
	Respiratory	• Acetone breath odor
	Gastrointestinal	• Weight loss in spite of increased appetite • Nausea, vomiting
	Genitourinary	• Impotence in men • Amenorrhea • Frequent bladder and vaginal infections
	Neurological	• Depression • Confusion
Iron-Deficiency Anemia A decrease in the number of red cells caused by too little iron.	Integumentary	• Pale skin color (pallor) • Sore tongue • Brittle nails
	HEENT	• Frontal headache
	Respiratory	• Shortness of breath
	Cardiovascular	• Orthostatic hypotension
	Gastrointestinal	• Unusual food cravings (pica) • Decreased appetite (especially children)
	Neurological	• Fatigue

Common Abnormalities

ABNORMALITY	AREA	ASSESSMENT FINDINGS
Kwashiorkor A protein deficiency caused by inadequate dietary protein, malabsorption, cancer, or AIDS.	Integumentary	• Darkened, scaly skin • Hair depigmentation • Pitting edema
	Gastrointestinal	• Extreme abdominal swelling/bloating • Hepatomegaly
	Musculoskeletal	• Muscle atrophy
	Neurological	• Mental apathy • Developmental delays, retardation
Marasmus A severe protein and calorie deficiency that causes tissue to be sacrificed to meet energy needs. It is also called protein-calorie malnutrition. Other causes include severe infections, burns, eating disorders, chronic liver disease, cancer, and AIDS.	HEENT	• Facial appearance of an aged person
	Integumentary	• Wasting of subcutaneous fat and muscle
	Gastrointestinal	• Severe weight loss and emaciation • Potbellied appearance caused by swollen abdomen
	Musculoskeletal	• Growth retardation
	Neurological	• Mental apathy • Developmental delays, retardation

Summary

- Throughout the health assessment process, the nurse should be attuned to data related to nutrition.
- Nutrition is influenced by a myriad of factors. Basic information in the health history can identify the need to more thoroughly investigate nutritional status.
- Assessment of nutritional status involves eliciting data that is both directly and indirectly related to nutrition.
- Comprehensive nutritional assessment will provide specific data to enable the nurse to determine potential or actual nutritional health problems, to devise an appropriate plan of intervention, and to determine criteria for evaluation.

7

Spiritual Assessment

Before You Begin

INTRODUCTION TO SPIRITUAL ASSESSMENT

Historically, the practice of nursing has been based on holistic care of the client. This **holism** respects the interrelated nature of body, mind, and spirit. The body has been represented well by research and innovations in the care of physiological processes. Psychology and sociology have contributed to the understanding of the emotional processes.

More recently, an increased emphasis on holism is reflected in the increased importance given to the spiritual dimension. What is the spiritual dimension? **Spirituality** may be defined as the inherent quality of humans to believe in something greater than the self and in a faith that affirms life. Spirituality also involves interconnectedness between the self, nature, and others. Spirituality is larger than religion, although religion is a forum for expressing our spiritual nature. For example, the spiritual dimension encompasses how we feel when we see a new baby or a beautiful sunset. In essence, spirituality is all behavior that gives meaning to life and gives us strength. As a component of health, spirituality is characterized by meaning, hope, purpose, love, trust, forgiveness, and creativity.

Are you equipped to assist the client and family with issues that relate to spirituality? As with any physical system, the goal of a spiritual assessment is to detect strengths, potential problems,or dysfunction. You need adequate information in order to plan appropriate interventions. Assessing your client's spirituality is unique because the only "tools" needed are you and time. Your ability to listen actively is essential in obtaining a spiritual assessment.

Even so, your assessment will still follow a systematic approach. Although physical examination is not actually a part of the assessment, people often have physical symptoms that are related to underlying spiritual concerns. So spiritual assessment is a part of a holistic assessment, conducted along with the assessment of physiological and psychological systems.

Nursing is a humanistic science that focuses on caring for the whole person. Several authors have chosen to depict the nature of spirituality in different ways, but in each, the spiritual dimension is seen as all-encompassing or pervasive throughout a person's being. Nurses appreciate the interrelatedness and interconnectedness of all the dimensions of a person. As a result, we are especially suited to treat the client in a holistic manner. You may examine each system separately, but to achieve complete care, you must consider the client as a whole using the mind-body-spirit concept.

Brief Review of Spiritual Health

To adequately assess the spiritual dimension, you need to understand its general nature. Spiritual health and wellness reflect the spiritual nature of humans and are related to the client's overall health. Because humans are comprised of several aspects of interrelated function, you must assess and intervene in all these aspects to provide holistic and humanistic care. Many researchers believe that all human beings have three needs in common: the need for meaning and purpose, the need for love and belonging, and the need for forgiveness. When clients are having difficulty in these areas, the nurse is often the one who identifies the need for spiritual assistance.

When taking a client's history, your first questions about spirituality should focus on the basics. Ask the client the following questions:

- Do you identify with any organized religion? If so, what religion?
- If you do not identify with a particular religion, do you have a belief system that provides comfort and strength?
- Are you an **agnostic** or an **atheist**? If so, do you have any belief system that gives meaning to your life?

While asking these questions, keep in the back of your mind:

- What is the primary nature of the client's religion?
- Are people of this religion **monotheistic** (worshipping one God) or **pantheistic** (worshipping many gods)?

As you can see, not all these questions have easy answers. To best serve your client's spiritual needs, you must remain open and nonjudgmental when assessing him or her.

HELPFUL HINT

Recognizing your own spiritual beliefs and biases will help you be as open as possible when assessing your client's spirituality.

Developmental, Cultural, and Ethnic Variations

The development of the spiritual dimension is closely linked to intellectual, psychological, and sociological factors. In addition, you must also consider your client's age and culture. Intellectual factors often depend on physiologic factors such as brain development. Psychological and sociological factors are greatly influenced by family dynamics and environment.

Infants

Infants are dependent on their parents and other caregivers. They are capable of feeling trust or mistrust but are incapable of the abstract thought necessary for spiritual faith. So when assessing and caring for infants, you must consider the spiritual needs of the family and other caregivers and listen actively to their concerns.

When the client is an infant, ask the parents or caregivers the following questions:

- What concerns do you have about your child's illness?
- How can I help support your use of religious practices (e.g., by referral to the hospital chaplain or hospital meditation room)?

Ask yourself the following questions:

- Do parents ask why their child is ill?
- Do they see the infant's illness as a religious punishment?
- Are they practicing religious rituals?

Toddlers and Preschoolers

Toddlers learn values by mimicking others and by receiving positive or negative feedback in response to their behavior. Toddlers who participate in their family's celebrations of religious ceremonies or rites will begin to incorporate those aspects of spiritual development. They also learn values, including the importance of respect for life and others. These interactions set the stage for further spiritual development. Toddlers and preschoolers are just beginning to develop language and intellectual skills and an appreciation for cause and effect. A true understanding of the nature of spiritual or religious values is not possible at this level; however, the young child is aware of the interconnectedness of family.

When the client is a preschooler, ask the following questions:

- How do you feel about what is happening to you?
- Whom do you talk to when you are in trouble, sad, lonely, or scared?
- What makes you feel better when you are scared, sad, or lonely?

Ask yourself the following questions:

- Does the child express concerns or show anxiety about illness and dying?
- Does he or she speak of being punished by a deity for "being bad?"
- Is he or she practicing religious rituals, such as saying bedtime prayers?

School-Age Children

Once a child begins school, he or she is influenced by peers as well as family. Development of a spiritual awareness parallels cognitive and emotional development. The younger school-age child often believes in the magic value of religious ritual, whereas the older school-age child may begin to understand the abstractness of faith. To have faith in a power bigger than yourself requires abstract thought—which is usually not common in children before age 11 or 12.

Children begin to question spiritual issues as they explore their world. Although the loss of a loved one at this time is difficult for a child to grasp because he or she can see no benefit to the death, nurses who work with dying children often find that they are mature beyond their years regarding spiritual concerns. If the conditions are right, spiritual development and awareness can appear at almost any age. Therefore, do not dismiss the need for assessment of spiritual needs in children.

When the client is a school-age child, ask the same questions as were used with toddlers and preschoolers.

Adolescents

Adolescents are searching, trying to form a unique identity for themselves. Consequently, they begin examining their parents' beliefs in all aspects of life. In the area of spiritual development and awareness, they may review, critique, rebel, search for alternatives, and sometimes embrace their parents' values and beliefs as their own. This phase may continue into young adulthood. Do not assume that the adolescent is without spiritual concerns because of his or her behavior.

When the client is an adolescent, ask the following questions:

- How do you feel about what is happening to you?
- Whom do you usually go to for support?
- What gives your life meaning? Has this changed since you got sick?

Also ask yourself the following questions:

- Does the adolescent express concerns about dying or the seriousness of his or her illness?
- Does he or she practice any religious rituals?
- Does he or she verbalize his or her own beliefs and values?

Young Adults

Young adults are a diverse group, and so each person may be in a different stage of spiritual development. Some young adults may be very spiritual with a well-developed sense of religious commitment or a commitment to something more personal, such as music or the arts. Others appear to have no sense of spirituality and may live just for the moment, focusing on survival. Significant life events, such as the death of a friend, a close brush with death, or the beginning of a new relationship may be the nucleus for the start of a spiritual awakening.

The experience of pregnancy and birth may have profound effects on spiritual growth and development. Impending parenthood is often the impetus for a deepening of existing spirituality or an awakening of new feelings. The responsibility of parenting and the desire to transmit beliefs and values to a new generation often stimulates a search to clarify those beliefs and values and find answers to spiritual questions. As the family grows and matures, parents' lives usually revolve around their children. First, they strive to impart values to young children; then eventually they deal with adolescents beginning to question these values.

When the client is a young adult, ask the same questions as you would an adolescent (see previous section).

Older Adults

As people grow older, they may cling more tightly to their connection with spirituality. Older adults are confronted with resolving the developmental task of integrity vs. despair. Those who find a sense of meaning and purpose to their lives and enjoy the interconnectedness with others that may be found in a place of worship are successfully working through this stage of development.

When the client is an older adult, ask the same questions as you would an adolescent or a young adult. However, older clients often suffer many losses and therefore have fewer support systems, and so you may need to make referrals to community services.

People of Different Cultures or Ethnic Groups

Culture is a multidimensional factor in human development. It includes shared values, beliefs, and practices of a group that are transmitted from one generation to another. Culture often guides the way in which a group of people thinks and acts. Values, beliefs, and practices related to spiritual issues are also part of culture and are passed on to each generation. Just as it is important to be aware of physiologic variations when assessing a client, it is important to be aware of variations among people's spiritual and/or religious values, beliefs, and practices.

Spirituality develops from a person's worldview, which is often strongly influenced by cultural background. Before you can assess your client's spirituality, familiarize yourself with his or her cultural domain. This will help you choose the right questions to ask, depending on the client's age. The following are important areas to consider:

- Use of prayer: Learn about the use of prayer, meditation, and other activities or symbols that help people of this cultural or ethnic group reach fulfillment.
- Meaning of life and individual sources of strength: Know what gives meaning to life for the client's cultural group. Identify the client's individual sources of strength.
- Spiritual beliefs and healthcare practices: Become familiar with the way in which spiritual beliefs affect this cultural group's healthcare practices (Table 7–1).

Table 7–1 How Culture Affects Spirituality

CULTURE	DOMINANT RELIGIONS/ USE OF PRAYER	MEANING OF LIFE/ SOURCES OF STRENGTH	SPIRITUAL BELIEFS/ HEALTHCARE PRACTICES
African-Americans	Majority are Baptists and Methodists. Strong belief in prayer.	Sickness and pain are weaknesses coming from Satan, whereas God is a source of inner strength.	Sickness is a separation from God. God is the Supreme Healer.
Amish	No national church hierarchy; local leaders are chosen from community. Silent prayer before and after meals is important.	Share view of most Christians, but emphasis is on community, not individual.	May seek counsel from religious leaders on health issues, but final decision is made by immediate family.
Appalachians	Variety of religions, but most stress fundamentalism. Prayer is a primary source of strength.	Family and living right provide meaning.	Fatalistic view—illness is God's will.
Arab-Americans	Most are **Muslims**. Prayer 5 times a day is a duty.	Faith means submission to Allah and is a part of everyday life.	Religious practices are combined with medicine. Cleanliness essential before praying. Illness is seen as a punishment or a trial that is endured.
Chinese-Americans	Variety of religions, including Buddhism. Formal religious services are minimal. Pray alone rather than as a community. Prayer is a source of comfort.	Life viewed in terms of cycles and interrelationships. Life forces are a source of strength.	Cyclical explanation of life is connected to health.
Cuban-Americans	Most are Catholic, but practice is more personal than institutional.	Family is important source of strength.	Fatalistic, lack control, use of folk remedies.
Egyptian-Americans	**Islam** or Christian. Pray during illness.	Inner peace through practice of religious rituals.	When ill, you are at the mercy of God (Christian) or Allah (Islam).
Filipino-Americans	Most are Catholic. Prayer is important.	Strength comes from relationship with God.	Fatalistic—illness seen as God's will or induced by evil spirits.
French-Canadians	Mostly Catholic. Prayer is important.	Family is important source of strength, but divorce has affected this.	Little connection made between spirituality and health care. Spirituality still seen as religion.
Greek-Americans	Greek Orthodox faith and daily prayer very important.	Life has meaning through the different roles one performs.	Icons of family saint or Virgin Mary important when ill.

Table 7–1 How Culture Affects Spirituality

CULTURE	DOMINANT RELIGIONS/ USE OF PRAYER	MEANING OF LIFE/ SOURCES OF STRENGTH	SPIRITUAL BELIEFS/ HEALTHCARE PRACTICES
Iranian-Americans	Islam influence. Prayer is important.	Accepting Allah's will is source of strength, as are family and friends.	Fate and Allah's will explain illness.
Irish-Americans	Most are Catholic. Prayer is individual and private.	Church is a source of strength.	Somewhat fatalistic. Religion is important when ill. Sacraments and religious medals may provide solace.
Jewish-Americans	Monotheistic belief in God. Pray alone or in groups.	Preservation of life is most important; therefore, good health is very important.	Caring for the sick takes precedence over keeping Sabbath.
Mexican-Americans	Mostly Catholic. Prayer is important and individualized.	Family is most important.	When ill, important to talk about soul or spirit.
Navajo Indians (Native Americans)	Spirituality based on harmony with nature.	Strength comes from inner self and being in harmony with surroundings.	Illness results from not being in harmony. Healing ceremonies help restore mental, physical, and spiritual harmony.
Vietnamese-Americans	Most are Buddhists. Prayer and offerings may be made at altar in home or temple.	Family and religion are important.	Harmony and order influence perspective of illness that is characterized by self-control, acceptance of one's destiny, and fatalism.

Source: Data from Purnell and Paulanka, 1998.

CRITICAL THINKING ACTIVITY #1

Consider the different cultures described in Table 7–1. How might your client's culture influence your approach to planning his or her care?

CRITICAL THINKING ACTIVITY #2

What questions should you ask your client to help identify the impact of spirituality on his or her health care?

CRITICAL THINKING ACTIVITY #3

For each of the cultures described in Table 7–1, identify interventions that would incorporate the client's spiritual belief into his or her health care.

ALERT

Although many ethnic groups are linked with a particular spiritual viewpoint or religion, do not assume a client's spiritual perspective by his or her ethnic background alone. Assess each client as a unique being.

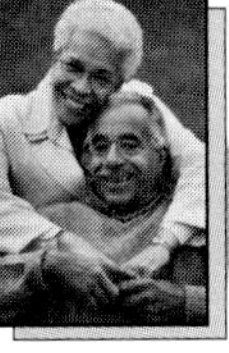

Introducing the Case Study

January Mays is a 68-year-old retired schoolteacher. She lives in a single, two-story home in a small town in Pennsylvania. Her husband died last year, and her only child, a daughter, lives in California with her husband and two sons. Her sister lives across the street. Mrs. Mays was admitted to the hospital after apparently suffering a "flare-up" of congestive heart failure. As you begin your interview, she states, "I don't know why people are making so much fuss."

Performing the Assessment

Data for a spiritual assessment are obtained during the health history. Before conducting the history, you can also make preliminary observations related to the client's behavior, relationships, and environment that may result in a more thorough spiritual assessment. You will also take a spiritual history that specifically relates to the client's spiritual needs and identifies potential or actual problems.

Health History

First, obtain the client's biographical data; then ask questions about his or her current health history, past health history, family history, and psychosocial profile.

Biographical Data

A review of the client's admission sheet may reveal basic religious information such as church or temple affiliation. Be sure to ask questions to clarify this information because religious affiliation may range from being in name only to being a very involved relationship.

ALERT

Be aware that the absence of religious identification does not mean that the client has no spiritual needs.

Other helpful information includes marital status and contact person. This provides clues about the state of connectedness of the client to others. A client who has not listed relatives may have spiritual needs that a client with a strong family network doesn't. Age is another indicator of spiritual needs. Older adults with an identified connection to organized religion may find that connection to be a source of comfort and support.

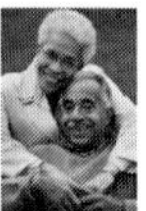

Case Study Findings

Reviewing Mrs. Mays' biographical data:

- 68-year-old African-American woman
- Husband died 1 year ago
- One grown daughter who lives in California with her husband and two sons, ages 4 and 6
- Lives in two-story home; sister lives across the street in her own home
- Born in Grady Falls, Pennsylvania
- Methodist Episcopal religion
- MS in education, retired from teaching elementary school
- Has Medicare with supplemental HMO from teacher's union
- Hospital admission for congestive heart failure
- Good historian; alert and seems reliable

Current Health Status

Your client's current physical health and spiritual health are intertwined. A sense of spirituality is influential during periods of physical and/or mental illness for the client or a significant other. For some, acceptance of losses is easier because life as a whole has been full of meaning; for others losses are seen as punishment for a life that could have been lived differently.

Although anyone may have spiritual needs, clients with chronic or terminal diseases are especially prone to spiritual distress. Exploring the connection between medical diagnosis and spiritual needs is an ongoing process, because as time passes, your client's experience and situation change.

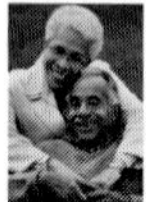

Case Study Findings

Mrs. Mays' current health status includes:

- Difficulty breathing at rest, lower extremity edema, change in sleep patterns, uses two pillows
- Currently hospitalized for exacerbation of congestive heart failure
- Also has hypertension
- Current medication lisinopril (Prinivil), 10 mg/day, for hypertension.

Past Health History

Health problems that occurred in your client's past can have long-lasting physical and spiritual effects. The past health history will give you clues about your client's overall health up to this point in his or her life. If he or she has been relatively healthy until now, an acute illness may precipitate spiritual distress. Or a series of past health problems may have tested and strengthened the client's spirituality. Whatever the case, you need to explore the connection between your client's health and spiritual needs.

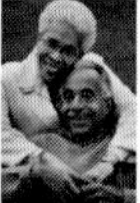

Case Study Findings

Mrs. Mays' past health history reveals:

- Congestive heart failure, treated for 3 to 5 years
- Hypertension, treated for 15 years

Family History

The family history is invaluable in identifying familial problems that pose a threat to your client's health. This in turn may affect his or her spiritual needs. The family history can also be helpful in identifying supports and relationships.

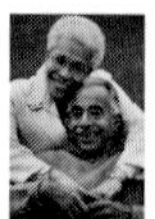

Case Study Findings

Mrs. Mays' family history reveals:

- Father died of heart failure at age 89.

- Mother died at age 70 from complications of cardiovascular accident (CVA, stroke).

Psychosocial Profile

The psychosocial profile reveals patterns in the client's lifestyle that affect spiritual health. Begin by examining your client's typical day. Are there any activities that reflect spirituality, such as praying or attending religious services? Dietary preferences may also be influenced by religious practices. For example, some religions have dietary restrictions that need to be considered when caring for your client, such as **kosher** diet for clients of Jewish faith.

The psychosocial history also identifies relationships and support systems. These supports can be within the family or the community. Organized religion can also be a source of support for your client. The amount of stress in your client's life and his or her ability to deal with it can be greatly influenced by spirituality. Spirituality can be a source of comfort and coping.

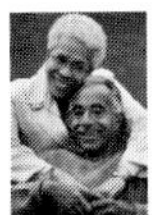

Case Study Findings

Mrs. Mays' psychosocial profile includes the following:

- **Typical day:** Arises at 7 AM, makes her bed, eats breakfast, and reads the paper. Usually does light housework, such as dusting and washing breakfast dishes. She then rests because the activity leaves her short of breath. She generally calls her sister to come over for lunch and watch soap operas. Sister leaves by 4 PM to get dinner for her husband. Mrs. Mays usually eats a light supper and then does needlework until 10 PM, when she watches the news. She goes to bed at 10:30 PM.
- **Nutrition:** Eats three meals a day. Lunch is her main meal, and she enjoys it most because she usually has her sister for company. Doesn't like to cook just for herself, so eats a light supper.
- **Activity and Exercise:** Until last week she walked to the corner store for her daily paper. She now has it delivered because the walk is too difficult. She is also unable to walk to services at her church, which is three blocks away. She does not drive.
- **Sleep and Rest:** Goes to bed at 10:30 PM and arises at 7 AM. Not sleeping well because of breathing problems caused by congestive heart failure (CHF).
- **Self-Care Activities:** Sees her doctor regularly for hypertension and CHF.
- **Roles/Relationships:** Sister lives across the street and spends most weekday afternoons with client. Client's only child and two grandchildren live in California. They talk on the phone weekly, but she sees them rarely. Attended church and taught Sunday school and vacation Bible school until recently.
- **Occupational Activities:** Retired teacher.
- **Hobbies:** Needlepoint, reading, watching television.
- **Environmental Risks:** Lives in 2-story house with bedroom on second floor.
- **Personal Habits:** Has never smoked; doesn't drink alcohol.
- **Stress and Coping:** Says she doesn't like to make a "big fuss" over her health problems or "burden anyone" with them.

CRITICAL THINKING ACTIVITY #4

List all the strengths and areas of concern that have a bearing on Mrs. Mays' health status.

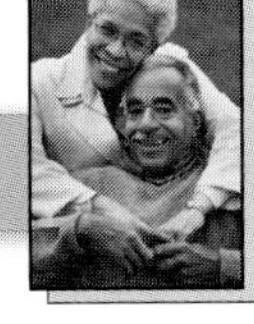

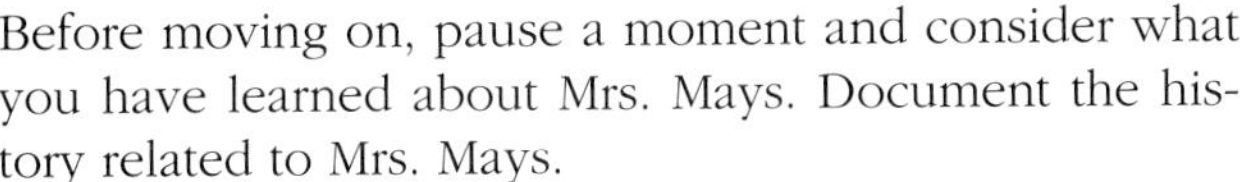

Case Study Evaluation

Before moving on, pause a moment and consider what you have learned about Mrs. Mays. Document the history related to Mrs. Mays.

To assess your client's spiritual health, focus your attention in four particular areas—behavior, verbal communication, relationships, and environment—and ask yourself questions in the following areas.

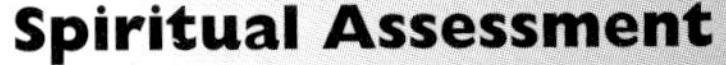

Spiritual Assessment

A person's spirit cannot be "measured," so you must rely on other evidence to make nursing diagnoses in the spiritual dimension. For example, emotional and physical behaviors often signal underlying spiritual disturbances.

Assessing Behavior

Is the client:

- Praying or meditating?
- Shutting others out?
- Constantly complaining?

- Having sleep difficulties?
- Pacing?
- Requesting frequent pain or sleep medication without apparent need?

Assessing Verbal Communication

Is the client talking about:

- God or another deity?
- Church, temple, mosque, or other place or worship?
- Prayer, hope, faith, or the meaning of life?
- The effect of the diagnosis on his or her quality of life?

Assessing Relationships

Does the client:

- Have many visitors? Who are his or her visitors (family, friends, clergy, or other spiritual support people)?
- Interact with them well?

Assessing Environment

Does the client have:

- A ***Bible, Koran (Qur'an),*** or other religious reading material?
- Religious jewelry or symbols, such as a **cross, Star of David,** prayer cap or shawl, flowers from a church altar, or religious greeting cards?

Additional Questions

Assessing the previous four areas will help you pinpoint your client's spiritual resources. In addition, also ask these questions:

- Who are your support people?
- What provides you with strength and hope?
- What gives your life meaning and purpose?
- How has your life changed since you became ill?

Phrase these questions carefully so that you do not offend the client or seem to be unduly prying. If a specific religious affiliation was listed on the admission record, be sure you have a general understanding of its perspective. For example, is the religion monotheistic, such as **Christianity** or **Judaism;** pantheistic, such as **Hinduism;** or **nontheistic,** such as **animism** or **New Age**? You need to know basic similarities and differences to be able to assist the client in the best possible way. Answers to the broad questions can then be used to further refine questions that are in line with the client's belief system. Examples might be:

- What is important to you?
- How is your religion, deity, or faith important to you?
- Is prayer important?
- What accommodations can be made to assist you in continuing any spiritual practices (e.g., religious symbols and/or dietary needs)? (Table 7–2).

Table 7–2 How Belief Systems Influence Health Care

BELIEF SYSTEM	SIGNIFICANT BELIEFS AND SYMBOLS	EFFECTS ON HEALTH CARE
Christianity		
Roman Catholic 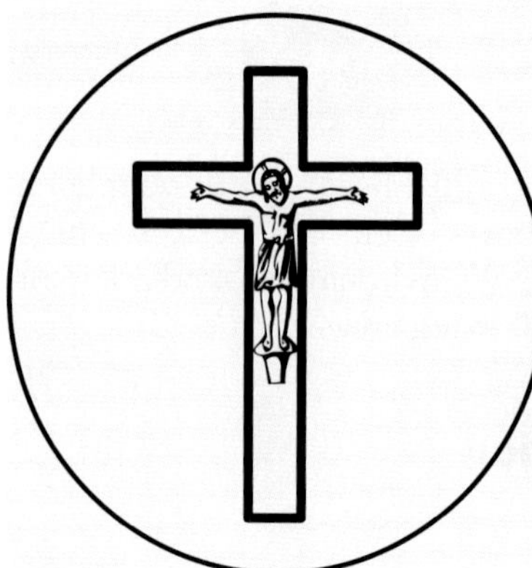 **Crucifix**	Important religious rites: baptism, holy communion, and anointing of the sick. **Crucifix** and **rosary** (beaded chain with small crucifix) are important symbols. ***Missal*** and *Bible* are important reading materials. Abstain from meat during Lent and other holy days.	Modern health care accepted, but many rely on a strong sense of faith for healing. Healing services may be held. Rites may be requested in the hospital as needed. Stillborn or critically ill infants are baptized as soon as possible after delivery. Prayers for and by ill person are encouraged. Presence of symbols often a source of comfort. Opposed to abortion and most forms of birth control.

Table 7–2 How Belief Systems Influence Health Care

BELIEF SYSTEM	SIGNIFICANT BELIEFS AND SYMBOLS	EFFECTS ON HEALTH CARE
Eastern Orthodox 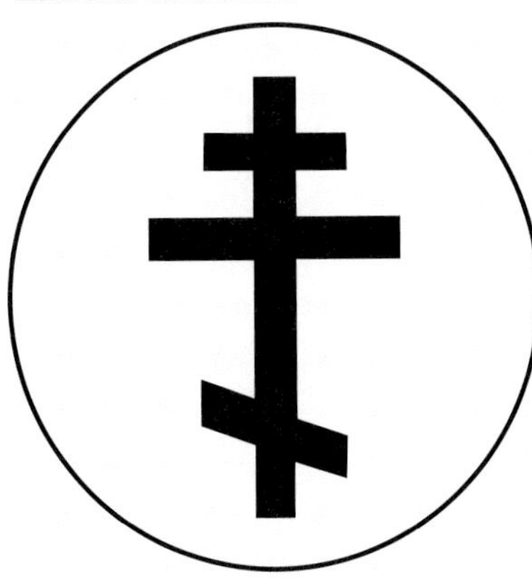 **Orthodox cross**	Practices same rites as Roman Catholic and Anglican Church: baptism, holy communion and anointing of the sick. **Orthodox cross** has a diagonal cross bar near the bottom of the upright bar and two cross bars at the top. Wearing this cross is important to the religious person. Parishes are often established along ethnic/national lines (e.g., Greek, Russian, Ukrainian). Church follows different liturgical calendar, so most high holy days are celebrated at different times than rest of Christian world.	Generally accepts modern health care. Disapproves of birth control and strongly opposes abortion. Orthodox priest may be called on for blessings, exorcisms, and direct healing. Having religious symbols near is a source of faith and comfort. Organ donation is acceptable.
Episcopalian or Anglican 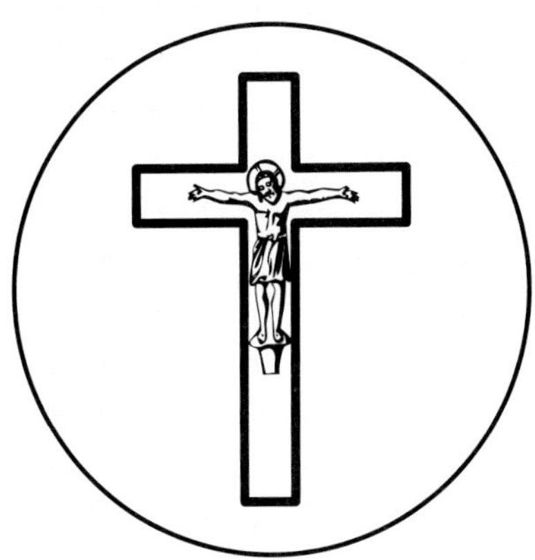 **Crucifix**	Important religious rites: baptism, holy communion and anointing of the sick. Both crucifix and plain cross are used. ***Book of Common Prayer*** and *Bible* are important reading materials.	Similar to Roman Catholics. Some Episcopal parishes practice healing by laying on of hands and prayers of special intention.
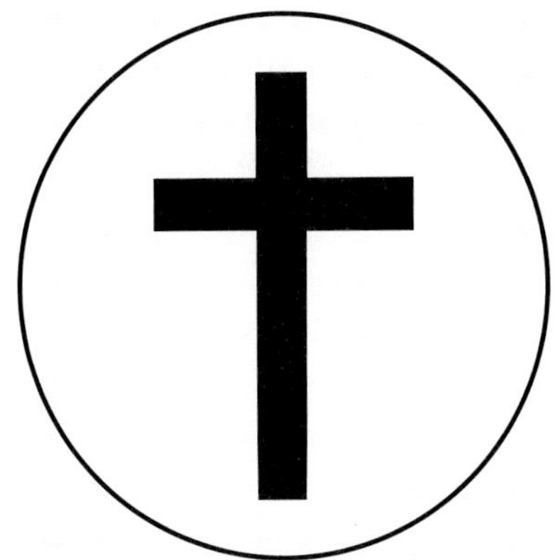 **Plain cross**	Fast on high holy days and abstain from meat on Fridays in Lent.	Rites may be requested in the hospital as needed. Stillborn or critically ill infants are baptized as soon as possible after delivery. Prayers for and by ill person are encouraged. Responsible family planning and free choice are important. No sanctioned restrictions on birth control or abortion.

(Continued)

Table 7–2 How Belief Systems Influence Health Care *(Continued)*

BELIEF SYSTEM	SIGNIFICANT BELIEFS AND SYMBOLS	EFFECTS ON HEALTH CARE
Other Protestant Denominations 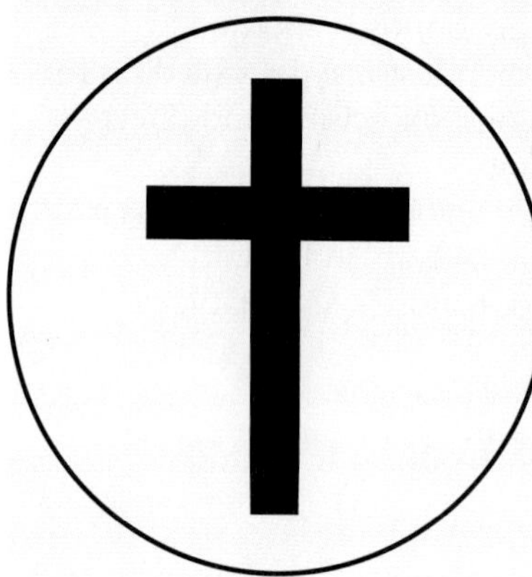 **Plain cross**	Wide range of practices found among a diversity of denominations (e.g., Baptist, Pentecostal, Lutheran, Methodist). A plain cross and *Bible* are symbols common to almost all Protestant denominations. When practiced, baptism is usually reserved for older children or adults. Holy communion is practiced infrequently, if at all. Special prayers for sick are a more common practice than anointing.	Because there are many different denominations, nurse must ask questions that address specific religious practices that may affect client's health and health care (i.e., dietary restrictions). Use of prayers and healing by "laying on of hands" varies. Strict Christian Scientists reject all medical treatment and rely on prayer for healing. Interpretation of biblical scripture within each denomination determines acceptance of such practices as blood transfusions (forbidden by Jehovah's Witnesses), abortion, or organ transplantation.
Judaism 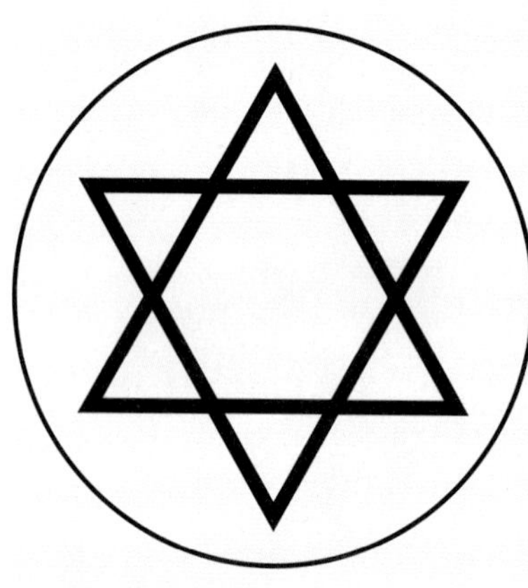 **Star of David**	Encompasses three groups of believers with different practices: Orthodox (most traditional), Reform (most liberal) and Conservative (has elements of both traditional and liberal practices). Common symbols are the Star of David and the ***Torah***, the first five books of the *Bible* written on scrolls. It contains guidelines for life. A prayer book may be carried for reading of special prayers. Services held after sundown on Friday and/or before sundown on Saturday. Male infants usually circumcised at 8 days old in a religious ceremony known as a **bris**. Orthodox and some Conservative Jews keep kosher dietary laws. Men may wear a **yarmulke**, a small skull cap. Cap is often worn in temple by all men but may be worn at all times.	Be sure to ask questions about diet and religious practices, such as, "Do you follow any dietary rules that we should know about while you are here in the hospital?" Prayer is important to all groups. Observation of Sabbath and other holy days is important. Some clients may refuse treatment on those days or refuse to eat on traditional days of fasting. Kosher food is available in most hospitals. Religious law provides for the individual's responsibility to stay healthy, both physically and mentally. Traditional medicine is valued as well as prayer for relief of suffering. Organ transplants are allowed, but donation of organs from dying people is not permitted without the donor's consent.
Islam	Islam faith is based on teachings of Mohammed. In North America, adherents of Islam may be either traditional ethnic Muslims or members of the Nation of Islam, a primarily African-American	Caregivers must be of the same gender to protect modesty. Women may continue to wear traditional head scarf with or without face veil while hospitalized. Traditional hospital gowns may be unacceptable.

Table 7–2 How Belief Systems Influence Health Care

BELIEF SYSTEM	SIGNIFICANT BELIEFS AND SYMBOLS	EFFECTS ON HEALTH CARE
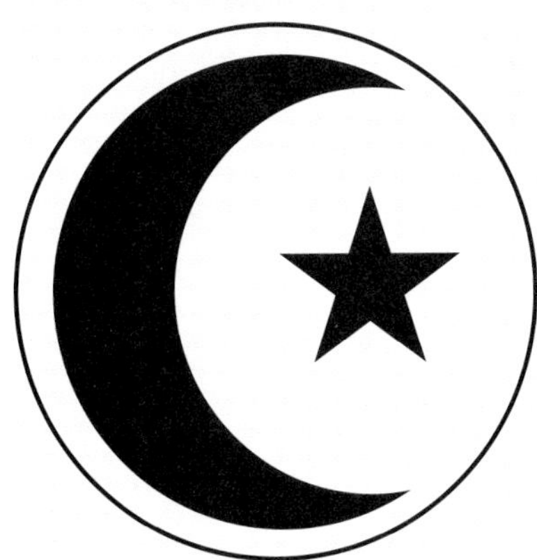 **Crescent moon**	group. The *Qur'an* (*Koran*) is the sacred book of Islam. Many have a special prayer rug that they carry. Symbols vary, but generally include a **crescent moon** in some position. Ritual prayer, five times a day while kneeling and facing toward Mecca (in Middle East) and specific dietary restrictions are common to all members. Alcohol and pork are forbidden. Many practice fasting during the month of Ramadan. Women dress with clothing that hides the body.	Some have a fatalistic view of health and may refuse treatment. Islam has rituals related to all aspects of life and death. Be aware of these needs and show sensitivity for the client and family. Medications that have an alcohol base, such as elixirs and cough syrups, may be unacceptable.
Hinduism 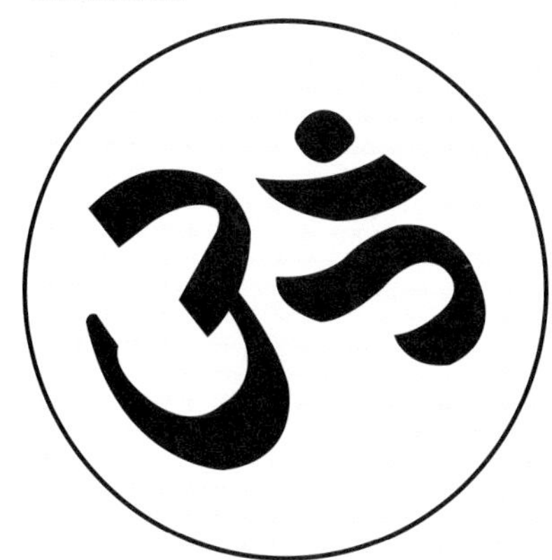 **Om symbol**	Ancient religion originating in India. Many Indians now living in North America continue to follow their religion. Universal symbol is the **om symbol**. A major tenet is achieving a state of oneness with the universe. Prayer is important to achieve oneness. Many gods have power over the individual. Religious shrines are often erected in the home. Killing any living creature is forbidden, so many sects are vegetarians.	Clients may want to set up a small shrine in the hospital room. Although the traditional sari is not religion-based, some women may wish to wear it while in the hospital. It is a long length of soft cloth that is wrapped around the body like a long skirt, with the loose end draped over the head like a scarf. The belief in *karma* (unchangeable fate) may influence the approach to self-care and the seeking of health care.
New Age 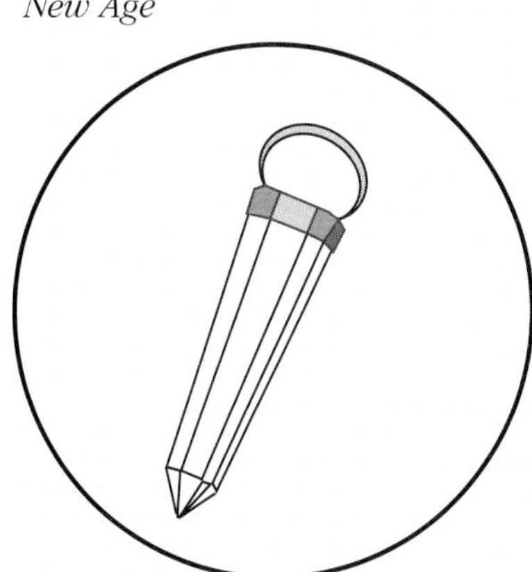 **Crystal**	Although not a religion, this belief system is growing in popularity. Beliefs are borrowed from Buddhism, Native Americans, humanism, physics, and occultism, among others. Objects such as pyramids and **crystals** are thought to impart strength and healing energy. There is great diversity of thinking, but some common beliefs are that all people are divine, right and wrong is determined by the individual, and reality can be controlled.	The *crystal* is a common symbol. It is thought to impart healing energy and may be rubbed over the skin in close proximity to diseased tissue. Nurses need to recognize the crystal as a possible belief object and not as jewelry. No clergy, but several believers may meditate with client to increase healing power. These beliefs do not usually prevent the client from seeking traditional therapies.

(Continued)

Table 7–2 How Belief Systems Influence Health Care *(Continued)*

BELIEF SYSTEM	SIGNIFICANT BELIEFS AND SYMBOLS	EFFECTS ON HEALTH CARE
Nonreligious		
Agnostic	Believes that it is impossible to know if God or other supreme being exists.	Diverse and individual influences on health care. Assess each client individually.
Atheist	Does not believe in any God but may have beliefs that are of the spiritual dimension.	Diverse and individual influences on health care. Must assess each client individually.
No organized religion	People who believe in a supreme being that is unidentified may avoid an organized religion but still have spiritual beliefs and needs.	Diverse and individual influences on health care. Must assess each client individually.

Assessment Instruments

Several assessment surveys have been developed to help in the identification of spiritual needs. Some of the surveys are biased toward a Judeo-Christian viewpoint and are not suitable for all clients. Some of the surveys are long or designed for self-report; they may be difficult to use with an acutely ill client. Some healthcare facilities have developed their own spiritual assessment tools and included them on their overall nursing assessment instrument. You may find the spiritual assessment questions in the previous section and other questions in this chapter more helpful than using any one survey. Box 7–1 provides a scale for assessing spiritual well-being.

Keep in mind that people need to understand the meaning of their existence and need to be connected to other human beings regardless of the presence or absence of organized religious affiliations.

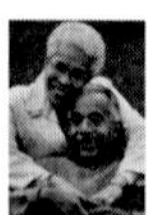

Case Study Findings

Mrs. Mays' focused spiritual assessment findings include:

- Behavior
  - Lies in bed with her face turned away from the door.
  - BP remains elevated despite medication.
  - Eyes are closed but her hands are folded and her lips move silently.
- Verbal Communication
  - Asks if anyone from church has called for her when she was off the floor for a test.
  - Asks why she is sick. States that when she was teaching she felt alive and useful. "What use am I now?"
- Relationships
  - No visitors have been noted for Mrs. Mays since her admission 2 days ago.
  - Client wonders why her sister hasn't visited or even called.
- Environment
  - A well-worn *Bible* is on Mrs. Mays' nightstand
  - She wears a small gold cross around her neck. States that it was a confirmation gift from her godparents many years ago.
- Additional questions
  - Who are your support people?
    Client states: "I usually rely on my sister, but I don't want to burden her. My daughter is so far away, and it's expensive for her to come back here. Besides, she has her own family."
  - What provides you with strength and hope?
    Client states: "I usually find strength in my church, the services are so beautiful. The people are great, too. We're just like a family. I haven't been able to get there recently, and I really miss it. I guess they don't know I'm here yet. Our pastor recently left, and we have a temporary right now. I don't know him very well."
  - What gives your life meaning and purpose?
    Client states: "Teaching the children was my first love after my husband and daughter, of course. Those little ones were so eager to learn, you know. I retired 3 years ago. My husband and I were only able to travel to California one time

Box 7–1 Jarel Spiritual Well-Being Scale©

Directions: Please circle the choice that *best* describes how much you agree with each statement. Circle only *one* answer for each statement. There are no right or wrong answers or good or bad scores. The purpose of this scale is to help the client talk about his or her spirituality in a nonthreatening way and to give you a sense of the importance of spirituality in your client's life so that you can plan appropriate interventions.

	Strongly Agree	Moderately Agree	Agree	Disagree	Moderately Disagree	Strongly Disagree
1. Prayer is an important part of my life.	SA	MA	A	D	MD	SD
2. I believe I have spiritual well-being.	SA	MA	A	D	MD	SD
3. As I grow older, I find myself more tolerant of others' beliefs.	SA	MA	A	D	MD	SD
4. I find meaning and purpose in my life.	SA	MA	A	D	MD	SD
5. I feel there is a close relationship between my spiritual beliefs and what I do.	SA	MA	A	D	MD	SD
6. I believe in an afterlife.	SA	MA	A	D	MD	SD
7. When I am sick, I have less spiritual well-being.	SA	MA	A	D	MD	SD
8. I believe in a Supreme Power.	SA	MA	A	D	MD	SD
9. I am able to receive and give love to others.	SA	MA	A	D	MD	SD
10. I am satisfied with my life.	SA	MA	A	D	MD	SD
11. I set goals for myself.	SA	MA	A	D	MD	SD
12. God has little meaning in my life.	SA	MA	A	D	MD	SD
13. I am satisfied with the way I am using my abilities.	SA	MA	A	D	MD	SD
14. Prayer does not help me in making decisions.	SA	MA	A	D	MD	SD
15. I am able to appreciate differences in others.	SA	MA	A	D	MD	SD
16. I am pretty well put together.	SA	MA	A	D	MD	SD
17. I prefer that others make decisions for me.	SA	MA	A	D	MD	SD
18. I find it hard to forgive others.	SA	MA	A	D	MD	DS
19. I accept my life situations.	SA	MA	A	D	MD	DS
20. Belief in a Supreme Being has no part in my life.	SA	MA	A	D	MD	SD
21. I cannot accept changes in my life.	SA	MA	A	D	MD	SD

Source: Adapted from J. Hungelmann et al., 1987.

to see our daughter and her family before he got so sick. My, how he suffered. I miss him terribly."

- How has your life changed since you became ill? *Client says:* "Since I retired, I have taught Sunday school and vacation Bible school. It keeps me young to be around the children. But since I've been bothered by this pesky heart, I don't even have the energy to walk to church let alone handle teaching. I guess I'll have to find something else to do. Why has this happened to me now? What is God thinking?"

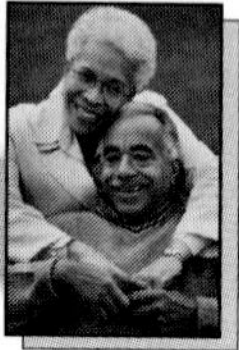

Case Study Analysis and Plan

Now that your assessment of Mrs. Mays is complete, document your key history and key spiritual assessment findings.

List key history findings and spiritual assessment findings that will help you formulate your nursing diagnoses.

Nursing Diagnoses

The next step is to analyze the data from Mrs. Mays' spiritual assessment and develop nursing diagnoses. The following are possible nursing diagnoses for this client. Cluster the supporting data for each.

1. **Spiritual Distress, related to current life situation**
2. **Hopelessness, related to chronic illness**
3. Social Isolation

Identify any additional nursing diagnoses.

CRITICAL THINKING ACTIVITY # 5

Now that you have identified some nursing diagnoses for Mrs. Mays, select one from the above list and develop a nursing care plan and a brief teaching plan.

Research Tells Us

Limited research has been done in the spiritual realm. Some researchers have shown that spiritual well-being is closely associated with states such as hope (Fehring, Miller, & Shaw, 1997; Mickley, Soeken, & Belcher, 1992) and hardiness (Carson & Green, 1992). Strengthening a person's sense of spiritual well-being also has been shown to help people cope with illness (Carson & Green, 1992). On the other hand, a reduced sense of spiritual well-being is associated with increased depression, anxiety, and anger (Fehring, Miller, & Shaw, 1997). Although the above studies were done with ill adults, Fehring, Brennan, and Keller had similar results in 1987 with healthy college students. The relationships appear to hold true over time.

Summary

- Because the body, mind, and spirit are interrelated, illness can have an impact on your client's spiritual well-being.
- The opposite is also true—your client's spirituality can have a positive or a negative effect on his or her illness.
- Performing a spiritual assessment involves listening closely and compassionately and knowing what questions to ask. It also involves performing a systematic assessment.
- Armed with this information, you can then formulate appropriate nursing diagnoses to help your client cope with his or her illness.

UNIT III

Systems Physical Assessment

8

Assessing the Integumentary System

Before You Begin

INTRODUCTION TO THE INTEGUMENTARY SYSTEM

The integumentary system, consisting of the skin, hair, and nails, is the largest organ of the body and the easiest of all systems to access. It provides invaluable information about all other bodily systems. The skin, hair, and nails provide clues about general health, reflect changes in environment, and signal internal ailments stemming from other organs. Because integumentary system cells reproduce rapidly, changes in the skin, hair, and nails may be an early warning of a developing health problem. Yet the importance of carefully assessing the integumentary system for subtle changes is often overlooked. A thorough assessment of this system may help you detect actual or potential problems, not only in the skin but also in underlying systems.

Anatomy and Physiology Review

Before you begin your assessment, you need a basic understanding of the integumentary system, including its general function and purpose. A knowledge of normal functions and structures will enable you to detect and interpret any abnormalities.

Structures and Functions of the Integumentary System

The structures of the integumentary system are the skin, hair, nails, sweat glands, and sebaceous glands. Their functions are described in the following paragraphs.

The Skin

The skin is a layer of tissue that covers all exposed body surfaces. Although similar to the mucous membranes, the skin also includes appendages such as hair follicles and sebaceous glands. Its thickness varies according to location or site. The **epidermis,** the outer visible layer, contains keratin, an extremely tough, protective protein substance that can cause tissue to become hard or horny. The deeper **dermis** is made up of proteins and **mucopolysaccarides,** thick, gelatinous material that provides a supporting matrix for nerve tissue, blood vessels, sweat and sebum glands, and hair follicles. Beneath the dermis lies the **subcutaneous layer,** made up of fatty connective tissue. Together, the layers of the skin protect underlying structures from physical trauma and ultraviolent radiation. The skin is essential to maintaining body temperature, fluid balance, and sensation. It is involved in absorption and excretion, immunity, and the synthesis of vitamin D from the sun. (Fig. 8–1).

The Hair

The hair is also made up of keratinized cells. Hair is found over most of the body. It grows from hair follicles supplied by blood vessels located in the dermis. **Vellus,** which is short, pale, and fine hair, is located over all of the body. **Terminal hairs,** which are dark and coarse, are found on the scalp, brows, and, after puberty, on the legs, axillae, and perineum. The texture and color of hair are highly variable. Hair provides protection by covering the scalp and filtering dust and debris away from the nose, ears, and eyes.

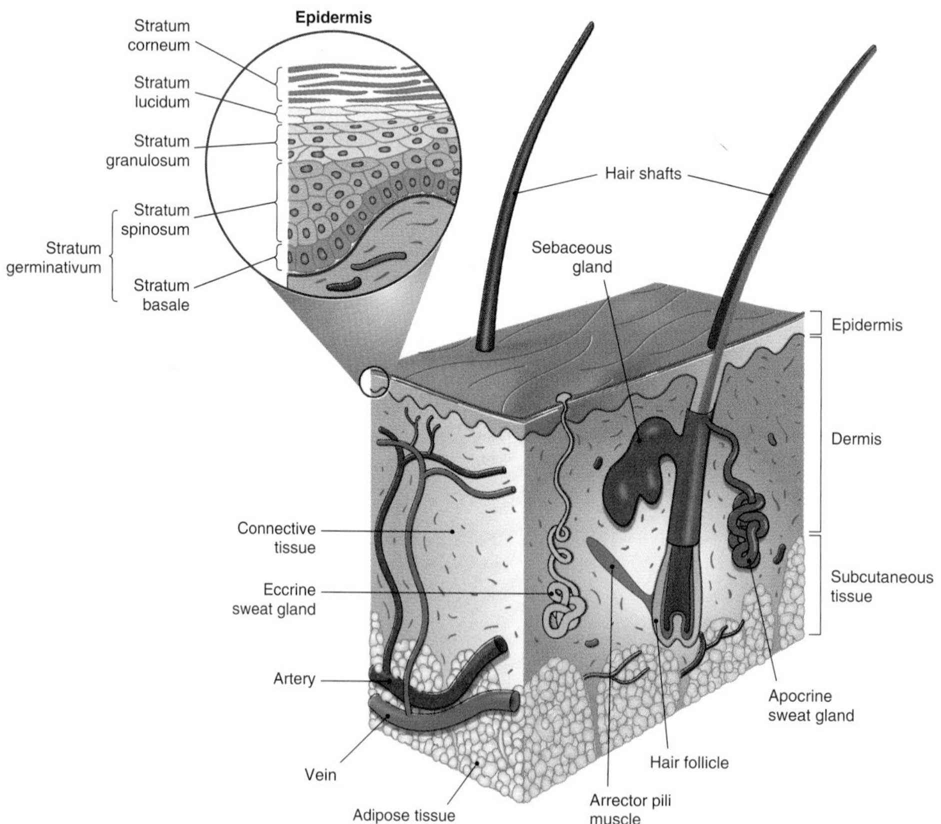

FIGURE 8–1. Structures of the skin.

Structures and Functions of the Skin

STRUCTURE	FUNCTION
Epidermis	Covers, protects, and waterproofs. Contains four main layers: stratum corneum, stratum lucidum, stratum granulosum, and stratum germinativum.
Stratum corneum	Keratinized layer. Prevents loss or entry of water; protects against pathogens and chemicals.
Stratum lucidum	Translucent layer of dead cells with eleidin, precursor of soft keratin. Found only on palms of hands and soles of feet; protects against ultraviolet sun rays to prevent sunburn.
Stratum granulosum Contains:	Keratinization begins at this layer.
• Keratohyaline	Precursor of soft keratin.
• Keratinocytes	Secrete interleukin-1, which affects skin T-cell maturation.
• Langerhans' cells	Identify foreign substances (antigens), initiating the immune response.
Stratum germinativum:	Continually produces new cells to replace worn-off surface cells. Includes stratum spinosum and stratum basale.
Stratum spinosum	Has polyhedral cells (spinelike projections) that block entry to bacteria.
Stratum basale	Has single layer of columnar or cuboidal cells and melanocytes, which produce melanin. Production of new cells occurs at this layer; site of basal cell carcinoma; melanin production increases with UV light exposure; melanin determines pigmentation and protects from UV light.
Dermis	Contains collagen, reticular and elastic fibers. Adds strength and elasticity to skin. Contains papillary layer, reticular layer, sweat glands, sebaceous glands, cholesterol, and arterioles.
Papillary layer	Contains capillaries that supply the stratum germinativum; also contains nerve endings, touch receptors, and fingerprint pattern; double layer on hands and feet.
Reticular layer	Contains connective tissue with collagen and elastic fibers, blood and lymphatic vessels, nerves, free nerve endings, fat cells, sebaceous glands and hair roots, deep pressure receptors, and smooth muscle fibers.
Sweat glands (sudoriferous)	Most numerous on palms of hands and soles of feet. Two types are eccrine and apocrine glands.
Eccrine glands	Respond to external temperature and psychological stress; found over most of body but most numerous on palms of hands and soles of feet; secrete sweat, which helps regulate body temperature and, to a lesser degree, excretes wastes such as urea.
Apocrine or odoriferous glands	Found in axilla and genital area; respond to stress; secrete pheromones, a barely perceptible odor; when apocrine secretions react with bacteria, body odor results. *Ceruminous glands* are a type of apocrine gland found in the external ear canal. They secrete cerumen, which prevents drying of the ear drum and traps foreign substances.
Sebaceous glands	Produce sebum, which lubricates and protects skin and hair.
Cholesterol	Converts to vitamin D when exposed to UV lights.
Arterioles	Dilate when hot to increase heat loss and constrict when cold to conserve heat; constrict in response to stressful situations to shunt blood to vital organs.
Hypodermis/ Subcutaneous	Contains connective tissue and adipose tissue.
Connective tissue	Connects skin to muscles; contains white blood cells.
Adipose tissue	Contains stored energy, cushions bony prominences, provides insulation.

Structures and Functions of the Hair

STRUCTURE	FUNCTION
Shaft: Portion that protrudes	Scalp hair provides insulation, protection from heat and cold; eyebrows cushion and protect eyes from glare and perspiration; eyelashes protect eyes from foreign substances; nasal hair traps foreign particles.
Medulla has soft keratin, central core	
Cortex has hard keratin	Pigment found in cortex gives hair color.
Cuticle has hard keratin, outer layer	
Root: Portion embedded in skin	Cellular mitosis occurs here.
Bulb is composed of a matrix of epithelial cells enclosed by a follicle	
Arrector pili muscle	Causes hair to stand up (as in "goosebumps") and squeezes sebum from sebaceous glands.

The Nails

Nails are made up of hard, keratinized cells and grow from a nail root under the cuticle. Other nail structures include the free edge, which overhangs the tip of the finger or toe; the nailbed, or epithelial layer of skin; and the **lunula,** the proximal part of the nail. The nailbed's vascular supply gives the nail a pink color, although the nail itself is generally transparent. The purpose of the nails is to protect the distal portions of the digits and to aid in picking up objects (Fig. 8–2).

Other Structures

Other appendages to the integument include the **sweat glands** and **sebaceous glands.** There are two types of sweat glands: **eccrine glands,** which are distributed over much of the body, and **apocrine glands,** which are limited to the genitalia, axillae, and areolae. Sebaceous glands are located near hair follicles, over most of the body. They secrete **sebum,** which lubricates the hair shaft.

Interaction with Other Body Systems

Changes in the integumentary system may reflect a problem in any of the systems described in the following paragraphs.

The Respiratory System

The respiratory system is responsible for obtaining the oxygen necessary for cellular metabolism, as well as for eliminating the carbon dioxide produced through the metabolic processes. If the process of respiration is impaired, alterations in the skin are most often evident through the development of **cyanosis,** a bluish discoloration, as hemoglobin becomes unsaturated with oxygen. Central cyanosis occurs when oxygen saturation is

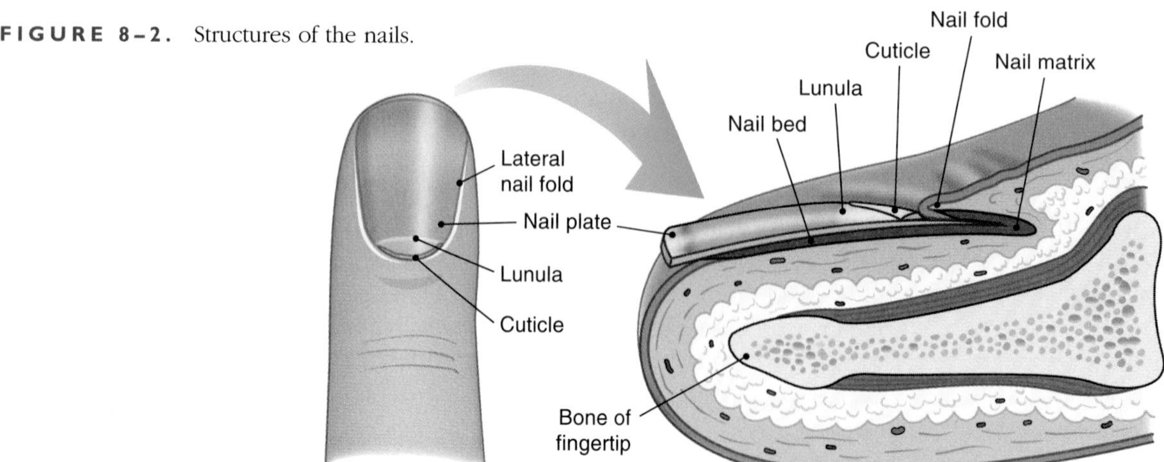

FIGURE 8–2. Structures of the nails.

less than 80 percent and results in diffuse changes in the skin and mucous membranes. In contrast, peripheral cyanosis, which occurs in response to decreased cardiac output, is evident in areas of the body such as the nailbeds and lips, which are cooler than other regions; it may also be evident when an individual is chilled. In severe and chronic cardiopulmonary diseases, clubbing of the nails occurs due to hypoxia (Fig. 8–3).

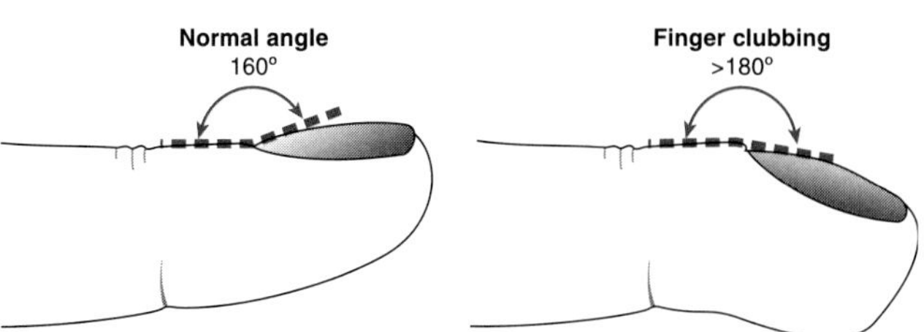

FIGURE 8–3. Nail clubbing.

The Cardiovascular System

The skin layer also contains a network of blood vessels, which contribute to its ability to regulate temperature and to obtain nourishment. Alterations in the cardiovascular system can lead to circulatory impairment and changes in skin coloring and temperature, as well as to the development of **lesions, ulcerations,** and **necrosis.** When cardiac output is decreased, cyanosis may develop.

The Gastrointestinal System

The primary roles of the gastrointestinal (GI) system are the conversion of food to absorbable nutrients and the elimination of wastes. When GI disorders impair the body's ability to excrete toxins, the accumulation of toxins may become evident in the skin. For instance, when bile excretion is impaired so that bile builds up, **jaundice,** a yellow discoloration, often results. When dietary lipids accumulate, **xanthomas,** which are lipid deposits, or **papules** may develop. Nutritional deficits, which may stem from gastrointestinal problems, are often evident in the skin. For example, deficits in vitamin A, riboflavin, vitamin C, iron and protein may all result in skin, hair, or nail alterations.

The Urinary System

The urinary system is primarily responsible for filtering the blood, but it is also involved in the production of red blood cells and regulation of electrolyte and fluid status. When renal function is altered and filtration decreases, toxins and fluids build up in the body. The toxins often include **pigmented metabolites,** which alter the skin coloring. For example, an increased concentration of urea may lead to a residue of urea on the skin, which is called **uremic frost.** Toxins are also responsible for the development of **pruritus,** or itching. Calcium deposits may lead to **excoriations** of the skin. Altered hematologic status may be evident through **ecchymoses** and **hematomas.** Increased fluid volume associated with diminishing renal function may result in edema.

The Neurological System

The skin contains an intricate system of sensory and autonomic nerve fibers and serves as the body's largest sensory organ. Not only does this network of fibers permit sensation of touch, temperature, pressure, vibration, and pain; the autonomic nervous system fibers control the skin's blood vessels and glands, regulating the skin's temperature, moisture, and oiliness. Alterations in the nervous system can have profound effects on the skin, placing it at risk for injury or discomfort. For instance, if sensation is decreased, a person is more likely to experience trauma to the skin because he or she is less likely to detect the need to withdraw from potentially dangerous objects or activities. Irritated nerves can produce disagreeable sensations in the skin, such as burning. Alterations in the autonomic nervous system can result in drying of the skin.

The Endocrine System

Alterations of the endocrine system may affect the skin in a myriad of ways. Diabetes leads to alterations in skin integrity through complex processes involving changes in the immune, vascular, and neurological systems. Diabetic foot ulcers are examples of altered skin associated with diabetes. When thyroid disease occurs, the skin is often affected. In hypothyroidism, the skin is often dry and cool and becomes puffy, with nonpitting edema. It may develop a yellow hue as **carotene** accumulates. The hair is affected, becoming dull, brittle, and sparse. In contrast, hyperthyroidism causes the skin to be warmer, sweatier, and smoother than usual. The nails are thin and brittle and may separate from the nail plate. The hair is fine and silky, with patchy hair loss. Adrenal diseases affect the skin, hair, and nails. Hypofunction of the adrenals can result in hyperpigmentation of the skin (a bronze color) and alopecia (baldness). Hyperfunction results in thin and fragile skin, petechiae, plethora, bruises, and poor wound healing.

The Lymphatic/Immune System

The immune system is involved in protecting the body from both external and endogenous factors. Impairments in the immune system are reflected in the skin when infectious diseases result in their typical rashes or lesions. Abnormalities of the immune system can also result in hypersensitivity and the development of **atopic,** or **allergic,** skin changes, including pruritus or rashes such as

ENDOCRINE

Thyroid affects growth and texture of skin, hair and nails.

Hormones stimulate sebaceous glands.

Sex hormones affect hair growth and distribution, fat and subcutaneous tissue distribution and activity of apocrine sweat glands.

Adrenal hormones affect dermal blood supply and mobilize lipids from adipocytes.

LYMPHATIC/IMMUNE

Skin is first line of defense.

Langerhan cells and macrophages resist infection.

Mast cells trigger inflammatory responses.

Lymphatic system protects skin by sending more macrophages and lymphocytes when needed.

RESPIRATORY

Provides oxygen to and removes carbon dioxide from integumentary system.

Color of skin and nails can reflect changes in respiratory system.

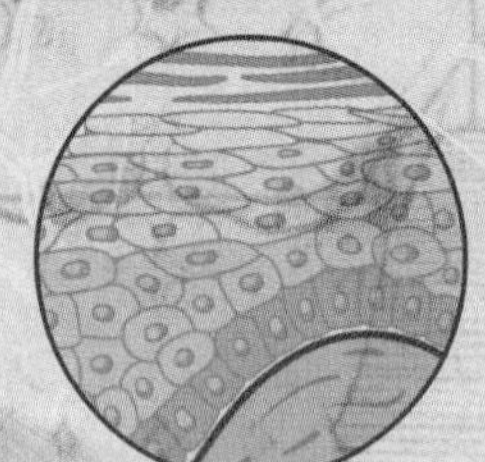

URINARY

Kidneys remove waste and maintain normal pH.

Skin helps eliminate water and waste.

Skin prevents excess fluid loss.

DIGESTIVE

Skin synthesizes vitamin D for calcium and phosphorous absorption.

Supplies nutrients while skin stores lipids.

CARDIOVASCULAR

Mast cell stimulation produces localized changes in blood flow and capillary permeability.

CV system provides nutrients and removes wastes.

Delivers hormones and lymphocytes.

Provides heat for skin temperature.

MUSCULAR

Skin synthesizes vitamin D needed for calcium absorption for muscle contraction.

Gives shape to and supports skin.

Contraction of facial muscles allows communication through expressions.

REPRODUCTIVE

Provides sensory receptors for sexual stimulation.

NEUROLOGICAL

Sensory receptors in dermis to touch, temperature, pressure, vibration and pain.

Provides communication with external environment.

Controls blood flow and sweating through thermoregulation.

SKELETAL

Skin synthesizes vitamin D needed for calcium and phosphorus absorption.

Skeletal system provides a framework for skin.

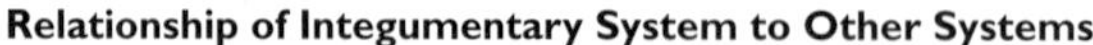

Relationship of Integumentary System to Other Systems

atopic dermatitis or **psoriasis.** Skin changes are also common in some systemic autoimmune disorders such as **lupus erythematosus.**

Developmental, Cultural, and Ethnic Variations

Infants

Various differences can be noted in the newborn skin. Infants have very smooth skin, partly because of their lack of exposure to the environment, but also there is less subcutaneous tissue. Color changes can be readily seen. Newborns often appear pinker or redder because of the lack of subcutaneous tissue. Physiologic jaundice may occur 2 to 3 days after birth as a result of the breakdown of excessive red blood cells at birth and immature functioning of the liver. Newborns have little or no coarse terminal hair. They shed their hair at approximately 3 months and it is soon replaced. Eccrine sweat glands begin to function within a month after birth. The immature sweat glands lead to poor thermoregulation. With no functioning **apocrine** sweat glands, babies' skin is less oily than adults' and lacks offensive odor. The secretion of **sebum** by the sebaceous glands can result in cradle cap. Numerous skin lesions may also be seen on the newborn, such as **mongolian spots, nevus flammeus** (port wine stains), **capillary hemangiomas** (stork bites), **hemangioma simplex** (strawberry marks), **milia,** and **erythema toxicum neonatorum.**

Adolescents

Adolescence is a time of rapid hormonal change that may affect the integumentary system. During adolescence, the apocrine glands begin to enlarge and to function. At this time, young people develop increased axillary sweating and the potential for a more pronounced body odor. The sebaceous glands increase sebum production and the skin becomes more oily, leading to the onset of **acne.** During adolescence, pubic and axillary hair and male and female body hair patterns become apparent.

Pregnant Women

During pregnancy, there is increased blood flow to the skin, particularly to the hands and feet, as peripheral vessels dilate and the number of capillaries increases to dissipate heat. Along with this increased flow, there is an increase in sweating and sebaceous activity. The skin thickens and separates with stretching, with the appearance of **striae.** Hormonal changes result in hyperpigmentation. The pigmentary changes occur on the face resulting in **chloasma,** on abdominal midline (the **linea alba** becomes the **linea nigra**) and on the nipples, areolae, axillae, and vulva.

Menopausal Women

During menopause, hormonal fluctuations result in hot flashes, often accompanied by flushing of the skin and increased pigmentation. There may be an increase in facial hair and some degree of scalp hair loss. Chloasma may occur. The incidence of skin tags increases at menopause.

Older Adults

With age, the skin atrophies. There is a decrease in production of sebum and sweat. The skin becomes drier and flattens, often becoming paperlike. The elasticity decreases and wrinkles develop. There is a decreased *melanocyte* function, so that the hair grays and the skin becomes more pale. Target areas of increased melanocyte function result in "age spots." There is a decrease in axillary, pubic, and scalp hair. Women may experience increased facial hair as estrogen function is lost; men experience an increase in nasal and ear hair growth. The nails grow more slowly and become thicker and more brittle. Furthermore, specific skin lesions are more common in elderly persons, including: **actinic keratoses, basal cell carcinomas, seborrheic keratoses, stasis ulcers, senile pruritus,** and **keratotic horns.**

People of Different Cultures and Ethnic Groups

Cultural and ethnic variations can readily be seen in the integumentary system. Genetic factors determine the skin color. The greater the amount of melanin, the darker the skin color. Assessing for subtle changes in the skin becomes more of a challenge the darker the skin color. The oral mucosa is best for assessing color changes in dark-skinned people. Also, assessing the sclera for jaundice is more accurate than assessing the skin in an Asian person. Fair-skinned persons of Irish, German, or Polish descent have an increased risk for skin cancer with prolonged sun exposure. African-Americans have a higher incidence of **keloids. pseudofolliculitis,** and **mongolian spots.**

Differences in hair can also be readily seen with different ethnic groups. Asians often have black, straight, silky hair, and Chinese men have very little facial hair. The hair texture of African-Americans is often thick and kinky. Cultural variations may also be noted in the amount of sweat production. For example, Asians produce less sweat and therefore have less body odor. Be alert to your client's ethnicity when assessing the integumentary system; changes may be culturally related rather than an indication of pathology.

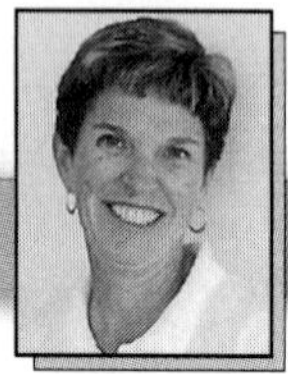

Introducing the Case Study

As a nurse in a community health setting, you have volunteered to participate as an examiner in a community skin cancer screening program. Eva Green, a 48-year-old woman with fair, freckled skin, presents for a total skin assessment. She states that several of her relatives have been diagnosed with skin cancer and she is very much afraid that she might have it. She goes on to say that because she has always had very freckled skin that "easily blemishes," she has difficulty determining what is normal and what should be a concern. As part of the screening program, you will complete a health history and physical examination that focuses on the integumentary system.

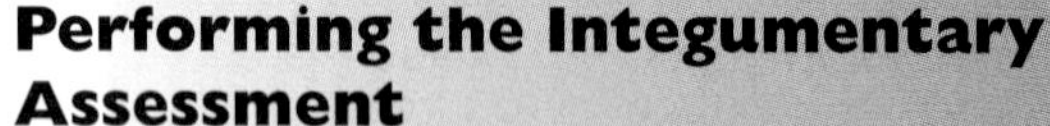

Performing the Integumentary Assessment

Assessment of the integumentary system includes a comprehensive health history and physical examination. The history identifies any symptoms related to the integumentary system, risk factors for skin problems, and the presence of diseases in other systems that would contribute to skin problems. The physical examination identifies the current condition of the integument, including any abnormal function. Throughout the assessment, be attentive to signs or symptoms of both actual and potential problems of the integument.

Health History

The health history includes obtaining biographical data and asking questions about the client's current health, past health, and family and psychosocial history. It also involves a review of systems.

Biographical Data

Briefly review all biographical data. Identify your client's age; skin function varies by age, and certain skin diseases are more likely to develop at particular ages. For example, **papules, vesicles,** and **pustules** associated with **impetigo** are mostly seen in children; acne frequently occurs during puberty, and **plaques** and malignancies are more common in older adults. Your client's occupation and recreational activities can provide clues regarding the potential for exposures to harmful chemicals, trauma, or environmental hazards. Exposure to chemicals may cause a **contact dermatitis.** Excessive sun exposure from either work or play may increase the risk for skin cancer. Similarly, the client's living situation can suggest environmental exposures to factors that might be harmful to the skin.

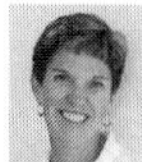

Case Study Findings

Reviewing Mrs. Green's biographical data:

- 48-year-old woman, married, with two adult children (27 and 22 years old)
- Works part-time in retail sales
- Born in the United States, of English-Scottish descent
- Protestant religion
- Husband is accountant and provides insurance through his employer.

Current Health Status

If the client has a specific skin complaint, analyze it as you begin your history, using the PQRST system. The major complaints to be alert for include: changes in moles or other lesions, nonhealing sore or ulcer or chronic irritation, pruritus/itching, and rash, a very common complaint. Because the integumentary system also includes the hair and nails, a symptom analysis should focus on changes in these areas. Generally, the problems that trigger integumentary complaints are of a stable nature and not life-threatening, and so you will be able to proceed with the full history and physical. If the client is overly distressed by the symptoms (for instance, severe itching or fear of malignancy), focus first on the presenting problem and perform a comprehensive history at a later time.

HELPFUL HINT

- Remember, skin, hair, and nails cells reproduce rapidly, and so changes are often seen when a serious acute heath problem occurs or with use of chemotherapeutic agents.
- Changes in skin, hair, and nails are often seen with underlying endocrine problems.

Symptom Assessment

Symptom Analysis tables for all the symptoms described in the following paragraphs are available on the Web for viewing and printing. In your Web browser, go to *http://www.fadavis.com/detail.cfm?id=0882-9* and click on Symptom Analysis Tables under Explore This Product.

Change in Mole or Lesion

Skin cancer is the most common type of cancer, and changes in a mole **(nevus)** or skin lesion can often evoke fear in the client. Although there are many types of

Age-Related Skin Disorders

Age	Disorders
Children	Impetigo Atopic dermatitis or eczema Pityriasis rosea Juvenile plantar dermatosis Rashes secondary to bacterial or viral infections Pediculosis capitis Varicella
Adolescents/ Young Adults	Acne Pityriasis rosea Tinea versicolor
Adults	Psoriasis Seborrheic dermatitis Malignant melanoma Herpes simplex virus type 2 (HSV2) Tinea cruris Seborrheic interigo Rosacea
Older Adults	Actinic keratosis Seborrheic keratosis Basal cell carcinoma Squamous cell carcinoma Xerosis Herpes zoster
Children and Adults	Nummular eczema/dermatitis Scabies Insect bites, poisonous plants Contact dermatitis Herpes zoster Tinea pedis

lesions, most of which are benign, it is important to be able to detect skin cancer at its earliest stages, when treatment yields the best results. There are three types of skin cancer: basal cell and squamous cell carcinomas, which affect the epidermal keratinocytes, and melanoma, which affects the melanocytes of the basal layer of the epidermis. Sun exposure is a risk factor in all types.

The majority of skin cancers are basal cell. Basal cell carcinomas are directly related to sun exposure, with 90 percent of lesions occurring on the head and neck. Basal cell carcinomas are easily treated and relatively benign. Squamous cell carcinoma is often preceded by **actinic keratosis** (premalignant macule or papule of rough, sandpaper texture, caused by excessive UV exposure). Sixty-six percent of these lesions occur on sun-exposed areas and respond well to treatment. Even though melanoma occurs less frequently than basal cell and squamous cell carcinomas, it is the most deadly type of skin cancer. Congenital nevi and **dysplastic** nevi may be precursor lesions to melanoma.

Unfortunately, there are usually no symptoms associated with skin cancers unless the lesion has metastasized regionally or distantly. In these cases, various symptoms might be present related to whether a lesion, for instance a malignant melanoma, had metastasized to another organ such as the bowel, lung, liver, or brain.

Nonhealing Sore or Chronic Ulceration

When your client's history includes a sore that won't heal or a chronic ulceration, the routine symptom analysis questions will provide a good picture of the lesion and any previous self-treatment applied. Keep in mind that a nonhealing wound or chronic irritation is often associated with an underlying disease. The most common types of nonhealing wounds or chronic skin ulcerations are caused by vascular disease or pressure or by diabetes.

Pruritus

Pruritus is severe itching. It may be localized or generalized and caused by a dermatologic problem or underlying systemic problem. Pruritus is often accompanied by a rash. Itching, when not associated with a rash, may be indicative of significant systemic disease or simply dry skin.

Itching arises from free nerve endings (nonmyelinated), which are especially abundant in the flexor aspects of the wrist and ankles. It occurs as a result of a spinal reflex and external stimuli, such as heat, dryness, inflammation, and vasodilation. Psychological factors, such as depression, can influence the perception of itching, which explains the varied responses to it. A thorough symptom analysis will help you to pinpoint the underlying cause.

Rashes

Rashes, like itching, may be localized or generalized, acute or chronic, and caused by an obvious dermatologic problem or an underlying systemic problem. A thorough symptom analysis will help you to pinpoint the problem and direct your physical assessment.

Seasonal Skin Disorders

Certain skin disorders are more common during one time of year than others. Seasonal skin problems include those caused by temperature fluctuations, air humidity, and exposure to contaminants. It is important to remember, though, that although these problems may be more common at certain times of the year, they may appear at any time.

Hair Changes

Hair loss **(alopecia)** is probably the most distressing change in hair that can occur because of its cosmetic effect. Alopecia not only refers to scalp hair but also body hair. Normally hair growth is cyclical, with 85 to 90 percent of scalp hair in the growth phase **(anagen),** and the remaining 10 to 15 percent in the resting phase **(telogen).** Scalp hair grows about 0.25 mm/day, and about

Seasonal Skin Disorders

Season	Skin Disorders
Spring	Pityriasis rosea Chickenpox Acne flare-ups
Summer	Contact dermatitis Tinea *Candida* Impetigo Insect bites
Fall	Senile pruritus/winter itch Pityriasis rosea Urticaria Acne flare-ups
Winter	Contact dermatitis of hands Senile pruritus/winter itch Psoriasis Eczema

100 strands of hair are lost per day. Hair loss can occur for many reasons. Alopecia can be classified as scarring or **cicatricial** (resulting from injury such as burns, radiation, or traction with irreversible damage to the hair follicles) and nonscarring or **noncicatricial** (resulting from hormonal changes, medications, infectious diseases, or thyroid disease, in which the follicles remain intact with a potential to reverse the process.

Nail Changes

Changes in the nails also often reflect an underlying systemic problem. Changes in color and texture are frequent complaints. A symptom analysis will help you identify any underlying problems.

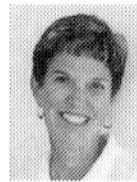

Case Study Findings

Mrs. Green's current health status includes:

- Feels she is in very good health. No current problems.
- Has recently started taking estrogen and progesterone (Prempro) daily for menopause symptoms. Is tolerating therapy well.
- Occasionally takes aspirin or acetominophen for headache or back and shoulder discomfort, but not monthly.

Past Health History

The past health history allows you to determine what illnesses or problems the client has had in the past, including those related to the skin, hair, or nails. It additionally permits you to determine episodes of illnesses involving other systems that might have an impact on the integument.

Past Health History

RISK FACTORS/ QUESTIONS TO ASK	RATIONALE/SIGNIFICANCE
Childhood Illnesses	
Do you have a history of infectious diseases such as chickenpox or rubella?	Explains scarring from rashes and degree of immunity for diseases that have skin eruptions.
Did you have asthma or allergies as a child?	History of asthma/allergic disorders commonly associated with skin problems such as eczema or psoriasis.
Did you have frequent skin problems or chronic skin illness?	Explains scarring or chronic changes to skin and potential for recurrence.
Surgery/Injuries	
Have you ever had surgery, biopsies, or a major traumatic injury?	History of surgery/trauma helps explain scars. Keloids may also develop on scar tissue. Biopsies may signal history of skin cancer or other malignancies associated with skin changes.
Hospitalizations/Diagnostic Procedures	
Have you have been hospitalized or had procedures such as electrophysiologic studies or scans?	Helps identify previous disorders that might be associated with skin condition. History of diagnostic procedures provides information on major problems that might influence integumentary system.
Allergies	
Are you allergic to foods, drugs, chemicals, or environmental agents? If yes, what type of reaction?	Skin changes are often related to substances that are ingested, applied, or come into contact with skin.

Past Health History

RISK FACTORS/ QUESTIONS TO ASK	RATIONALE/SIGNIFICANCE
Other Medical Problems	
Do you have a history of skin cancer, eczema, or psoriasis?	Consider potential for recurrence.
Do you have a history of asthma?	Often associated with atopic problems including atopic dermatitis, psoriasis.
Do you have a history of diabetes, thyroid disease, respiratory disorders, liver disease, or heart disease?	May be reflected in skin's appearance. Diabetes causes poor wound healing; hyperthyroidism, moist skin and skin necrosis; hypothyroidism, dry, scaly skin, hair loss, brittle nails and transverse ridges; chronic lung disease, cyanotic color changes; liver disease, jaundice and itching; and cardiovascular disease, color changes, edema, leg ulcers.
Exposures to Infectious or Contagious Illnesses	
Have you recently been exposed to any infectious or contagious disease?	Impetigo, chickenpox, herpes, and other contagious disease cause skin rashes.
Have you been exposed to anyone with lice or scabies?	Exposures to infestations can cause skin and hair problems.
Immunizations	
What immunizations have you had; for example, MMR, varicella, hepatitis A and B?	Identifies likelihood of immunity against vaccine-preventable diseases that have associated skin changes.
Medications	
Are you taking any prescribed or OTC medications? Do you use recreational drugs?	Any medications can cause adverse skin reactions and allergic dermatitis. See box, Drugs That Adversely Affect the Integumentary System. Antimalarials may cause pigmentary changes; many others result in photophobia, rashes, or other skin effects. Use of specific medications points to diseases of other organs that may be associated with skin changes. For instance, insulin indicates a diagnosis of diabetes. Provides information on client's understanding of currently prescribed treatments.

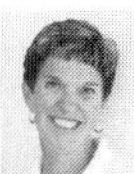

Case Study Findings

Mrs. Green's past health history reveals:

- Usual childhood diseases, without sequelae
- One miscarriage at 10 weeks' pregnancy, age 22
- Hospitalized for two childbirths, with uncomplicated vaginal deliveries and a cholecystectomy 2 years ago
- No history of allergies, skin disorders
- No recent exposures to persons with infections
- Unsure about immunization status. Received all immunizations in youth, but cannot recall later tetanus, others

Drugs That Adversely Affect the Integumentary System

Drug Class	Drug	Possible Adverse Reactions
Adrenocorticosteroids	methylprednisolone, prednisone	Urticaria, skin atrophy and thinning , acne, facial erythema, striae, allergic dermatitis, petechiae, ecchymoses
Anticonvulsants	carbamazepine	Pruritic rash, toxic epidermal necrolysis, Stevens-Johnson syndrome
	lamotrigine	Same as carbamazepine
	valproate	Alopecia
	phenytoin sodium	Morbilliform (measleslike) rash, excessive hair growth
	ethosuximide	Urticaria, pruritic (itchy) and erythematous (reddened) rashes
Antimalarial	chloroquine phosphate	Pruritus; pigmentary skin changes, eruptions resembling lichen planus (with prolonged therapy)

(Continued)

Drugs That Adversely Affect the Integumentary System *(Continued)*

Drug Class	Drug	Possible Adverse Reactions
Antineoplastic agents	bleomycin sulfate	Skin toxicity may be accompanied by hypoesthesia that may progress to hyperesthesia, urticaria, erythematous swelling, hyperpigmentation, patchy hyperkeratosis, alopecia
	busulfan	Cheilosis, melanoderma (increased melanin in the skin), urticaria, dry skin, alopecia, anhidrosis (absent or deficient sweating)
	cyclophosphamide	Skin and fingernail pigmentation, alopecia
Barbiturates	pentobarbital sodium, phenobarbital	Urticaria; maculopapular, morbilliform, or scarlatiniform rash
Cephalosporins	cefazolin sodium, cefoxitin sodium, cefuroxime sodium, ceftriaxone sodium, cefotaxime sodium	Rash, pruritus, urticaria, erythema multiforme
Gold salts	auranofin, gold sodium thiomalate	Rash, pruritus, photosensitivity, urticaria
Nonsteroidal anti-inflammatory agents	diflunisal	Rash, pruritus, erythema multiforme, Stevens-Johnson syndrome
	ibuprofen	Rash, erythema multiforme, Stevens-Johnson syndrome
	sulindac	Rash, pruritus, photosensitivity, erythema multiforme, Stevens-Johnson syndrome
Oral antidiabetic agents	all types	Photosensitivity, various skin eruptions
Penicillins	amoxicillin trihydrate, ampicillin, penicillin G potassium, penicillin V potassium, nafcillin, mezlocillin	Urticaria, erythema. maculopapular rash, pruritus
Phenothiazines	chlorpromazine hydrochloride, thioridazine hydrochloride, trifluoperazine hydrochloride	Dermatoses, pruritus, marked photosensitivity, urticaria, erythema, eczema, exfoliative dermatitis
Sulfonamides	co-trimoxazole, sulfamethoxazole, sulfasalazine, sulfisoxazole	Rash, pruritus, erythema nodosum, erythema multiforme, Stevens-Johnson syndrome, exfoliative dermatitis, photosensitivity
	griseofulvin	Rash, urticaria, photosensitivity, lupus erythematosus or lupuslike syndrome
Tetracyclines	demeclocycline hydrochloride, doxycycline hyclate tetracycline hydrochloride	Photosensitivity
Miscellaneous agents	allopurinol	Pruritic maculopapular rash, exfoliative dermatitis, urticaria, erythematous dermatitis
	captopril	Maculopapular rash, pruritus, erythema
	corticotropin (ACTH)	Urticaria, pruritus, scarlatiniform exanthema, skin atrophy and thinning, acne, facial erythema, hyperpigmentation
	oral contraceptives (estrogen	Chloasma or melasma, rash, urticaria, erythema
	thiazide diuretics	Photosensitivity
	lithium	Acne
	warfarin	Skin necrosis

Family History

The family history allows you to determine what, if any, integumentary problems are common to the client's family members. Diseases of the integument are as likely as others to have a familial predisposition. The history also helps to identify familial diseases that directly affect other systems and that might have some affect on the skin. This portion of the history also begins to explore the potential for problems stemming from the client's living environment.

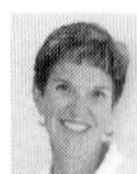

Case Study Findings

Mrs. Green's family history reveals:

- Mother died of breast cancer at age 65, had previously had 2 basal cell lesions removed.

Family History

RISK FACTORS/QUESTIONS TO ASK	RATIONALE/SIGNIFICANCE
Skin Disorders Do you have a family history of skin cancer, psoriasis, or eczema?	Identifies familial predisposition for skin disease that can be inherited.
Cardiovascular Disorders Do you have a family history of heart anomaly, output disorders, or peripheral vascular disease?	Identifies familial disorders that might affect skin.
Pulmonary Disorders Do you have a family history of asthma or other chronic lung diseases?	
GI Disorders Do you have a family history of liver or gallbladder disease?	
Endocrine Disorders Do you have a family history of diabetes or thyroid disorders?	
Immune Disorders Do you have a family history of allergies or autoimmune diseases such as lupus erythematosus?	Identifies familial tendencies and environmental triggers
Infectious/Contagious Diseases in Family Has anyone in your family recently had which an infectious or acontagious disorder?	Identifies contagious diseases to client has been exposed.

- Brother (45) has hypertension and a history of childhood asthma.
- Father (73) has "borderline high blood pressure" and adult onset diabetes but is in generally good health. He also had two basal cell cancers on his face and has several "sun spots."
- Two older siblings (49 and 50) are in generally good health, although one had a small malignant melanoma between two toes, which was surgically removed 3 weeks ago, with no lesions or spread detected.
- Children are both in good health.

Review of Systems

The review of systems is extremely important when exploring a complaint related to the integumentary system. It helps you identify problems in other systems that directly affect the skin, hair, and nails. Health problems directly affecting many systems can have profound effects on the integument. The review of systems is also useful in prompting the client to identify problems that he or she previously felt were not related or worth mentioning.

Review of Systems

SYSTEM/QUESTIONS TO ASK	RATIONALE/SIGNIFICANCE
General Health Survey Have you noticed a change in your energy level? Do you have fevers, weight changes or sweats?	Helps identify problems that are relatively nonspecific to any one system. Many endocrine and immune diseases present with this type of complaint.
Head, Eyes, Ears, Nose, and Throat (HEENT)/*Head/Neck/Throat* Do you have swollen glands/nodes, congestion, nasal discharge, sore throat, or sneezing?	Swollen glands or nodes may be associated with infectious or malignant cause of skin problems. Congestion and sore throat are common symptoms of several viral illnesses that typically cause skin changes.

(Continued)

Review of Systems *(Continued)*

SYSTEM/QUESTIONS TO ASK	RATIONALE/SIGNIFICANCE
Eyes	
Do you have watery or itchy eyes?	Congestion with watery/itchy eyes is common in atopic disorders that may be associated with urticaria, eczema, and other skin problems.
Respiratory	
Do you have a cough, wheezing, tightness in your chest, or difficulty breathing?	Chronic lung disorders such as emphysema and bronchitis may limit oxygenation to the point of cyanosis. Reversible airway disease (asthma) may be associated with atopic disorders of the skin.
Cardiovascular	
Do you have pain in your legs when walking (**claudication**), shortness of breath, difficulty breathing (**dyspnea**), chest pain, or palpitations?	Dyspnea, palpitations, and chest pain are seen with cardiac disease and result in poor output, which contributes to cyanosis. Claudication is common in vascular disorders and results in discoloration, hair loss, and ulceration of skin over lower extremities.
Gastrointestinal	
Do you have abdominal pain, loss of appetite, nausea/vomiting, jaundice, changes in bowel habits or in color of stool?	Abdominal pain, anorexia, nausea, changes in bowel habits and clay-colored stools occur with liver diseases. Liver disease can result in jaundice and pruritus.
Genitourinary	
Have you noticed a change in the color of your urine?	Dark orange urine is often seen with obstructive jaundice.
Do you have increased urination or burning?	UTIs are frequently seen in type II diabetes, which can lead to skin changes.
Are you incontinent?	Can cause dermatitis.
Female Reproductive	
When was your last menstrual period? Are they regular periods?	Menstrual irregularities are often found in endocrine disorders, including hypothyroidism and glucose intolerance.
Are you pregnant?	Pregnancy may explain localized changes in skin pigmentation.
Do you practice safe sex? Do you have any vaginal discharge?	Unprotected sex increases the risk for sexually transmitted diseases (STDs). Discharge may be associated with STD and may also cause skin lesions of genitalia or other skin.
Male Reproductive	
Do you practice safe sex? Do you have any penile discharge or rashes?	Unprotected sex increases the risk for STDs. Discharge may be associated with STD, which may also cause lesions on genitalia or other skin.
Musculoskeletal	
Do you have joint pain, swelling, or redness?	Common in some autoimmune disorders such as lupus and in infectious syndromes, such as Reiter's syndrome, that affect the skin. Gout is associated with development of **tophi**, uric acid deposits beneath the skin
Neurological	
Do you have numbness, tingling, or burning?	The altered sensation found in neuropathic disorders can predispose to skin injuries. Altered sensation is also found in some neurological disorders that result in skin dryness.
Immune/Hematologic	
Do you have any bleeding disorders, or are you on any anticoagulants?	Bleeding disorders or use of anticoagulants may result in vascular lesions such as petechiae, purpura, and ecchymosis.
Are you on any immunosuppressive drugs?	Immunosuppressive drugs can cause skin changes. For example, steroids can cause acne, decreased wound healing, ecchymosis, thinning of skin, hirsutism and petechiae.

Review of Systems *(Continued)*

SYSTEM/QUESTIONS TO ASK	RATIONALE/SIGNIFICANCE
Immune/Hematologic *(Continued)*	
Do you have any immune disorders?	Immune diseases such as lupus or HIV often have skin manifestations, such as Kaposi's sarcoma.
Endocrine	
Do you have increased thirst, frequent urination, fatigue, or weight loss?	Polyuria, polydipsia, polyphagia, fatigue and weight loss are common symptoms in diabetes, which alters the healing ability of the skin and promotes other changes through alterations in circulation and sensation.
Have you gained weight? Do you have energy loss or dry skin?	Fatigue and weight gain are commonly found in hypothyroid disorders, which result in dry skin and pruritus.

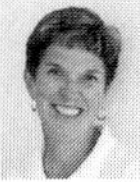

Case Study Findings

Mrs. Green's review of systems reveals:

- Feels well overall.
- Skin is somewhat dry; itches occasionally. No sores or rashes. Reports no changes in hair and nails.
- No problems with shortness or breath, congestion, dizziness, chest pain, runny nose/itchy eyes, cough, abdominal discomfort or nausea, joint pain (except mild after extensive gardening), change in urination or bowel habits.
- Last menstrual period was about 1.5 years ago. Before that they were regular until the final year, when they fluctuated a little.

Psychosocial Profile

The psychosocial profile serves several purposes. It provides important information regarding dietary and other habits, as well as occupational, social, and recreational activities that could influence the condition or health of the skin, hair, and nails. It provides an opportunity to explore the client's self-care and social activities, which may identify his or her response to an integumentary system problem.

Psychosocial Profile

CATEGORY/QUESTIONS TO ASK	RATIONALE/SIGNIFICANCE
Health Practices and Beliefs	
Do you get yearly physical exams?	Determines if your client takes preventative measures concerning skin care. Health promotion activities such as annual exams, self-examinations, and use of sunblock are proactive measures.
Do you examine your skin regularly for any unusual lesions, or changes in moles?	Helps determine health promotion and protective patterns. May identify teaching needs.
Self-Care Activities	
Do you use sunblock?	
How often do you bathe and shampoo your hair? What products do you normally use? How do you care for your nails? Do you use detergents or hair dyes?	Certain products or overuse of products can result in altered integrity or appearance of the skin, hair, and nails. Poor hygiene can also alter skin, hair, and nail integrity.
Typical Day	
How would you describe your typical day?	Identifies frequent exposure to chemicals, light, or temperature variations that affect skin.
Nutritional Patterns	
What did you eat and drink in the past 24 hours? What is your usual fluid intake?	Nutritional deficits and inadequate hydration can affect the skin. **Anorexia nervosa** can cause loss of hair and blotchy, sallow skin.

(Continued)

Psychosocial Profile *(Continued)*

CATEGORY/QUESTIONS TO ASK	RATIONALE/SIGNIFICANCE
Nutritional Patterns *(Continued)*	
What did you eat and drink in the past 24 hours? What is your usual fluid intake?	Diets high in yellow vegetables can cause **carotemia** (yellow-orange color of skin). Iron deficiency anemia can cause spoon nails and pallor.
What dietary supplements do you use?	Dehydration can cause dry skin.
Activity/Exercise Patterns	
Do you exercise routinely? What type of exercise do you do?	Exercise patterns may explain skin calluses, abrasions, potential for injuries and the need for education regarding safety and use of protection.
Recreation, Pets, Hobbies	
What type of recreational activities do you do?	Outdoor activities increase sun exposure and risk for skin cancers. Assess use of protection, such as sunscreens, hats.
Do you have any pets? What kind?	Allergies are frequently associated with animals. Pets may also be carriers of fleas and ticks, which can lead to infestation and skin irritations and disease.
Hobbies?	Chemicals associated with some hobbies may result in contact dermatitis.
Sleep/Rest Patterns	
How many hours of sleep do you get daily? Are you having any sleep problems?	Itching and other skin symptoms may result in altered sleep habits. Difficulty sleeping may also help identify other problems that might be associated with skin changes, including thyroid or renal diseases.
Personal Habits	
Do you smoke cigarettes? If so, how many/day and for how many years?	Tobacco causes vascular impairment with related skin changes. Cigarette smoking increases wrinkling of skin, and nicotine stains fingers and nails yellow.
Do you use recreational drugs or alcohol?	Alcohol abuse is a contributing factor for liver disease and related skin changes. Illegal drug use increases risk for hepatitis B, HIV, and other infectious diseases with associated skin changes.
Occupational Health Patterns	
What type of work do you do? Are you exposed to chemical irritants?	Identifies potential risks associated with client's occupation, as well as his or her understanding of proper use of protective devices and equipment.
Socioeconomic Status	
Do you have health insurance?	Determine available resources for client and determine if it has impact on his or her health care.
Environmental Health Patterns	
How would you describe your home environment?	Important in determining potential for exposures, including infestations of mites, lice, etc.
What type of heating and cooling do you use?	Ability to properly heat and cool a home or work setting influences skin integrity.
Roles/Relationships/Self-Concept	
Do you participate in group activities?	Groups increase risk for contracting contagious diseases.
Have any changes in your skin, hair, or nails affected your personal relationships?	Because skin, hair, and nails are so evident, alterations may cause some people to withdraw from or limit interaction with others.
Stress and Coping	
How much stress do you routinely have? How do you cope with stress?	Stress can trigger changes in skin, hair, and nails. Persons with alterations in the skin, hair, or nails may be embarrassed about their appearance, and this can add to usual stressors.

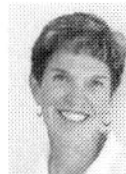

Case Study Findings

Mrs. Green's psychosocial profile includes:

- She bathes or showers daily, usually with very warm water. She shampoos her hair every other day and rarely uses any hair spray, mousse, or other products. She keeps her nails closely filed and wears clear polish. She wears cosmetics daily and has never had problems tolerating any brand. She colored her hair in the past, but does not do so at this time.
- She is often out in the Florida sun as she walks and gardens, but only occasionally wears sunscreen. She does not reapply the product when she has been out for an extended time, which often occurs. She thought that skin cancer was something she would worry about in old age; however, now that her sister has had skin cancer she has been worried about any damage she may have done to her skin.
- Typical day starts at 7 AM, when her alarm awakens her. On days when she works (2 to 3 days a week), she showers, dresses, eats breakfast, then works from 9 AM to 5 PM. On her off days, she cleans her house, works in the yard/garden when weather permits, and just "keeps busy" until about 5 PM. She then fixes dinner and watches TV or does needlework in the evening. She generally goes to bed at 10:30 to 11:00 PM.
- She eats three meals daily, including foods from all categories. She feels that she should lose 10 to 15 lb, which she has gradually gained over the past 10 years. She tries to remember to drink several glasses of water daily, but sometimes only drinks one or two 8-oz glasses.
- Gardening is one of her main forms of exercise. She also walks 2 or 3 miles a day, 3 or 4 times a weeks.
- She sleeps very well, with rare interruptions to void (2 to 3 times/week).
- Her only medications are those mentioned earlier. She drinks 1 cup of coffee and 4–5 glasses of iced tea daily. She rarely drinks colas. She has never smoked but used to be exposed to cigarette smoke until her husband quit 5 years ago. She does not drink alcohol or use recreational drugs.
- She is not exposed to chemicals or unusual environmental situations at work. She uses various chemicals in her gardening (fertilizers, pesticides, weed killers) and doesn't always wear gloves, masks, or other protective equipment.
- She has no pets. She has lived in her current home, a ranch style, for 12 years. The home is very adequate for her needs, and has central heat and air conditioning.
- She enjoys meeting customers at work and has several close friends with whom she often has lunch or shops. She and her husband have a very close and caring relationship. She has good relationships with her two children, who live nearby. Her father and siblings live 600 miles away, but she sees them 2 or 3 times a year for an enjoyable visit. She is not currently involved in any specific community group and rarely attends church.

▸ Focused Integumentary History

If your client's condition or time prohibits a detailed integumentary history, ask the following questions:

- Do you have any changes in your skin, hair, or nails? (If yes, ask questions following the PQRST format.)
- Do you have any food, drug, or environmental allergies?
- Do you have any medical problems?
- Are you on any medications, prescribed or over-the-counter?

Case Study Evaluation

Before you proceed with the physical examination of the skin, hair, and nails, document the key information you have learned from Mrs. Green's health history and the integumentary history related to her.

CRITICAL THINKING ACTIVITY #1

What history findings put Mrs. Green at risk for skin problems?

CRITICAL THINKING ACTIVITY #2

What strengths can you identify that will help Mrs. Green adapt to or prevent skin disorders?

Physical Assessment

Once you have taken the history, proceed to collect objective data through your physical examination. Even though the skin, hair, and nails are easily accessible and we look at them every day, you still need to be very objective and attentive to details that could easily be overlooked.

Approach

The techniques used in the examination of the integument are inspection and palpation. As you conduct the assessment, along with your sense of sight and touch, use your sense of smell to note any unusual odors. It is important to inspect all areas of skin, including **intertriginous** areas, which lie between or under folds of skin. Throughout the examination, compare symmetrical parts. Also be aware of the "feel" of the skin, hair, and nails. You can inspect the skin in one of three ways:

1. Using a head-to-toe approach
2. Observing all skin on the anterior, posterior, and lateral surfaces of the body
3. Inspecting the skin by regions, as you examine the cardiovascular, respiratory, and other systems

Regardless of your approach, a complete examination is necessary and a systematic approach will help you avoid omissions. During the examination, keep in mind the underlying structures or organs because they may explain changes in the overlying skin. Also compare exposed to unexposed areas. Variations might be signs of "wear and tear," poor alignment or injury, or they may indicate the need for further history.

Toolbox

The tools necessary for this assessment include gloves, a flexible transparent ruler, a marker, a penlight, a glass slide, and a magnifier. Good overall lighting is important. The examination area must be adequately screened to provide privacy, and the person must be adequately covered or draped with only the area being immediately examined exposed at any particular time. Also make sure the room temperature is comfortable. Examination in an overly warm or cold environment may alter the skin's condition. For example, if the room is cold, it can change the surface texture of the skin or lead to peripheral cyanosis; if the room is too warm, the skin may become flushed.

Performing a General Survey

A general survey of the integumentary system is typically done while obtaining the health history. Be attentive to any signs that suggest alterations in the integrity of the skin, hair, and nails. During the early observation phase, note general skin coloring, as well as any obvious variations by region. Coloring is a highly variable feature, even among people of the same race or ethnic background. Variations can indicate sun or chemical exposure, emotional responses, illness, or just a personal characteristic. Also observe the general distribution of the hair, including its condition, color, and sheen. Note the general condition of the nails. The examination also relies on your sense of smell and touch. Be attentive for any unusual odors. As you shake the client's hand or take vital signs, check the temperature and moisture of the skin.

In addition, consider the client's overall skin condition in comparison with his or her stated age. If the skin appears chronologically older, it may have been aged by chronic illness, substance use, or environmental exposures. Exposure to sunlight increases the risk of malignancy; exposure to chemicals increases the risk for various forms of dermatitis.

Also do the following:

- Determine the client's overall nutritional status. Signs of nutritional deficiencies are often evident on inspection of the skin, hair, or nails.
- Note the client's apparent emotional status. This provides insight into his or her ability to cope with any real or perceived disfigurement associated with alterations in the integument. It may also suggest the likelihood that lesions might be self-inflicted
- Be aware of the client's overall body habitus—weight distribution, posture, and muscle mass. Besides providing information on nutritional status, this suggests other health problems that influence the skin. For instance, a person who has truncal obesity and a tripod posture (sitting leaning forward on elbows) may have chronic lung disease requiring systemic corticosteroid treatment. Lung disease may be reflected by nail clubbing and cyanosis; corticosteroid therapy may cause the skin to thin and become friable.
- Obtain the client's vital signs. Elevations in temperature may indicate an infection that might be accompanied by a rash or other skin lesion.

Performing a Head-to-Toe Physical Assessment

Next, do a head-to-toe survey, checking for more specific signs of diseases affecting other organ systems that might alter the skin, hair, or nails.

Performing a Head-to-Toe Physical Assessment

SYSTEM/NORMAL FINDINGS	ABNORMAL FINDINGS/RATIONALE
General Health Survey *INSPECT* Awake, alert, and oriented.	*Confusion and irritability:* May indicate hypoxia due to cyanosis.

Performing a Head-to-Toe Physical Assessment *(Continued)*

SYSTEM/NORMAL FINDINGS	ABNORMAL FINDINGS/RATIONALE
Memory intact. Able to provide adequate history.	*Inability to recall information/ provide history:* May indicate neurological disorders that cause impaired judgment and altered sensation, placing skin at risk for injury. *Lethargy/somnolence?* May indicate a variety of disorders including disease of thyroid, liver, kidney, or cardiovascular or neurological systems, which may be reflected in skin.
HEENT/*Head* *INSPECT/PALPATE* Facial movements symmetrical	Facial expression and movements often reflect neurological or psychological diseases. For example, pruritus may be associated with depression and neurotic excoriations. Depression may also show in the client's facial expression.
HEENT/*Neck* No neck vein distention	*Neck vein distention:* Altered cardiac function that could be reflected with cyanosis of skin.
No unexplained hypertrophy of neck accessory muscles	*Hypertrophy of neck muscles:* Normal in a person who lifts weights. Otherwise, suggests chronic pulmonary disease, with potential for cyanosis or ruddy skin.
No palpable or visible cervical nodes	*Palpable/visible nodes:* May indicate infectious process or malignancy that could cause skin rashes, pruritus.
Thyroid not palpable	*Palpable thyroid:* Hyper- or hypothyroidism, both of which cause integumentary changes.
Eyes • Clear and bright; no lesions or edema	*Sclera icterus (yellow sclera):* Jaundice. *Exophthalmos:* Hyperthyroidism with associated skin changes.
Nose/Throat Nares patent, nasal mucosa pink, no nasal drainage, oral mucous membranes pink	*Red, swollen mucous membranes:* Allergy or infection. Infections

(Continued)

Performing a Head-to-Toe Physical Assessment *(Continued)*

SYSTEM/NORMAL FINDINGS	ABNORMAL FINDINGS/RATIONALE
Nose/Throat (Continued)	such as streptococcal infection or or mononucleosis can cause a macular rash.
Respiratory *INSPECT/PALPATE/PERCUSS/AUSCULTATE* Respiratory rate within normal limits. Respiratory movements symmetrical and unlabored. Breath sounds clear without adventitious sounds. Percussion tones resonant and palpable. Fremitus within normal range.	*Tachypnea:* Respiratory distress. *Asymmetrical or labored respiratory movements:* Pneumothorax or chronic restrictive lung diseases. *Crackles, wheezes, rhonchi, or bronchial breath sounds:* Altered pulmonary function. *Dull percussion tones/increased fremitus:* Consolidation within pulmonary tissue. *Hyperresonant percussion tones and decreased/absent fremitus:* Emphysemic changes. All of these respiratory alterations have the potential to impair oxygenation and cause cyanosis. Chronic cardiopulmonary disease with hypoxia can result in clubbing.
Cardiovascular *INSPECT* Extremities pink, warm, and dry, +2 pulses, no edema.	*Thin, shiny, hairless, cool skin with decreased pulses:* Arterial insufficiency. *Peripheral edema, leathery skin with cyanosis and brownish discoloration:* Venous insufficiency.
AUSCULTATE Radial and apical pulses within normal limits. S_1 and S_2 present and regular. No extra or adventitious heart sounds.	*Tachycardia:* Respiratory with impaired oxygenation, causing cyanosis. *Irregular heart rate/extra or adventitious heart sounds:* Cardiovascular disease impairs cardiac output and/or peripheral oxygenation, causing altered skin appearance and integrity, such as diaphoresis and cyanosis.
Gastrointestinal *INSPECT/PALPATE* Abdomen round, soft, nondistended, nontender, no organomegaly, positive bowel sounds.	*Hepatomegaly:* May cause jaundice and pruritus.

Performing a Head-to-Toe Physical Assessment *(Continued)*

SYSTEM/NORMAL FINDINGS	ABNORMAL FINDINGS/RATIONALE
Reproductive	
INSPECT	
External genitalia pink, intact, no lesions.	*Genital warts (acuminatum condyloma):* human papillomavirus.
INSPECT	
External genitalia pink, intact, no lesions.	*Burning, itching, vesicles:* Herpes simplex II.
Musculoskeletal/Neurological	
Grade 5 muscle strength, no atrophy, sensations intact, +2 deep tendon reflexes (DTR).	*Decreased sensation/DTR:* Associated with neuropathy, which increases risk for injury to skin.

Case Study Findings

Before you proceed to a focused examination of the integumentary system, review what you discovered during your general survey and head-to-toe assessment of Mrs. Green.

Mrs. Green's physical assessment findings include:

- **General Health Survey:** Well-developed, 48-year-old, fair-skinned woman, appearance consistent with stated age. Awake, alert, oriented × 3, memory intact. No signs of distress, appears comfortable and provides history with no difficulty.
- **Vital Signs:** Height 5'4"; weight 138 pounds; temperature 97.4 F; pulse 82 and regular; respirations 14 and unlabored; BP 134/82, left arm.
- **HEENT:** No neck vein distention; thyroid not palpable; no palpable nodes; eyes clear and bright; nares patent; mucous membranes pink and intact, no drainage.
- **Respiratory:** Lungs clear to auscultation (CTA), no adventitious sounds.
- **Cardiovascular:** +2 pulses, heart/rhythm regular, no extra sounds.
- **Gastrointestinal:** Positive bowel sounds; abdomen soft, nontender; liver nonpalpable.
- **Reproductive:** External genitalia skin intact with no lesions.
- **Musculoskeletal/Neurological:** +5 equal muscle strength, sensations intact, no edema.

Performing a Focused Integumentary Assessment

Once the general survey and head-to-toe assessment arecompleted, begin the focused examination of the skin, hair, and nails, using inspection and palpation. For purposes of simplicity, inspection and palpation are discussed separately below. However, rather than inspecting all areas of skin, hair, and nails, and then palpating all areas and suspicious lesions, you are more likely to inspect and palpate specific areas almost simultaneously. As you read the following information, keep in mind that areas that vary from normal should be explored using palpation.

Assessing the Skin

Use inspection and palpation to examine the skin.

Inspection

Examine the client's skin, noting color, odor, and the presence of lesions. Once you have determined the client's overall skin coloring, take a moment to decide if the coloring suggests something other than a normal variation.

Assessing Color

In addition to alterations in general coloring, it is normal for various *regions* of a person's skin to differ in color, depending primarily on the amount of exposure to light. These variations are generally symmetrical. If you notice that one area—for instance, the shoulders or arms—is darker than other areas—such as the anterior chest or buttocks—make sure that the difference is symmetrical or explained. For instance, a long-distance truck driver's left arm might be darker than the right because that arm receives greater sun exposure during daylight driving hours.

Inspection of the Skin

ASSESS/NORMAL VARIATIONS	ABNORMAL FINDINGS/RATIONALE
Color Uniform skin color with slightly darker exposed areas. Ethnic/racial differences account for many variations in skin color. Mucous membranes and conjunctiva pink.	Color changes may be benign or indicate underlying pathology

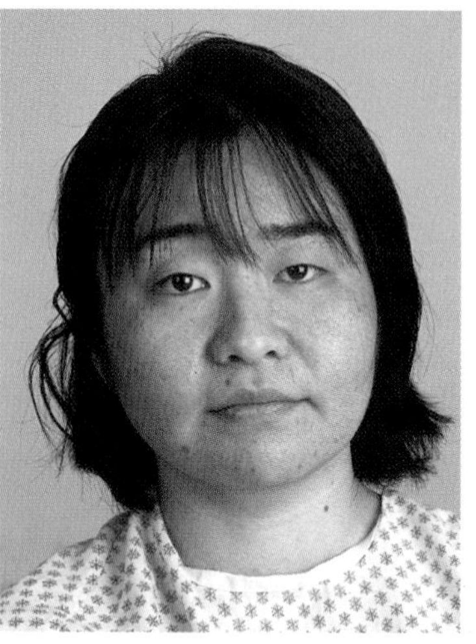

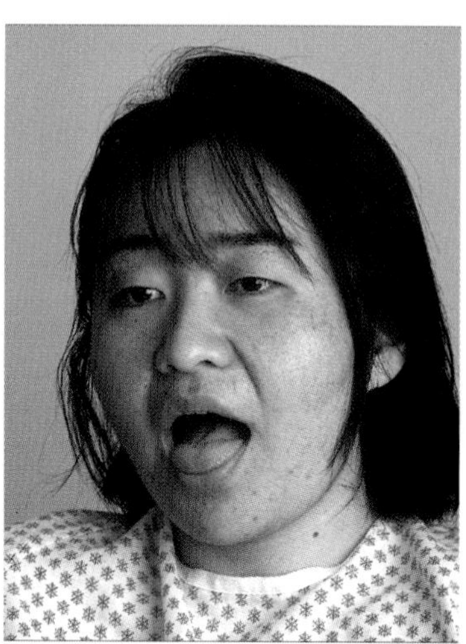

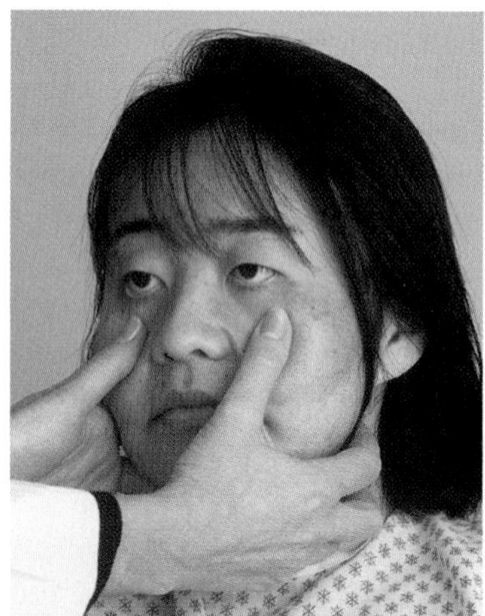

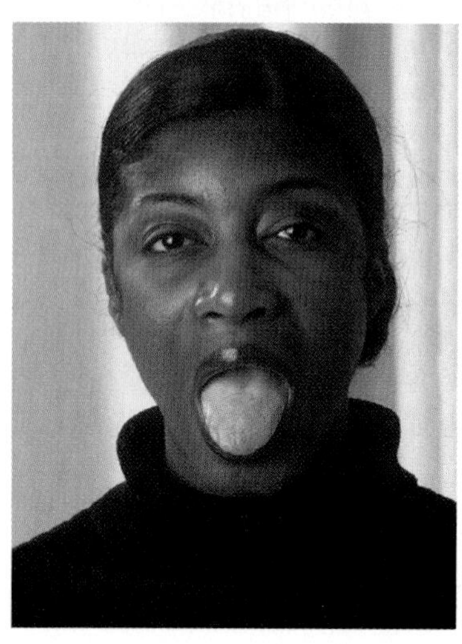

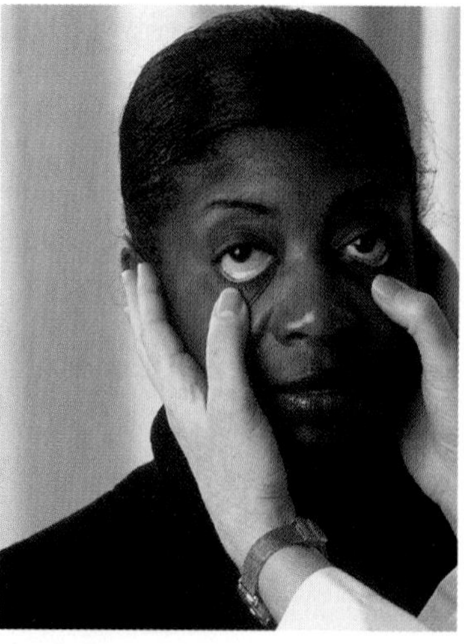

HELPFUL HINT

When assessing for color changes in dark-skinned clients, check oral mucous membranes.

Inspection of the Skin

ASSESS/NORMAL VARIATIONS	ABNORMAL FINDINGS/RATIONALE
Odor No unusual odor	*Unusual body odor:* Poor hygiene or underlying disease. If from poor hygiene, may be related to self-care deficit that warrants nursing intervention. *Odors from excessive sweating (hyperhydrosis):* Possible thyrotoxicosis. *Odors from night sweats:* Possible tuberculosis. *Urine odor:* Incontinence problem. Stale urine odor may be associated with uremia. *Mousy odor:* Liver disease.
Lesions No skin lesions No vascular lesions	Classify lesion as primary or secondary. Primary lesion is an initial alteration in the skin. Secondary lesion arises from a change in a primary lesion. A thorough description of lesions should include: *Morphological (clinical) description:* Size Shape Color Texture Surface relationship Exudate Tenderness *Configuration* *Location and Distribution* *For vascular lesions, also note:* Pulsations Blanching

Skin Color Variations

Color/Cause/Description | **Example**

Bronzing/Tanning
- Addison's disease/adrenal insufficiency: generalized, most evident over exposed areas
- Hemochromatosis: Generalized, may be gray-brown coloring

Tan
- Chloasma: "Mask of pregnancy" (on face)
- Lupus: Butterfly rash on face
- Scleroderma: Generalized tanning/yellowing of skin, associated with loss of elasticity

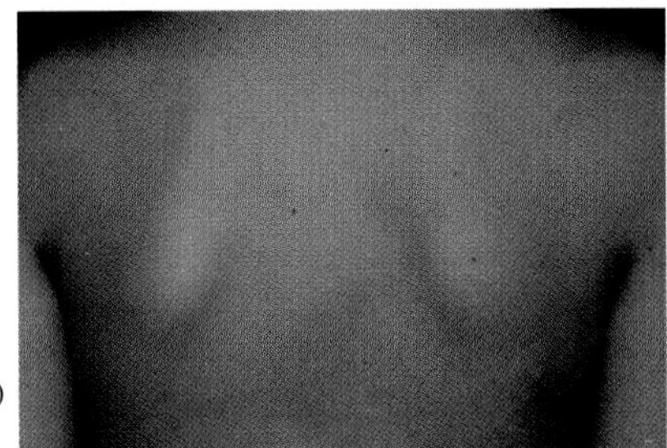

Addison's disease

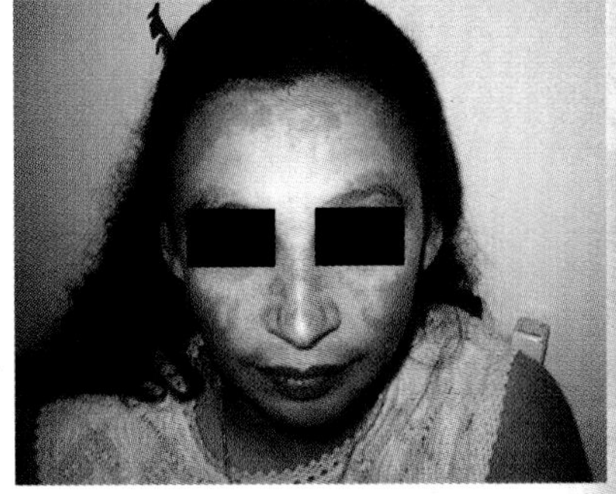

Chloasma

(Continued)

Skin Color Variations *(Continued)*

Color/Cause/Description | **Example**

Tan *(Continued)*
- Ichthyosis: With coarse scaliness
- Sprue: Tan/brown patches of any area
- Tinea versicolor: Fawn color or yellow patchy

Yellow
- Uremia: Generalized
- Liver disease, such as hepatitis, cirrhosis, liver cancer, gallbladder disease with obstructive jaundice: Generalized
- Carotemia: Not found in conjunctiva or sclera

Dusky Blue
- Arsenic poisoning: Paler spots on trunk and extremities
- Central cyanosis with hypoxia; peripheral cyanosis from vasoconstriction: caused by cold exposure or vascular disease

HELPFUL HINTS
- Jaundice from liver disease is seen in the sclera and conjunctiva, whereas pseudojaundice—yellow color variations associated with carotemia—is seen on the skin but not in the eyes.
- When differentiating peripheral cyanosis (caused by vasoconstriction or decreased circulation) from central cyanosis (caused by hypoxia), check the oral mucous membranes and conjunctiva. Cyanotic mucous membranes and conjunctiva indicate a central process.

Pallor
- Anemia: Also on conjunctiva and mucous membranes
- Vitiligo: Patchy
- Albinism: Generalized

Red
- Polycythemia
- Erythema: Dilated superficial capillaries, such as rosacea

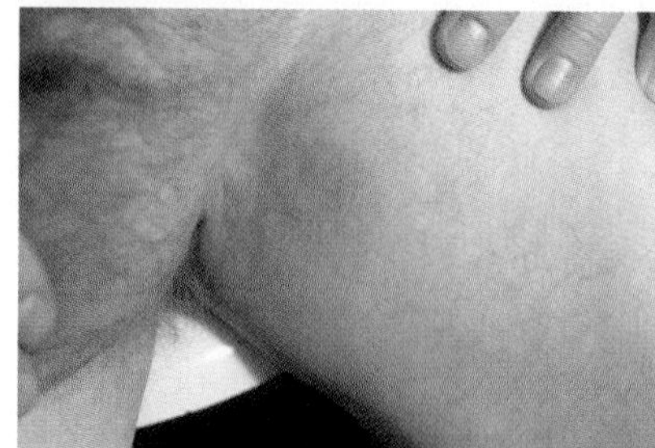
Tinea versicolor

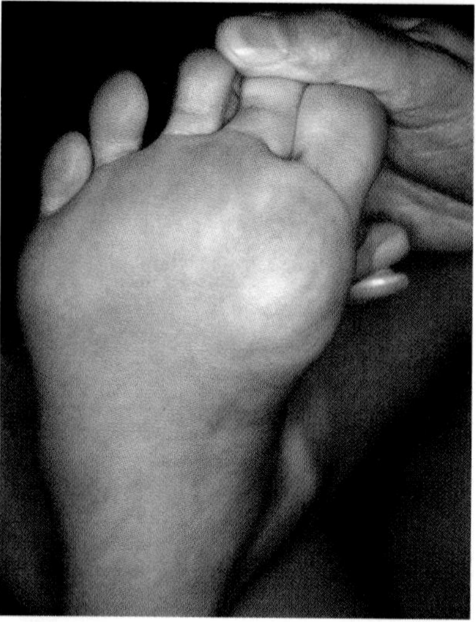
Carotemia

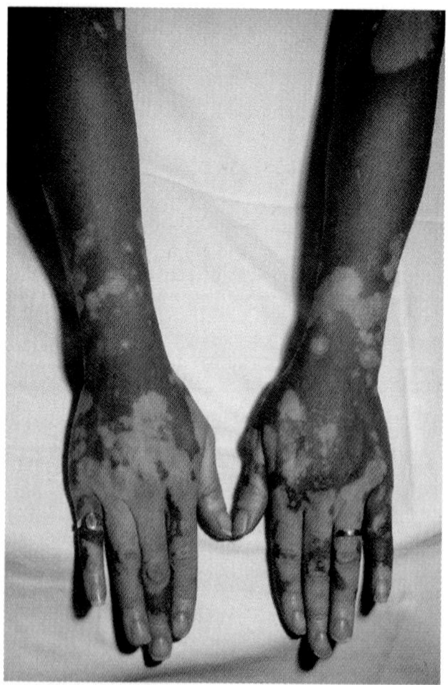
Vitiligo

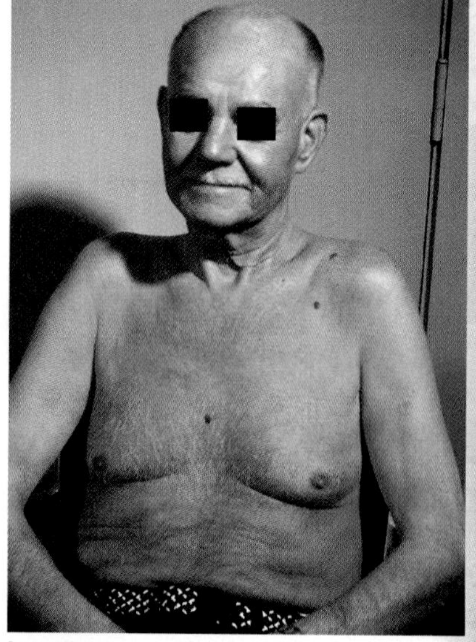
Jaundice

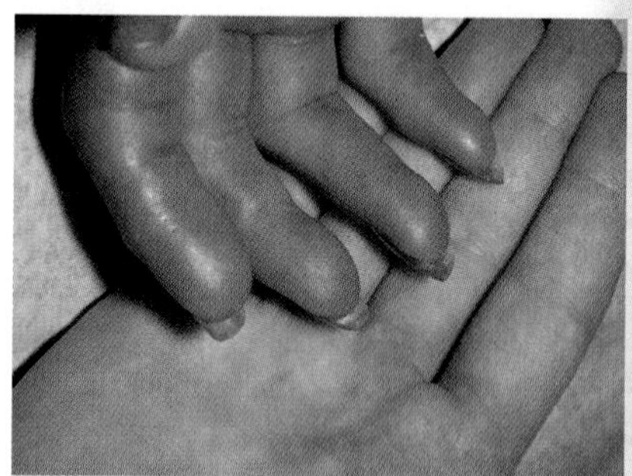
Cyanosis

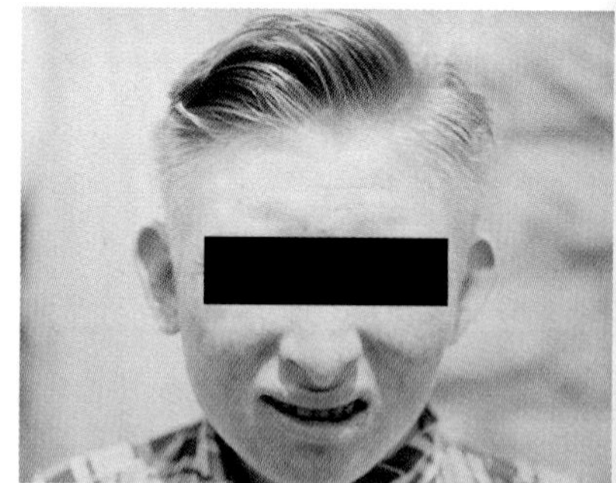
Albinism

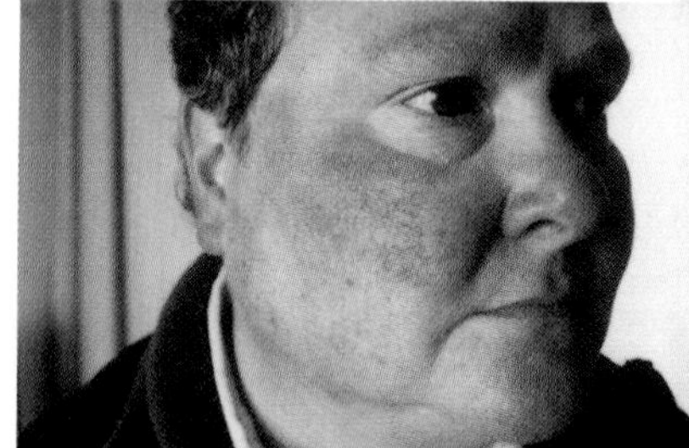
Erythema

Assessing Lesions

The skin should be a continuous tissue, and so note breaks, erosions or lesions. Document localized and/or pigmented variations, including moles, freckles, or vascular lesions, and examine them closely.

Use a flashlight or penlight and a magnifier to determine the surface, pigmentary, or border characteristics of many lesions, particularly when they are small. Besides providing brighter light to a specific skin area, the penlight or flashlight can also be used to shed tangential or oblique light to a lesion. *Tangential lighting* will cause the distal edge of the lesion to cast a shadow if the lesion is raised. Another use of the light is to transilluminate a lesion. For very small lesions, you will need either a small beam penlight or transilluminator attachment for an otoscope or ophthalmoscope. Transillumination of a raised lesion helps determine whether the lesion is solid or fluid filled. Fluid-filled lesions have a yellow or pink glow, whereas solid lesions do not.

Use a transparent ruler with centimeter markings to measure any lesions you detect. Clean the ruler after each use, using the method recommended by your facility. Either the transparent ruler or a glass slide can be used as a diascope to determine whether or not a vascular lesion blanches. Press the ruler or slide gently against the lesion, noting whether it blanches or pales with the pressure. Vascular lesions are red to purple in color. They may be caused by an **extravasation** of blood into the skin tissue or by visible superficial vascular irregularities.

Continues on page 163

Clinical Description of Lesions

Characteristic	Significance
Size	Major determinant of correct category for primary lesions. Pigmented lesions are typically <0.5 cm. If larger, consider potential for malignancy. Depth of pressure ulcers is major determinant of assigned grade (see box, Staging Criteria for Pressure Ulcers, pages 163–164)
Shape	Macules, wheals, and vesicles are circumscribed. Fissures are linear. Irregular borders are associated with melanoma.
Color	Varies widely, and many changes are diagnostic of specific skin diseases. Variegated-colored lesions may signal melanoma. Pustules are usually yellow-white. New scars are red and raised; old scars, white or silver. Petechiae are red. Purpura are red to purplish. Vitiligo is white
Texture	Macules are smooth. Warts are rough. Psoriasis is scaly.
Surface Relationship	Surface characteristics help differentiate potential causes of a change and between various primary and secondary lesions. *Flat (nonpalpable):* Macules, patches, purpura, ecchymoses, spider angioma, venous spider. *Raised (palpable) solid:* Papules, plaques, nodules, tumors, wheals, scale, crust. *Raised (palpable) cystic:* Vesicles, pustules, bullae, cysts. *Depressed:* Atrophy, erosion, ulcer, fissures. *Pedunculated:* Skin tags, cutaneous horns.
Exudate	*Clear or pale, straw-yellow exudate:* Serous oozing/weeping from noninfected lesion. *Thicker, purulent discharge:* Infected lesion. Clear serous exudates: Vesicles, as seen with herpes simplex; or bullae, larger than vesicles, as seen with second-degree burns. *Yellow pus exudates:* Pustules, as seen with impetigo or acne.
Tenderness or Pain	Tenderness or pain associated with a lesion depends on the underlying cause. May be associated with bullae from a burn or ecchymoses (bruise).

Vascular Lesions

Lesion/Causes/Description	Example
Ecchymosis • Extravasation of blood into skin layer • Caused by trauma/injury • Does not blanch	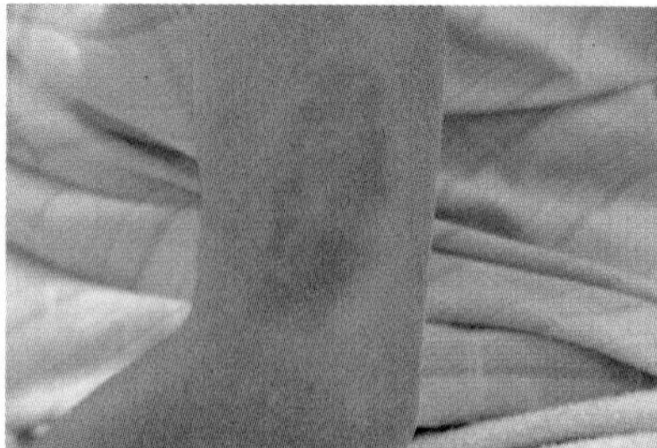 Ecchymosis
Petechiae or purpura • Extravasations of blood into skin • Caused by steroids, vasculitis, systemic diseases • Does not blanch	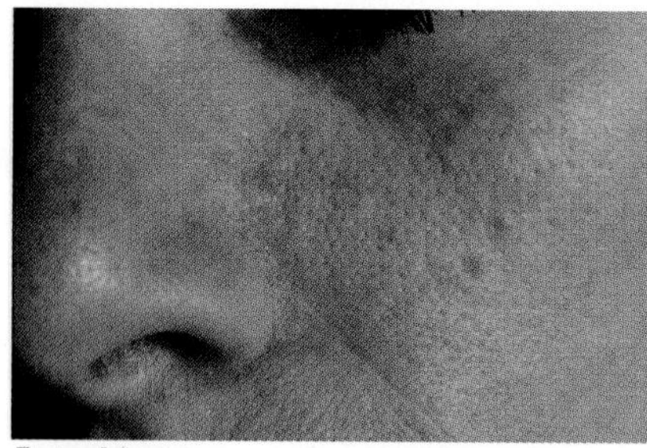 Petechiae
Venous star • Blue color • Irregularly shaped, linear, spider • Does not blanch • Cause by increased pressure on superficial veins	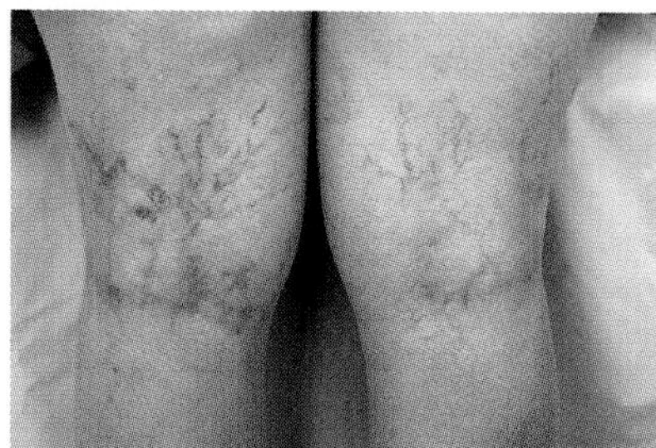 Venous star
Telangiectasia • Red color • Very fine and irregular vessels • Blanches • Seen with dilation of capillaries	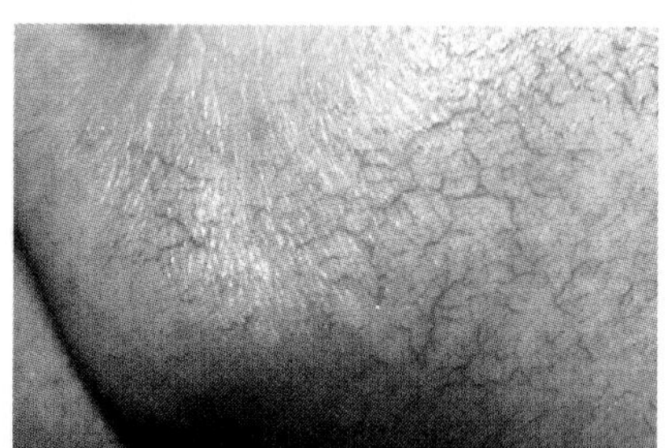 Telangiectasia
Spider angioma • Red color, type of telangiectasis • Looks like a spider, with central body and fine radiating legs • Blanches; seen in liver disease, vitamin B deficiencies, idiopathic origin	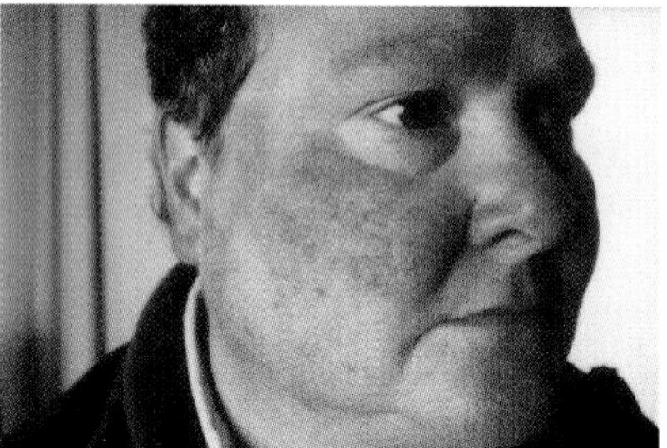 Spider angioma
Capillary hemangioma • Red color • Irregular-shaped macular patch	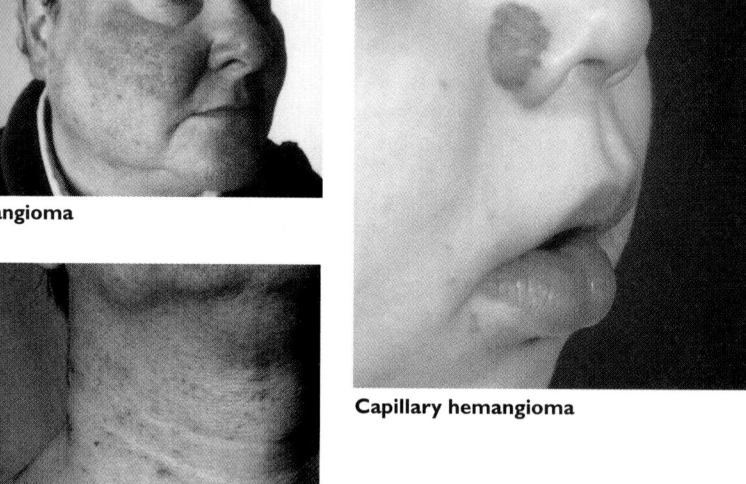 Capillary hemangioma
Port-wine stain • Red color • Does not blanch • Seen with dilation of dermal capillaries	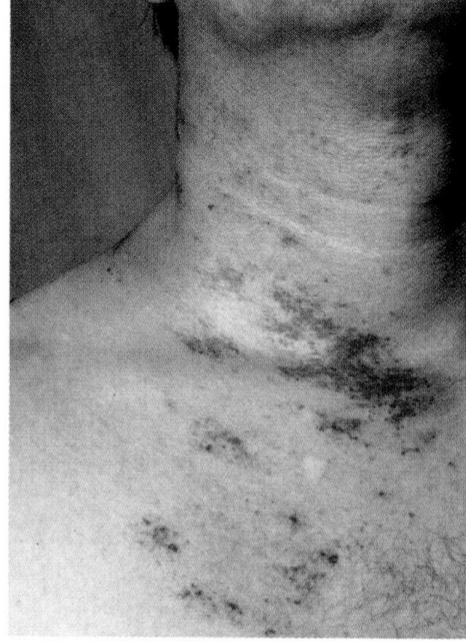 Port-wine stain

HELPFUL HINT

Pressure ulcers often develop over bony prominences, such as the sacrum and heels, so inspect these areas carefully.

ALERT

Extensive undermining often occurs, extending through the dermal layer to the bone. The visible pressure ulcer may be only the tip of the iceberg.

RISK FACTORS FOR PRESSURE ULCERS

- Impaired mental status
- Impaired nutritional status
- Sensory deficits
- Immobility
- Mechanical forces
- Shearing and friction
- Excessive exposure to moisture from bodily secretions

Staging Criteria for Pressure Ulcers

Stage	Appearance	Characteristics
Stage I	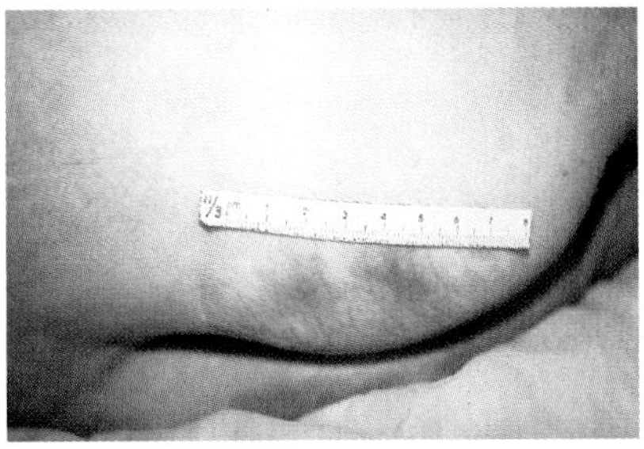	Nonblanchable erythema of intact skin; indicates potential for ulceration.
Stage II	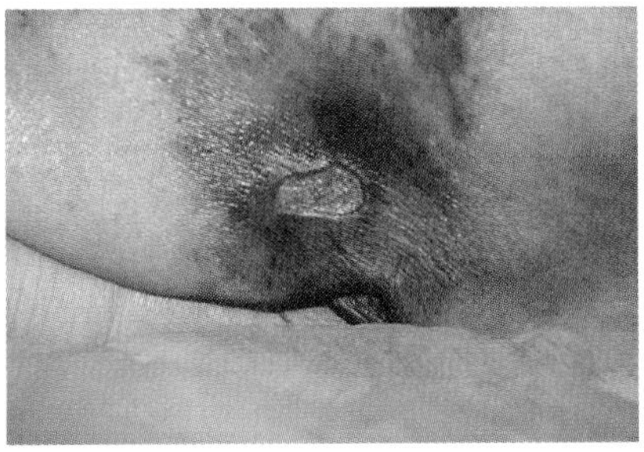	Partial thickness loss involving both epidermis and dermis. Ulcer is still superficial and appears as a blister, abrasion, or very shallow crater.
Stage III	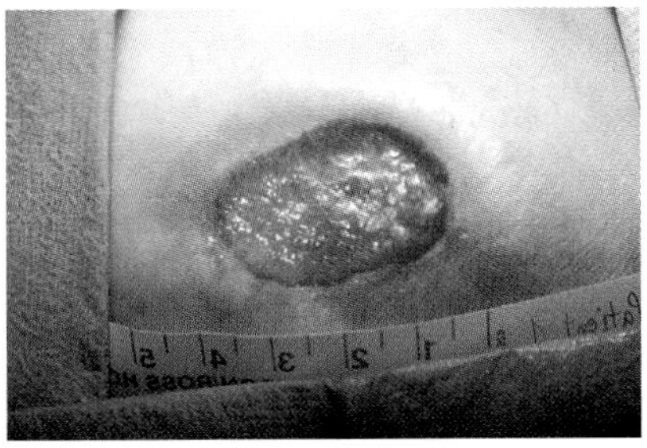	Full-thickness loss involving subcutaneous tissue. Ulcer may extend to but not through fascia. A deep crater that may undermine adjacent tissues.

(Continued)

Staging Criteria for Pressure Ulcers *(Continued)*

Stage	Appearance	Characteristics
Stage IV		Full-thickness loss with extensive involvement of muscle, bone, or supporting structures. This deep ulcer may involve undermining and sinus tracts of adjacent tissues.
Stage V		Ulcers that are covered with eschar cannot be staged without débridement.

If you detect a lesion, inspect it closely and palpate it to determine its characteristics. Decide whether it represents a primary or secondary skin lesion. A *primary lesion* is one that appears in response to some change in the internal or external environment of the skin and is not altered by trauma. Primary lesions are categorized by whether or not they are raised and by their overall dimensions. Different sources use different dimensions (0.5 cm or 1.0 cm) to determine the "cutoff" at which a lesion is given one label or another. This text uses 1.0 cm as the dimension at which lesions are differentiated.

Continues on page 167

Primary Lesions

Surface Characteristics	Lesion	Example
Flat, nonpalpable *Examples:* Cherry angioma Freckle Flat mole Lentigines Melanoma Petechiae Scarlet fever	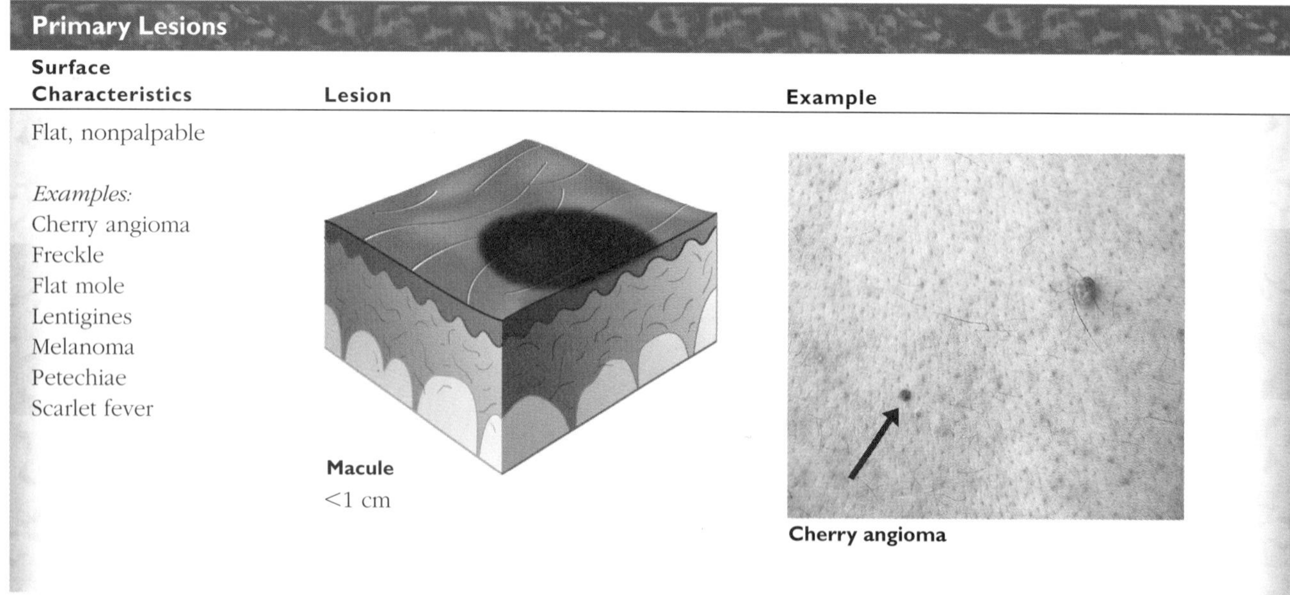 **Macule** <1 cm	**Cherry angioma**

Primary Lesions *(Continued)*

Surface Characteristics	Lesion	Example
Flat, nonpalpable *(Continued)* *Examples:* Birthmark Café-au-lait spot Chloasma Mongolian spot Port-wine stain Tinea versicolor Vitiligo	Patch >1 cm	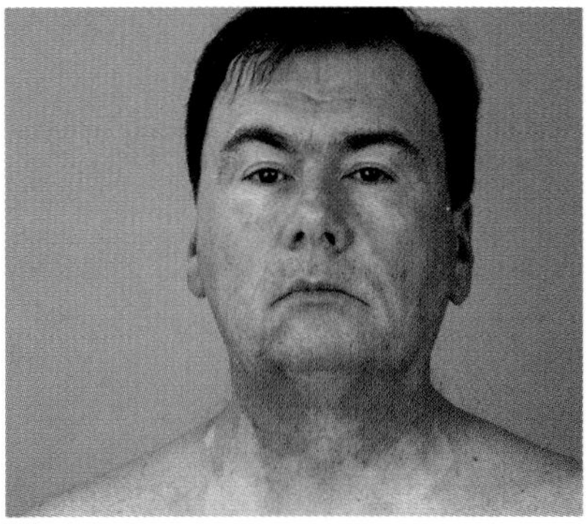 **Vitiligo**
Palpable, raised, but superficial *Examples:* Baisal cell carcinoma Kaposi's sarcoma Lichen planus Psoriasis Raised mole Seborrheic keratosis	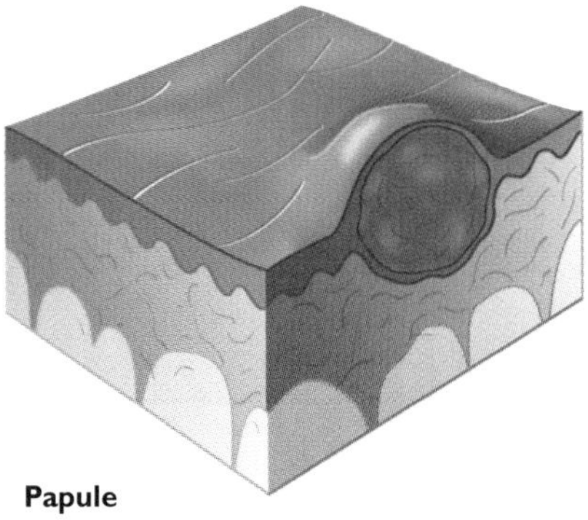 **Papule** <1 cm	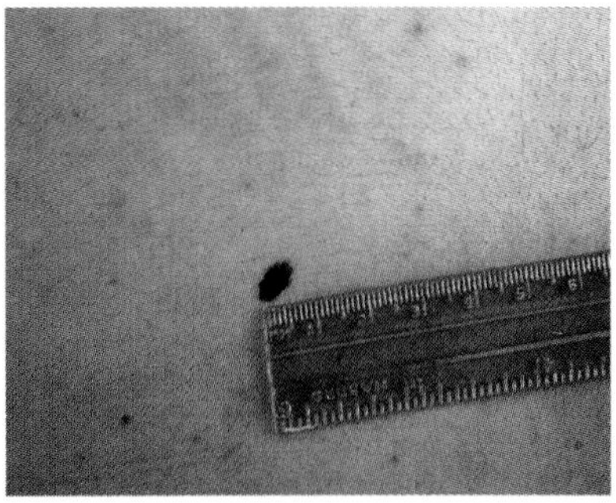 **Mole**
	Plaque >1 cm	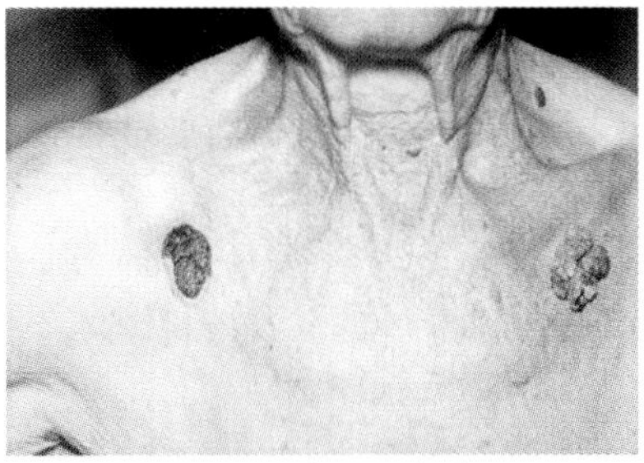 **Seborrheic keratosis, psoriasis**
Raised, superficial *Examples:* Allergic reaction Hives (urticaria) Insect bite	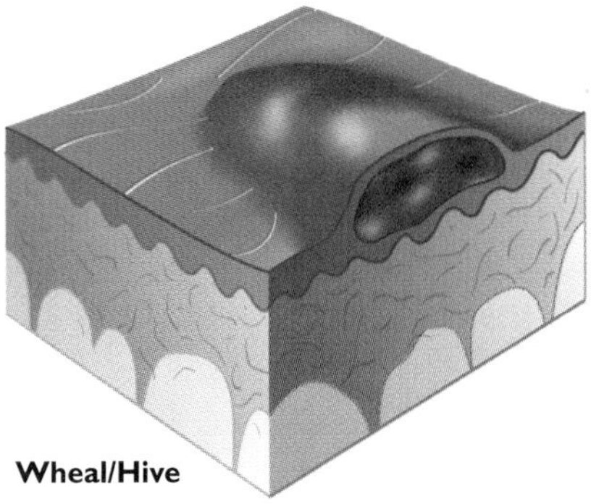 **Wheal/Hive**	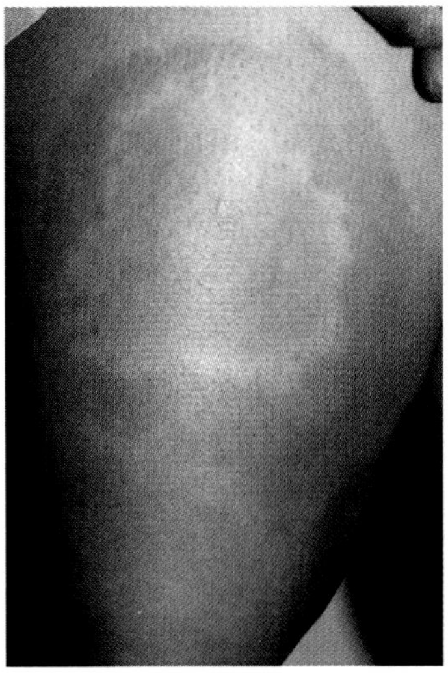 **Transient lesion (hive)**

(Continued)

Primary Lesions *(Continued)*

Surface Characteristics	Lesion	Example
Palpable, solid with depth into dermis *Examples:* Bartholin's cyst Erythema nodosum Keratogenous cyst Lipoma Xanthoma	Nodule <2 cm If fluid filled and encapsulated, called a cyst 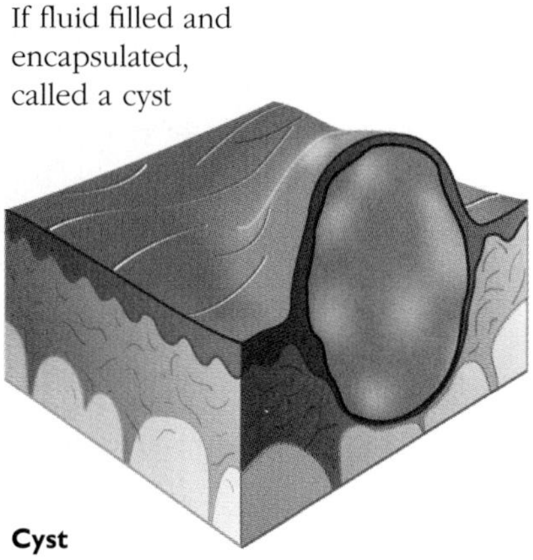 **Cyst**	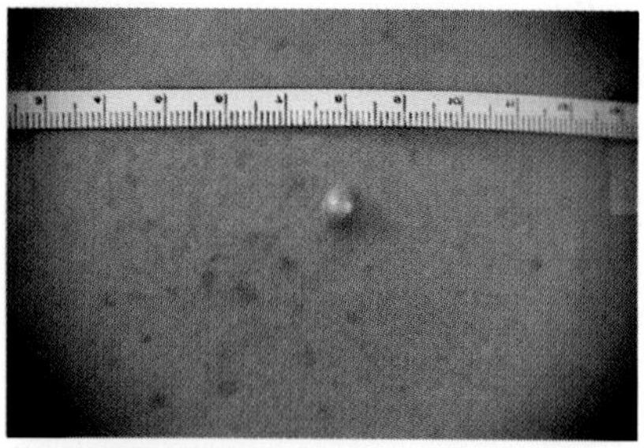 **Keratogenous cyst**
	Tumor >2 cm	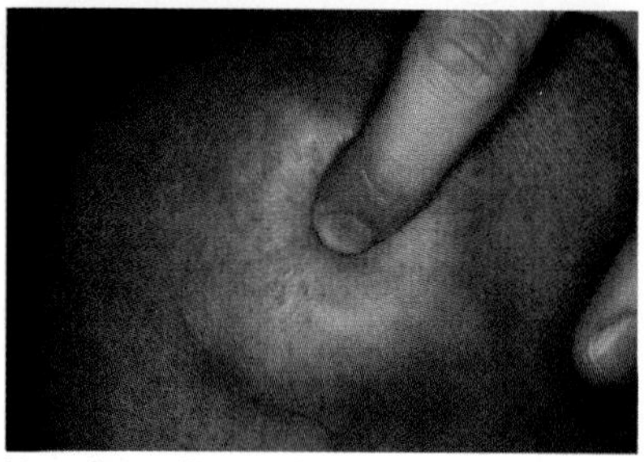 **Neoplasm (lipoma)**
Palpable, fluid filled *Examples:* Blister Contact dermatitis Herpes simplex	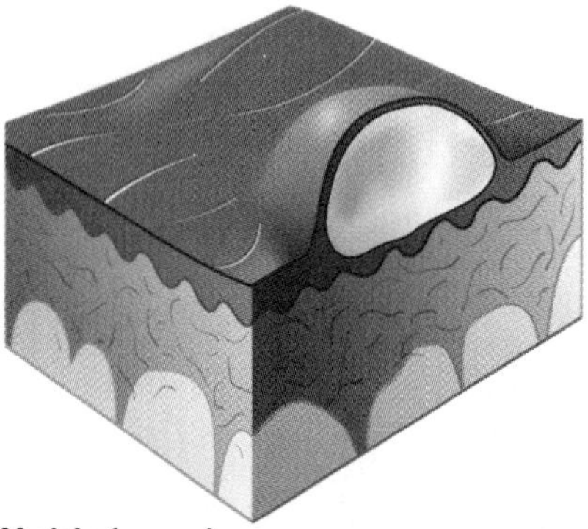 **Vesicle (serous)** <1 cm	Blister, herpes simplex, contact dermatitis 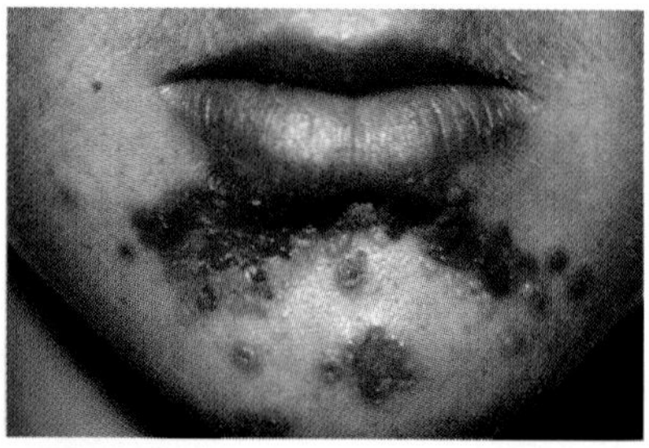 **Herpes simplex**
Examples: Blister Burn Contact dermatitis	Bulla (serous) >1 cm	Blister, contact dermatitis, burns 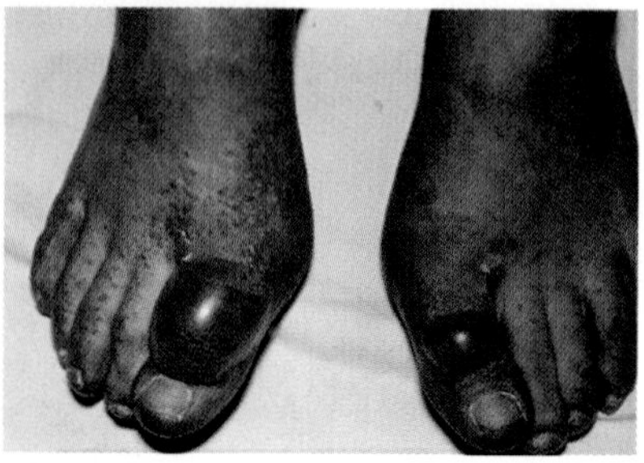 **Blister**

Primary Lesions *(Continued)*

Surface Characteristics	Lesion	Example
Palpable, fluid filled *(Continued)* *Examples:* Acne vulgaris Folliculitis Impetigo	**Pustule (pus filled)**	**Acne vulgaris**

Secondary lesions result from changes in primary lesions. They either add to or take away from an existing primary lesion.

Secondary Lesions

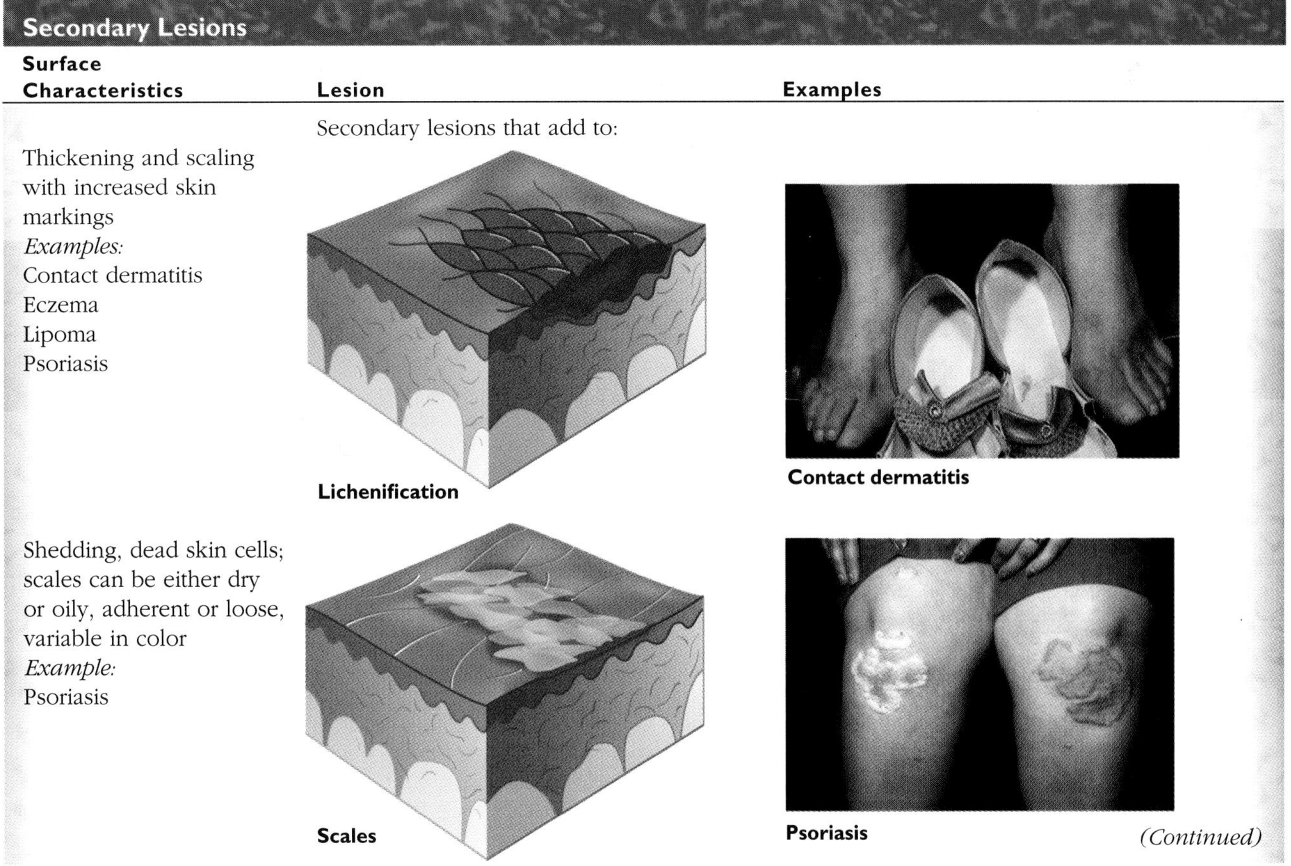

Surface Characteristics	Lesion	Examples
	Secondary lesions that add to:	
Thickening and scaling with increased skin markings *Examples:* Contact dermatitis Eczema Lipoma Psoriasis	**Lichenification**	**Contact dermatitis**
Shedding, dead skin cells; scales can be either dry or oily, adherent or loose, variable in color *Example:* Psoriasis	**Scales**	**Psoriasis**

(Continued)

Secondary Lesions *(Continued)*

Surface Characteristics	Lesion	Example
Dried exudates *Examples:* Dried herpes simplex Impetigo	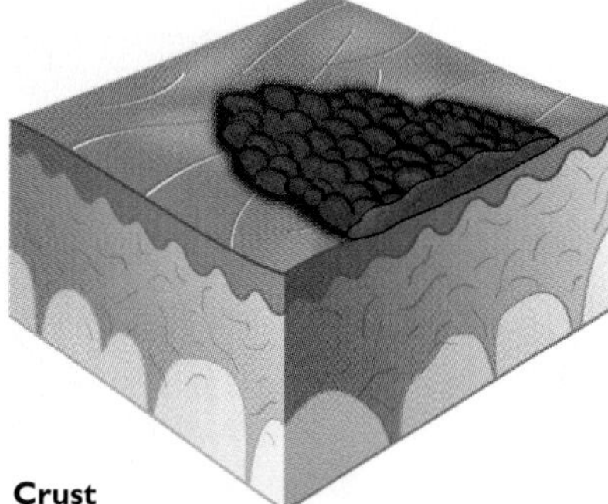 **Crust**	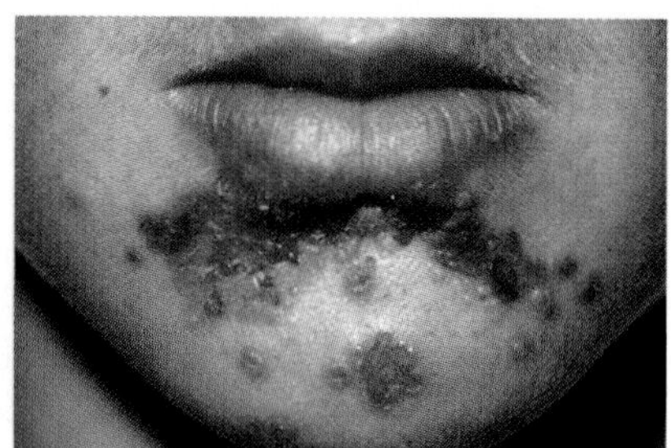 **Dried herpes simplex**
Replacement connective tissue formations *Examples:* Surgical site Trauma site	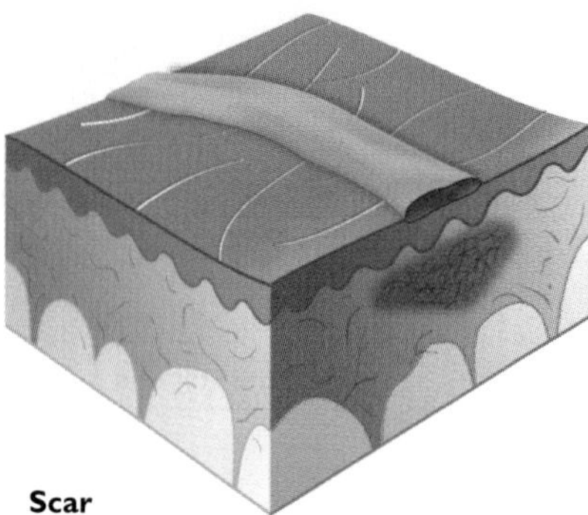 **Scar**	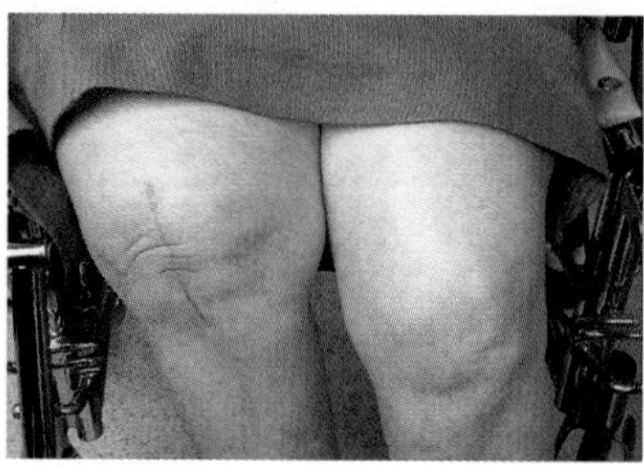 **Surgical site**
Hypertrophic scarring because of excess collagen formation; raised and irregular *Examples:* Ear piercing site Keloids Surgical site Tattoo	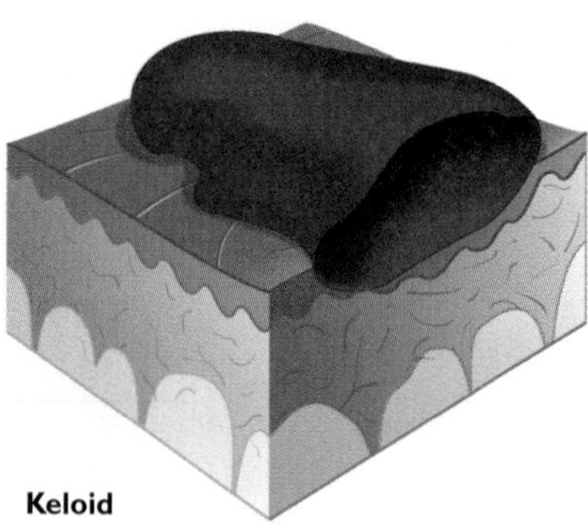 **Keloid**	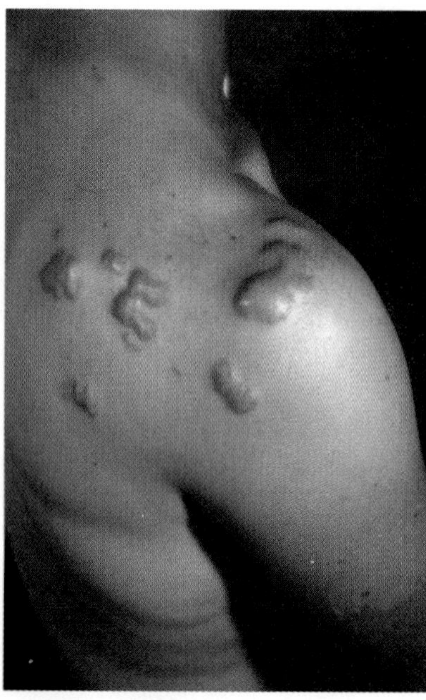 **Keloids**

Secondary Lesions *(Continued)*

Surface Characteristics	Lesion	Example
	Secondary lesions that take away from:	
Abrasion or other loss that does not extend beyond the superficial epidermis *Examples:* Atopic dermatitis Excoriations (scratch marks) Insect bite Scabies Stasis dermatitis Vascular rupture site	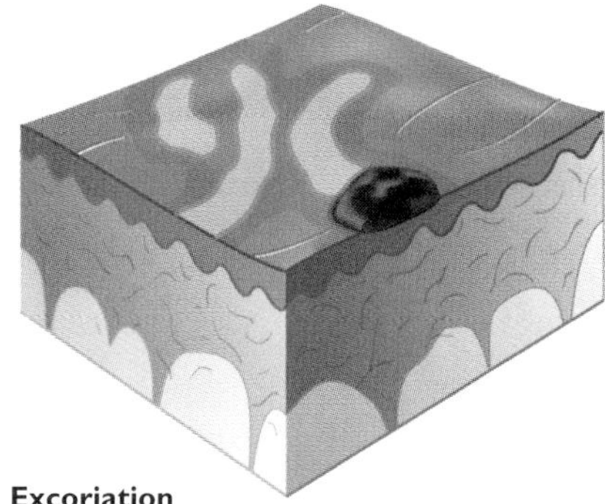 **Excoriation**	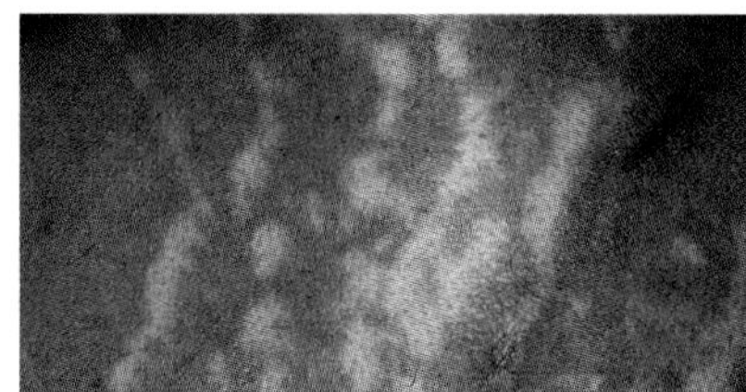 **Excoriation from uremic pruritus**
Loss of superficial epidermis *Examples:* Abrasion Candidiasis erosion Dermatophyte infection Fragile skin Impetigo Intertrigo	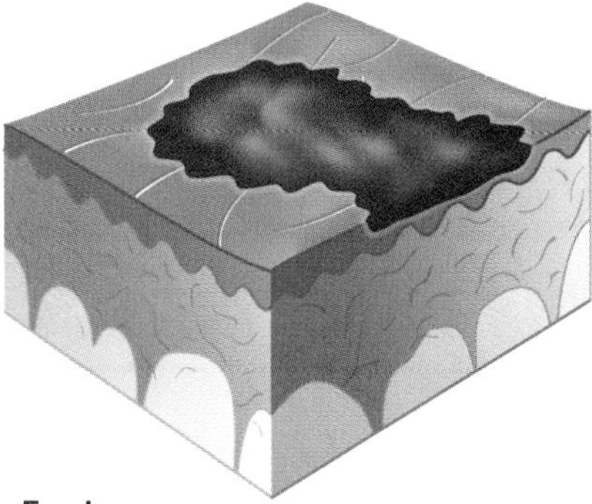 **Erosion**	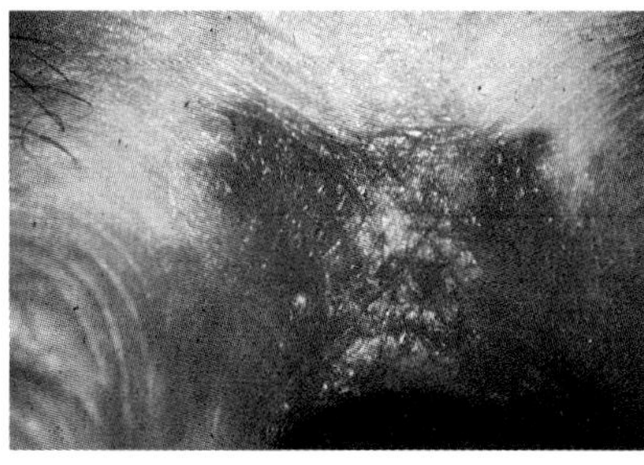 **Candidiasis**
Linear breaks in the skin with well-defined borders, may extend to the dermis *Examples:* Athlete's foot Cheilitis Hand dermatitis (chapped hands) Syphilis	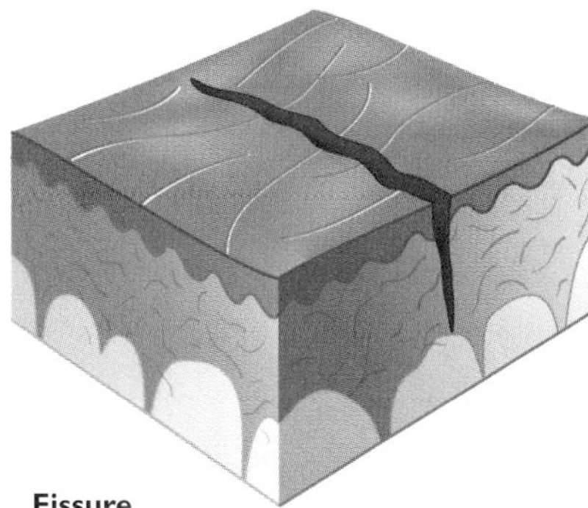 **Fissure**	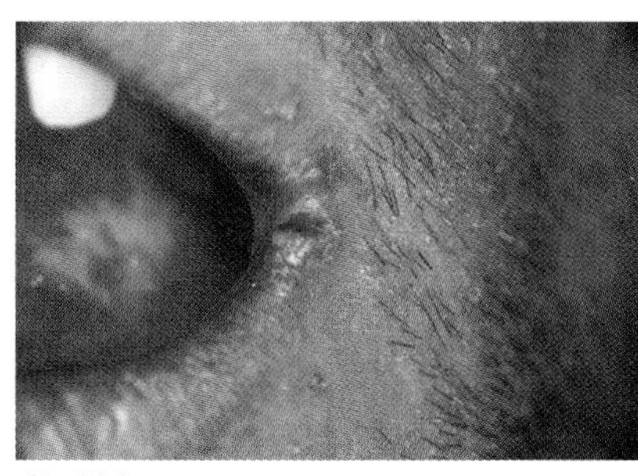 **Cheilitis**
Irregularly shaped loss extending to or through the dermis; may be necrotic *Examples:* Pressure ulcer Stasis ulcer	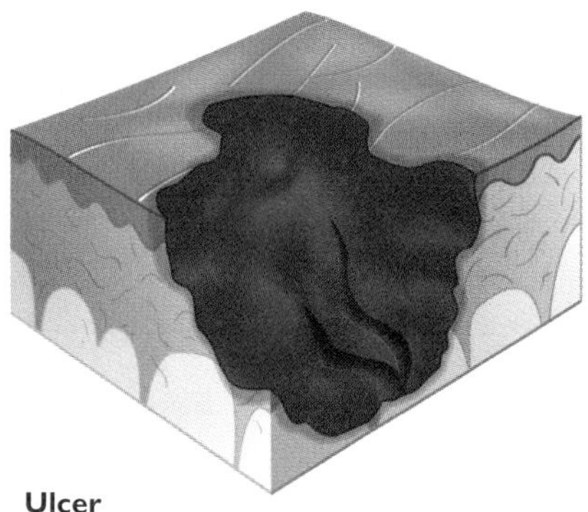 **Ulcer**	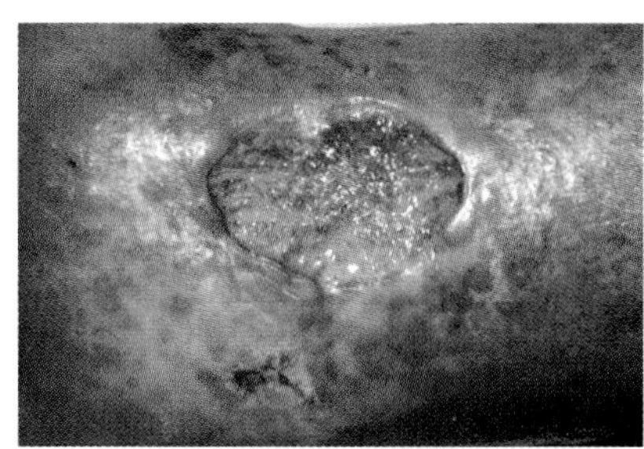 **Stasis ulcer**

(Continued)

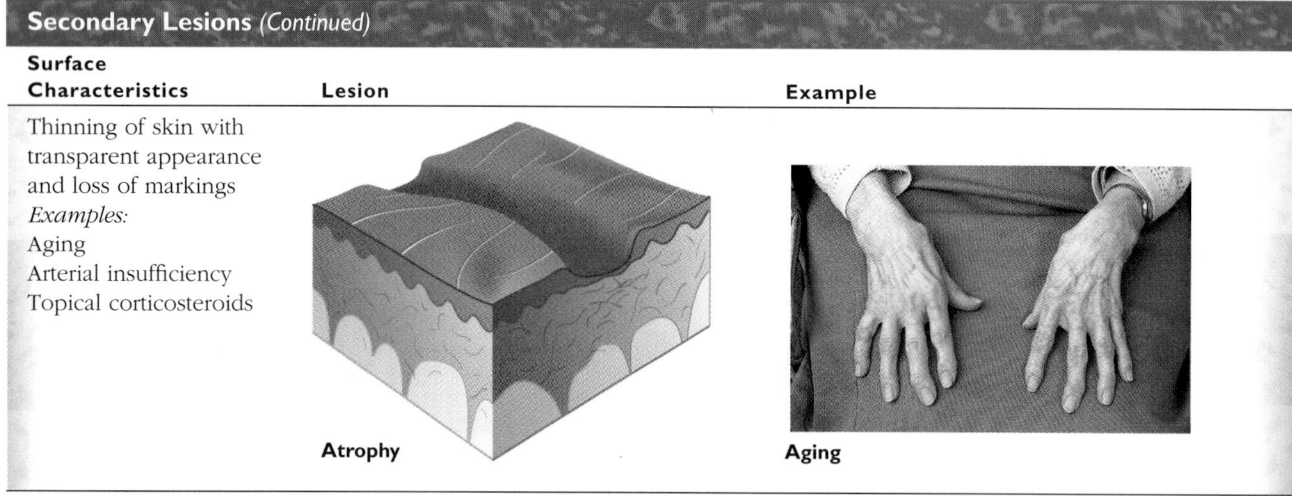

Secondary Lesions *(Continued)*

Surface Characteristics	Lesion	Example
Thinning of skin with transparent appearance and loss of markings *Examples:* Aging Arterial insufficiency Topical corticosteroids	Atrophy	Aging

Lesions may also be categorized according to their pattern, configuration, and distribution.

Pattern and Configuration of Lesions

Pattern	Description	Example
Round/oval	Coin or oval-shaped, as in nummular eczema.	
Discrete	Lesions that remain separate and apart are common in many skin disorders. Moles (nevi) are an example.	
Grouped	Lesions that are grouped, or clustered, such as herpes simplex.	

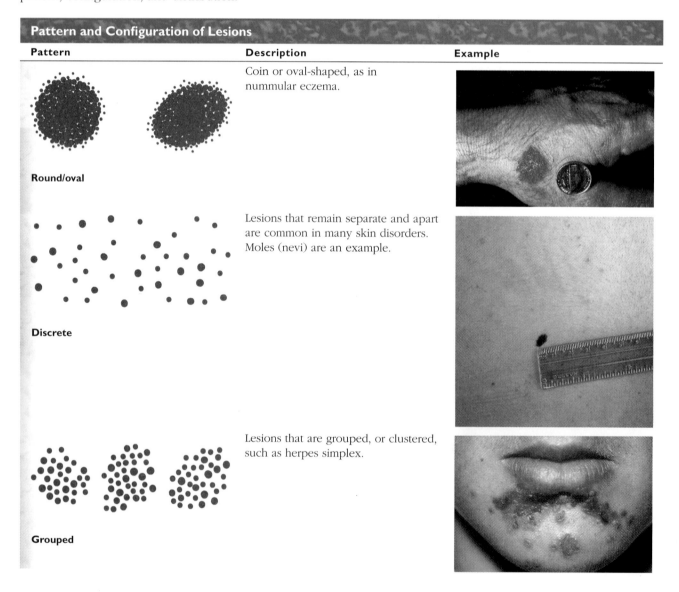

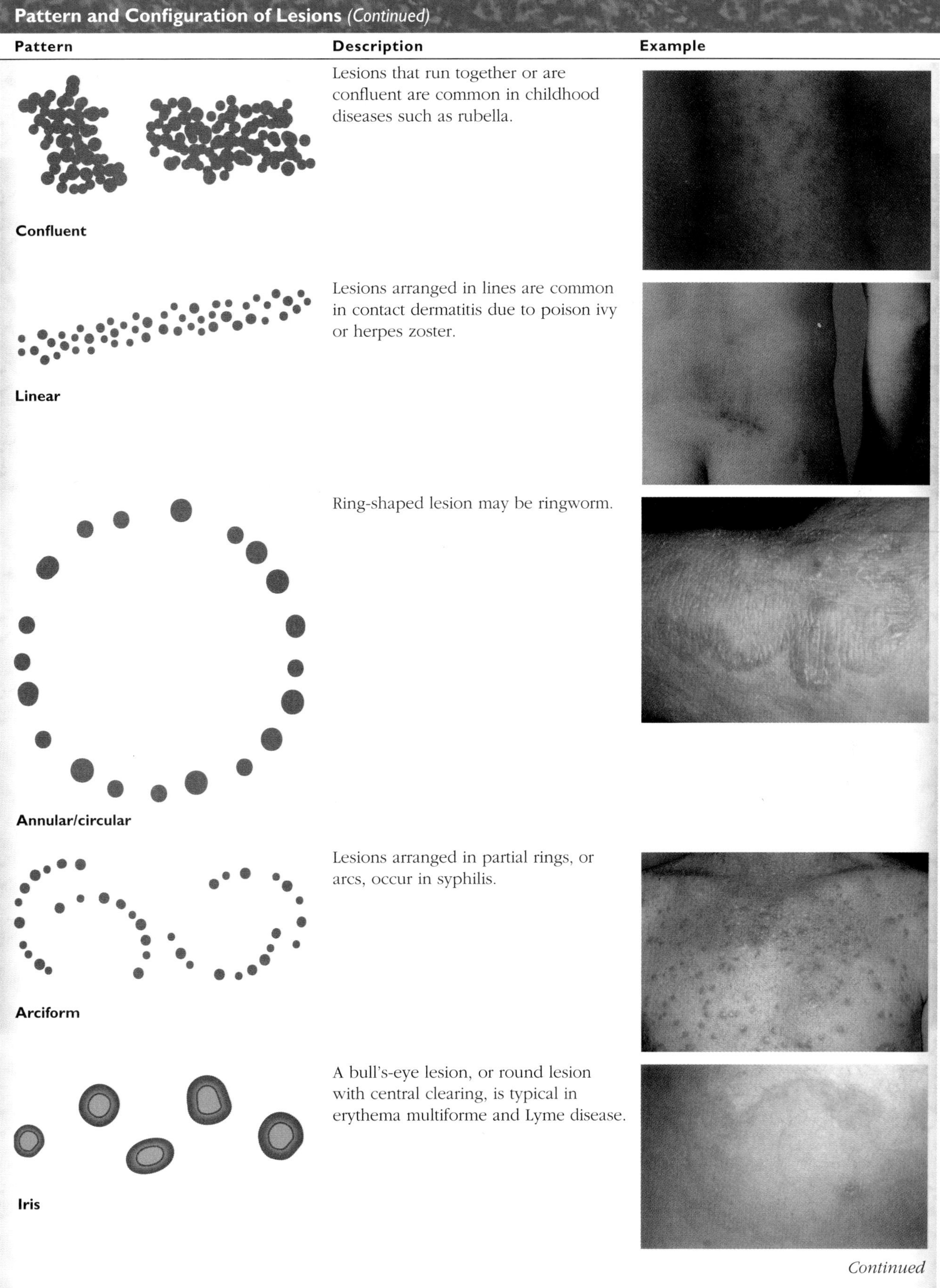

Pattern and Configuration of Lesions *(Continued)*

Pattern	Description	Example
Confluent	Lesions that run together or are confluent are common in childhood diseases such as rubella.	
Linear	Lesions arranged in lines are common in contact dermatitis due to poison ivy or herpes zoster.	
Annular/circular	Ring-shaped lesion may be ringworm.	
Arciform	Lesions arranged in partial rings, or arcs, occur in syphilis.	
Iris	A bull's-eye lesion, or round lesion with central clearing, is typical in erythema multiforme and Lyme disease.	

Continued

Pattern and Configuration of Lesions *(Continued)*

Pattern	Description	Example
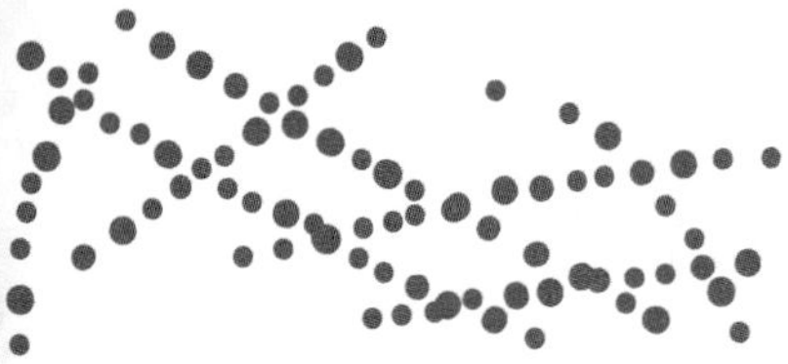 Reticular	Meshlike pattern as in lichen planus.	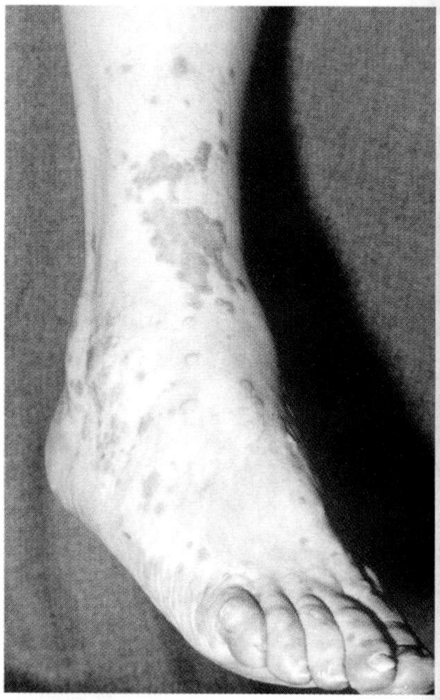
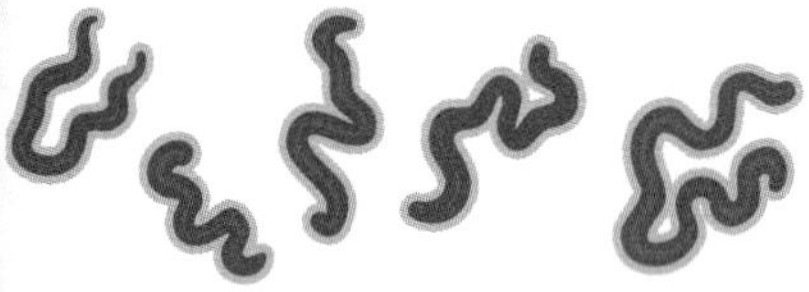 Gyrate	Lesions have serpentine configuration as in gyrate erythema.	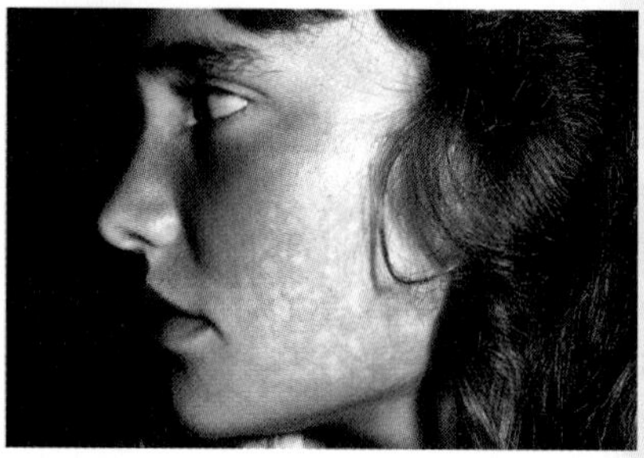
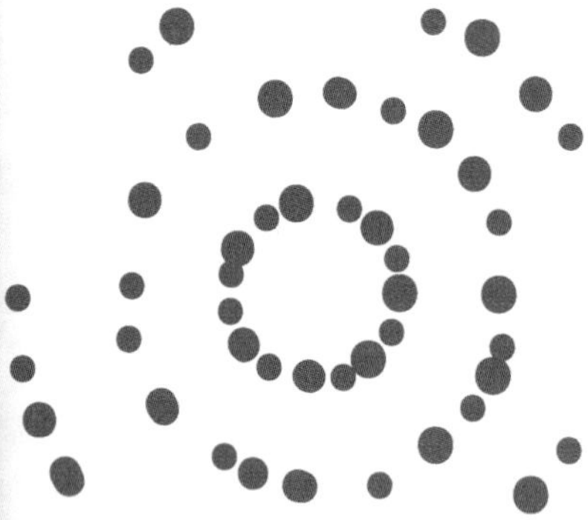 Polycyclic	Coalesced, concentric circles such as urticaria.	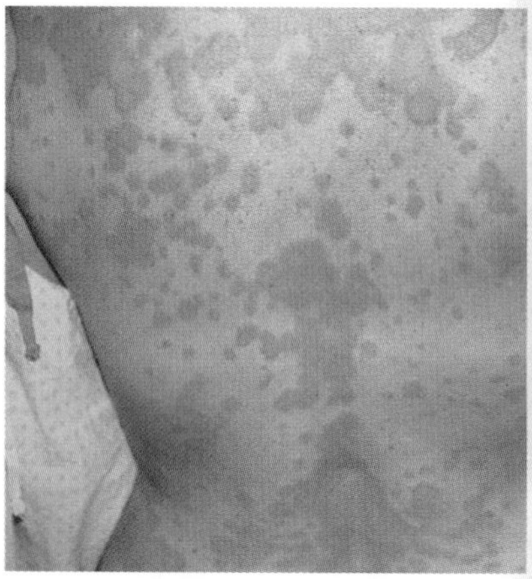

Distribution of Skin Lesions

Area	Description	Example
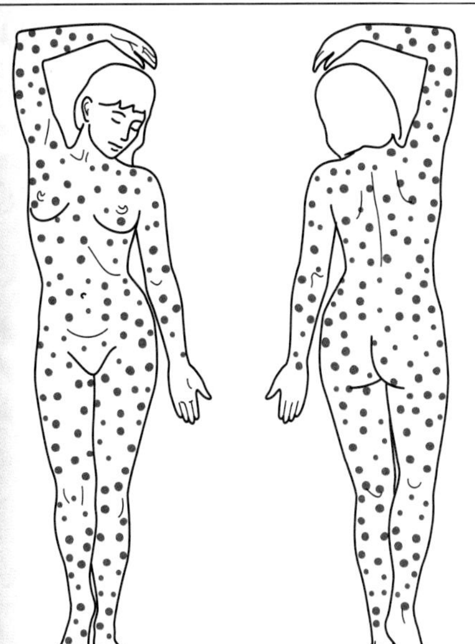  **Diffuse/generalized**	Lesions distributed over entire body, as in urticaria from allergic reactions	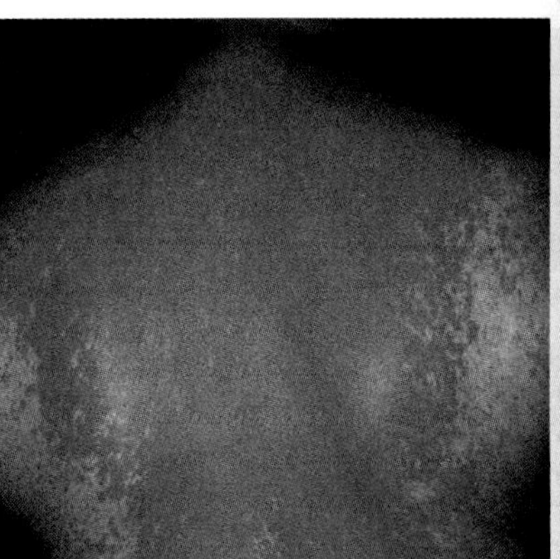
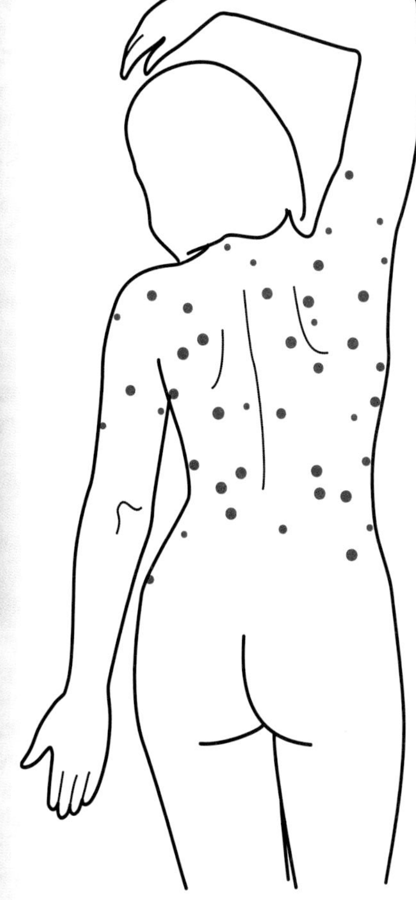 **Scattered**	Lesions that are sparsely distributed, as in seborrheic keratosis	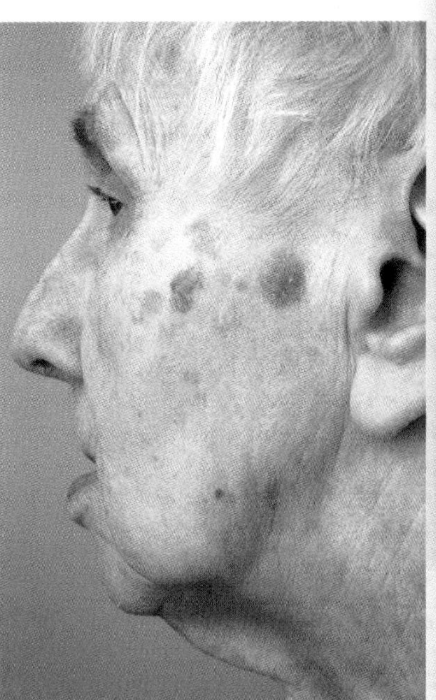

Continued

Distribution of Skin Lesions *(Continued)*

Area	Description	Example
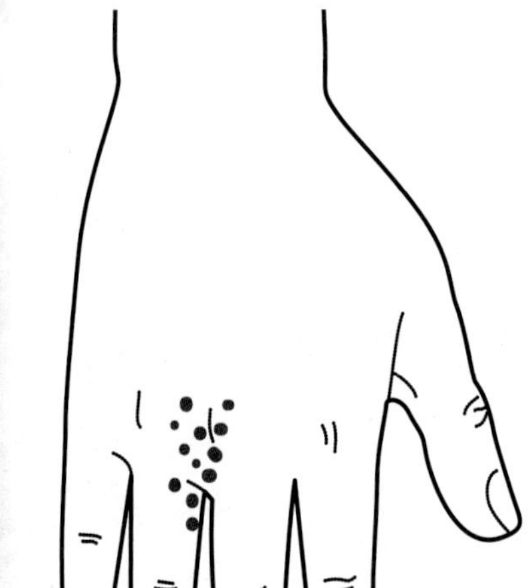 **Localized**	Lesions in a very limited, discrete area Location may indicate contact with an allergen or a wheal from insect bite	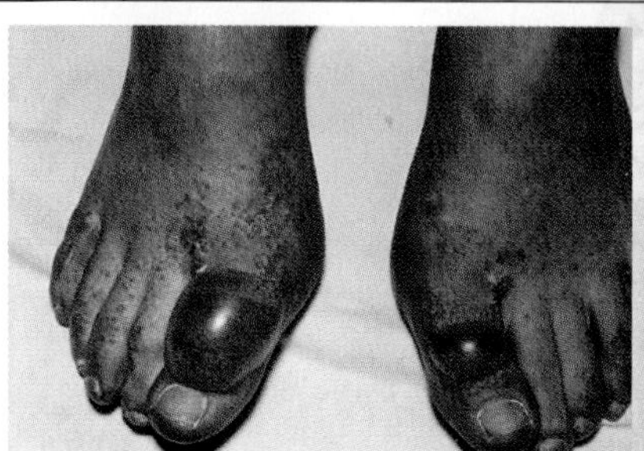
Regional 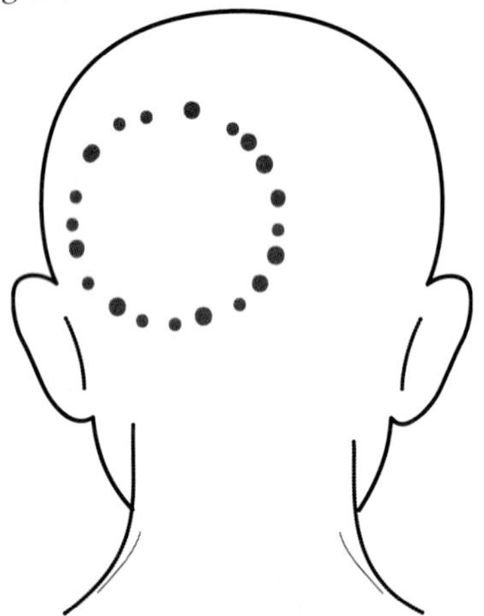 **Head**	Confined to a specific body area: Tinea capitis	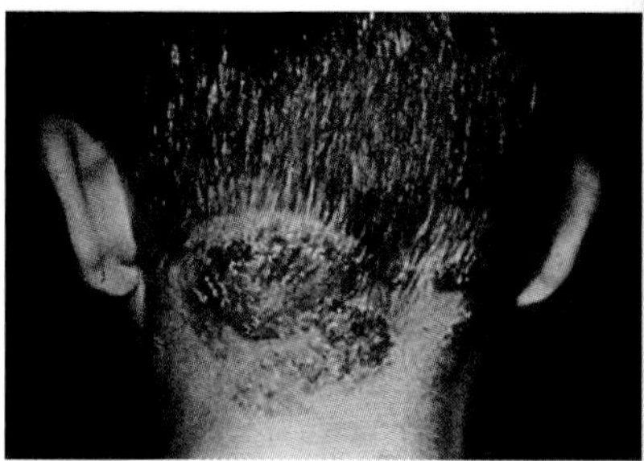
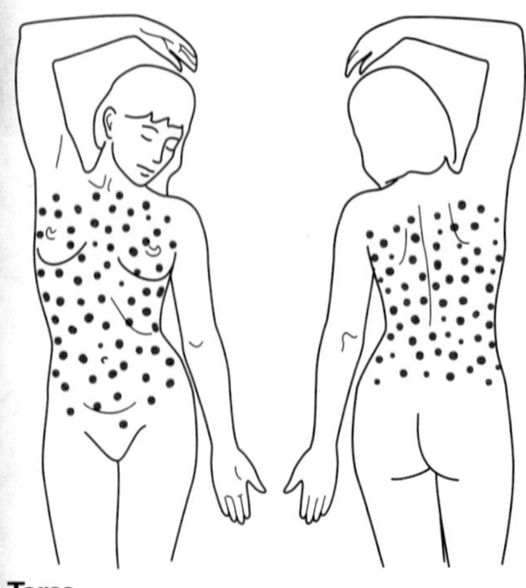 **Torso**	Pityriasis rosea	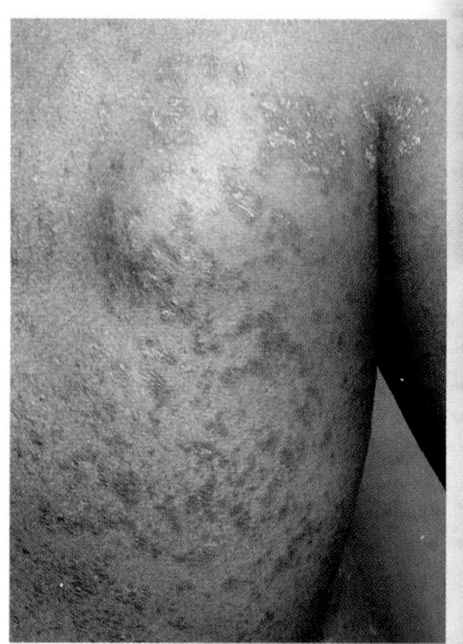

Distribution of Skin Lesions *(Continued)*

Area	Description	Example
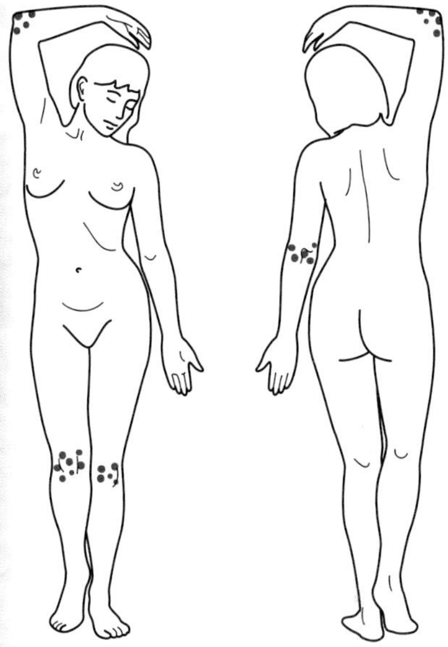 **Extensor surfaces**	Psoriasis	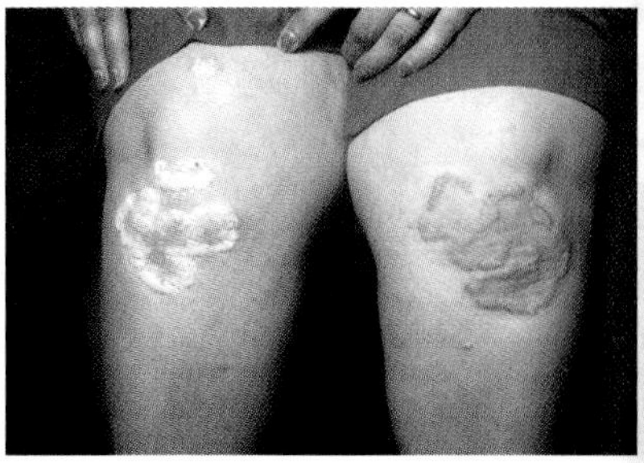
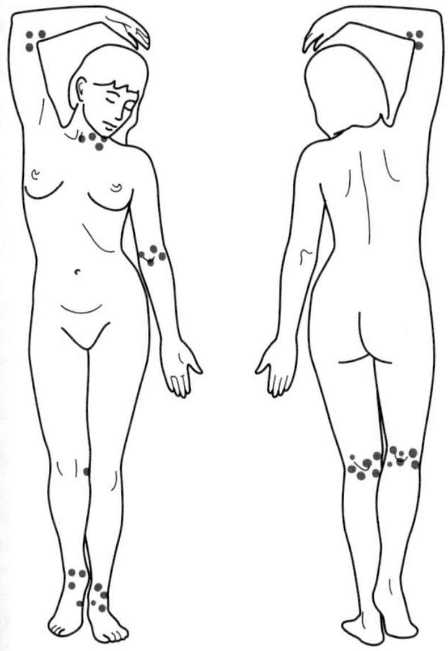 **Flexor surfaces**	Intertrigo	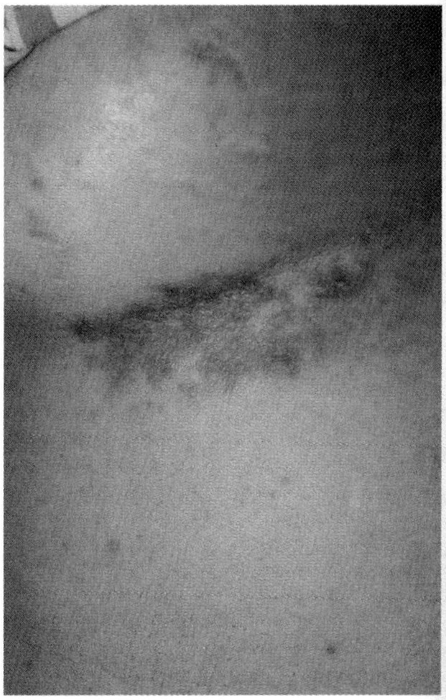
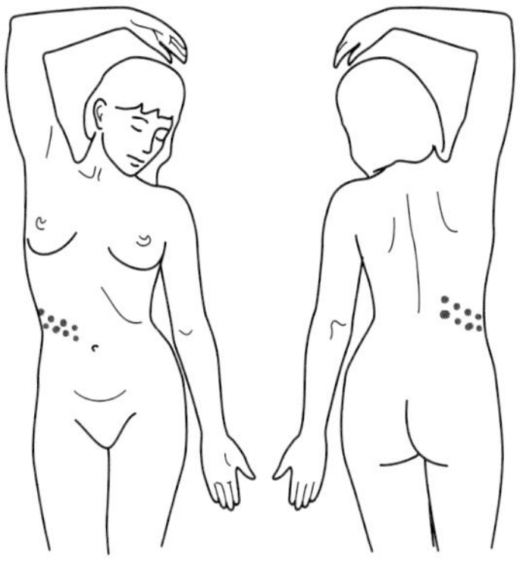 **Dermatome**	Herpes zoster	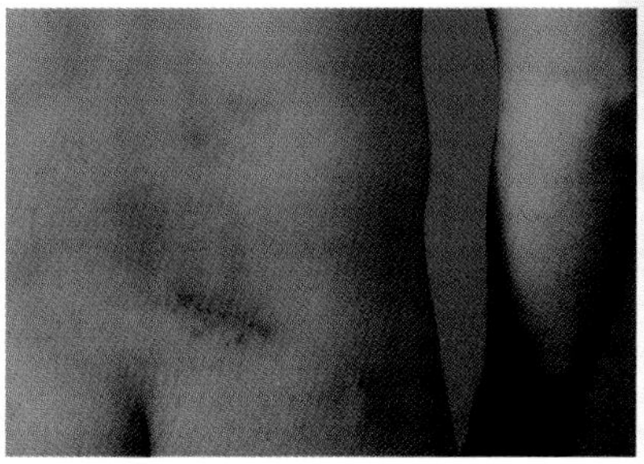

Continued

Distribution of Skin Lesions *(Continued)*

Area	Description	Example
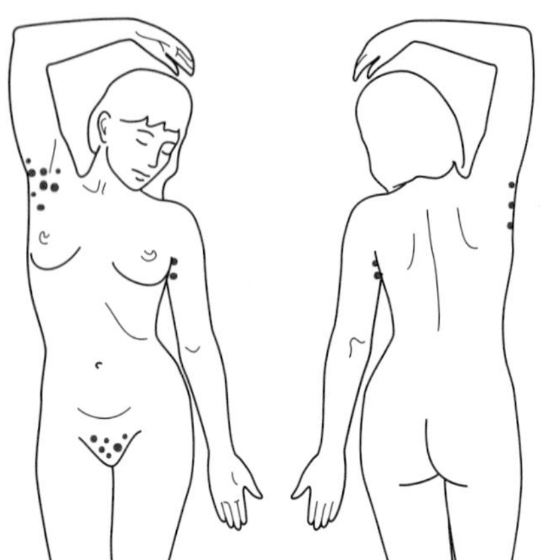 **Hairy areas**	Herpes II, pediculosis pubis	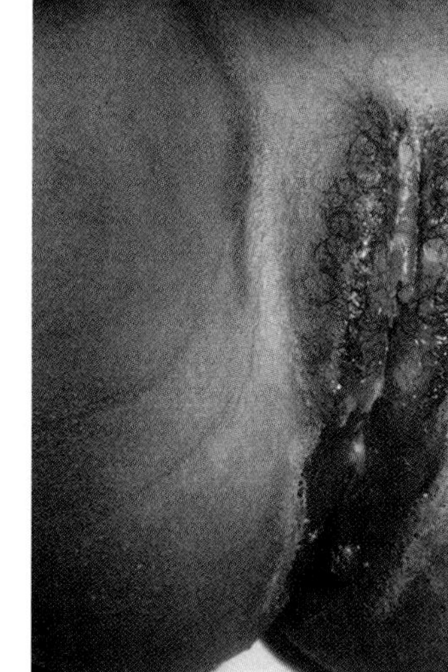
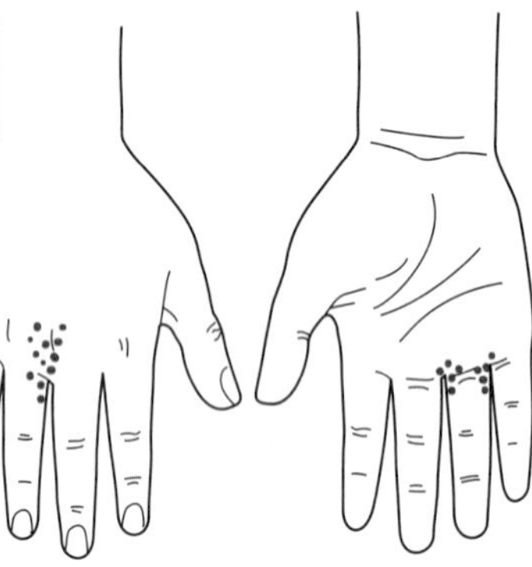 **Intertriginous areas (folds of skin)**	Contact dermatitis, diaper rash, intertrigo (erythema and scaling of body folds) 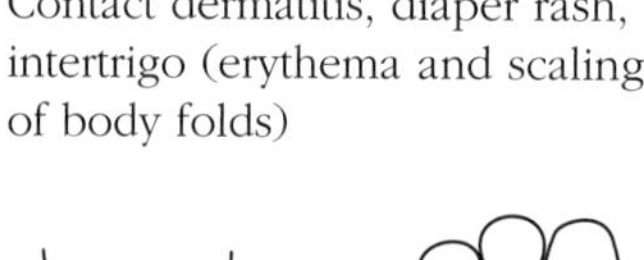 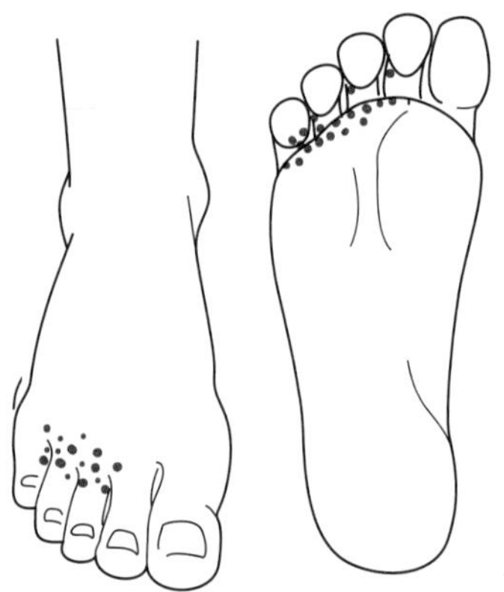	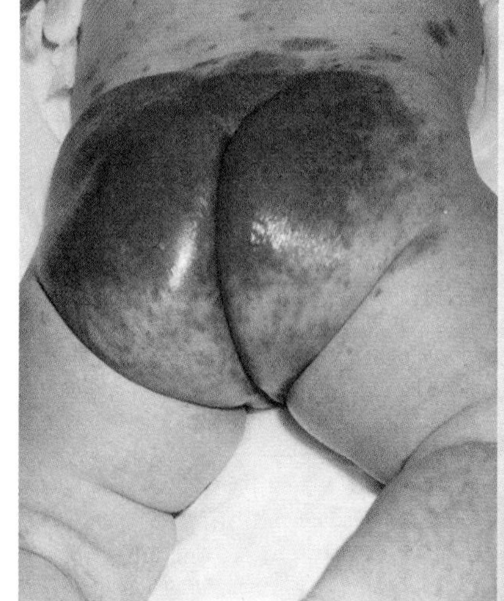
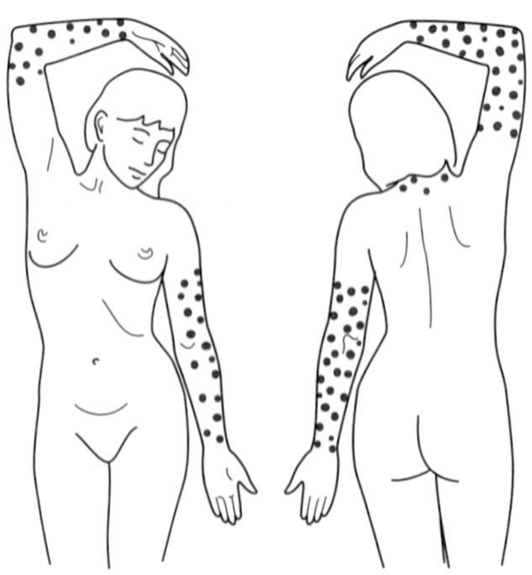 **Sun-exposed areas**		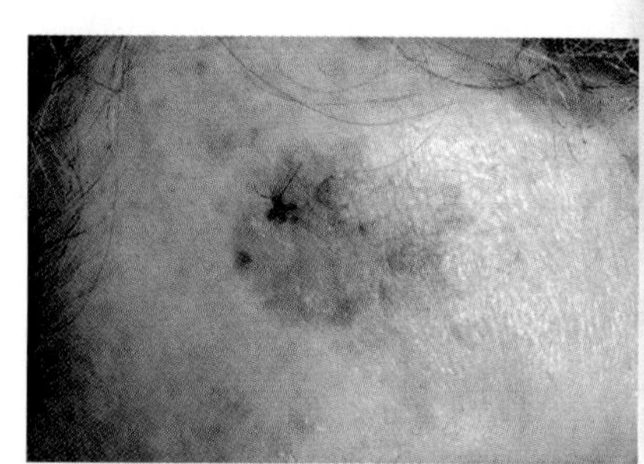

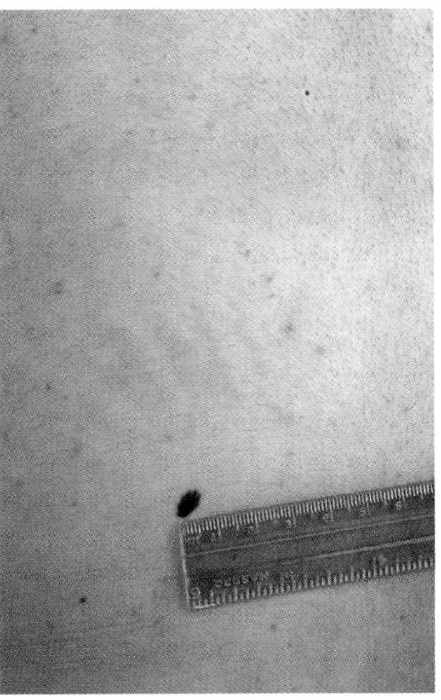

FIGURE 8–4. Moles (nevi). Moles are generally uniformly tan or brown, round or oval in shape, and have well-defined borders. Moles tend to look very similar to one another. They usually start out flat and, with time, become raised. They should be less than 0.5 cm in diameter. A person may normally have ten to forty scattered moles, which generally appear above the waist. When a mole changes in appearance, it needs evaluation, including biopsy, to rule out malignant melanoma.

Always be attentive to the signs of malignant melanoma when assessing a skin lesion. The warning signs are easily recalled using the mnemonic "ABCD." Any time a client indicates that a pigmented area has newly developed or changed significantly from its original appearance, you must be alert to the potential for malignancy. In addition to malignant melanomas, there are several other types of skin malignancies that are less aggressive and less likely to be fatal (Figs. 8–4 and 8–5).

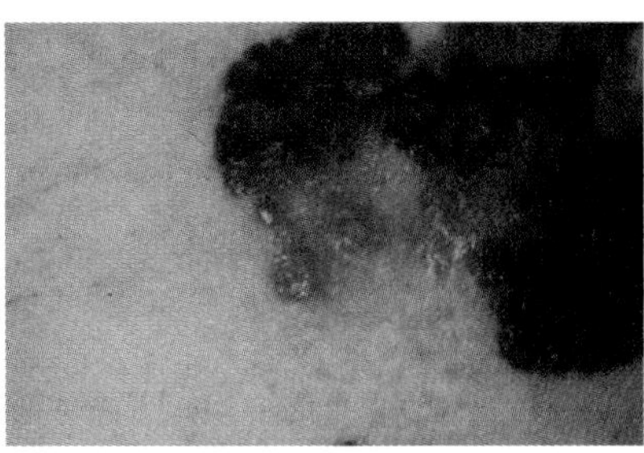

FIGURE 8–5. Warning signs of malignant melanoma. When assessing for malignant melanoma, think of the acronym "ABCD." A is for asymmetry, B is for border irregularity, C is for color variations, and D is for diameter >0.5 cm.

Palpation

After inspecting the skin, explore any findings through palpation. Palpation is used to determine the skin's temperature, moisture, texture, and **turgor.** It can also help to determine whether a localized lesion is raised, indented, or **pedunculated** and its surface characteristics.

As you palpate for temperature, you will find that the dorsal part of your hands and your fingers are most sensitive to temperature variations. Remember to wear gloves when palpating any potentially open areas of the skin.

The skin's moisture varies among body parts, as well as with changes in the environmental temperature, physical activity, or body temperature. Perspiration is produced to cool the body. In the winter, the skin tends to be drier because of the lower ambient temperature and decreased humidity in the environment.

Turgor is assessed as an indication of elasticity. To determine turgor, pinch a fold of skin over an unexposed area, such as below the clavicle, or on the abdomen or sternum. You may also use the forearm. Do not test turgor on the dorsal hand or other areas where the skin is noticeably loose or thin. As you pinch the skinfold, it should feel resilient, move easily, and return to place quickly when released.

(text continues on page 179)

Palpation of the Skin

ASSESS/NORMAL VARIATIONS	ABNORMAL FINDINGS/RATIONALE
	Local area with increased temperature: Inflammatory process, infection, or burn, caused by increased circulation to area. *Generalized increase in temperature:* Fever.

(Continued)

Palpation of the Skin *(Continued)*

ASSESS/NORMAL VARIATIONS	ABNORMAL FINDINGS/RATIONALE
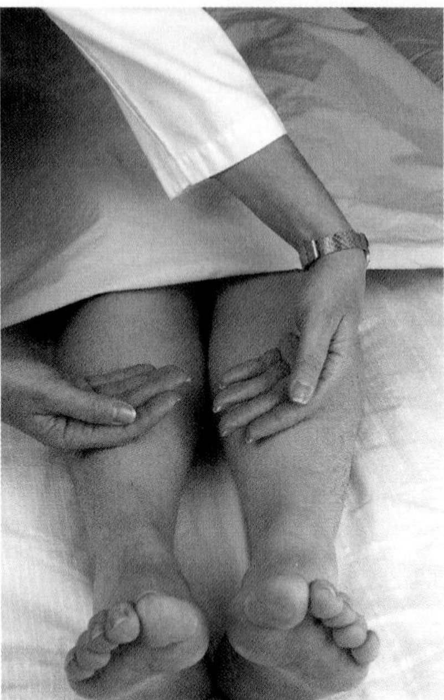	*Local area with decreased temperature:* Decreased circulation to area, as with arterial occlusion. *Generalized decrease in skin temperature:* Exposure or shock.
Temperature Skin warm. Temperature varies depending on area being assessed; for example, exposed areas may be cooler than unexposed areas.	

HELPFUL HINT

When assessing for temperature changes, always use the dorsal aspect of your hand and compare from one side to the other.

ASSESS/NORMAL VARIATIONS	ABNORMAL FINDINGS/RATIONALE
Moisture Depends on environmental conditions and client's age. Elderly people have drier skin because of decreased sweat production. Exposed areas are usually drier than unexposed areas. Also, moisture varies according to body area; for example, the axillae are usually more moist than other areas.	*Increased moisture:* Fever or thyrotoxicosis. *Decreased moisture:* Dehydration, myxedema, chronic nephritis.
Texture Varies from soft and fine to coarse and thick, depending on area assessed and client's age.	*Coarse, thick, dry skin:* Hypothyroidism. *Skin that becomes more fine-textured:* Hyperthyroidism.
Exposed skin usually not as soft as unexposed.	*Smooth, thin, shiny skin:* Arterial insufficiency.
Extensor surfaces, such as elbows, have coarser skin.	*Thick, rough skin:* Venous insufficiency.
Usually, the younger the client, the softer the skin, so infants have very soft skin.	

Palpation of the Skin *(Continued)*

ASSESS/NORMAL VARIATIONS

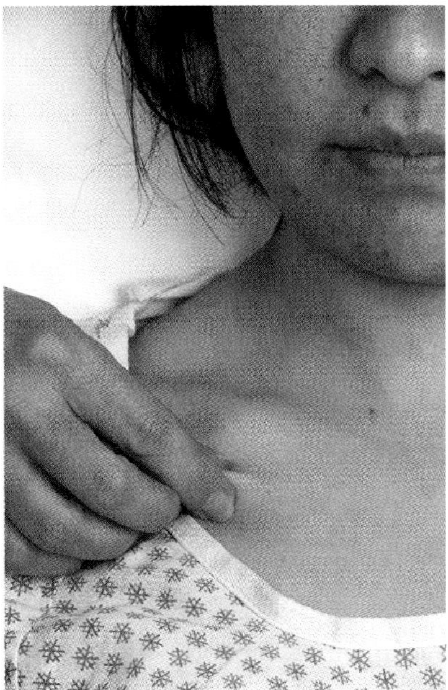

Turgor

Elasticity decreases with age.
Exposed areas may have less turgor.

HELPFUL HINT

Turgor is often used to assess hydration status. But because turgor decreases with age, it is not a useful tool for assessing hydration status in elderly people.

ABNORMAL FINDINGS/RATIONALE

Decreased turgor or tenting: Dehydration or normal aging.

With scleroderma, the turgor is actually increased and the tension does not allow the skin to be pinched upward. This may also be seen with edema.

Assessing the Nails

Assess the nails through inspection and palpation.

Inspection

The condition of the nails often provides important clues about the client's overall health status. Inspect the color and shape of the nails. The color beneath the nails should be similar to the overall skin coloring, although somewhat rosier. There should be no hemorrhage. Nail texture should be uniform and not brittle. Note any grooves or lines in the nail or nailbed.

Also assess for **clubbing,** or loss of the normal angle (Lovibond's angle) between the nail base and finger. When no clubbing is present, the nailbed is firm. You can further assess for clubbing by having the client place the dorsal aspect of two opposite distal fingers together, so that the nails rest against one another. In the absence of clubbing, you should be able to detect a window of light caused by the space created by Lovibond's angle.

Inspection of the Nails

ASSESS/NORMAL VARIATIONS

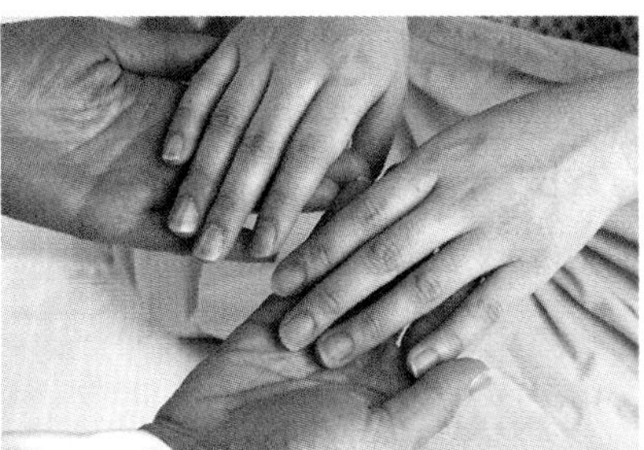

Color

ABNORMAL FINDINGS/RATIONALE

Color changes in nails may indicate a local or systemic problem.

Yellow nails: Cigarette smoking, fungal infections, psoriasis

Very distal band of reddish-pink or brown covering <20% of nail (Terry's nails): Cirrhosis, disorders causing disorders hypoalbuminemia

(Continued)

Inspection of the Nails *(Continued)*

ASSESS/NORMAL VARIATIONS

Normal nails vary from pink in light-skinned clients to light brown in darker-skinned clients.

Shape

Angle of attachment 160 degrees; nails convex

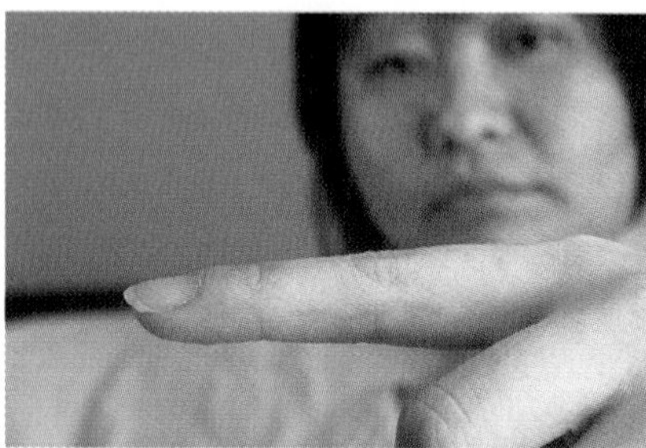

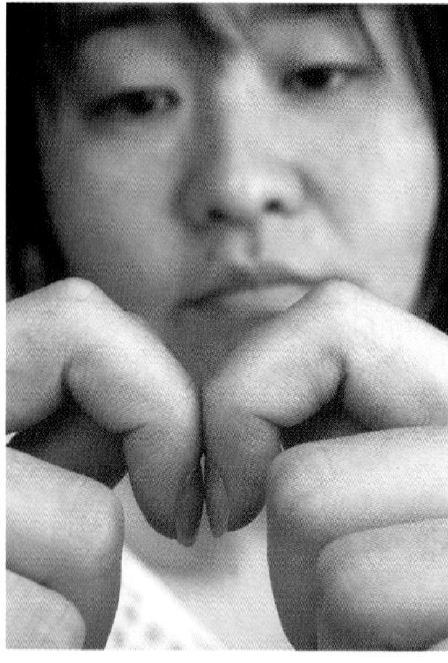

ABNORMAL FINDINGS/RATIONALE

Distal band of reddish-pink or brown covering 20–60% of nails (Lindsay's nails or half-and-half nails): Renal disease, hypoalbuminemia

Blue (cyanotic) nails: Peripheral disease or hypoxia

White nails (leukonychia): Trauma; cardiovascular, liver, or renal disease

Black nails: Trauma

Splinter hemorrhages: Bacterial endocarditis or trauma

Angle of nail attachment 180 degrees or more: Clubbing associated with diseases that affect level of oxygenation, such as congenital heart disorders, cystic fibrosis, and chronic pulmonary diseases.

Spooning or concave nail ***(koilonychia):*** Severe iron deficiency anemia, hemochromatosis, thyroid and circulatory diseases, in response to some skin diseases and local trauma

Onycholysis, separation of the nail from nailbed: Fungal infections, psoriasis, thyrotoxicosis, eczema, systemic diseases, following trauma, or as allergic response to nail products/contactants

Pitting: Psoriasis

Red and inflamed perionychium (paronychia): Infection or ingrown nail

tuberculosis.

Nail Abnormalities: Inspection

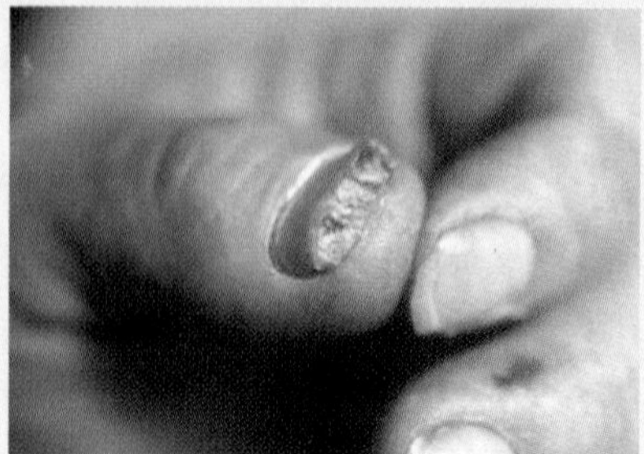

Fungal infection

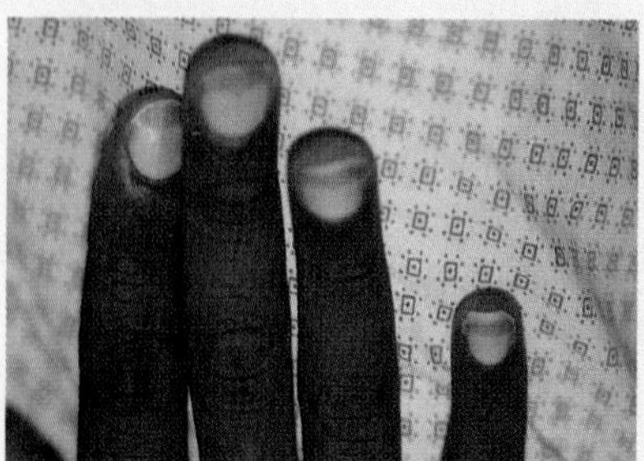

Half-and-half nails

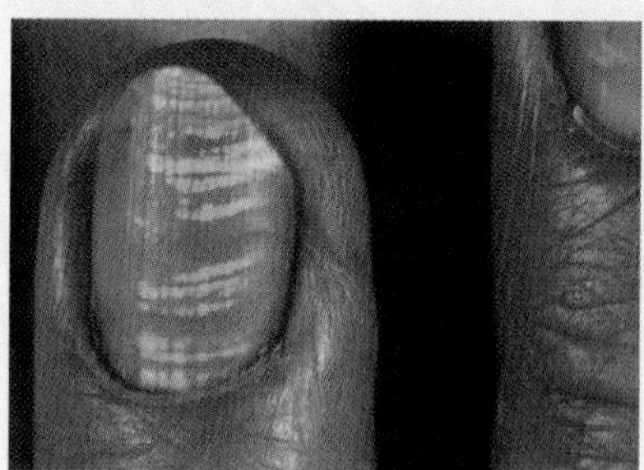

Leukonychia

Inspection of the Nails *(Continued)*

Nail Abnormalities: Inspection *(continued)*

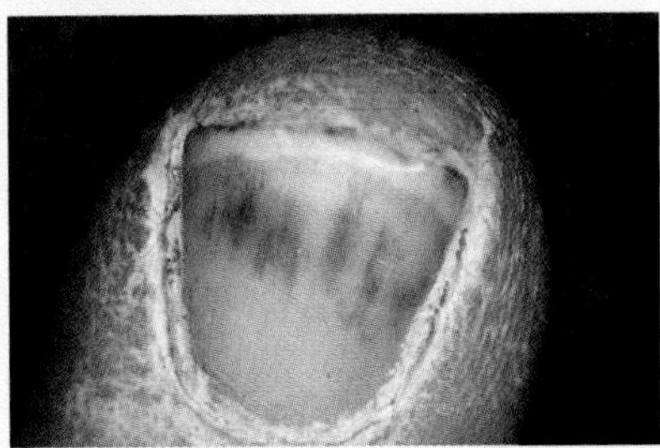

Splinters hemorrhages

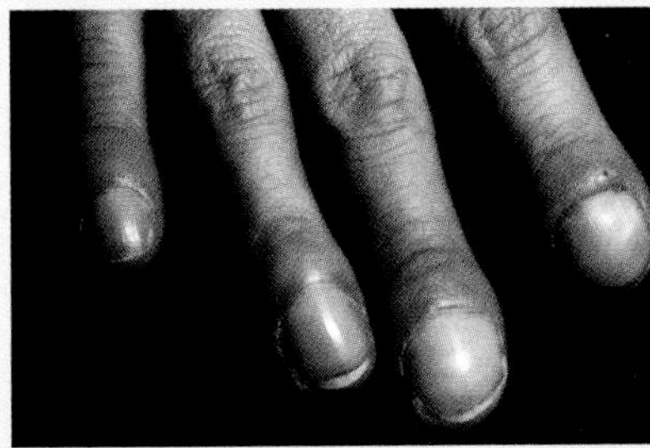

Blue nails

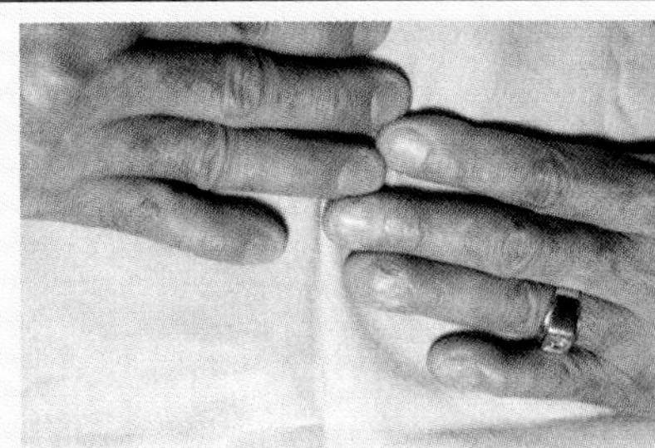

Onycholysis

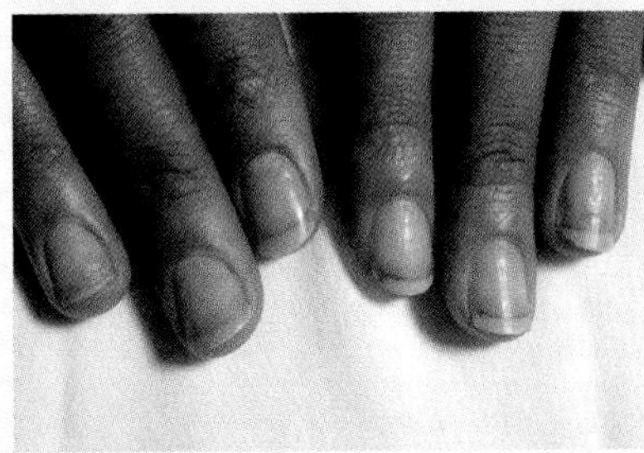

Psoriasis

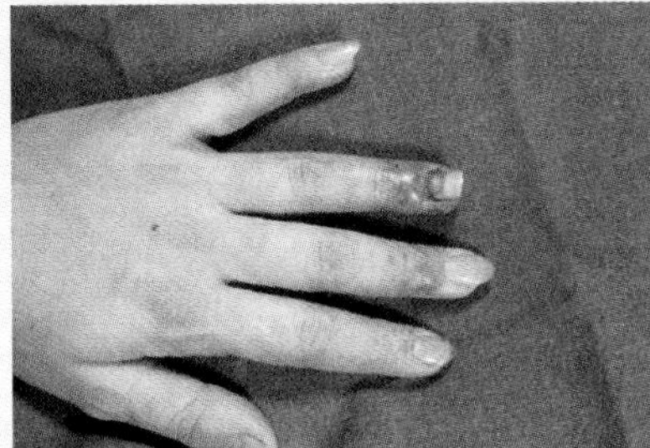

Paronychia

Palpation

Palpate the nail for texture and refill. Nail texture should be uniform and not brittle. Note any grooves or lines or pitting in the nail or nailbed. To check for capillary refill, press on the tip of the nail. It should blanch, and upon release the color should return within 3 seconds.

Palpation of the Nails

ASSESS/NORMAL VARIATIONS

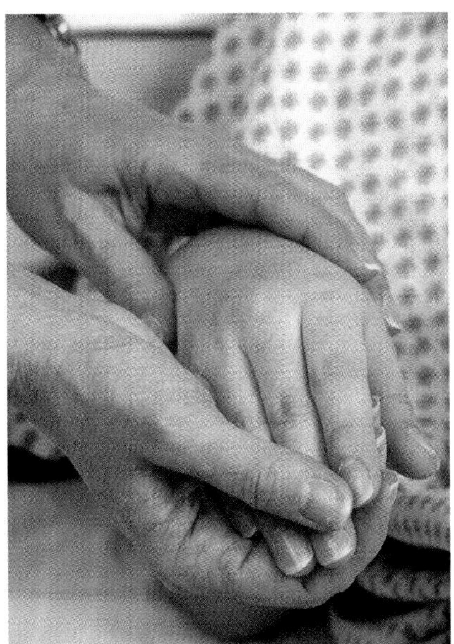

Texture

ABNORMAL FINDINGS/RATIONALE

Soft, boggy nails: Clubbing caused by poor oxygenation

Brittle nails: Hyperthyroidism, malnutrition, calcium and iron deficiency, repeated use of harsh nail contactants or products.

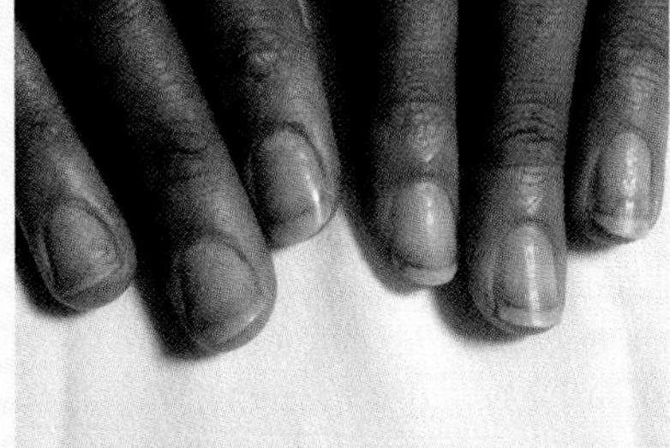

Pitted nails

Pitted nails: Psoriasis, eczema, alopecia areata

(Continued)

Palpation of the Nails *(Continued)*

ASSESS/NORMAL VARIATIONS	ABNORMAL FINDINGS/RATIONALE
Firm Longitudinal ridges usually benign	*Beau's lines (transverse ridges):* Serious illness that causes nail growth to slow or halt

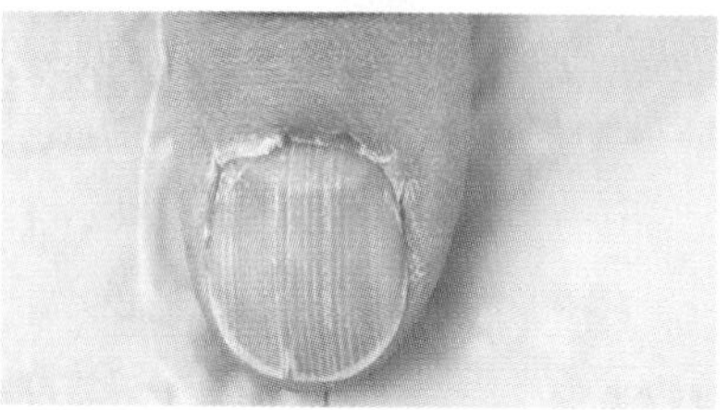

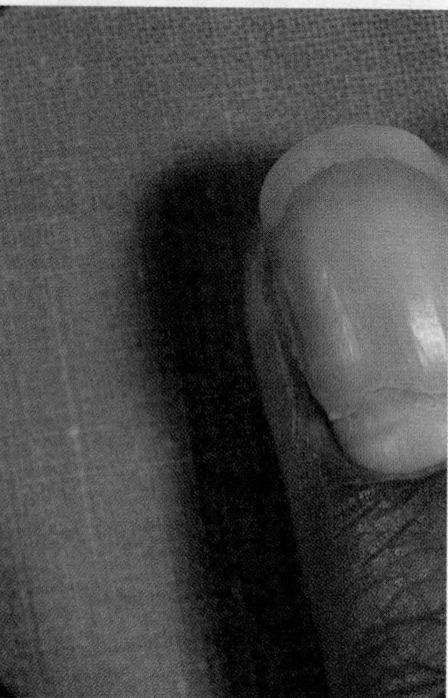

Beau's lines

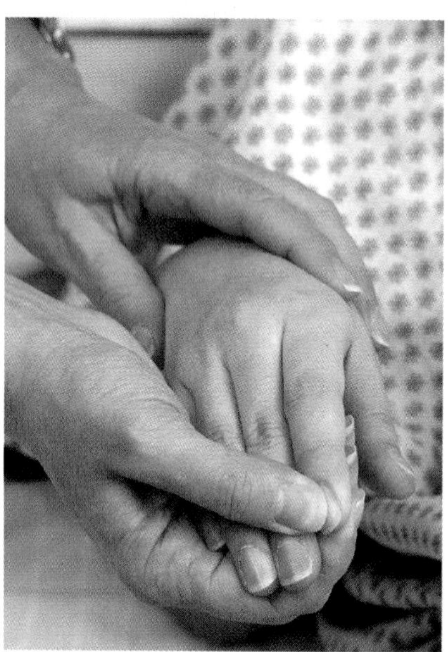

Pressing nail **Releasing pressure**

ASSESS/NORMAL VARIATIONS	ABNORMAL FINDINGS/RATIONALE
Capillary refill Positive capillary refill may be affected by cold temperatures	*Poor capillary refill:* Cardiopulmonary problems or anemia

Assessing the Hair

Assessing the hair is done by inspection and palpation.

Inspection

Inspect the hair for distribution, color, and condition of the scalp. Note any increased hair growth or areas of thinning or **alopecia.** Also, assess the body for normal distribution of hair. The color of the hair can be very difficult to assess, primarily because so many people color their hair. Inspect the scalp as you would any area of skin, assessing any lesions for size, relationship to the overall scalp plane, color, and surface integrity. A morphological description of individual lesions often provides clues to their cause. Almost any of the common skin disorders can affect the scalp.

Note whether there is any adherent material on the hair. Small 1- to 2-mm white eggs are found with lice or **pediculosis,** which occurs on the hairs of the scalp, beard, axillae, or pubic areas. Although head lice can be seen with the naked eye, they are quite small and mobile and their eggs, called nits, are easier to see. Nits are deposited near the base of the hair shaft, so that fresh nits are usually found within 1/8 inch of the scalp or skin. When an infestation of lice has persisted for some time, or if nits were not removed from an earlier infestation, they will be found along a greater portion of the hair shaft because the hair will have grown during the period. Nits found 1/4 of an inch or more from the skin have probably already hatched.

Inspection of the Hair

ASSESS/NORMAL VARIATIONS

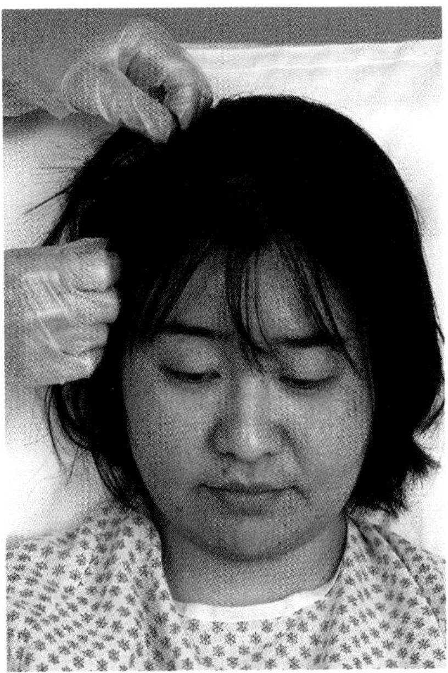

Scalp-hair distribution

Gender, age, and genetics affect hair distribution. Hair should be evenly distributed; exceptions are normal balding patterns common to men or persons of advanced age. Hair thins with age.

Assess areas for the pattern. Note whether there is actual hair loss, with smooth skin beneath, or whether hair has been broken off near the scalp, with palpable stubble over the skin. True hair loss occurs in many conditions.

ABNORMAL FINDINGS/RATIONALE

Generalized hair loss: Nutritional deficiencies, hypothyroidism, lupus erythematosus, thyroid disease, and in response to disorders or situations that stress the integumentary system, such as serious illnesses or side effects of medications.

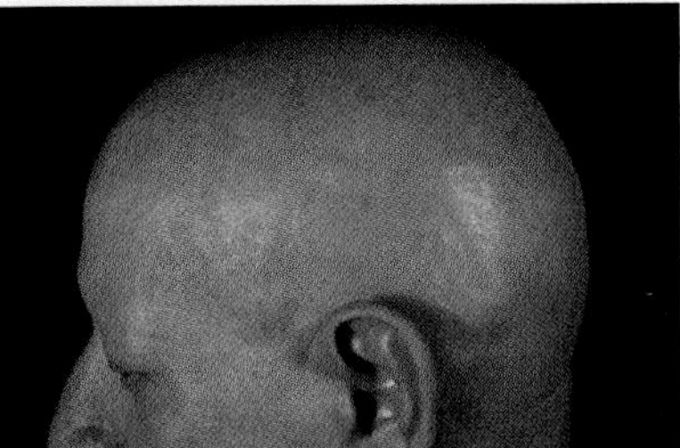

Alopecia

Patchy alopecia associated with alopecia areata, trichotillomania, and fungal infections such as tinea capitis.

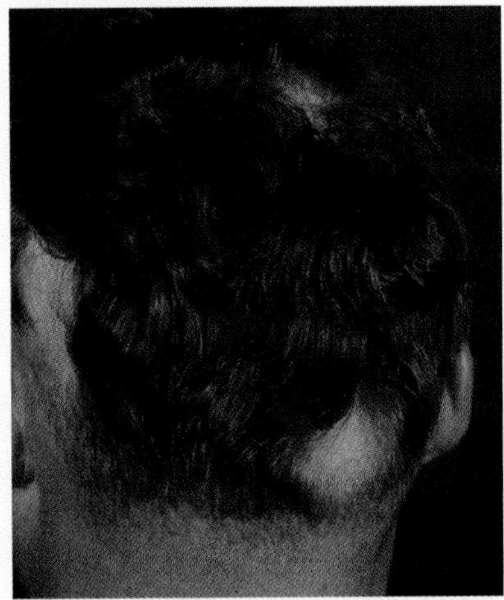

Alopecia areata

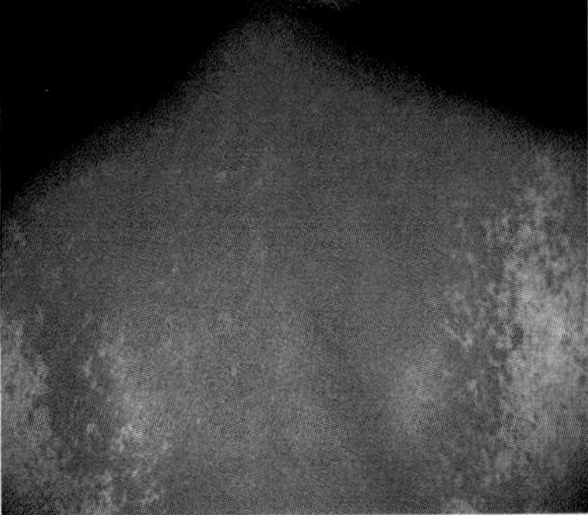

Tinea capitis

(Continued)

Inspection of the Hair *(Continued)*

ASSESS/NORMAL VARIATIONS	ABNORMAL FINDINGS/RATIONALE
Body hair Fine body hair (vellus) noted over body. Gender, age, and genetics influence amount of body hair. Men usually have more hair on chest. Puberty marks the onset of pubic hair growth and increased growth on legs and axillae.	Hirsutism, usually caused by endocrine disorders or medications such as steroids, is hair in male patterns in a female; for instance, excess facial or trunk hair. 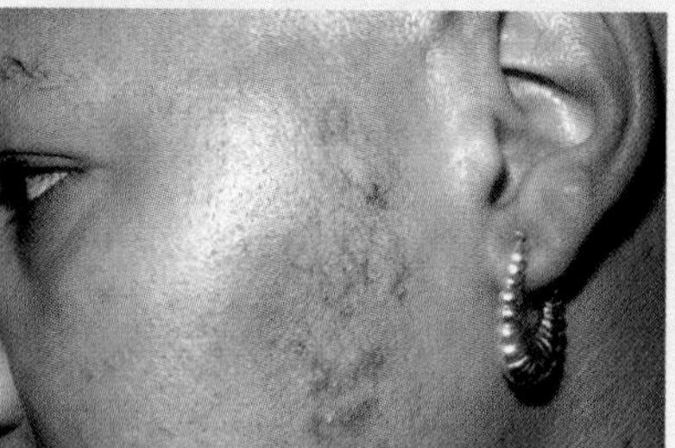 **Hirsutism**
Color Wide range of normal color variations. Gray coloring occurs with aging. Condition of scalp Scalp intact and free of lesions and pediculosis.	*Localized areas of white or gray hair:* In clients recovering from alopecia areata and in those with vitiligo and piebaldism. *Diffuse white hair:* Albinism. *Green hair:* Copper exposure and pernicious anemia. *Scaling of scalp:* Dandruff, seborrhea, psoriasis, certain tineas, and eczema (atopic dermatitis).

Palpation

Palpate the texture of the hair. If it is unusually coarse or fine, consider a thyroid disorder.

Palpation of the Hair and Scalp

ASSESS/NORMAL VARIATIONS	ABNORMAL FINDINGS/RATIONALE
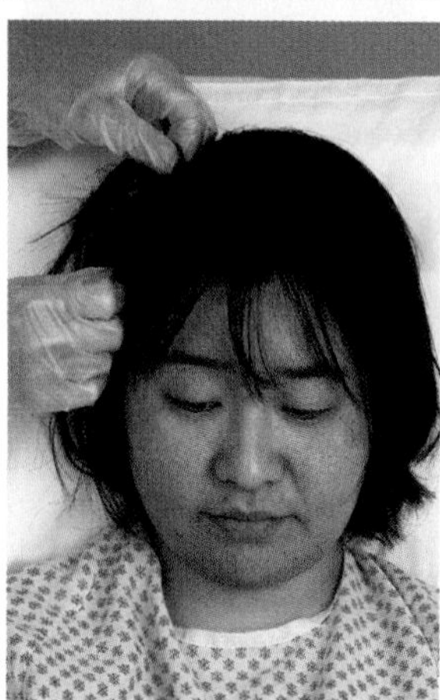 **Texture** 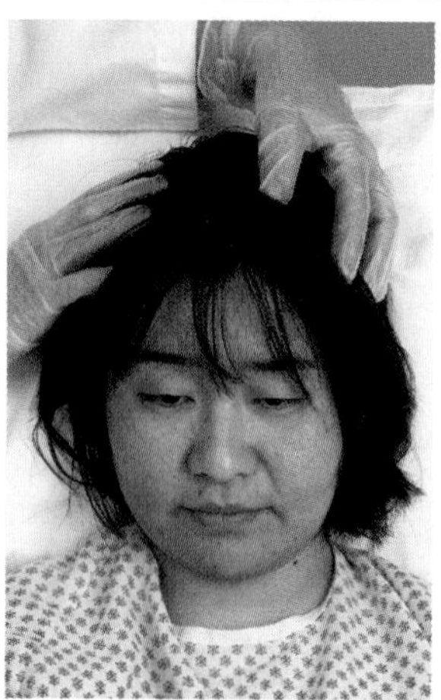 **Scalp** Genetics influence hair texture Scalp mobile, nontender	*Dry, coarse hair:* Hypothyroidism *Fine, silky hair:* Hyperthyroidism *Tenderness:* May indicate a localized infection

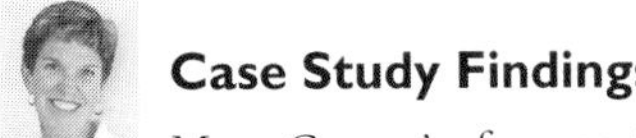

Case Study Findings

Mrs. Green's focused physical assessment findings include:

- Skin:
  - Warm, with good turgor indicated by brisk recoil
  - Generally intact, with smooth texture
  - Coloring symmetrical: pale pink on unexposed areas, moderately tanned on exposed areas with diffusely scattered freckles, consistently light brown in color and all 0.2 to 0.4 cm in diameter.
  - Approximately 30 moles, 0.2 to 0.4 cm in diameter, with well-circumscribed, regular borders. All are very dark brown and consistent in color.
  - Three patches of slightly pink, scaly, flat skin, approximately 0.8 cm each (2 right forearm, 1 left forearm). No telangiectasia or ulcerations of the sites, no changes in surrounding skin.
- Nails:
  - Short, with smooth edges
  - Coat of clear, glossy polish present
  - Nail bed pink, firm to palpation
  - No hemorrhages or discoloration of nails or surrounding tissues
  - No clubbing
- Hair:
  - Generally brown with scant amount of gray interspersed and distributed evenly over scalp.
  - Shortly cut and well-groomed.
  - Shiny, with no signs of damage.
  - No areas of excess hair growth on body.

Case Study Analysis and Plan

Now that your examination of Mrs. Green is complete, document your key history and physical examination findings.
List key history findings and physical examination findings that will help you formulate your nursing diagnoses.

CRITICAL THINKING ACTIVITY #3

List the strengths and areas of concern that you have identified related to Mrs. Green's current health status.

Nursing Diagnoses

Next, consider all of the data you have collected during your assessment of Mrs. Green. Use this information to identify a list of nursing diagnoses. Some possible nursing diagnoses are provided below. Cluster the supporting data.

1. Health-Seeking Behaviors, related to the fear of skin cancer
2. Skin Integrity, Risk for Impaired
3. Fear, related to family history of skin cancers

Identify any additional nursing diagnoses.

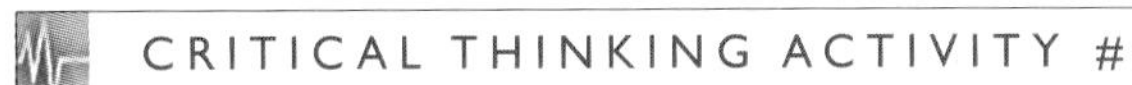

CRITICAL THINKING ACTIVITY #4

Now that you have identified some nursing diagnoses for Mrs. Green, select one diagnosis from above and create a nursing care plan and a related teaching plan including learning outcomes and teaching strategies.

AREA/SYSTEM	SUBJECTIVE DATA
General	*Ask about:* Changes in energy level Weight changes Fevers
HEENT *Head and Neck*	*Ask about:* Lumps or swelling in neck Difficulty swallowing History of endocrine problems
Eyes	*Ask about:* Watery eyes and allergies Changes in eye color
Ears, Nose and Throat	*Ask about:* Ear, throat or sinus infections Sore throats Nasal discharge
Respiratory	*Ask about:* Cough, breathing difficulty History of respiratory disease
Cardiovascular	*Ask about:* History of cardiovascular disease Leg pain
Gastrointestinal	*Ask about:* History of liver disease Nausea/vomiting, loss of appetite Change in stool to clay color
Genitourinary/ Reproductive	*Ask about:* Changes in urine color Urinary tract infections Incontinence History of STDs Safe-sex practices
Musculoskeletal	*Ask about:* History of joint disease, rheumatoid arthritis
Neurological	*Ask about:* Loss of sensation
Endocrine	*Ask about:* History of thyroid disease, diabetes
Immune/ Hematologic	*Ask about:* Immune disorders Use of immunosuppressive drugs Bleeding Use of anticoagulants or aspirin

AREA/SYSTEM	OBJECTIVE DATA
General	*Inspect for:* Signs of distress *Measure:* Vital signs Height and weight
HEENT *Head and Neck*	*Inspect for:* Facial expression Neck vein distention Enlarged accessory muscles *Palpate for:* Lymph node enlargement Thyroid gland enlargement
Eyes	*Inspect for:* Red eyes Icteric eyes
Ears, Nose and Throat	*Inspect for:* Red, swollen nasal and oral mucous membranes
Respiratory	*Inspect for:* Signs of hypoxia Asymmetrical chest movement *Auscultate for:* Abnormal/adventitious breath sounds
Cardiovascular	*Inspect for:* Signs of impaired circulation Skin changes in extremities *Palpate for:* Pedal pulses Edema *Auscultate for:* Irregular rhythms, rates and extra sounds
Gastrointestinal	*Inspect for:* Ascites *Palpate for:* Liver enlargement, tenderness *Percuss for:* Liver size
Genitourinary/ Reproductive	*Inspect for:* Lesions on external genitalia skin
Musculoskeletal	*Inspect for:* Joint deformity Decreased ROM Skin changes over joints
Neurological	*Test for:* Sensory perception changes, both superficial and deep sensations Deep tendon reflexes
Immune/ Hematologic	*Inspect for:* Ecchymoses or petechiae

Assessment of Integumentary System's Relationship to Other Systems

Research Tells Us

Skin cancer is the most common form of malignancy in the United States. A projected one-third of Caucasians born in the U.S. after 1994 will develop at least one skin cancer. In the past, there was limited empirical evidence showing that ultraviolet light exposure actually caused skin cancers, rather than simply stimulating existing cancers. However, a recent study by the National Institute of Arthritis and Musculoskeletal and Skin Diseases of clients receiving ultraviolet treatments for psoriasis showed that those who received initial high doses of ultraviolet light, even when later treatments were at lower doses, continued to develop new skin cancers, both squamous and basal cell types. The investigators interpreted their findings as supporting the theory that ultraviolet light was capable of actually starting the cancers. Based on these findings, the institute finds strong support for using sun protection, including using a sunscreen (SPF $\geq$ 15); wearing long sleeves, pants, and wide-brimmed hats; avoiding sunlight during peak hours (10 AM to 3 PM); and seeking protection under shaded areas.

Some day there may be added measures to prevent skin cancer. Recent studies revealed that mice fed a COX-2 inhibitor (celecoxib) developed squamous cell cancers at only half the rate of mice that did not receive the drug. Further studies might find that COX-2 inhibitors or other drugs help prevent skin cancer. But for the time being, avoiding sun exposure is very important (NIH, 2000).

Health Concerns

Facts about Melanoma

- The incidence of malignant melanoma has greatly increased over the past several decades. In 1997, the overall incidence of melanoma in the United States was 14.3/100,000, up from 7.6/100,000 in 1977.
- The exact cause of the increase is not known, but sun exposure is a major contributing factor.
- The rate is higher in whites (19.3/100,000) than in blacks (0.9/100,000) and increases with age. For instance, the incidence is 10.1/100,000 for all people under age 65 and 45.5/100,000 for those aged 65 and older.
- The 5-year survival rate for persons from 1989 to 1996 averaged 88.3 percent. However, when melanoma is diagnosed at an early stage when it presents as a local site, the 5-year survival rate is 98.3/100,00. It drops to 12.5/100,000 when it has spread distally.

Common Abnormalities

ABNORMALITY	ASSESSMENT FINDINGS
Acne vulgaris Caused by sebaceous gland overactivity with plugging of hair follicles and retention of sebum, resulting in comedones, papules and pustules. Onset is typically at puberty, but acne may last into advanced age. Greater incidence in males.	• Pimples present as papules or pustules. • Cysts may develop and leave extensive scarring. • Most common on face, back, and shoulders. • Bacillus is cause. • Lesions may be sore and painful. • Aggravated by emotional distress, greasy topical applications (cosmetics) and certain medications (oral contraceptives, isoniazide,rifampin, lithium, phenobarbital) 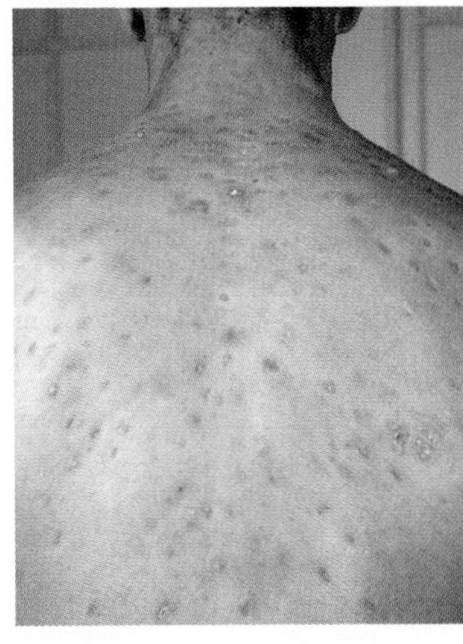

(Continued)

Common Abnormalities *(Continued)*

ABNORMALITY	ASSESSMENT FINDINGS
Actinic keratosis Causes reddish, irregular, slightly raised lesions that have a rough, gritty surface. Sign of sun-damaged skin. Precancerous lesion, may progress to squamous cell cancer.	• Typically less than 1 cm in diameter. • Generally on sun-exposed areas of face, head, neck and hands. 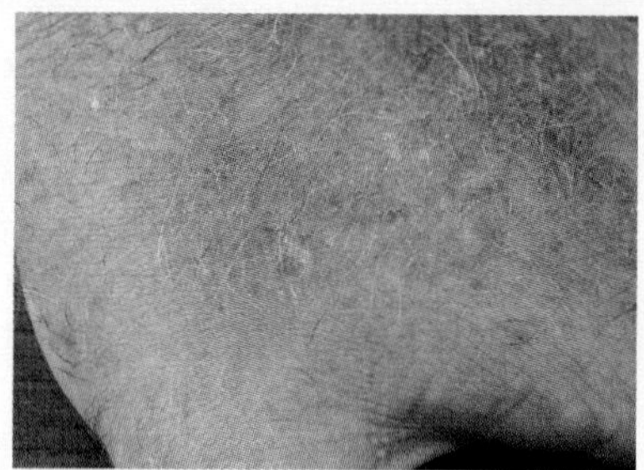
Basal cell carcinoma An epidermoid cancer, one of the most common malignant skin diseases, but rarely metastatic.	• Typically has pearly, flesh-colored or transparent "rolled" border. • Central area develops telangiectasia and may ulcerate. • Variations can present with nodular, sclerotic, and/or pigmented appearance. • Usually occurs on sun-exposed surfaces, especially the face. 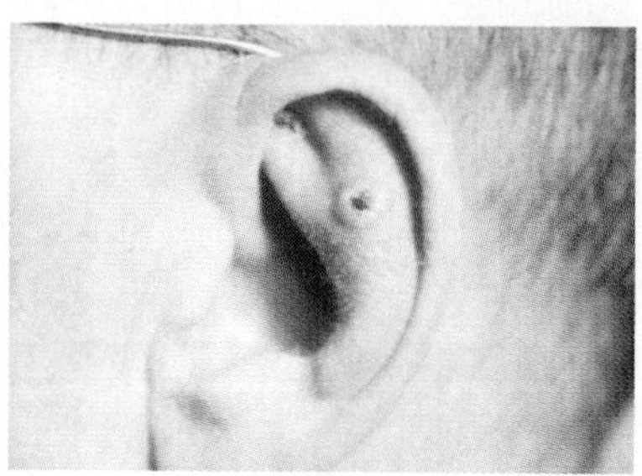
Contact dermatitis Localized skin irritation, inflammation, and pruritus from contact with an irritating substance. Can occur as an additive effect of multiple irritants (soaps, detergents, or chemicals) or allergy to a specific agent (topical to a specific agent (topical medication, plant oils, or metals). Secondary infections may occur at the site.	• Edema may occur, with development of vesicles and bullae. • Vesicles or bullae may rupture, causing crusting. • Edema maybe very significant, particularly when face or genitalia are involved. • Person may have history of previous reaction to agent and recent exposure. 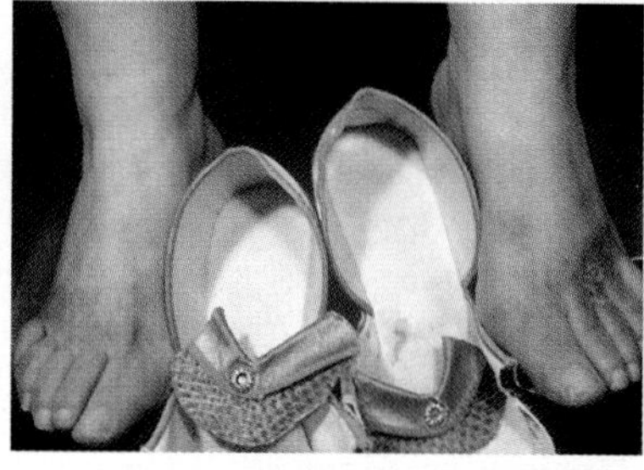
Eczema/atopic dermatitis Causes redness, pruritus, scratching, and skin lesions in a person with a predisposition to skin irritations	• Red to red-brown, slightly scaly lesions. • Lichenification with increased skin markings common. • Exudative • As sites resolve, skin pigmentation is often permanently altered. • Common sites include face, neck, upper truck, wrists, hands, and flexor surfaces (folds) of knees and elbows. 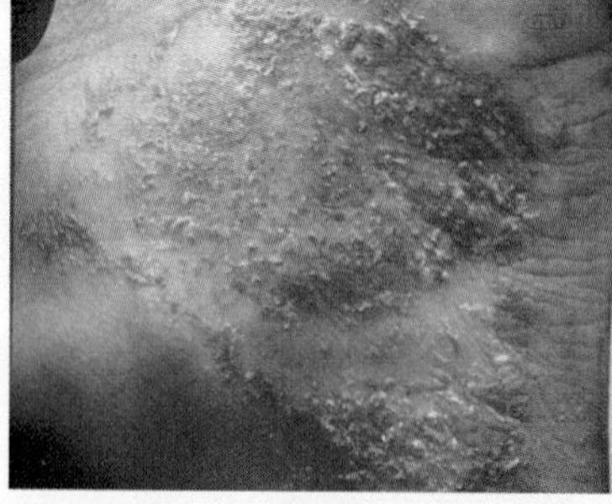 • Lesions on face, neck, and upper trunk are called "monk's cowl." • Person also often has asthma or allergic rhinitis; family history is often positive for asthma, rhinitis, eczema, or other allergy problems. • Itching can be quite severe. • Sites may develop secondary infection. • May be triggered by changes in temperature, emotional stress, or food allergies.

Common Abnormalities *(Continued)*

ABNORMALITY | **ASSESSMENT FINDINGS**

Herpes simplex

A common, contagious disease caused by the herpes simplex virus type 1. More prevalent in women than in men.

- Recurrent clusters of small vesicles on erythematous base.
- Sites burn and sting; neuralgia often occurs.
- Typically found on perioral and genital areas.
- May initially follow a minor infection.
- Later recurrences may be triggered by trauma, stress, or sun exposure.
- Often associated with lymphadenopathy of regional nodes.

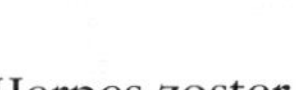

Herpes zoster

Also called "shingles"; an acute, infectious disease caused by the varicella zoster virus. Postzoster neuralgia discomfort can last for months. Ocular involvement can lead to blindness.

- Pain along a nerve dermatome is often the first symptom.
- Discomfort followed in 2–4 days by erythematous area that develops papules or plaques followed by painful grouped vesicles unilaterally along the dermatome.
- Vesicles or bullae rupture with crusting.
- Most common sites are face and trunk.
- Most common in people over age 60 and those with impaired immunity.

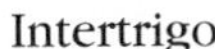

Intertrigo

A superficial dermatitis in the skinfolds. It is caused by heat, moisture, and friction, and is most common in obese people.

- Pink to reddened skin in body folds (between and beneath buttocks, beneath fatty abdominal pad, or beneath pendulous breasts).
- Areas in folds develop erythema, fissures, and denudation.
- Lesions may itch, burn, or sting.

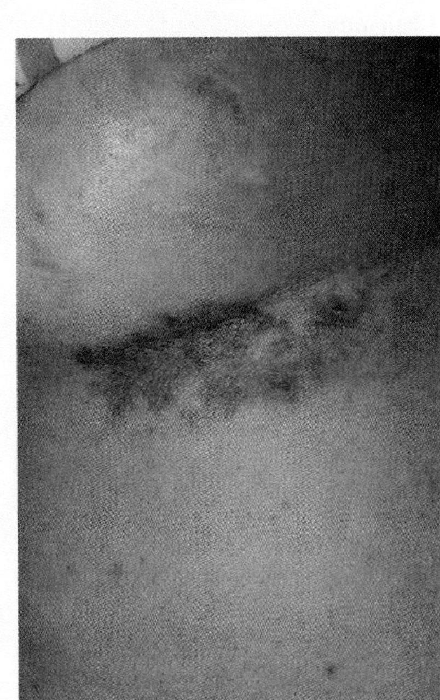

(Continued)

Common Abnormalities *(Continued)*

ABNORMALITY	ASSESSMENT FINDINGS
Kaposi's Sarcoma A type of malignant skin cancer seen most often in people who are HIV positive	• Purple-blue to red papules • Mild scaling of surface that progresses to ulcerate and bleed • Dissemination common, with widespread involvement of skin and mucosa 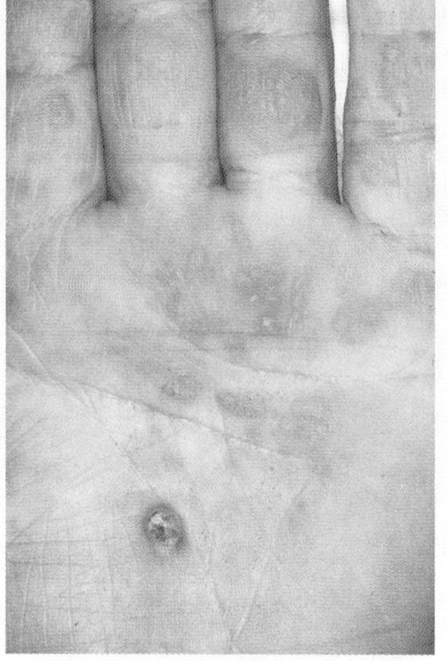
Malignant Melanoma An invasive, cancerous skin tumor with strong potential for metastasis to both regional and distant sites and organs.	• Commonly presents as a black or purple nodule. • Other color variations include pink, tan, brown, red, or even "normal" tones. • May also be flat or pedunculated. • Erythema or halo of coloring may surround lesion. • May ulcerate or become friable. • May be found on any location, including sun-exposed areas, palms, or soles.
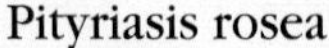 **Pityriasis rosea** A common, mild, acute inflammatory skin disease occurring most often in the spring and fall.	• Herald (or mother) patch usually precedes onset of smaller fawn-colored, oval, scaly eruptions 1–2 weeks later. • Later rash has individual oval lesions with a diagonal orientation. Often described as "Christmas tree" rash because of shape. • Rash may last 4–8 weeks. • Can be intensely pruritic. • As lesions exfoliate, they develop a "crinkly" scale and clear centrally so that they may mimic tineas. • Believed to be caused by viral infection. 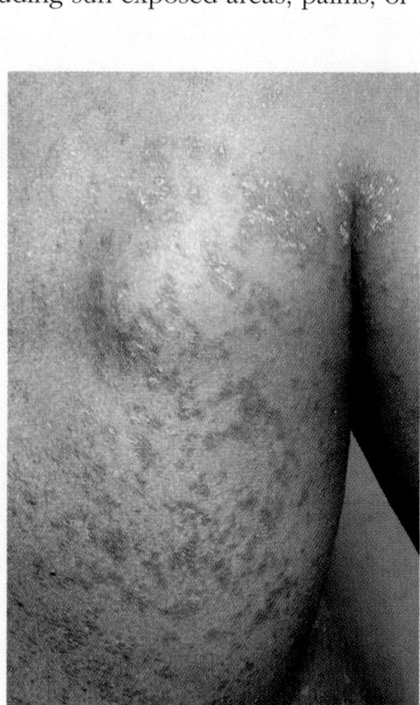

Common Abnormalities *(Continued)*

ABNORMALITY | **ASSESSMENT FINDINGS**

Psoriasis

A common dermatitis that has genetic causes and may begin at any age

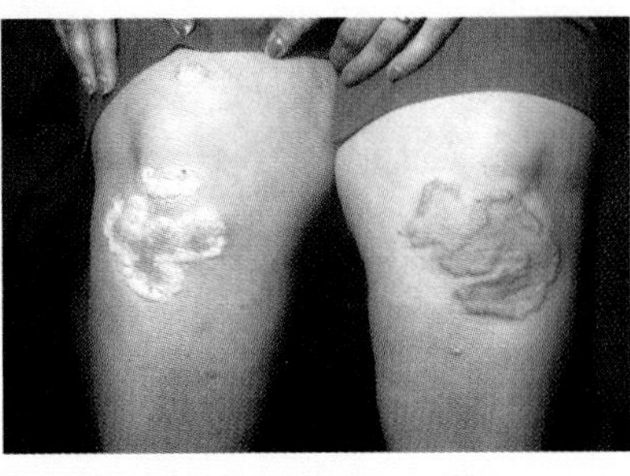

- Silvery scales on bright red papules.
- Scales generally thick; area beneath bleeds if scale is removed.
- Usually occurs on extensor surfaces of knees, elbows, and scalp.
- Can occur elsewhere, including between buttocks.
- Nails may develop a stippled, "pitted" appearance and separations.
- Itching may be mild or severe.
- A genetic predisposition is suggested by family history.
- May occur with arthritis.

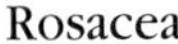

Rosacea

A chronic disorder of unknown cause that occurs mainly on the face

- Vascular component with erythema and telangiectasias.
- Acne component with papules, pustules, and seborrhea.
- Glandular component with hyperplasia of soft tissue of nose (rhinophyma).
- Usually rosy hue is diagnostic.
- Onset usually in 40s and 50s.
- May be aggravated by alcohol, caffeine, chocolate, heat, and spicy foods, as well as by situations that promote flushing.

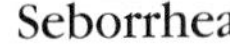

Seborrhea

A disorder of the sebaceous glands that causes an increase in the amount of sebaceous secretion and may also alter its quality

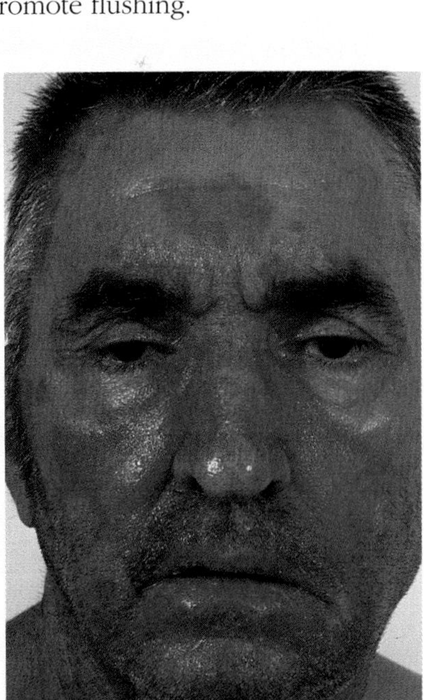

- Greasy scales may have underlying, flat erythema site.
- Some degree of papules and pustules possible.
- Typical sites include scalp, face (between brows, along sides of nose, at mustache/beard areas) and on presternal, interscapular, and umbilical regions.
- Genetic tendency, with family history possible.
- Itching may be present.
- Fissuring is possible with secondary infections.
- "Super dandruff" is common term because it occurs along sites with greater hair distribution.

(Continued)

Common Abnormalities *(Continued)*

ABNORMALITY	ASSESSMENT FINDINGS

Seborrheic Keratosis

A benign skin tumor that may be pigmented

- Sharply demarcated lesions.
- Brown to black pigmentation.
- Rough, dry surface.
- Elevation, with pasted or stuck-on appearance.
- Surrounding skin generally normal.
- Incidence increases with age.
- Generally found on trunk, although potentially can occur anywhere.

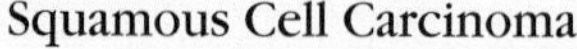

Squamous Cell Carcinoma

A form of skin cancer occurring mainly in the squamous cells

- Pink, scaly, elevated lesions.
- Base of lesions may be inflamed.
- Scablike appearance is common.
- Typically on sun-exposed surfaces, including scalp, hands, lips, and ears.

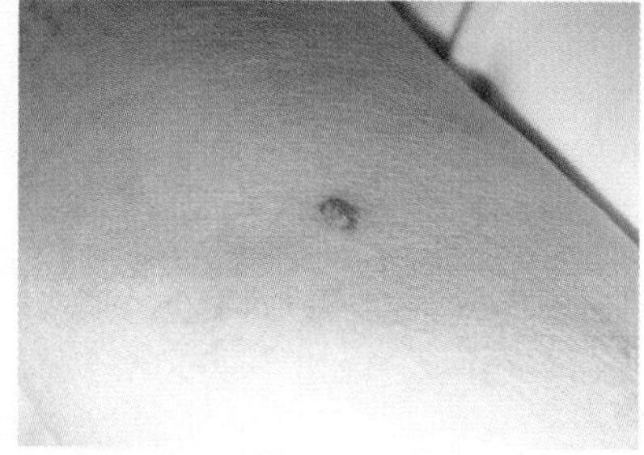

Stasis Dermatitis

Eczema of the legs with pigmentation, edema, and, at times, chronic inflammation resulting from venous insufficiency. **Stasis ulcer** is associated with stasis dermatitis and develops from venous insufficiency.

- Red, scaly patch often initial sign.
- Site develops vesicles and crusts.
- Ulcer may develop as a result of trauma, edema, or infection.
- When site does not progress to ulceration, reddish-brown hyperpigmentation may develop.
- Caused by poor circulation, which can be related to peripheral vascular diseases, obesity, or poor nutrition.

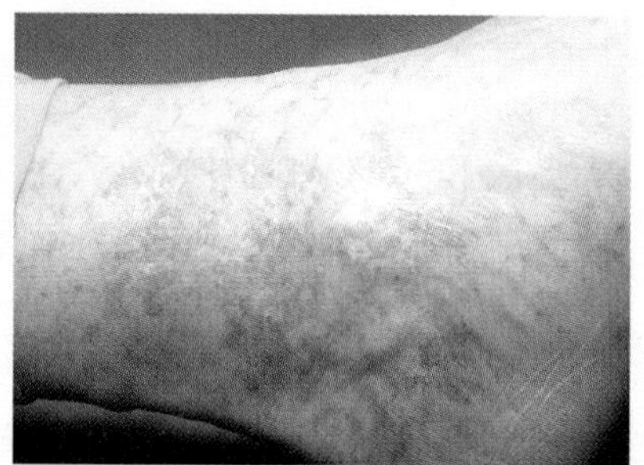

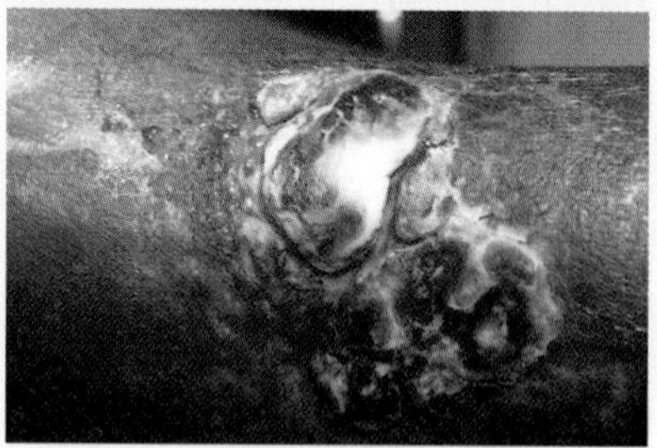

Tinea capitis

A fungal infection of the scalp

- Well-demarcated, reddened area
- Scaling, itching
- Dry, brittle hair

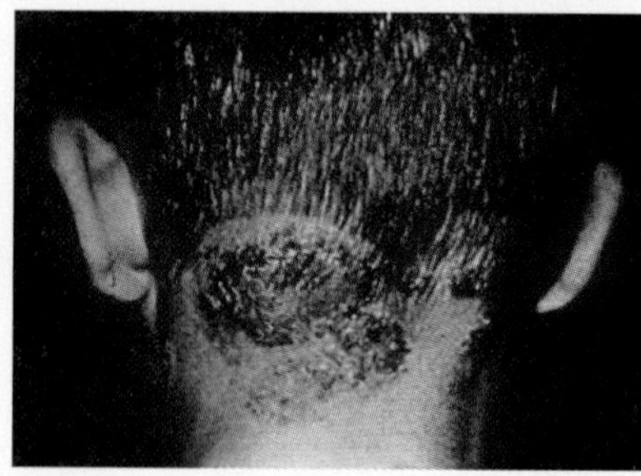

Common Abnormalities *(Continued)*

ABNORMALITY	ASSESSMENT FINDINGS
Tinea corporis Ringworm, a fungal skin disease occurring anywhere on the body	• Ring-shaped erythematous lesions on body • Central clearing • Advancing border with small vesicles • Pruritic • Most often on exposed surfaces
Tinea cruris "Jock itch," a fungal skin disease occurring in the genital and anal areas in males	• Sharply demarcated, reddened areas. • Central clearing. • Severe pruritus. • Intertriginous area in groin. • When it occurs on scalp, proper term is tinea capitis.
Tinea pedis "Athlete's foot," a fungal skin disease occurring in the foot. Tinea manum occurs on the palms or soles.	• Exfoliating, fissuring, macerated area of erythema. • Sites itch, burn, and/or sting. • Tinea manum occurs in interdigital folds of fingers or on palms. • Tinea pedis occurs in interdigital folds between toes or on soles of feet
Vitiligo Characterized by white patches of skin surrounded by areas of normal pigmentation. Progresses slowly and is more common in dark-skinned people.	• Irregular areas of depigmentation. • May have hyperpigmented border. • Flat, nonraised, with smooth surface. • Most common sites are face, hands, and feet. • Probably autoimmune cause; also associated with various endocrine disorders. 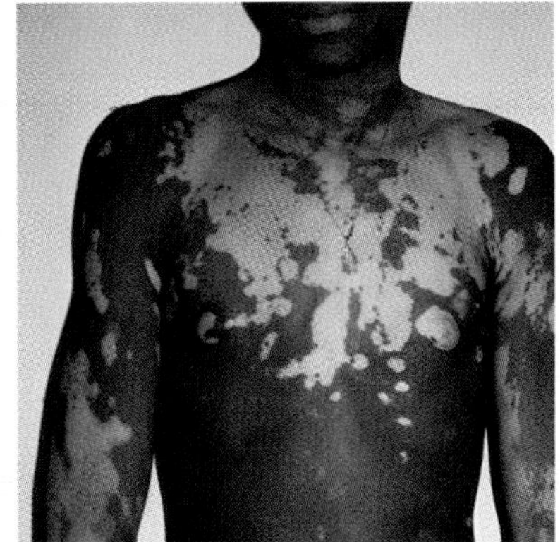

Summary

- The integumentary system provides invaluable information about your client's overall health status. Therefore it is important that you learn to objectively assess the skin, hair, and nails and be aware of the wide range of normal variations, which further differ according to age, race, and ethnic background.
- During your assessment, use a consistent approach and make careful observations about the overall integrity of the tissues, as well as any specific areas of abnormality.

CHAPTER 9

Assessing the Head, Face, and Neck

Before You Begin

INTRODUCTION TO THE HEAD, FACE, AND NECK

The head, face, and neck form a large portion of what is often referred to as the head, eyes, ears, nose, and throat (HEENT) system. This is actually a complex set of varied organs, combined during assessment because of their proximity to one another and the integration among the components of the system. The HEENT encompasses almost all of the systems: integumentary, respiratory, cardiovascular, gastrointestinal, musculoskeletal, neurological, endocrine, and lymphatic. The vascular, neurological, and musculoskeletal components of the HEENT, as well as the eyes and ears, are covered in separate chapters. The components addressed in this chapter include the head, face, nose, sinuses, neck, mouth, and pharynx. These components are complex in their actions and are involved in expression, communication, nourishment, respiration, and sensation, among other functions. Furthermore, disorders involving the head and face can be devastating to clients because they can greatly affect appearance. Even minor disorders involving the head, face, or neck can be perceived as disfiguring by clients.

Anatomy and Physiology Review

Before you begin your assessment, you need an understanding of these complex structures, their basic anatomy (Figs. 9–1 through 9–10) and function, the ways in which they relate to other systems, and expected normal findings.

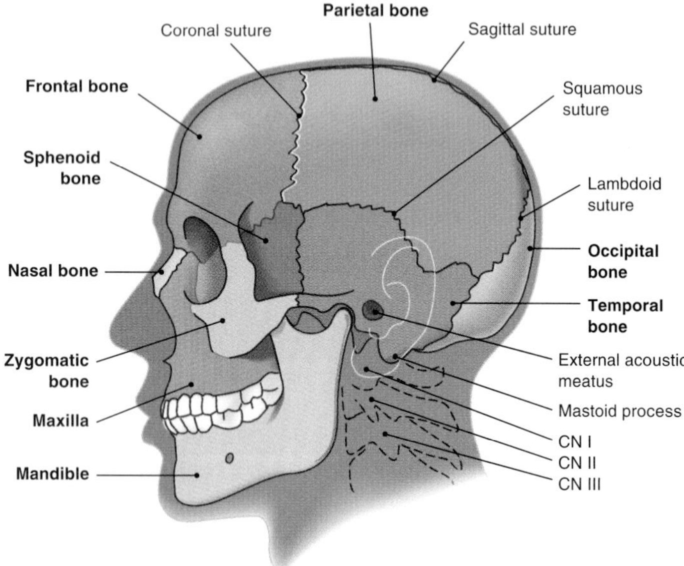

FIGURE 9–1. Skull.

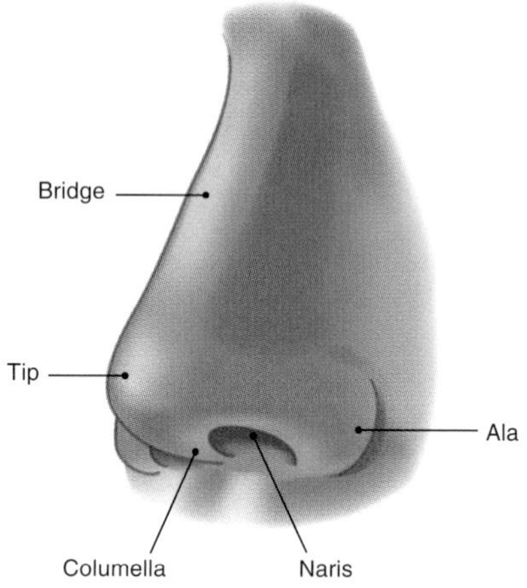

Bridge
Tip
Ala
Columella
Naris

FIGURE 9–2. External nose.

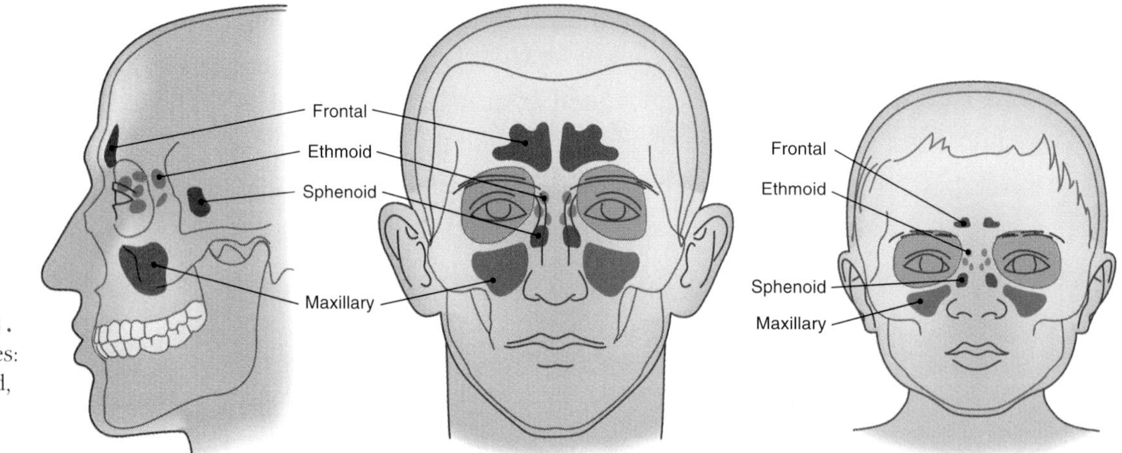

FIGURE 9–3. Paranasal sinuses: Frontal, ethmoid, sphenoid, and maxillary.

Head, Face, and Neck Structures and Functions

STRUCTURE	FUNCTION
Skull	
Cranial Skull: Parietal, temporal,occipital, frontal, sphenoid, and ethmoid	Protects and supports the brain.
Facial Skull: Maxillary, zygomatic, lacrimal, nasal, inferior nasal concha, palatine, mandible, and vomer	Forms facial framework.

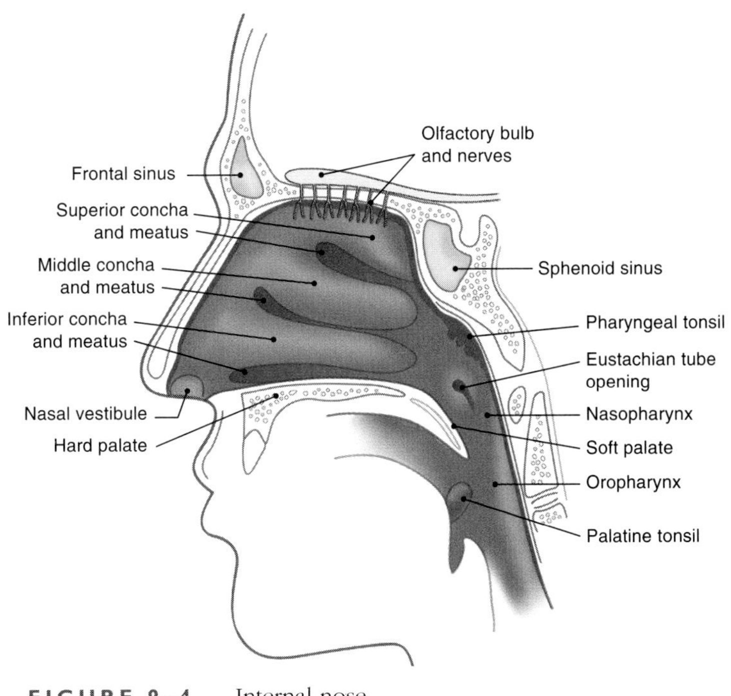

FIGURE 9–4. Internal nose.

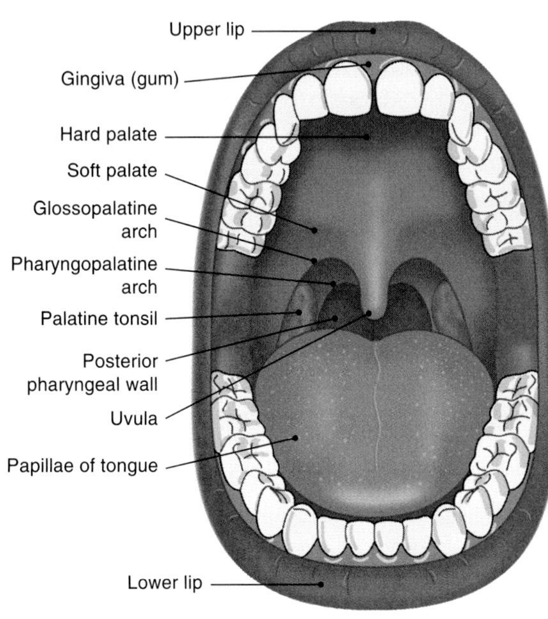

FIGURE 9–5. Structures of the mouth.

Head, Face, and Neck Structures and Functions

STRUCTURE	FUNCTION
Skull *(Continued)*	
Joints: The sutures: coronal, lambdoid, sagittal, and squamous	Immovable joints that connect cranial bones. (Bones are joined at birth by pliable membranes called fontanels, which permit delivery through the birth canal and allow the brain to grow and develop.)
Temporomandibular Joint (TMJ)	Joins mandible and temporal bone, allowing movement of the mandible
Paranasal Sinuses	Air cavities that add resonance to the voice and lighten the weight of the head. Lined with mucous membranes, the sinuses drain through the meatus, located beneath the turbinates on the lateral aspects of the nasal cavity.
Nose	
Nares (Nostrils) and Vestibul	Nares provide access to the nasopharynx through structures lined with mucous membranes, which are rich with blood vessels and covered with cilia (see below).
Nasal Mucosa	Ciliated epithelium cells with goblet cells produce mucus, which traps bacteria and air pollutants.
Nasal Septum	Composed of the ethmoid bone and vomer, divides the nasal cavities.
Cilia	Small hairs that filter air.
Turbinates: Superior, middle,	Bony conchae (folds) of the internal nasal walls that increase the surface area for and inferiorair to be filtered, warmed, and humidified before entering the lungs.
Olfactory Nerve (CN I)	Controls sense of smell. Stimulated by olfactory receptor cells located in upper nasal cavities.

(Continued)

Head, Face, and Neck Structures and Functions *(Continued)*

STRUCTURE	FUNCTION
Mouth	
Lips	Muscular folds that surround the mouth; contain sensory receptors and are very sensitive. Lips assist with eating, expression, and speech.
Superior and Inferior Labial Frenulum	Connect the lips to the gums.
Buccal Mucosa	Moist mucous membrane of the cheeks that assists with eating.
Teeth: 20 deciduous, 32 permanent	Needed for chewing; also have esthetic value.
Gingiva (Gums)	Help to anchor teeth, part of oral mucosa, cover alveolar bone.
Tongue	Muscle controlled by CN XII; needed for chewing, swallowing, and speech. Sensory (taste) CN VII and CN IX.
Lingual Frenulum	Attaches the tongue to the floor of the mouth.
Pharynx: Nasopharynx, oropharynx, and laryngopharynx	The pharynx is a muscular tube. Contraction of the oropharynx and laryngopharynx is part of swallowing reflex. The nasopharynx is the uppermost portion behind the nasal cavity. The adenoids are located on the posterior nasopharynx. The eustachian tubes open into the nasopharynx. The oropharynx is a part of the oral cavity and the palatine tonsils located on the lateral walls. The laryngopharynx is the most posterior portion of the pharynx. The anterior portion opens into the larynx; the posterior portion opens into the esophagus.
Tonsils: Palatine, lingual, and pharyngeal	Lymphatic tissue that prevents infection. The palatine tonsils lie laterally on each side of the soft palate between the palatoglossal and palatopharyngeal arches. The lingual tonsils are at the base of the tongue, and the pharyngeal tonsils (adenoids) are behind the nose in the posterior pharyngeal wall.
Hard Palate	Forms the floor of the nasal cavity.
Soft Palate	Posterior to hard palate, elevates during swallowing to prevent food and saliva from entering the nasopharynx.
Uvula	Fleshy conelike structure in the center of the soft palate that prevents food from entering nasal passages.
Salivary Glands	Secrete saliva, which contains amylase to convert starch to maltose.
Parotid Glands	Salivary glands anterior to the ear. Secretions help lubricate food to facilitate chewing and swallowing.
Stensen's Duct	Drains parotid gland, enters oral cavity through buccal mucosa, opposite the second molar.
Submandibular Glands	Located at posterior corner of mandible.
Sublingual Glands	Located below the floor of the mouth.
Wharton's Duct	Drains submandibular and sublingual salivary glands, enters oral cavity under the tongue on the floor of the mouth.
Neck	
Thyroid Gland	Controls metabolism and helps regulate calcium. The thyroid is the largest endocrine organ and produces thyroxine (T4) and triiodothyronine (T3), which are largely involved in the body's metabolism as well as cardiovascular, gastrointestinal, and neuromuscular functions. The thyroid also produces calcitonin, which lowers calcium and phosphate blood levels.
Parathyroid Glands	Located on the posterior side of the thyroid; increase blood calcium levels.
Cervical Lymph Nodes	Part of the lymphatic system. Drain the structures of the head and neck.

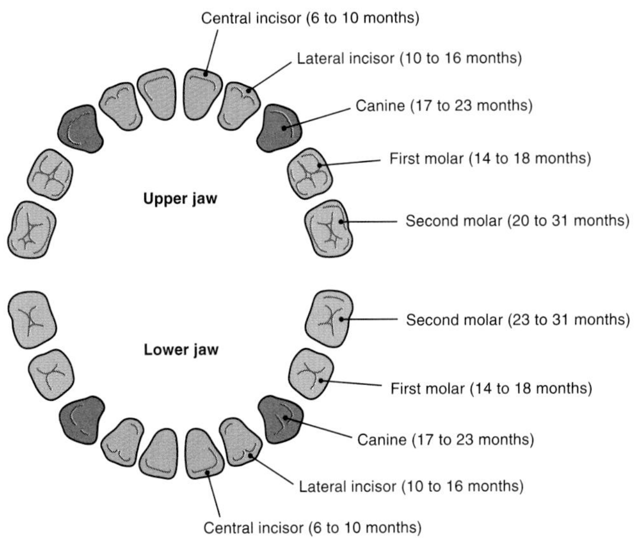

FIGURE 9–6. Deciduous teeth.

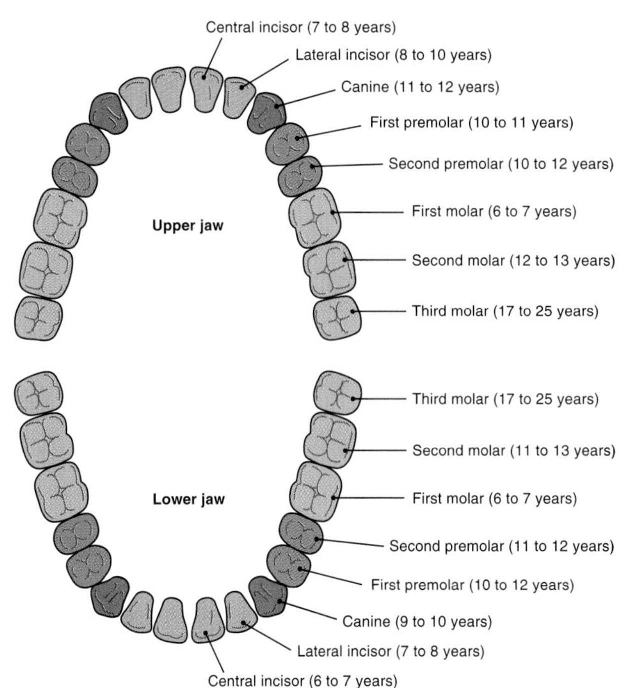

FIGURE 9–7. Permanent teeth

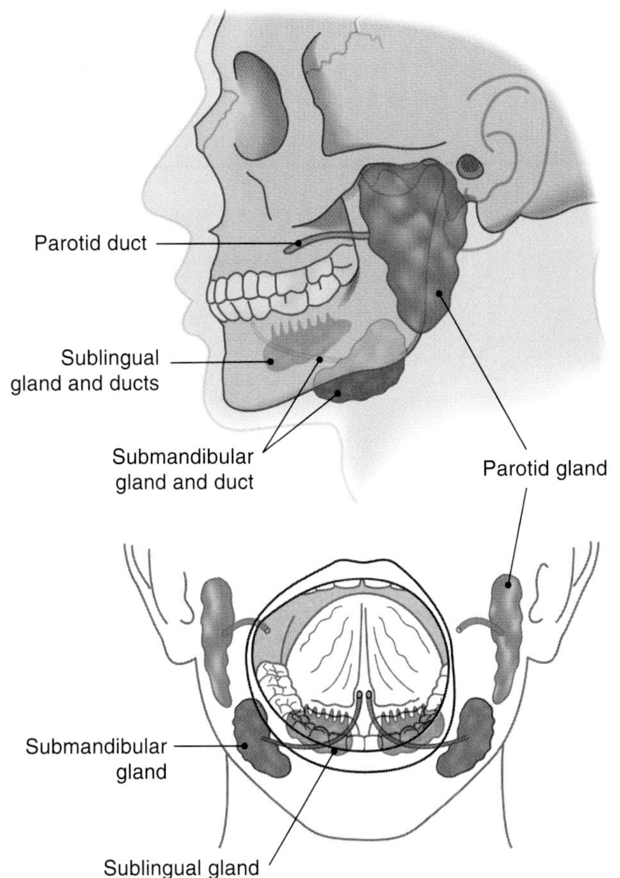

FIGURE 9–8. Salivary and parotid glands.

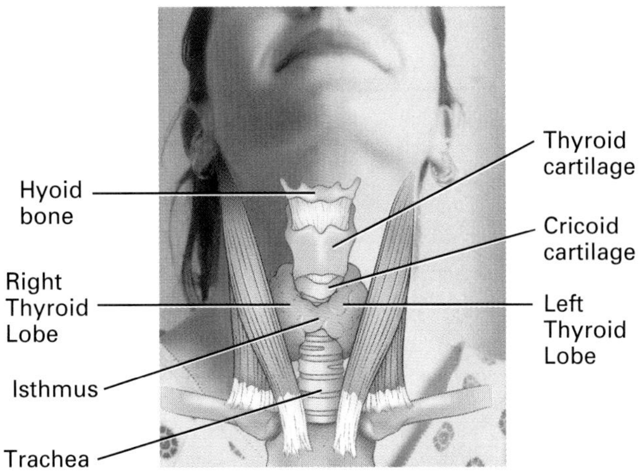

FIGURE 9–9. Thyroid gland.

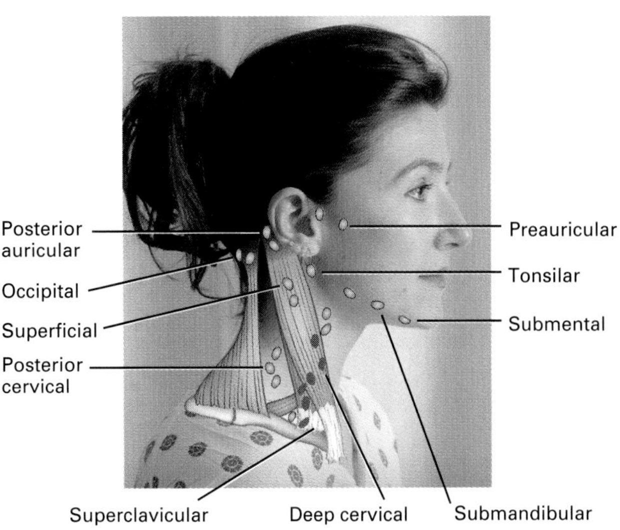

FIGURE 9–10. Cervical lymph nodes.

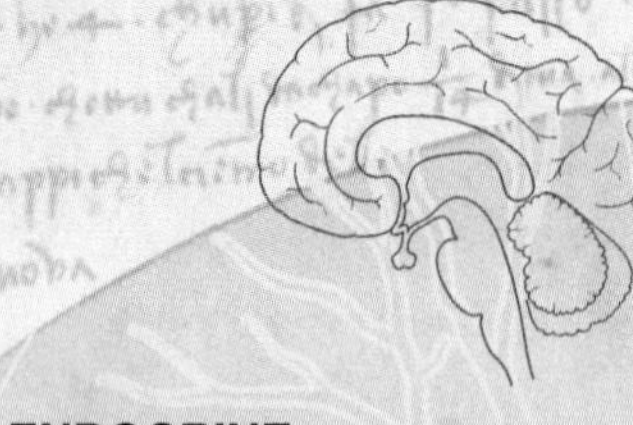

NEUROLOGICAL

Cranial nerves located in head, face and neck.

Cranial nerves influence ability to communicate both verbally and nonverbally and to eat.

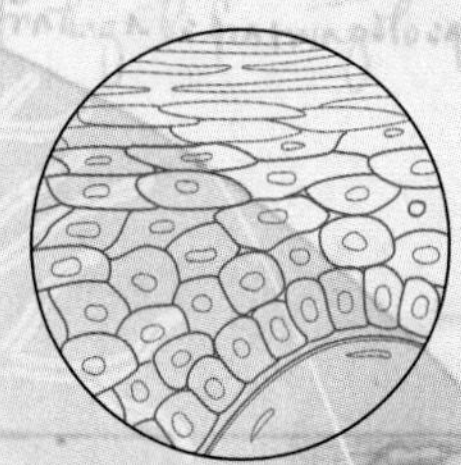

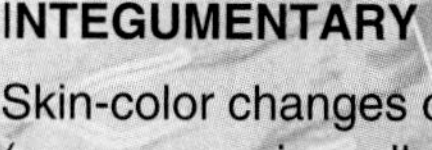

ENDOCRINE

Thyroid and parathyroid glands located in neck.

INTEGUMENTARY

Skin-color changes on face (e.g., cyanosis, pallor, jaundice) may indicate systemic problems.

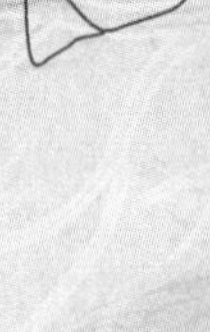

RESPIRATORY

Respiratory tract begins at nasal and oral cavities.

Injuries to head and face can affect breathing.

Respiratory infections often begin in upper airways of nose and throat.

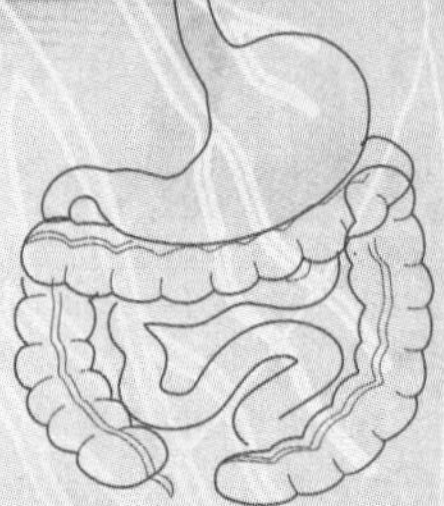

DIGESTIVE

Mouth is beginning of digestive tract.

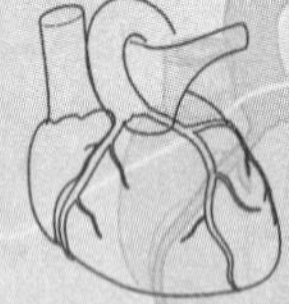

CARDIOVASCULAR

Temporal and carotid arteries located in head and neck.

Neck and jaw pain may indicate cardiovascular disease.

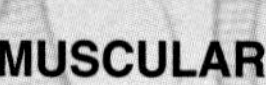

MUSCULAR

Facial muscles needed for expression, communication and nutrition.

URINARY

Changes in face (e.g., edema or uremic frost) may reflect renal problems.

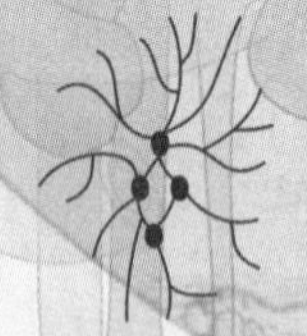

LYMPHATIC

Cervical lymph nodes located in neck.

Tonsils located in pharynx.

Mast cells located in pharynx.

SKELETAL

Skull protects brain.

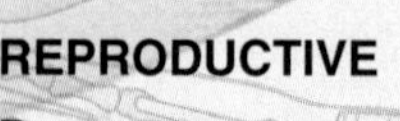

REPRODUCTIVE

Pregnancy can cause changes in facial color (chloasma).

Lips and mouth are erogenous areas.

Relationship of Head/Face/Neck to Other Systems

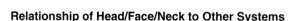

Interaction with Other Body Systems

The head, face, and neck include many structures with highly varied functions. Disruption or disease of several other systems can affect the organs of the head, face, and neck. These other systems include those described in the following paragraphs.

The Respiratory System

The nasal and oral cavities are entry points to the respiratory system. Injuries or diseases of these two structures can result in impaired ability to breathe. The ears, nose, and pharynx form the upper respiratory system. These structures communicate with the lower respiratory system through the trachea, so that infections in one area can be transmitted to the other.

The Cardiovascular System

Many structures of this system receive rich vascular supply. The mucosa of the nasal cavity includes a plexus of vessels that bleed easily. The temporal arteries are assessed during the examination of the face, as are the carotids during the examination of the neck. Disorders of the cardiovascular system may be reflected in the structures of the head, face, and neck. Infarct or ischemic pain may radiate to the jaw or throat. Facial edema can reflect fluid retention.

The Musculoskeletal System

The muscles of the face (Fig. 9–11) are highly involved in expression, communication, and nourishment. Diseases of the musculoskeletal system can have profound effects on these actions. Inflammatory changes of the TMJ can cause limited jaw motion and jaw pain and can be unilateral or bilateral; disorders of the cervical vertebrae or strain or inflammation of supporting structures can have profound effects on neck comfort and motion.

The Neurological System

The head, face, and neck are highly involved in many sensory processes. The neurological system includes the structures responsible for olfaction and taste as well as for sensation in the face and related structures. Dysfunction of the neurological system can have intense effects on these senses. Furthermore, the neurological system is involved in the complex movements necessary for speech, feeding, and expression. Altered neurological function is often evident in these actions. For example, Bell's palsy, an inflammatory paralysis of the trigeminal nerve, has a profound effect on the function of the motor components on the affected side.

The Endocrine System

The neck houses the thyroid gland, a major endocrine organ. Dysfunction of the thyroid is often accompanied

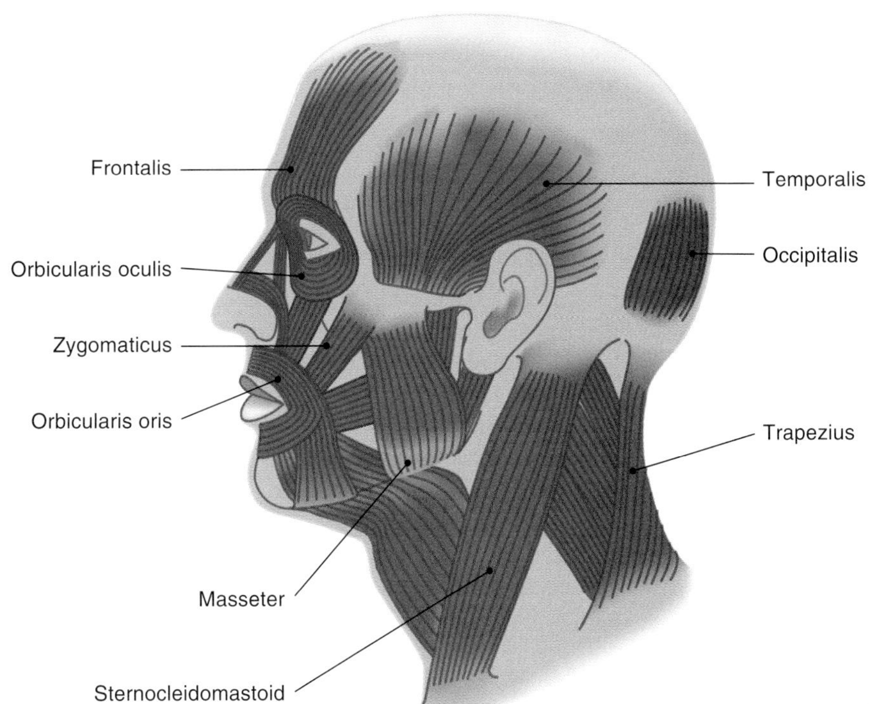

FIGURE 9–11. Facial muscles.

by organ hypertrophy, or enlargement, regardless of whether the dysfunction results in hyperactivity or hypoactivity of the thyroid gland. Enlargements, called goiters, are evident during the examination of the neck. Many endocrine disorders have typical facies. For example, when hypocalcemia develops from parathyroid disease, Chvostek's sign, a facial spasm, may be an early symptom.

The Lymphatic/Hematologic System

The nasopharynx and oropharynx are rich with mast cells, responsible for allergic control symptoms. After exposure to allergens, the mast cell and basophil mediators are triggered, with resulting inflammatory responses responsible for the typical sneezing, itching, and secretions of the nasal, nasopharyngeal, oropharyngeal, and other linings. The ultimate result can include congestion, drainage, and secondary infections involving additional structures including the sinuses. The cervical nodes are sensitive to infection or inflammatory changes in the regions they drain, with resulting enlargement of nodes often signaling a disorder.

Because of the rich vascular supply of the nasal and oral mucosa, hematologic changes may first be reflected here. For instance, thrombocytopenia may first cause petechiae of the mucous membranes or bleeding of the gums or nose. Anemia may be accompanied by pallor of the mucosa or glossitis.

Developmental, Cultural, and Ethnic Variations

Infants and Children

Head: The head, at birth, is often molded into a less than round shape during vaginal delivery, yet assumes a symmetrical, rounded shape in several days. The fontanels (anterior, posterior, anterolateral, and posterolateral), which are the openings between the skull bones, remain open for growth, but close over the first year of life. The head circumference is an important measurement because a large head can indicate hydrocephaly, whereas a small head can indicate a developmental delay. In comparison to the head of an adult, the head of an infant or toddler is large in proportion to its body.

Nose and sinuses: Only the ethmoid and maxillary sinuses are fully developed at birth. Others develop over the first 7 years. Children have a tendency to place small objects in their noses. Unilateral purulent drainage often results.

Teeth: The number of teeth varies, depending on a child's age. Infants get their first incisors at approximately 6 months of age. At age 6 or 7 years, they gradually begin to lose the 20 deciduous teeth, which are replaced with 32 permanent ones.

Throat and neck: The tonsils, which are small in infancy, may become larger during childhood. They often become smaller again by approximately age 12. The neck muscles of an infant are weak, and the infant must develop control of them to control the head. The thyroid of infants and children is not palpable. It is not unusual for young children to have palpable, small, "shoddy" cervical nodes.

Older Adults

Teeth: With proper care and improved products, teeth should now last through advanced age. However, it is not unusual for older people to lose at least some of their teeth. They often have dental prostheses. Dentition plays a significant role in the nutrition of elderly people.

Mouth and Nose: Older people tend to have decreased production of salivation. With age, the senses of olfaction and taste may be diminished, which can affect nutritional status.

Pregnant Women

Neck: Pregnant women may have palpable thyroids because the gland is stimulated by estrogen and develops increased vascular supply.

Face: A brownish pigmentation (chloasma or "the mask of pregnancy") may occur.

Mouth: Hypertrophy of the gums may occur during pregnancy.

People of Different Cultures and Ethnic Groups

You need to consider your client's cultural background when assessing the head, face, and neck. What might be considered an abnormal finding in one cultural group may be a normal cultural variation for another.

Face: Facial skin color can vary greatly depending on cultural background. Remember, cyanosis or jaundice may be difficult to assess in clients with dark skin tones. Cultural variations can also be seen in skin textures and hair growth patterns. For example, African-Americans may develop facial pseudofolliculitis (razor bumps) and Chinese-Americans normally have little facial hair. Irish-Americans have a greater incidence of skin cancer, so be sure to thoroughly assess sun-exposed areas, especially the face and ears. The shape and position of the eyes and nose may also have cultural variations. Chinese-Americans have Mongolian traits, and Filipino-Americans have almond shaped-eyes, mildly flared nostrils, and a low, flat nose bridge.

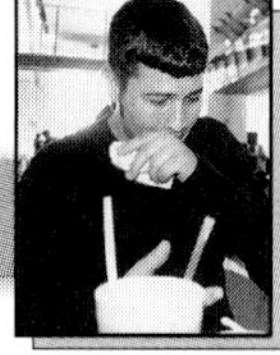

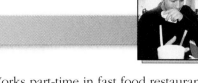

Introducing the Case Study

John Henck, a 17-year-old high school senior, is required to have a physical examination before participating in a deep-sea diving course and receiving certification. He is very excited about spending his spring vacation diving. You plan to complete both a health history and physical examination. Because of the requirement that John be able to tolerate use of the diving equipment, a major emphasis of the examination is on the head, face, and neck.

Performing the Head, Face, and Neck Assessment

Assessment of the head, face, and neck involves obtaining a complete health history and performing a physical examination. As you perform the assessment, be alert for signs and symptoms of actual and potential problems of the various components of the head, face, and neck.

Health History

The health history identifies any related symptoms or risk factors and the presence of diseases involving the head, face, and neck. It must also detect any other disorders that may affect these structures. Your history will include obtaining biographical data and asking questions about the client's current health, past health, and family and psychosocial history. It also includes a review of systems (ROS).

Biographical Data

Review the client's biographical information. Note your client's age—certain diseases are more prevalent in specific age groups. For example, children tend to have more upper respiratory problems and pharyngitis than older adults. Also ask about your client's occupation. Does he or she have a job that puts him or her at risk for head injury? Does he or she spend long hours at a computer terminal (may result in tension headaches)? Questions like these will help to identify the potential for exposures to physical and environmental situations that could harm the head, face, and neck structures.

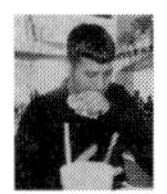

Case Study Findings

Reviewing John's biographical data:

- 17-year-old unmarried male.
- Works part-time in fast food restaurant.
- Born in the United States, was adopted immediately after birth.
- Protestant religion.
- Father is computer salesman and mother is radiology technician.
- Source: Self, reliable.

Current Health Status

Determine whether the client has any specific presenting complaints related to the head, face, or neck. Some common complaints include headaches, jaw pain, neck pain or stiffness, masses, nasal congestion, epistaxis, mouth or dental pain, mouth lesions, sore throat, and hoarseness. Any such complaints, as well as others that you might identify later, should be explored and developed using an organized system of symptom analysis, such as the "PQRST" format. Because disorders of several systems can influence the head, face, and neck, it is important to determine the client's overall health status. There will be times, however, when the client's presenting problems are particularly acute or distressful, and the initial history and physical will have to be very focused.

Symptom Analysis

Symptom Analysis tables for all of the symptoms described in the following paragraphs are available on the Web for viewing and printing. In your Web browser, go to *http://www.fadavis.com/detail.cfm?id=0882-9* and click on Symptom Analysis Tables under Explore This Product.

Head Pain

Head pain can be associated with a variety of problems, including migraines, tension, systemic infections, and trauma.

Jaw Tightness and Pain

When a client presents with jaw tightness and/or pain, the cause may be TMJ syndrome, but it could also be trauma or infection/inflammation in the structures near the jaw. An important consideration for jaw discomfort is whether it might be caused by cardiovascular disease. Always ask clients if they have a personal or family history of heart disease.

Neck Pain and Stiffness

Neck pain and stiffness can stem from musculoskeletal problems as well from infections. Symptom analysis can help identify any forgotten trauma or physical exertion that might explain the complaint.

Neck Mass

When a client complains of a neck mass, it might be a goiter of the thyroid gland or enlarged lymph nodes. Enlarged nodes may signal either an infectious or malignant disorder.

Nasal Congestion

Nasal congestion is usually caused by an upper respiratory infection or allergy.

Nosebleed

Epistaxis, or nosebleed, is usually self-limited and has relatively benign causes. However, it can be cased by coagulopathies or other hematologic disturbances, malignancies, hypertension, or trauma.

Mouth Lesions

A mouth lesion can be caused by a malignancy, trauma, nutritional deficit, or poorly fitted dentures or orthodontic appliances.

Mouth and Dental Pain

Mouth pain can be caused by ischemic heart disease, musculoskeletal disorders, or dental problems.

Sore Throat

When a client complains of a sore throat, the most common cause is a bacterial or viral illness. However, throat discomfort can be associated with throat masses, including thyroid hypertrophy or malignancies, foreign objects in the throat, and other causes.

Hoarseness

Another common complaint is hoarseness. Hoarseness may be caused by overuse of the voice, for example, prolonged periods of shouting or loud speech. It can also be an indication of gastroesophageal reflux, malignancies, neuromuscular disorders, or other health problems.

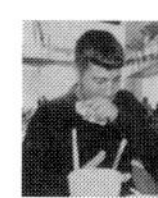

Case Study Findings

John's current health status includes:

- Describes current health as excellent. Says he is "health directed" and wishes to maximize health.
- No current complaints, although he does have "hay fever" in spring and fall. He is not currently experiencing any symptoms, but generally has several weeks of sneezing, runny nose, itching eyes, and head congestion. Antihistamines generally control the symptoms. On rare occasions at times other than the fall or spring, he has symptoms that last several hours, but he is not sure what triggers them.

Past Health History

Once you have investigated the client's chief complaint, explore the past health history. This portion of the history includes childhood and adulthood illnesses, surgeries, or major injuries; hospitalizations; major diagnostic procedures; exposures to infectious diseases; and allergies; as well as an immunization and medication history.

Past Health History

CATEGORY/QUESTIONS TO ASK	RATIONALE/SIGNIFICANCE
Childhood Illnesses	
As a child, did you have frequent respiratory infections, such as strep throat, sinus infections, or tonsillitis? Did you have allergies or asthma?	Asking these questions identifies the potential for recurrence of problems that have existed since youth and for surgical or diagnostic procedures that should be explored. It also identifies the potential for rhinitis, which is commonly associated with other **atopic** disorders.
Hospitalizations	
Have you ever been hospitalized? What for? Have you had radiation to the neck; biopsies of the head, face, and neck; or other procedures?	This further explores the existence of health problems that may be related to the head, face, and neck or other problems that might have an influence on these structures. It may identify disorders or previous syndromes that are still unidentified.

Past Health History

CATEGORY/QUESTIONS TO ASK	RATIONALE/SIGNIFICANCE
Surgeries/Serious Injuries	
Have you ever had surgery? If so, what kind? For example: Tonsillectomy, adenoidectomy, thyroidectomy, or rhinoplasty?	This may explain physical findings, such as scars or the presence or absence of palatine tonsils. Both past surgeries and traumatic injuries may suggest the potential for chronic problems.
Serious/Chronic Illnesses	
Have you ever been diagnosed with or experienced thyroid disease, a malignancy, headaches, Bell's palsy, rhinitis, sinusitis, frequent upper respiratory infections, or TMJ syndrome?	These questions point out diseases of the head, face or neck that have a potential for recurrence or **sequelae** or that should be evaluated during current examination. They also inform you about treatment at the time of incidence and the client's understanding of the diagnosis and treatment.
Immunizations	
Are your immunizations up to date? Have you ever had a flu shot or pneumovax? If so, when? When was your last tetanus/diphtheria vaccination?	This allows you to document immunization history, especially influenza and diphtheria vaccines, which are of special significance to the upper respiratory tract.
Allergies	
Have you ever had an adverse reaction to medications, foods, chemicals, or environmental agents?	This allows you to record previous allergic reactions so that they can be avoided in the future. A history of one atopic disorder, such as asthma or eczema, causes higher incidence of others, such as allergic rhinitis. A common allergic reaction is **angioedema** (benign swelling of skin, mucous membranes, or viscera).
Medications	
Are you currently taking any prescribed or over-the-counter (OTC) medications? What are they?	Medications can cause reactive symptoms, including a sense of throat tightness from angioedema or adverse reactions such as ototoxicity. Knowing all agents the client is using alerts you to potential for interactions with new agents. Chemotherapy often causes stomatitis, and superimposed fungal infections often occur with antibiotic therapy. Other medications, such as steroids, may have side effects that affect the head, face, and neck (e. g., moon face or hirsutism). See box, Drugs That Adversely Affect the Head, Face, and Neck, on page 206.
Recent Travel/Military Service/ Exposure to Infections or Contagious Diseases	
Are you aware of any recent exposures to infectious or contagious illnesses? Have you traveled to foreign countries? Shared a glass or eating utensils with anyone?	Identifies the potential for pending problem and presents an opportunity to determine the client's understanding of protection from infections. Drinking water and eating in foreign countries can expose client to parasitic infections. Knowing previous exposure to infectious disease may initiate further investigation of symptoms and prompt diagnostic testing to assist with a differential diagnosis. Note dates of possible exposure. Teens on sports teams may share water bottles and pass on infectious disease.

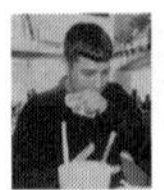

Case Study Findings

John's past health history reveals:

- Usual childhood illnesses, without complications.
- Tonsils and adenoids removed at age 4, after frequent throat infections.
- Tympanoplasty at age 3 after frequent bouts of ear infections.
- Immunizations up to date. Tetanus updated last year when he stepped on a piece of glass while wading on a shoreline.
- Seasonal hay fever since childhood.
- Takes over-the-counter antihistamines when he has no prescribed antihistamines on hand, but usually takes Claritin during seasonal allergy attacks. Has always taken one multivitamin daily. Takes no other medications.
- No recent exposures to known infections, but notes that he works in a busy restaurant and attends public school, so could be exposed to "whatever's going around."

Family History

The purpose of the family history is to identify health problems that are familial or genetic. The history should

Drugs That Adversely Affect the Head, Face, and Neck

When obtaining a health history to assess a client's head and neck, the nurse must ask about current drug use. Many of the commonly used drugs listed below can produce adverse reactions in the head and neck, including gingivitis (gum inflammation), alopecia (hair loss), and epistaxis (nosebleed).

Drug Class	Drug	Possible Adverse Reactions
Anticholinergics	atropine, scopolamine, glycopyrrolate, propantheline, belladonna alkaloids, dicyclomine, hyoscyamine	Decreased salivation, dry mouth
Anticonvulsants	phenytoin sodium	Gingival hyperplasia
Antidepressants	tricyclics, including amitriptyline and nortriptyline, paroxetine	Dry mouth
Antihistamines	diphenyhydramine, brompheniramine, chlorpheniramine	Dry mouth
Antihypertensives	guanabenz, clonidine, methyldopa, nifedipine	Dry mouth
	(all calcium channel blockers)	Gingival hyperplasia
Antilipemics	clofibrate	Dry brittle hair, alopecia
Antineoplastics	bleomycin sulfate	Ulcerated tongue and lips, alopecia
	dactinomycin	Mouth lesions, alopecia
	melphalan	Mouth lesions
	mitomycin	Mouth lesions, alopecia
	methotrexate	Gingivitis, mouth lesions, alopecia
	cyclophosphamide	Mouth lesions, alopecia
	vincristine sulfate	Mouth lesions, alopecia
	chlorambucil	Mouth lesions
	uracil mustard	Mouth lesions
	cisplatin	Gingival platinum line, alopecia
	hydroxyurea	Mouth lesions
	fluorouracil	Alopecia, epistaxis
	doxorubicin	Mouth lesions, alopecia
	cytarabine	Mouth lesions, alopecia
	daunorubicin	Mouth lesions, alopecia
	etoposide	Alopecia
Cardiac agents	disopyramide phosphate	Dry mouth
Genitourinary smooth-muscle relaxants	flavoxate, oxybutynin, propantheline	Dry mouth
Gold salts	gold sodium thiomalate	Gingivitis, mouth lesions
	auranofin	Mouth lesions
Nonsteroidal anti-inflammatory agents	indomethacin	Gingival lesions
	ibuprofen	Dry mouth, gingival lesions
Miscellaneous agents	lithium salts	Dry mouth, dry hair, alopecia
	metoclopramide	Dry mouth, glossal or periorbital edema
	penicillamine	Mouth lesions
	isotretinoin	Inflamed lips, epistaxis, dry mouth
	allopurinol	Alopecia
	propranolol	Hyperkeratosis and psoriasis of the scalp, alopecia
	guanethidine sulfate	Nasal stuffiness, dry mouth
	edrophonium	Increased salivation
	pyridostigmine	Increased salivation, increased tracheobronchial secretions
	fluorides	Staining or mottling of teeth
	warfarin sodium	Epistaxis with excessive dosage
	amphetamines	Dry mouth, continuous chewing or bruxism (tooth grinding) with prolonged use
	tetracycline	Enamel hypoplasia and permanent yellow-gray to brown tooth discoloration in children under age 8 and in offspring of pregnant clients
	cyclosporin	Gingival hyperplasia
	valproic acid	Alopecia

include information on close relatives, both living and dead. The focus should be on problems that either have a genetic component or are attributed to environmental/living situations shared with the client. The genogram described in earlier chapters is a helpful way to organize the information obtained through the family history.

Family History

RISK FACTORS/ QUESTIONS TO ASK	RATIONALE/SIGNIFICANCE
Head and Neck Disorders	
Do you have a family history of migraine, cluster, or other headaches? Neck masses, thyroid disease, or malignancies?	Headache syndromes are often found in several family members. Identify the history of neck masses or enlargements, including thyroid goiter and lymphadenopathy associated with lymphomas or other malignancies.
Nose/Sinus Disorders	
Do you have a family history of rhinitis or nasal polyps?	Rhinitis has a familial component. A family history of rhinitis, like other allergic problems, may have environmental triggers.
Mouth/Throat Disorders	
Do you have a family history of cancers of the mouth or throat?	This may indicate an increased likelihood of similar problems.
Respiratory Disorders	
Is there a history of asthma in your family?	A family history of asthma increases the client's chance of having rhinitis or other atopic diseases.
Cardiovascular Disorders	
Do you have a family history of heart disease or hypertension?	A family history of coronary artery disease or cardiovascular disease is particularly important if the client presents with neck or jaw pain unrelated to trauma, chewing, strain, or epistaxis.
Hematologic Disorders	
Is there any history of clotting or bleeding disorders among your close relatives?	Familial bleeding disorders are significant when the client has a history of bleeding gums or nosebleeds.
Neurological Disorders	
Do you have a family history of strokes, neuritis, or other neurological disorders?	A family history of neurological disorders might help explain facial weakness or sensory disturbances, such as alteration of olfaction or taste.
Endocrine Disorders	
Do you have a family history of thyroid disease, acromegaly, or other endocrine diseases?	Thyroid disease and other endocrine disorders have familial components. Acromegaly, a pituitary disorder, may be responsible for altered bone structure or soft tissue hypertrophy causing appearance changes. Many other endocrine disorders, such as Cushing's syndrome, present with typical facial changes.
Musculoskeletal Disorders	
Do you have a family history of arthritis or osteoporosis?	A predisposition to arthritic disorders or osteoporosis is important when assessing pain of the neck or jaw.
Lymphatic Disorders	
Is there a family history of allergies or autoimmune disorders of the thyroid or other organs?	Allergic disorders, which can be inherited, are a crucial consideration when assessing the nose and throat. Autoimmune disorders, such as rheumatoid arthritis or Sjögren's syndrome, are reflected in changes of the head, face, and neck.
Infectious or Contagious Disorders	
Have you recently been exposed to an upper respiratory infection or any other potentially contagious infection from family members or close friends?	Identify the potential that any current symptoms might be related to contagious illness.

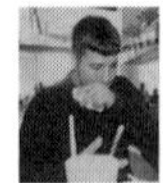

Case Study Findings

John's family history reveals:

- Biological family history unknown; would like to know his family health history, but has been told this is not available.
- Adoptive parents are both in good health.

Review of Systems

The review of symptoms (ROS) allows you to explore each body system to determine whether the client has a complaint that might affect the head, face, or neck. Ask the client about problems that commonly affect the head, face, and neck, as well as all other systems. Although exploring the client's presenting complaint will already have alerted you to the potential for many symptoms, this review has the potential to trigger the client to recall symptoms that he or she might otherwise have forgotten or to relate symptoms that he or she previously thought were unimportant.

Review of Systems

SYSTEM/QUESTIONS TO ASK	RATIONALE/SIGNIFICANCE
General Health Survey	
Has your energy level or weight changed? Have you had fevers or sweating?	Endocrine and lymphatic system disorders often result in nonspecific symptoms, which are best elicited through the general review of systems. Examples include thyroid disorders and allergies, both of which are important to the assessment of the head, face, and neck.
Integumentary	
Have you had any itching, rashes, sores, or other skin changes? Has the texture of your skin, hair, or nails changed?	People with allergic rhinitis often have allergies affecting other systems, including the skin, and could have atopic rashes or pruritus. Sores or lesions might cause enlarged lymph nodes. Changes in the texture of skin, hair, and nails commonly occur with thyroid disorders.
Have you noticed any changes in your skin, hair, or nails, such as texture changes or an increase in facial hair?	Color changes may be associated with endocrine disorders, such as the bronze color change of Addison's disease. Hirsutism (increase in facial or body hair growth) may be a result of Cushing's disease or a side effect of steroids.
HEENT	
Head/Neck	
Have you had head or neck pain, neck masses, or swollen nodes?	Although the symptom analysis and other history addresses symptoms of the head and neck, the ROS should again focus on that system in order to identify additional problems.
Eyes/Ears	
Have you noticed any changes in your vision or hearing? Have you had any drainage from your eyes or ears? Any itching in your eyes or ears? Any eye or ear pain?	Because of their proximity, disorders that affect the eyes and ears may also affect other organs of the head, face, and neck. The ears communicate with the rest of the upper airways, so infections involving one structure may move to the other. Allergic disorders causing rhinitis often involve the ears and/or eyes as well.
Nose/Mouth	
Have you had nasal congestion, nasal drainage, sinus pain, or nosebleeds? Mouth sores, dental pain, or jaw pain?	The ROS should also include the nose and mouth to ensure that all potential problems have been explored.
Respiratory	
Have you had a cough or sputum or phlegm production? Do you ever wheeze or feel as though your chest is tight? Do you ever have trouble breathing?	The upper and lower respiratory tracks are closely related, so infections in one often influence the other. People with asthma have a high incidence of allergic rhinitis.
Cardiovascular	
Have you had shortness of breath, chest pain, or palpitations?	Cardiovascular disorders can result in fluid imbalances that cause facial edema. Veins may become distended and arterial pulses may be bounding. Extreme

Review of Systems

SYSTEM/QUESTIONS TO ASK	RATIONALE/SIGNIFICANCE
Cardiovascular *(Continued)*	
Do you have high blood pressure? How well do you tolerate activity?	elevations in blood pressure can cause nosebleeds. Other symptoms of cardiac ischemia may help to explain jaw, tooth, or neck discomfort. Thyroid disorders have profound cardiovascular effects, including tachycardia and/or arrhythmias.
Gastrointestinal	
Have you had abdominal pain, appetite changes, nausea, vomiting, diarrhea, or constipation?	Thyroid disorders can alter bowel habits. Infections that involve the upper respiratory tract, particularly viral ones, are often associated with nausea, abdominal discomfort, vomiting, and/or diarrhea.
Genitourinary	
Do you have any history of kidney disease?	Chronic renal failure may cause periorbital edema. Uremic frost may be seen on the face in end-stage renal disease.
Female Reproductive	
When was your last normal menstrual period? Have your periods been irregular? Have you ever been pregnant? When? Do you have vaginal discharge or sores? Changes in sexual drive?	Thyroid disorders frequently alter the menstrual pattern. Pregnancy may cause nasal congestion. Oral lesions and pharyngitis may be found in people with sexually transmitted diseases (STDs). Decreased libido is associated with both hypothyroid and hyperthyroid disease.
Male Reproductive	
Do you have penile discharge or sores? Changes in sexual drive?	Oral lesions and pharyngitis may be found in people with STDs. Decreased libido is associated with both hypothyroid and hyperthyroid disease.
Musculoskeletal	
Have you had joint pain or swelling, muscle aches, or limitations in motion? Do you ever have weakness?	Joint and muscle symptoms suggest arthritic or neuromuscular disorders that would cause head, face, and neck discomfort or limit motion. Infectious diseases affecting the head, face, and neck may also cause generalized aches and pains. Hypothyroidism can result in an overall sense of fatigue or weakness; hyperthyroidism causes weakness of the proximal muscle groups of the extremities.
Neurological	
Do you have numbness, tingling, or muscle weakness? Nervousness, changes in level of consciousness, trouble staying focused, forgetfulness, headaches, or history of head trauma?	Neurological disorders can cause head pain and neck pain/stiffness. **Paresthesias**, paralysis, or weakness from neurological disorders may have a profound influence on facial expressions and ability to swallow. Thyroid disease may manifest as neurological symptoms. Nervousness, fine tremors, restlessness, and **labile** moods are associated with hyperthyroidism, apathy, lethargy; forgetfulness, slowed speech, and slowed mental processes are associated with hypothyroidism. A history of head trauma or headaches may also explain physical findings.
Endocrine	
Has your shoe size or ring size changed recently? Have your appearance or features changed significantly? Do you tire easily? Has your weight changed recently? Do you feel nervous or have trouble sleeping?	Acromegaly, a pituitary hypersecretory disorder, causes enlargement and hypertrophy of bone and connective tissues, with profound alterations in facial structures and headaches. Fatigue, nervousness, altered sleep patterns, and weight changes are associated with thyroid disorders. Including these questions in the ROS ensures that issues missed by earlier history will be detected.
Lymphatic/Hematologic	
Do you have unusual bruising or bleeding?	Disorders of the hematologic system may become evident through bleeding of other structures and help to explain nasal or oral bleeding.

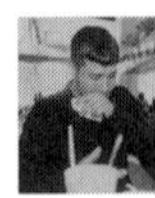

Case Study Findings

John's review of systems includes:

- **General Health Survey:** States that health is usually good. No changes in weight or energy level.
- **Integumentary:** No changes in skin, hair, and nails. No skin rashes.
- **HEENT:** No swollen nodes or masses in head or neck. "Allergy attack" causes ear fullness; nasal congestion and clear drainage; postnasal drip; sneezing; and scratchy/itchy throat, eyes, and nose. Vision 20/20, no problems reported.
- **Respiratory:** No cough, SOB, or wheezing.
- **Cardiovascular:** No chest pain or history of cardiovascular disease.
- **Gastrointestinal:** Appetite good, no dietary restrictions, no nausea or vomiting, has daily bowel movement.
- **Genitourinary:** No history of renal disease.
- **Reproductive:** Heterosexual, not currently sexually active, is aware of safe sex practices.
- **Musculoskeletal:** No weakness reported.
- **Neurological:** No headaches, dizziness, tremors or paresthesia.
- **Endocrine:** No changes in weight or shoe size (11).
- **Lymphatic/Hematologic:** Positive seasonal allergies, no bleeding disorders.

Psychosocial Profile

The psychosocial profile provides information about the client's occupation, social involvement, recreational interests, and daily activities and habits in order to identify factors that can influence the health of the head, face, and neck. It determines risks associated with exposure to hazards, provides information about the client's support system, and helps identify the client's ability to perform self-care activities and obtain and carry out recommended treatments.

Psychosocial Profile

CATEGORY/QUESTIONS TO ASK	SIGNIFICANCE/RATIONALE
Health Practices and Beliefs/ Self-Care Activities	
What is your usual bathing and toiletry routine? What toiletries or cosmetics do you usually use?	Makeup and other toiletries may alter the skin integrity over the face.
Typical Day	
How do you usually spend the day?	Knowledge of typical daily activities identifies potential exposures to hazards and habits that might adversely affect the head, face, and neck.
Nutritional Patterns	
What have you eaten in the past 24 hours? What types of foods do you usually eat? How much water and other fluids do you usually drink? What, if any, dietary supplements or vitamins do you take?	Many nutritional deficits can affect the mucous membranes; for example, a "beefy" tongue is associated with pernicious anemia. Foods and additives may be sources of allergens. Nutrition influences many of the diseases that affect the head, face, and neck. Changes in appetite and weight are often associated with thyroid disease. Decreased appetite, nausea and vomiting, and weight gain are associated with hypothyroidism; increased appetite and thirst and weight loss are associated with hyperthyroidism.
Activity and Exercise Patterns	
Do you exercise? What type of exercise do you do?	Information on the ability to exercise and exercise tolerance helps to provide a picture of any limitations presented by diseases such as rhinitis, headache, and neck pain. On the other hand, the type of exercises and activities performed may explain complaints such as headache or neck pain and stiffness. Thyroid disorders affect activity tolerance.
Recreation/Pets/Hobbies	
What do you do for recreation and hobbies? Do any of these activities involve exposure to extreme environmental conditions, chemicals, noise, or other harmful situations? What, if any, protective equipment do you use in your recreational activity?	Chemicals, environmental extremes, and noise can affect the head, face, and neck.

Psychosocial Profile

CATEGORY/QUESTIONS TO ASK	SIGNIFICANCE/RATIONALE
Sleep and Rest Patterns How many hours of sleep do you usually get? Do you have problems with rest or sleep? Do you usually awaken feeling rested?	Nasal congestion; sore throat; and other head, face, and neck complaints may limit or impair sleep. People with sleep apnea have altered sleep patterns and feel sleepy throughout the day. The need to nap during the daytime may suggest a poor night's sleep. Hypothyroidism often causes an increase in amount of sleep required; hyperthyroidism often interferes with ability to rest or sleep.
Personal Habits Do you smoke cigarettes or use any other form of tobacco? If so, what type and quantity do you usually use daily? Do you drink alcohol? If so, what do you usually drink and how much? Do you use recreational drugs? If so, which ones, how often, and in what amount?	Tobacco affects the nose and sinuses. Smokeless tobacco is associated with oral cancers. Excessive alcohol use is associated with throat cancer. Drugs such as cocaine that are inhaled affect the nasal mucosa and erode the nasal septum.
Occupational Health Patterns What type of work do you do? Does your daily work involve exposures to loud noises, environmental extremes or chemicals? What, if any, protection do you use in your work?	Many occupations expose people to injury from either sound or trauma. These questions help to determine the client's access to, understanding of, and use of protective equipment.
Environmental Health Patterns Are you able to keep your home clean? Do you have problems with pests or dust? Is your home adequately heated and cooled?	The home environment presents potential allergens. Humidity and temperature affect the mucous membranes. Roach excrement is an important allergen for people with asthma.
Roles/Relationships/Self-Concept Do you participate in any group activities? Have changes in your health recently affected your personal relationships?	The face, head, nose, mouth, and neck are very visible features. Any alteration may result in withdrawal from social activities because of depression or embarrassment.
Stress and Coping How much stress do you usually experience? How do you usually deal with it?	Stress and tension can trigger tension neck aches and headaches. Coping mechanisms are an important consideration for all clients.

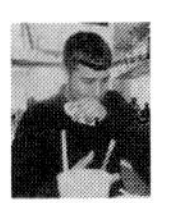

Case Study Findings

John's psychosocial profile includes:

- Bathes daily; uses no cosmetics on face other than occasional over-the-counter acne medication; sees doctor and dentist for checkup once a year.
- Typical day starts at 6:45 AM, when his mother awakens him to get ready for school. Attends school from 8 AM until 3:15 PM on weekdays, and works 5 PM until 11 PM Monday and Friday nights and noon until 6 PM on Saturday. Goes to bed at 11:30 PM on school nights and 1 AM on weekends.
- Eats three meals plus one or two snacks daily. Breakfast consists of cereal, milk, and juice. Lunch is fast food, obtained between classes. Dinner is usually a cooked meal, shared with his parents. No specific dietary restrictions or food intolerances.
- Plays baseball and competes on swim team; practices 1 to 2 hours a day, depending on time of year. Wears protective gear while playing baseball.

- Tolerates swimming well, wearing goggles. Does some amount of physical activity daily, and this is well tolerated.
- Normally sleeps well and awakens rested. During "allergy season" sometimes has sleep difficulty. When he takes OTC antihistamines, they make it difficult to sleep and he wakes frequently through the night. If he takes no antihistamines or decongestants, he often awakens with congestion and/or sinus pressure.
- No medications other than seasonal use of antihistamines and daily vitamin. Uses no recreational drugs. Admits to rare use of alcohol (beer).
- Works 5 PM until 11 PM Monday and Friday nights and noon until 6 PM on Saturday. Exposed to second-hand smoke in the restaurant where he works; otherwise not generally around smokers or exposed to any known chemicals. Tries to avoid exposure to smoke, as he is concerned about the potential health hazards.
- Lives in a single-family, two-story home described as "more than adequate" for his family.
- Has many friends and enjoys spending time with groups. Dates, but has no steady girlfriend.
- Does well in school and has been accepted to the state university. No major yet chosen.
- Not currently sexually active.

Focused Head, Face, and Neck History

If a detailed history is either not feasible or inappropriate, be sure to ask the following basic questions. Remember that you must pursue a symptom analysis (PQRST) for any complaint identified during this focused history.

- Do you have problems or complaints related to your head, face, nose, mouth, throat, or neck? Some examples are head pain, nasal congestion, nosebleeds, nasal discharge, mouth sores or pain, sore throat, postnasal drip, difficulty swallowing, and neck pain.
- Do you have allergies to any medications, foods or environmental factors?
- What, if any, health problems do you have?
- What, if any, over-the-counter or prescribed medications do you take?
- Is there anything specific that you think I should know related to your overall health or this specific complaint?

Case Study Evaluation

At this point, you should review what you have learned about John. The information from your client history will be important to consider before and during your physical examination. Document the head, face, and neck history related to John.

 CRITICAL THINKING ACTIVITY #1

Based on his history, is John at risk for any problems of the head, face, or neck?

 CRITICAL THINKING ACTIVITY #2

What strengths can you identify that will help John prevent or adapt to any problems of the head, face, or neck?

Anatomical Landmarks

Before you begin your physical assessment of the head, face, and neck, you need to visualize the underlying structures and identify landmarks. Two landmarks on the face that are useful in determining symmetry of facial features are the **palpebral fissures** and the **nasolabial folds** (Fig. 9–12). The palpebral fissure is the distance between the upper and lower eyelid. The nasolabial fold is the distance from the corner of the nose to the edge of the lip. This is the facial crease that is often seen when someone smiles.

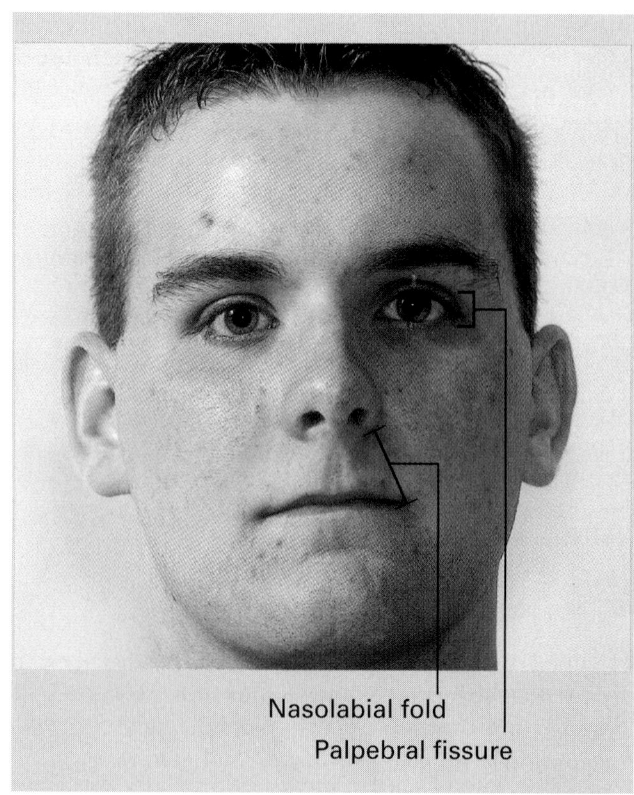

FIGURE 9–12. Palpebral fissures and nasolabial folds.

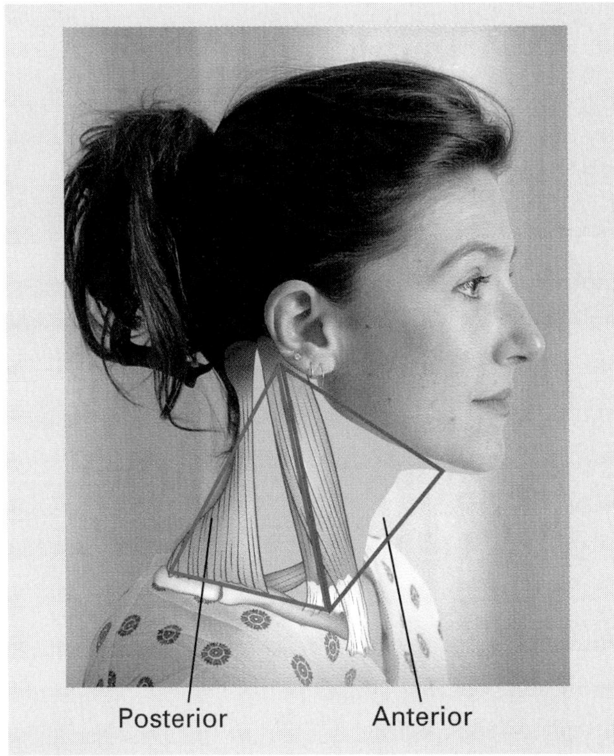

FIGURE 9–13. Anterior and posterior triangles.

The anterior and posterior triangles (Fig. 9–13) are important landmarks of the neck. The **sternocleidomastoid** and **trapezius** muscles form the triangles. Both triangles are helpful in locating the underlying structures of the neck.

Physical Assessment

During the history, you probably developed a sense of the client's concerns and may have begun to cluster the data obtained to help guide your physical examination. You should have an awareness of any physical limitations or discomfort that will influence the physical examination. Throughout the history, you observed the client's body posture, fluidity of movements, facial expressions, and speech—all of which are important observations for the head, face, and neck. Now, as you approach the physical examination, you must be very objective in your observations as you inspect the internal structures of the nose, mouth, and throat.

Approach

All four techniques of physical assessment are used in the examination of the head, face, and neck: inspection, palpation, percussion, and auscultation. Some structures, like the throat and internal nose, can only be inspected; generally only the sinuses are percussed, and only the vessels of the neck and thyroid are auscultated. The cranial nerve (CN) assessment is generally incorporated in the examination of the face, mouth, nose, throat, and neck. The assessment of the arteries and veins is also incorporated into the examination of the neck and face. Although there is no "right" sequence to follow for the examination of these structures and organs, you should develop, practice, and adhere to a set routine in order to avoid omitting a test. One common sequence is the head-to-toe approach that begins with inspection of the shape and general placement of the head and facial structures, followed by a thorough inspection of the facial muscles and then the neck. Some examiners prefer to examine the nose, mouth, and throat along with the face, whereas others do this only after they have completed the examination of the neck. No matter what sequence you use, always take into consideration the structures' symmetry during your examination.

Toolbox

The tools that will be necessary to examine the head, face, nose, mouth, throat, and neck are a penlight or otoscope for focused light, tongue blades, gauze, stethoscope, transilluminator, cup of water, and gloves. If you are using an otoscope as a light source, you will want a wide-tipped speculum. Another piece of equipment that can be useful is a nasal speculum. Lighting is very important, and some examiners prefer also using a "gooseneck lamp" or headlamp when examining the mouth and throat.

Performing a General Survey

The first step of the physical examination is a general survey, although in many cases this is accomplished during history taking. Besides providing early information regarding speech and movements, the general survey allows you to detect clues about the client's emotional status, nutritional status, and overall posture. During the general survey, obtain vital signs. Altered pulse can be associated with thyroid disease. Respiratory rate changes can be related to an altered airway, including the nose, mouth, or pharynx. The temperature is an important consideration for infection. Blood pressure elevations may explain epistaxis. Aside from the vital signs, be alert for other signs that may indicate underlying problems with the head, face, and neck. For example:

- Note facial expression. Is it appropriate? Nervousness or a flat expression may be associated with thyroid disease. A masklike expression is seen with Parkinson's disease.
- Note any gross abnormalities, such as exophthalmus, which is seen with thyroid disease.
- Consider dress and grooming. Are they appropriate? Temperature intolerance associated with thyroid disease may cause people to overdress or underdress.

- Note speech and thought processes. Are responses appropriate? Are thought process intact? Problems with focusing may be related to thyroid disorders.
- Look for changes in weight or weight distribution. A "**buffalo hump**" (fat pads on the lower midcervical and upper thoracic areas) is associated with Cushing's disease or steroid use.

Performing a Head-to-Toe Physical Assessment

The head, face, and neck reflect many different systems, so look for changes that may indicate underlying pathology. Next, perform a head-to-toe physical assessment, checking for specific signs of disease in other organ systems that might be reflected in the head, face, and neck.

Performing a Head-to-Toe Physical Assessment

SYSTEM/NORMAL FINDINGS	ABNORMAL FINDINGS/RATIONALE
General Health Survey *INSPECT* Awake, alert, oriented	Altered mental status may indicate meningeal infection, which could be associated with head or neck pain or stiffness.
Memory intact, able to provide adequate history	Forgetfulness or slow mental processes are associated with hypothyroidism; mood lability, personality changes, and restlessness are associated with hyperthyroidism.
Integumentary/*Skin* *INSPECT/PALPATE* Skin color varies according to racial and genetic makeup. Oral mucosa pink, skin warm, moist, intact, with good turgor. Should have stippled appearance, resembling orange peel.	Color changes can readily be seen in mucous membranes. For example, cyanosis related to hypoxia, jaundice related to liver dysfunction, pallor related to anemia, or bronze/tan discoloration related to Addison's disease. Dry, thick, cool skin with poor turgor is associated with hypothyroidism; warm, smooth, moist skin is associated with hyperthyroidism.
Integumentary/*Hair* Hair evenly distributed. Texture dependent on racial and genetic makeup.	Dry, sparse, coarse hair seen with hypothyroidism; patchy alopecia, and fine, silky hair, with hyperthyroidism. Increased facial hair in women is associated with Cushing's disease or steroid use.
Integumentary/*Nails* Nails pink and firm.	Thick, brittle nails seen with hypothyroidism; thin, brittle nails with hyperthyroidism.
HEENT/*Eyes* *INSPECT* Conjunctiva moist and pink. No drainage.	Conjunctival redness and drainage suggest infection or

Performing a Head-to-Toe Physical Assessment

SYSTEM/NORMAL FINDINGS	ABNORMAL FINDINGS/RATIONALE
HEENT/*Eyes (Continued)* *INSPECT*	allergy, both of which may involve the nose and sinuses.
Palpebral fissures equal. No lid lag.	Exophthalmos and lid lag are associated with hyperthyroidism.
HEENT/*Ears* Hearing intact. Tympanic membrane gray; light reflex intact.	Hearing changes and altered appearance of tympanic membrane and landmarks associated with fluid accumulations behind the tympanic membrane (serous otitis) or infection (otitis media), both of which may affect the nose or throat.
Landmarks visible. No drainage or bleeding.	Bleeding from the ear and nose signals possible skull fracture.
Respiratory *INSPECT/AUSCULTATE* Normal respiratory rate. Respirations regular and unlabored. No cough. Clear breath sounds; no adventitious sounds.	**Tachypnea**, cough, and wheezing may indicate asthma, which is highly related to other atopic diseases, such as allergic rhinitis or a respiratory infection that may also involve the upper respiratory tract. Masses or lesions in the nose, mouth, or throat can influence respiratory status.
Cardiovascular *AUSCULTATE* Apical and radial pulses within normal limits. S_1, S_2 present and regular, with no adventitious or extra heart sounds. Pulses +2/4.	Bounding temporal arteries paired with temporal pain suggests **temporal arteritis**, an explanation for head pain.
No bruits.	Bruits of the carotid arteries are detected during the examination of the neck and may indicate carotid stenosis. Proper examination should differentiate between bruits of the carotids and vascular sounds over the thyroid.
Gastrointestinal *INSPECT/PALPATE/PERCUSS/AUSCULTATE* Abdomen round, soft. Positive bowel sounds. Nontender, no organomegaly.	The mouth is the beginning of the GI tract, so oral problems may affect the GI system. Jaundice can be seen on the palate. *(Continued)*

Performing a Head-to-Toe Physical Assessment *(Continued)*

SYSTEM/NORMAL FINDINGS	ABNORMAL FINDINGS/RATIONALE
Genitourinary *INSPECT* External genitalia pink, intact, no lesions.	Oral lesions may be caused by STDs.
Musculoskeletal Full range of motion (ROM). No tenderness. Strength 5/5 (see Chapter 18). No joint deformities.	Limitations of motion, pain, and/or joint deformities are found with various forms of arthritis and may affect the TMJ and cervical joints. Weakness can be a sign of thyroid disorder, as well as of various neuromuscular disorders that may affect expression, speech, and eating. Limited ROM of the neck and **nuchal rigidity** (resistance to neck flexion) are associated with meningitis.
Neurological Intact cranial nerves and sensation. Coordinated movements.	Cranial nerves innervate most structures of the head, face, and neck and affect their function. Changes in sensation and coordination indicate neurological disorders that influence function of the nose (olfaction) and muscles of facial expression, eating, and speech.

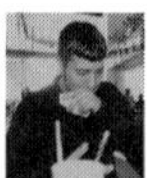

Case Study Findings

Before you proceed to a focused examination of the head, face, and neck, review what you discovered during your general survey of John:

- **General Health Survey:** Well-developed 17-year-old male, tanned skin, healthy appearance consistent with stated age. No apparent distress, projects a confident and comfortable affect, provides history with ease.
- **Vital Signs:** Temperature 97.8°F; pulse 62; respirations 14; BP 100/72, left arm; height 5′10″; weight 160 lb.
- **HEENT:** Eyes clear, bright, with no discharge, redness, or swelling. Facial movements are symmetrical.
- **Respiratory:** Lungs clear bilaterally, with no adventitious sounds.
- **Cardiovascular:** Pulses 2+, apical pulse regular with no extra or adventitious sounds.
- **Gastrointestinal:** Abdomen soft, nontender, positive for bowel sounds; liver nontender.
- **Genitourinary:** External genitalia intact, no lesions.
- **Musculoskeletal:** Coordinated and smooth movements. Full ROM of extremities, strength +5/5, no deformities or tenderness.
- **Neurological:** Alert, oriented × 3, memory apparently intact.

Performing a Focused Physical Assessment

After the general survey and head-to-toe assessment, perform a physical examination that focuses on the head, face, and neck. Although inspection and palpation are discussed separately below, they are not distinct, sequential activities. They are actually performed almost in concert. Although you inspect an area or structure before touching or moving it, this takes only a moment and is usually followed immediately by touching or palpating the area. The only area of the head, face, and neck to be percussed is the sinus area, and this generally occurs after you have applied pressure over the sites during palpation. The only areas to be auscultated are the carotids and jugulars and, if it is enlarged, the thyroid.

Assessing the Head and Face

Examination of the head and face involves inspection and palpation.

Inspection

Have clients remove hats, wigs, or hair ornaments if present. Put on gloves in case there are open lesions under the hair. Begin with inspection. Identify the prominences of the brows, cheeks, **mastoids,** and **occiput.**

Inspection of the Head and Face

ASSESS/NORMAL VARIATIONS	ABNORMAL FINDINGS/RATIONALE
Head Size 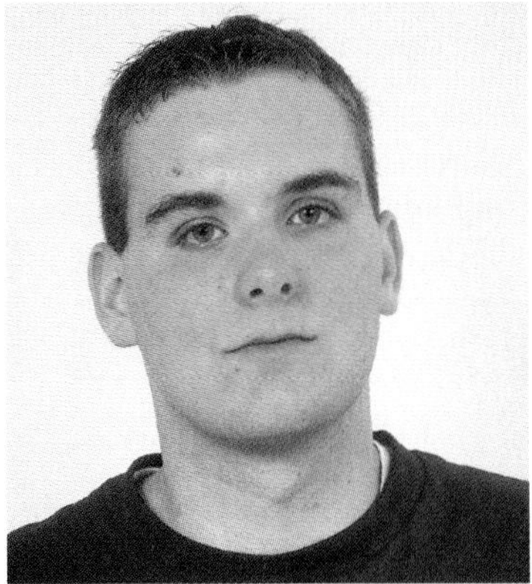 **Inspecting head size and shape and symmetry of facial features** • **Variation** is wide, between and within gender and racial/ethnic group.	*Head increasing abnormally in size in young child:* May indicate hydrocephalus. *Inconsistently large head size in adolescent or adult:* May indicate acromegaly. 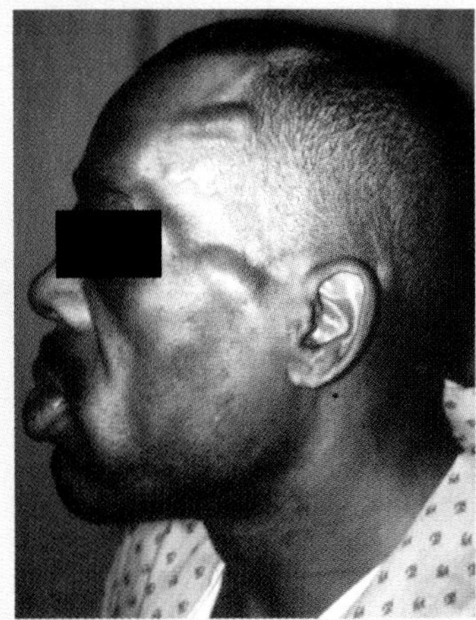 **Acromegaly**
Head Shape Variation is wide, although shape should be symmetrical and contour rounded.	*Asymmetry of shape and contour:* Previous trauma, surgery, or congenital deformity. **HELPFUL HINT** Abnormal shapes or flat occiputs in infants and small children may result from positioning during the first year of life.
Facial Appearance Facial appearance varies by gender, age, and racial/ethnic group. However, there should be symmetry of features and movement.	*Facial appearance inconsistent with gender, age, or racial/ethnic group:* May indicate an inherited or chronic disorder with typical facies, such as Graves' disease, hypothyroidism with **myxedema**, Cushing's syndrome, or acromegaly.

(Continued)

Inspection of the Head and Face *(Continued)*

ASSESS/NORMAL VARIATIONS	ABNORMAL FINDINGS/RATIONALE
Facial Appearance *(Continued))*	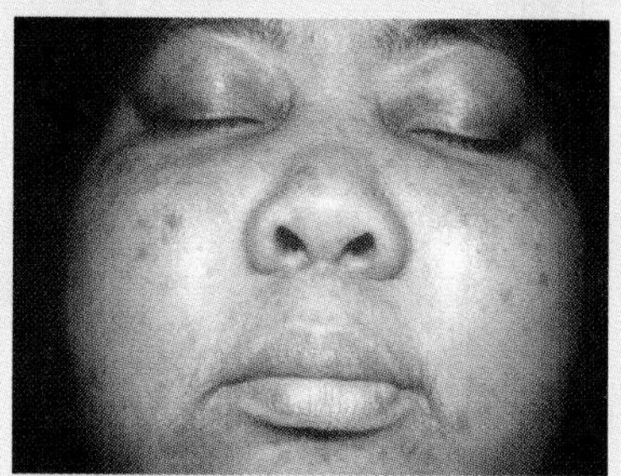 **Cushing's syndrome**
	Asymmetry of features: Previous trauma, surgical alterations, congenital deformity, paralysis, or edema. Asymmetry is also seen with Bell's palsy and cerebrovascular accident (CVA).
HELPFUL HINT Two good places to inspect for symmetry of facial features are the palpebral fissures and the nasolabial folds.	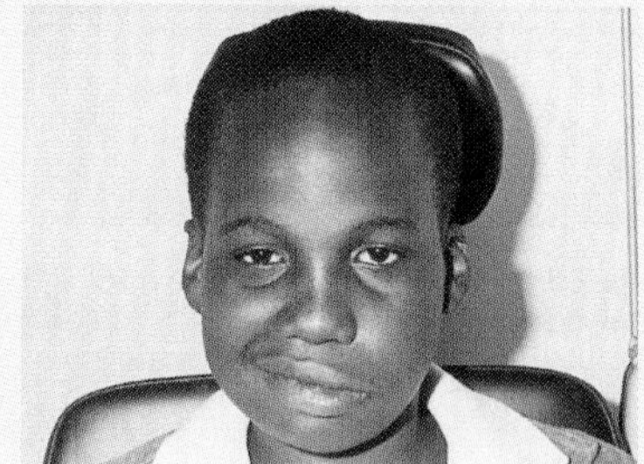 **Bell's palsy**
	Asymmetry of movement: Suggests neuromuscular disorder or paralysis. **Tics**, or spastic muscular contractions,usually occur in the head and face.

Palpation

Next, palpate the head and face. There should be no tenderness and, except in infants, no soft areas in the head. As you palpate the TMJ, ask the client to open and close his or her mouth and deviate his or her jaw from side to side. Determine sensation, motion, and strength of the face, as described in Chapter 19, and assess the temporal artery, as described in Chapter 13.

Assessing the Sinuses

Assessment of the sinuses includes inspection (with transillumination), palpation, and percussion. Only the frontal and maxillary sinuses are readily accessible for assessment. Envision the areas of the face that overly the sinuses. Remember, the frontal sinuses are located above the eyebrows and the maxillary sinuses are located below the eyes.

Inspection

The sinus areas are inspected for edema and discoloration. If you suspect a sinus problem after regular inspection, palpation, and percussion, you can also transilluminate the sinuses. A transilluminator should be used; however, either a penlight or an otoscope with a speculum attached are good alternatives. Transillumination requires a darkened room. To transilluminate the frontal sinuses, hold the light source so that the light is directed upward from just below the brows. A glow of light may be detected over the brow. To transilluminate the maxillary sinuses, have the client open his or her mouth and position his or her head so that you can observe the roof of the mouth. Place the light source below the eyes and above the cheek, with the client's mouth opened, and look for a glow on the roof of the mouth. Absence of transillumination suggests sinus fullness or thickening. Any glow noted with transillumination of either the frontal or maxillary sinus should be symmetrical. However, absence of transillumination may not always indicate pathology. It may simply be a normal variant caused by the thickness of the bones overlying the sinuses or underdevelopment of the sinuses.

Palpation of the Head and Face

ASSESS/NORMAL VARIATIONS	ABNORMAL FINDINGS/RATIONALE

Head Contour/Facial Structures

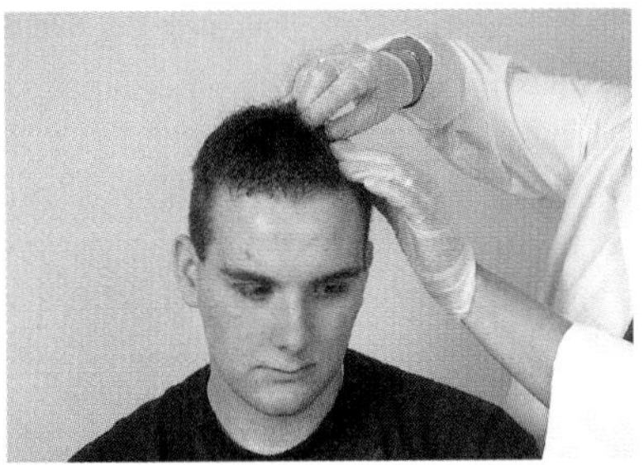

Palpating the head

Relatively smooth with no unexpected contours or bulges.

Contour abnormalities, including bulges or projections: Previous trauma, surgery, or congenital deformity.

No tenderness or lesions.

Tenderness: Trauma, TMJ, temporal arteritis or inflammatory process.

TMJ

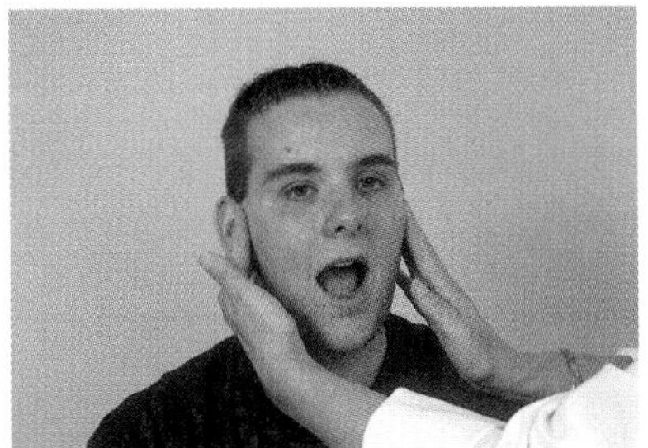

Palpating the TMJ

Smooth, symmetrical motion, with no pain, crepitus, or clicking.

Irregular or uneven movement, pain with motion or crepitus/popping: TMJ syndrome.

Inspection of the Sinuses

ASSESS/NORMAL VARIATIONS	ABNORMAL FINDINGS/RATIONALE

Frontal and Maxillary Sinuses

No periorbital edema or discoloration.

Periorbital edema and dark undereye circles: Sinusitis.

Frontal and Maxillary Sinuses by Transillumination

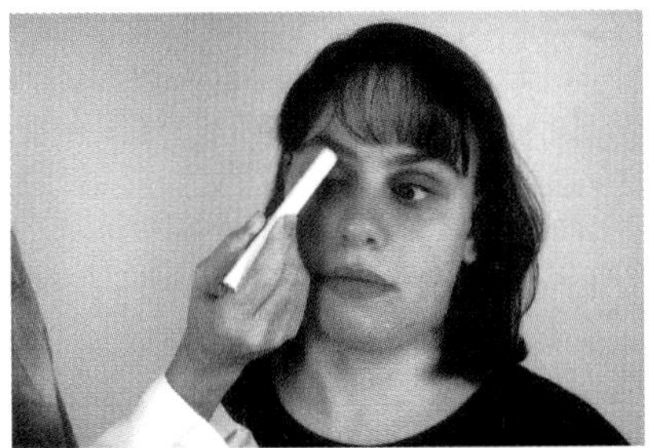

Transilluminating frontal sinuses

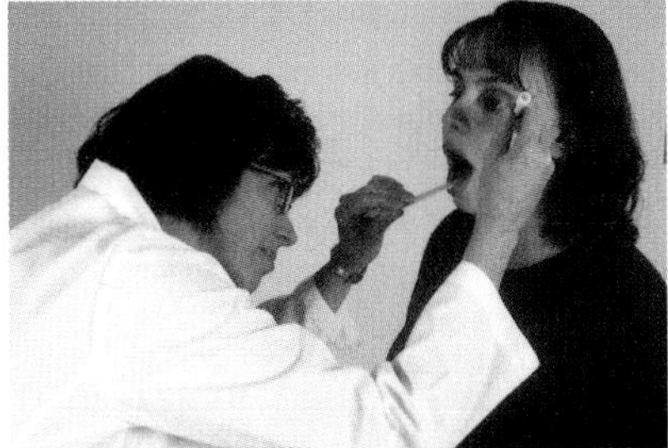

Transilluminating maxillary sinuses

Frontal sinus: Normally red glow noted above eyebrow.

Maxillary sinus: Normally red glow noted on roof of mouth.

Expected variations include absence of transillumination because the ability to transilluminate is dependent on the thickness of the bones overlying the structure examined.

Absence of transillumination over one sinus when opposite structure transilluminates: Mucosal thickening or sinus fullness with sinusitis.

Absence of transillumination must be considered with other findings.

Palpation

Palpate the sinuses for tenderness. To palpate the frontal sinuses, press upward just below the medial third of each eyebrow. To palpate the maxillary sinuses, apply pressure to the lower portion of the cheeks, below the eyes.

Percussion

Percussion is performed to further assess for sinus discomfort. If tenderness is elicited with palpation, omit percussion over that area. Otherwise, you should percuss the sinuses by tapping over these same areas. Direct percussion, using the tapping finger to strike directly over the bony prominence, is most frequently used. Because the sinuses are normally filled with air, percussion should elicit somewhat of a resonant tone.

Assessing the Nose

To examine the nose, inspect the external structures, palpate the external structures, and then inspect the internal structures (nasal cavity).

Inspection

Inspection of the internal structures includes the septum, nasal mucosa, and medial and inferior turbinates. If you are using an otoscope with a wide-tipped speculum, stabilize the client's head with one hand and then slowly and gently insert the speculum into the **naris.** If you are using a penlight and nasal speculum, insert the closed speculum and then gently open it once it is in the nose, being careful not to open it too much. Take care not to scrape or press on the central septum because this area is sensitive. During your assessment, take note of any sounds the client is making with his or her nose, such as sniffing or snorting.

Palpation of the Sinuses

ASSESS/NORMAL VARIATIONS

Frontal and Maxillary Sinuses

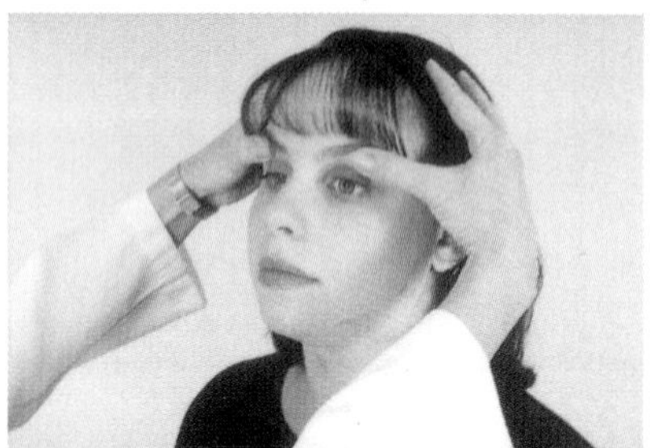

Palpating frontal sinuses

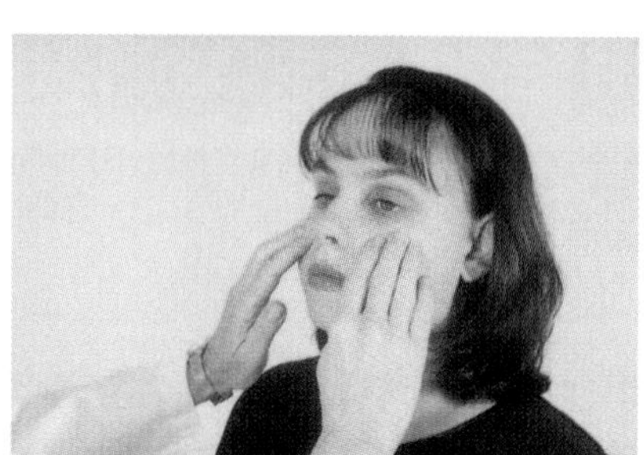

Palpating maxillary sinuses

No tenderness

ABNORMAL FINDINGS/RATIONALE

Tenderness: May indicate infectious or allergic sinusitis.

Percussion of the Sinuses

AREA/NORMAL VARIATIONS

Frontal and Maxillary Sinuses

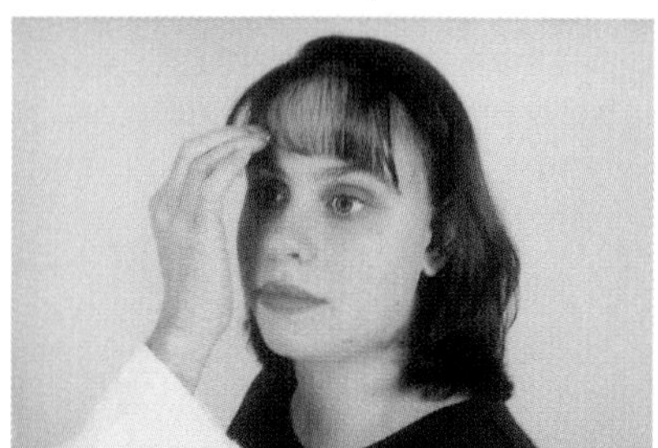

Percussing frontal sinus

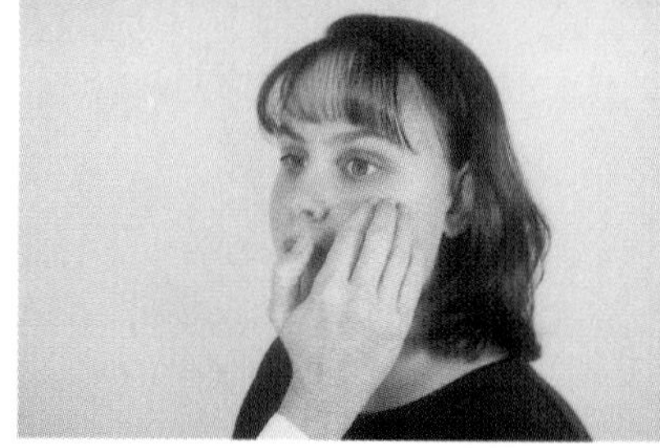

Percussing maxillary sinus

No tenderness. Resonant tone.

ABNORMAL FINDINGS/RATIONALE

Tenderness: Suggests sinusitis.

Dull tone: Indicates thickening or fullness of sinus cavity or cavities, associated with chronic or acute sinusitis.

Inspection of the Nose

ASSESS/NORMAL VARIATIONS	ABNORMAL FINDINGS/RATIONALE
External Nose	
Midline placement. Shape symmetrical and consistent with age, gender, and race/ethnic group.	*Misalignment of nose or shape inconsistent with client's biographic information:* Previous trauma, congenital deformity, surgical alteration, or mass. Abnormal shape also associated with typical facies, including acromegaly or Down syndrome.
No nasal flaring.	*Nasal flaring:* Suggests respiratory distress, especially in infants, who are obligatory nose breathers.
No drainage.	*Clear, bilateral drainage:* Allergic rhinitis. *Clear, unilateral drainage:* May be spinal fluid as a result of head trauma or fracture. *Clear, mucoid drainage:* Viral rhinitis. *Yellow or green drainage:* Upper respiratory infection. *Bloody drainage:* Trauma, hypertension, or bleeding disorders.
Internal Nasal Mucosa 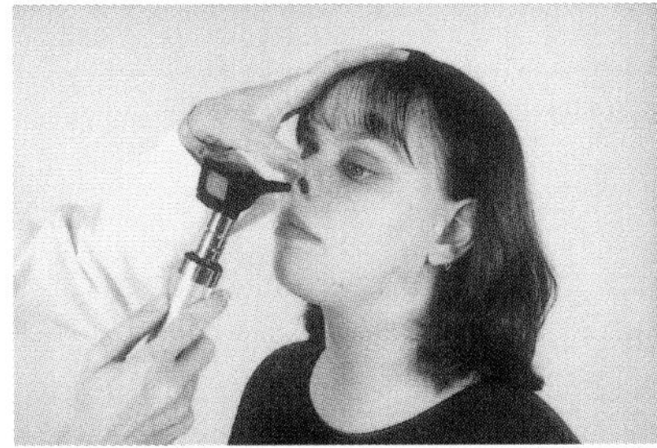 **Inspecting nasal mucosa** Pink, variations consistent with ethnic group/race and with oral mucosa. Moist, with only clear, scant mucus present. Intact, with no lesions or perforations. No crusting or polyps.	*Bright red mucosa:* Inflammation from rhinitis or sinusitis; also suggests cocaine abuse. Pale or gray mucosa: Allergic rhinitis. *Copious or colored discharge:* Allergic or infectious disorder, epistaxis, head or nose trauma. Clustered vesicles: Herpes infection. *Ulcers or perforations:* Chronic infection, trauma, or cocaine use. *Dried crusted blood:* Previous epistaxis. Polyps (elongated, rounded projections): Allergies. 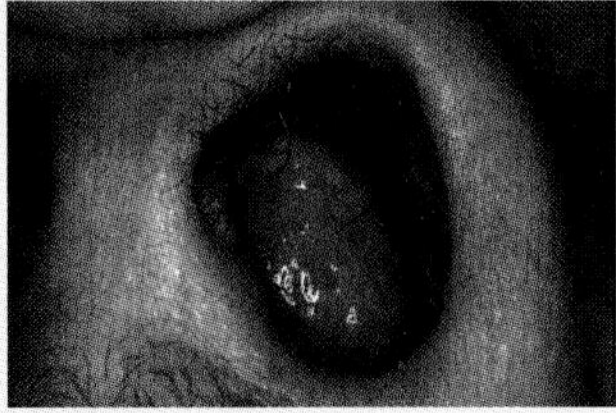 **Polyps**

(Continued)

Inspection of the Nose

ASSESS/NORMAL VARIATIONS	ABNORMAL FINDINGS/RATIONALE
Internal Nasal Mucosa *(Continued)* Septum located midline.	*Deviated septum:* Normal variant or following trauma

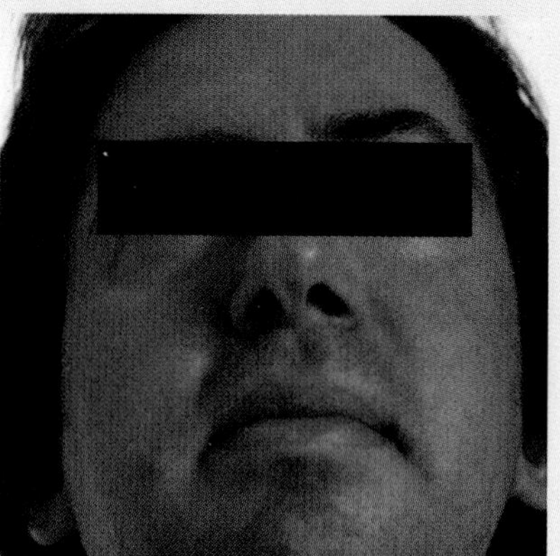

Deviated septum

ALERT

A deviated septum is cause for concern if breathing is obstructed.

ASSESS/NORMAL VARIATIONS	ABNORMAL FINDINGS/RATIONALE
Turbinates Medial and inferior turbinates visible, symmetrical and shape/size consistent with general features of client. Overlying mucosa coloring consistent with other mucous membranes.	*Enlarged, boggy turbinates:* Allergic disorder. *Pale or gray mucosa overlying turbinates:* Allergic disorder.

Palpation

Palpate the bony ridge and soft tissues of the external nose. The cartilaginous, distal two-thirds of the nose should be mobile, without pain. Gently occlude one nostril at a time and have the client inhale through the nose to determine patency.

Assessing the Mouth and Throat

The mouth and throat are components of both the respiratory and digestive tracts. Assessment involves inspection and palpation. The assessment begins with examination of the lips, then the structures of the mouth and throat. Remember to wear gloves when examining the internal structures of the mouth. You will also need a penlight and tongue depressor to perform the examination.

HELPFUL HINT

Because the mucous membranes reproduce cells rapidly, mouth lesions tend to heal quickly with treatment. Therefore any persistent lesion requires medical attention.

Inspection

Inspect the lips, gingiva, buccal mucosa, tongue, and pharynx for color, lesions, and exudates. Note the color, number, condition, and occlusion of the teeth. The upper and lower molars should approximate with the jaw closed. The front teeth should slightly override the lower ones. Observation of the teeth with a physical assessment does not replace a dental examination, so remind the client of the importance of maintaining routine dental care.

Using the tongue blade to displace the cheeks and lips, first inspect the **buccal mucosa.** The **Stensen's ducts,** openings for the parotid glands, are located on the buccal mucosa at the point of the second molars. The **Wharton's ducts,** openings for the submandibular glands, are located on either side of the **frenulum.**

Inspect all aspects of the tongue: dorsal, ventral, and lateral edges. Note the color, moisture, and surface texture and observe for any swelling. Observe the frenulum and the mobility of the tongue.

Palpation of the Nose

ASSESS /NORMAL VARIATIONS	ABNORMAL FINDINGS/RATIONALE
External Nose	*Deviations or masses:* Previous trauma or infection.

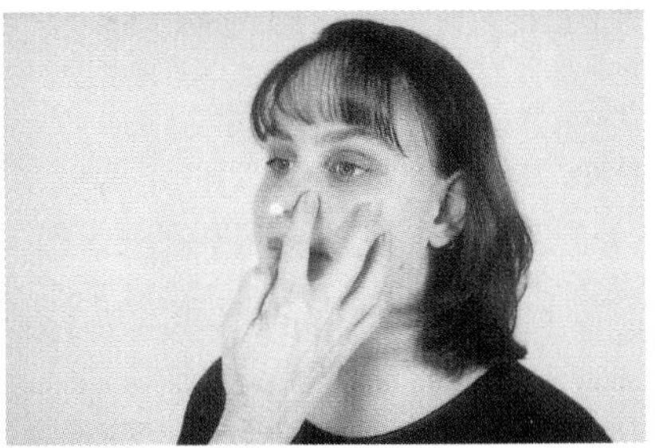

Palpating nostril

Cartilaginous portion is slightly mobile. Nontender, no masses. Nares patent.

Inspection of the Mouth and Throat

ASSESS/NORMAL VARIATIONS

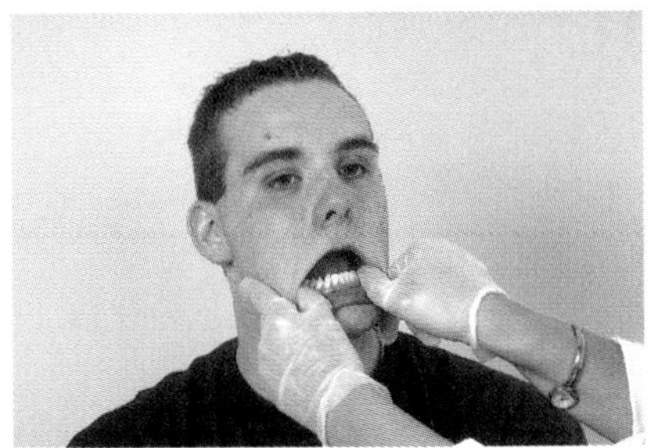

Lips

Midline, symmetrical, skin intact, pink and moist.
Coloring consistent with ethnic group/race.
No unusual odors

ABNORMAL FINDINGS/RATIONALE

Asymmetry of placement: Congenital deformity, trauma, paralysis, or surgical alteration.
Pallor: Anemia.
Redness: Inflammatory or infectious disorder.
Cyanosis: Vasoconstriction or hypoxia.
Lesions: Infectious or inflammatory disorder.
Cheilitis (inflammation of lips), drying and cracking: Dehydration, allergy, lip licking.
Cheilosis (fissures at corners of lips): Deficiency of B vitamins or maceration related to overclosure.
Chancre: Single, painless ulcer of primary syphilis.
Angioedema: Allergic response.
Herpes simplex (clustered area of fullness/nodularity that forms vesicles, then ulceration): Herpes viral infection.
Halitosis: Infections or GI problems.

Abnormalities of the Lips

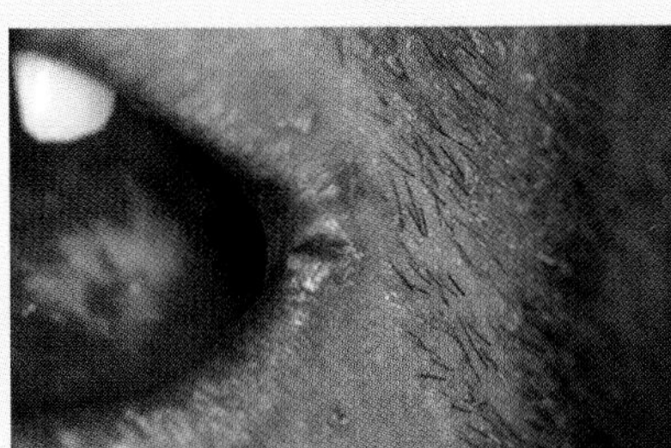

Cheilitis and cheilosis

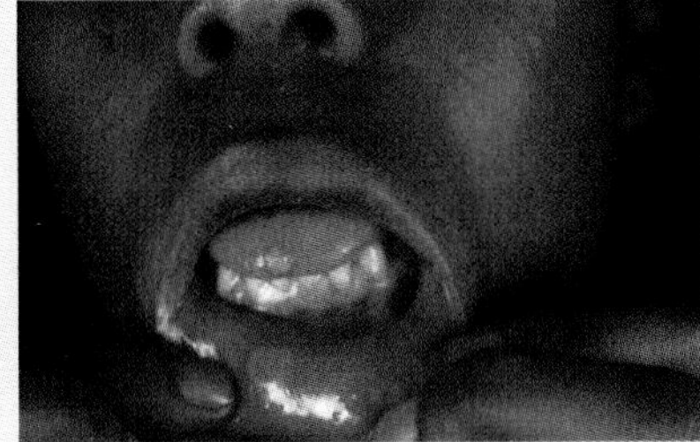

Chancre

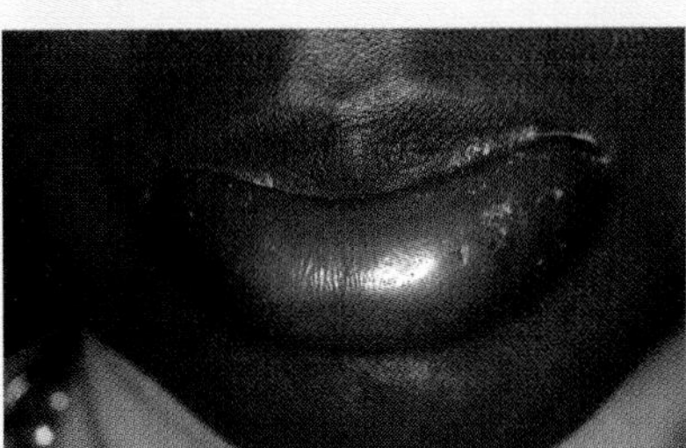

Angioedema: Allergic response

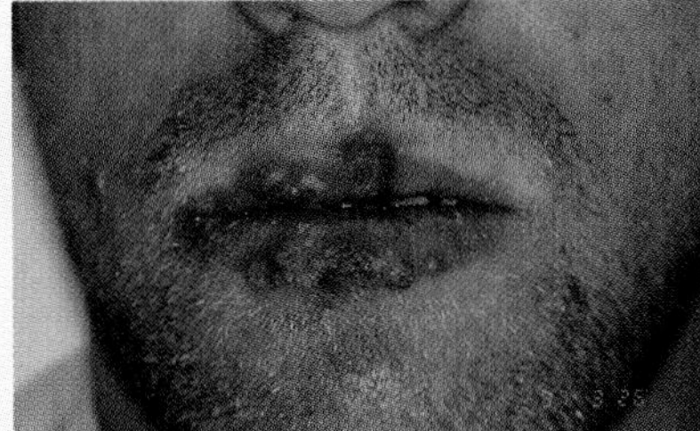

Herpes viral infection

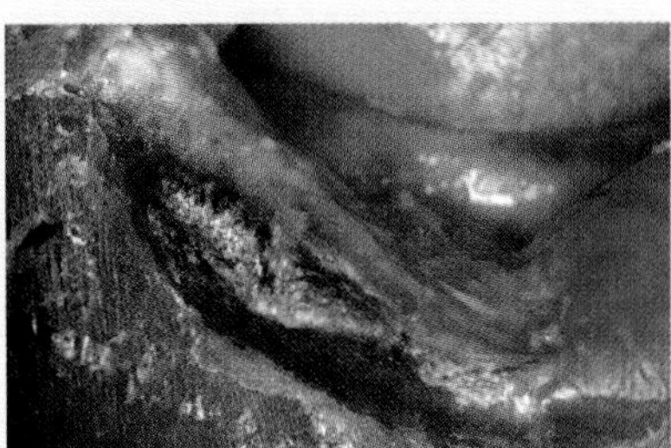

Cancer on lip

(Continued)

Inspection of the Mouth and Throat *(Continued)*

ASSESS/NORMAL VARIATIONS

Teeth and Bite

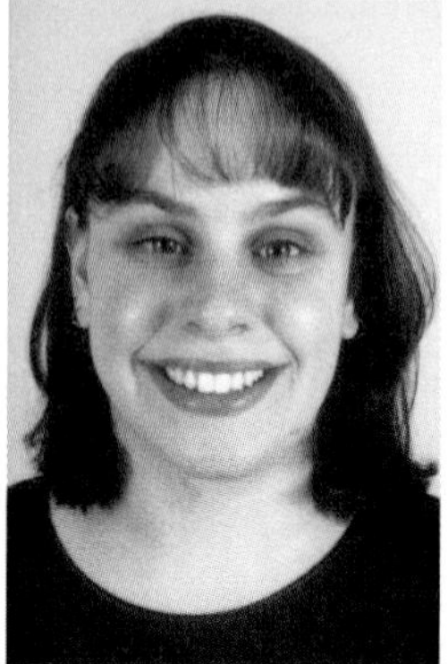

Inspecting teeth and bite

Most adults have 28 teeth, or 32 if the four third molars or "wisdom teeth" are erupted. (However, they are usually impacted or extracted.)

Teeth should be white, not loose, with good occlusion, and in good repair.

ABNORMAL FINDINGS/RATIONALE

Various abnormalities include loose, poorly anchored teeth, malalignment, dental caries.

Discoloration of teeth: Chemicals or medications (tetracycline may discolor teeth gray if administered before puberty).

Mottled enamel: Fluorosis (excessive fluoride).

Abnormalities of Teeth

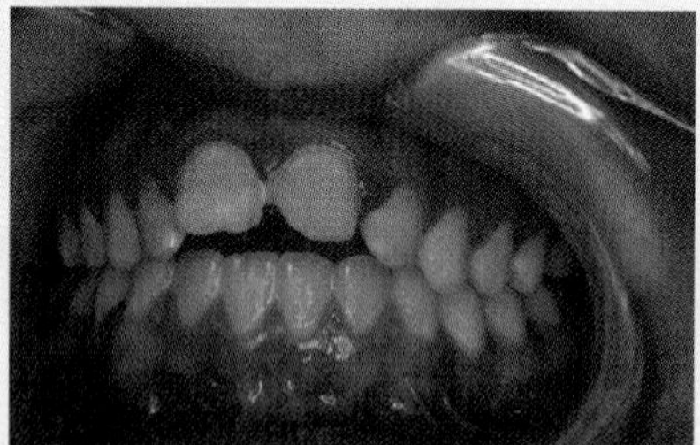

Malocclusion

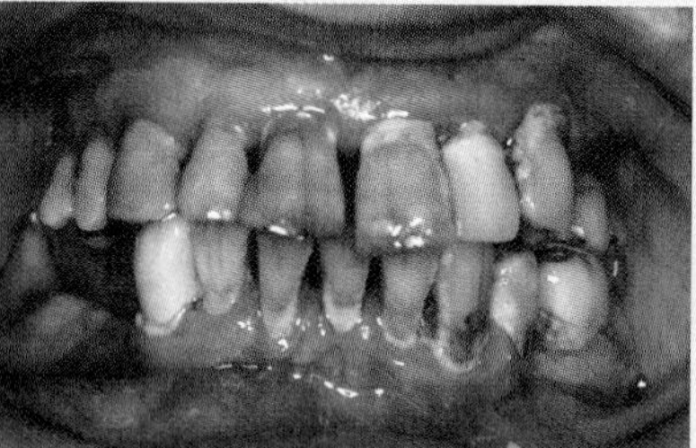

Dental caries

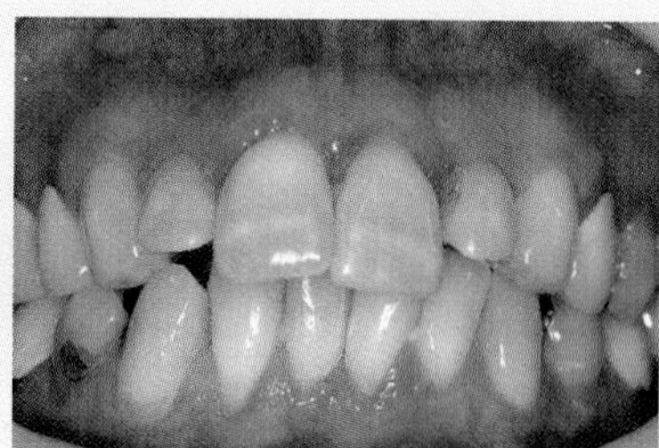

Tetracycline staining

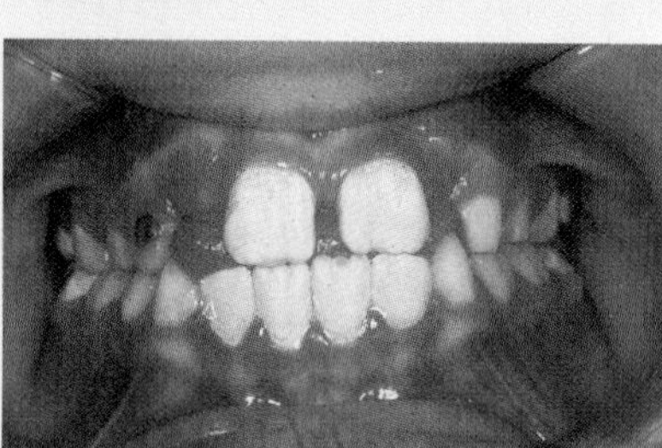

Fluorosis

Oral Mucosa and Gums

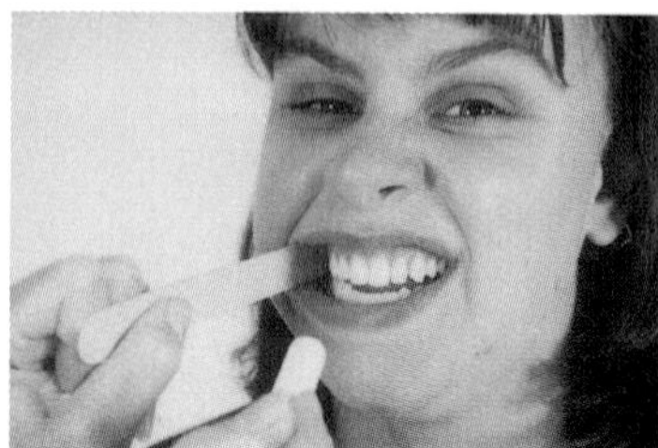

Inspecting oral mucosa and gums

Pink, moist, intact mucosa. Color variants acceptable if consistent with client's ethnic group/race—for instance, dark stippling in dark-skinned clients.

Hyperplasia of gums: Side effect of medications, such as dilantin or calcium channel blockers.

Gum recession or inflammatory gum changes (gingivitis/ periodontal disease): Poor dental hygiene or vitamin deficiency.

Pale or gray gingivae: Chronic gingivitis.

Inspection of the Mouth and Throat

ASSESS/NORMAL VARIATIONS

Oral Mucosa and Gums *(Continued)*

Gums consistent in color with other mucosa and intact, with no bleeding

Abnormalities of Oral Mucosa and Gums

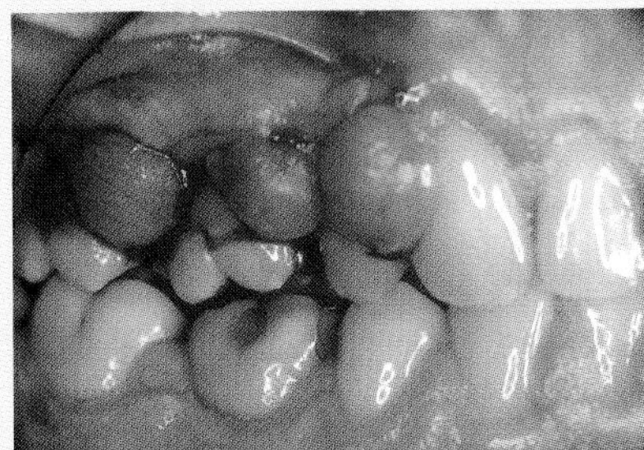
Gum hyperplasia

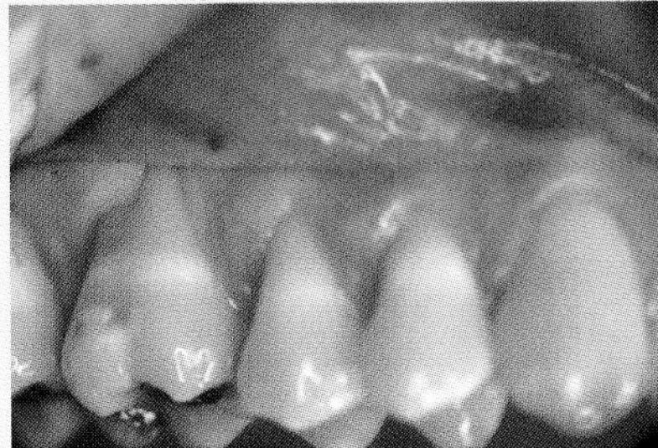
Gingival recession

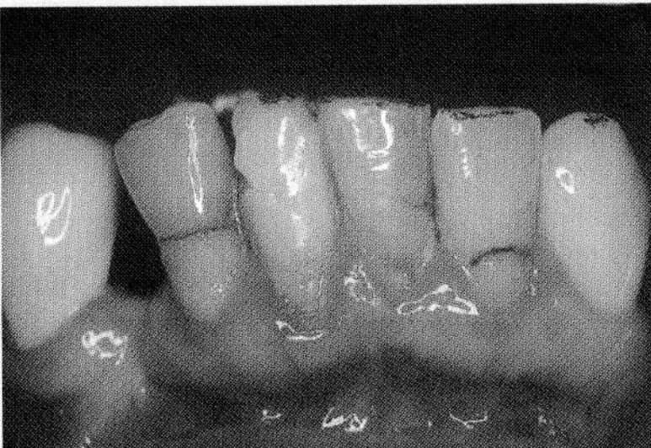
Chronic gingivitis

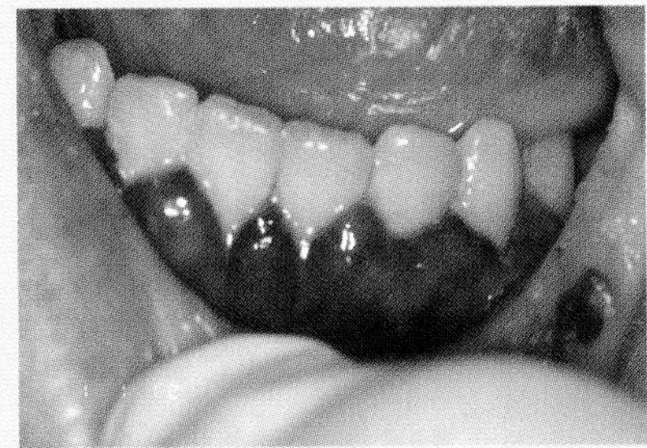
Leukemia

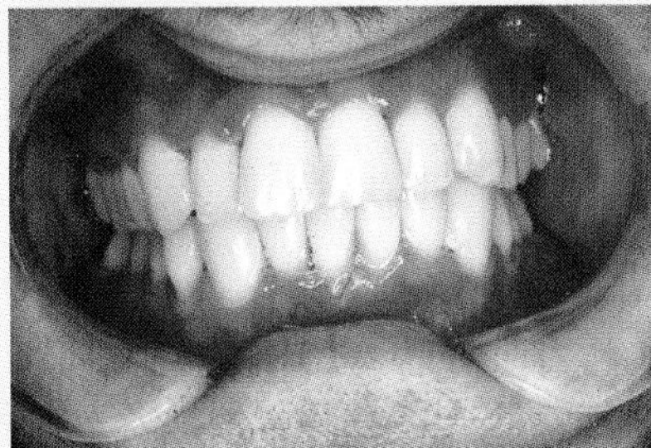
a. Early HIV periodontitis

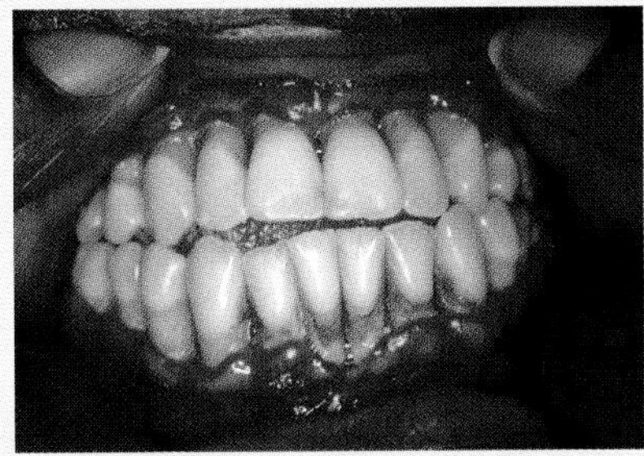
b. Advanced HIV periodontitis

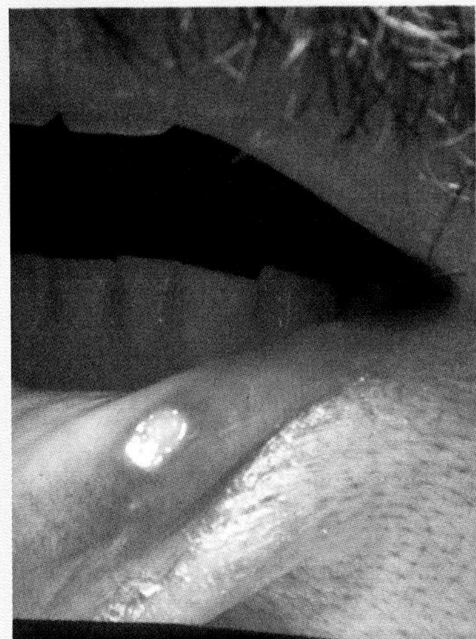
Aphthous ulcer

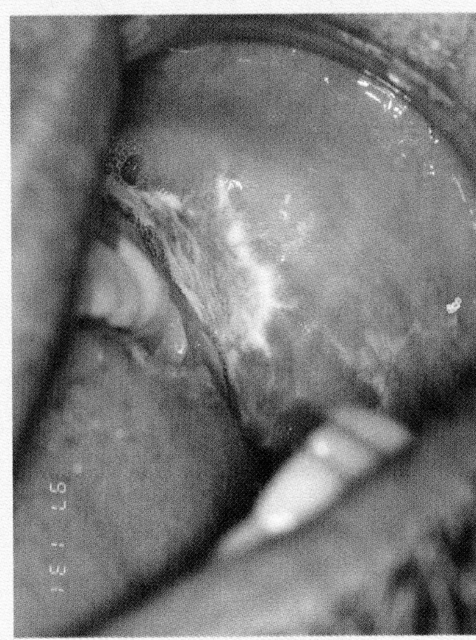
Lichen planus

ABNORMAL FINDINGS/RATIONALE

Abrasions, erosion of underlying mucosa: In denture wearers, poorly fitted dentures. Inflamed, bleeding gingivae may also be seen with leukemia and HIV.

Painful, reddened mucosa, often with mildly adherent white patches: Candida albicans.

Reddened, inflamed oral mucosa, sometimes accompanied by ulcerations: Allergic stomatitis.

Small, painful vesicles that often have a reddened periphery and a white or pale yellowish base: Aphthous ulcer, believed to be caused by viral infection, stress, or trauma.

Nodular, macular, or papular lesions widely involving the integument and often evident on the oral mucosa: Kaposi's sarcoma. Incidence has increased with the development of AIDS.

Inflammatory changes of the integument, often found on oral mucosa as chronic gray, lacy patches with or without ulceration: Lichen planus. May progress to neoplasm.

Reddened mucosal change that may progress to form cancer: Erythroplakia

White, adherent mucosal thickening: Leukoplakia. May progress to cancer.

Oral cancer on lip or oral mucosa: Cancers can be found on the lips, gums, oral mucosa or other areas of the mouth and are associated with tobacco use and alcohol abuse.

Enlarged sebaceous glands on buccal mucosa, white/yellow raised lesions: Fordyce granules (very common).

Medication reactions can cause a variety of changes to oral mucosa, as can infections.

(Continued)

Inspection of the Mouth and Throat *(Continued)*

ASSESS/NORMAL VARIATIONS | **ABNORMAL FINDINGS/RATIONALE**

Oral Mucosa and Gums *(Continued)*

Abnormalities of Oral Mucosa and Gums *(Continues)*

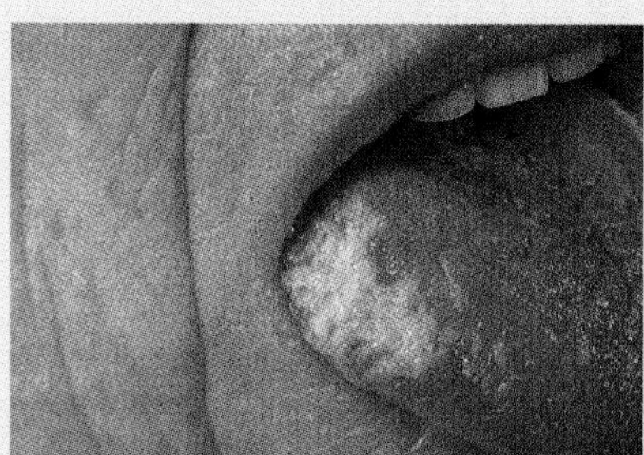

Leukoplakia

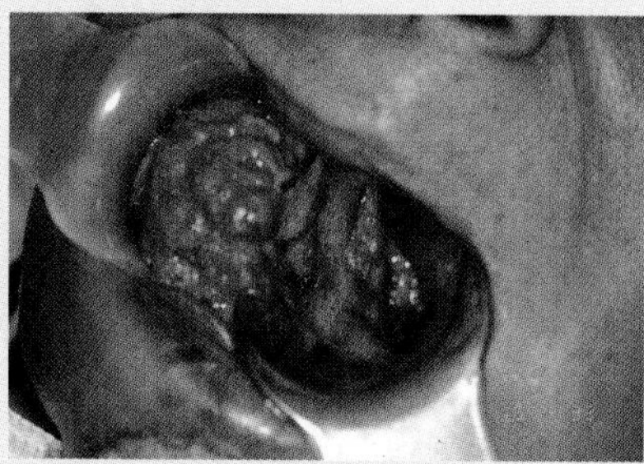

Cancer on oral mucosa

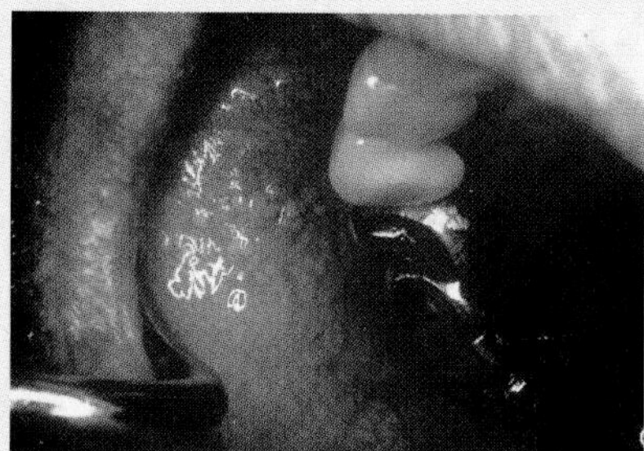

Fordyce granules

Hard and Soft Palate

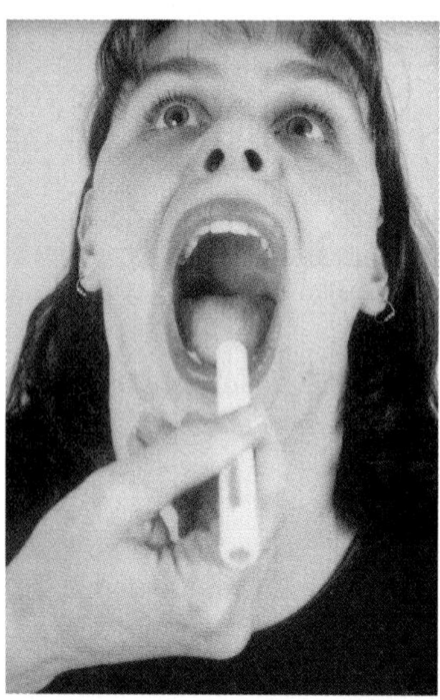

Inspecting palate

Palate intact, smooth, pink.

Bony, mucosa-covered projection on the hard palate (torus palatinus) or on floor of mouth (torus mandible) are normal variations.

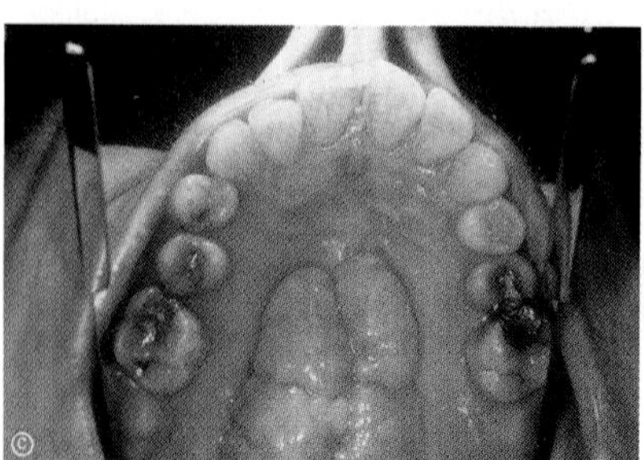

Torus palatinus

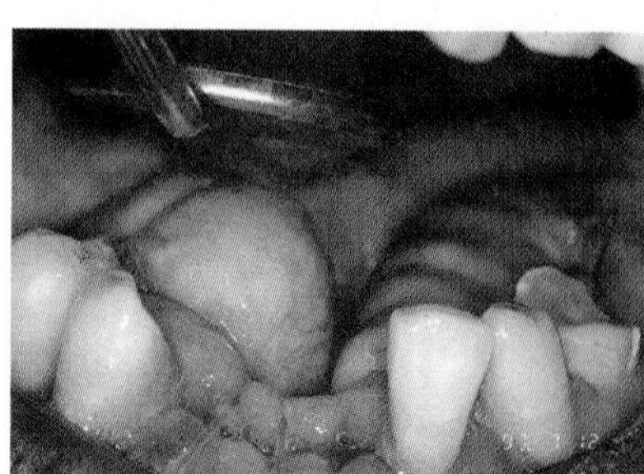

Torus mandible

Perforation: Congenital or from trauma or drug use.

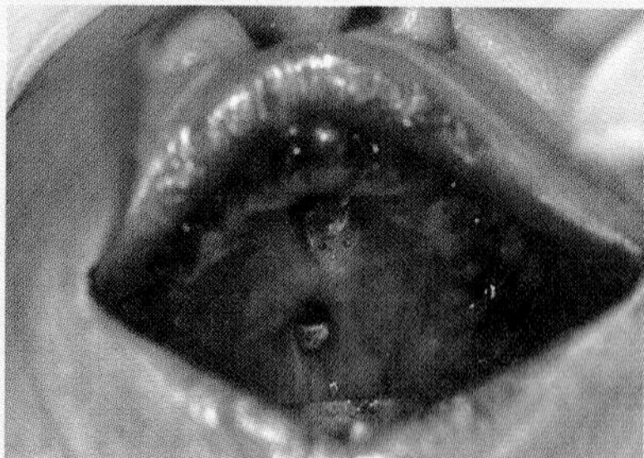

Cocaine use

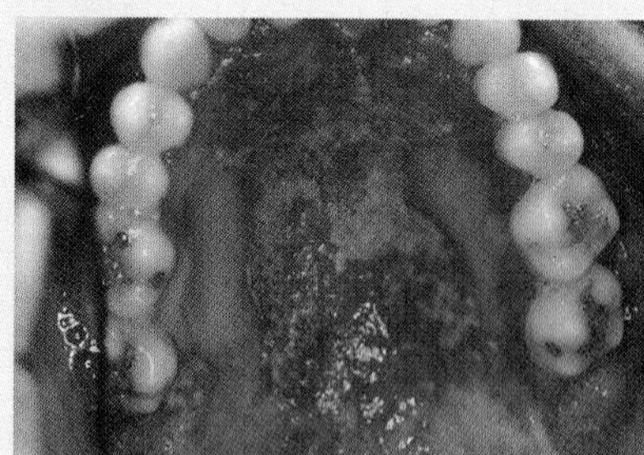

HIV palatal candidiasis

Inspection of the Mouth and Throat

ASSESS/NORMAL VARIATIONS	ABNORMAL FINDINGS/RATIONALE

Salivary Ducts

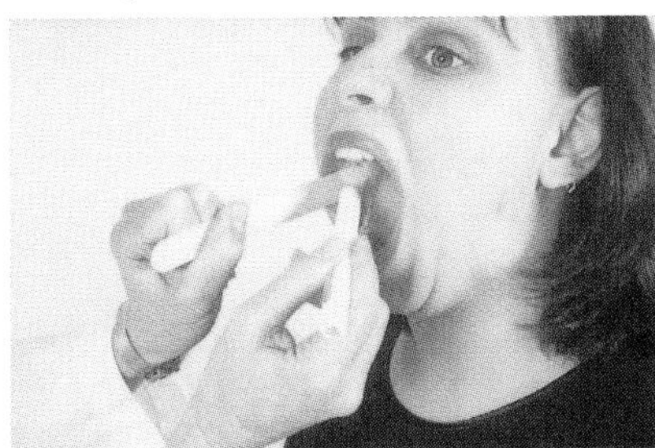

Inspecting Stensen's ducts

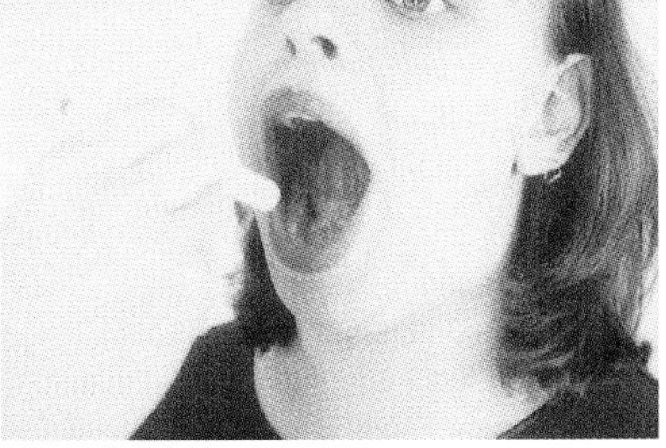

Inspecting Wharton's ducts

Stensen's duct intact at buccal mucosa at level of second molars.
Wharton's duct intact at either side of frenulum.
Both ducts with moist and pink mucosa; no lesions, swelling, or nodules.

Fullness or inflammatory changes of glands: Blockage of duct by calculi, infection, malignancy. Parotitis is inflammation of parotid glands.

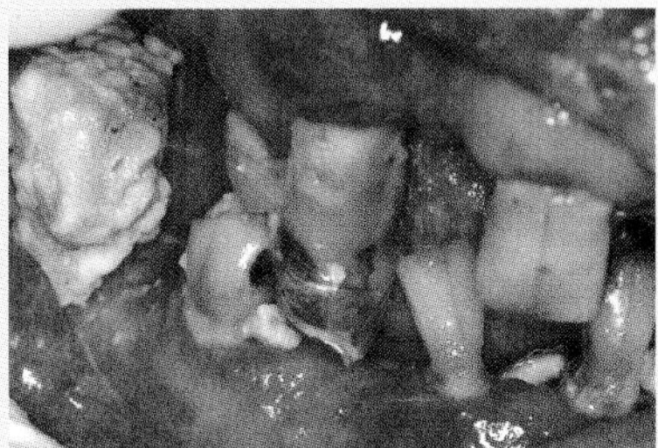

Parotitis

Tongue

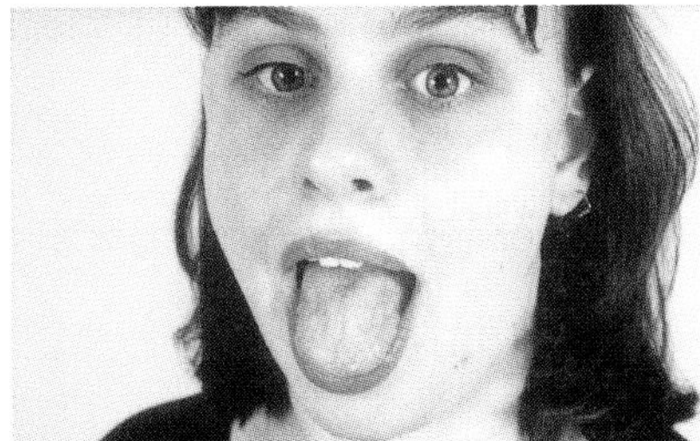

Inspecting the tongue

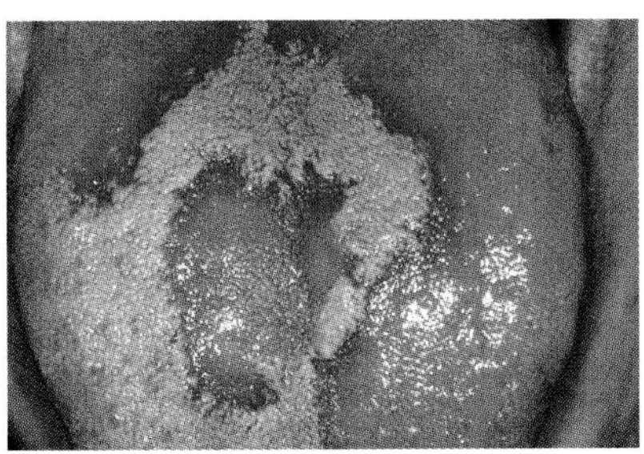

Geographic tongue

Pink and moist.
Coloring may vary consistent with ethnic group/race.
Mucosa intact with no lesions or discolorations.
Papillae intact. Tongue is freely and symmetrically mobile (CN XII intact).
Geographic tongue is a normal variation.

Absence of papillae, reddened mucosa, ulcerations: Allergic, inflammatory, or infectious cause.

Color changes: May indicate underlying problems; for example, red "beefy" tongue is seen with pernicious anemia. *Black, hairy tongue:* Fungal infections.

Hypertrophy and discoloration of papillae: Antibiotic use.

Reddened, smooth, painful tongue, with or without ulcerations (glossitis): Anemia, chemical irritants, medications.

Cancers may form on the tongue and on other oral mucosa.

Abnormalities of the Tongue

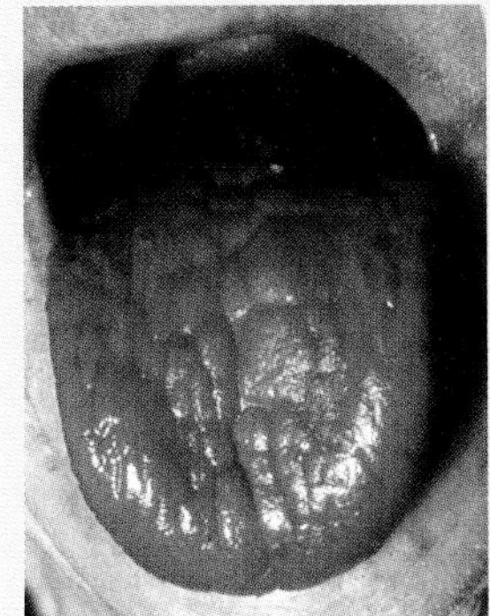

Red "beefy" tongue

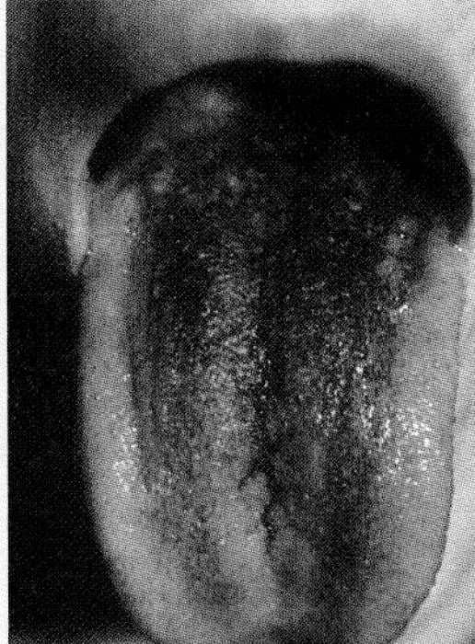

Black, hairy tongue

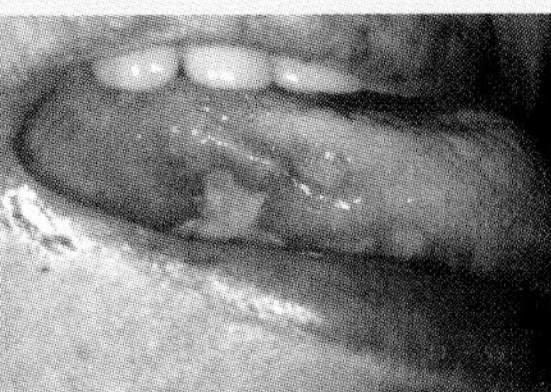

Glossitis

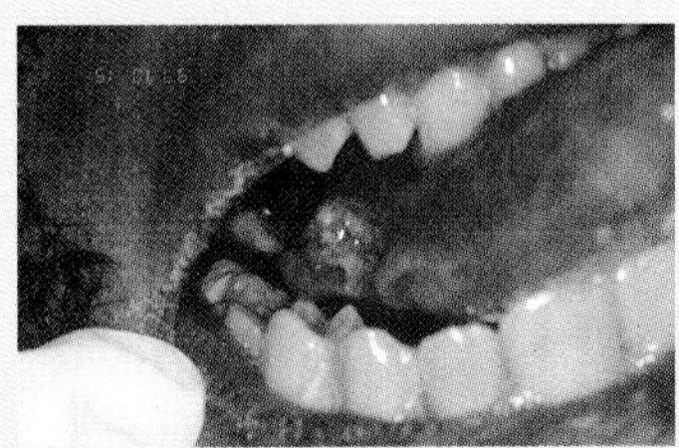

Cancer of the tongue

(Continued)

Inspection of the Mouth and Throat *(Continued)*

ASSESS/NORMAL VARIATIONS	ABNORMAL FINDINGS/ SIGNIFICANCE
Oropharynx 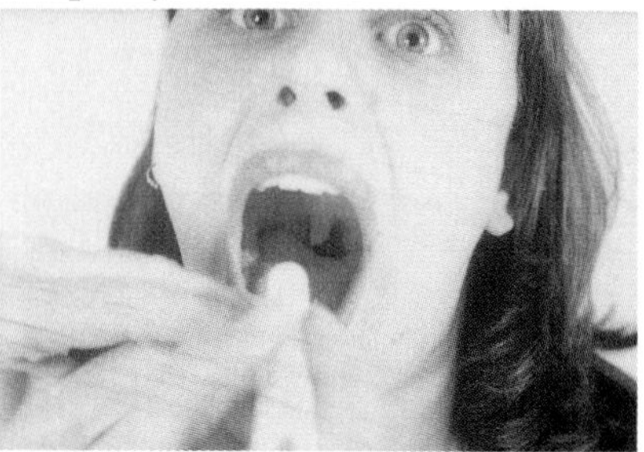 **Inspecting the oropharynx** Mucosa is pink, moist, intact. The lymphoid-rich posterior wall may have a slightly irregular surface. No lesions, erythema, swellings, exudate, or discharge.	*Yellowish or green streaks of drainage on the posterior wall:* Postnasal drainage. *Gray membrane/adherent material:* Diphtheria. *White or pale patches of exudates with erythemic mucosa:* Infection, including streptococcal bacterial infection or mononucleosis viral infection. Gonorrhea and chlamydia are also associated with exudative pharyngitis. *Erythema:* Inflammatory response, typically associated with infectious pharyngitis; also common in smokers. Scattered vesicles/ulcerations: Herpangioma. 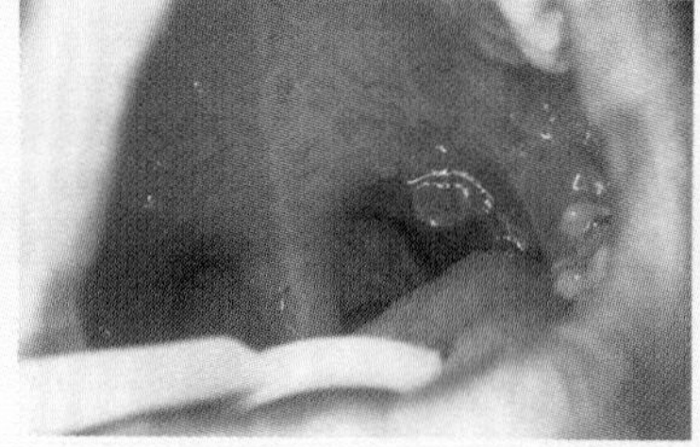 **Herpangioma**
Tonsils Symmetrical, pink, clean crypts. Crypts may have normal variation of small food particles (tonsilar pearls) or scant amounts of white cellular debris.	*Bulges adjacent to the tonsilar pillars:* Potential peritonsillar abscess. *Reddened, hypertrophic tonsil, with or without exudates:* Acute infection or tonsillitis. Lymphoid cobblestoning. Enlarged tonsils with exudates. 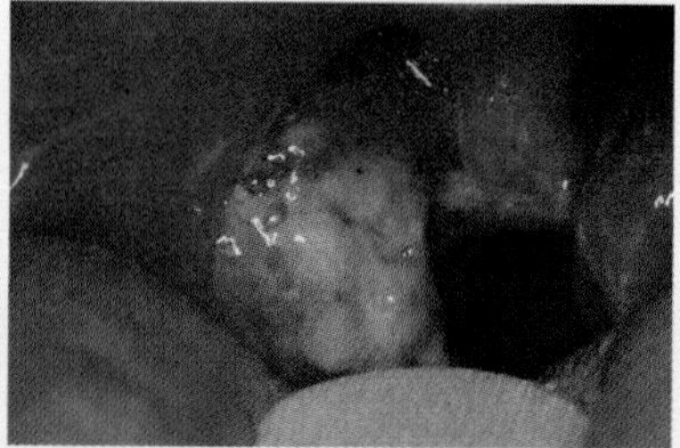 **Enlarged tonsils with exudates. See box for specific tonsil grades.**
Uvula Midline, pink, moist, without lesions.	*Erythema, exudate, lesions:* Infectious process.
Symmetrical rise of the uvula (CN IX, glossopharyngeal, and CN X, vagus, intact).	*Asymmetrical rise of the uvula:* Problem with CN IX and CN X.

Tonsil Grading Scale

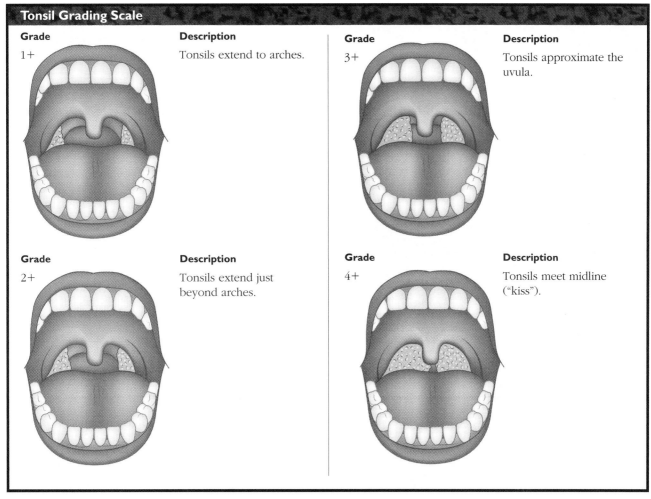

Grade	Description
1+ 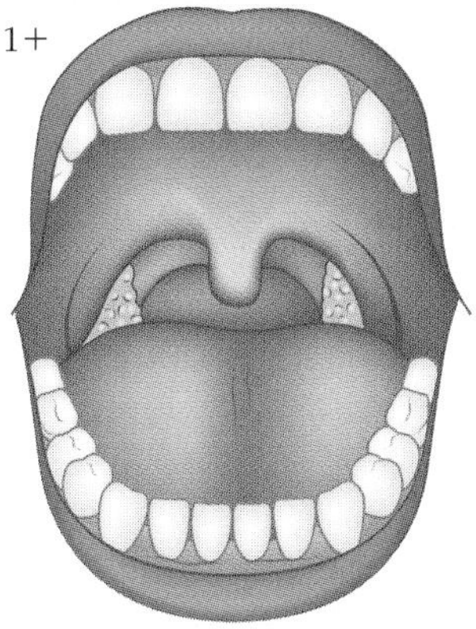	Tonsils extend to arches.
2+ 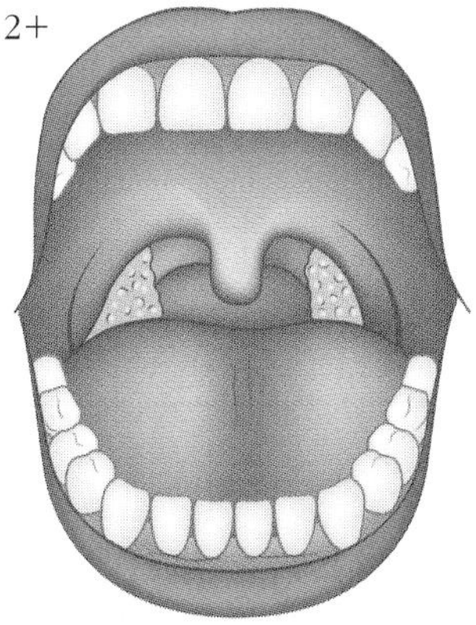	Tonsils extend just beyond arches.
3+ 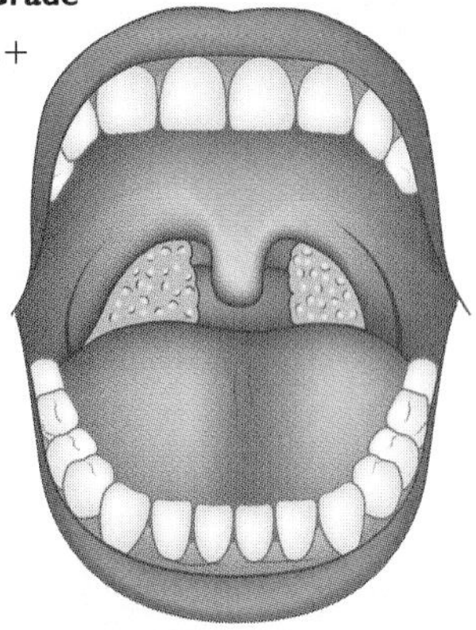	Tonsils approximate the uvula.
4+ 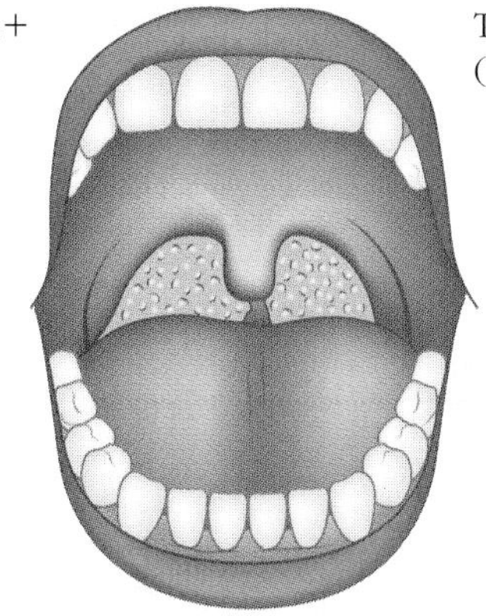	Tonsils meet midline ("kiss").

Palpation

Palpate the tongue for nodules or areas of thickening. Palpate the floor of the mouth for nodules or masses. To palpate the floor of the mouth, use your nondominant hand to press upward beneath the client's chin to provide support while palpating downward with a gloved hand inside the mouth. The support provided externally helps to ensure that the examining hand actually palpates a mass and does not merely push it away. The use of two hands will help to assess any mass, examining the dimensions, consistency, tenderness, and texture.

The parotid, submandibular, and sublingual glands should also be palpated for enlargement and tenderness. The parotid glands are located anterior to the ear and the submandibular and sublingual glands are located under the mandible.

HELPFUL HINT

If the salivary glands are enlarged, palpate very gently because they may be very tender.

Palpation of the Mouth and Throat

ASSESS/NORMAL VARIATIONS	ABNORMAL FINDINGS/RATIONALE
Lips 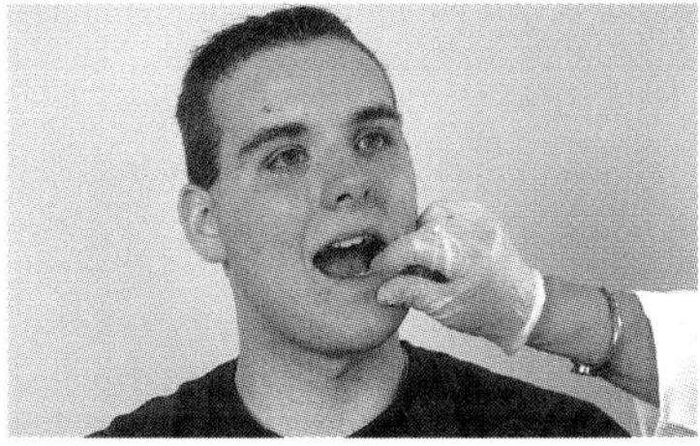 **Palpating the lips** Soft, nontender, no masses.	*Areas of induration, thickening, nodularity, or masses:* Neoplasm. *Tender induration that soon develops vesicles:* Herpes simplex.

(Continued)

Palpation of the Mouth and Throat *(Continued)*

ASSESS/NORMAL VARIATIONS	ABNORMAL FINDINGS/RATIONALE
Tongue Tissue is soft, without masses, nodules, thickenings, or tenderness.	*Areas of induration, thickening, nodularity:* Potential malignancy.
Tissue is soft, supple, without nodules, thickenings, masses, or tenderness. Sublingual glands may be palpable under the tongue but should be nontender, soft, and supple.	*Areas of unexpected induration, thickening, nodularity or other mass:* Malignancy.
Glands (Parotid, Submandibular, and Sublingual)	

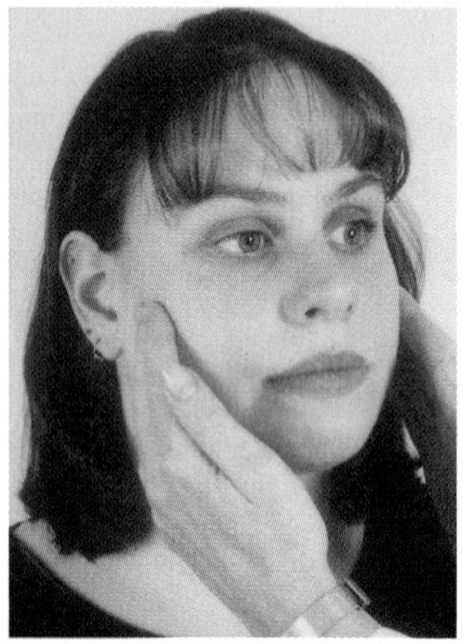

Palpating the submandibular gland

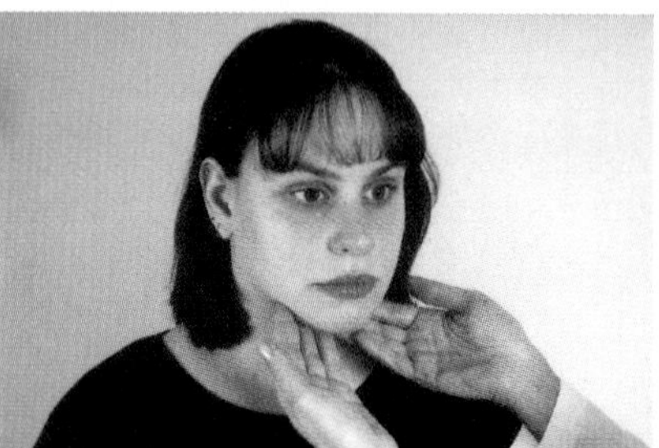

Palpating the sublingual gland

ASSESS/NORMAL VARIATIONS	ABNORMAL FINDINGS/RATIONALE
Parotid glands are nonpalpable and nontender. Submandibular and sublingual glands may be palpable but should be nontender, supple, and soft.	*Enlarged, tender parotid glands:* Parotitis, blocked ducts, infection, or malignancy.

COMMON FINDINGS/COMPLAINTS WITH ORAL CANCER

- Nonhealing lip or mouth sore
- Swelling or mass in the mouth or throat
- Erythroplakia/leukoplakia
- Unusual bleeding in the mouth
- Unusual sensation, such as pain or numbness, in the mouth
- Chronic sore throat
- Foreign body sensation in the throat
- Dysphagia
- Voice change
- Ear pain

Assessing the Neck

Examination of the neck integrates components of the vascular, respiratory, musculoskeletal, neurological, lymphatic, and endocrine systems. This chapter will focus on the lymphatic and endocrine systems, primarily on assessment of the cervical lymph nodes and the thyroid through inspection, palpation, and auscultation.

Inspection

You will be inspecting the cervical lymph nodes and thyroid gland. Remember, lymph nodes drain toward the center of the body. When examining the thyroid gland, focus your attention on the middle to lower third of the anterior neck, checking for enlargements.

Inspection of the Neck

ASSESS/NORMAL VARIATIONS	ABNORMAL FINDINGS/RATIONALE
Neck, Lymph Nodes, and Thyroid	
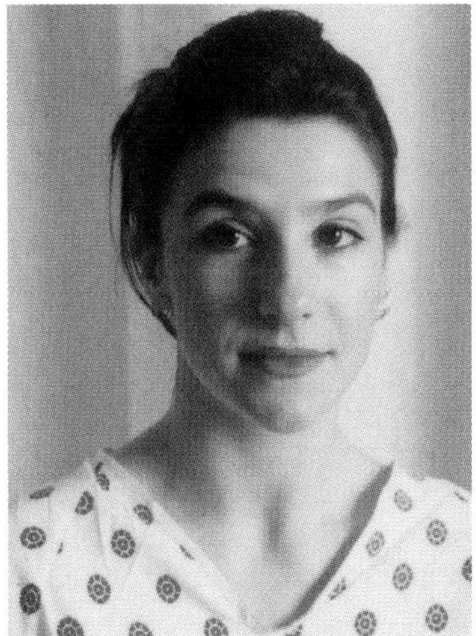 a. Inspecting neck from neutral position 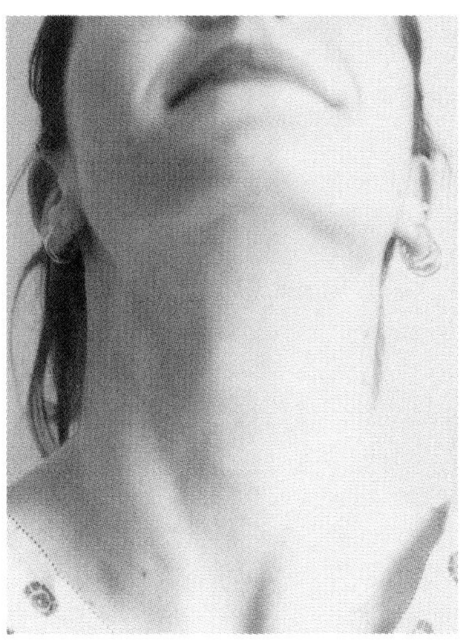 b. Inspecting neck when hyperextended 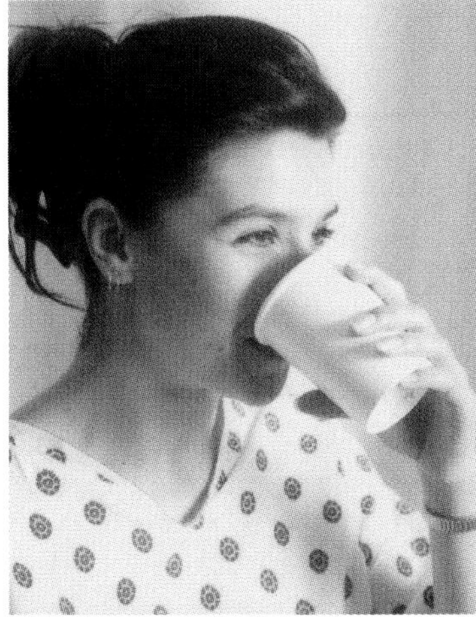 c. Inspecting neck when client swallows water Neck erect, midline, no lumps, bulges, or masses.	*Enlargements:* Lymphadenopathy, lymphoma, or other malignancy. *Torticollis (deviation of neck to one side caused by spasmodic contraction of neck muscles):* Scars, tonsillitis, adenitis, disease of cervical vertebrae, enlarged cervical glands, cerebellar tumor, rheumatism retropharyngeal abscess. 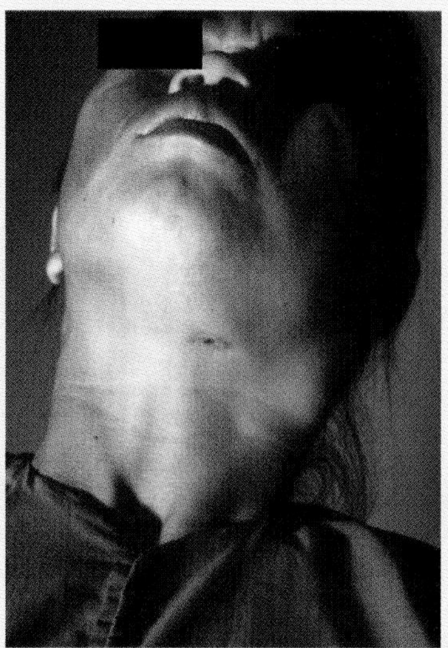 **Cervical adenitis**
Thyroid not visible. No masses, swelling, or hypertrophy in mid to lower half of anterior neck.	*Enlarged, visible thyroid:* Goiter or malignant mass.

Palpation

The order in which you palpate the cervical lymph nodes is not important, although it is best to develop a sequence and be consistent to ensure that you do not omit a group. One common sequence is to start with the preauricular nodes, followed by the postauricular nodes, then move to the tonsillar, submandibular, and submental nodes along the mandible. Next, palpate the occipital area, followed by the superficial and deep cervical, posterior cervical, and supraclavicular nodes. Palpate node groups gently with one or two fingers, applying alternate pressure. Palpate any identified nodes between two fingers to establish their dimensions, texture, consistency, and shape.

Although the lymph nodes are generally not palpable, it is not unusual to identify them at 1 cm or less in size. Palpable lymph nodes should be described according to their location, size, shape, consistency, mobility, and tenderness. Palpable small nodes should be soft to rubbery in consistency and be freely mobile, distinct, round, and nontender. The term used to describe enlarged nodes (greater than 1 cm in diameter) is **lymphadenopathy.** Lymphadenopathy can be regional (involving one or two groups) or more generalized (involving three or more groups).

HELPFUL HINTS

- Lymphatic tissue is largest in childhood and decreases in size with age. Normal palpable nodes are more likely to be found in children than in adults.
- Clients who present with a sore throat often complain about "swollen glands." They are actually feeling their submandibular salivary glands. To distinguish between salivary glands and lymph nodes, remember: A normal lymph node is either small (<1 cm), round, soft to rubbery, movable, and nontender or tender and enlarged with infection. Submandibular glands are larger, soft, glandular, and not freely movable.
- A palpable normal node is more likely to be a superficial node than a deep cervical one. Deep cervical nodes are normally nonpalpable.

To palpate the thyroid, use an anterior or posterior approach. Some examiners combine both approaches when assessing a thyroid nodule or enlargement. Both approaches are depicted here, so that you can determine which works best for you. Begin by locating the thyroid gland.

Although the thyroid is usually nonpalpable, you may be able to feel the isthmus, which connects the two lobes and lies below the cricoid cartilage. The lobes are located behind the sternocleidomastoid muscle. The likelihood of palpating the isthmus increases with very thin or pregnant clients. You may be able to feel the edge of the gland, especially in women, who have larger thyroid glands than men.

The thyroid gland moves as the individual swallows. Therefore, have the client drink water while you palpate the gland, to facilitate detection. Instruct him or her to take a sip from the cup and hold it in the mouth until you ask him or her to swallow. Do this at least twice, as you examine both the left and right thyroid lobes.

To use the posterior approach, stand behind the client and ask him or her to flex his or her neck slightly forward and to the left. This relaxes the muscles and the skin overlying the left side of the neck, making it easier to detect the tissue of the left thyroid lobe. Using the fingers of your left hand, locate the cricoid process. Push the trachea slightly to the left with your right hand as you palpate just below the cricoid process and between the trachea and the sternocleidomastoid muscle with your left hand. As you palpate, ask the client to swallow the water he or she is holding in the mouth. Now, repeat the steps with the client's head flexed slightly forward and to the right. This time, displace the trachea slightly to the right with your left hand and palpate the right lobe of the thyroid with your right hand.

To use the anterior approach, stand in front of the client and ask him or her to flex the neck slightly forward and in the direction you intend to palpate. Place your hands on the neck and apply gentle pressure to one side of the trachea while palpating the opposite side of the neck for the thyroid. The client should take a sip of water during this approach as well.

Differentiating Lymph Nodes

Characteristics	Normal	Infection	Malignancy
Size	<1 cm	Enlarged	Enlarged
Shape	Round	Round	Irregular
Consistency	Soft to rubbery	"Boggy"	Hard
Delimitation	Well defined	Well defined	Irregular borders
Mobility	Mobile	Mobile	Immobile
Tenderness	Nontender	Tender	Nontender

Palpation of the Neck

ASSESS/NORMAL VARIATIONS	ABNORMAL FINDINGS/RATIONALE
Neck Supple, nontender, no masses	*Masses:* Lymphadenopathy, malignancies, thyroid masses.
Cervical Nodes	*Palpable nodes (1 cm or greater)*: Malignancy, inflammatory, or infectious process of glands or area they drain.

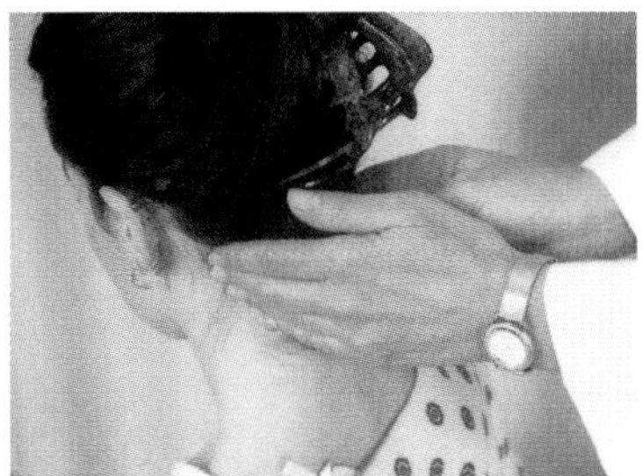

a: Occipital

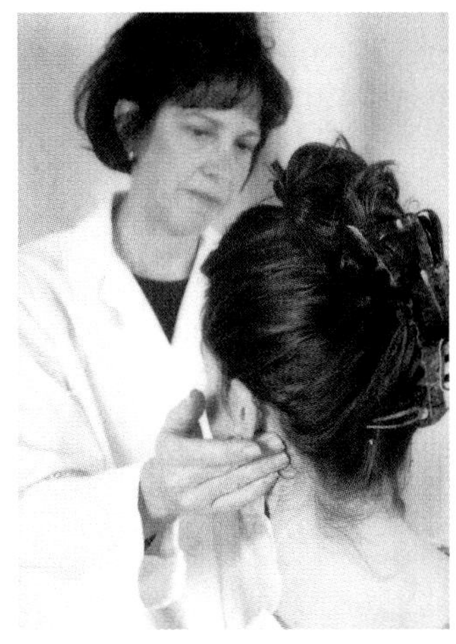

b: Postauricular

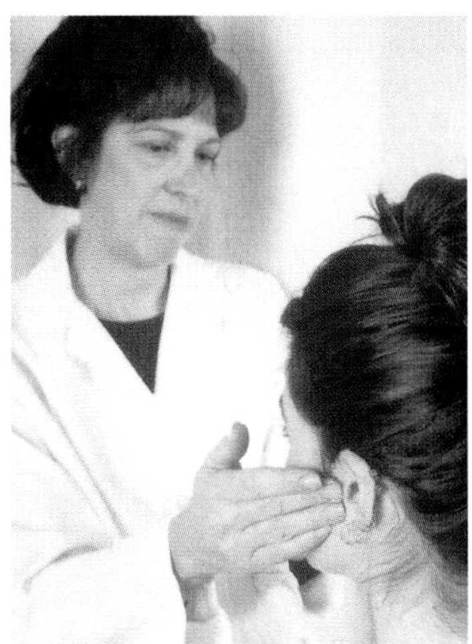

c: Preauricular

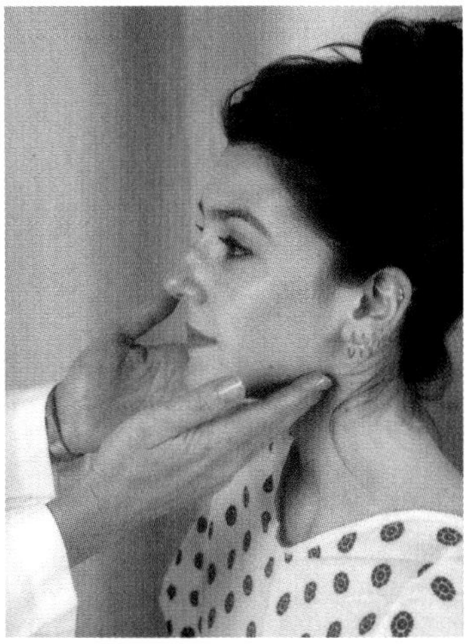

d: Tonsilar

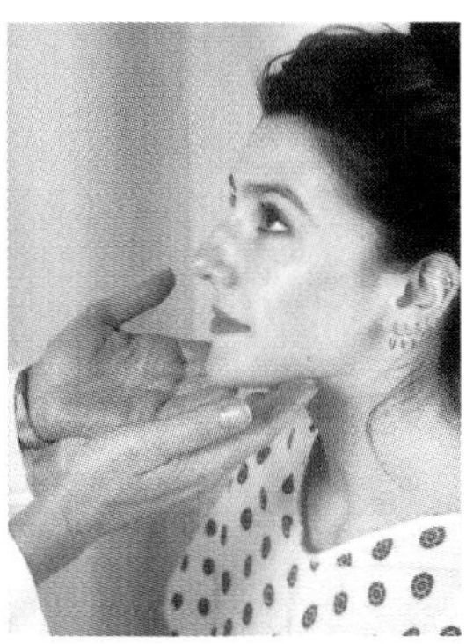

e: Submandibular

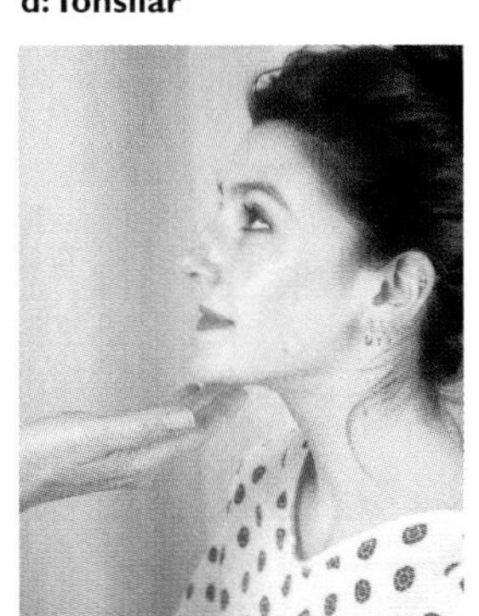

f: Submental

Nonpalpable or palpable, small, 1 cm mobile, soft, nontender

(Continued)

Palpation of the Neck *(Continued)*

ASSESS/NORMAL VARIATIONS	ABNORMAL FINDINGS/RATIONALE

Cervical Nodes *(Continued)*

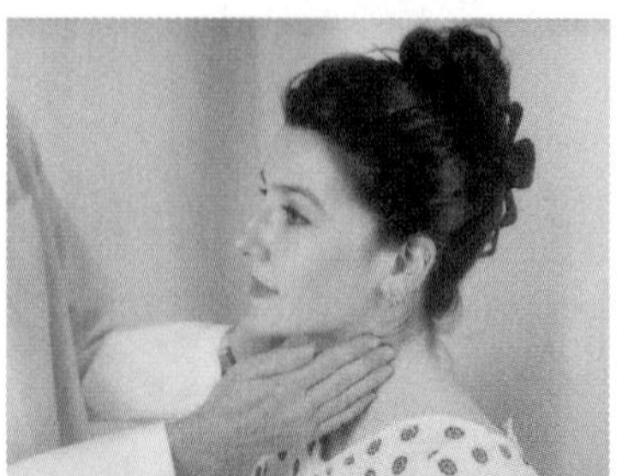
g: Superficial cervical

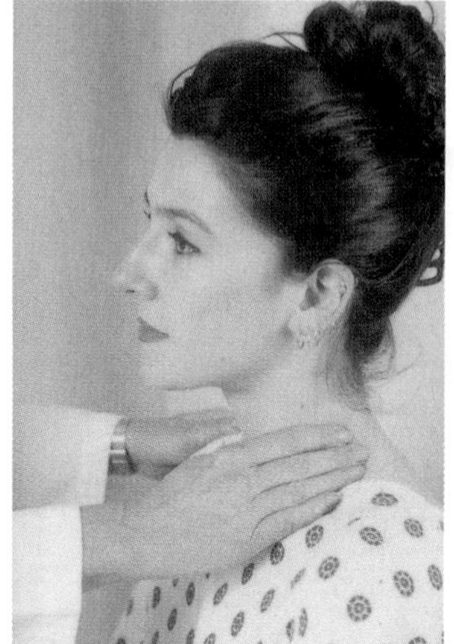
h: Posterior cervical

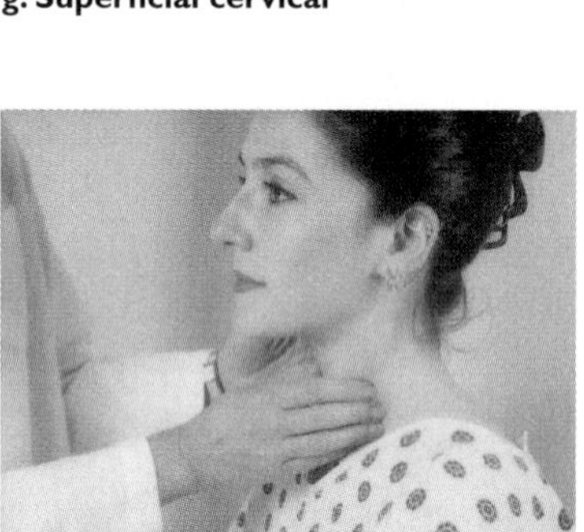
i: Deep cervical

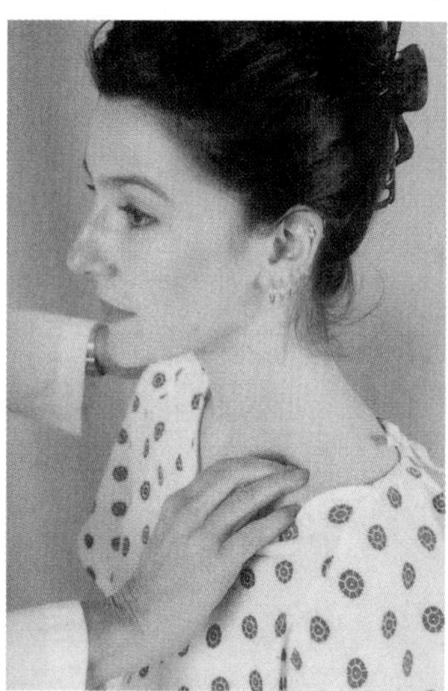
j: Supraclavicular

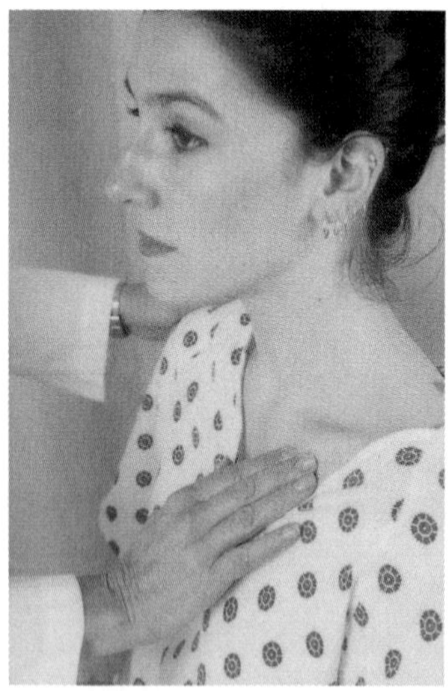
k: Infraclavicular

Palpation of the Neck

ASSESS/NORMAL VARIATIONS	ABNORMAL FINDINGS/RATIONALE
Thyroid	*Enlarged thyroid:* Tumor, goiter Nodular thyroid tissue. *Tender thyroid:* Inflammatory process such as acute thyroiditis.

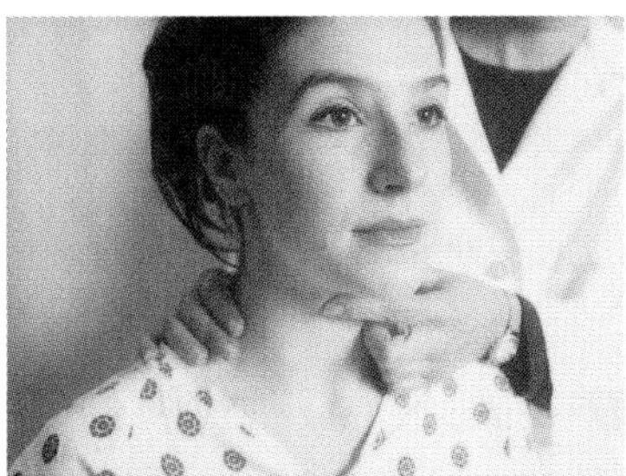
Landmarking thyroid

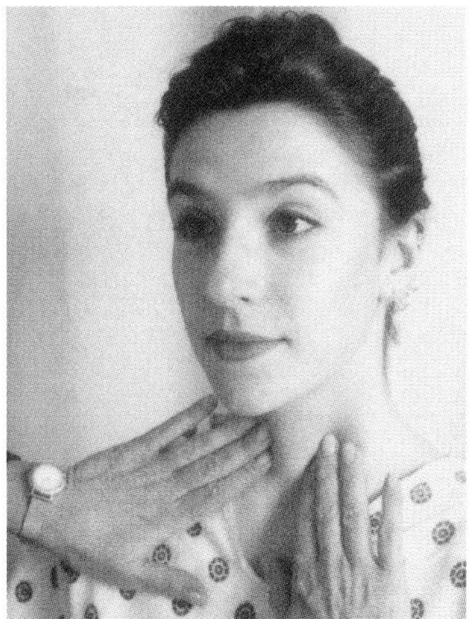
Palpating thyroid: Anterior approach

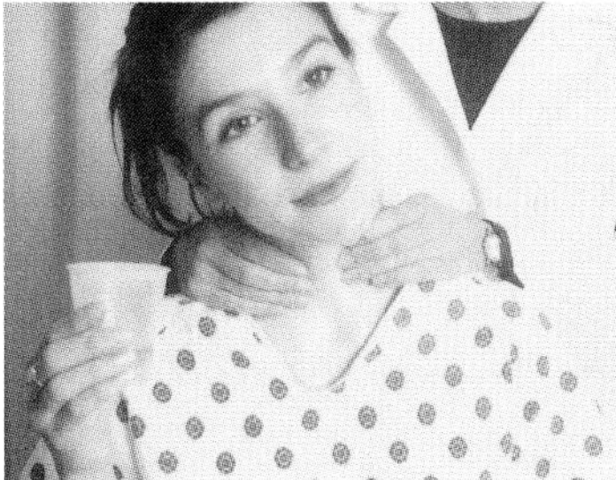
Palpating thyroid: Right posterior approach

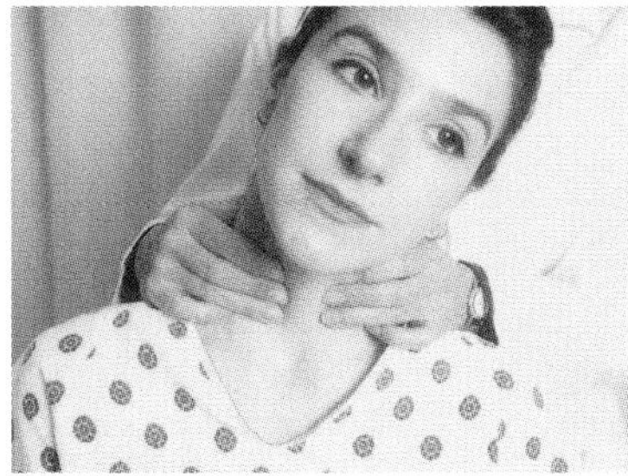
Palpating thyroid: Left posterior approach

Generally nonpalpable. If some tissue is palpable, (e.g., in very thin or pregnant clients), consistency is firm, smooth, and meaty, with no nodularity, enlargement, or tenderness.

Auscultation

The final portion of the neck examination, auscultation of the thyroid gland, is generally reserved for situations in which the thyroid is enlarged or a mass is palpated. To auscultate the gland, place the bell of your stethoscope over one lobe, then the other. Ask the client to briefly stop breathing as you auscultate, to optimize your ability to hear without the distraction of the tracheal breath sounds. There should be no thyroid sounds. Because the thyroid is a very vascular organ, vascular sounds are sometimes present in hyperthyroidism.

Auscultation of the Thyroid

ASSESS/NORMAL VARIATIONS	ABNORMAL FINDINGS/RATIONALE
Thyroid	*Bruit:* Increased vascularity of hyperthyroidism.

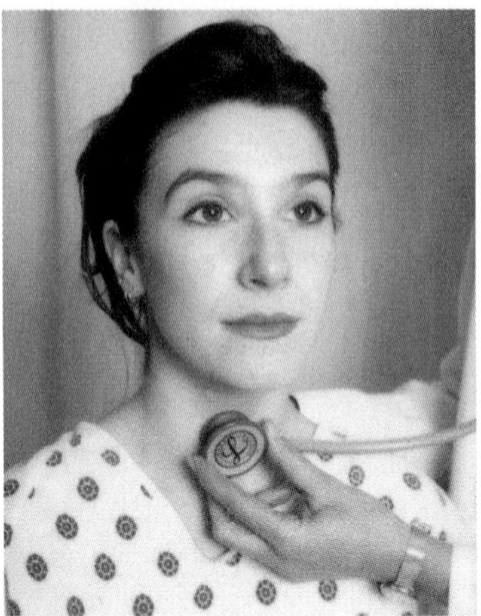

Auscultating thyroid

No sounds detected.

HELPFUL HINT

An enlarged thyroid gland may occur with either hyperthyroidism or hypothyroidism. If the gland is enlarged, further assessment of presenting signs and symptoms and thyroid function studies are warranted to determine the cause.

SIGNS AND SYMPTOMS OF HYPERTHYROIDISM AND HYPOTHYROIDISM

Hyperthyroidism

- Muscle weakness/tremors
- Irritability or emotional lability, manic behavior
- Decreased weight
- Sleep disturbance
- Thyroid enlargement, goiter
- Heat intolerance
- Irregular menses, amenorrhea
- Flushed skin, fine hair

Hypothyroidism

- Muscle weakness, aches and pain
- Apathy, agitation, paranoia, depression
- Increased weight
- Increased sleep
- Thyroid enlargement, goiter
- Cold intolerance
- Changes in menses
- Coarse, dry skin and hair

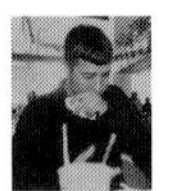

Case Study Findings

John's focused physical assessment findings include:

- Head and face
  - Head is normocephalic, with no abnormal contour, bulges, lesions, or tenderness.
  - Face is symmetrical at rest and at motion, with no lesions.
- Nose and sinuses
  - Sinuses are nontender, resonant to percussion, and maxillary/frontal sinuses transilluminate bilaterally.
  - External nose is midline, symmetrical, with no drainage or lesion.
  - Nasal mucosa is intact, slightly paler than oral mucosa, with no lesions or polyps.
  - Nares patent, no nasal flaring.
  - Septum is midline, mucosa intact and pink, with no deviation or perforation.
  - Turbinates symmetrical, slightly enlarged.
  - Scant clear, mucoid secretions.
- Mouth and teeth
  - Lips midline, symmetrical, close easily
  - 28 white teeth in good repair, good occlusion
  - Lips pink, supple, with no lesions or indurations
  - Oral mucosa uniformly deep pink, glistening, moist; no lesions or indurations
  - Tongue supple, freely mobile, pink mucosa with papillae intact, no lesions
  - Stensen's and Wharton's ducts with mucosa intact, no induration or swelling
- Pharynx
  - Tonsils symmetrical, small, pink, with clean crypts. No lesions or exudates
  - Uvula midline with symmetrical rise and pink mucosa

(Continued)

AREA/SYSTEM	SUBJECTIVE DATA
General	*Ask about:* Changes in energy level Weight changes Fevers Night sweats
Integumentary	*Ask about:* Changes in skin, hair and nails Rashes, itching
HEENT *Head and Neck*	*Ask about:* Head or neck pain Masses or swollen nodes
Eyes	*Ask about:* Vision changes, drainage, itching, pain
Ears, Nose and Throat	*Ask about:* Changes in hearing Ear drainage, itching, pain Nasal congestion, drainage, sinus pain Nosebleeds Mouth sores or dental pain Jaw pain
Respiratory	*Ask about:* Cough, congestion, wheezing, mucus production
Cardiovascular	*Ask about:* History of cardiovascular disease (e.g., CAD, HTN) Chest pain, palpitations
Gastrointestinal	*Ask about:* Changes in appetite Bowel changes Nausea, vomiting
Genitourinary/ Reproductive	*Ask about:* History of STD Changes in libido *Women:* Last menstrual period Menstrual changes Vaginal discharge or sores *Men:* Penile discharge, sores
Musculoskeletal	*Ask about:* Joint pain Muscle weakness Limited movement
Neurological	*Ask about:* Nervousness Difficulty staying focused Forgetfulness Changes in level of consciousness Numbness and tingling Headaches, head injury
Endocrine	*Ask about:* Changes in shoe size or ring size Changes in facial features Changes in energy level Weight changes Sleep problems
Lymphatic/ Hematologic	*Ask about:* Unusual bleeding, bruising Current/recent infection History of cancer

Assessment of the Head/Face/Neck's Relationship to Other Systems

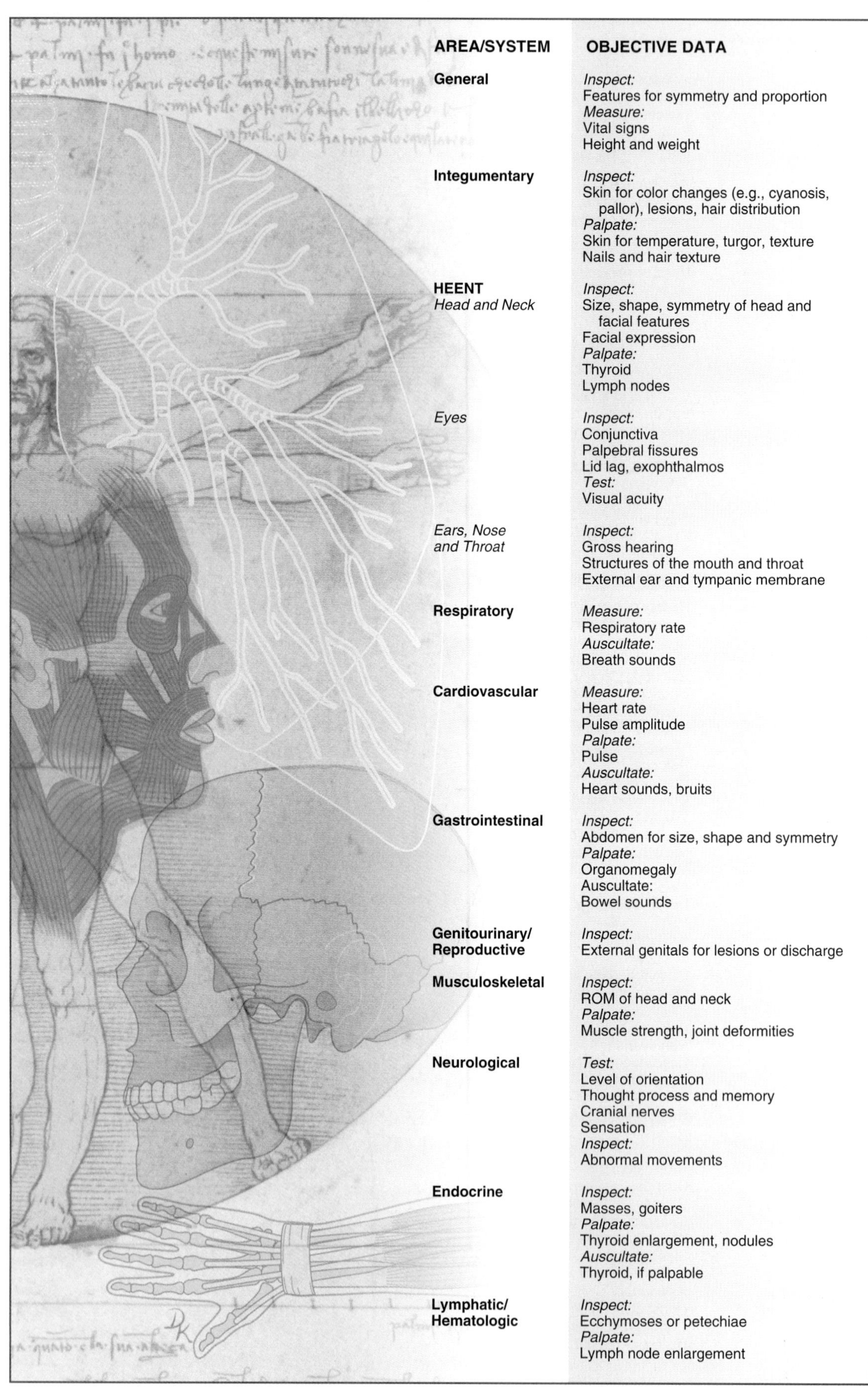

AREA/SYSTEM	OBJECTIVE DATA
General	*Inspect:* Features for symmetry and proportion *Measure:* Vital signs Height and weight
Integumentary	*Inspect:* Skin for color changes (e.g., cyanosis, pallor), lesions, hair distribution *Palpate:* Skin for temperature, turgor, texture Nails and hair texture
HEENT *Head and Neck*	*Inspect:* Size, shape, symmetry of head and facial features Facial expression *Palpate:* Thyroid Lymph nodes
Eyes	*Inspect:* Conjunctiva Palpebral fissures Lid lag, exophthalmos *Test:* Visual acuity
Ears, Nose and Throat	*Inspect:* Gross hearing Structures of the mouth and throat External ear and tympanic membrane
Respiratory	*Measure:* Respiratory rate *Auscultate:* Breath sounds
Cardiovascular	*Measure:* Heart rate Pulse amplitude *Palpate:* Pulse *Auscultate:* Heart sounds, bruits
Gastrointestinal	*Inspect:* Abdomen for size, shape and symmetry *Palpate:* Organomegaly Auscultate: Bowel sounds
Genitourinary/ Reproductive	*Inspect:* External genitals for lesions or discharge
Musculoskeletal	*Inspect:* ROM of head and neck *Palpate:* Muscle strength, joint deformities
Neurological	*Test:* Level of orientation Thought process and memory Cranial nerves Sensation *Inspect:* Abnormal movements
Endocrine	*Inspect:* Masses, goiters *Palpate:* Thyroid enlargement, nodules *Auscultate:* Thyroid, if palpable
Lymphatic/ Hematologic	*Inspect:* Ecchymoses or petechiae *Palpate:* Lymph node enlargement

Assessment of the Head/Face/Neck's Relationship to Other Systems (continued)

- Posterior wall moist, smooth pink, with no exudates or lesions
- ■ Neck
  - Head and neck erect. Neck supple, with full range of motion, no bulges or masses
  - Cervical nodes nonpalpable
  - Trachea midline and mobile
  - Thyroid nonpalpable, nontender

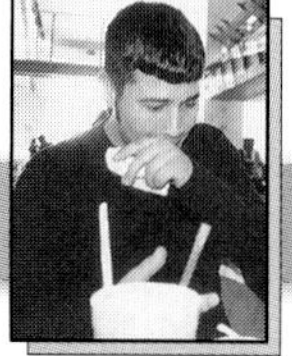

Case Study Analysis and Plan

Now that you have completed a thorough assessment of John Henck, document your key history and physical examination findings and key history findings that will help you formulate your nursing diagnoses.

CRITICAL THINKING ACTIVITY #3

What strengths and areas of concern have you identified related to John's current health status?

Nursing Diagnoses

Consider all of the data you have collected during your assessment of John Henck. Now, use this data to identify a list of nursing diagnoses. Below are some possible nursing diagnoses. Cluster the supporting data.

1. **Health-Seeking Behaviors, related to the desire to participate in recreational activities and to maintain overall health.**
2. **Trauma, risk for, related to frequent athletic activities, teenage driving, occasional alcohol intake.**
3. **Sleep Pattern, disturbed, related to adverse reaction to medication and/or sinus/nasal discomfort and congestion.**

Identify any additional nursing diagnoses.

CRITICAL THINKING ACTIVITY #4

Now that you have identified appropriate nursing diagnoses for John, design a nursing care plan and a brief teaching plan for one of the diagnoses identified above, including learning outcomes and teaching strategies.

Research Tells Us

An extremely dry mouth, or xerostomia, can be a symptom of several disorders, including Sjögren's syndrome and dehydration. It can also be an adverse effect of medications, including anticholinergics, antidepressants, and narcotic analgesics. It is unknown exactly what amount of saliva is necessary to maintain oral function; however, saliva is important in the maintenance of oral mucosa, initiation of digestion, and comfort.

Four objective findings are indicators of xerostomia: lip dryness; buccal mucosa dryness; decaying, missing, or filled teeth; and lack of salivary flow with gland palpation. Because mouth dryness is a relatively common symptom, work is being done to develop a subjective monitor of mouth dryness. An eight-item visual analog scale designed to measure clients' perceptions of eight symptoms associated with xerostomia is being tested. The researchers found that the eight indicators included on the scale had good reliability. Unfortunately, the validity of the tool was found to be inadequate for detecting acute changes in salivary production because subjective responses did not change significantly in response to acute, induced changes in salivary flow. Consequently, researchers recommend that the instrument be used to assess the subjective state associated with mouth dryness over time.

The visual analog scale features a series of eight 100-mm horizontal lines, each preceded by a subjective indicator of mouth dryness. The beginning and end of each line contain opposing ratings—for example, "none at all" and "very much." To complete the scale, clients mark the point along the 100-mm line that indicates their rating of each variable. The eight pairs of descriptors measure the client's rating of:

- Difficulty speaking caused by dryness
- Difficulty swallowing caused by dryness
- Amount of saliva in the mouth

- Dryness of the mouth
- Dryness of the throat
- Dryness of the lips
- Dryness of the tongue
- Level of thirst

Although the VAS is still being tested by the developers, it does identify several important questions that can be used to monitor the very disagreeable experience of mouth dryness (Pai, Ghezzi, & Ship, 2000).

Health Concerns

Facts About Disorders of the Head, Face, and Neck

Disorders affecting the head, face, and neck are quite common. At least 10 percent of the American population (26 million people) have allergic rhinitis, or hay fever. In 1996, allergic rhinitis accounted for 9.2 million healthcare visits and $6 billion in costs. Chronic sinusitis affects another 35 million Americans.

Thyroid disease is another common disorder. It affects an estimated 13 million Americans, with women up to eight times more likely to develop thyroid disease than men.

The vast majority of head and neck malignancies occur in the oral cavity. The most common sites are the floor of the mouth, the ventrolateral aspects of the tongue, and the soft palate. These generally occur after age 45. Most oral malignancies are of the squamous cell type, with tobacco (cigarettes, pipes, cigars, and chewing tobacco) and alcohol use the main risk factors. Another risk factor for cancer of the lip is sun exposure. Precancerous mucosal changes can often be detected and include leukoplakia (white patches) and erythroplakia (reddened patches). Another common form of head and neck cancer includes laryngeal malignancies, with over 12,000 cases diagnosed each year. In 1998, only 13 percent of people over age 49 had an annual examination for oral or pharyngeal cancer.

Projected Diagnosis and Deaths from Head and Neck Cancers, 2001

Site/Type of Malignancy	Projected New Diagnoses	Projected Related Deaths
Tongue	7100	1700
Mouth	10,500	1300
Pharynx	8400	1500
Other Oral	4100	1200
Larynx	10,000	4000
Thyroid	19,500	1300
Hodgkin's Lymphoma	7400	1300
Non-Hodgkin's Lymphoma	56,200	26,300

Source: Greenlee, R., Hill-Harmon, M.B., Murray, R., & Then, M. (2001). Cancer statistics 2001. *CA: A Cancer Journal for Clinicians, 51*(1), 15–36.

Common Abnormalities

ABNORMALITY	ASSESSMENT FINDINGS
Acute Cervical Adenitis Localized or regional enlarged and tender lymph nodes	• Affected area warm and erythematous • Fever • History of cat scratch, dental infection, URI, or other exposure
Acute Parotitis Inflammation of the parotid glands	• Pain over salivary gland site • Swelling with gland visible above jaw angle and anterior to earlobe • Swollen and tender over the duct • Firm consistency (hard growth that develops gradually may indicate malignancy) • Purulent discharge at duct orifice possible • Fever • Generalized overlying erythema possibly present
Acute Rhinitis, Viral Acute nasal congestion with increased mucus secretion	• Clear or mucoid drainage • Congestion • Fever • Mild scratchy sore throat • Mild dry cough • Sneezing
Acute Sinusitis Inflammation of the sinuses	• Mucopurulent nasal discharge • Postnasal drainage • Cough • Fever • Inflamed mucosa • Tenderness over sinuses • Periorbital swelling • Facial pain
Allergic Rhinitis Hay fever	• Sneezing • Rubbing nose and eyes • "Allergic salute" • Transverse nasal crease • Watery clear discharge • Allergic "black eye" • Periorbital puffiness • Single or clustered clear vesicles (1–10 mm) • Ruptured vesicles form ulcer with pale yellow base • Red, raised margins
Candidal Stomatitis Fungal inflammation of the mouth	• History of underlying condition (HIV, diabetes mellitus) or medication (corticosteroid, antibiotic) • Tongue usually involved • Erythematous mucosa • Thin, white plaques often present

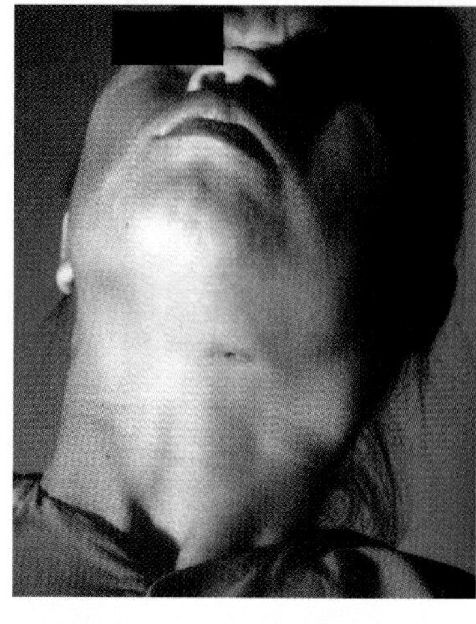

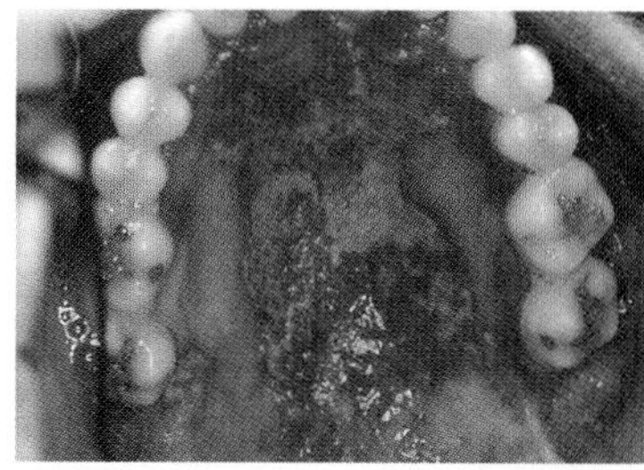

(Continued)

Common Abnormalities *(Continued)*

ABNORMALITY	ASSESSMENT FINDINGS
Chronic Sinusitis Chronic inflammation of the sinuses	• Nasal discharge • Congestion • Cough • Dull headache • Thick postnasal drainage • Ear pressure • Halitosis • Fatigue
Epistaxis Nosebleed	• History of trauma, local irritation, inflammation of nasal mucosa • Scant to significant bleeding • 90% of anterior bleeding at Kisselbach's plexus
Herpes Simplex Vesicular eruption caused by a virus	• Tender, enlarged lymph nodes • Clustered, small (3–4 mm) vesicles on mucosa • Vesicles rupture and form ulcers • Severe pain • Fever • History of previous episodes 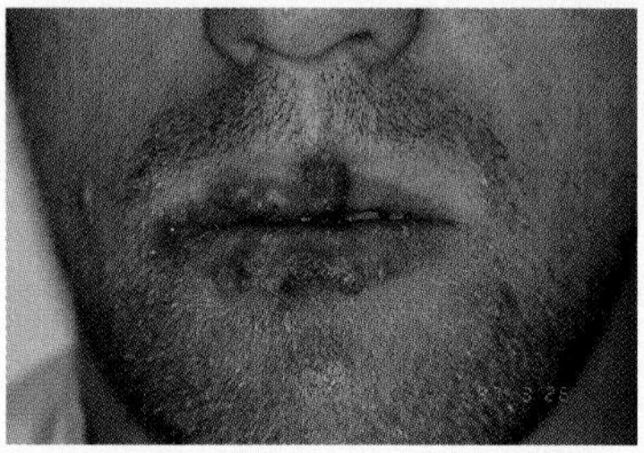
Ludwig's Angina A suppurative inflammation of subcutaneous tissue adjacent to a submaxillary gland	• History of dental disease • Cellulitis on floor of mouth (tender, red, swollen) • Fever • Systemic symptoms
Nasal Polyp A tumor with a pedicle, found in the nose	• Mobile (unlike fixed turbinates) • Pale, nontender rounded masses • Pale coloring • Variable size • Usually bilateral • History of atopic disease, chronic rhinitis, or chronic sinusitis 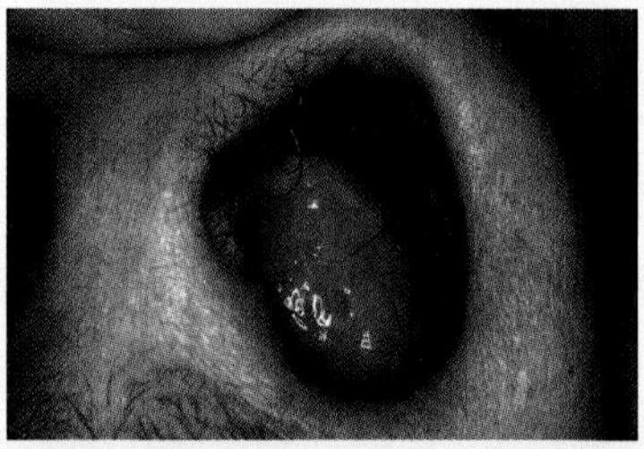
Periodontal Disease Disease of the supporting structures of the teeth	• Loose teeth • Inflamed gingiva • Bleeding • Edema of gums • Possible tooth loss 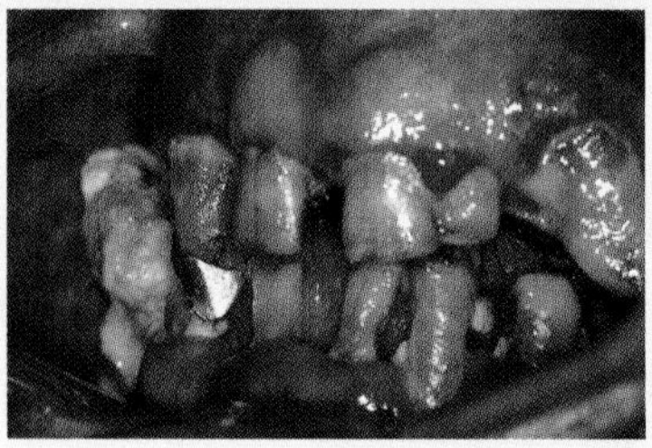
Pharyngitis Inflammation of the pharynx	Throat pain • Upper respiratory infection symptoms • Tender anterior cervical nodes • Posterior pharyngeal erythema • Fever • Scant white or yellow exudate possibly present
Pharyngitis, Mononucleosis Inflammation of the pharynx caused by mononucleosis	Same symptoms as pharyngitis, plus: • Increased fever • Fatigue • Enlarged lymph nodes • Palatal petechiae

Common Abnormalities

ABNORMALITY	ASSESSMENT FINDINGS
Pharyngitis, B Streptococcal Inflammation of the pharynx caused by streptococci	Same symptoms as pharyngitis, plus: • Increased fever • Dysphagia • Abdominal pain, nausea and/or vomiting • Headache • No upper respiratory symptoms • Increased exudate • "Sandpaper" rash
Tonsillitis Inflammation of the tonsils	Same symptoms as pharyngitis, plus: Exudative tonsils • Tonsils enlarged 2+ to 4+ • Dysphagia
Torus Palatinus A benign exostosis located in the midline of the hard palate	• Midline bony growth projecting outward from the hard palate • Covered with normal mucosa • May have multiple "lobules"

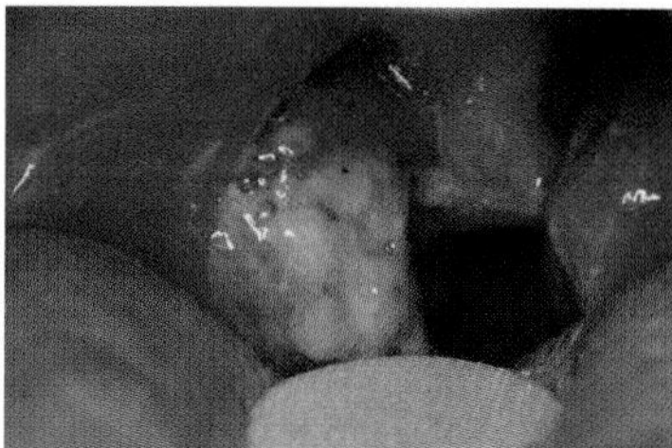

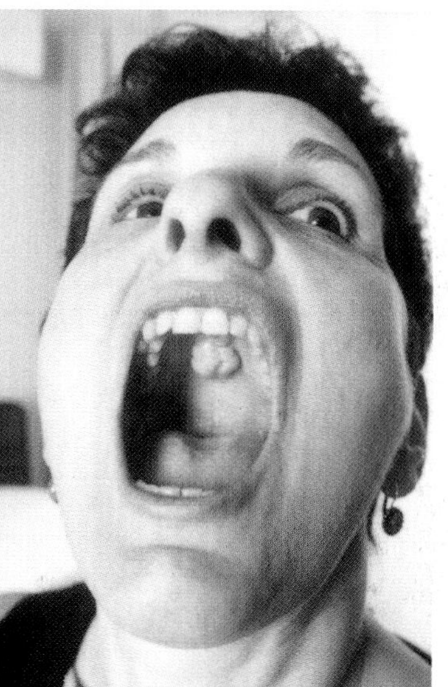

Summary

- Disorders of the head, face, and neck have the potential to exert profound influence over the morbidity and mortality of clients.
- The physical changes associated with these disorders can have devastating effects.
- The structures and function of the head, face, and neck are greatly influenced by changes in other systems.
- It is essential that nurses be skilled in performing examinations of this system and differentiating between normal and abnormal findings.

10

Assessing the Eye and Ear

Before You Begin

INTRODUCTION TO THE EYE AND EAR

The eye and ear are sensory structures that connect us with the environment. They allow us to perceive our surroundings through sight and sound. Disorders of the eye and ear can range from minor annoyances to life-threatening problems. Most problems do not result in acute illness; however, they may be associated with more serious neurological conditions such as brain tumor, stroke, or head injury.

No matter what the cause, visual and hearing problems can have a major impact on physiological functioning as well as psychological and social well-being. Early detection reduces the likelihood of problems related to social interaction.

Determining whether a client has adequate vision and hearing is crucial before assessing mental status or providing instructions. The eyes and ears are common sites of injury; they also exhibit structural variations as a result of age, cultural background, and genetic influences. Although, for the sake of clarity, the eyes and ears are covered separately here, they are usually examined along with the head and neck because of their location.

A thorough assessment of the eyes and ears includes vision and hearing screenings and examination of the external and internal structures. The assessment provides not only specific data about the eyes and ears but also vital information on the health status of other systems.

Before you begin your assessment, an understanding of the anatomy and physiology of the eyes and ears is essential. You need to be able to identify normal structures before you can identify abnormal findings, accurately perform the assessment, and correctly interpret your findings. This chapter covers assessment of the eyes first and then assessment of the ears.

Anatomy and Physiology Review: The Eye

The primary function of the eye is vision, including central and peripheral vision, near and distance vision, and differentiation of colors. To accomplish these tasks, the external and internal structures of the eye work together to receive and transmit images to the occipital lobe of the brain for interpretation. Visual difficulties can result from disease or injury to any of the structures involved in the visual pathway.

Structures and Functions of the Eye

The eye consists of internal and external structures that support or protect it (Figs. 10-1 through 10-5).

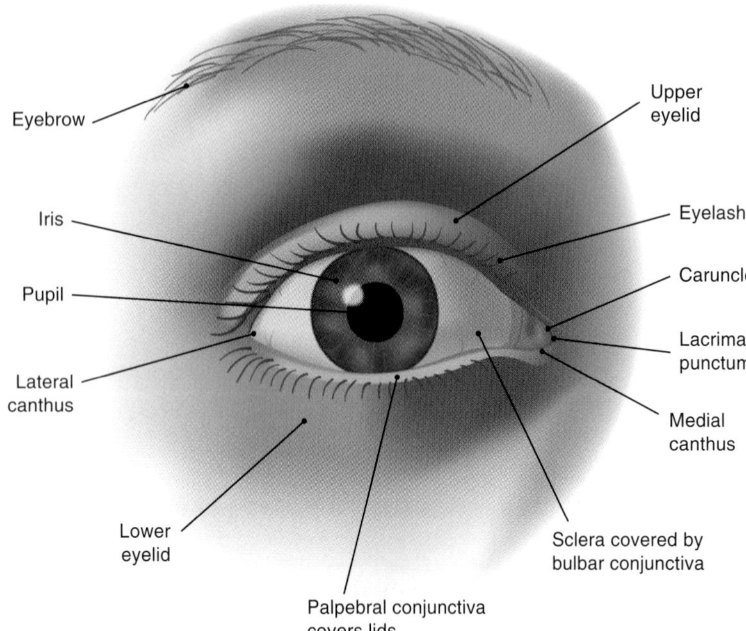

FIGURE 10–1. Frontal view of eye and eyelid.

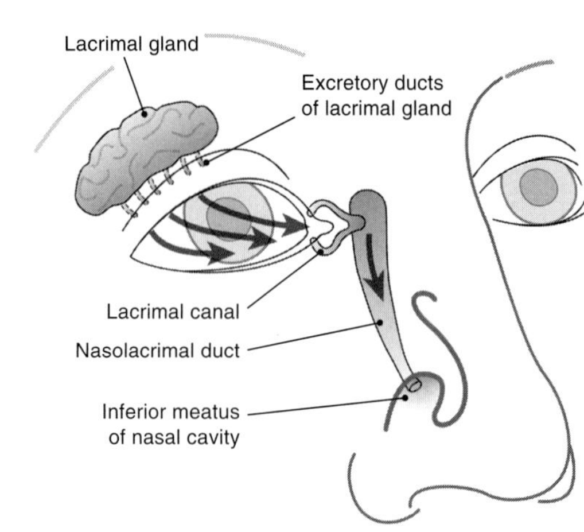

FIGURE 10–2. Lacrimal glands and ducts.

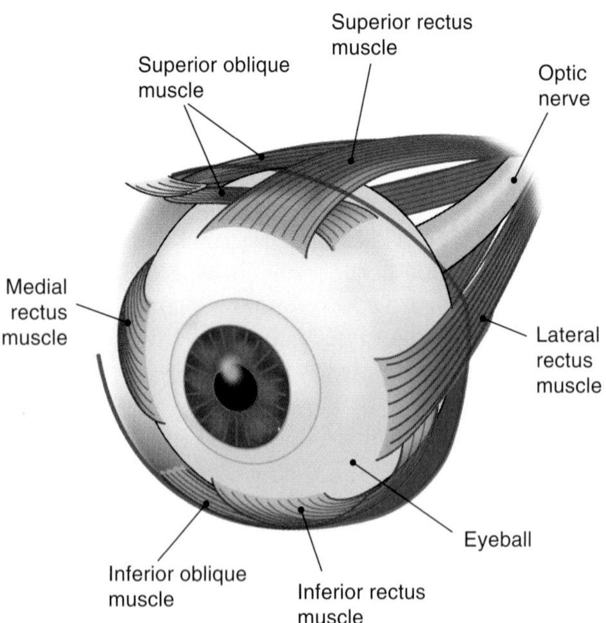

FIGURE 10–3. Eye globe with attachment of extraocular muscles.

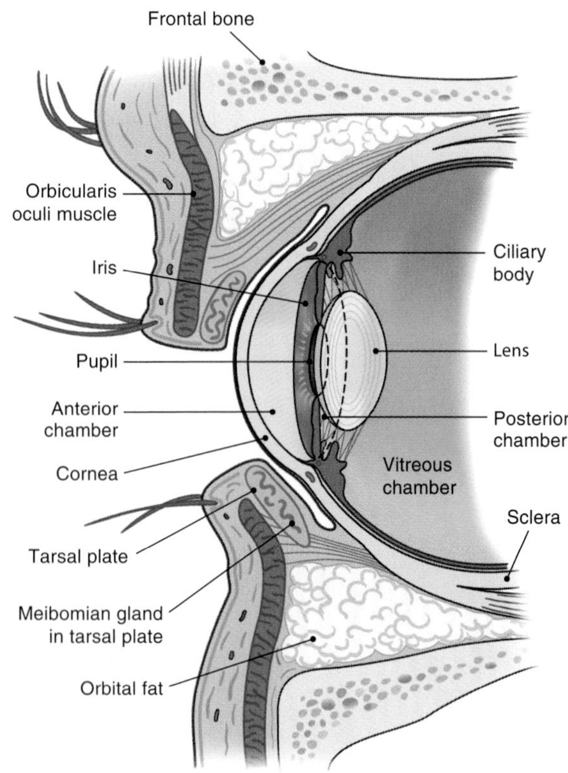

FIGURE 10–4A. Cross section of the eye showing anterior and posterior chambers.

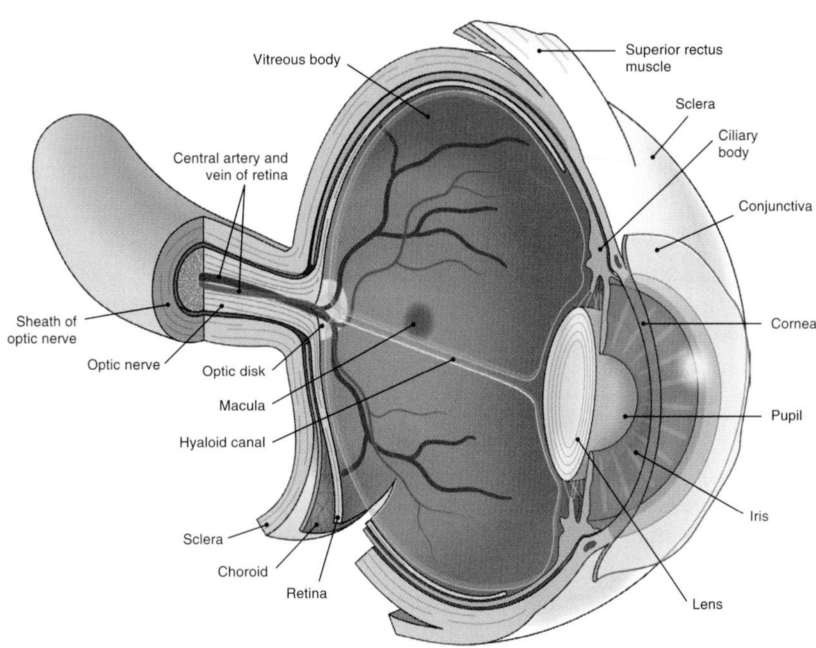

FIGURE 10–4B. Cross section of the eye showing choroid layer.

Structures and Functions of the Eye

STRUCTURE	FUNCTION
Eyelid	Protects eye from injury and distributes lubrication over the eye globe. Lid margins contain meibomian glands, which lubricate the lid margins.
Orbicularis Oculi Muscle	Closes the eyelid. Is innervated by cranial nerve (CN) VII (facial).
Levator Palpebrae	Raises the eyelid. Is innervated by CN III (oculomotor).
Eyelashes	Protect eyes from injury from foreign bodies.
Medial Canthus	Contains the punctum, which drains the lacrimal gland fluids (tears) into the nasolacrimal sac.
Nasolacrimal Sac	Located alongside the nasal bridge. Receives excessive tears from the lacrimal gland and drains them into the inferior meatus in the nose.
Lacrimal Gland	Located in the upper lid just below the orbital rim. Produces tears to moisturize the globe and wash away foreign bodies.
Conjunctiva	A mucous membrane that lines the eyelids (palpebral conjunctiva) and the outermost portion of the globe (bulbar conjunctiva). Contains goblet cells that secrete fluids to lubricate the eyes.
Cornea	The anterior outermost layer of the eyeball, which covers the pupil and iris and extends to the limbus. Contains sensory innervation for pain, thus providing an early warning system for eye injury. Avascular and transparent.
Sclera	Underlies the bulbar conjunctiva and gives the eyeball its white color. A tough avascular layer that gives the eye its structure and shape, which is important for transmission of visual images to the back of the eye for interpretation.
Iris	A circular, muscular tissue that forms the colored part of the eye. The aperture of the iris forms the pupil and controls the amount of light entering the retina.

(Continued)

Structures and Functions of the Eye *(Continued)*

STRUCTURE	FUNCTION
Extraocular Muscles	A set of six muscles, innervated by cranial nerves, that move the eyes in a conjugate (parallel) manner (see figure).Superior rectus: Rolls eyeball upward, innervated by CN III Inferior rectus: Rolls eyeball downward, innervated by CN III Lateral rectus: Rolls eyeball laterally, innervated by CN VI Medial rectus: Rolls eyeball medially, innervated by CN III Superior oblique: Rolls eyeball downward and laterally, innervated by CN IV Inferior oblique: Rolls eyeball upward and laterally, innervated by CN III
Anterior Chamber	The area between the cornea and the iris. Filled with a clear fluid called aqueous humor.
Posterior Chamber	Space between the iris and lens; contains aqueous humor.
Aqueous Humor	Clear fluid produced continuously by the ciliary processes. Circulates between the posterior and anterior chambers and is drained by a collecting vessel called Schlemm's canal. Supplies the lens and cornea with nutrition.
Ciliary Body	A muscle attached around the lens via zonules that change the shape of the lens when constricted. Produces aqueous humor and some vitreous humor.
Schlemm's Canal	Pathway in the sclerocorneal region that provides drainage for aqueous humor. Opening for canal is located in the anterior chamber. Pressure in the eye is regulated by filtration of aqueous humor through Schlemm's canal, where it is recirculated into the blood supply of the conjunctiva.
Lens	A biconvex disc through which light and images pass. Lies behind the pupil and is partly covered by the iris. The shape of the lens flattens when focusing on far objects and returns to its natural convex shape when focusing on near objects (accommodation).
Zonules	Tough fibers that hold the lens in place and facilitate adjustment of the lens shape for seeing near and far objects.
Vitreous Humor	The area behind the lens of the eye. Filled with a clear, jellylike substance called vitreous humor that serves to cushion the retina and maintain the eye's shape and pressure.
Choroid Layer	Highly vascular middle layer of the eye, which is continuous with the posterior wall of the posterior chamber. Provides nourishment for the eye and dissipates heat produced by the light energy that enters the eye.
Retina	The sensory network of the eye located on the inner surface of the posterior chamber. It contains photoreceptors (rods and cones) that transform light and color impulses into electrical impulses and transmit them to the brain.
Optic Disc	Yellow-orange disc where nerves and blood vessels enter and leave the eye. Serves as a reference point for measuring and locating other structures on the retina.
Physiological Cup	Lighter whitish/yellow area of optic disc area located near center of the disc. Diameter of cup is not more than half of the optic disc's diameter.
Macula	An indistinct, darker, avascular area on the retina responsible for night, color, and central vision and motion detection. Located 2 disc diameters temporally from the optic disc.
Fovea Centralis	A slight depression in the center of the macula that appears as a light reflection during ophthalmoscope examination. Contains a high concentration of cones for color and bright light vision.
Arteries	Emerge from the center of the optic disc. Supply retina with oxygen and nutrients. Arteries are about 1/3 smaller than veins, are brighter red, and display a light reflex as a thin streak of light reflecting off each artery.
Veins	Emerge from the center of the optic disc. Remove waste products from retina. Are larger, darker and duller in color than arteries, and show no light reflex.

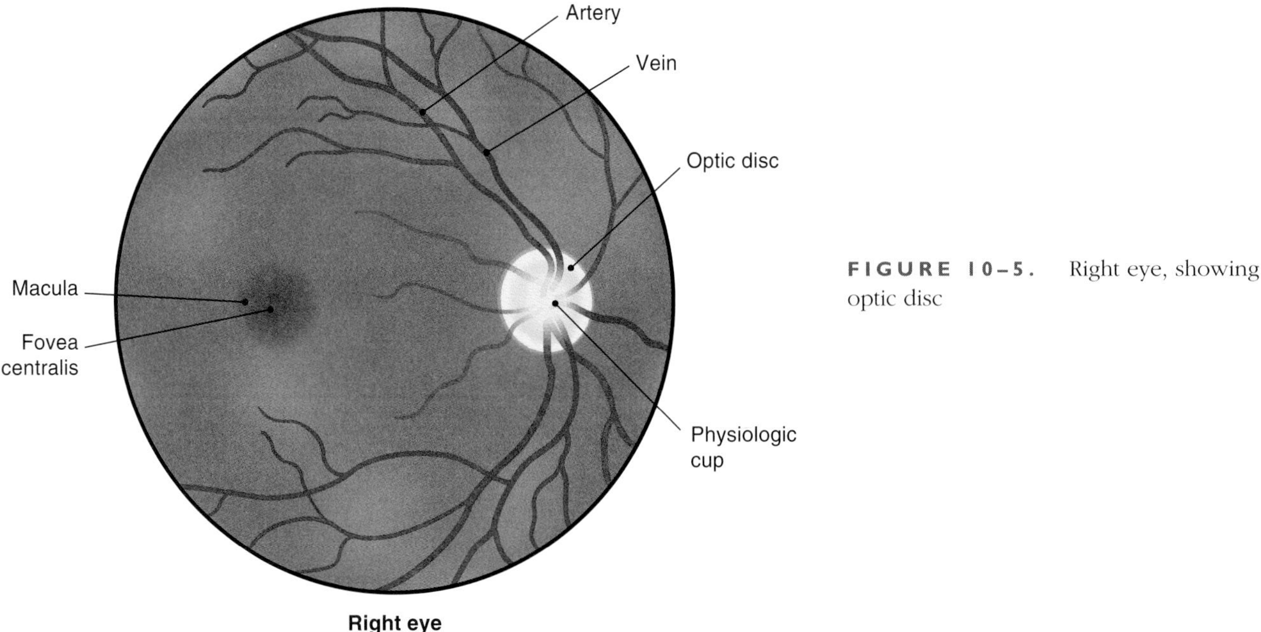

FIGURE 10–5. Right eye, showing optic disc

How We See

The ability to see objects in the environment is dependent on light waves that reflect off images. Natural lighting produces gradations of shading that help to determine an object's shape and position in the environment. The light rays pass through the cornea, anterior chamber, pupil, lens, and posterior chamber to the back of the eye (retina). The pupil, which is actually created by the aperture of a muscular layer of tissue called the iris, dilates or constricts to allow more or less light onto the retina. The lens, an elastic biconvex disc, bends the light waves entering the eye by either flattening or increasing the lens curvature. The precise functioning of the pupil and iris together allows a clear image to focus on the retina.

Several conditions result from variations in how or where the light rays entering the eye converge and focus. People with myopia (nearsightedness) need to hold objects close to the eye to see them clearly. In the myopic eye, the globe is elongated, causing light rays to focus in front of the retina. When the globe is shorter than normal, light rays focus at a point beyond the retina producing a condition called hyperopia (farsightedness). People with hyperopia must move close objects farther away to see them clearly. Astigmatism is an irregular curvature of the lens or cornea that causes light rays to scatter, blurring images on the retina (Fig. 10–6).

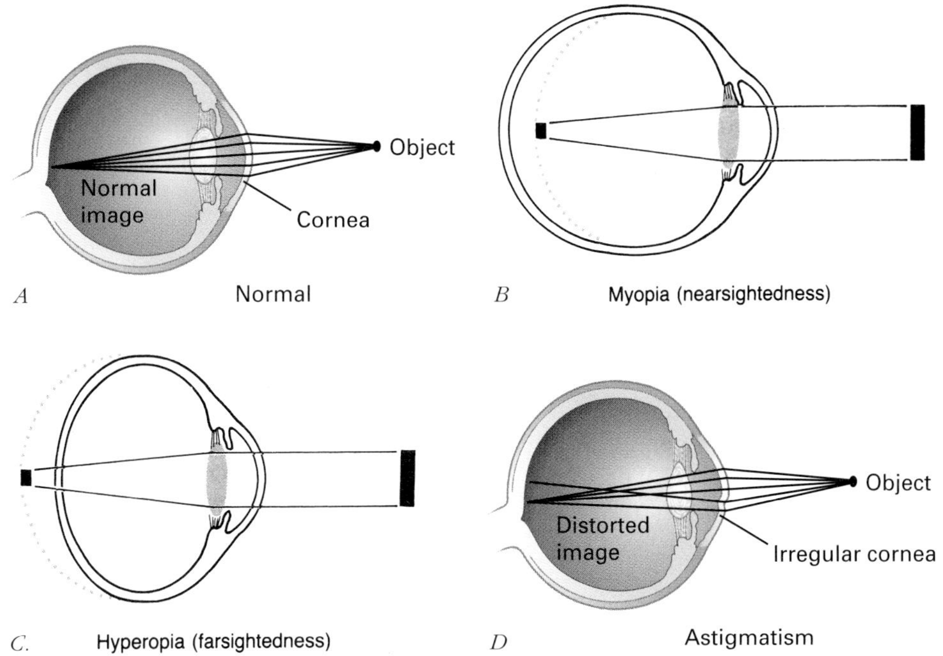

FIGURE 10–6. *A*. Normal eye; *B*. Myopia; *C*. Hyperopia; *D*. Astigmatism. (From Scanlon, V. C., and Sanders, T. (1999). Essentials of Anatomy and Physiology (3rd ed.). Philadelphia: F. A. Davis, with permission).

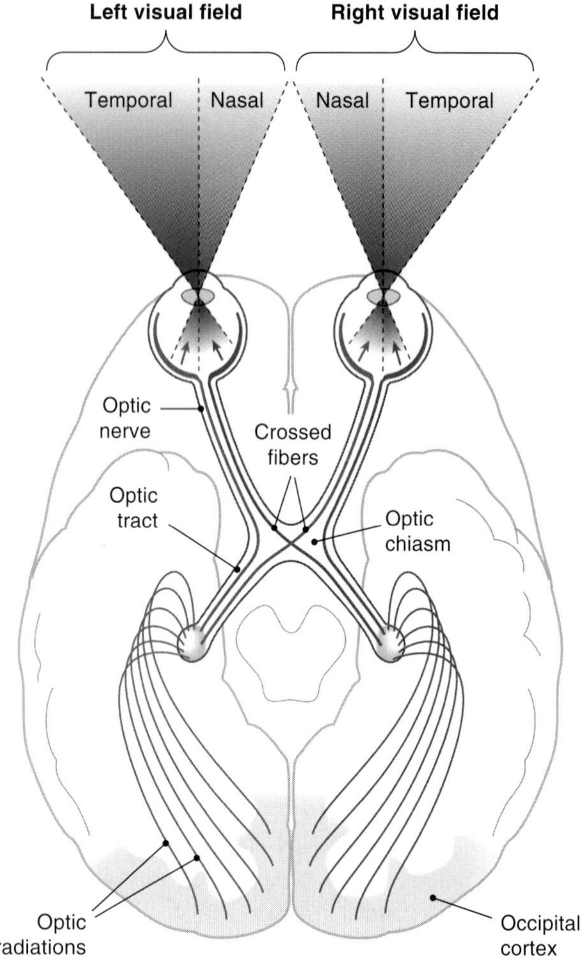

FIGURE 10–7. Optic pathways and visual fields.

The retina is rich in sensory neurons, which are necessary for reception and transmission of accurate images. The retina contains specialized nerve cells called rods, which are sensitive to dim light, and cone cells, which are sensitive to bright light and color. From the rods and cones of the retina, the visual image is transmitted to the optic disc, where the nerve fibers of the retina converge to enter the optic nerve.

Nerve fibers from the optic disc join to form the optic nerve. The neural impulses are then transmitted by the optic nerve to the optic track and optic radiations, where they are interpreted by the visual cortex. Nerve fibers from the nasal portion of each eye cross over to the opposite side of the brain at the optic chiasm. Fibers from the temporal portion of the retina of each eye do not cross over before being received by the visual cortex in the occipital lobe of the brain (Fig. 10–7).

Interaction with Other Body Systems

The functions of the eyes are interconnected with those of the cardiovascular, musculoskeletal, and neurological systems.

The Cardiovascular System

The optic fundus is the only area in the body where blood vessels can be directly observed without using invasive techniques. Use of an ophthalmoscope provides direct visualization of the optic disc, where the vessels that supply the retina emerge. Changes in the optic disc, blood vessels, macula, and general background of the retina can reveal systemic problems with circulation as a result of chronic hypertension (HTN) or diabetes. Or they can reveal localized circulatory problems that occur with glaucoma, increased intracranial pressure, and other neurological problems.

The Musculoskeletal System

Movement of the eyes in a parallel or conjugate manner is made possible by the coordinated movement of the extraocular muscles. Each of the six extraocular muscles is responsible for rotating the eyes in a specific direction and maintaining the eyes' conjugate movement. Each extraocular muscle is innervated by a specific cranial nerve. The superior rectus, inferior rectus, medial rectus, and inferior oblique muscles are innervated by CN III. Damage to CN III can therefore result in limited range of movement in the upward, downward, nasal, and upper diagonal fields of vision. The remaining extraocular muscles, the lateral rectus and superior oblique, provide movement of the eye in the temporal lateral and nasal inferior direction, respectively. Damage to the nerves that innervate the lateral rectus muscle (CN VI) and the superior oblique muscle (CN IV) can result in limited eye movement in the corresponding directions.

Movement of the eyelid is controlled by another set of muscles, the orbicularis oculi and the levator palpebrae. The orbicularis oculi encircles the eyelids and is innervated by CN VII. Damage to the orbicularis oculi muscle or the part of the cranial nerve that innervates it results in inability to close the eyelid completely. The ability to raise or open the eyelid is dependent on an intact CN III, which innervates the levator palpebrae muscle.

Constriction and relaxation of the muscular tissue of the iris and ciliary body allows visual adaptation. In a darkened environment, contraction of the smooth muscle of the iris causes the aperture of the iris or pupil to dilate. As a result, more light enters the retina and night vision is enhanced. In brightly lighted environments, the retina does not need to receive additional light; as a result, the pupil is constricted.

The ciliary body, located posterior to the outer edge of the iris, alters the shape of the lens and allows the eye to adjust to near or far objects, an occurrence referred to as accommodation. Constriction of the ciliary body results in flattening of the normal convex shape of the lens. Flattening of the lens facilitates the eye's ability to focus on objects in the distance. Relaxation of the ciliary body

NEUROLOGICAL

CN II, III, IV and VI are responsible for vision and eye movement.

Changes in pupils can reflect changes in intracranial pressure.

Vision changes can reflect underlying neurological problems such as MS.

ENDOCRINE

Hyperthyroid disease may be seen in the eyes as exophthalmos.

Diabetes can cause visual changes that can be seen on fundoscopic examination.

LYMPHATIC/ HEMATOLOGICAL

Anemia can be seen as a pale conjunctiva.

RESPIRATORY

Pulmonary problems that result in hypoxia can be seen in the conjunctiva.

CARDIOVASCULAR

Xanthelasma (fat deposits) can be seen on the eyelids.

Vascular changes can be seen on fundoscopic examination.

DIGESTIVE

Jaundice from liver disease can be seen in the sclera.

MUSCULOSKELETAL

Eye muscles are needed for movement.

Rheumatoid arthritis can cause iritis and scleritis.

INTEGUMENTARY

Skin covers the lids.

Lashes protect the eyes.

URINARY

Renal disease can result in periorbital edema.

Relationship of the Eyes to Other Systems

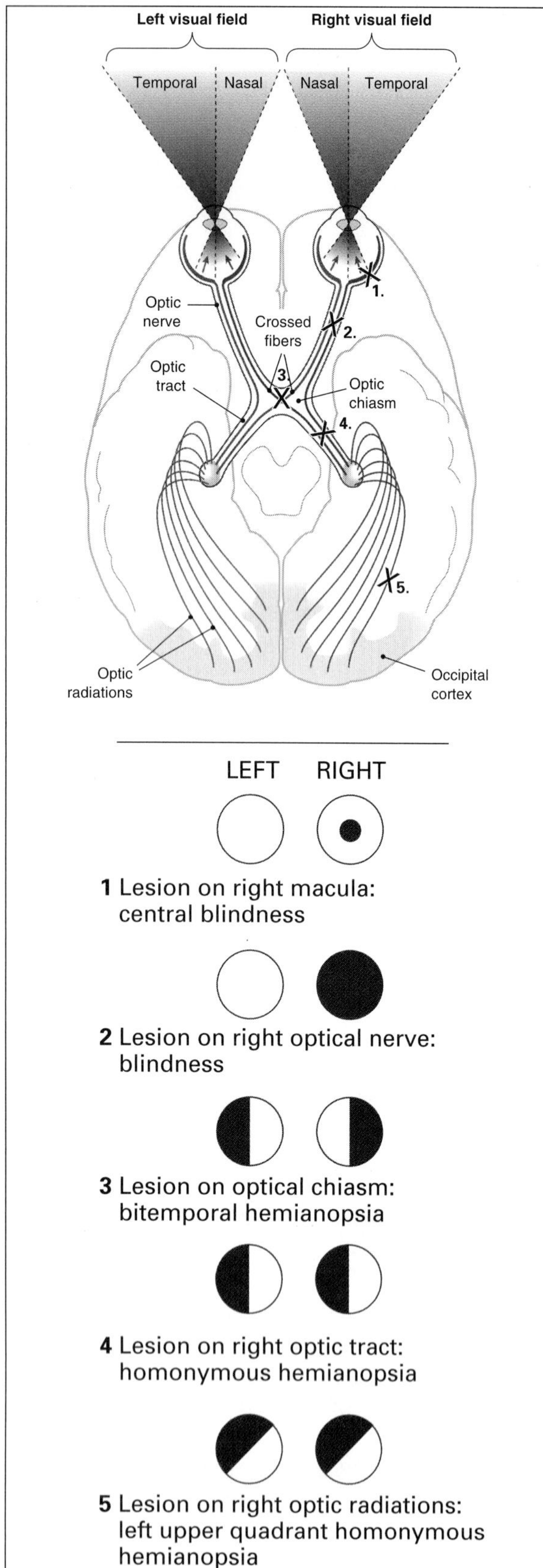

FIGURE 10–8. Optic nerve pathways visual fields and selected associated visual defects.

allows the lens to assume its normal convex shape and facilitates focusing on near objects. Both the iris and ciliary body can be affected by damage to CN III, resulting in pupil dilatation (mydriasis) and loss of accommodation.

The Neurological System

The ability to see images depends on an intact visual pathway. From the time when an image is received on the retina to the time when it is interpreted by the visual cortex, the neurological system plays a key role. Damage to the retina can result in diminished visual acuity or diminished color and night vision. Damage to the optic nerve, a source of retinal nervous tissue, can result in similar visual changes. Damage to specific points along the optic track or to the visual cortex can produce deficits in corresponding visual fields (Fig. 10–8).

The neurological system also innervates the extraocular eye muscles, which control the movement of the eyes, and the muscles of the eyelids, which control the opening and closing of the eyes. The cranial nerves responsible for innervation of each of the six extraocular muscles include CN III (oculomotor), CN IV (trochlear) and CN VI (abducens) (Fig. 10–9). Inability of these muscles to function properly is largely caused by damage to the nerves that innervate the muscles.

Increased intracranial pressure from intracranial tumors, head injuries, or severe intracranial hemorrhage may impinge on CN II (optic), CN III, CN IV, or CN VI, causing specific eye changes. The optic nerve innervates the retina and is surrounded by a meningeal sheath that is continuous with the meninges of the brain. When intracranial pressure increases, the pressure is transmitted from the brain to the optic disc, where swelling occurs. Pressure on a specific part of the optic nerve tract can produce visual loss (hemianopia) on the ipsilateral (same side) or contralateral (opposite side) visual field, depending on the location of the injury or lesion.

Developmental, Cultural, and Ethnic Variations

Infants

Several variations may be noted in the eyes of infants. The shape, slope, spacing, and color of the eyes should be noted. Normal shape is oval. Slope is determined by drawing an imaginary line through the inner canthus to the occiput. Except in people of Asian descent, the slope line transects the outer canthus. Measurement of the distance between various structures of the eye can be plotted on a growth chart. Normal spacing measurements are plotted between the 10th and 90th percentile.

Infants usually open their eyes when held upright, permitting inspection of the iris, pupil, and sclera. The

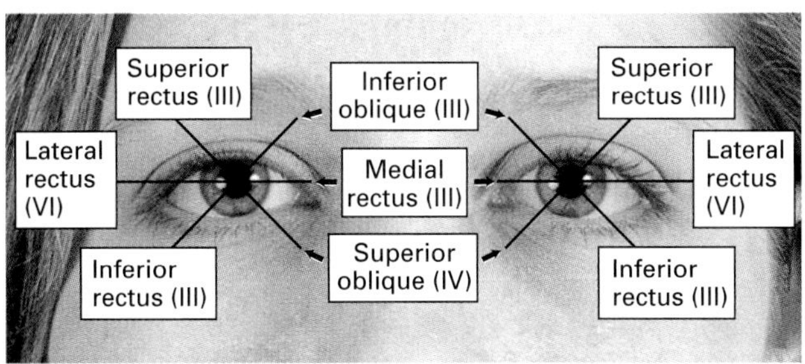

FIGURE 10–9. Cranial nerves and eye muscles.

color of the iris after birth is normally blue-gray in light-skinned infants and brown in darker-skinned infants. Permanent eye color is usually established by 9 months of age. White specks in the iris called Brushfield spots can be a normal variant or a sign of Down syndrome. Edema of the eyelids and irritation of the conjunctiva may be caused by birth trauma or silver nitrate prophylaxis. The sclera is very thin at birth, so it may have a slightly blue undertone.

A gross assessment of visual acuity is made by testing for pupillary light reflexes and also by noting the infant's behavior. The pupils should normally constrict to light. After three weeks, if no pupillary light reflex is present, blindness is indicated. However, the presence of pupillary reaction alone does not confirm an infant's ability to see. A blink reflex in response to bright light and observing the infant for ability to follow objects or light with the eyes confirms that some degree of vision is intact. By 2 to 4 weeks, an infant should be able to fixate on an object, and by 1 month, to fixate and follow an object. An infant's visual acuity is usually about 20/200; 20/20 vision is usually achieved by school age.

During the first 1 to 2 months, infants' eye movements are often disconjugate (not working in unison), making screening for strabismus difficult. Persistence of disconjugate eye movements after this time may indicate strabismus and warrants referral to a specialist. In infants, the fundoscopic examination is difficult but still important. The internal structures of the eye should be examined regularly during the first few years of life. One of the first things to note is the presence of a red reflex, which is a normal finding. Absence of a red reflex may indicate congenital cataracts or retinal detachment. The general background in infants is typically paler than in adults, because the blood vessels to the area are not fully developed. The macula also is not fully developed until about 1 year of age.

Toddlers

Visual acuity in toddlers is determined by the Allen test, which uses picture cards of seven common objects. The child should successfully identify three of the seven objects at a distance of 15 feet. If the child cannot do so, move closer until he or she is able to do so.

The corneal light reflex can provide an initial, rapid screening test for strabismus that can be followed by additional measures as the child grows. Untreated strabismus can lead to permanent visual damage. Eventually, the brain suppresses information from the affected eye, and visual acuity in that eye deteriorates.

Preschool Children

By age 3 to 5, the Snellen E chart, which uses various sizes of E's facing in different directions, can usually be used to determine visual acuity. Normal visual acuity for a 3-year-old is approximately 20/40 or better. By the time the child is 4 years old, visual acuity should be about 20/30 or better.

School-Age Children

By the time a child is about 5 to 6 years old, normal visual acuity approximates that of the adult—20/20 in both eyes. You should continue using the Snellen E chart until the child has acquired reading skills and can easily verbalize the letters seen on the Snellen chart.

Children should be screened for defects in color perception (color blindness) between 4 and 8 years of age. Though many forms of color blindness exist, most cases involve inherited, recessive X-linked traits in males that affect the ability to distinguish red and green.

Older Adults

Many changes in the structure and function of the eye occur with aging. Both central and peripheral visual acuity may be diminished with advanced age. Changes in near vision occur around the fourth and fifth decades, often resulting in decreased ability to focus clearly on near objects (presbyopia). The adult may compensate for these changes by holding near objects farther away.

External structures of the eye also undergo significant changes with advanced age. Tissues of the eyelids lose elasticity and fatty deposits, causing the eyes to appear sunken. The lower eyelid may sag away from the globe. The latter condition, called ectropion, is significant because the punctum, which drains the tears, is no longer in contact with the globe, resulting in constant tearing. The laxity that develops in the eyelids may also lead to an inward turning of the eyelids, referred to as entropion. With entropion, the punctum also may not be able to drain tears. In addition, the eyelashes may rub the conjunctiva and cornea, causing pain and injury to the cornea. Older adults also may experience dry eyes because of a decrease in tear production.

Changes in the internal structures of the eye are also common with aging. The lens becomes more opaque and yellowish, obscuring the transfer of light rays to the retina. This clouding of the lens is referred to as senile cataract. Arcus senilis, a white opaque ring around the edge of the cornea resulting from fat deposits, is a common benign finding. The older adult's pupil size at rest is generally smaller than that of younger adults. Pupillary reaction to light and accommodation slows because of decreased ability to constrict and relax. The general background is paler, and the blood vessels of the eye may show signs of the same atherosclerotic processes that are occurring elsewhere throughout the body. Visual fields may be less than normal. Other visual changes that occur with aging reflect degeneration of the rods and cones. Color vision may be less vivid as a result of degeneration of the cones, and night vision may be impaired because of degeneration of the rods.

Several eye diseases also occur more commonly in older adults. Macular degeneration and glaucoma, the two leading causes of blindness in older adults, show a significant increase with aging.

People of Different Cultures and Ethnic Groups

Differences in physical characteristics of the eye and differences in the risk of certain eye diseases are found in various ethnic groups. People of Asian origin typically have an epicanthal fold at the medial canthus, giving the eyes an almond-shaped appearance. The outer canthus also may slant in an upward direction. In blacks and others with normally dark skin, brown pigmented spots on the sclera, referred to as muddy sclera, are common. In dark-skinned people, the color of the optic disc is also typically darker orange, and the retinal background is darker red than in fair-skinned people. A black person's sclera also may have a blue-gray appearance or a yellowish cast at the peripheral margins.

The incidence and severity of glaucoma is greater in blacks than in people of other races. Cataracts also occur with greater frequency in people living in sunny climates.

Introducing the Case Study

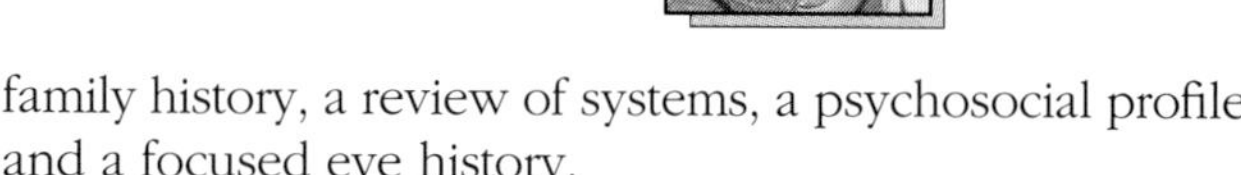

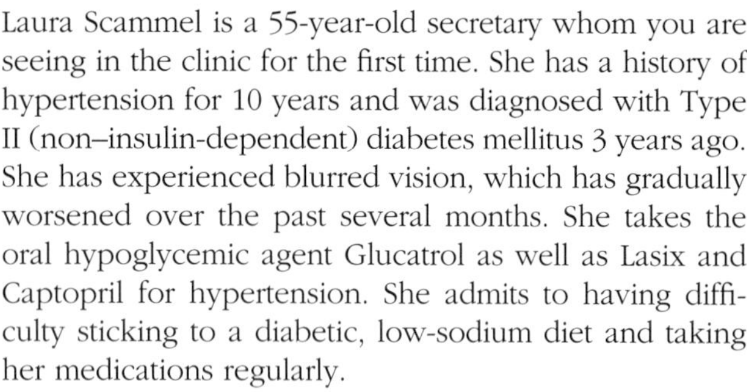

Laura Scammel is a 55-year-old secretary whom you are seeing in the clinic for the first time. She has a history of hypertension for 10 years and was diagnosed with Type II (non–insulin-dependent) diabetes mellitus 3 years ago. She has experienced blurred vision, which has gradually worsened over the past several months. She takes the oral hypoglycemic agent Glucatrol as well as Lasix and Captopril for hypertension. She admits to having difficulty sticking to a diabetic, low-sodium diet and taking her medications regularly.

Performing the Eye Assessment

Assessment of the eye includes taking a thorough health history and performing a physical examination. Data obtained are combined and analyzed to determine the client's existing health status and to identify potential health risks and disorders of the eye.

Health History

The health history addresses the client's personal and family history of eye diseases and diseases that affect the eye. A comprehensive health history also allows the nurse to identify areas of the physical examination that require more or less depth. The health history will include biographical data, current health status, past health history, family history, a review of systems, a psychosocial profile and a focused eye history.

Biographical Data

First, review the client's medical records, intake surveys, and other sources of data to identify his or her age, occupation, gender, and ethnic background. This information will help you decide what questions to ask and to interpret subsequent history and examination findings. For example, the way you measure visual acuity and interpret the findings differs greatly with the client's age. The client's occupation can be a source of environmental risk for eye injury. Gender may be a factor in certain disorders such as color blindness, which is more common in males. Knowledge of the client's race or ethnic group is useful when interpreting many physical examination findings.

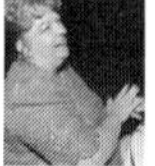

Case Study Findings

Reviewing Mrs. Scammel's biographical data:

- 55-year-old Caucasian widow and mother of one child, age 30.
- Works full-time as a secretary at a large law firm.
- Has major medical insurance coverage through her employer. Does not have coverage for dental or vision examinations.
- Catholic religion, of Irish/Italian descent.

CRITICAL THINKING ACTIVITY #1

Considering Mrs. Scammel's age, what eye changes might you expect to see?

Current Health Status

Begin by asking about the person's chief complaint, asking him or her to describe the problem in his or her own words. Use the PQRST format to probe further about any symptoms reported. If the person has an eye problem, focus your questions on the eye symptoms prioritized below.

Symptom Analysis

Symptom Analysis tables for all of the symptoms described in the following paragraphs are available on the Web for viewing and printing. In your Web browser, go to *http://www.fadavis.com/detail.cfm?id=0882-9* and click on Symptom Analysis Tables under Explore This Product.

Vision Loss

Vision loss refers to the inability to see the shape, size, position, or color of objects. Vision loss may be complete, resulting in the inability to perceive light from dark, or incomplete, causing the person to see objects with varying degrees of detail.

ALERT

Acute primary angle closure (closed) glaucoma is a medical emergency.

Eye Pain

Eye pain is a subjective sensation of discomfort in the eye that may be caused by trauma, irritation, infection, or neurological conditions.

Double Vision

Double vision (diplopia) refers to seeing two overlapping images because of the inability of the eyes to focus on an object and move in a conjugate manner. Double vision can be caused by a variety of conditions, including diseases of the cerebellum, cranial nerves, and extraocular muscles.

Eye Tearing

Tears are normally produced by the lacrimal gland, located along the upper outer orbit of the eye, and are distributed over the eye by blinking. Tearing is a discharge of clear, watery fluid as a result of the inability of the tears to drain through the punctum and into the nasolacrimal duct. Tearing occurs in a variety of conditions such as infections; irritation; and exposure to chemicals, irritants, or allergens.

Dry Eyes

Dry eyes occur when there is insufficient lubrication of the eye and the bulbar and palpebral conjunctiva become less moist. It often results in a subjective sensation of irritation, a gritty sensation or discomfort, especially during blinking. Dryness occurs from trauma to the eye surface or facial trigeminal nerve paralysis, in certain systemic diseases, or after taking certain medications.

Eye Drainage

Drainage from the eyes is abnormal and is commonly associated with eye infections or allergies.

Eye Appearance Changes

Changes in the appearance of the external eye, such as in the iris, anterior chamber, and sclera, can signal a variety of problems, including trauma, infection, and systemic disorders.

Blurred Vision

Blurred vision refers to an object's shape and detail being indistinct and fuzzy. It can occur for near objects as well as distant ones.

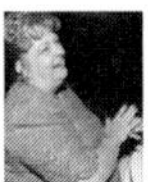

Case Study Findings

Mrs. Scammel's current health status includes:

- Complains of blurred vision that has increased over the past month. Blurred vision is constant and worsened by fatigue. States that nothing seems to cause the problem or has helped relieve it. Wonders if she needs new glasses.
- Typically works at a computer for at least 4 hours each day.
- Blurred vision has not prevented her from caring for herself at home; however, it is difficult to read the material she is typing on the computer screen, even with reading glasses.
- Denies tearing, eye pain, drainage, double vision, sensitivity to light, or changes in the appearance of the eyes. Currently takes Lasix 20 mg bid, Captopril 25 mg bid, Glucatrol 5 mg bid, and 400 to 600 mg of ibuprofen as needed for joint pain nearly every day.

Past Health History

This section of the health history focuses on gathering relevant information about the client's past eye health and any injuries, diseases, or medications that could affect the eyes. The following are specific areas that should be explored related to the eye.

Past Health History

RISK FACTORS/QUESTIONS TO ASK	RATIONALE/SIGNIFICANCE
Childhood Illnesses	
Were you ever diagnosed with strabismus?	Uncorrected strabismus results in disuse of affected eye and eventual blindness in that eye.
Surgeries/Serious Injuries/ Hospitalizations	
Have you had surgery for strabismus, cataracts, or vision correction? Have you had corneal abrasions or chemical burns?	May explain physical findings such as scarring.
Serious/Chronic Illnesses	
Do you have a history of hypertension, diabetes, hyperthyroidism, or multiple sclerosis?	May explain physical findings. Vascular changes associated with HTN and diabetes can be seen on fundoscopic examination. Exophthalmos is seen with hyperthyroidism (Graves' disease). Visual changes associated with multiple sclerosis (MS) include temporary vision loss, patchy blindness (scotomas), diplopia, blurred vision, nystagmus, and optic disc atrophy.
Immunizations	
Are your immunizations up to date?	Communicable diseases such as varicella can affect eyelids and conjunctiva.
Allergies	
Do you have any allergies? If so, what are you allergic to and how do you react?	May explain physical findings.
Medications	
Are you taking any medications, including prescription drugs and over-the-counter or herbal supplements? If so, what is the dosage? How often do you take them? How long have you been using these medications? When was your last dose?	Determines medications used to treat eye disorders and those that have secondary effects on the eyes. Mydriatic and cycloplegic medications, used for eye examinations and treatment of uveitis and keratitis, dilate the pupil and prevent accommodation, respectively. See box, Drugs That Adversely Affect the eyes on page 257. Miotics to constrict the pupil are used to treat glaucoma. Drug interactions with secondary effects on the eye include pupillary constriction from narcotics and pupil dilatation from marijuana and atropine.
Recent Travel/Military Service	
Have you been exposed to sun or infectious/contagious diseases through recent travel? Or been exposed to irritants, chemicals or projectiles in military service?	Sun (ultraviolet) exposure is associated with cataracts. May explain examination findings or identify health promotion or teaching needs.

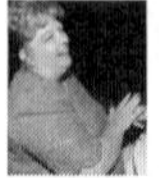

Case Study Findings

Mrs. Scammel's past health history reveals:

- History of hypertension for past 10 years and poorly controlled adult-onset diabetes diagnosed 3 years ago.
- Denies trauma or surgery affecting the eyes or hospitalizations except for childbirth. One child, no abortions.
- Denies allergies to foods, drugs, or environment.
- Last physical examination 10 months ago; last eye examination 5 years ago. Mammogram and Pap smear negative.

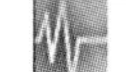

CRITICAL THINKING ACTIVITY #2

What part of the assessment would reveal the effects of hypertension and diabetes mellitus on Mrs. Scammel's vision?

Family History

When gathering information on your client's family history, consider familial conditions that may affect the eyes.

Drugs That Adversely Affect the Eyes

Drug Class	Drug	Possible Adverse Reactions
Aminoglycosides	All aminoglycosides	Optic neuritis with blurred vision, **scotomas**, enlargement of the blind spot
Antiarrhythmics	Quinidine sulfate	Blurred vision, color perception disturbances, night blindness, mydriasis, **photophobia**, diplopia, reduced visual fields, scotomas, optic neuritis
	Flecainide acetate	Blurred vision, difficulty focusing, spots before eyes, diplopia, photophobia, **nystagmus**
Anticholinergic agents	All types	Blurred vision, **cycloplegia**, **mydriasis**, photophobia
Anti-infectives	Chloramphenicol	Optic neuritis, decreased visual acuity
	Norfloxacin	Visual disturbances
	Sulfisoxazole	Periorbital edema, conjunctival and scleral injection
Antineoplastics	Cisplatin	Optic neuritis, **papilledema**, cerebral blindness
	Methotrexate	Conjunctivitis
	Tamoxifen	Retinopathy, corneal opacities, decreased visual acuity
Antitubercular agents	Isoniazid, pyrazinamide, ethambutol	Optic neuritis, decreased visual acuity, loss of red-green color perception, central and peripheral scotomas (ethambutol only)
Cardiotonic glycosides	Digitalis leaf, digoxin, digitalis	Altered color vision, photophobia, diplopia, halos or borders on objects
Diuretics	Amiloride	Visual disturbances
	Hydrochlorothiazide	Altered color vision, transient blurred vision
Genitourinary smooth muscle relaxants	Flavoxate	Blurred vision, disturbed accommodation
	Oxybutynin	Transient blurred vision, cycloplegia, mydriasis
Glucocorticoids	Prednisone and others	**Exophthalmos**, increased intraocular pressure, cataracts, increased susceptibility to secondary fungal and viral eye infections
Antipsychotics	All phenothiazines	Abnormal corneal lens pigmentation
	Chlorpromazine	Cataracts, retinopathy, visual impairment
	Quetiapine	Lens changes
Miscellaneous agents	Carbamazepine	Blurred vision, transient diplopia, visual hallucinations
	Oral contraceptives (estrogen with progesterone)	Worsening of myopia or astigmatism, intolerance to contact lenses, neuro-ocular lesions
	Iotretinoin	Conjunctivitis, dry eyes, corneal opacities, eye irritation
	Loxapine	Blurred vision, pigmentary changes
	Metrizamide	Diplopia, amblyopia, photophobia, eye flickering, blurred vision
	Pentazocine hydrochloride	Blurred vision, focusing difficulty, nystagmus, diplopia, **miosis** Photophobia, calcific conjunctivitis (with vitamin D intoxication)

Family History

RISK FACTORS/QUESTIONS TO ASK	RATIONALE/SIGNIFICANCE
Familial/Genetic Eye Disorders	
Does anyone in your family have vision problems such as blindness, cataracts, glaucoma, or color blindness?	Person with family history of these problems has greater risk of developing them. Color blindness is an X-linked recessive disorder.
Familial/Genetic Disorders That Affect Eyes	
Does anyone in your family have a history of hypertension, diabetes, or MS?	Person with family history of these problems has a greater risk of developing them.

Review of Systems

AREA/SYSTEM QUESTIONS TO ASK	RATIONALE/SIGNIFICANCE
General Health Survey	
How have you been feeling? How would you describe your general health?	Changes in usual state of health may reflect underlying problems that can affect the eyes.
Integumentary	
Do you have any rashes or lesions?	Rashes or lesions may be associated with irritation, infection, or allergies that cause eye irritation. May explain physical findings or source of symptoms.
HEENT	
Do you have a history of headaches or migraines?	May be associated with disorders of visual acuity. Visual aura often precedes migraines.
Do you have a history of head trauma?	Visual changes are early sign of increased intracranial pressure.
Do you have watery eyes or runny nose?	Associated with environmental allergies or upper respiratory infections.
Respiratory	
Do you have a history of COPD or other respiratory problems?	Cyanosis can be seen in the conjunctiva.
Cardiovascular	
Do you have a history of cardiac problems, such as hypertension or stroke?	May be responsible for changes in the blood vessels of the eye and the retinal background. Linked to deficits in visual fields or damage to the optic track.
Gastrointestinal	
Do you have a history of liver disease?	Jaundice may be seen as icteric sclera.
Genitourinary	
Do you have a history of kidney disease?	Periorbital edema may be seen with renal disease.
Reproductive	
Do you have a history of sexually transmitted diseases (STDs), discharge, or lesions?	Cross-contamination may transmit infections to eyes. Newborns may be exposed to STDs during delivery through the birth canal.
Musculoskeletal	
Do you have joint pain, joint deformity, or rheumatoid arthritis?	**Episcleritis** and **keratoconjunctivitis** are associated with rheumatoid arthritis.
Neurological	
Do you have MS, myasthenia gravis, trigeminal neuralgia or Bell's palsy?	MS may produce visual disturbances such as partial blindness, diplopia, or nystagmus as a result of demyelinization of nerve fibers. Myasthenia gravis may cause ptosis. Trigeminal neuralgia may cause orbital pain. Bell's palsy may cause orbital dryness and risk of injury caused by inability to blink.
Endocrine	
Do you have hyperthyroidism?	Results in exophthalmos and may be associated with visual acuity changes and diplopia.
Do you have diabetes mellitus?	Damages the eye vessels, resulting in retinal hemorrhages, exudate, and changes in visual acuity.
Lymphatic	
Do you have a history of HIV/AIDS, recent immunotherapy, or chemotherapy?	Toxoplasma and cytomegalovirus infection of the retina occur frequently in immunosuppressed clients.

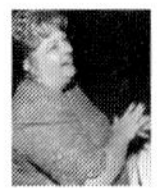

Case Study Findings

Mrs. Scammel's family history reveals:

- One child, age 30, alive and well.
- One brother, deceased 2 years ago at age 50 from a myocardial infarction.
- Father deceased, history of colon cancer and died of heart attack at age 56.
- Mother, age 78, lives in nursing home and has history of NIDDM, multiple sclerosis, and stroke 4 years ago.
- No family history of glaucoma or vision loss.

Review of Systems

Changes in the structure and function of the eye may relate to every other system of the body. The review of systems (ROS) will help you identify problems in other systems that directly affect the eye and allow you to pick up on symptoms that you might have missed in your health history by triggering your client's memory.

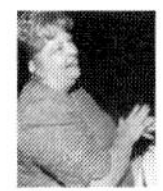

Case Study Findings

Mrs. Scammel's review of systems includes:

- **General Health Survey:** States that she is usually in good health.
- **Integumentary:** No skin lesions or allergies.
- **HEENT:** No eye tearing or drainage. No history of headache or head injury. No symptoms of upper respiratory infection.
- **Respiratory:** No history of respiratory disease.
- **Cardiovascular:** No history of cardiac symptoms; positive history of hypertension.
- **Gastrointestinal:** No history of liver or renal disease.
- **Musculoskeletal:** No joint pain or deformity or rheumatoid arthritis.
- **Neurological:** No muscle weakness, paresthesia, MS, or myasthenia gravis
- **Endocrine:** Positive history Type II diabetes; no history of thyroid disease.
- **Lymphatic:** No history of HIV, chemotherapy, or immunotherapy.

Psychosocial Profile

The psychosocial profile may reveal patterns in the client's lifestyle that affect health, increase the risk of health problems, or influence adaptation to health problems. Obtaining a psychosocial profile includes asking the client about activities of daily living, personal habits, relationships, roles, coping, and home and work environment.

Psychosocial Profile

CATEGORY/QUESTIONS TO ASK	RATIONALE/SIGNIFICANCE
Health Practices and Beliefs/Self-Care Activities	
How often do you have your eyes examined? When was your last exam? If you wear contact lenses, what special eye care practices do you follow? Do you wear eye makeup?	Identifies risk factors and teaching needs of client. Adults with normal vision shouldhave eye exam every 2 years and begin screening for glaucoma at age 40. Eye makeup can be a source of eye irritation or infection. It should be changed every 6 months.
Typical Day	
What activities do you engage in regularly? Has your ability to engage in these activities changed recently because of your eye problem?	Helps identify activities that pose a danger to the client's health or safety. Or may clarify progression of the condition.
Nutritional Patterns	
What did you eat in the past 24 hours? Does your diet include sources of vitamin A (leafy green vegetables, yellow fruits and vegetables, liver, milk, cheeses, and egg yolks)?	Vitamin A deficiency can result in night blindness and keratomalacia. Vitamin A excess can result in exophthalmos.
Activity and Exercise Patterns	
Does your eye problem limit your ability to exercise or perform the usual activities?	People with diminished visual acuity may be unable to exercise as usual and may be at increased risk for injury from falls or other trauma.

(Continued)

Psychosocial Profile *(Continued)*

CATEGORY/QUESTIONS TO ASK	RATIONALE/SIGNIFICANCE
Recreation/Pets/Hobbies	
Does your eye condition affect your ability to read, watch television, use equipment such as computers, or engage in other hobbies?	Difficulty engaging in hobbies may affect the client's sense of well-being and satisfaction.
Sleep/Rest Patterns	
Has your eye condition affected the amount of uninterrupted sleep you get?	Pain may cause interrupted sleep and increased fatigue.
Personal Habits	
Do you use street drugs?	Marijuana causes pupil dilation. Crack cocaine, heroine and opioids cause pupil constriction.
Occupational Health Patterns	
Does your occupation expose your eyes to irritants, chemicals, or the sun? Do you work at a computer?	Awareness of occupational hazards helps identify the client's health risk factors and teaching needs such as wearing protective goggles. Long hours at computer monitors can result in eyestrain.
Environmental Health Patterns	
Are you exposed to chemicals, light, heat, or projectile objects?	Greater risk of injury to the eye. May indicate health teaching needs related to ultraviolet protection and protective goggles.
Are you around environmental irritants, pollutants, tobacco smoke, or allergens?	May cause eye irritation, producing tearing and redness of the conjunctiva.
Family Roles and Relationships	
Has your eye condition affected your ability to interact with others or to assume your usual roles (parent, employee, student, and so forth)?	Eye problems may result in a loss of self-esteem if the client is no longer achieving satisfaction in roles.
Cultural Influences	
Do you have any cultural influences that affect your healthcare practices?	It is important to identify cultural influences that may affect your client's healthcare practices.
Religious Influences	
Do you have any religious practices /beliefs that influence your healthcare practices?	It is important to identify religious practices/beliefs that may affect healthcare practices.
Social Supports	
If you are visually impaired, does it curtail your social activities?	Visual changes or losses may cause client to withdraw from social activities and become isolated.
Stress and Coping	
If you are visually impaired, how are you dealing with it?	Need to identify client's ability to deal with vision changes .

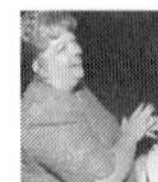

Case Study Findings

Mrs. Scammel's psychosocial profile includes:

- Last physical 10 months ago; last eye exam 5 years ago. Gets yearly mammograms and Pap tests.
- Typical day includes: Rises at 6:30 AM, showers and dresses, has breakfast (bagel and coffee), leaves for work at 8 AM. Works 8:30 AM to 5 PM Monday through Friday. Eats lunch (sandwich) at diner most days. Usually returns home by 6 PM unless she runs errands or shops for groceries. Rarely cooks a full dinner unless her son visits. Watches TV or reads after dinner. Goes to bed at 11 PM. Spends weekends gardening in warm weather, visiting mother in nursing home, visiting son, running errands, doing housework. Goes to movies with friends occasionally.

- Admits difficulty following prescribed diabetic and low-sodium diets. Tries to eat regularly but has a limited appetite and finds it difficult to cook balanced meals for one person.
- Main source of exercise is gardening and yard work.
- Since loss of her husband, has tried to become more involved in her favorite hobbies: reading, watching TV, and gardening.
- Generally sleeps 8 hours a day without napping.
- Drinks socially 3 to 4 times a year. Smoked 1 pack of cigarettes a day since age 18 until 10 years ago when diagnosed with high blood pressure.
- Was a full-time homemaker during her 22-year-marriage, but returned to workforce after husband died of a heart attack 2 years ago. Now works full-time as a secretary, with occasional overtime. Reports using computers for an average of 4 hours a day.
- Lives in a rural community just outside of town, in her own home. Commutes 30 minutes to and from work.
- Sees son once a week (lives in a neighboring town). Visits mother in nursing home once a week.
- Is Catholic, but is not currently active in church. Denies any specific ethnic or cultural practices.
- Main social supports are friends from neighborhood and son and daughter-in-law.
- Stress and coping mechanisms include gardening and talking over problems with son and longtime friends from neighborhood.

Focused Eye History

If the severity or acuity of the person's condition prohibits obtaining a detailed eye history, take a focused eye history. The person's responses will allow you to obtain the most relevant and crucial information. Follow up any key symptoms with additional questioning, using the PQRST format. Ask these questions:

- Have you noticed any changes in your vision?
- Do you wear glasses or contact lenses?
- Have you ever had an eye injury?
- Have you ever had eye surgery?
- Have you ever had blurred vision?
- Have you ever seen spots or floaters, flashes of light, or halos around lights?
- Do you have a history of frequent or recurring eye infections, styes, tearing or dryness?
- When was your last eye examination?
- Do you have a history of diabetes or high blood pressure?
- What medications are you currently taking?
- Do you use any prescription or over-the-counter eye drops?

Case Study Evaluation

Before you move on to the physical examination, review and summarize the key information from Mrs. Scammel's health history and document the eye history related to Mrs. Scammel.

CRITICAL THINKING ACTIVITY #3

Considering Mrs. Scammel's health history, how might her visual problem affect her?

CRITICAL THINKING ACTIVITY #4

What special needs might Mrs. Scammel have because of the problems with her eyes?

CRITICAL THINKING ACTIVITY #5

What strengths does Mrs. Scammel possess that will help her cope with and manage her health problems?

CRITICAL THINKING ACTIVITY #6

What factors from her health history might affect her eyes?

Anatomical Landmarks

Before beginning your physical assessment of the eye, review the anatomical landmarks of the external eye (Fig. 10–10).

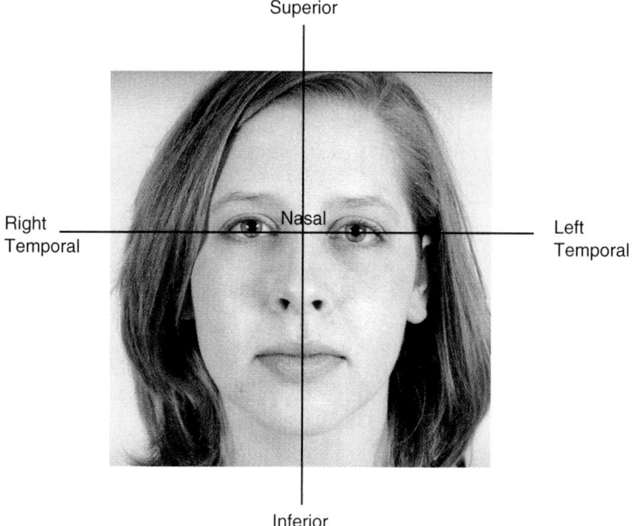

FIGURE 10–10. Front view of eyes with fields.

Physical Assessment

During the physical examination, you will assess the functions and structures of the body, including a focused examination of the eye. You will use the information obtained in the health history to guide you and help determine what body structures and functions should be focused upon. After you have explored the client's key health history information and determined what aspects should be explored, begin the physical examination. The purpose of the physical examination is to identify normal, age-appropriate structures and functions of the eye as well as potential and actual health problems.

Approach

To assess the eye, use the techniques of inspection and palpation. Begin by testing visual acuity and performing other assessments that can be completed while you stand at a distance from the client. For visual acuity, test and record the findings for each eye separately and then together. Standard abbreviations for recording findings are OD for the right eye, OS for the left eye, and OU for both eyes.

HELPFUL HINTS

- Perform the ophthalmic examination last to avoid eye fatigue and tearing, which would interfere with assessment of visual acuity, eye movements and inspection of the external eye.
- To guard against having the client memorize the eye chart, keep it out of visual range until ready to use. Test each eye separately, having the client cover one eye and then the other. Then test both eyes together. If the client wears glasses or contact lenses, test visual acuity first without corrective lenses, then with corrective lenses.

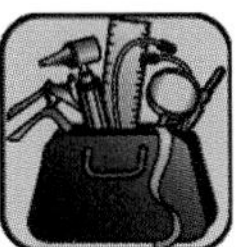

Toolbox

To perform the physical assessment, you'll need the following tools: visual acuity charts (Snellen and Snellen E chart, Allen cards, Jaeger chart), color vision chart (Ishihara's cards), ophthalmoscope, penlight, cotton swab, and cotton ball.

Performing a General Survey

Before performing the eye assessment, perform a general survey, noting the client's overall appearance. Observe nutritional status, emotional status, and body habitus, noting changes that would relate to the eyes. Then inspect for use of corrective lenses; noticeable visual deficits; and gross eye abnormalities such as ptosis, exophthalmos, edema, and redness.

Also take vital signs. A temperature elevation may indicate an infection and give the eyes a glazed appearance. High blood pressure should alert you to look for vascular changes when performing the fundoscopic examination.

Performing a Head-to-Toe Physical Assessment

Now examine the client for more specific signs of diseases affecting other organ systems that might have an impact on the eyes and vision.

Performing a Head-to-Toe Physical Assessment

SYSTEM/NORMAL FINDINGS	ABNORMAL FINDINGS/RATIONALE
General Health Survey *INSPECT* Awake, alert, and oriented to time, place and person	*Changes in mental status:* Head injury or conditions that cause an increase in intracranial pressure. *Changes in eyes (e.g., in pupils):* Early sign of increased intracranial pressure (ICP).
Integumentary *INSPECT* Eyelids and eyelashes intact	*Xanthelasma, chalazion, and other skin lesions:* Eyelids are covered by skin, so they are vulnerable to various skin lesions.

Performing a Head-to-Toe Physical Assessment

SYSTEM/NORMAL FINDINGS	ABNORMAL FINDINGS/RATIONALE
General Health Survey	
HEENT/*Head* *INSPECT/PALPATE* Head symmetrical, nontender	*Changes in pupil reaction and papilledema:* Head trauma, which can result in increased ICP and is readily detected in the eye.
HEENT/*Ear/Nose/Throat* No drainage from ears or nose, mucous membranes pink and intact.	*Watery* eyes: Upper respiratory infection or ear infection.
HEENT/*Neck* No neck masses	*Exophthalmos and eyelid lag:* Hyperthyroid disease.
Respiratory Lungs clear	*Pale, cyanotic conjunctiva:* Hypoxia associated with respiratory disease.
Cardiovascular Regular heart rate/rhythm +2 pulses	*Vascular changes (e.g., cotton wool, AV nicking, retinal hemorrhages) on fundoscopic examination:* Cardiovascular disease.
Gastrointestinal Abdomen soft, no hepatomegaly	*Yellow sclera:* Jaundice associated with liver disease.
Reproductive External genitalia pink, moist, and intact	Eye infections can be caused by cross-contamination.
Musculoskeletal Equal muscle strength, full ROM, no joint deformity	*Ptosis, episcleritis and keratoconjunctivitis:* Muscle weakness associated with rheumatoid arthritis.
Neurological Movements smooth, sensory function intact	*Ptosis:* Myasthenia gravis and Bell's palsy. *Visual problems and fundoscopic changes:* MS.

Case Study Findings

Before you proceed to a focused physical examination of the eye, review what you learned in your general survey/head-to-toe assessment of Mrs. Scammel.

Mrs. Scammel's physical assessment findings include:

- **General Health Survey:** Moderately obese 55-year-old female, alert and oriented ×4, affect pleasant but anxious
- **Vital Signs:** Height 5′2″; weight 170 pounds; temperature 98.2°F; BP 170/108; pulse 96; respirations 24
- **Integumentary:** Skin pink, moist, no lesions noted

- **HEENT:** Normocephalic, thyroid not palpable, no palpable lymph nodes, mucous membranes pink and moist
- **Respiratory:** Lungs clear to auscultation
- **Cardiovascular:** Heart rate and rhythm regular, +S4, pulses +2
- **Gastrointestinal:** Abdomen large, round, soft, nontender; positive bowel sounds; negative organomegaly
- **Genitourinary:** External genitalia intact, no lesions
- **Musculoskeletal:** +5 muscle strength; full range of motion; no deformities, redness, or swelling of joints
- **Neurological:** Awake, alert, and oriented to time, place, and person (AAO × 3); affect appropriate, cerebellar function intact, light and deep sensations intact, CN I through XII intact

Performing a Focused Physical Assessment

A comprehensive physical examination of the eye involves assessing the functions, such as vision (distant, near, color, and peripheral), eye muscle functioning, and pupil reflexes, as well as inspecting the external and internal eye structures. The sequence for testing visual acuity progresses from testing done at a distance, such as the visual acuity examination, to observations made at close range, such as the ophthalmic examination. Proceeding in this sequence allows the client to become comfortable with the nurse before examination at close range is performed. It also allows the nurse to establish the client's degree of visual functioning, which establishes a baseline for conducting the remainder of the examination. The ophthalmic examination often requires administration of mydriatic or pupil-dilating eye drops.

HELPFUL HINTS

- Mydriatic drops should be administered toward the end of the examination to prevent interference with visual acuity and pupillary reflex testing.
- If the client wears corrective lenses, first test his or her vision without the lenses, and then with them. This reduces the likelihood that the measurement without correction will be influenced by reading the chart with corrective lenses.

ALERT

If mydriatics are administered for the examination, instruct the client to wear sunglasses to protect the eyes until the medication wears off.

Visual Acuity Testing

Visual acuity testing involves determining distant, near, peripheral, and color vision. The Snellen eye chart is used to test distant vision in adults and children of school age. The client stands 20 feet from the chart, covers one eye, and reads the smallest line of print. He or she continues reading successively smaller lines until he or she reads them incorrectly (no more than two mistakes

Testing Visual Acuity

ASSESS/NORMAL VARIATIONS

Distance

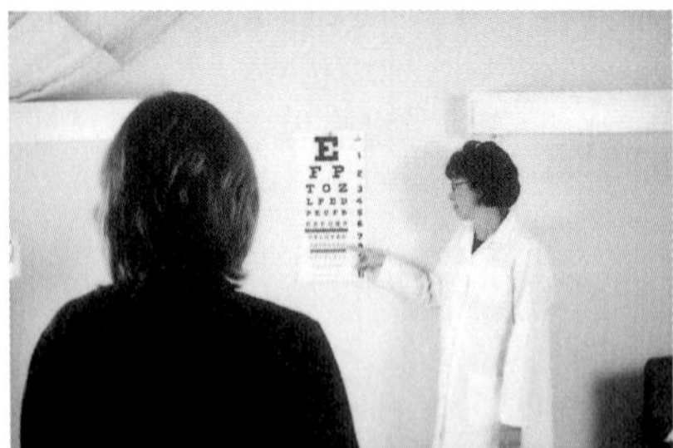

Using Snellen chart

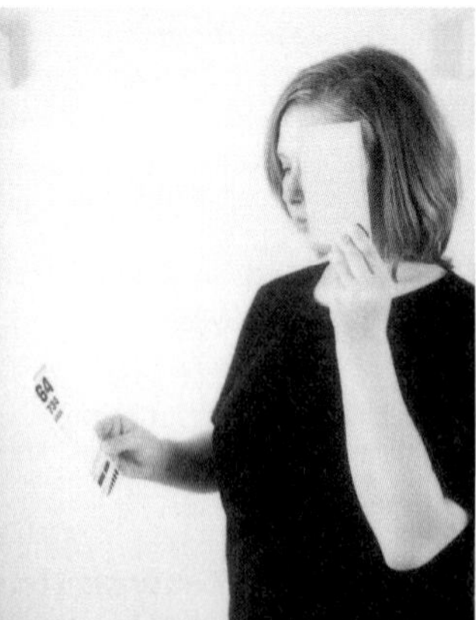

Using pocket vision screener

Reads letters without correction on Snellen chart or Snellen E chart corresponding with 20/20 in OS, OD, and OU. (Use Snellen E chart for children who do not know the alphabet, people who cannot read, and those who do not read English.)

ABNORMAL FINDINGS/RATIONALE

A smaller fraction (e.g., 20/40): Person standing 20 feet from chart can see lines of print that a normal eye can read at 40 feet. Indicates diminished distant vision or myopia (nearsightedness).

Testing Visual Acuity

ASSESS/NORMAL VARIATIONS

Near Vision

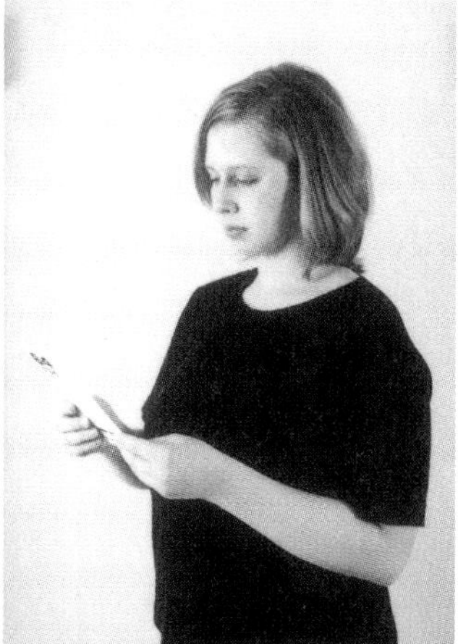

Reading newsprint

Adult reads newsprint or Jaeger cards easily at a distance of 14 inches (recorded as 14/14 OS, OD, and OU).

Color Vision

Correctly identifies embedded figures in the Ishihara cards or identifies colored bars on the Snellen eye chart.

Visual Fields

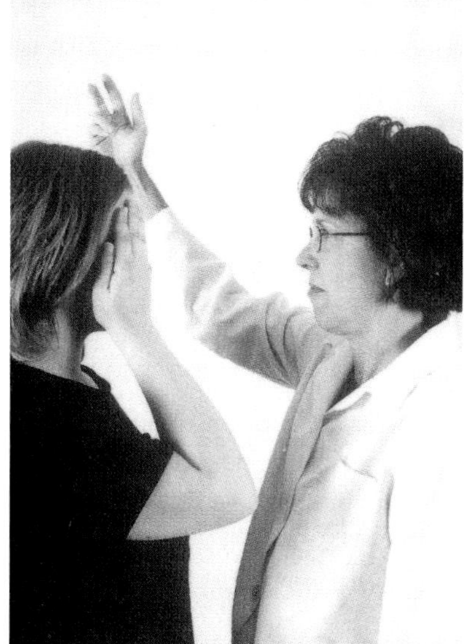

Examiner coming in from periphery

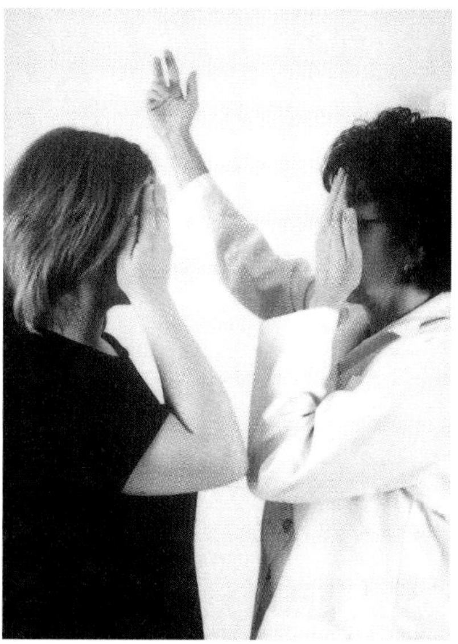

Comparing patient to examiner

HELPFUL HINT

Go slowly. If you move your hands too rapidly into the client's visual field, it will be difficult to obtain an accurate measure of peripheral vision.

ABNORMAL FINDINGS/RATIONALE

A smaller fraction (e.g., 14/18): Person must hold print farther away to see clearly because of decreased ability of lens to accommodate to near objects. Indicates diminished near vision, called hyperopia (farsightedness) or presbyopia if it occurs with aging.

Inability to detect the embedded number or letter in the Ishihara test cards: Defect in color perception (color blindness). Often inherited in an X-linked recessive pattern, predominantly affecting males. Also results from macular degeneration or other diseases that affect the cones that mediate color vision.

Diminished visual fields: Chronic glaucoma or stroke.

allowed per line) or says that the print is too blurry to distinguish letters. Record the fraction next to the smallest line of letters that the client read. The top number or numerator indicates the distance in feet from the chart, and the bottom number or denominator indicates the distance in feet that a person with normal vision would be able to read the chart. The higher the denominator or bottom number, the worse the person's distant vision.

Have the person cover the opposite eye and repeat the procedure. After testing each eye individually, test both eyes simultaneously and record the fraction next to the smallest line read. A pocket vision screener may also be used. The letters are scaled down and simulate the Snellen chart, but the card is held only 14 inches from the client.

HELPFUL HINT

If the client wears corrective lenses, first test his or her vision without the lenses, and then with them. This reduces the likelihood that the measurement without correction will be influenced by reading the chart with corrective lenses.

Near vision is tested using Jaeger cards, in which lines of text are repeated in progressively smaller fonts. Test each eye separately by having the client cover one eye and read the smallest line of text while holding the card at a distance of 14 inches. If Jaeger cards are not available, an alternative method is to have the client read a newspaper and then record how far away he or she holds it.

Color vision is tested using Ishihara's embedded colors test, which consists of a series of cards displaying colored dots that contain an embedded colored figure or number. The client is asked to identify the figure in each card. An alternative measure is to point to one of the red or green colored bars on the Snellen eye chart and ask the client what color he or she sees (Fig. 10–11).

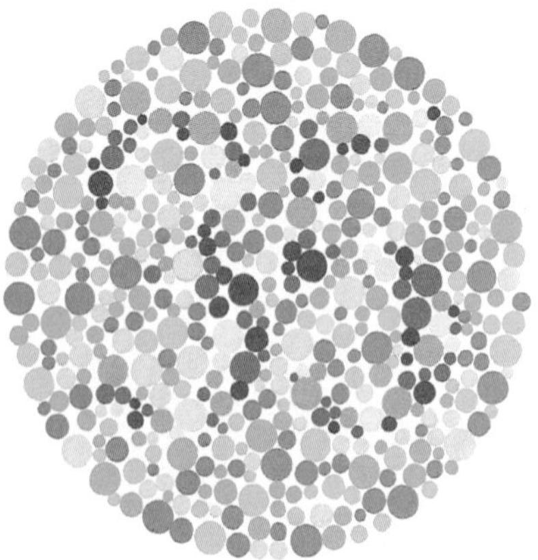

FIGURE 10–11. Card from Ishihara's embedded colors test. (From Scanlon, V. C., and Sanders, T. (1999). Essentials of Anatomy and Physiology (3rd ed.). Philadelphia: F. A. Davis, with permission).

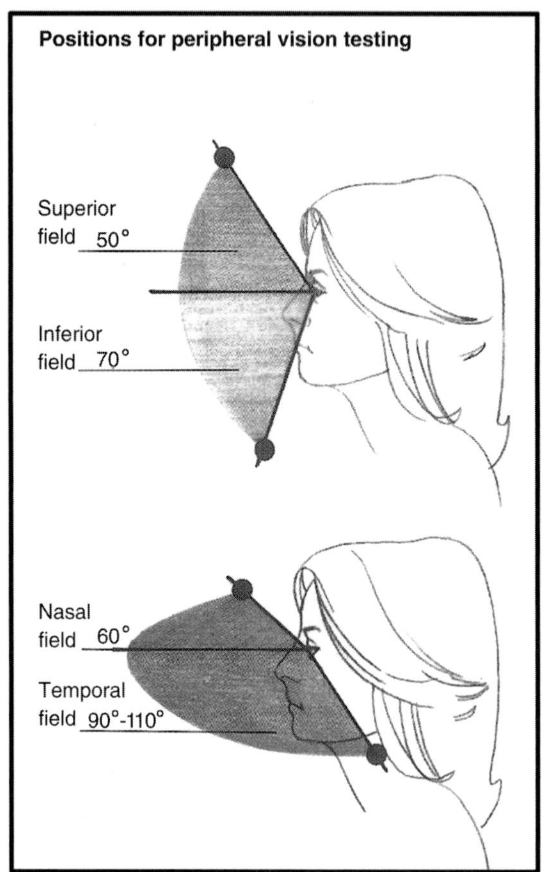

FIGURE 10–12. Positions for peripheral vision testing.

Peripheral vision in each eye is measured on two planes—horizontal and vertical—and in four directions—superior, inferior, medial (nasal) and lateral (temporal), using the confrontation test. The client and nurse stand face to face, about 1 to 1–1/2 feet apart. Ask the client to fix his or her gaze straight ahead and cover one eye at a time, using his or her hand or an opaque cover. Then wiggle your fingers or bring a pen or other small object from the periphery to the center of the visual field. Tell the client to say "now" as soon as your hand or the object enters his or her peripheral vision.

Repeat this procedure in each of the four visual fields, moving in a clockwise direction. Be sure to start testing from positions that are outside the normal peripheral vision range; then slowly move your hand or the object into each of the four peripheral fields. Measure the degree of peripheral vision using the client's fixed gaze as a base (Fig. 10–12).

You can also test peripheral vision by comparing the client's peripheral vision to yours. This is helpful in detecting gross peripheral deficits, but the method is somewhat subjective because you have to assume that you have normal peripheral vision.

Assessment of the Extraocular Muscles

To perform the corneal light reflex test, instruct the client to fix his or her gaze straight ahead. Shine a penlight at the bridge of the nose and note where the light reflects on the cornea of each eye. Using the face of a clock as a guide, determine if the light reflex appears at the same clock position in each eye. The corneal light reflex test determines if the eyes are being maintained in a conjugate position.

The cover/uncover test helps determine if there is a weakness in the eye muscles of one or both eyes that can result in disconjugate eye movement. To perform the test, have the client fix his or her gaze straight ahead. Stand in front of the client, cover one of his or her eyes with a piece of paper, and observe the uncovered eye for movement indicating re-fixation of the gaze. Remove the cover and observe the previously covered eye for movement indicating re-fixation of the gaze. Repeat the procedure for the other eye. The gaze should remain steady in each eye throughout the test.

Further testing of the extraocular muscles is done by testing for symmetrical (conjugate) rotation of the eyes, symmetrical movement of the upper eyelid, and nystagmus in the six cardinal fields of gaze test. The six cardinal fields of gaze tests the cranial nerves III, IV and VI and the extraocular muscle. To perform this test, stand in front of the client and instruct him or her to look straight ahead and follow your finger as you move slowly through the six cardinal fields. The client should hold his or her head still and move only his or her eyes. Observe for smooth, symmetrical movement of the eyes and eyelids.

Assessment of the External Structures

The next phase of the eye examination involves inspection and palpation of external eye structures. Careful inspection and palpation can reveal a variety of eye disorders as well as systemic disorders that affect the eye.

Assessing the Extraocular Muscles

ASSESS/NORMAL VARIATIONS

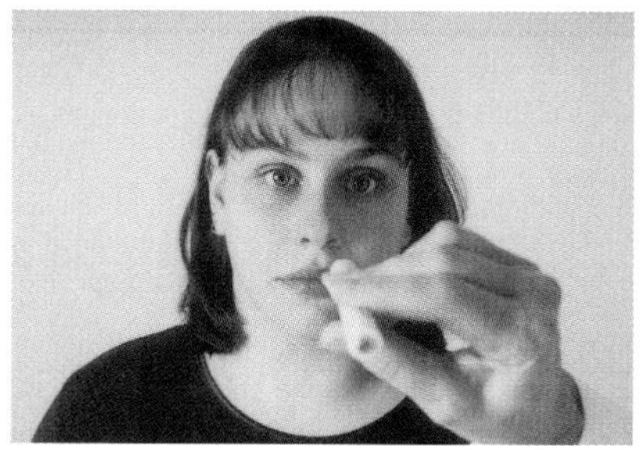

Corneal light reflex test

HELPFUL HINT

As you shine the light in your client's eyes, look for the sparkle. That is the light reflecting off the cornea.

Light should be seen symmetrically on each cornea.

ABNORMAL FINDINGS/RATIONALE

Asymmetrical corneal light reflex: Weak extraocular muscles or strabismus.

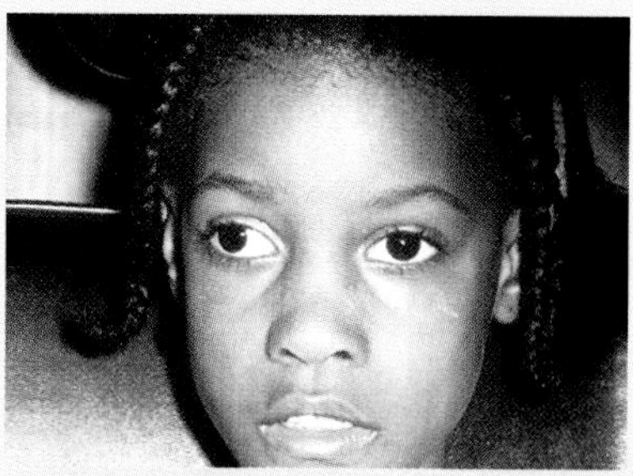

Exotropia (divergent strabismus)

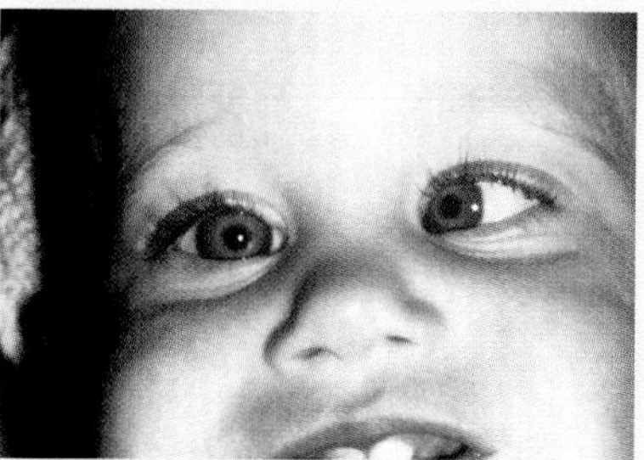

Congenital exotropia

(Continued)

Assessing the Extraocular Muscles *(Continued)*

ASSESS/NORMAL VARIATIONS

Cover/Uncover Test

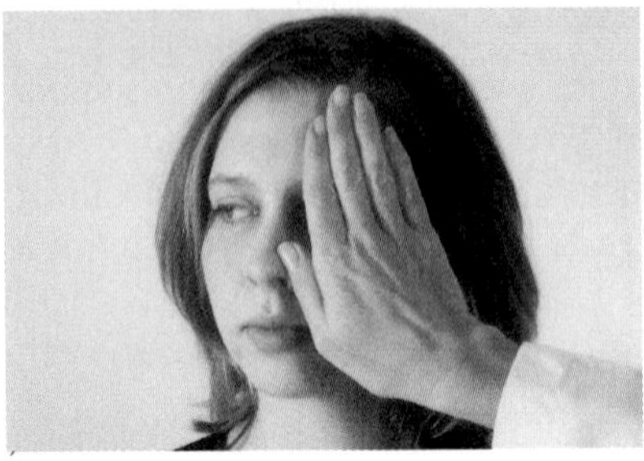

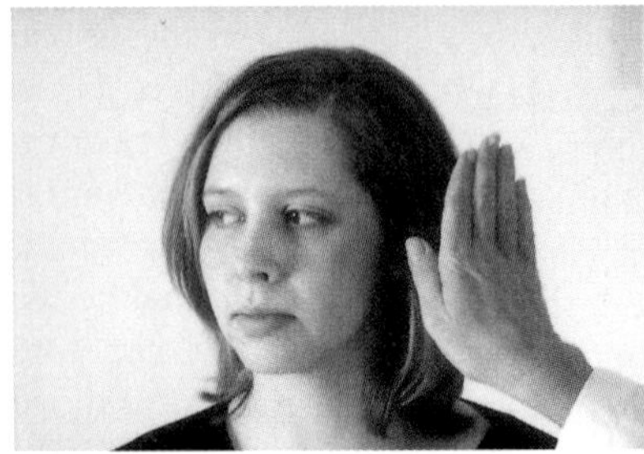

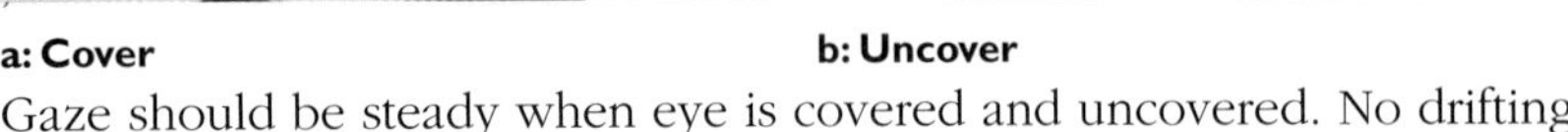

a: Cover **b: Uncover**

Gaze should be steady when eye is covered and uncovered. No drifting.

Cardinal Fields of Gaze Test

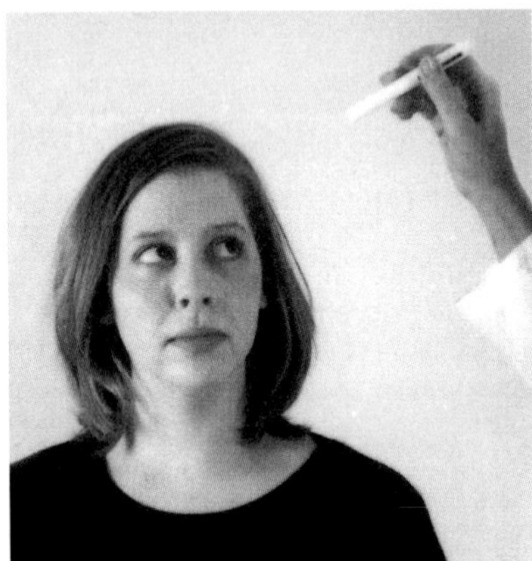

a: Up

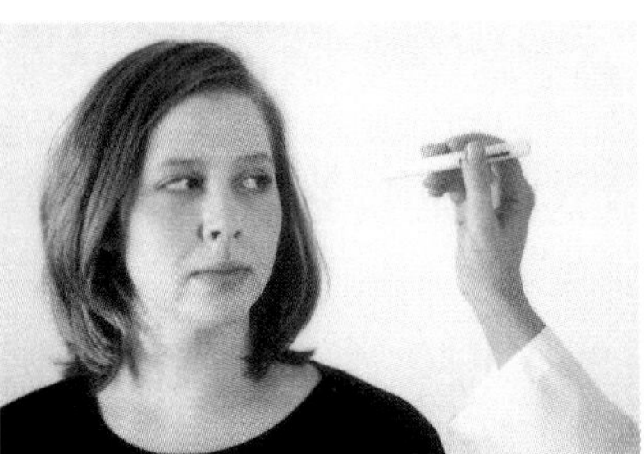

b: Side

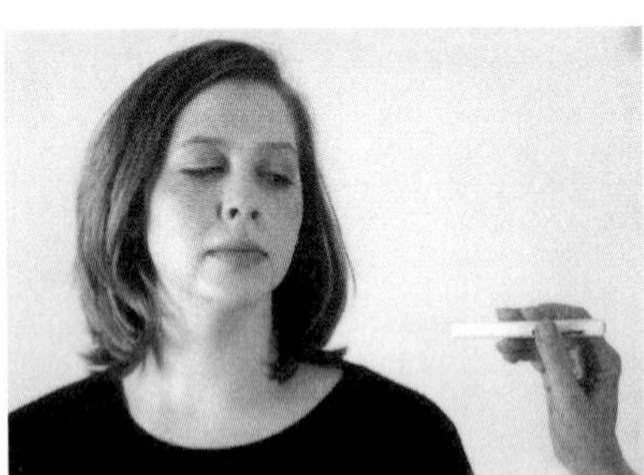

c: Down

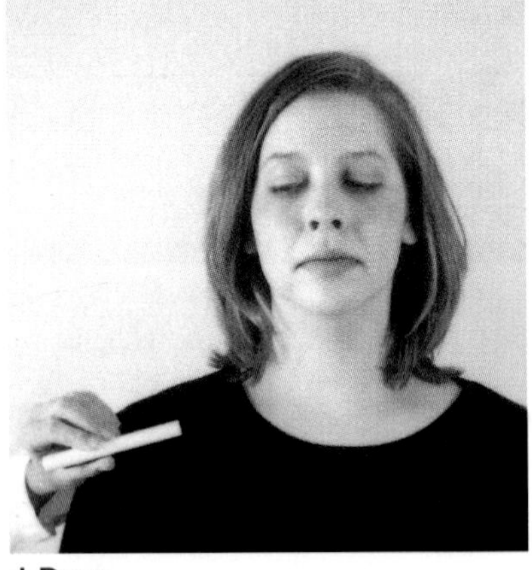

d: Down

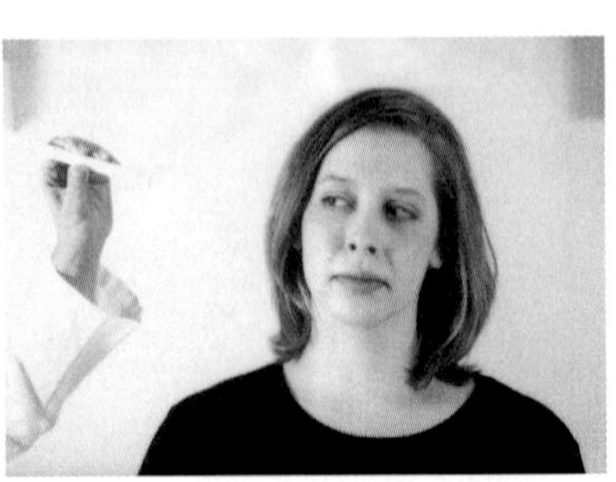

e: Side

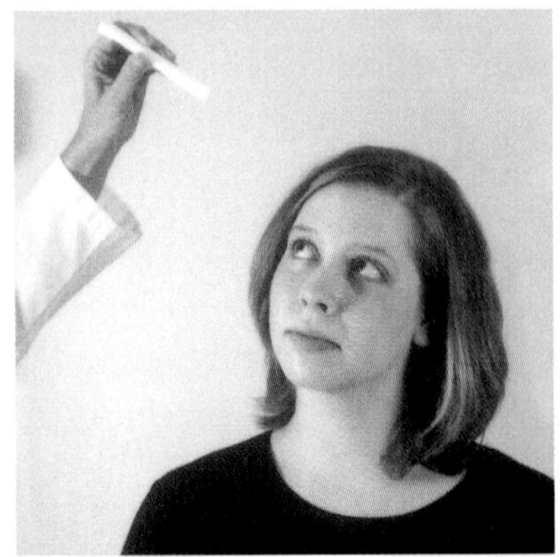

f: Up

ABNORMAL FINDINGS/RATIONALE

Shift in gaze: Weak eye muscle or muscles. If uncovered eye shifts in response to covering opposite eye, covered eye is dominant. If covered eye shifts after being uncovered, that eye is weak.

Movement of eyes to refocus gaze: Weakness of extraocular muscles or CN III, IV, and VI, which innervate extraocular muscles.

Assessing the Extraocular Muscles

ASSESS/NORMAL VARIATIONS	ABNORMAL FINDINGS/RATIONALE
Cardinal Fields of Gaze Test *(Continued)* Smooth, conjugate (parallel) movement of eyes in all directions, equal palpebral fissures without eyelid lag. Nystagmus or horizontal jerking eye movements noted only in extreme lateral gaze. EOM intact.	*Limited or disconjugate movement in one or more fields of gaze, nystagmus in fields other than extreme lateral, ptosis (drooping of upper eyelid) and eyelid lag:* Damage, irritation, or pressure on corresponding extraocular muscle or cranial nerve that innervates the muscle.

Testing the pupils to determine reaction to light is important for evaluating neurological function of the optic nerve. Increased intracranial pressure from a head injury, tumor, or stroke may manifest in specific pupillary changes. Other conditions such as hypoxia or brain death or the use of certain medications also can affect the pupillary light reflex.

To test pupillary reflex, observe for direct (same side) and consensual (opposite side) response to a focused beam of light. Darken the room if possible. Then, using a penlight, flashlight, or ophthalmoscope light, shine the light onto one eye as you observe whether the pupil constricts (referred to a direct response). Repeat the procedure and note whether the other eye exhibits a consensual response or constriction to light. Repeat the test for the opposite eye.

Inspection of the anterior chamber of the eye can reveal a variety of conditions including infection, trauma and risk for glaucoma. The shadow test is useful in identifying a shallow anterior chamber, which is commonly seen in glaucoma. To inspect the anterior chamber using this test, have the client look straight ahead. Hold your penlight at the temporal side of one eye at a 90-degree angle across the anterior chamber. Without moving the penlight, shine the light across the limbus of the eye, toward the nose. A crescent-shaped shadow on the nasal side of the iris indicates a shallow anterior chamber.

Inspecting the External Structures

ASSESS/NORMAL VARIATIONS | **ABNORMAL FINDINGS/RATIONALE**

General Appearance

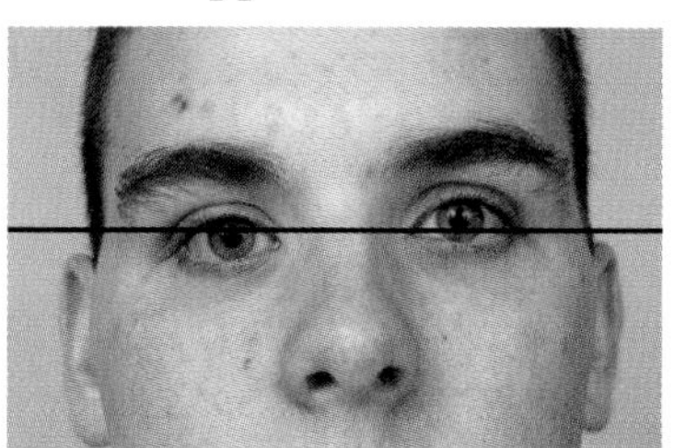

Check that eyes are in parallel alignment

Eyes clear and bright, in parallel alignment. Note presence of contact lenses.

Glazed eyes: Febrile state.

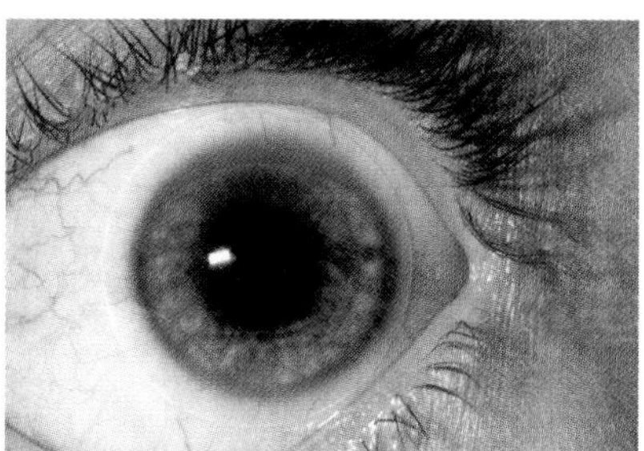

a: Soft contact lenses;

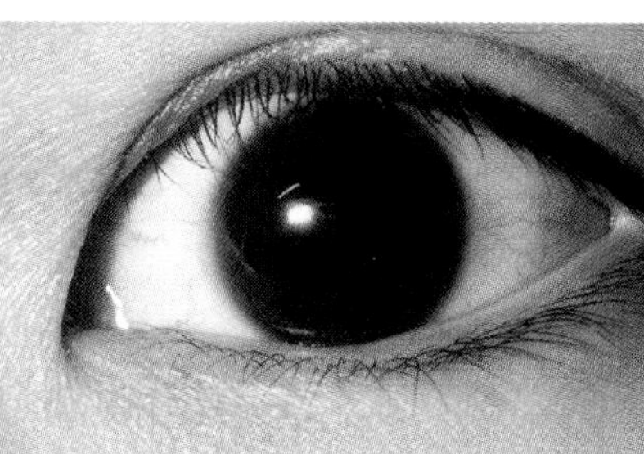

b: Hard contact lenses

(Continued)

Inspecting the External Structures *(Continued)*

ASSESS/NORMAL VARIATIONS

Eyelashes

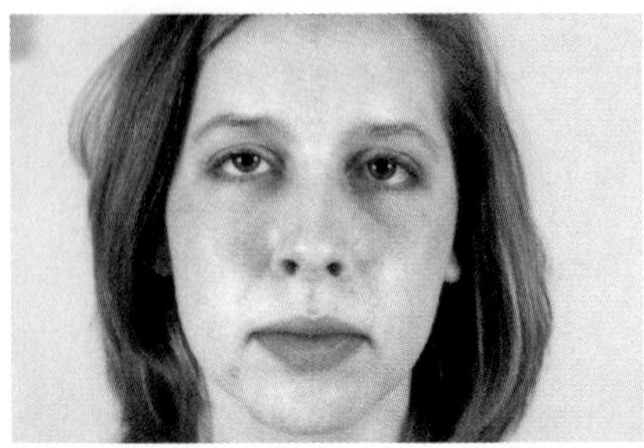

Inspecting eyelashes

Present and curving outward.
No crusting or infestation.

Eyelids

Upper eyelid normally covers 1/2 of upper iris.
Palpebral fissures symmetrical. Eyelids in contact with eyeball.
No lesions.

ABNORMAL FINDINGS/RATIONALE

Absence of eyelashes: Alopecia universalis.
Lice or ticks at base of eyelashes: Infestation.
Inflammation: Blepharitis—inflammation of edge of eyelids involving hair follicles and meibomian glands of eyelids.
Inverted eyelashes: Entropion; can scratch cornea.
Everted eyelashes: Ectropion; can lead to excessive drying of eyes.
Visible sclera between iris and upper lid (exophthalmos): Seen in hyperthyroidism and hydrocephalus ("setting-sun eyes").
Asymmetry of lids: CN III damage, CVA.
Ptosis of both eyelids: Myasthenia gravis.
Lesions on eyelids: Basal cell carcinoma, squamous cell carcinoma, xanthelasma, chalazion, hordeolum.

Inspecting the External Structures

ASSESS/NORMAL VARIATIONS | **ABNORMAL FINDINGS/RATIONALE**

Abnormalities of the Eyelids and Eyelashes

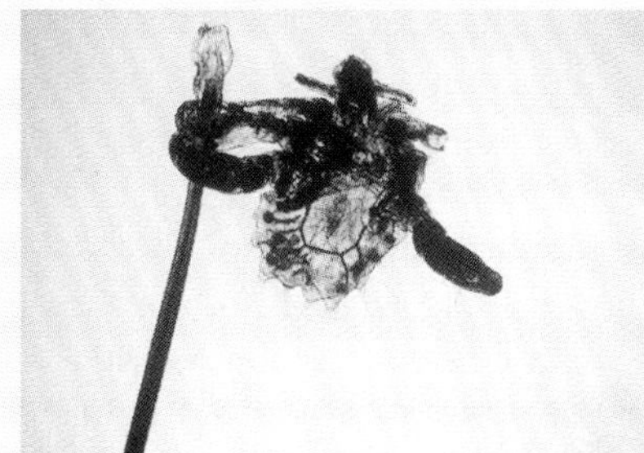

Lice

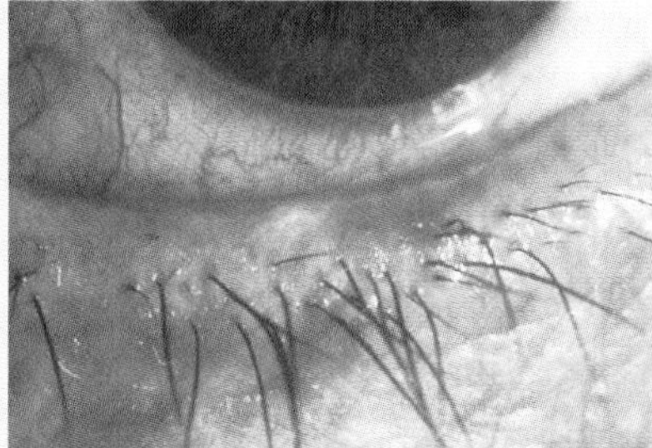

Blepharoconjunctivitis

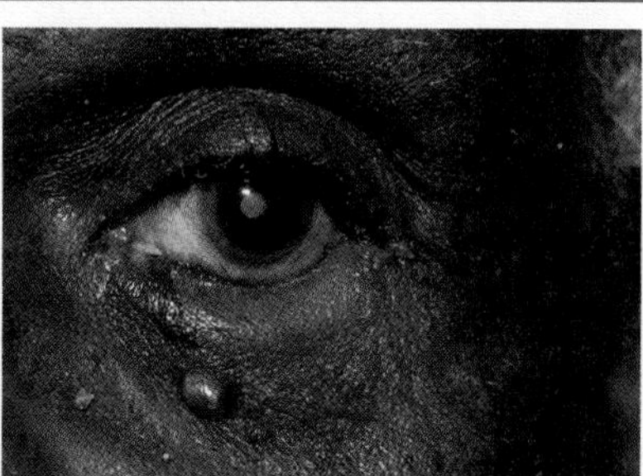

Entropion

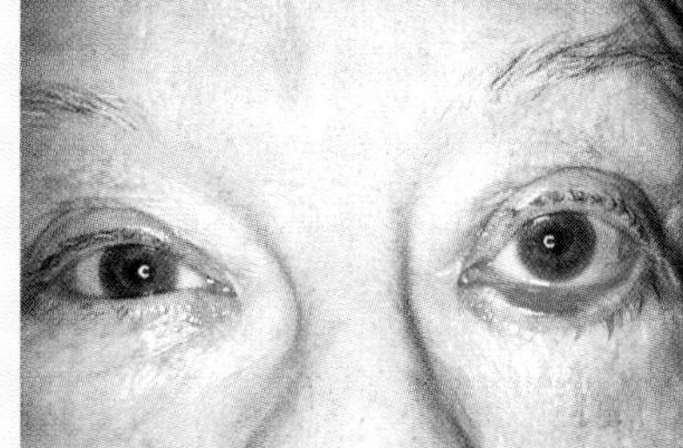

Ectropion

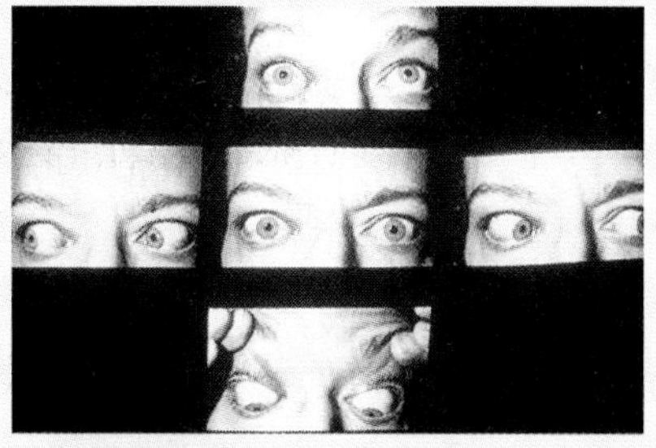

Exophthalmos

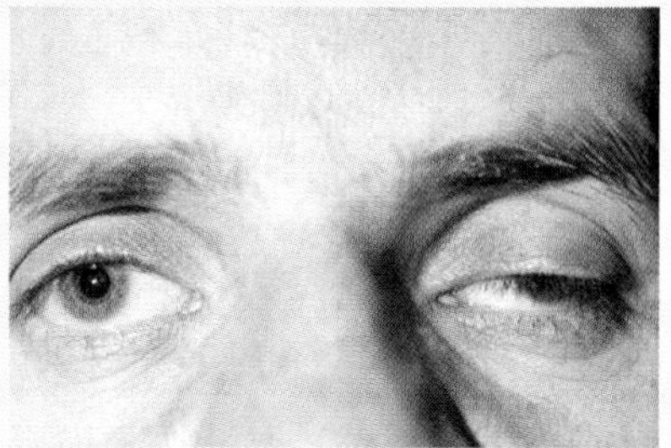

Ptosis

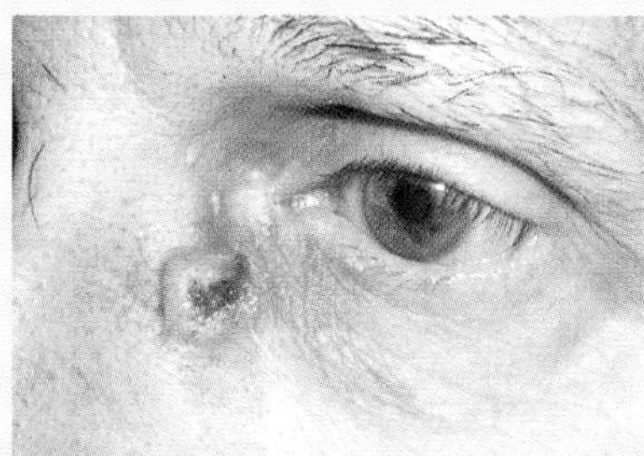

Basal cell carcinoma

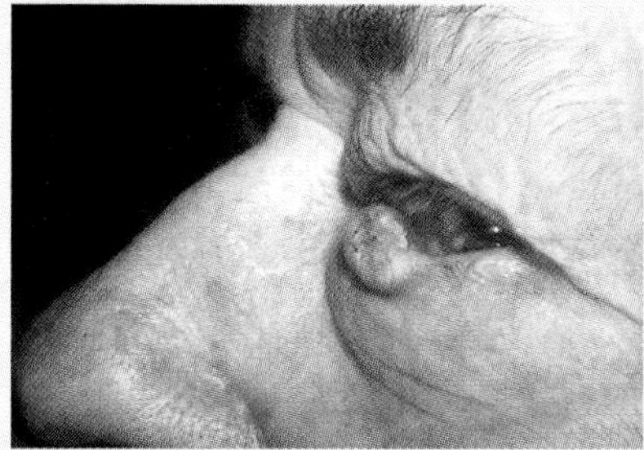

Squamous cell carcinoma

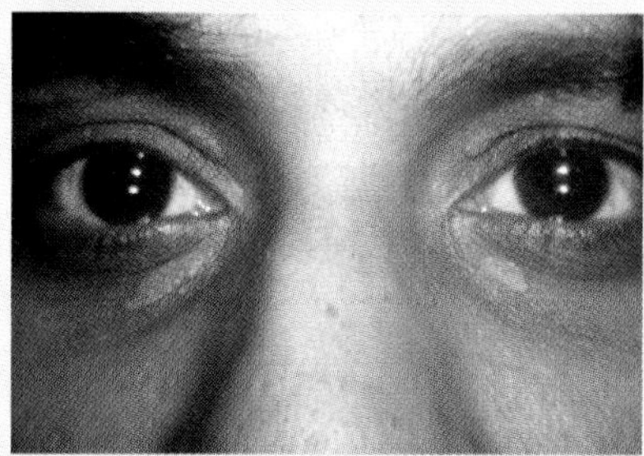

Xanthelasma

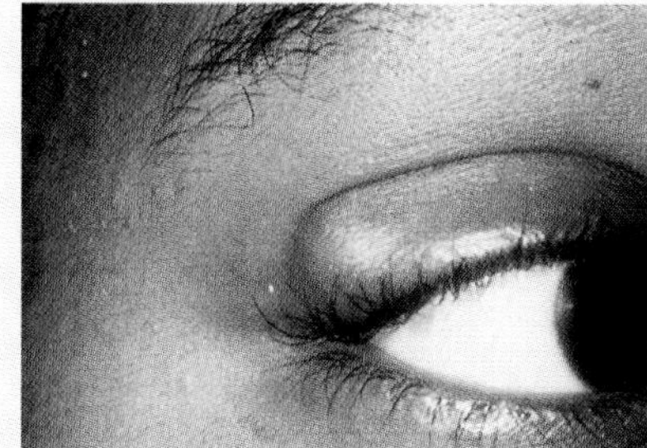

Chalazion

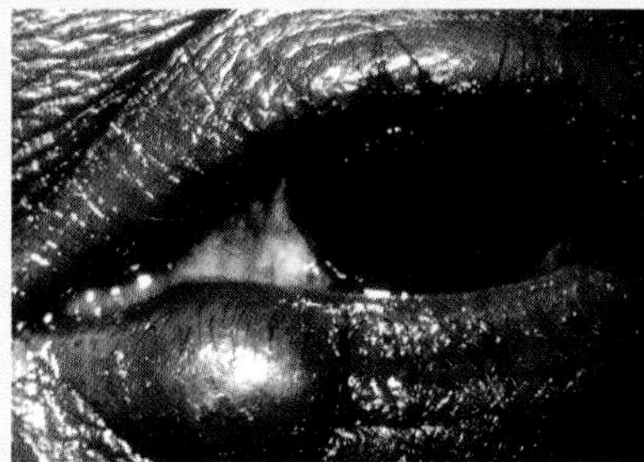

Hordeolum

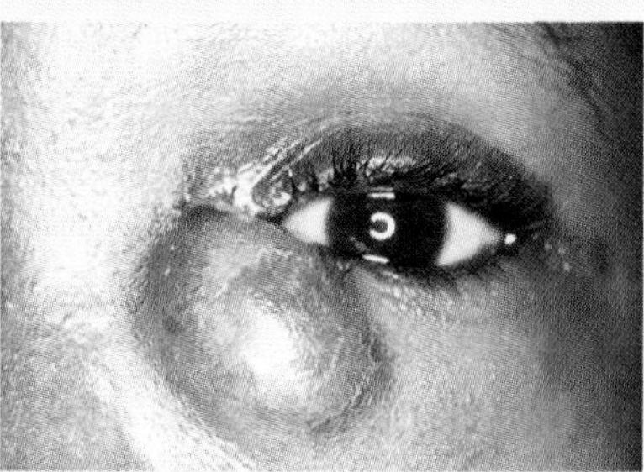

Dacryocystitis

(Continued)

Inspecting the External Structures *(Continued)*

ASSESS/NORMAL VARIATIONS

Eyeball

Normally doesn't protrude beyond frontal bone. Mild protrusion seen in some African-Americans.

Lacrimal Gland and Nasolacrimal Duct

No swelling, redness, or drainage.

Conjunctiva

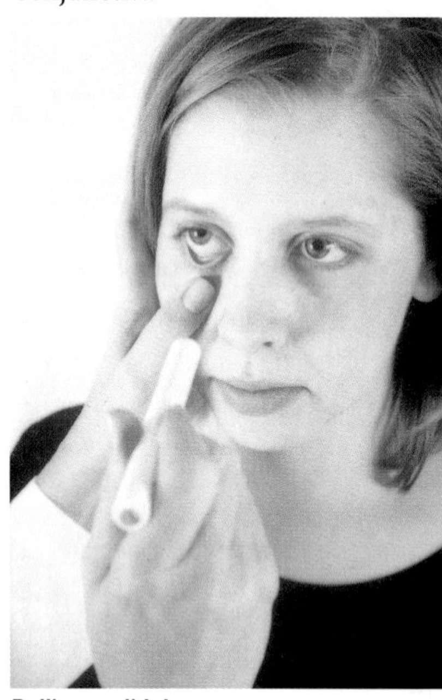

Pulling eyelid down

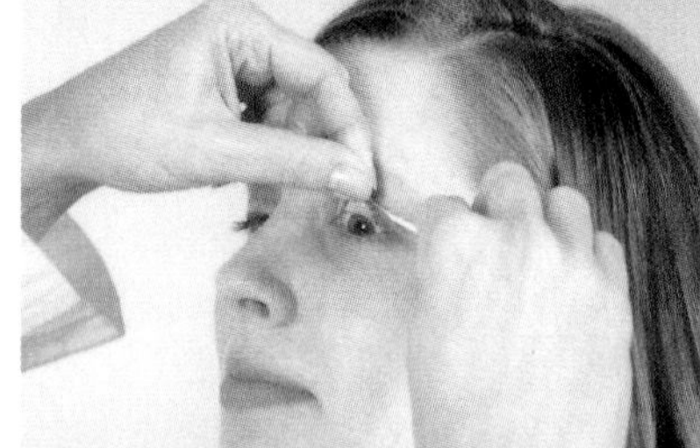

Rolling eyelid up

Palpebral conjunctiva is smooth, glistening, pinkish-peach color, with minimal blood vessels visible. Bulbar conjunctiva over globes are clear, with few underlying blood vessels and white sclera visible.

Sclera

Should be smooth, white, glistening. Dark-skinned clients may have a yellowish cast to the peripheral sclera with whiter sclera at the limbus or small brown spots called "muddy sclera."

ABNORMAL FINDINGS/RATIONALE

Protrusion: Hyperthyroidism or inherited disorders of mucopolysaccharide metabolism.

Swelling, redness, drainage, tenderness: Obstruction or inflammation.

Red palpebral and bulbar conjunctiva: Conjunctivitis.

Pale pink conjunctiva: Anemia.

Growth or thickening of conjunctiva from inner canthal area toward iris: Pterygium or pinguecula.

Subconjunctival hemorrhage: Eye injury.

Benign pigmented congenital discoloration: Nevus

Benign growth: Papilloma.

Bluish sclera: Osteogenesis imperfecta.

Icteric (yellow) sclera at the limbus: Elevated bilirubin (jaundice).

Inspecting the External Structures

ASSESS/NORMAL VARIATIONS | **ABNORMAL FINDINGS/RATIONALE**

Conjunctiva *(Continued)*

Abnormalities of the Conjunctiva and Sclera

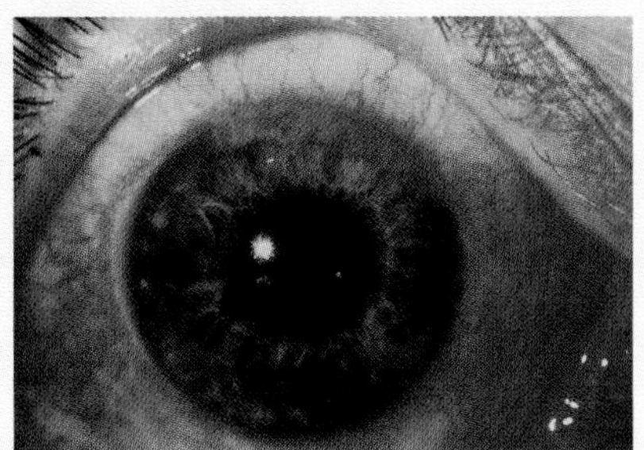
Acute allergic conjunctivitis

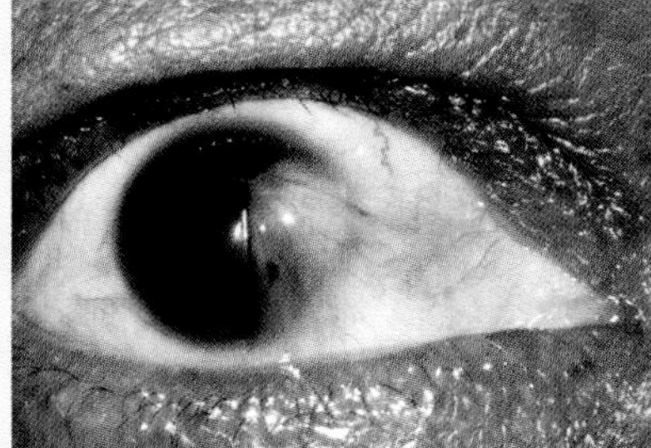
Pterygium

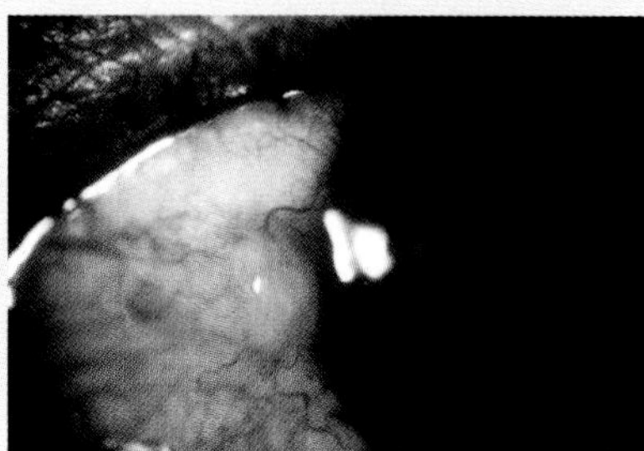
Pinguecula

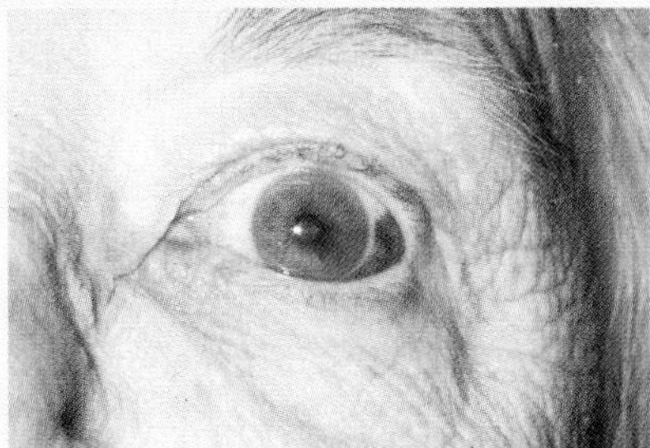
Subconjunctival hemorrhage

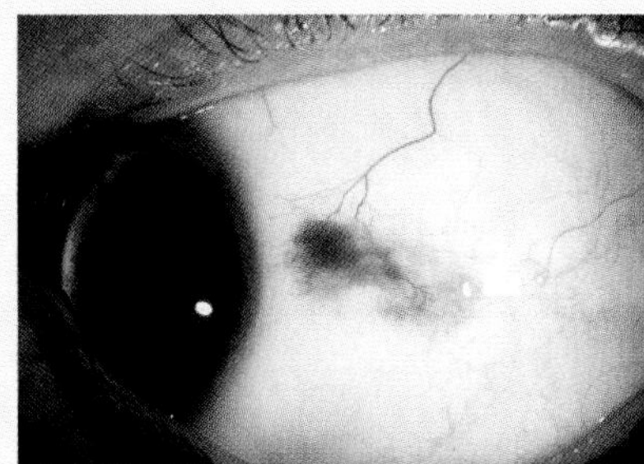
Nevus

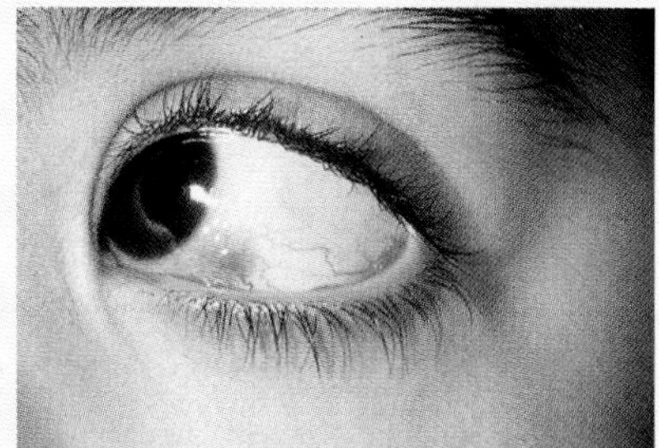
Papilloma

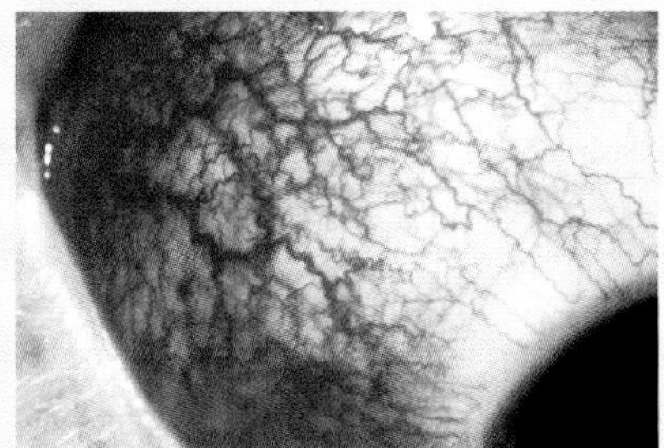
Diffuse episcleritis

(Continued)

Inspecting the External Structures *(Continued)*

ASSESS/NORMAL VARIATIONS

Cornea and Lens

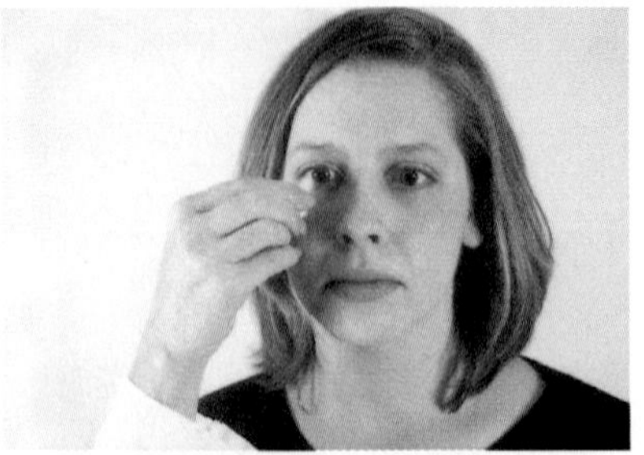
Corneal reflex with cotton ball

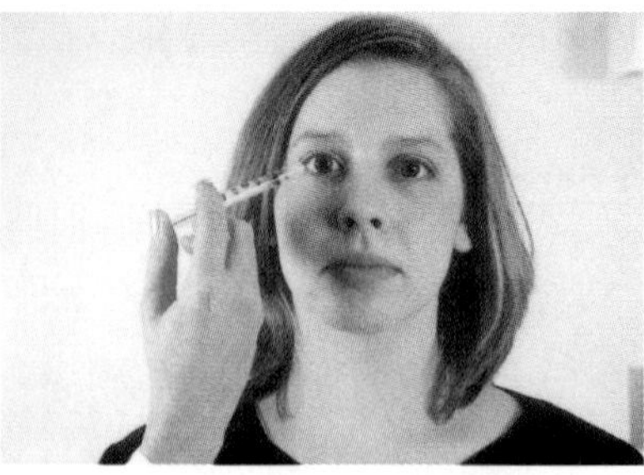
Corneal reflex with puff of air

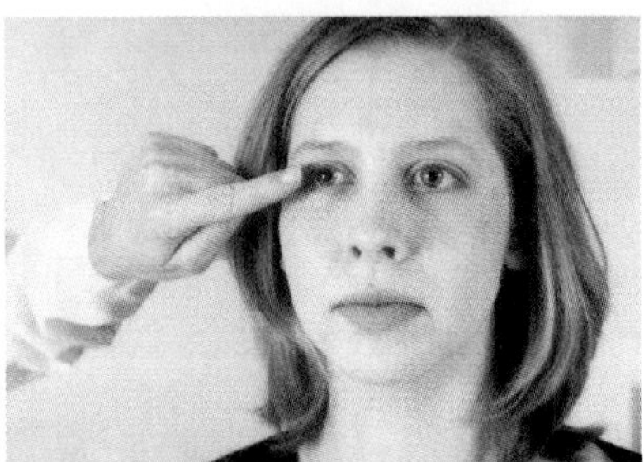
Blink reflex

Corneal reflex positive.

Cornea and lens clear, smooth, and glistening. White ring encircling outer rim (arcus senilis) is a normal variant in older adults.

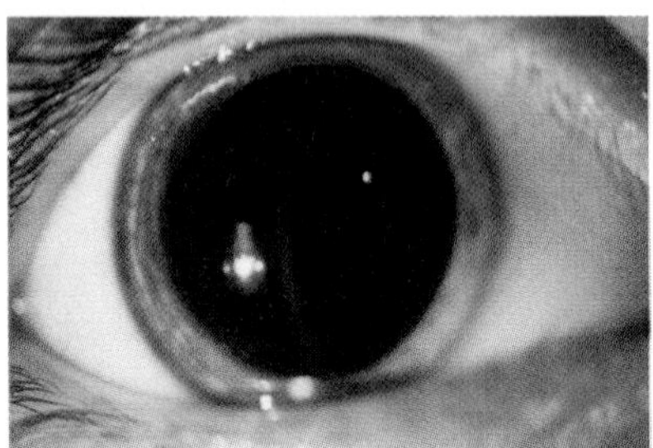
Normal lens

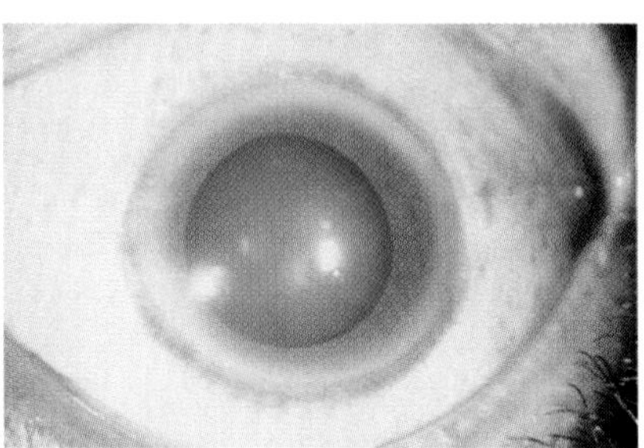
Arcus senilis

ABNORMAL FINDINGS/RATIONALE

Cloudy cornea: Vitamin A deficiency; infection, which may be accompanied by hypopyon (pus in anterior chamber).

Roughness or irregularity of cornea: Corneal abrasions and ulcers.

ALERT

Corneal scratches or abrasions may not always be visible with the naked eye.

*Yellow ring in outer margin (Kayser-Fleischer ring):*Wilson's disease, characterized by increased copper absorption.

Lens opacities: Cataracts.

Negative corneal reflex: May indicate neurological problem, CN V and VII, but also may be absent or diminished in people who wear contact lenses.

Abnormalities of the Cornea and Lens

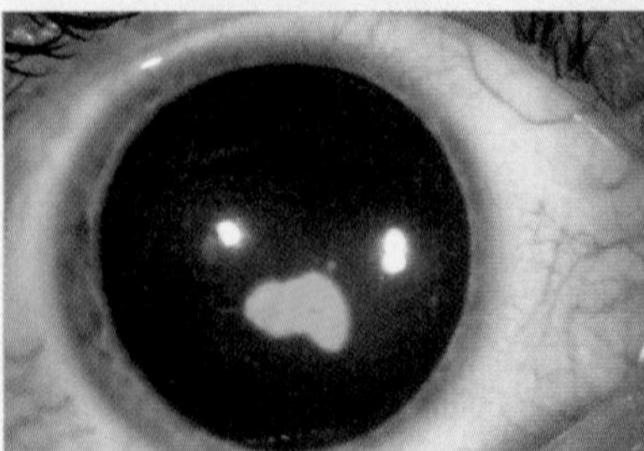
Corneal abrasion

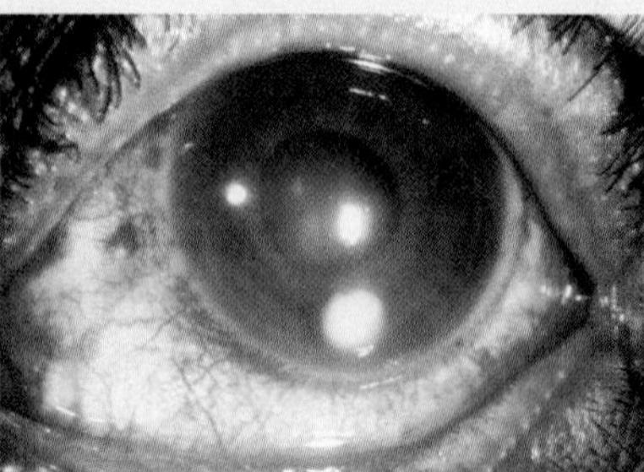
Healing corneal ulcer

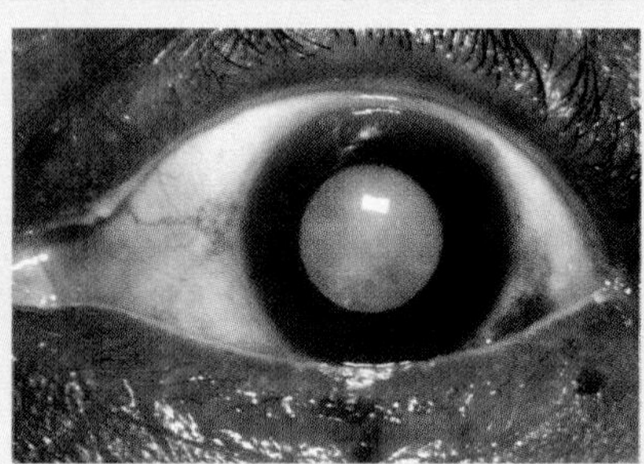
Mature cataract

Inspecting the External Structures

ASSESS/NORMAL VARIATIONS

Iris

Color should be normal variations of blue, green, or brown.

Different iris color or different in one section of iris can be a normal variant.

Shape should be circular.

Pupils

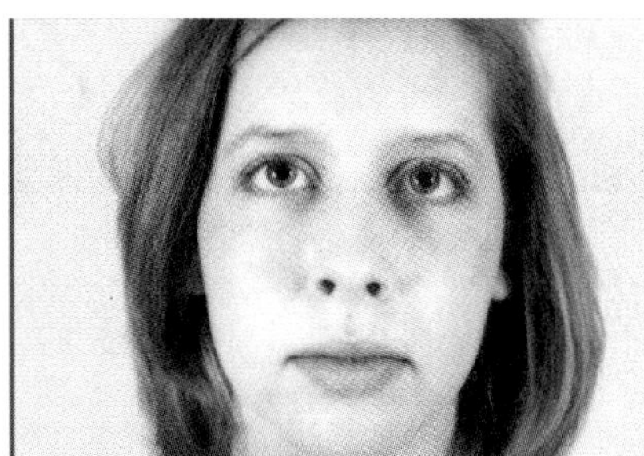

Checking pupil size

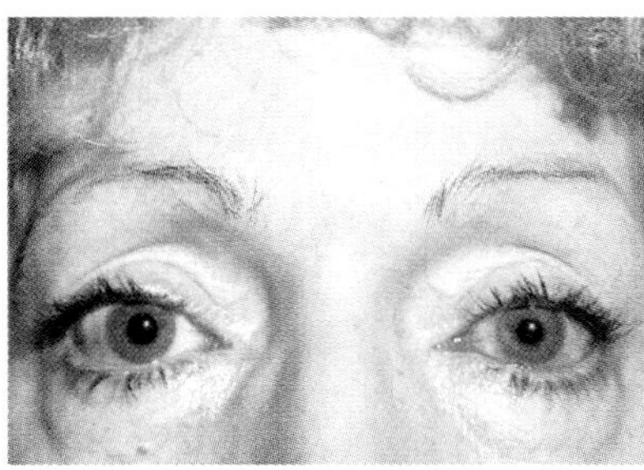

Anisocoria

Should be round and equal bilaterally. Size is larger in children, smaller in older adults. Normal range is 3–5 mm in adults (usually 3 mm).

Unequal pupils (*anisocoria*) can be a normal variation if difference is less than 0.5 mm.

Shape is round.

ABNORMAL FINDINGS/RATIONALE

White specks (Brushfield spots): Common in Down syndrome.

Bloodshot appearance of vessels: Iritis.

New blood vessel on anterior surface: Diabetes.

Different-colored irides (heterochromia iridis): Previous damage in lighter-colored eye or (rarely) Waardenburg syndrome.

Absence of part or all of iris (aniridia): Congenital problem.

Keyhole wedges in iris: Previous eye surgery.

Small, pinpoint pupils (miosis): Brain injury to the pons; use of narcotics, atropine, and other drugs.

Larger, dilated pupils (mydriasis): Brain herniation, anoxia, or use of marijuana and mydriatic eye drops.

Unequal pupils (anisocoria): CN III (oculomotor) damage, dilated pupil, ptosis, and later deviation of affected eye; unilateral brain herniation or increased ICP.

Unilateral large pupil (tonic pupil) that reacts to light slowly (benign): Adie's pupil.

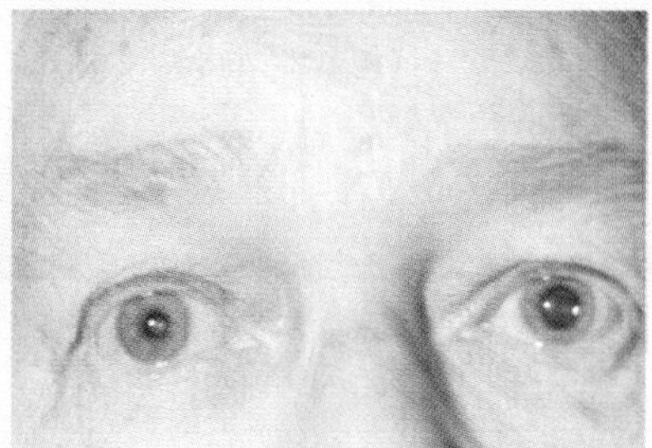

Adie's pupil

Unequal pupils; affected pupil small but reacts to light and has ptosis on affected eye related to sympathetic nerve lesion: Horner's syndrome.

(Continued)

Inspecting the External Structures *(Continued)*

ASSESS/NORMAL VARIATIONS

Pupils *(Continued)*

Light Reactions

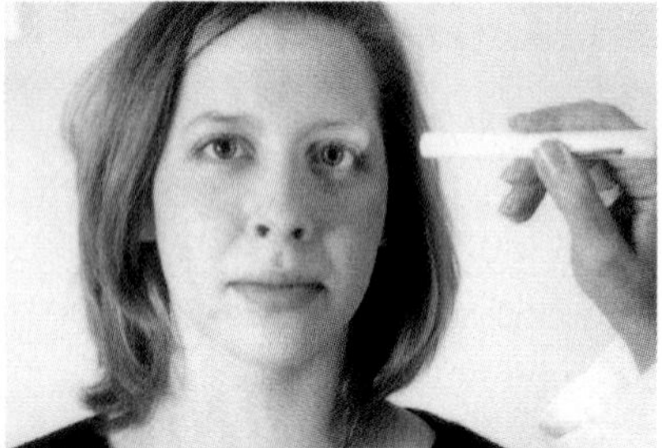

Checking pupillary response to light

HELPFUL HINT

Pupils constrict in response to looking at a near object, so shine light from temporal side, not directly in front of client's line of vision. This ensures that pupil constriction you observe is a result of pupillary light reflex and not focusing on a near object.

Normal direct and consensual pupillary response to light is brisk constriction of the pupil to about 1 mm or less.

ABNORMAL FINDINGS/RATIONALE

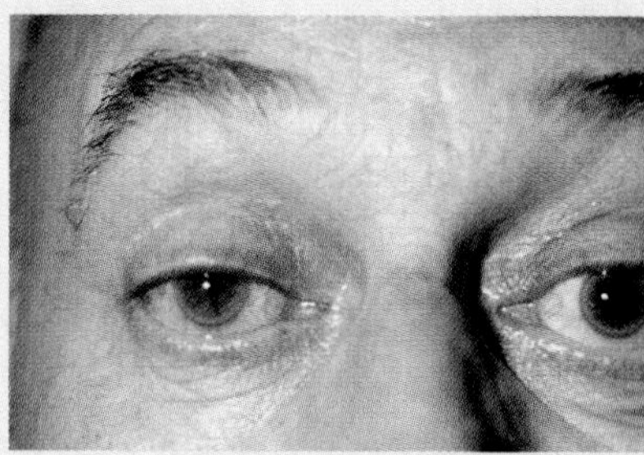

Horner's syndrome

Argyll Robertson pupil—pupils small and irregular with no reaction to light or accommodation, associated with neurosyphilis.

Oval pupils may occur early in head injury. Irregularly shaped pupils may be caused by certain eye surgeries.

Sluggish or fixed pupil reaction pupil to about 1 mm or less. *to light:* Lack of oxygen to optic nerve or brain or topical or systemic drug effects.

Absence of consensual response: Seen in conditions that compress or deprive those areas of oxygen.

Absent light reflex but no change in power of contraction during accommodation (Argyll Robertson pupil): Paralysis and locomotor ataxia caused by syphilis.

Inspecting the External Structures

ASSESS/NORMAL VARIATIONS	ABNORMAL FINDINGS/RATIONALE

Accommodation (adjustment of eye for various distances)

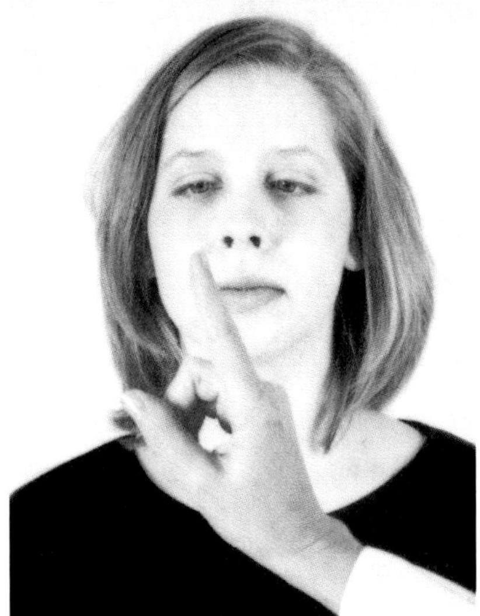

Checking accommodation

Convergence of eyes and constriction of pupil to focus on a near object and dilation of pupil when looking at a far object. Accommodation may be sluggish in advanced age.

One or both pupils fail to dilate or constrict to near or distant objects: May reflect a problem with CN III or extraocular eye muscles. Clients with hyperthyroidism (exophthalmos) also have poor convergence.

Sluggish accommodation not caused by advanced age: Drug effect, as from anticholinergics.

Anterior Chamber

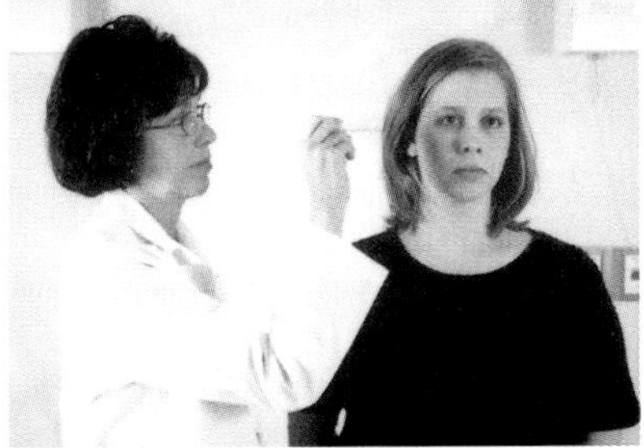

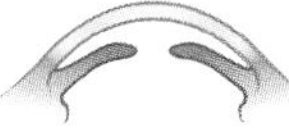

Checking anterior chamber

Absence of pus or blood.

Absence of a shadow when light is shined across the eye at the limbus area.

Crescent-shaped shadow may be a normal variant.

Pus (hypopyon): Corneal ulcer or other infection.

Blood in anterior chamber (hyphema): Trauma or intraocular hemorrhage.

Crescent-shaped shadow on nasal side of iris: Protrusion of iris into anterior chamber from increased intraocular pressure, seen in narrow-angle glaucoma.

Abnormalities of the Cornea and Lens

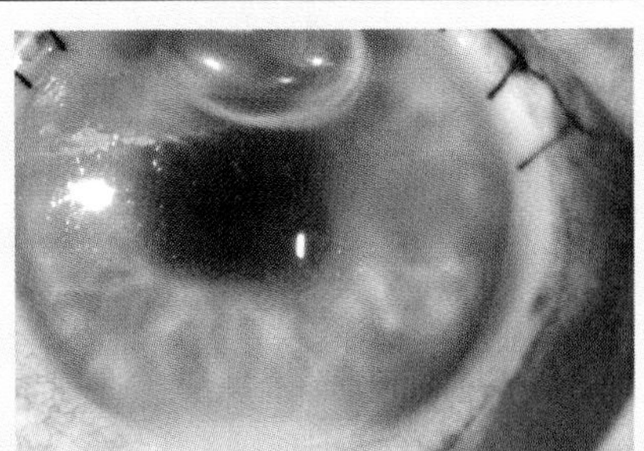

Hypopyon

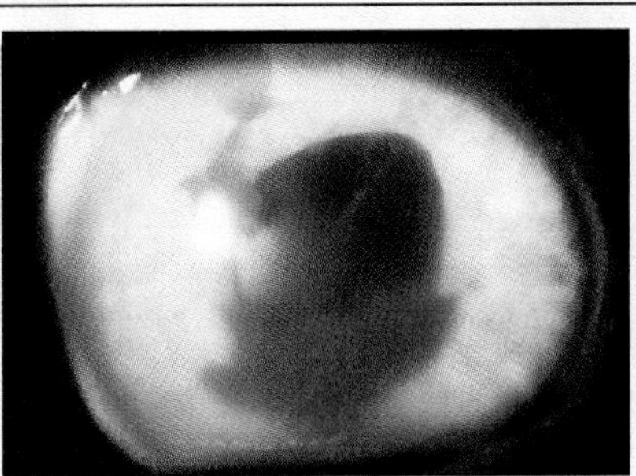

Hyphema

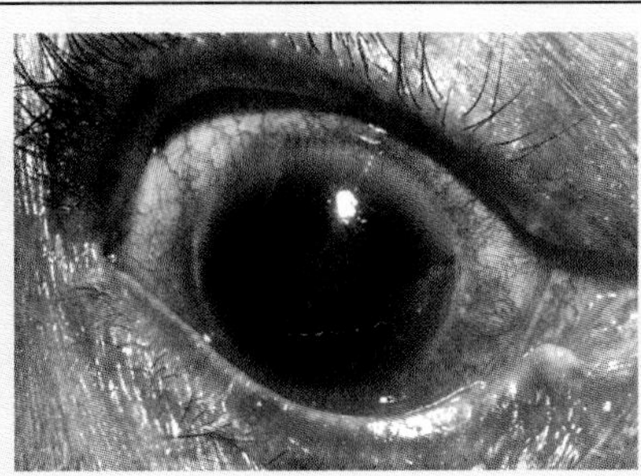

Acute angle closure

CRITICAL THINKING ACTIVITY #7

Conjunctivitis or "pink eye" is an inflammation of the conjunctiva. If your client has this condition, how would you explain that, even though it is called conjunctivitis, the sclera is actually what appears pink?

Palpating the External Structures

ASSESS/NORMAL VARIATIONS	ABNORMAL FINDINGS/RATIONALE
Eyeball	*Excessively firm or tender globe:* Glaucoma.

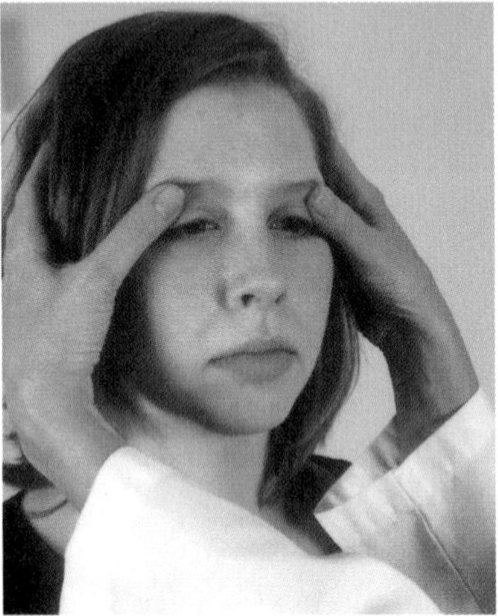

Palpating eyeballs

ALERT

Do not palpate eyeball in clients with eye trauma or known glaucoma.

Globe is firm and nontender.

ASSESS/NORMAL VARIATIONS	ABNORMAL FINDINGS/RATIONALE
Lacrimal Glands and Nasolacrimal Ducts	Swelling and tenderness indicate inflammation.

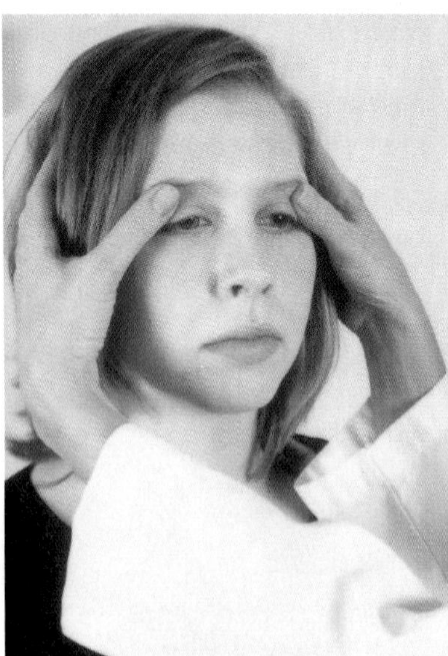

a: Palpating glands

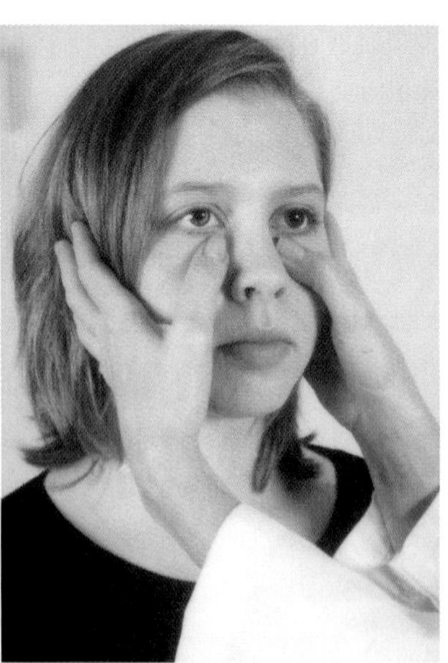

b: Palpating ducts

Nontender; gland nonpalpable

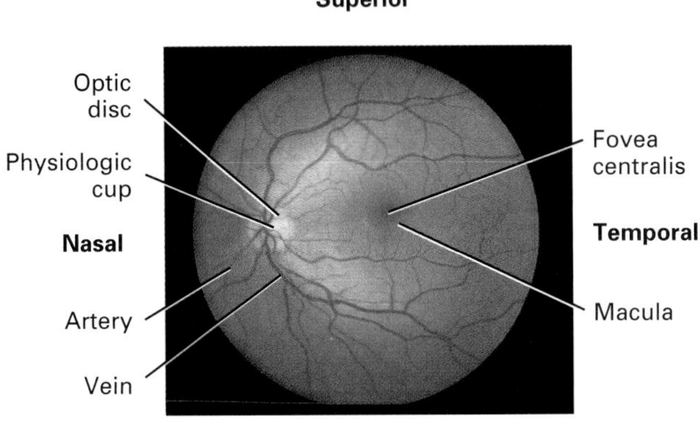

FIGURE 10–13. Normal fundoscopic structures of the left eye with fields (Courtesy of Wills Eye Hospital, Philadelphia, PA).

Assessment of the Internal Structures

The internal structures of the eyes are examined last. Using the ophthalmoscope permits the visualization of the red reflex, optic disc, blood vessels, general background, and macula (Fig. 10–13). Changes in the appearance of these structures can indicate localized eye disorders and eye trauma as well systemic health problems.

The first thing you should see with the ophthalmoscope is a red reflex over the pupil area, which is the reflection of light off the retina. Note the color and clarity of the red reflex. Now gradually move closer to the client while holding the red reflex in sight. When you are approximately 2 inches from the eye, you should see either blood vessels or the general background of the retina. Follow the blood vessels nasally back to their origin at the optic disc. Now examine the optic disc for color, shape, discreteness of the disc margins, and a paler area near the center called the physiological cup. The optic disc is located nasally and has a yellow to yellow-orange color, with sharp distinct edges except for the nasal side, which may be slightly blurred.

Note the size of the physiological cup compared to the size of the optic disc (cup/disc ratio). The cup should be half the size of the disc or less. The cup is normally lighter or white in color. Follow the vessels as they leave the optic disc. Note the size of the arteries compared to the veins (A/V ratio). Arteries will appear smaller and brighter red than veins and will have a light streak reflecting off them. Also note constriction of the vessels and whether or not any nicking is noted when vessels cross. Inspect the general background for color and lesions. Color should be a uniform yellow orange red color, depending on individual skin tone. The lighter the skin tone, the lighter the background. After inspecting the optic disc, vessels, and general background, examine the macula. The macula is a circular area of slightly darker pigmentation located about two disc diameters (DD) temporally from the optic disc. It is the site of central vision and the source of one the most common causes of blindness, macular degeneration. The macula is difficult to see, especially through undilated pupils. To see it, have the client look directly into the ophthalmoscope light. This places the macula into direct view.

HOW TO USE THE OPHTHALMOSCOPE

Because the ophthalmic portion of the eye examination is conducted in a darkened room, you need to be familiar with the parts of the instrument and feel comfortable manipulating the lens and aperture discs while holding the scope in one hand. Hold the ophthalmoscope in the palm of your hand with the brow rest facing toward you. Keep your index finger free so that you can use it to adjust the focusing disc and the light aperture disc. When examining undilated eyes, use the smallest white light aperture. This will cause less constriction of the pupils.

Start with the small round light and the lens focus set at "0." Stand about 1 foot from the client at a 15-degree lateral angle from his or her line of vision. With the client's vision fixed straight ahead, shine the light at the pupil to obtain a red reflex. Hold the scope up to your brow, and move closer to the client while maintaining the red reflex, until you are only a few inches from him or her. Use your right eye to examine the client's right eye and your left eye to examine the client's left eye. As you move toward the client, place your free hand on his or her head near the eye you are examining to stabilize yourself and provide a sense of direction as you approach the eye.

If the retinal structures are not focused, use your index finger to adjust the lens focus. The lens is measured in diopters and indicated as black and red numbers. The black diopters or positive numbers are convex lenses that help you to focus closer; the red diopters or negative numbers are concave lenses that help you to focus farther away. Turn the lens focus disc clockwise to select a positive diopter for farsighted people (indicated with black numbers in the illuminated lens indicator), or rotate the lens focus counterclockwise to use the negative diopters for nearsighted people (usually indicated in red numbers). The amount and degree of focusing needed depend on the combined refractive state of both you and the client.

Ophthalmoscope Apertures

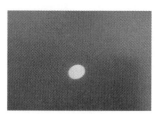

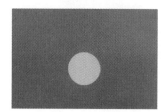

Aperture Type	Purpose
 Small white aperture	Best for examining the undilated eye. Start the eye examination with this setting
 Large white aperture	For general examination of the eye and when pupils are dilated.
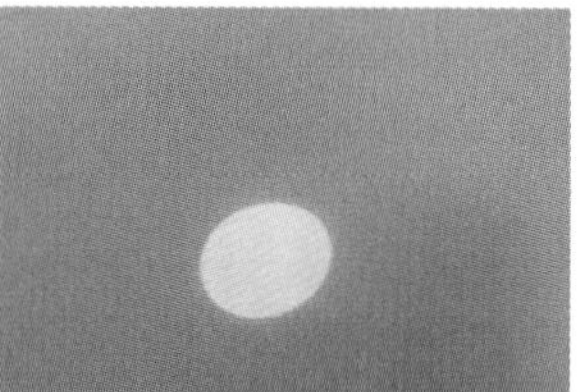 Red-free filter	A green light differentiates hemorrhages, which appear black, from melanin, which looks gray. Also differentiates arteries, which appear black, from veins, which appear blue.
 Blue light	When fluorescein dye is injected into client intravenously, blue filter enables examiner to see movement of dye into eye vessels. Useful for detecting hemorrhages, leaking vessels,or vessel abnormalities.
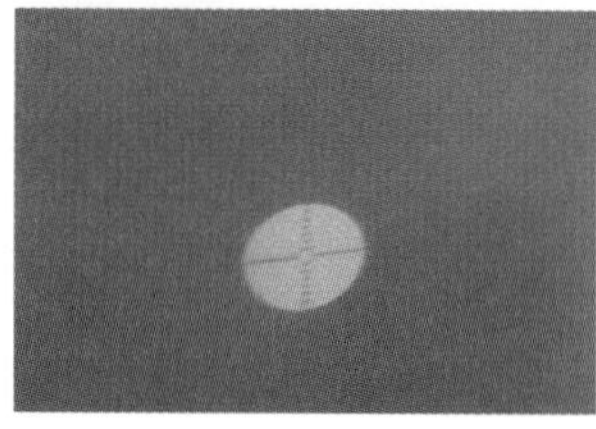 Grid	Used to measure the size or location of lesions.
 Slit or streak	Used to determine levels or depth of lesions.

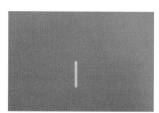

Performing an Ophthalmic Examination

AREA/NORMAL VARIATIONS

Red Reflex

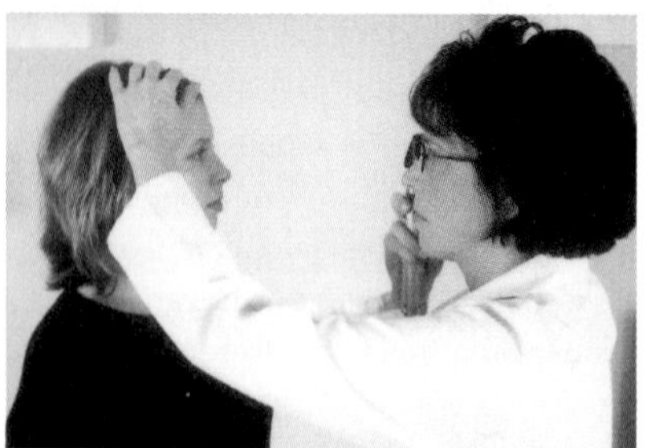

Checking red reflex

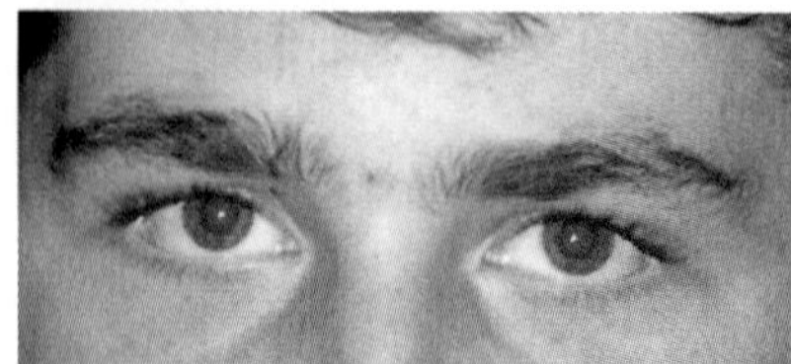

Red reflex over pupil area

ABNORMAL FINDINGS/RATIONALE

Blackened/opaque areas: Cataracts

Dark spots or shadows that interrupt red reflex: Opacities in lens or vitreous humor.

Whitish/gray color: Partial or complete death of optic nerve (optic atrophy).

Blurred margins other than nasally: Hypertension, glaucoma, or papilledema.

Cup-disc ratio greater than 1/2: Open-angle glaucoma.

Large arteriovenous (A/V) ratio: Hypertension.

Narrowed arteries: Severe hypertension, retinitis pigmentosa, and central retinal artery occlusion.

Performing an Ophthalmic Examination

AREA/NORMAL VARIATIONS

Optic Disc

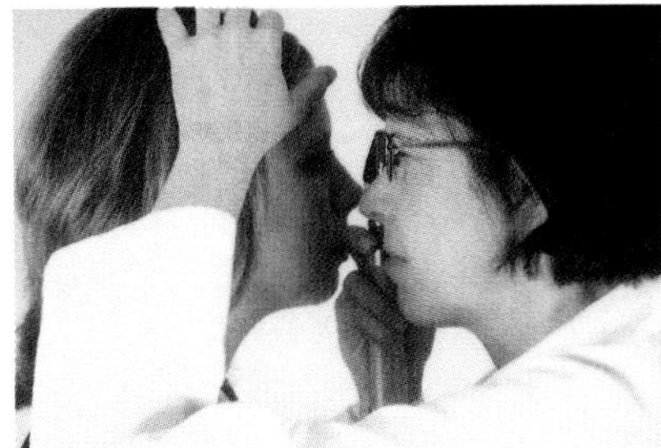

Examining optic disc

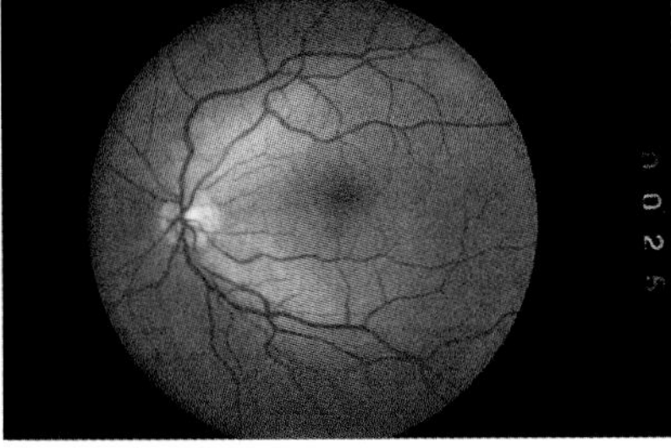

Normal fundus

Yellow-peach color in fair-skinned people, orange in dark-skinned people. Round or oval shape

Disc margins sharply demarcated; nasal edge may be slightly blurred.

Cup-disc ratio: Cup is 1/2 the DD or less. When visible, cup is located centrally in disc and is a lighter color than rest of disc.

Blood Vessels

Arteries and veins are paired.

Arteries are bright red with a light reflex; artery-vein size ratio is 2:3 or 4:5.

Arteries and veins may cross paths within 2 DD of optic disc if no nicking or interruption of blood flow occurs.

General Background

Color ranges from yellow to orange red. Color is even throughout and corresponds with client's skin pigmentation. Light-skinned clients have lighter retinas; dark-skinned clients have darker retinas.

Macula

HELPFUL HINT

The macula is the area of most acute vision and is very sensitive to light, so always examine it last.

Indistinct but darker circular area located 2 DD temporal to the optic disc. Size is about 1 DD.

May see the foveal light reflex, a tiny white dot indicating the ophthalmoscope light shining on the macula.

ABNORMAL FINDINGS/RATIONALE

AV crossings more than 2 DD from optic disc or nicking or pinching of underlying vessel: Hypertension.

White spots with indistinct edges (cotton wool spots): Microinfarctions that occur with diabetes, hypertension, lupus, and papilledema.

Deep intraretinal hemorrhages (dot hemorrhages): Diabetes.

Flame-shaped, superficial hemorrhages: Hypertension.

Excess or clumped pigment: Trauma or retinal detachment.

Hemorrhage or exudate in macula: Macular degeneration. See page 282 for illustrations.

(*Continued*)

Performing an Ophthalmic Examination *(Continued)*

AREA/NORMAL VARIATIONS | **ABNORMAL FINDINGS/RATIONALE**

Abnormalities of the Optic Disk

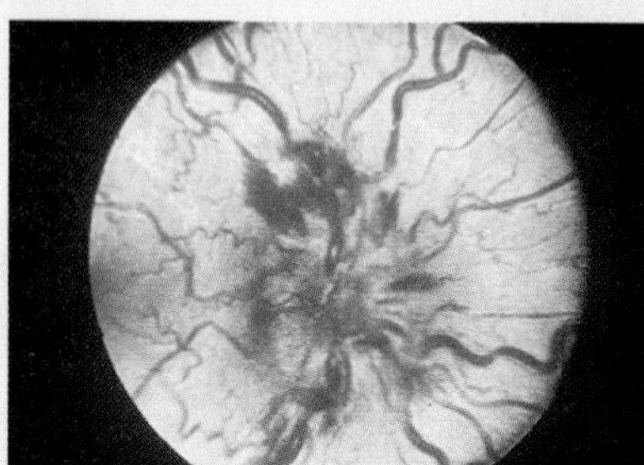
a: Acute papilledema

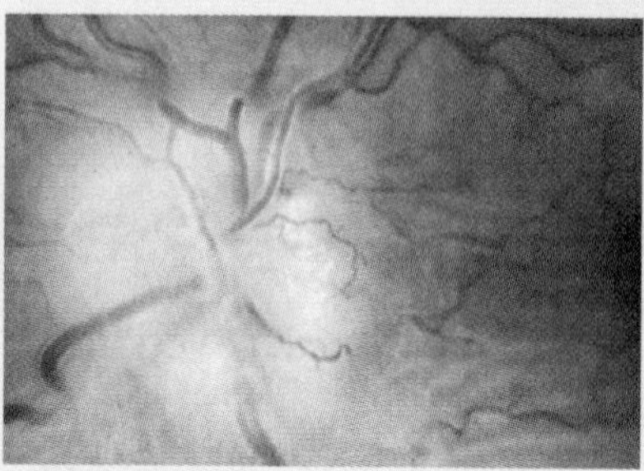
b: Chronic papilledema

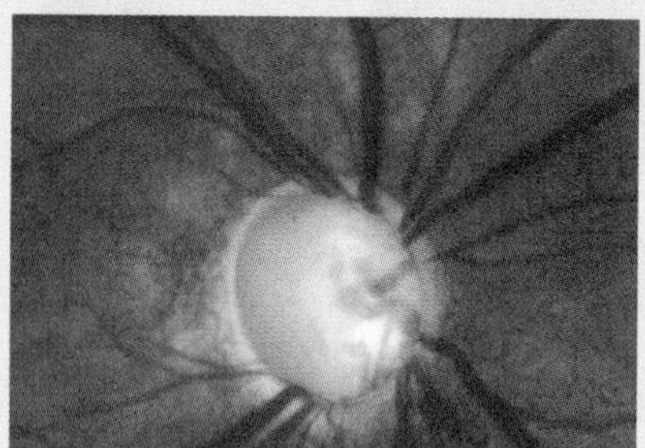
Glaucomatous optic nerve

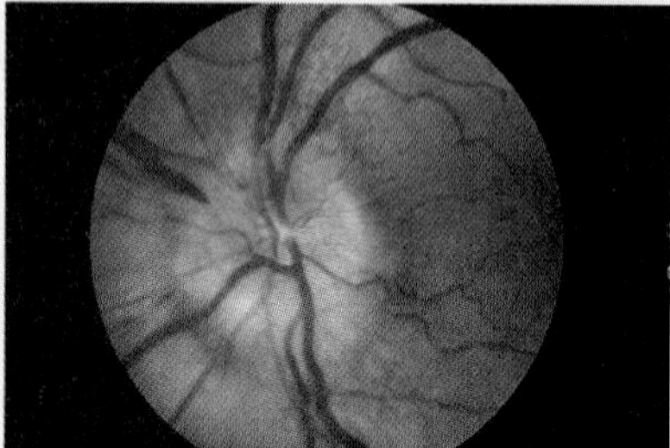
Optic neuritis

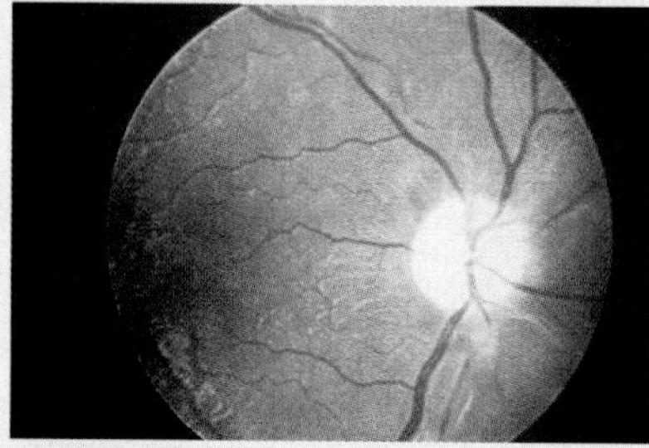
Optic nerve pallor

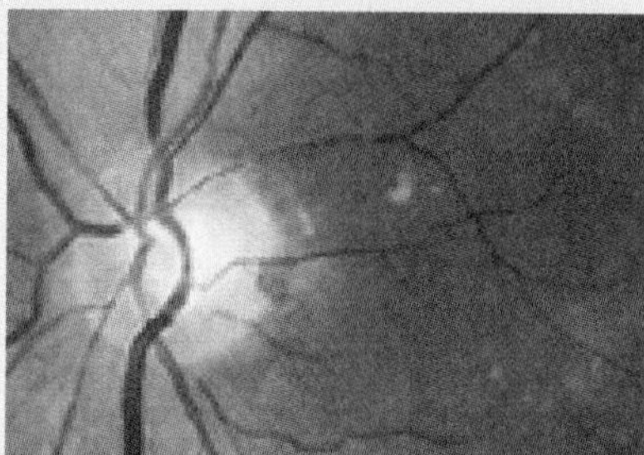
Hypertensive changes

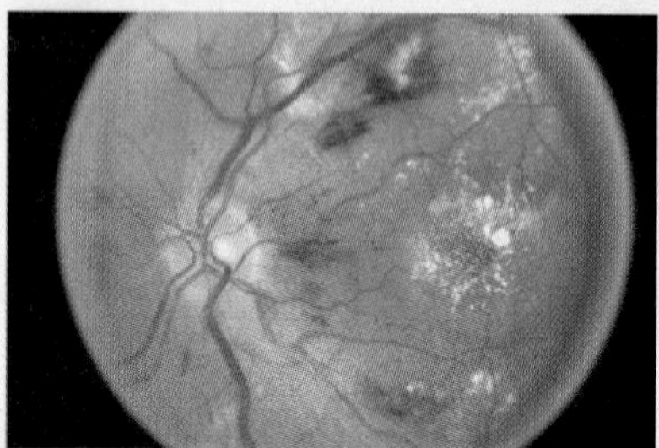
Diabetic retinopathy

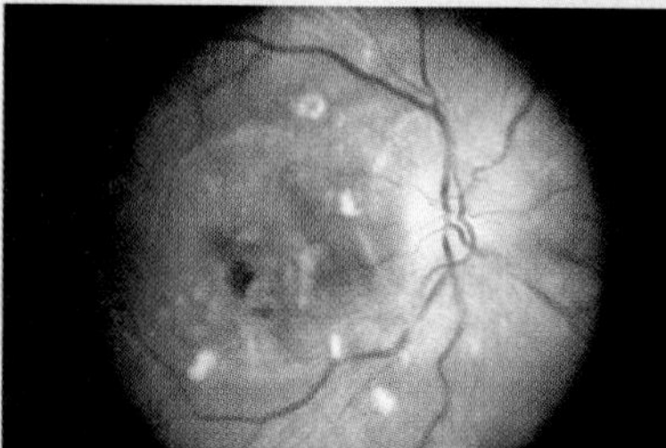
Malignant hypertension

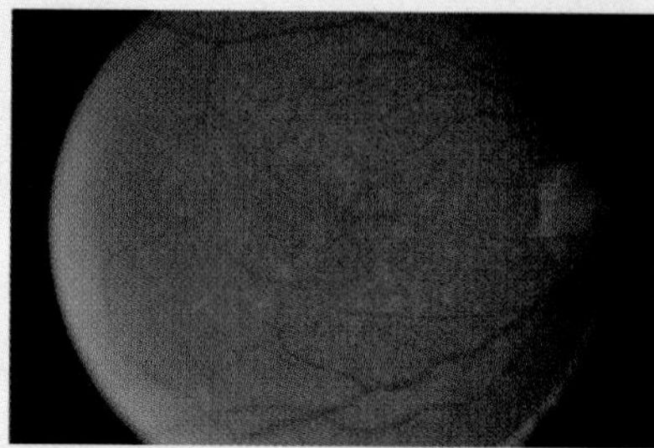
Age-related macular degeneration ("dry")—vision 20/20

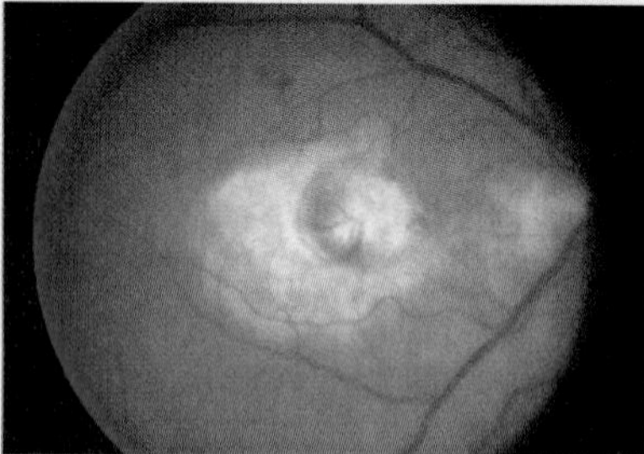
Advanced macular degeneration ("wet")—vision 20/400

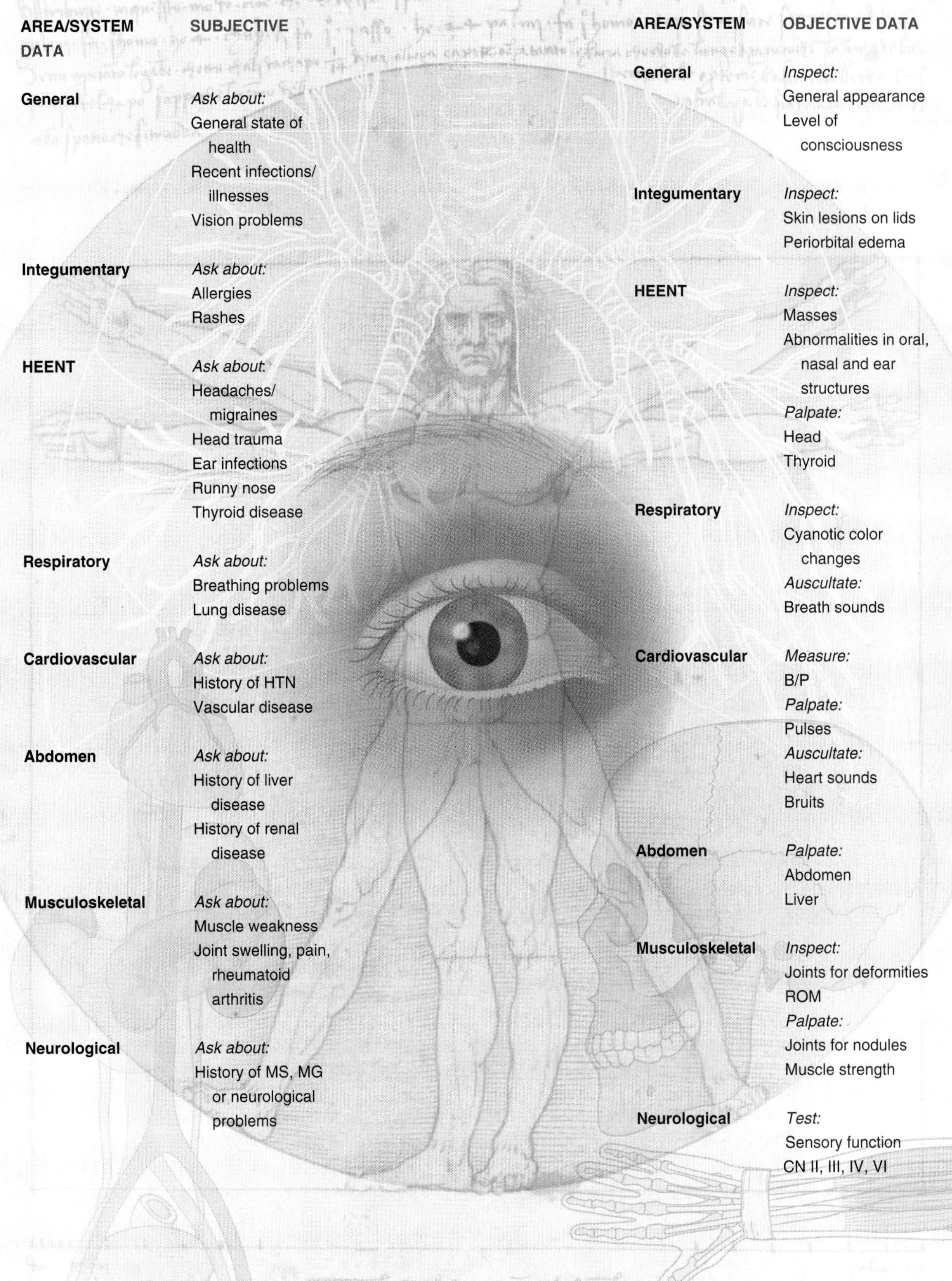

AREA/SYSTEM	SUBJECTIVE DATA
General	*Ask about:* General state of health Recent infections/ illnesses Vision problems
Integumentary	*Ask about:* Allergies Rashes
HEENT	*Ask about:* Headaches/ migraines Head trauma Ear infections Runny nose Thyroid disease
Respiratory	*Ask about:* Breathing problems Lung disease
Cardiovascular	*Ask about:* History of HTN Vascular disease
Abdomen	*Ask about:* History of liver disease History of renal disease
Musculoskeletal	*Ask about:* Muscle weakness Joint swelling, pain, rheumatoid arthritis
Neurological	*Ask about:* History of MS, MG or neurological problems

AREA/SYSTEM	OBJECTIVE DATA
General	*Inspect:* General appearance Level of consciousness
Integumentary	*Inspect:* Skin lesions on lids Periorbital edema
HEENT	*Inspect:* Masses Abnormalities in oral, nasal and ear structures *Palpate:* Head Thyroid
Respiratory	*Inspect:* Cyanotic color changes *Auscultate:* Breath sounds
Cardiovascular	*Measure:* B/P *Palpate:* Pulses *Auscultate:* Heart sounds Bruits
Abdomen	*Palpate:* Abdomen Liver
Musculoskeletal	*Inspect:* Joints for deformities ROM *Palpate:* Joints for nodules Muscle strength
Neurological	*Test:* Sensory function CN II, III, IV, VI

Assessment of the Eyes' Relationship to Other Systems

Case Study Findings

Mrs. Scammel's focused physical assessment findings include:

- Near vision blurred, Snellen deferred, can see fingers at 10 feet, peripheral vision 70 degrees temporally, other fields within normal limits.
- Cardinal fields of gaze without nystagmus or eyelid lag.
- Eyelids without lesions, conjunctiva pink without excessive tearing or drainage.
- No periorbital edema; lacrimal gland nonpalpable.
- Cornea hazy in OD, clear in OS, smooth bilaterally, arcus senilis bilaterally.
- Iris and pupil within normal limits (wnl); pupils equal, round, react to light and accommodation (PERRLA).
- Ophthalmic exam OD: red reflex obscured, disc margins blurred, AV ratio 2:3 with nicking noted 1–1/2 DD inferiorly at 5 o'clock. OS: Red reflex present, disc margins blurred, nicking noted superiorly 1 1/2 DD at 2 o'clock. OU: scattered dot hemorrhages throughout, deep pigmentation of macula, no fovea light reflex.

Case Study Analysis and Plan

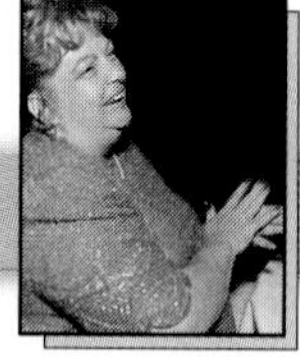

Now that you have completed a thorough assessment of Mrs. Scammel, document your key history and physical examination findings. List key history findings and key physical examination findings for Mrs. Scammel that will help you formulate your nursing diagnoses. Cluster the supporting data and list possible additional nursing diagnoses.

CRITICAL THINKING ACTIVITY #8

Identify some nursing diagnoses for Mrs. Scammel, select one, and develop a brief nursing care plan and a teaching plan for her, including learning outcomes and teaching strategies.

Research Tells Us

The Food and Drug Administration (FDA) has approved a new therapy for the wet form of macular degeneration, the most severe form. A type of photodynamic therapy, it involves the use of a light-activating drug called Visudyne. After the drug is administered, a nonthermal laser beam is aimed at the abnormal blood vessel. The laser stimulates the light-activating drug and causes destruction of the abnormal blood vessel. Unlike conventional laser therapy, the cool laser causes very little damage to the areas surrounding the blood vessel, thus avoiding additional visual loss. The therapy does not restore lost vision but does prevent additional vision loss. Familiarity with this photodynamic therapy will help the nurse provide and reinforce pre- and postoperative education for the client receiving this therapy.

Source: Hoglund, T. (2000). Food and Drug Administration approves photodynamic therapy in the treatment of wet AMD. The Foundation Fighting Blindness (Available online at *http://www.blindness.org*)

Health Concerns

The American Academy of Ophthalmology recommends a comprehensive vision examination including visual acuity and glaucoma by an ophthalmologist:

- Every 3 to 5 years for African-Americans ages 20 to 39
- Every 2 to 4 years for anyone ages 40 to 64 regardless of race
- Every 1 to 2 years starting at age 65
- Yearly for anyone with diabetes (Department of Health and Human Services, 1998)
- Strabismus screening is done in preschool because, if undetected or left untreated in a child before the age of 4 to 6, blindness can result from disuse. Color vision screening is usually done for boys between the ages of 4 and 8.

Common Abnormalities

ABNORMALITY	ASSESSMENT FINDINGS
Astigmatism Refraction of light rays diffused rather than sharply focused on retina	• History of blurred vision • Corneal irregularity
Cataract Abnormal, progressive opacity of the lens	• Pupil may appear cloudy. • Red reflex absent or darkened.
Conjunctivitis Irritation and inflammation of bulbar and palpebral conjunctiva One of most common sources of eye discomfort Typically caused by allergies, viruses, or bacterial infections	• Manifests as redness of the palpebral conjunctiva and bloodshot sclera • Purulent drainage usually present if caused by infection
Cranial Nerve Palsy	• Limited range of motion in one or more cardinal fields of gaze • May have eyelid lag, asymmetrical palpebral fissures, or unequal pupil size
Glaucoma Second leading cause of blindness worldwide	• Changes in optic disc and visual fields. • Signs and symptoms include protrusion of posterior chamber into anterior chamber, crescent shadow, firm eyeball, blurred optic disc margins, loss of peripheral vision and depth perception, contrast sensitivity.
Two main types: primary open angle glaucoma (POAG) and primary angle closure glaucoma (PACG)	• May be asymptomatic. • POAG associated with loss of central vision and elevated eye pressure, but excessive eye pressure is not required for diagnosis. • Acute PACG may present with acute symptoms including red eye, dilated pupil, nausea, vomiting, eye pain, and halos around lights. Assessment of the anterior chamber with oblique flashlight test often reveals forward bowing of iris.
Iritis Inflammation of iris that manifests as cloudy or reddened iris with	• Symptoms include severe eye pain, tearing, sensitivity to light (photophobia), and, in severe cases, diminished visual acuity. • If untreated, scarring and permanently diminished vision occur.

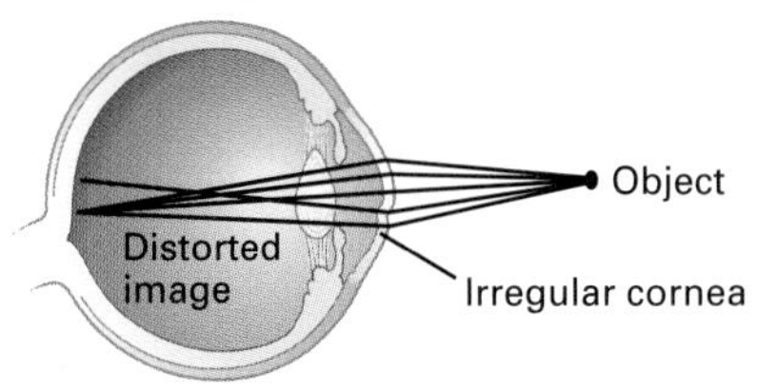

Astigmatism

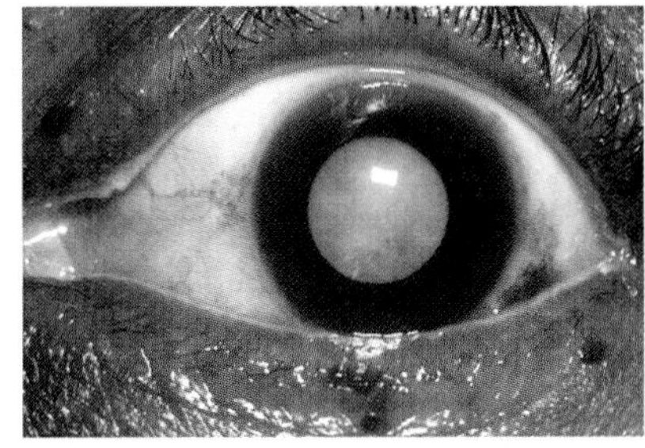

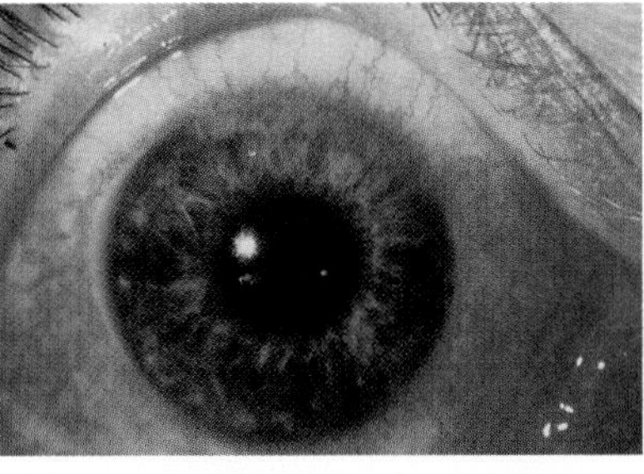

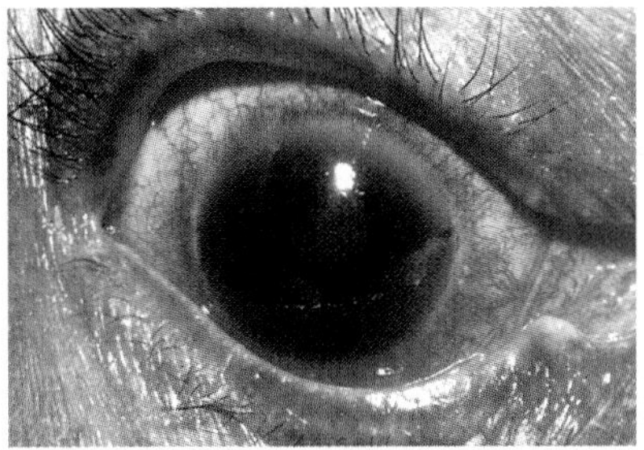

(Continued)

Common Abnormalities *(Continued)*

ABNORMALITY	ASSESSMENT FINDINGS
Iritis ***(Continued)*** constricted pupil. Blood vessels may be visible in iris.	
Macular Degeneration	• Diminished visual acuity • Loss of central vision • Increased pigmentation of macula 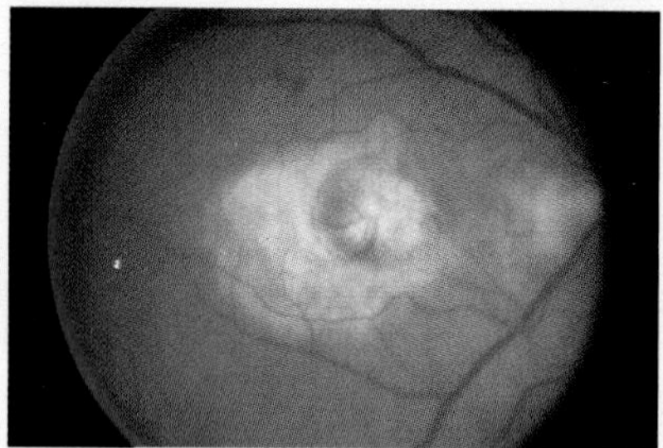
Pinguecula Painless yellow nodule caused by thickening of bulbar conjunctiva	• Usually located nasally • Often caused by exposure to sunlight or wind 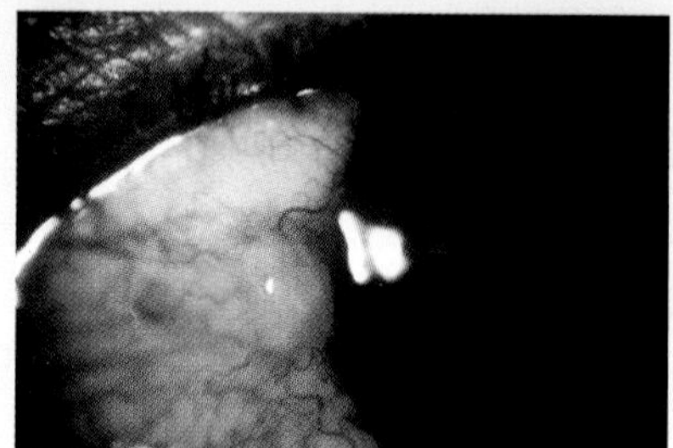
Presbyopia Occurs with aging	• Decreased elasticity of the lens • Results in decreased ability to focus on near objects
Pterygium Triangular growth of the bulbar conjunctiva from the nasal side of the eye toward the pupil	• Can obstruct vision if growth occludes the pupil 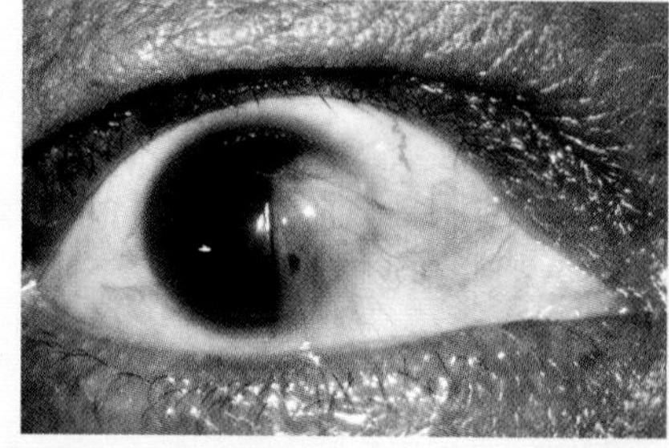
Retinal Detachment Separation of retinal layer and choroid layer in back of eye	• Signs usually develop gradually. • Initial symptoms include seeing large numbers of floaters (resolves after several days), seeing flashing lights when the eyes move, and seeing a slowly expanding shadow in the lateral fields of gaze. • Untreated retinal detachment results in irreversible blindness.
Retinitis Pigmentosa Degeneration of retina. Begins in childhood and may progress to blindness by middle adulthood. Photoreceptors in retina, known as rods, are initially affected, followed by the cones.	• Earlier signs may include night blindness, reduced visual fields, pigmentation of the retina, and macular degeneration.
Sjögren's Syndrome Immunologic disorder in which lacrimal, salivary, and other glands do not produce enough moisture	• Causes dryness of the mouth, eyes, and other mucous membranes. • Damage to external eye tissues, such as the cornea and conjunctiva, may result from excessive and prolonged dryness.

Common Abnormalities

ABNORMALITY	ASSESSMENT FINDINGS
Strabismus Axis of eye deviates and does not fixate on an object Also called crossed or wall eye Caused by weak intraocular muscles or a lesion on the occulomotor nerve Types: Convergent strabismus (esotropia) and divergent strabismus (exotropia)	• Causes disconjugate vision (one eye deviates from fixated image). • Initially, diplopia results as each eye transmits the images received. • Eventually, brain suppresses images received from deviating or weak eye. • After a period of disuse, visual acuity in the weak eye deteriorates and loss of vision results. • Treatment before age 6 is necessary to prevent permanent damage.

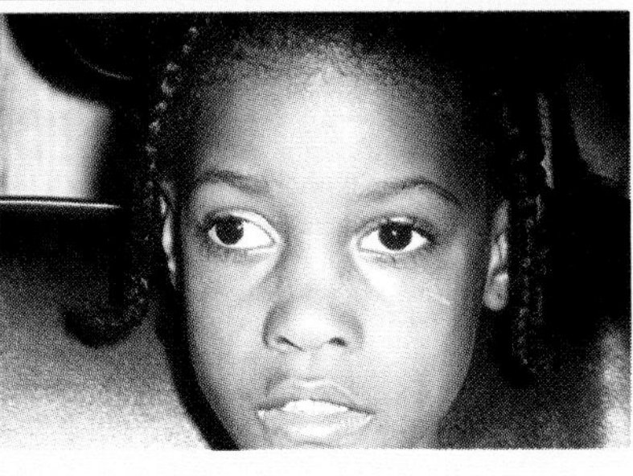

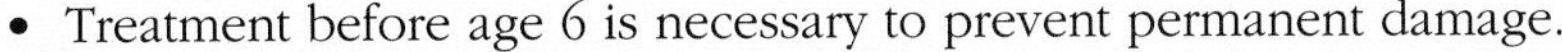

Summary

- A thorough health history provides direction for the physical examination, including exploration of factors that may be related to eye health.
- Information from both the history and the physical examination is then analyzed to determine appropriate nursing diagnoses.
- The eyes are complex sensory organs that provide specialized functions crucial to neurosensory development in infancy; the development of psychosocial, motor, and cognitive skills in childhood; and the maintenance of those skills in adulthood.
- A comprehensive history and physical examination enable early detection and treatment of sight problems.

Anatomy and Physiology Review: The Ear

The main functions of the ears are hearing and equilibrium. Hearing requires an intact and unobstructed external canal, middle and inner ear, vestibulocochlear nerve (CN VIII), and temporal lobe (Figs. 10–14 and 10–15). Sound waves move through the external, middle, and inner ear, where they stimulate the vestibulocochlear nerve and transmit the impulses to the temporal lobe for interpretation. Maintaining normal equilibrium requires proper functioning of the structures in the inner ear.

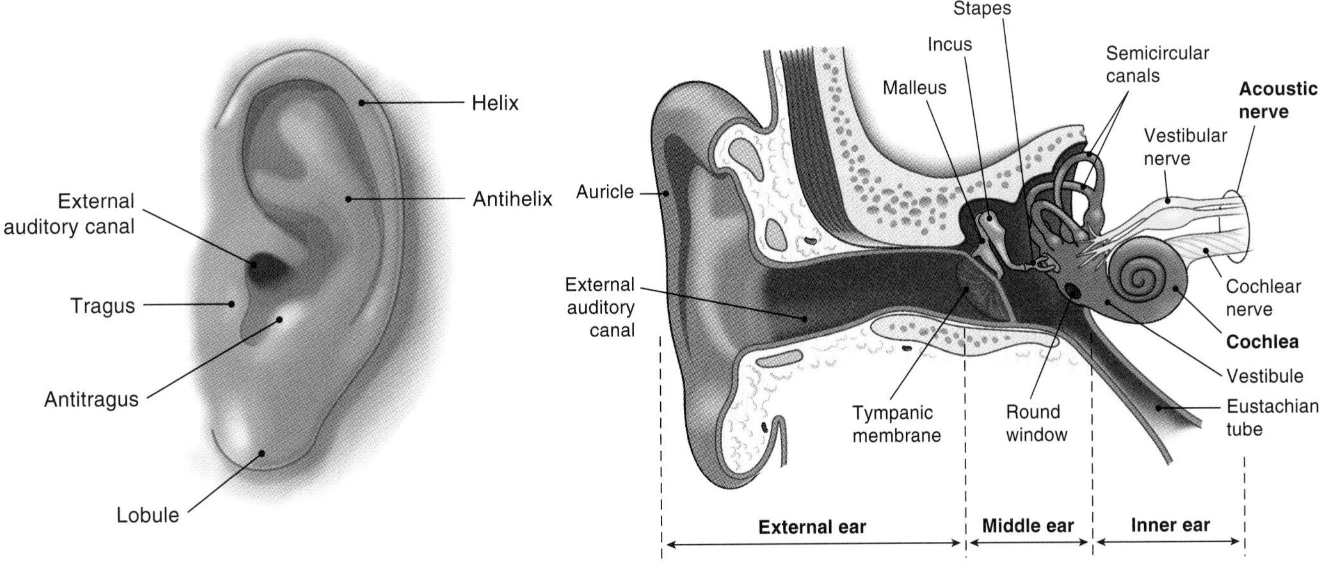

FIGURE 10–14. External ear.

FIGURE 10–15. Cross section of ear.

Structures and Functions of the Ear

The three parts of the ear—external, middle, and inner—contain anatomical structures that work together to allow us to hear.

Structures and Functions of the Ear

STRUCTURE	FUNCTION
External Ear	
Auricle	Cartilaginous external ear whose shape is useful in collecting and conveying sound waves to the middle ear.
External Ear Canal (Meatus)	One-inch (2.5-cm) canal that connects the auricle to the tympanic membrane. Outer third is cartilage; inner two-thirds covers the temporal bone. Contains fine hair and glands that secrete cerumen (ear wax). Fine hair and cerumen protect the canal from insects and foreign matter. Cerumen also keeps canal lubricated. Canal protects tympanic membrane from external environmental factors, such as temperature and humidity changes, that might affect the elasticity of the drum.
Middle Ear	
Tympanic Membrane (Eardrum)	Thin, fibrous, pearl-gray membrane that separates the external ear from the middle ear. Slightly concave and pulled in near the center by the malleus. Conducts sound waves to ossicles.
Tympanic Cavity	Small, air-filled space in temporal bone that contains the ossicles. Contains the oval and round windows. The eustachian tube also opens into the middle ear.
Eustachian Tube	The auditory tube from the middle ear to the nasopharynx that maintains equal pressure on both sides of the tympanic membrane.
Auditory Ossicles (Malleus, Incus, and Stapes)	The smallest bones of the body, they transmit sound waves to the inner ear.
Inner ear	
Bony Labyrinth	Contains the vestibule, the central chamber of the labyrinth, which in turn contains the utricle and saccule, sacs filled with endolymph and sensory receptors. Three semicircular canals that contain receptor structures called crista ampullaris. The utricle, saccule, and semicircular canals affect equilibrium.
Cochlea	Shell-like structure containing perilymph-filled scala vestibuli and scala tympani and endolymph-filled scala media. Transmits sound vibrations.
Spiral Organ of Corti	Organ of hearing composed of supporting cells and hair cells that transmit to CN VIII (vestibulocochlear nerve).

Understanding Sounds and Sound Waves

Hearing occurs by air conduction and bone conduction of sound waves. Sound waves are characterized by differences in pitch and loudness. Frequency, the number of sound waves per second, determines the pitch of the sound. Intensity or loudness is determined by the size of the sound waves. Sound waves can be classified on a continuum from high-pitched to low-pitched—for example, the high-pitched sounds of a whistle blowing or the screech of chalk on a chalkboard or the low-pitched sounds of a deep drum, thunder, or an explosion. The highness or lowness of pitch is a function of frequency or how fast or slow a sound wave vibrates. The frequency of a sound wave is measured in waves per seconds or hertz (Hz). Low-frequency sound waves are interpreted by the brain as low-pitched sounds and higher frequency waves are interpreted as high-pitched sounds.

The loudness of a sound wave is measured in a scale of units called decibels (dB). The structures on the inner ear are especially sensitive to loudness. Although we tolerate conversation, which is typically around 60 dB, exposure to excessive or repeated noise above 80 dB such as traffic or machinery noise or exposure to rock music concerts at 120 dB or more can cause damage to the hearing structures and result in permanent hearing loss.

How We Hear

Air conduction is the primary mechanism of hearing and involves carrying sound waves through the external auditory canal to the tympanic membrane. There the sound vibrations cause the tympanic membrane and the malleus (hammer), incus (anvil), and stapes (stirrup) bones to move, thus transmitting the vibrations to the inner ear structures.

Bone conduction provides an additional pathway whereby sound waves vibrate the skull bones and transmit the vibrations to the inner ear structures. Both air and bone conduction use a common final pathway involving transmission of the vibrations to the inner ear structures, then on to the cranial nerve and the temporal lobe (Fig. 10–16).

Interaction with Other Body Systems

The Musculoskeletal System

Normal hearing involves proper functioning of certain skeletal structures. Hearing by air conduction involves the transmission of sound waves that vibrate the tympanic membrane, which in turn transfers the vibrations

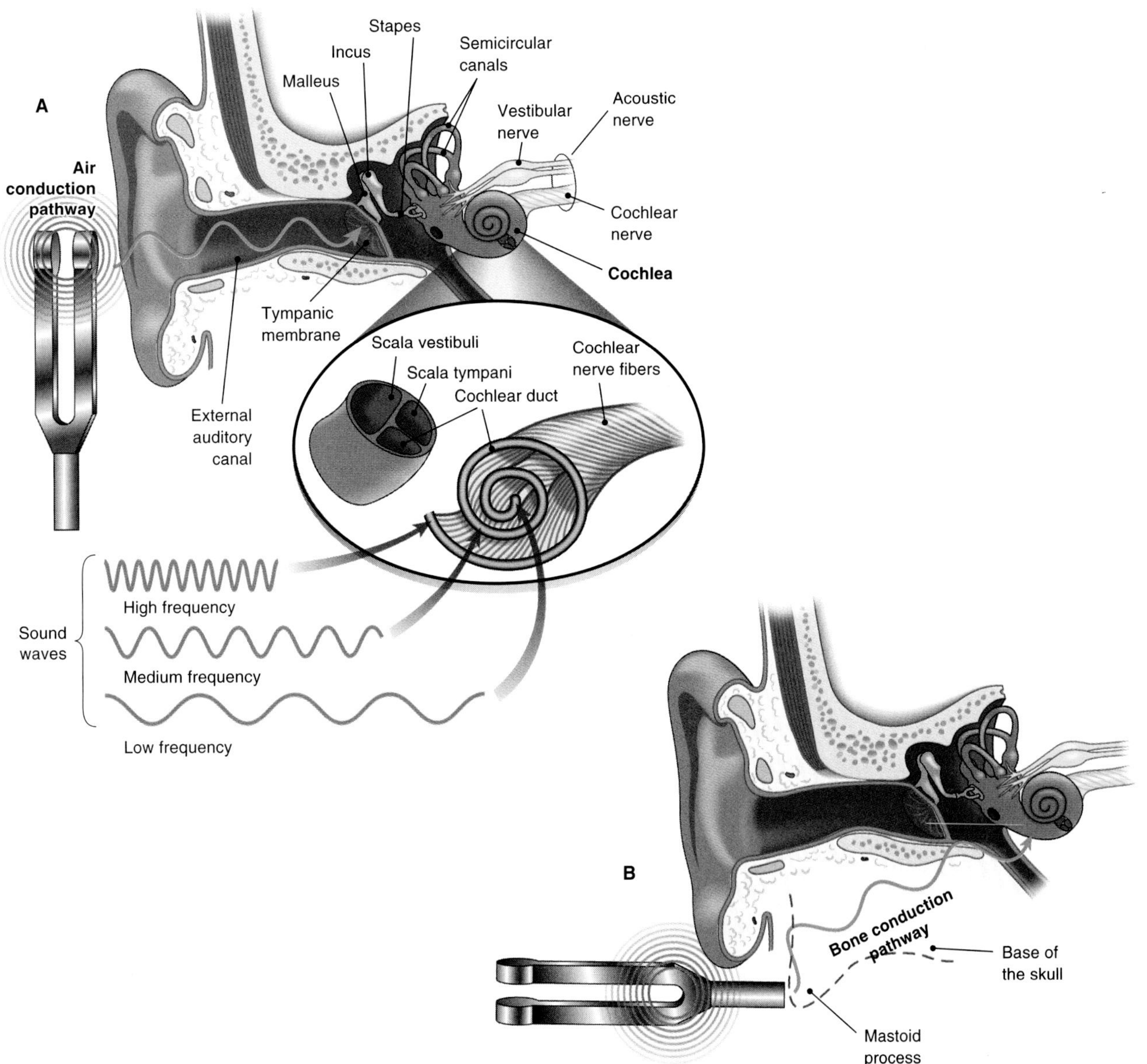

FIGURE 10–16. Transmission of sound. *A*. Air conduction, *B*. Bone conduction.

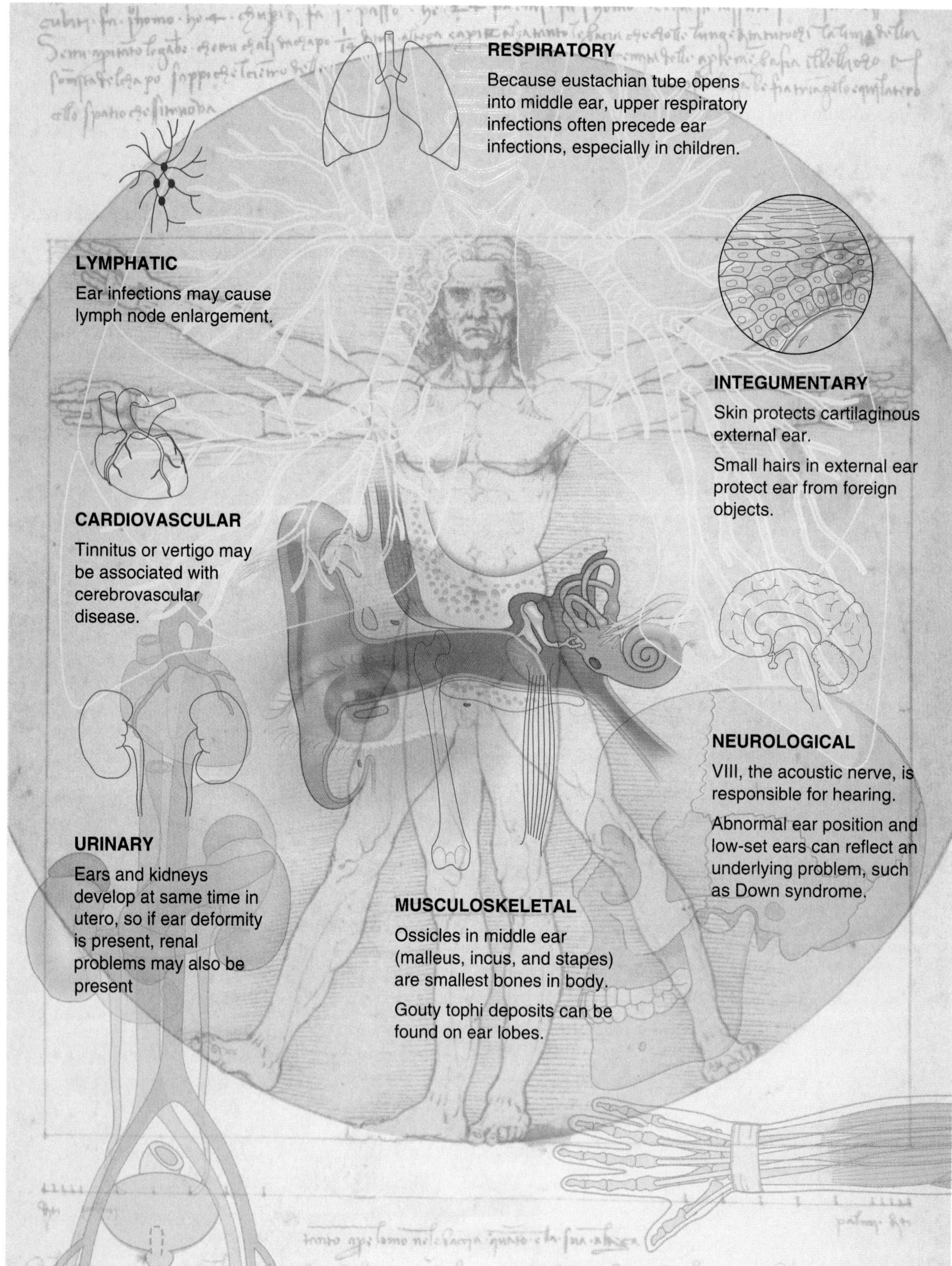

RESPIRATORY
Because eustachian tube opens into middle ear, upper respiratory infections often precede ear infections, especially in children.
LYMPHATIC
Ear infections may cause lymph node enlargement.
INTEGUMENTARY
Skin protects cartilaginous external ear.
Small hairs in external ear protect ear from foreign objects.
CARDIOVASCULAR
Tinnitus or vertigo may be associated with cerebrovascular disease.
NEUROLOGICAL
VIII, the acoustic nerve, is responsible for hearing.
Abnormal ear position and low-set ears can reflect an underlying problem, such as Down syndrome.
URINARY
Ears and kidneys develop at same time in utero, so if ear deformity is present, renal problems may also be present
MUSCULOSKELETAL
Ossicles in middle ear (malleus, incus, and stapes) are smallest bones in body.
Gouty tophi deposits can be found on ear lobes.

Relationship of the Ears to Other Systems

to the three auditory ossicles. First, the malleus, which is in direct contact with the tympanic membrane, receives the vibrations. The malleus then transfers the vibrations to the incus and then to the stapes, which transmits it directly to the oval window in the inner ear.

Hearing by bone conduction is much less precise and is dominant only when hearing by air conduction is not possible because of obstruction or perforation of the tympanic membrane, fluid behind the membrane, or otosclerosis of the auditory ossicles. Nevertheless, hearing by bone conduction also relies on an intact skeletal structure, the temporal bone, to transmit vibrations to the inner ear. Cooperation between the neurological and skeletal systems is necessary to provide precise and accurate hearing.

The Neurological System

The primary functions of the ears, hearing and equilibrium, rely strongly on an intact and functioning neurological system. Whether hearing occurs solely by air conduction or bone conduction, the sound waves must eventually travel to the inner ear, where they are picked up by the organ of Corti, the sensory organ for hearing. Hair cells in the organ of Corti bend and mediate the vibrations into electrical impulses that are conducted to the vestibulocochlear nerve (CN VIII). The process of picking up sound waves, transmitting them, converting them to electrical impulses, and transmitting them to the brain represents only the first of three levels of auditory functioning.

The second level involves the interaction of both ears and the brainstem in determining the location of the sound in space. When a sound is heard, the vestibulocochlear nerve from each ear sends electrical impulses to each side of the brainstem. The brainstem pinpoints the origin of the sound by evaluating factors such as head position, intensity and timing of the information received from each ear.

The cortex of the brain, specifically the temporal lobe, is involved in the third level of auditory function, interpretation of the sound. Once sound waves have been converted to electrical impulses, they are received in the temporal lobe, where they are identified on the basis of past experience. Impulses are then sent to motor areas of the brain so that an appropriate response to the sound can be made. This level of response allows us to differentiate a telephone ring from a doorbell and take the action needed to either pick up the phone or answer the door. As for maintaining equilibrium, the vestibule of the inner ear plays a crucial role. The vestibule is involved in sensing and perceiving how the body is moving in space. The vestibule also orients the body to maintain a vertical position, stabilizes the position of the head, and helps to maintain the center of gravity.

Disorders of equilibrium can result from two primary causes. The first is chronic loss of vestibular information caused by eighth cranial nerve and vestibular hair cell degeneration related to aging or neurotoxicity. The second is distortion of information produced by disruption of the fluid dynamics in the labyrinth of the inner ear. With chronic degeneration, problems with balance are more constant and the person can adapt to them to some degree if the terrain remains constant. However, persons with disorders involving disruption or distortion tend to have symptoms more intermittently and unpredictably, thus preventing the person from adapting as readily. In addition, movement of the head may trigger the vestibular receptors to signal the brain that the head and body are moving when in fact they are not.

Developmental, Cultural, and Ethnic Variations

Infants and Children

The structures needed for hearing are predominantly developed in utero during the first trimester. During this time, damage to the structures from genetic, congenital, and infectious processes can cause hearing problems. Assessment of the ear is especially important in infancy. Observing the appearance of the external ear and noting behaviors that indicate intact hearing are important ways to screen for potential problems that can cause developmental delays or indicate genetic conditions. Abnormalities in the structure and positioning of the ears are more common in infants who have a hearing deficit. Low-set ears, ears that are positioned at greater than a 15-degree angle, and malformed ears are often associated with genetic disorders and developmental delays.

Infants and children are more prone to inner ear infections than adults. One reason is that the eustachian tube, which opens from the nasopharynx to the middle ear, is shorter, wider, and more horizontal than in adults, making migration of bacteria from the nasopharynx common. Infants also have greater amounts of lymphoidal tissue surrounding the lumen of the eustachian tube, which can occlude and trap bacteria. By school age, the external auditory canal has assumed a straighter, more adult configuration, which is less prone to infection (Fig. 10–17).

Young and Middle-Aged Adults

Conductive hearing loss caused by excessive or chronic exposure to noise damages the cochlear structures of the inner ear that are involved in conduction of vibrations to the eighth cranial nerve. Noise-induced hearing loss from

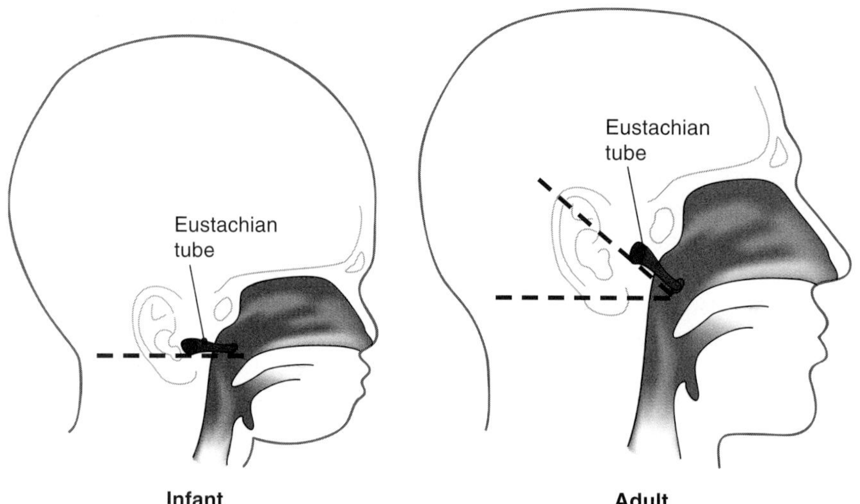

FIGURE 10–17. *A.* Infant ear canal, *B.* Adult ear canal.

exposure to loud music or machinery is the most common cause of hearing loss for the 20-to-40 age group.

Older Adults

Hearing loss in older adults is extremely common and can be associated with sensorineural loss or conductive loss. Hearing loss associated with aging, referred to as presbycusis, occurs around the fifth decade and gradually progresses. Typically, presbycusis involves hearing loss for high-pitched sounds such as consonants and affects men more often than women.

Older adults are prone to stiffening of the cilia in the external canal. This impedes the transmission of sound waves to the tympanic membrane and causes cerumen to accumulate more readily and obstruct the membrane. Excess accumulation of cerumen impairs hearing by air conduction and is one of the most common correctable causes of conductive hearing loss in older adults.

People of Different Cultures/Ethnic Groups

Several variations in ear structure and disorders of the ear are known to occur in certain ethnic groups. Otitis media, or middle ear infection, is a relatively common affliction in infants as a result of bottle feeding and exposure to second-hand smoke. However, the incidence and severity of otitis media for Native American, Hispanic, and Alaskan infants is higher than for infants in the general population.

The characteristics of cerumen, or ear wax, also vary with different ethnic groups. Cerumen can be of two types—dry, white, and flaky, as seen in the majority of Asians and Native Americans; or brown, wet, and sticky as seen in the majority of blacks and whites. People living in highly industrialized communities are routinely exposed to sounds above 80 dB, such as traffic and occupational machinery, and are more prone to hearing loss. In the United States, conductive hearing loss caused by noise affects more than one million people and is one of the most prevalent occupational disorders.

Introducing the Case Study

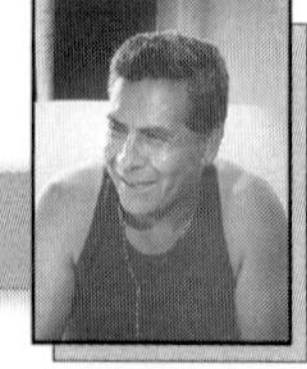

Pablo Arnez is a 50-year-old constuction supervisor. He is the sole support of his two teen-aged children (ages 14 and 16) and his physically disabled wife. He has worked in construction for 15 years. He has a clinic appointment to discuss "problems with my ears" that make it increasingly difficult for him to function in the work environment.

Performing the Ear Assessment

Assessment of the ear involves obtaining a complete health history and performing a physical examination. As you perform the assessment, be alert for signs and symptoms of actual or potential problems in the various structures of the ear.

Health History

The health history identifies any related symptoms or risk factors and the presence of diseases involving the ear. It must also detect any other disorders that may affect the ear. Your history will include obtaining biographical data and asking questions about the client's current health, past health, and family and psychosocial history. It also includes a review of systems and a focused ear history. If your client has severe hearing problems, you may have to communicate by writing or have a family member answer questions.

Biographical Data

Review the client's biographical data to identify age, occupation, gender, and ethnic background. Use these client characteristics to guide the types of health history questions that you ask and facilitate your interpretation of subsequent history and examination findings. For example, the techniques used to examine an infant's ear differ from those used to inspect an adult's ear. The types of assessments you perform for hearing acuity also vary greatly with the client's age. Knowledge of the client's cultural and ethnic heritage can provide information on potential language barriers and can facilitate the evaluation of physical examination findings that vary with different groups. Knowing the client's occupation can provide information about environmental risk for ear trauma and can help identify areas for health promotion education.

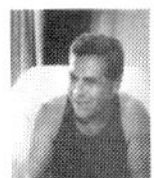

Case Study Findings

Reviewing Mr. Arnez's biographical data:

- Married, 50-year-old father of two (ages 14 and 16).
- Full-time construction supervisor with bachelor's degree.
- Family's main source of financial support; wife is disabled.
- Carries HMO insurance through his employer that covers entire family.
- Native American and Spanish descent; practicing Catholic.
- Source of biographical data is client, who appears reliable.

Current Health Status

First, ask the client to describe the chief complaint in his or her own words. Next, use the PQRST format to investigate further about any symptoms reported. If your client reports an ear problem, focus your questions on the ear symptoms presented in the following section.

HELPFUL HINT

- If a hearing deficit is known to exist, determine whether the client can be interviewed orally, or if written questioning would be more effective. If you use oral questioning, be sure to face the client at all times while asking questions and have your face adequately illuminated.
- Hearing impairment in older adults tends to involve high-tone frequency loss. To facilitate communication, use a deeper tone of voice.

Symptom Analysis

Symptom Analysis tables for all of the symptoms described in the following paragraphs are available on the Web for viewing and printing. In your Web browser, go to *http://www.fadavis.com/detail.cfm?id=0882-9* and click on Symptom Analysis Tables under Explore This Product.

Hearing Loss

Hearing loss is a diminished ability to perceive sounds. It may be a result of problems that affect transmission of sound waves to the middle ear (conductive loss) or problems involving interpreting the sound and converting it to neurological impulses (sensorineural loss). Hearing loss may be sudden or gradual, unilateral or bilateral, and may be limited to sounds of certain frequencies or pitches.

Vertigo

Vertigo is a subjective feeling of the body moving or swaying in space or of stationary objects moving or spinning in space. Vertigo most often results from a disturbance of structures involved with equilibrium and balance, which includes the inner ear and central nervous system.

Tinnitus

Tinnitus is a subjective perception of a high-pitched ringing or buzzing sound in one or both ears. It occurs in certain disorders of the external, middle, and inner ear.

Ear Drainage (Otorrhea)

Drainage from the ear is abnormal. Purulent drainage indicates infection; drainage that is clear or contains CSF or blood indicates trauma.

Earache (Otalgia)

Ear pain, known as earache or **otalgia,** is a common symptom of ear disorders, particularly ear infections.

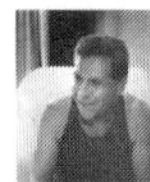

Case Study Findings

Mr. Arnez's current health status includes:

- Chief complaint is intermittent fullness and pressure in both ears for past 2 weeks.
- Denies precipitating factors such as recent upper respiratory infection or recent altitude changes.
- Related symptoms include intermittent, bilateral hearing loss described as "like hearing in a tunnel" and intermittent dizziness.
- Rates severity of his ear fullness and pressure as 7 on a 10-point scale.
- Denies ear pain, drainage, or recent trauma to the ears.

Past Health History

During this section of the health history interview, focus on gathering relevant information about the client's childhood illnesses and injuries, adult illness and injuries, and medication use as they relate to the ears.

Past Health History

RISK FACTORS/QUESTIONS TO ASK	RATIONALE/SIGNIFICANCE
Childhood Illnesses	
Do you have a history of frequent ear infections?	May result in damaged tympanic membrane (ruptured or scarred) and hearing loss.
Were you exposed to second-hand smoke as a child?	Contributes to more frequent ear infections in infants and children.
Hospitalizations/Surgeries/Serious Injuries	
Have you ever had a severe head injury? A stroke?	May explain reports of tinnitus and client's difficulty interpreting speech.
Have you ever received intravenous antibiotics?	Use of aminoglycosides, antineoplastics, and loop diuretics may cause hearing loss and tinnitus.
Serious and Chronic Illnesses	
Do you have a history of tinnitus? Vertigo?	Increased risk of injury from falls.
Immunizations	
Are your immunizations up to date?	Mumps can cause sensorineural deafness.
Allergies	
Do you have any allergies? If so, what are they and how do you react?	May explain physical findings.
Medications	
What medications are you taking? What dosage? How often do you take them? For how long?	Ototoxic drugs in high doses can cause tinnitus, vertigo, and hearing loss. See box, Drugs That Adversely Affect the Ear, on page 295.
Military Service/Exposure to Irritants	
Were you ever in the military? Have you ever been exposed to loud noises?	Noise pollution from guns can cause hearing loss.

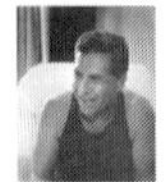

Case Study Findings

Mr. Arnez's past health history reveals:

- History of frequent ear infections as an infant and young child. Treated with antibiotics.
- Hospitalized once at age 3 with pneumonia and concurrent bilateral otitis media.
- Denies asthma, diabetes, or hypertension.
- Received polio, measles/mumps/rubella, tetanus, and diphtheria vaccinations.
- Allergic to sulfa, penicillin, dust, and pollen.
- Current medications include an over-the-counter allergy medication.

Drugs That Adversely Affect the Ear

Drug Class	Drug	Possible Adverse Reactions
Aminoglycosides	All aminoglycosides	Tinnitus, vertigo, hearing loss
Anti-inflammatory agents	All nonsteroidal anti-inflammatory agents (such as diflunisal, ibuprofen, and indomethacin)	Tinnitus, vertigo, hearing loss
Antimalarials	Quinine	Tinnitus, vertigo, hearing loss
Diuretics	Furosemide and bumetanide	Tinnitus, vertigo, hearing loss (with too-rapid I.V. administration)
Nonnarcotic analgesics and antipyretics	All salicylates and all combination products containing salicylates	Tinnitus, dizziness, hearing loss (with high dose or long-term therapy)
Miscellaneous agents	Capreomycin, cisplatin, erythromycin, ethacrynic acid, quinidine sulfate, and vancomycin	Tinnitus, vertigo, hearing loss

Family History

When gathering information on your client's family history, consider the following familial conditions that may affect the ears.

Family History

RISK FACTORS/ QUESTIONS TO ASK	RATIONALE/SIGNIFICANCE
Familial/Genetic Ear Disorders	
Is there a history of hearing loss in your family?	Many genetic disorders manifest with deafness as a feature.
Does anyone in your family have malformed or malpositioned ears?	Unusually shaped ears, low-set ears, or ears set at greater than a 10-degree angle are associated with genetic disorders and possible hearing loss.
Familial/Genetic Disorders That Affect the Ears	
Is there a history of family members with delayed development?	Tay-Sachs disease in Ashkenazi Jews causes developmental decline in infancy. Hypersensitivity to sound is an early sign.
Do any neurological disorders run in your family?	Williams' syndrome, a disorder of calcium metabolism, causes failure to thrive and hyperactivity. Affected people are often sensitive to loud noises. Charcot-Marie-Tooth disease, a slow, progressive syndrome causing lower extremity muscle weakness around age 10, later progresses to upper extremities. Renal problems often occur in early adulthood, and progressive sensorineural hearing loss begins in the teens.
Do you have any skeletal problems?	People with osteogenesis imperfecta (brittle bone disease) experience conductive hearing loss caused by damage to the ossicles. In Hunter's syndrome, growth rate in boys slows after toddler age. Joints stiffen, contractures develop, and facial features become coarse. Deafness is common. People with Treacher-Collins syndrome have facial deformities including a small mandible and maxillae. Half of them have small, malformed external ears and middle ears, causing conductive hearing loss. Waardenburg's syndrome is characterized by abnormalities of the upper limbs, eyes, and ears. Sensorineural deafness occurs in 1/4 of cases.

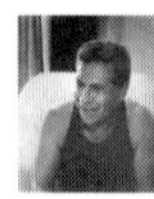

Case Study Findings

Mr. Arnez's family history reveals:

- Father, age 78, has controlled hypertension.
- Mother, age 70, diagnosed with MS at age 45, currently in remission.
- One sister, age 40, diagnosed with neurofibromatosis including acoustic neuroma.
- One brother, age 36, recently diagnosed with hypertension.
- Client has two teen-aged girls, ages 14 and 16, both alive and well.

Review of Systems

Changes in the structure and function of the ear may relate to every other system of the body.

The review of systems (ROS) will help you identify problems in other systems that directly affect the ear. Remember, the ROS allows you to pick up anything that you might have missed, and the findings will give meaning to the symptoms by relating them to the affected system.

Review of Systems

AREA/SYSTEM/ QUESTIONS TO ASK	RATIONALE/SIGNIFICANCE
General Health Survey	
How would you describe your general state of health? How have you been feeling?	Change in general health may indicate underlying problem that may affect the ears.
Integumentary	
Do you have any patches of skin that are darker colored?	Six or more brown patches of skin (café-au-lait spots) in the axillary region may signify neurofibromatosis, commonly associated with acoustic neuroma and hearing loss.
HEENT	
Do you have a history of environmental allergies? Head injury?	Can explain presence of ear examination findings.
Respiratory	
Have you had any recent respiratory infections or colds?	Ear infections often follow upper respiratory infections, especially in children.
Gastrointestinal	
Has your appetite decreased?	Children with ear infections often have a decrease in appetite.
Genitourinary	
Do you have a history of kidney disease?	The ears and kidneys are formed in utero during similar time periods.
Reproductive	
For female clients: Are you pregnant?	Increased vascularity may cause fullness and diminished hearing.
Musculoskeletal/Neurological	
Do you have any problems with balance or vertigo?	Indicates problem with inner ear or cerebellum. Tinnitus and balance problems may be associated with MS.
Lymphatic	
Have you had a recent ear infection?	Ear infections may cause lymph node enlargement.

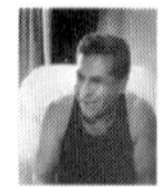

Case Study Findings

Mr. Arnez's review of systems reveals:

- **General Health Survey:** Denies fatigue or recent weight loss. Health is usually good.
- **Integumentary:** Denies rashes, lesions, or slow wound healing.
- **HEENT:** Denies ear pain, drainage, tinnitus, or ear trauma. Reports recent upper respiratory infection 4 weeks ago with earache, resolved with antibiotics. History of frequent childhood ear infections and occasional ear infections as an adult, occurring yearly or less. Environmental allergy to dust and pollen.

- **Gastrointestinal:** Denies nausea, vomiting, diarrhea, or recent changes in bowel habits.
- **Genitourinary:** Denies changes in bladder habits.
- **Neurological/Musculoskeletal:** Intermittent problem with balance since onset of ear pressure. Denies vertigo, muscle weakness, or paresthesia.

Psychosocial Profile

The psychosocial profile includes asking questions about the client's lifestyle, including a typical day, personal habits, medications, sleep patterns, and home and work environment. These factors affect the client's overall health.

Psychosocial Profile

CATEGORY/QUESTIONS TO ASK	RATIONALE/SIGNIFICANCE
Health Practices and Beliefs/ Self-Care Activities	
When was your last physical examination? When was your last hearing test and the results?	May indicate need for referral.
How do you clean your ears?	Use of Q-tips to clean ears may traumatize auditory canal or drum.
Do you have problems removing ear wax?	May need instructions on cerumen removal.
Typical Day	
How does your hearing/ear problem affect your ability to engage in usual activities such as work or school?	Ability to hear has major influence on how effectively and efficiently a person interacts and communicates with others.
Nutritional Patterns	
What did you eat in the past 24 hours? What is your usual diet?	It is important to identify nutritional patterns that may affect your client's overall health.
Activity/Exercise Patterns	
Do problems with hearing loss, tinnitus, vertigo, and balance adversely affect your ability to do your usual activities? To exercise?	Hearing loss and tinnitus may have a negative impact on ability to engage in sports or activities involving auditory communication. Vertigo and balance problems can make it difficult to navigate in a smooth manner.
Recreation/Pets/Hobbies	
Do your hobbies rely on a high degree of communication with others?	May be unable to enjoy hobbies, resulting in altered coping. Sense of social isolation may increase because of decrease in effective communication.
Do your hobbies include listening to music or playing musical instruments?	Exposure to loud music can result in permanent hearing loss.
Sleep/Rest Patterns	
Does the ear problem cause pain or discomfort that interferes with sleep patterns?	May result in fatigue and sleep deprivation. Tinnitus may interfere with ability to rest.
Personal Habits	
Do you smoke or are you exposed to second-hand smoke?	Children have an increased incidence of ear infection when exposed to second-hand smoke.
Occupational Health Patterns	
Are you exposed to loud noises or to continuous noise at lower decibels?	Exposure to noise levels higher than 80 dB results in varying degrees of permanent hearing loss depending on dB level and duration of exposure.
Environmental Health Patterns	
Are you exposed to loud noises in your home?	Living in areas of high traffic or where machinery is being used can result in permanent hearing loss.

(Continued)

Psychosocial Profile *(Continued)*

CATEGORY/QUESTIONS TO ASK	RATIONALE/SIGNIFICANCE
Family Roles and Relationships	
Has your ear disorder affected your ability to interact with others or to assume your usual roles (parent, employee, student)?	May affect self-esteem if client is not able to engage in usual roles and relationships.
Cultural Influences	
Do you have any cultural influences that affect your healthcare practices?	It is important to identify cultural influences that may affect your client's healthcare practices.
Religious Influences	
Do you have any religious practices/ beliefs that influence your healthcare practices?	It is important to identify religious practices/beliefs that may affect your client's healthcare practices.
Stress and Coping	
How do you usually deal with stress and resolve problems? What support systems do you have?	Loss of hearing may cause stress. Identifying coping mechanisms and supports can be used to help the client deal with hearing impairment.

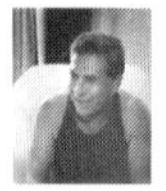

Case Study Findings

Mr. Arnez's psychosocial profile includes:

- Last physical examination was 6 months ago. Last ear exam was 4 weeks ago during recent ear infection. Denies ever having a hearing test.
- Typical day: Rises at 5:30 AM on workdays (works 7–3 shift). Showers, has breakfast (cereal and coffee), leaves for work by 6:15 AM. Eats quick lunch from sidewalk vendor. Returns home by 4 PM most days unless he has errands to run. Cooks dinner for wife and two daughters, then often drives daughters to various school or social activities. Spends evenings watching TV. Goes to bed by 10 PM. Spends weekends attending sporting events, running errands, chauffeuring daughters. (Wife cannot drive because of disability.)
- Generally eats a well-balanced diet, although lunch at work is rushed. Rarely exercises because of lack of time, fatigue, and intermittent balance problems.
- Ear pressure and fullness have caused intermittent problems in managing his household and socializing. States that he can usually compensate for the hearing loss at home (e.g., by turning up sound on TV and phone handset).
- Ear problems have not caused sleep difficulties. Usually gets 7 hours of sleep a night.
- States that hearing loss causes safety issues at work.
- Denies chronic or recent exposure to loud noise at home or at work.
- Main social supports are family, especially brother and father, and a few close friends at work.
- Has a hectic life with major family responsibilities and many stressors.Talking with friends and family is main coping mechanism.

Focused Ear History

If a detailed history is not feasible or appropriate, focus only on the most essential questions. Remember to do a symptom analysis (PQRST) for any positive symptom identified. Ask these questions:

- Do you have problems with your ears such as ringing? Do you have hearing problems?
- Do you have balance problems?
- Do you have drainage from your ears? If yes, how much and what color?
- Have you had recent head trauma?
- Do you have any health problems?
- Are you exposed to noise pollution at work or in your home environment?
- Are you on any prescribed or over-the-counter medications?
- Do you have allergies?

Case Study Evaluation

Before you proceed with the physical examination, review and summarize the key information from Mr.

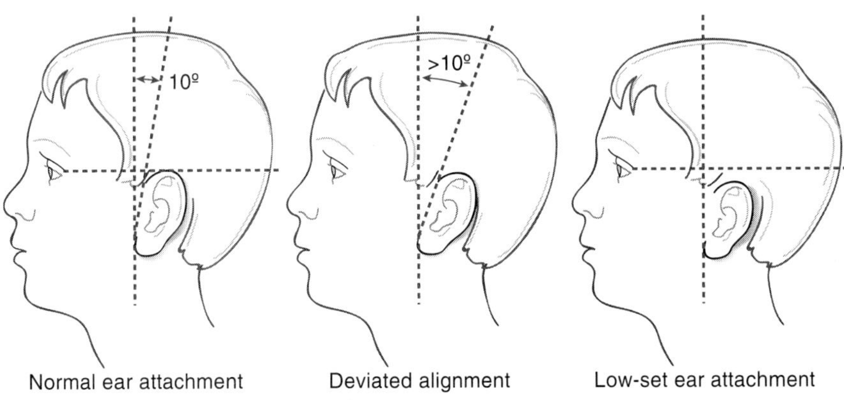

FIGURE 10–18. *A.* Normal ear attachment; *B.* Deviated alignment; *C.* Low-set ear attachment.

Arnez's health history. Document the ear history related to Mr. Arnez.

 CRITICAL THINKING ACTIVITY #9

What factors in Mr. Arnez's history may explain his hearing problem?

 CRITICAL THINKING ACTIVITY #10

Considering Mr. Arnez's history, how might this hearing problem affect him?

 CRITICAL THINKING ACTIVITY #11

What strengths does Mr. Arnez possess that will help him cope with and manage his health problems?

Anatomical Landmarks

Before beginning your physical examination of the ear, review the internal structures and normal positioning of the external ear (Figs. 10–18 and 10–19).

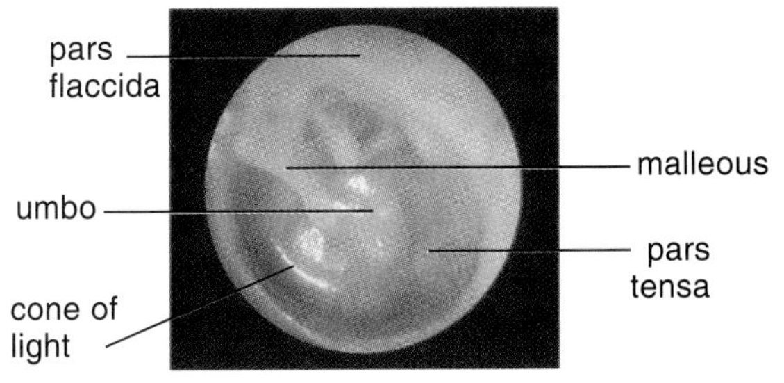

FIGURE 10–19. Tympanic membrane, left ear.

Physical Assessment

The health history has provided you with clues that will help direct your physical examination. When examining clients who have severe hearing deficits, you may need to explain what you are doing by some other means, such as writing.

Approach

Physical assessment of the ear entails screening for hearing deficits and examining the external ear and tympanic membrane. Keep in mind that ear problems may relate to other body systems, so assess for signs in every system. Examination of the ear involves inspection and palpation of the external ear and external auditory canal, followed by tests for hearing and equilibrium. Examination of the auditory canal and tympanic membrane are done early in the examination to ensure that structures for hearing are intact and unobstructed before testing hearing acuity.

The examination is usually performed with the person in a sitting position. However, when performing the otoscopic examination on a young child, it is better if the child is supine with the head turned to the side being examined. A quiet environment is essential when performing the hearing screening tests.

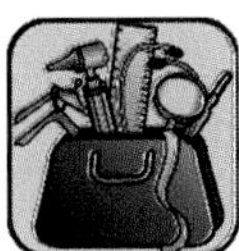

Toolbox

The tools needed for examination of the ears include a tuning fork (500 to 1000 cycles per second), an otoscope with pneumatic attachment, a thermometer, and a watch. Because examination of the ear involves inspection and palpation, you will need a keen eye and a gentle touch.

Performing a General Survey

Before assessing the ear, perform a general survey. Note the person's overall appearance, including nutritional

Performing a Head-to-Toe Physical Assessment

AREA/SYSTEM/NORMAL VARIATIONS	ABNORMAL FINDINGS/RATIONALE
General Health Survey *INSPECT* Alert, responds accurately when asked to identify person, place, and time.	*Behaviors similar to confusion or disorientation during conversation:* Hearing loss.
Integumentary/*External Ear* *INSPECT* External ear is pale, peach pink to dark brown color, depending on racial and genetic heritage.	*Axillary freckling, café-au-lait spots, acoustic neuroma, hearing loss:* Neurofibromatosis.
HEENT/*Eyes and Ears* *INSPECT/PALPATE* Eyes clear without tearing.	*Tearing eyes, ear fullness:* Environmental allergy.
HEENT/*Neck* Lymph nodes nonpalpable, nontender.	*Palpable, tender, warm lymph nodes:* Infection.
HEENT/*Nose* Pink or coral-colored nasal mucosa.	*Pale, boggy mucosa with watery drainage:* Environmental allergy.
No swelling or drainage.	*Purulent or mucoid discharge, often with concurrent otitis media:* Upper respiratory infection.
HEENT/*Mouth/Throat* Pharynx uniform pink coral without whitish exudate, tonsils +1 adults, +2 or less in children, without exudate.	*Reddened pharynx, whitish exudate on pharynx or tonsils or enlarged tonsils:* Upper respiratory infection, often with concurrent otitis.
Respiratory *INSPECT/AUSCULTATE* Equal bilaterally. No adventitious sounds or cough. Respiratory rate 12–20/minute for adults.	*Cough with sputum, crackles/wheezes:* Upper respiratory infection. (Ear infections often exist concurrently or as a precursor.)
Cardiovascular *AUSCULTATE* Heart: Regular, no extra sounds, no carotid bruits, +2 pulses.	*Tinnitus/vertigo:* Cardiovascular/cerebrovascular disease.
Musculoskeletal *INSPECT* Muscle strength strong and equal bilaterally. No tremors.	*Altered muscle strength, tremors, auditory problems, balance problems:* MS.
Neurological *INSPECT* Smooth movement of extremities, steady gait, sense of touch intact.	*Tinnitus/balance and gait problems:* MS; balance problems also may indicate problem with inner ear.

status, body habitus, and emotional status. Also take vital signs—temperature elevations may indicate an infection. Be especially alert for signs that suggest problems with the ear. Ask yourself these questions:

- Is the person guarding his or her ear? If the client is a child, is he or she tugging or rubbing the ear? These are signs of an ear infection.
- Is the client attentive and responding appropriately? Inappropriate responses or inattentiveness may result in hearing deficits.
- Is the client speaking loudly? People with hearing deficits tend to speak louder.
- Do you notice any problems with the client's ability to maintain balance? Balance problems are associated with inner ear problems.

Performing a Head-to-Toe Physical Assessment

Now scan your patient from head to toe. Check for more specific signs of diseases that involve other organ systems and that might affect the ears.

Case Study Findings

Before you focus on Mr. Arnez's ear examination, note the following findings from his general survey and head-to-toe assessment:

- **General Health Survey:** Well-developed, 50 year-old male in no acute distress. Alert and oriented ×4; pleasant and cooperative; good historian.
- **Vital signs:** BP 142/88; Pulse 78, strong and regular; Respirations 16/minute and regular; Temperature 98.8°F.
- **Integumentary:** Olive-colored skin, even skin tone throughout, axillary freckles and three café-au-lait spots on trunk.
- **Respiratory:** Lungs clear and equal bilaterally, no adventitious sounds.
- **Cardiovascular:** Heart rate regular, no extra sound or murmurs. Carotid pulse +2 bilaterally with no bruit. Radial and dorsal pedalis pulses +2 bilaterally. Capillary refill less than 3 seconds.
- **Gastrointestinal:** Abdomen soft, flat, nontender with normal bowel sounds in all 4 quadrants.
- **Musculoskeletal/Neurological:** Negative paresthesia, tremor, and muscle weakness.

Performing a Focused Ear Assessment

Now that you have completed your general survey and head-to-toe scan, you can focus on the ear. First, inspect and palpate the external structures of the ear. Then examine the internal ear with an otoscope. Finally, perform hearing acuity tests.

Focused Assessment of the External Ear

ASSESS/NORMAL VARIATIONS	ABNORMAL FINDINGS/RATIONALE
Inspection 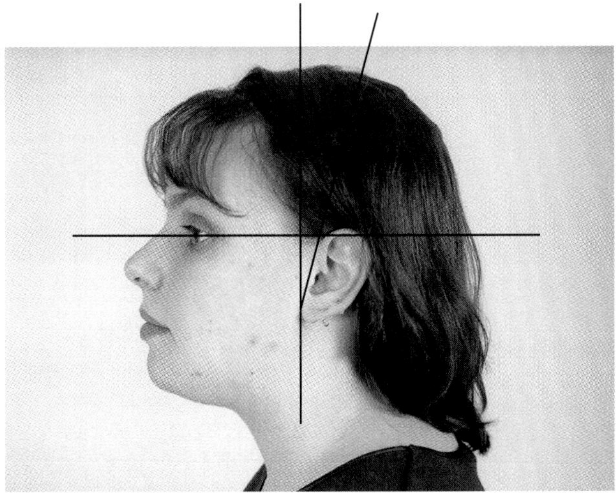 **Normal angle of attachment** Size greater than 4 cm and smaller than 10 cm. Normal shape and presence of landmarks: Helix, antihelix, antitragus, tragus, and lobule. Absence of pits, creases, or lesions. Darwinian tubercle is a benign protrusion on upper part of helix.	*Ears less than 4 cm vertical height in adults:* Microtia, seen in some genetic disorders. *Ears greater than 10 cm vertical height in adults:* Macrotia. *Missing or malformed landmarks:* Associated with hearing deficit. *Creased earlobe:* Associated with heart conditions. *Ear pits or sinuses usually located anterior to the tragus:* Associated with internal ear anomalies.

(Continued)

Focused Assessment of the External Ear *(Continued)*

ASSESS/NORMAL VARIATIONS	ABNORMAL FINDINGS/RATIONALE

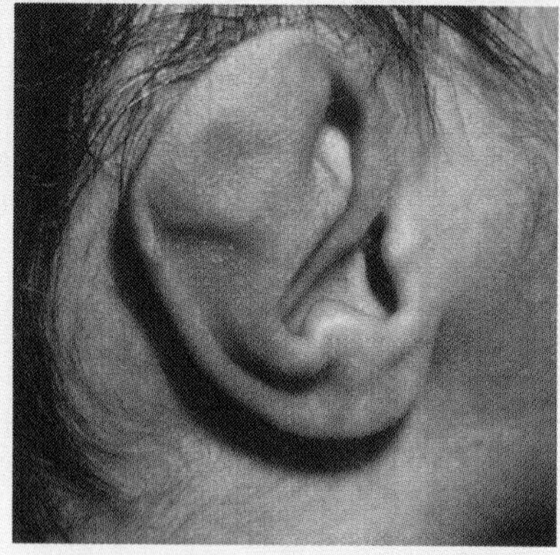

Congenital ear anomaly

Low-set ears or ears rotated posteriorly more than 15 degrees: Associated with mental retardation.

Position: Helix of ear is level with imaginary line drawn through inner and outer canthus to occiput. Ears should be rotated from 0–15 degrees posteriorly.

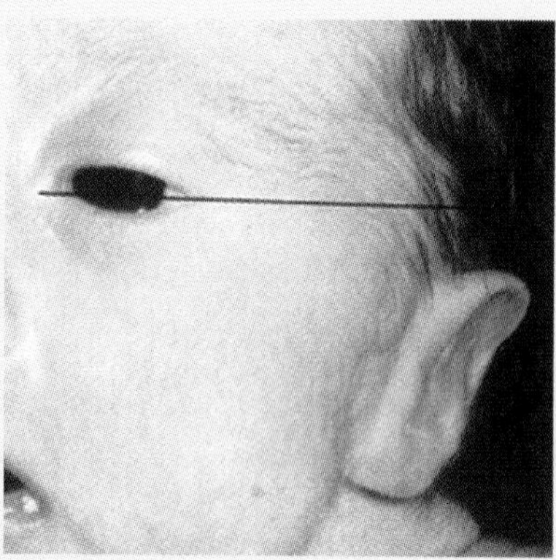

Low-set ears

Condition of skin: Intact, no lesions. Note if skin piercings are present.
Color: Consistent with skin color.
Drainage: Cerumen is the only normal drainage.
Darwinian tubercle is a benign protrusion on upper part of helix.

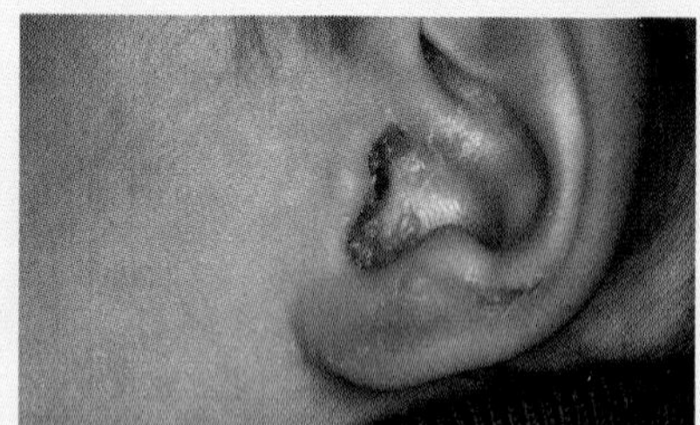

Impacted cerumen

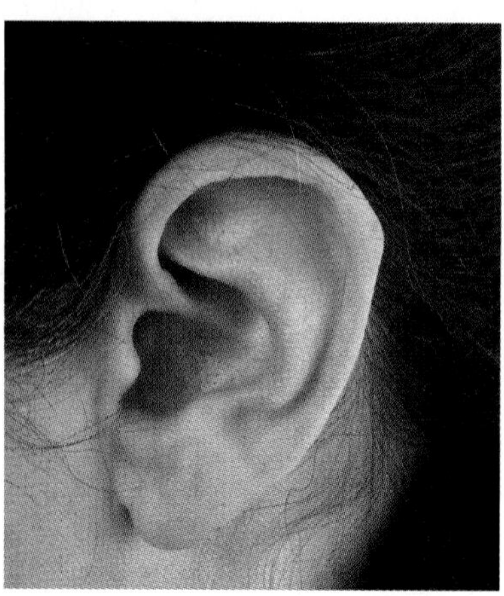

Darwinian tubercle

Drainage: Bloody drainage can result from trauma and purulent drainage from an infection. Clear drainage may be spinal fluid from a head injury.
Redness, inflammation may indicate infection, fever
Lesions— e.g., skin cancer from sun exposure
Cysts
Topic associated with gout

Focused Assessment of the External Ear *(Continued)*

ASSESS/NORMAL VARIATIONS	ABNORMAL FINDINGS/RATIONALE
Palpation Soft and pliable, nontender	*Tenderness of mastoid, helix, tragus or pinna:* Ear infections.

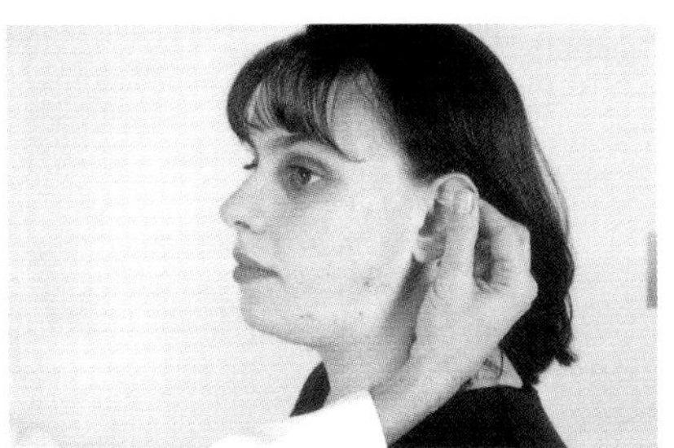
Palpating the ear

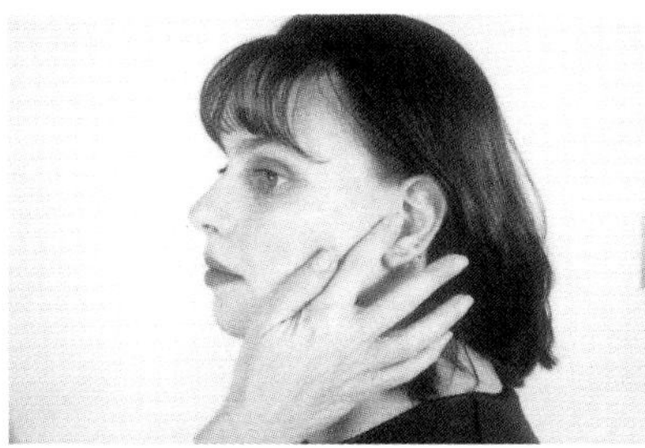
Palpating the tragus

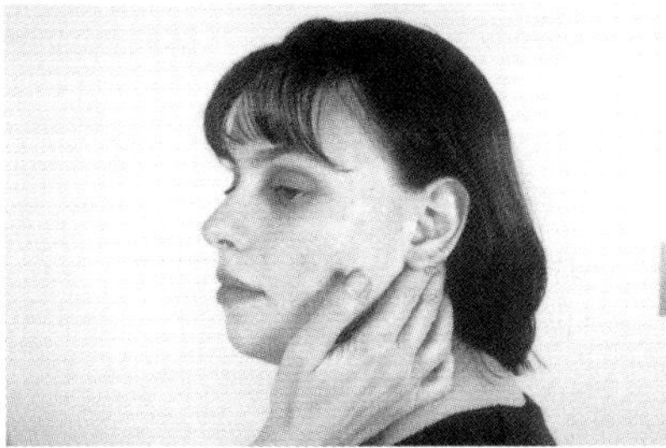
Palpating the mastoid

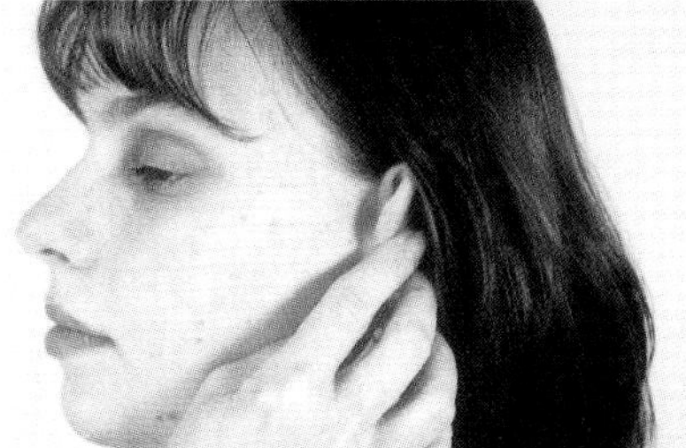
Pulling helix forward

Structures should be nontender, with no nodules or swelling.

Otoscopic Examination

The otoscope illuminates and magnifies the auditory canal and the tympanic membrane. The auditory canal is assessed for color, lesions, and foreign objects. The tympanic membrane is assessed for color, intactness, appropriateness of landmarks, and mobility of the drum. Select the largest and shortest speculum that will fit into the client's ear canal comfortably, and attach it to the head of the otoscope. Usually, a 4-, 5-, or 6-mm, 1/2 inch speculum is appropriate for an adult ear canal.

Turn the otoscope light on. Have the client tilt his or her head away from the side you are examining. Always look into the external canal before inserting the otoscope. Two insertion techniques may be used:

Technique #1: Hold the otoscope upside down like a pencil, with the magnifying lens facing the examiner. Pull the pinna of the ear up and back for adults or down for children under age 2. Brace your insertion hand on the client's head for stabilization. This technique is ideal for children, because if they move the head, your hand moves with it.

Technique #2: An alternative technique is to hold the otoscope handle upright and slowly and gently insert the scope along the axis of the external auditory canal (about 1/2 inch in an adult and 1/4 inch in a child). Be careful to enter only the outer third of the ear canal. With the scope inserted, put your eye up to the viewing lens. If you cannot visualize the tympanic membrane, do not move the otoscope. Instead, apply more traction, pull on the ear, or carefully adjust the angle of the otoscope more toward the client's nose. Do not release the traction on the ear until the speculum of the otoscope has been removed from the ear. Remove the speculum in the same angle as it was inserted, and then release the traction to the pinna.

ALERTS

- Before inserting the otoscope, palpate the tragus, mastoid, and helix. If any of these are tender, insert the scope very carefully.
- Always inspect the external canal for foreign objects before inserting the otoscope. Otherwise, you may inadvertently push an object farther up the canal.
- Insert the otoscope only in the outer third of the canal. The inner two-thirds of the ear canal are over the temporal bone and are very sensitive.

Performing an Otoscopic Examination

ASSESS/NORMAL VARIATIONS

External Auditory Canal

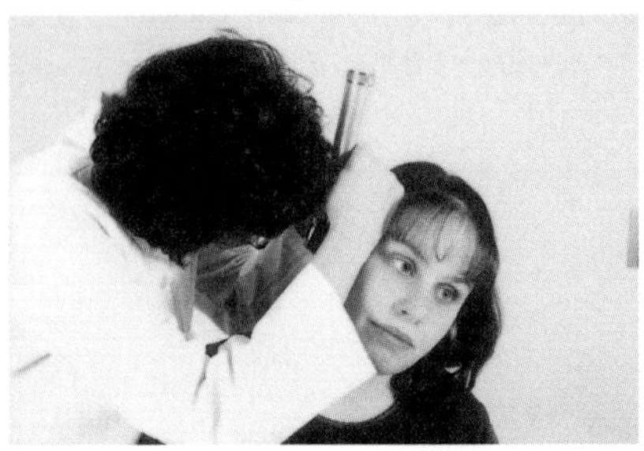

Otoscope insertion with handle up

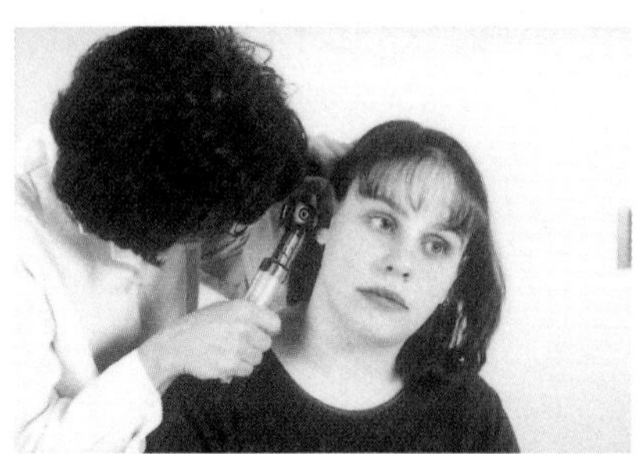

Otoscope insertion with handle down

No foreign objects. Canal patent. Free of redness and drainage.

Ear wax may be visible. Native Americans and Asians have higher rates of ear infections than Caucasians. Cerumen is white, dry, and flaky in clients of Asian and Native American descent vs. honey colored and sticky in whites and blacks.

Exostosis ("surfer's ear")—abnormal benign growth of bone in external auditory canal—often results from swimming in cold water.

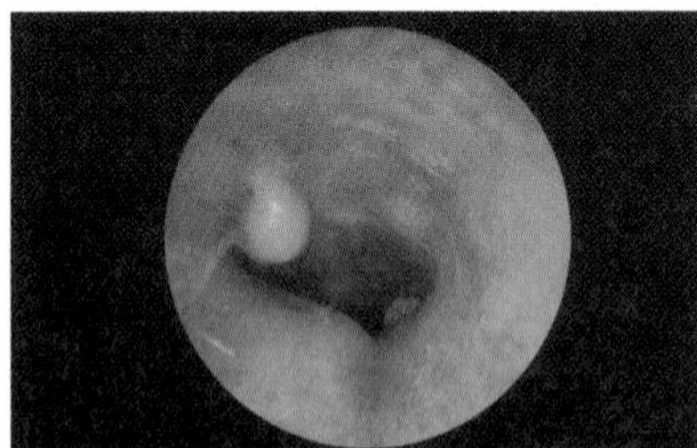

Exostosis

Tympanic Membrane (TM)

HELPFUL HINTS

- The ears are mirror images, so the cone of light, a triangular reflex, is at 5 o'clock in the right ear and 7 o'clock in the left ear.
- Assess drum mobility in pediatric patients with a pneumatic tube attachment to the otoscope.

Normally shiny, pearl gray, intact, and mobile. TM lighter colored in older adults. Bony landmarks of the umbo (the central depressed portion of the concavity on the lateral surface of the TM) and malleus should be visible. Capillaries may normally be seen on the malleus.

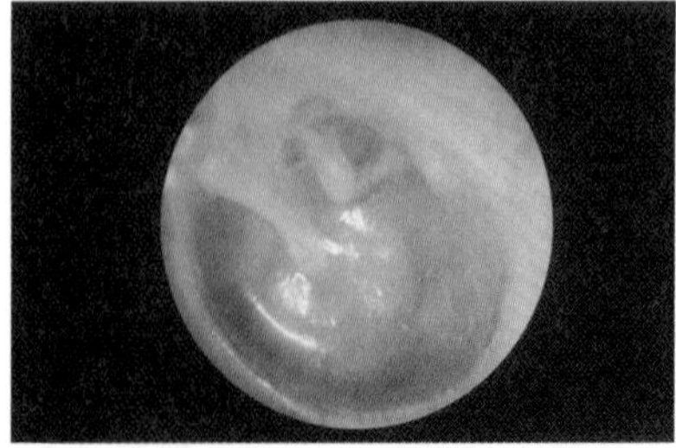

Normal tympanic membrane

ABNORMAL FINDINGS/RATIONALE

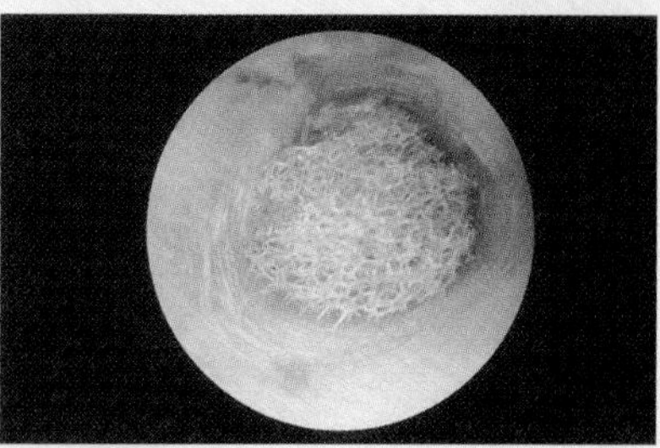

Foreign body

Reddened canal: Otitis externa.

Exudate and edema: "Swimmer's ear" or external otitis.

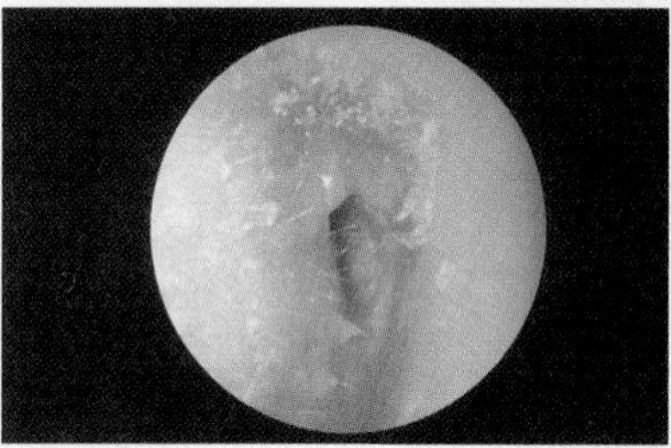

External otitis

Excessive impacted cerumen in older adults can contribute to conductive hearing loss.

Yellowish membrane with fluid and air bubbles visible behind TM: Serous otitis.

Reddish TM with absent ordistorted light reflex: Otitis media.

Round/oval dark area: Perforated TM.

White irregularly shaped area on TM: Scar tissue.

Change in position or shape of cone of light reflex and absence or exaggeration of bony landmarks: Imbalance in middle ear pressure. Bony landmarks more prominent if negative pressure in inner ear, less prominent in infections or conditions in which fluid or pus collects behind membrane.

Limited mobility of a drum: Associated with a bulging drum.

Blue to black TM from bleeding (hemotympanum): Usually results from trauma.

Performing an Otoscopic Examination

ASSESS/NORMAL VARIATIONS	ABNORMAL FINDINGS/RATIONALE
Tympanic Membrane (TM) *(Continued)*	*Golden-brown TM with caramel-color drainage that is thick and elastic like rubber cement (secretory, adhesive otitis media, also known as "glue ear")*: Associated with viral infection. *Cystic mass of epithelial cells that develops in middle ear (cholesteatoma)*: Complication of chronic otitis media. Tubes are placed in ear to promote drainage and equalize pressure.

Abnormalities of the Tympanic Membrane

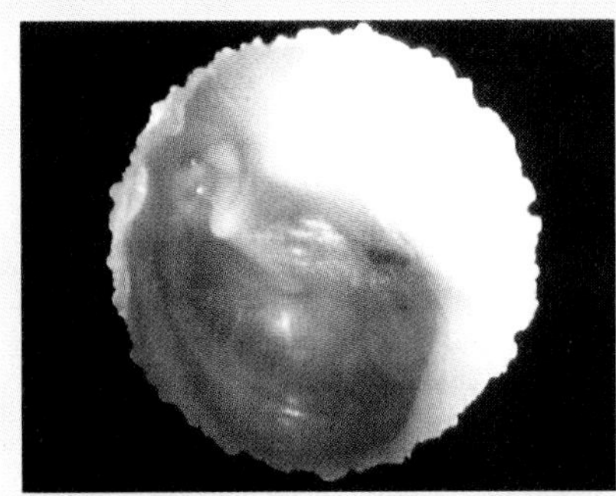

Serous otitis

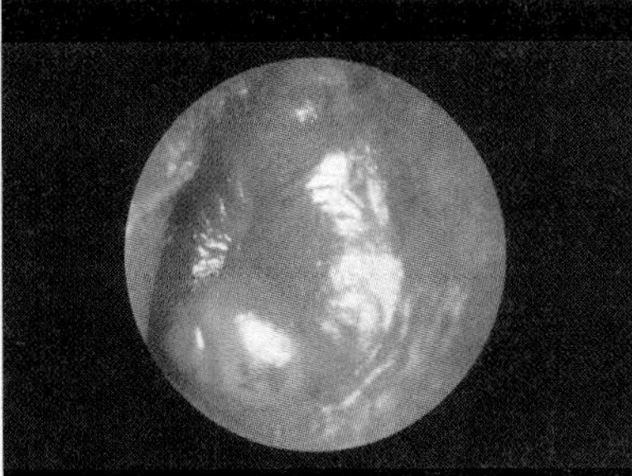

Otitis media

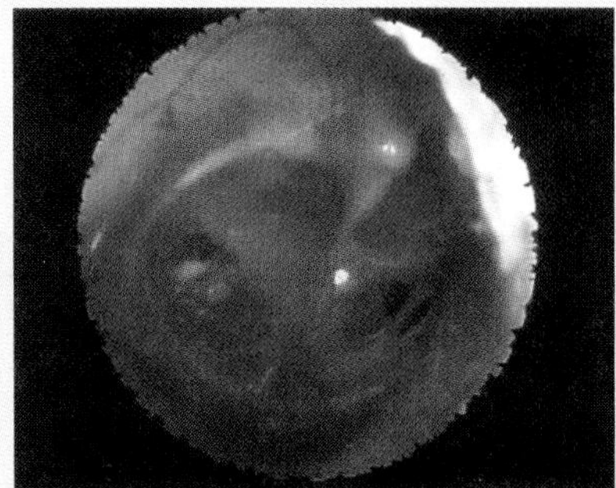

Perforated TM

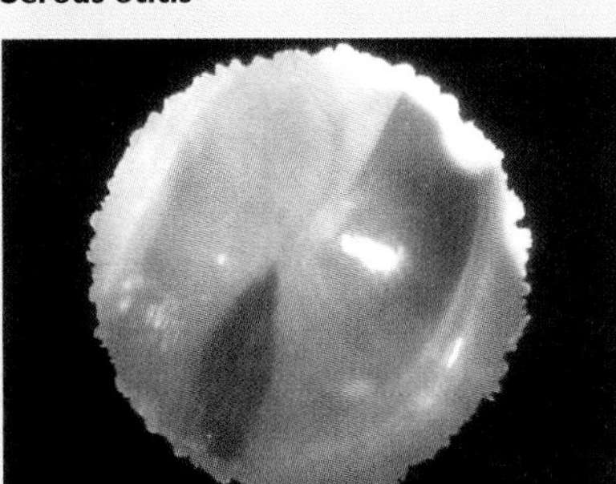

Hemotympanum

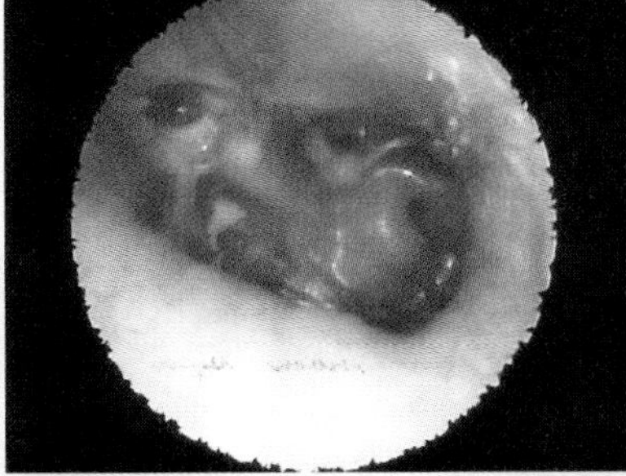

Adhesive otitis media

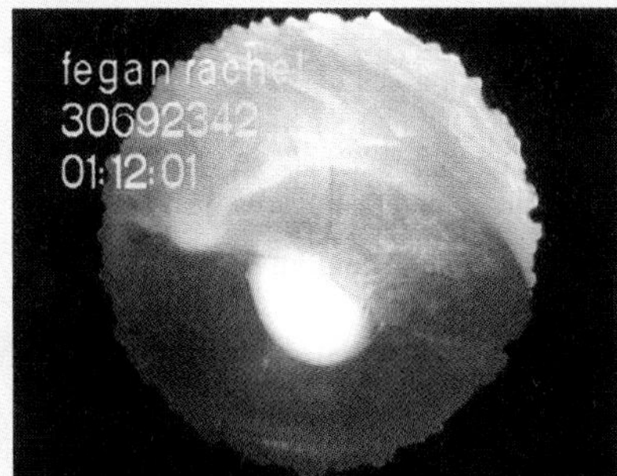

Cholesteatoma

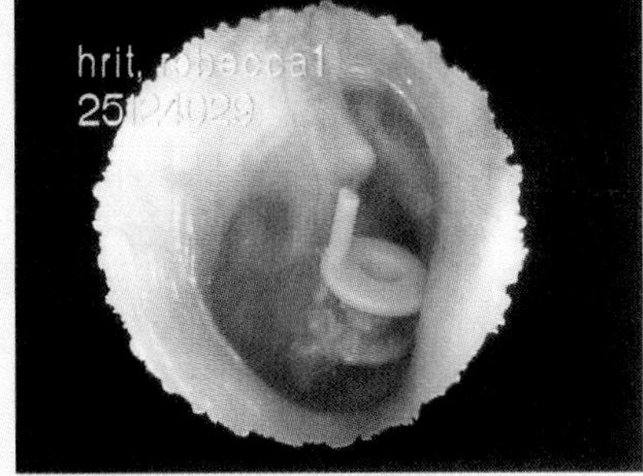

Pressure equalization tube

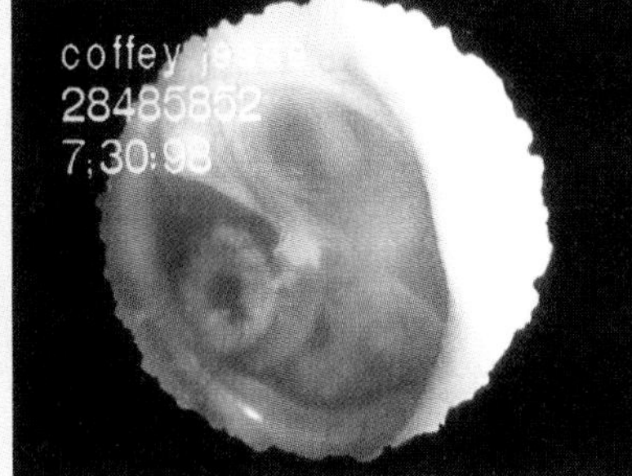

Tympanotomy

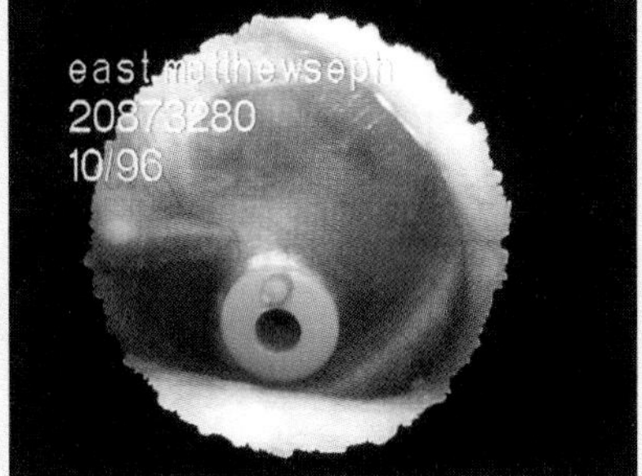

Intact patient pressure equalization tube

Hearing Tests

Examination of the ear includes conducting hearing tests for high-tone, low-tone, sensorineural, and conductive hearing loss. Typical tests include the following:

Watch tick test: This test determines the client's ability to hear high-pitched sounds and screen for high-tone hearing loss. To do this test, have the client obstruct one ear at a time by placing his or her index finger in the external canal. Using a ticking watch, hold it close to the unobstructed ear and slowly move it away until the client says that he or she can hear the watch tick (usually about 5 inches [13 cm]). Repeat the test on the other ear.

Whisper test: This test assesses low-pitch or low-tone hearing loss. Again, have the client obstruct one ear with the index finger. Then stand 1–2 feet behind and to the side of the client's unobstructed ear and whisper three or four unrelated words. Have the client repeat the words heard. Test the other ear in a similar fashion.

Tuning-fork tests: These tests check for intact sensorineural and conductive hearing. The Weber test assesses lateralization of sound. Sound transmission with the Weber test is both through bone conduction (BC) and air conduction (AC). To perform the test, place a vibrating tuning fork firmly on top of your client's head or forehead.

HELPFUL HINT

Hold the tuning fork by the stem and tap the prongs gently on your palm or thigh. Do not touch the prongs once they are vibrating; this will dampen or stop the vibrations.

Ask the client if the vibration sounds the same in both ears or different. Normally the vibration is heard equally in both ears. If the vibration is louder or more distinct in one ear than in the other, it has lateralized to that ear (positive lateralization). If there is conductive hearing loss, the sound lateralizes to the impaired ear; if there is sensorineural hearing loss, the sound lateralizes to the unaffected or good ear. Conductive hearing loss is usually caused by a problem with the external or middle ear, such as acute otitis media, perforated eardrum, or a blocked canal with cerumen. Sensorineural hearing loss is usually caused by a problem in the inner ear, such as acoustic nerve damage from ototoxic drugs.

Having a conductive loss in the lateralizing ear (e.g., as a result of accumulation of cerumen or a perforated eardrum) means that sound waves are not conducted effectively by air conduction to the inner ear. Thus, limited or no sound waves are received by AC. The only mechanism remaining for sound wave conduction in the lateralizing ear is by BC. But without competing AC, sound waves will be interpreted by the client as sounding louder. To test this yourself, create a temporary conductive hearing loss by occluding the external auditory canal and placing the vibrating tuning fork as described. In a person with normal hearing, sound will lateralize to the obstructed ear because you have blocked any competing AC sounds from being transmitted.

With a sensorineural hearing loss, the sound lateralizes to the good ear. The ear with sensorineural deafness is unable to transmit sound waves by AC or BC to the acoustic nerve to the brain. Consequently, the sounds transmitted to the opposite ear will be interpreted as louder, or lateralizing.

The Weber test can detect lateralization, but it cannot differentiate the cause. So if lateralization occurs, you will need to perform the Rinne test to establish if the problem is caused by a conductive hearing loss.

The Rinne test is a timed tuning fork test used to compare AC and BC. To perform this test, place a vibrating tuning fork on your client's mastoid process. When it is on the mastoid process, sound transmission is through BC to the inner ear. Ask the client to tell you when he or she no longer hears the vibrations. Record the amount of time the client heard the sound in seconds. When the sound is no longer heard, immediately place the vibrating fork about one inch in front of the external auditory canal and continue to time until your client can no longer hear the sound. When in front of the ear, sound transmission is through AC through the auditory canal, to the tympanic membrane, middle ear ,and inner ear. Avoid touching hairs in front of the ear with the vibrating tuning fork because this may provide a clue that the tuning fork is vibrating. Record the amount of time the client hears the vibrating tuning fork in seconds. Normally, sound transmission through air is twice as long as sound transmission through bone. If AC time is less than twice as long as BC time, it generally indicates hearing loss by AC. Inability to hear the tuning fork during BC indicates sensorineural hearing loss.

Hearing Tests

TEST/NORMAL VARIATIONS	ABNORMAL FINDINGS/RATIONALE

Whisper Test

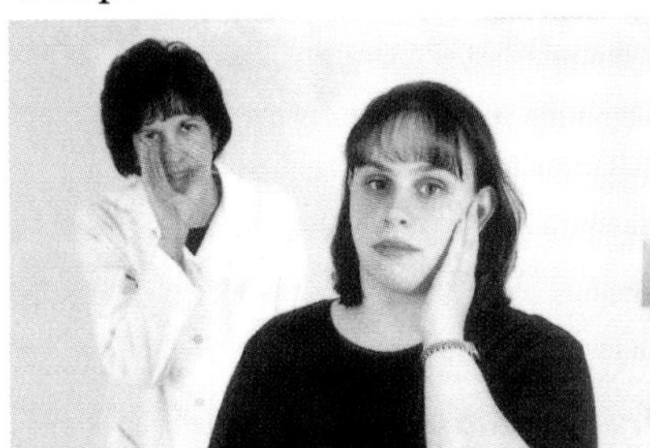

Performing whisper test

Watch Tick Test

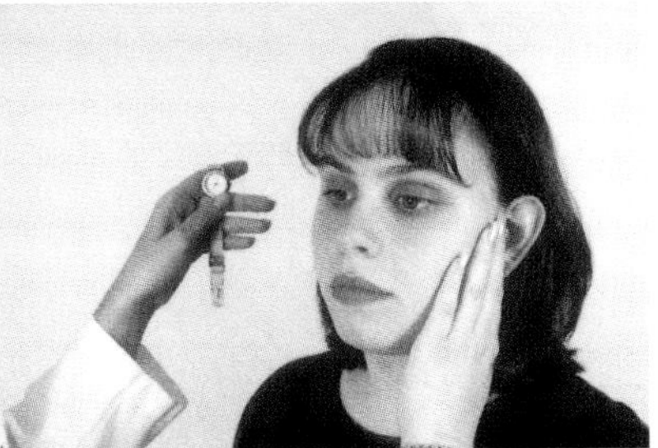

Performing watch tick test

Client repeats most words whispered in each ear at a distance of 1–2 feet.

Client hears tick of a watch in each ear at a distance of 5 inches.

Inability to repeat words: Low-tone frequency loss.

Inability to hear watch ticking: High-tone frequency loss.

Weber Test

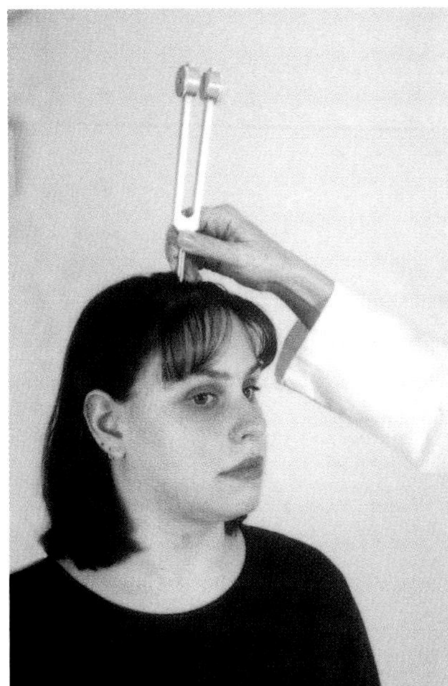

a:Performing Weber test on head;

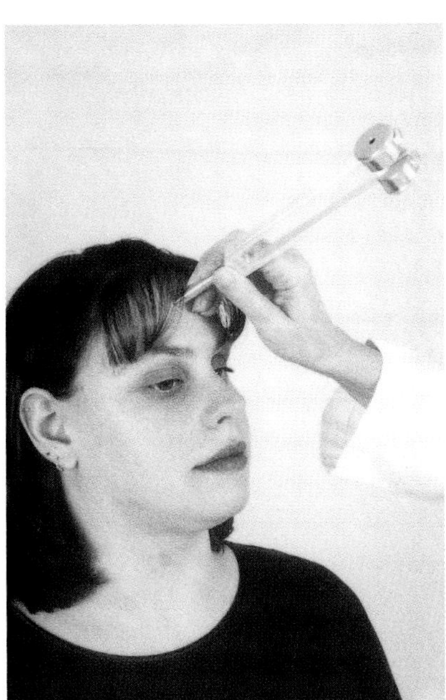

b: Performing Weber test on forehead

Vibrations should be felt or heard equally in both ears.

Lateralization of vibrations: Conductive or sensorineural loss.

(Continued)

Hearing Tests *(Continued)*

TEST/NORMAL VARIATIONS

Rinne Test

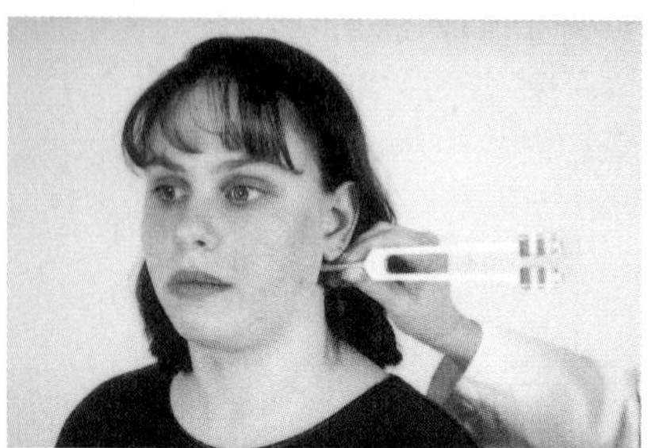

a: Performing Rinne test on mastoid

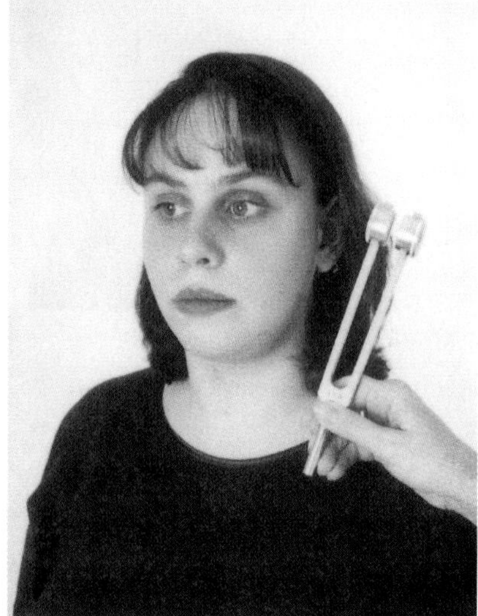

b: Performing Rinne test in front of ear

The length of time the client hears the vibrations by AC is normally twice as long as for BC.

The ratio of AC to BC is similar in both ears.

Romberg's Test

(Tests inner ear vestibular function)

Client stands with feet together and eyes closed. Maintains balance with minimal sway. (For more information, see Chapter 19.)

ABNORMAL FINDINGS/RATIONALE

AC to BC ratios that differ markedly in each ear: Unilateral hearing deficit.

AC less than twice BC: Hearing loss by AC, possibly caused by ear wax, otitis media, serous otitis, or damage to the ossicles of the middle ear.

Loss of balance: Inner ear disorder, cerebellar damage, or ingestion of intoxicants.

Case Study Findings

Mr. Arnez's focused physical assessment findings include:

- External ear normal shape, size, and position
- Mastoid, tragus, and pinna nontender
- External auditory meatus without drainage or lesions
- TM pearl gray with scattered white scar tissue and distorted light reflex
- No fluid or pus visible behind TM
- Hearing tests: Weber, no lateralizing; Rinne, AC 1.5 × BC bilaterally
- Dizziness with head rotation
- Positive sway with Romberg's test

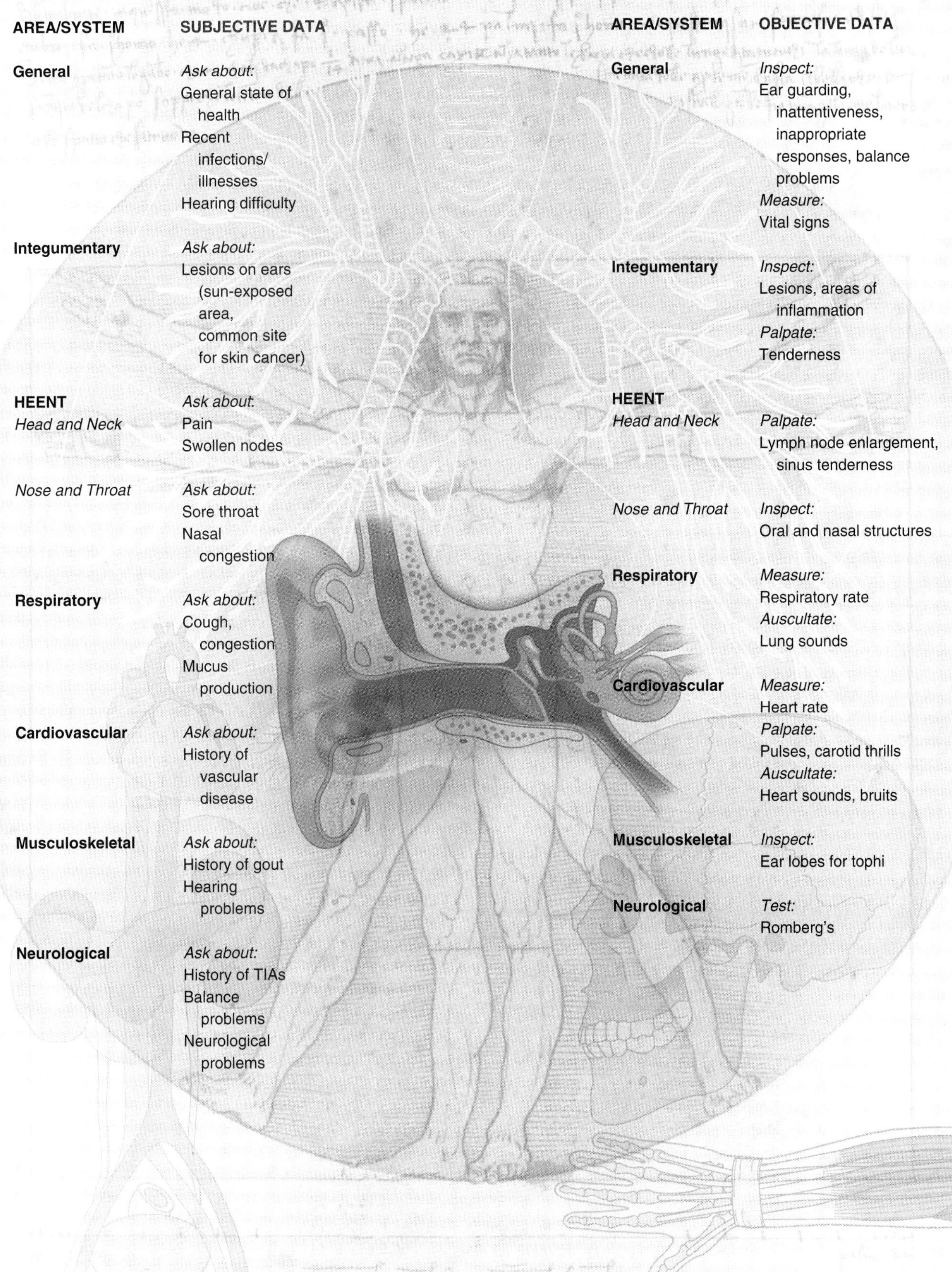

AREA/SYSTEM	SUBJECTIVE DATA
General	*Ask about:* General state of health Recent infections/ illnesses Hearing difficulty
Integumentary	*Ask about:* Lesions on ears (sun-exposed area, common site for skin cancer)
HEENT *Head and Neck*	*Ask about:* Pain Swollen nodes
Nose and Throat	*Ask about:* Sore throat Nasal congestion
Respiratory	*Ask about:* Cough, congestion Mucus production
Cardiovascular	*Ask about:* History of vascular disease
Musculoskeletal	*Ask about:* History of gout Hearing problems
Neurological	*Ask about:* History of TIAs Balance problems Neurological problems

AREA/SYSTEM	OBJECTIVE DATA
General	*Inspect:* Ear guarding, inattentiveness, inappropriate responses, balance problems *Measure:* Vital signs
Integumentary	*Inspect:* Lesions, areas of inflammation *Palpate:* Tenderness
HEENT *Head and Neck*	*Palpate:* Lymph node enlargement, sinus tenderness
Nose and Throat	*Inspect:* Oral and nasal structures
Respiratory	*Measure:* Respiratory rate *Auscultate:* Lung sounds
Cardiovascular	*Measure:* Heart rate *Palpate:* Pulses, carotid thrills *Auscultate:* Heart sounds, bruits
Musculoskeletal	*Inspect:* Ear lobes for tophi
Neurological	*Test:* Romberg's

Assessment of the Ears' Relationship to Other Systems

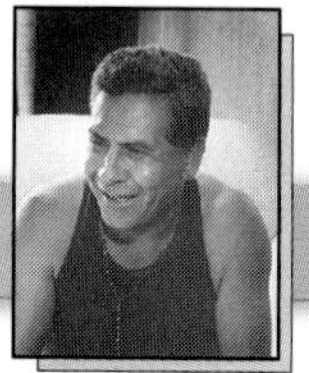

Case Study Analysis and Plan

Now that your examination of Mr. Arnez is complete, document your key history and physical examination findings.

List key history findings and key physical examination findings for Mr. Arnez that will help you formulate your nursing diagnoses.

Nursing Diagnoses

1. Sensory Perception, disturbed, auditory, related to ear pressure and fullness
2. Pain, chronic, related to ear pressure and fullness
3. Infection, risk for

Identify any additional nursing diagnoses.

CRITICAL THINKING ACTIVITY #12

Once you have identified appropriate nursing diagnoses for Mr. Arnez, select one from above and develop a nursing care plan and a brief teaching plan, including learning outcomes and teaching strategies.

Research Tells Us

Researchers have identified a new profile for neonates at risk of hearing disorders. In a study of 777 infants (431 males and 339 females) with a mean gestational age of 33.8 + or −4.3 weeks, 3 factors were found to be significant predictors of hearing problems. These were a family history of hearing loss, a history of bacterial infections, and craniofacial abnormalities. The nurse's assessment for these factors during the health history interview and physical examination can be useful for identifying infants at risk for hearing problems and can lead to early referral and intervention.

Source: Meyer, C., Witte, J., Hildmann, A., Hennecke, K., H., Schunck, K., U., Maul, K., Franke, U., Fahnenstich, H., Rabe, H., Rossie, H., Hartmann, S., & Gortner, l. (1999). Neonatal screening for hearing disorders in infants at risk: Incidence, risk factors, and follow-up. *Pediatrics, 104*(4), pp 900–904.

Health Concerns

Screening for hearing loss should begin in infancy. Because development of speech and psychosocial skills depend on adequate hearing, any child with a suspected developmental delay should be screened for hearing loss. Evaluate the environment and feeding habits of infants diagnosed with frequent ear infections. Chronic exposure to a smoker in the home and putting the child to bed with a bottle increase the incidence of ear infections. People exposed to loud noise should have regular hearing examinations and be instructed in ways to reduce their exposure, including the use of protective ear wear.

People receiving ototoxic medications should be evaluated for problems with balance, gait, vertigo, tinnitus and diminished hearing on a regular basis throughout therapy and be instructed to stay alert for signs of ototoxicity several weeks after therapy ends.

Common Abnormalities: Ears

ABNORMALITY	ASSESSMENT FINDINGS
Acoustic Neuroma Benign tumor that grows into auditory canal. Involves CN VIII	• Symptoms: tinnitus, progressive hearing loss, papilledema, headache, facial numbness and balance and gain problems (depending on the tumor's location and size).
Acute Otitis Media Inflammation or infection of middle ear	• Ear pain with reddened tympanic membrane. • Distorted cone of light reflex and signs of conductive hearing loss. 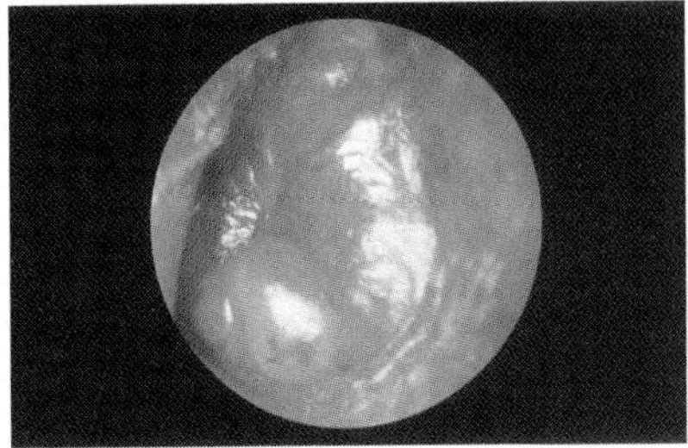
Cholesteatoma Cystlike sac of keratin debris caused by a congenital defect or chronic otitis media	• Can enlarge and obstruct middle ear. • Can release enzymes that erode. the ossicles. 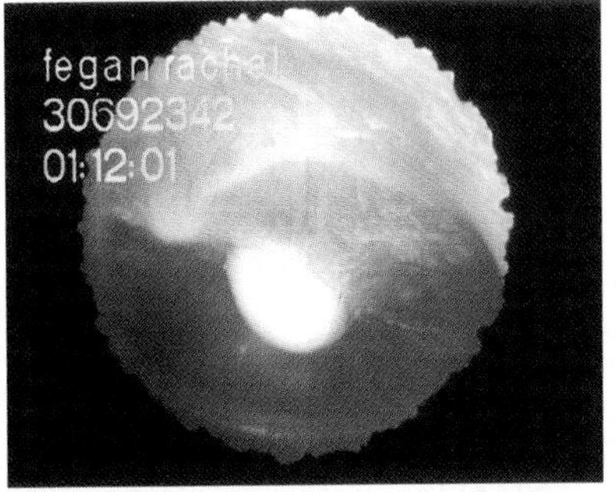
Hemotympanum Dark blue tympanic membrane caused by bleeding in middle ear behind it	• Sign of conductive hearing loss. • Evidence of recent head injury. 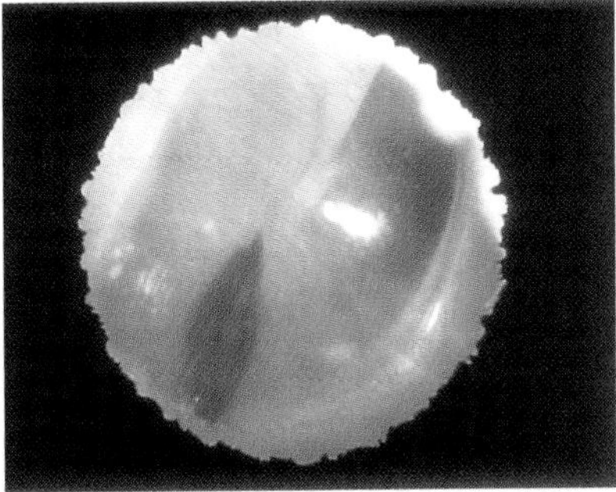
Ménière's Disease Chronic, progressive disease of inner ear that leads to permanent hearing loss	• Affects proprioception, the ability to accurately sense one's body position. • Characterized by a sensation of fullness or pressure in the ears and recurrent episodes of vertigo, tinnitus, and hearing loss, lasting from a few minutes to several hours. • Person may also experience nausea, vomiting, and profuse sweating. • Subjective sensation of ear fullness, vertigo, tinnitus. • Disturbance of balance and gait. • Positive sway with Romberg test.

(Continued)

Common Abnormalities: Ears *(Continued)*

ABNORMALITY	ASSESSMENT FINDINGS	
Otitis Externa Inflammation or infection of external ear, often caused by excessive swimming, chronic irritation, or removal of cerumen	• Ear pain, especially with movement of the tragus or pulling of ear lobe. • Redness of external auditory canal or auricle of external ear.	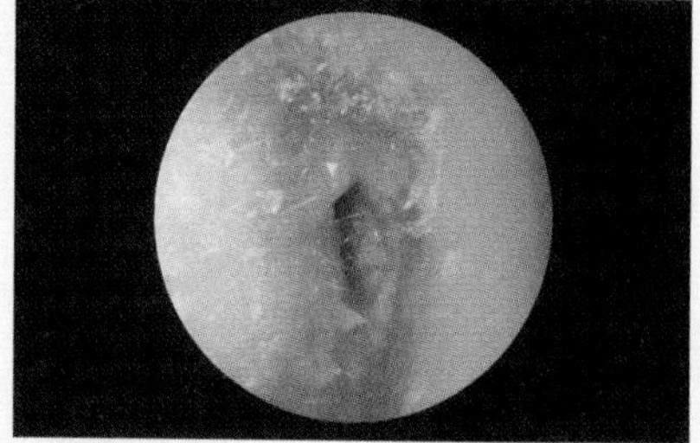
Presbycusis Diminished hearing acuity in older diminished for high-pitched sounds adults	• Hearing acuity especially • Diagnosed by watch tick test.	
Serous Otitis Media Yellowish tympanic membrane with serous fluid level or air bubble visible through membrane	• Cone of light reflex may be distorted. • Transient conductive hearing loss present.	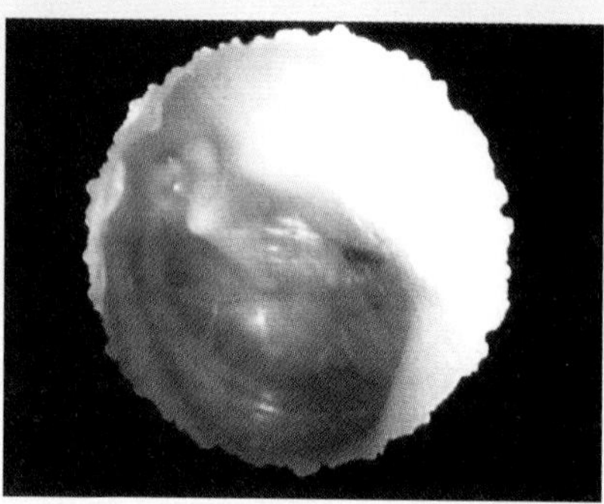

Summary

- A thorough health history provides direction for the physical examination to include exploration of factors that may be related to ear health. Information from both the history and the physical examination is then analyzed to determine appropriate nursing diagnoses.
- The ears are complex sensory organs that provide specialized functions crucial to neurosensory development in infancy and to the development of psychosocial, motor and cognitive skills in childhood, and the maintenance of those skills in adulthood.
- A comprehensive history and physical examination enable early detection and treatment of hearing problems.

11

Assessing the Respiratory System

Before You Begin

INTRODUCTION TO THE RESPIRATORY SYSTEM

Breathing is a natural function that most people never think about—unless it is impaired. As you will see, an ineffectively functioning respiratory system causes disruption throughout the body, just as changes in other body systems have a significant impact on the respiratory system.

Nurses can play a major role in preventing dysfunction or halting the progression of respiratory disease by identifying subtle changes. They can also identify people who are at risk because of unhealthy behaviors or genetic predisposition. Thus, the goal of a thorough respiratory assessment is early detection of risk factors, potential problems, or dysfunction of the system. With accurate and complete information, you will then be able to plan appropriate interventions—teaching health promotion/disease prevention and/or implementing treatment measures.

Anatomy and Physiology Review

Before you begin your assessment, you need to recognize normal respiratory function in order to distinguish abnormal findings. The anatomy will direct your assessment process. Visualizing the anatomical landmarks and underlying structures will enable you to perform the assessment accurately, and understanding the physiology will allow you to interpret your findings.

The primary function of the respiratory system is the exchange of oxygen and carbon dioxide through respiration. This system also plays a role in maintaining acid-base balance. The physiology of respiration consists of both mechanical and physiological processes.

The mechanical process of respiration is accomplished by pulmonary ventilation, the exchange of air between the lungs and the atmosphere. It consists of two phases—inspiration and expiration.

The physiological process occurs on three levels: external, internal and cellular:

- External respiration is the exchange of gases (oxygen and carbon dioxide) between the alveoli and the blood through the alveolar-capillary membrane.
- Internal respiration is the exchange of gases between the systemic capillaries and the tissue at the cellular level.
- The cellular physiological process is the exchange of gases within the cell.

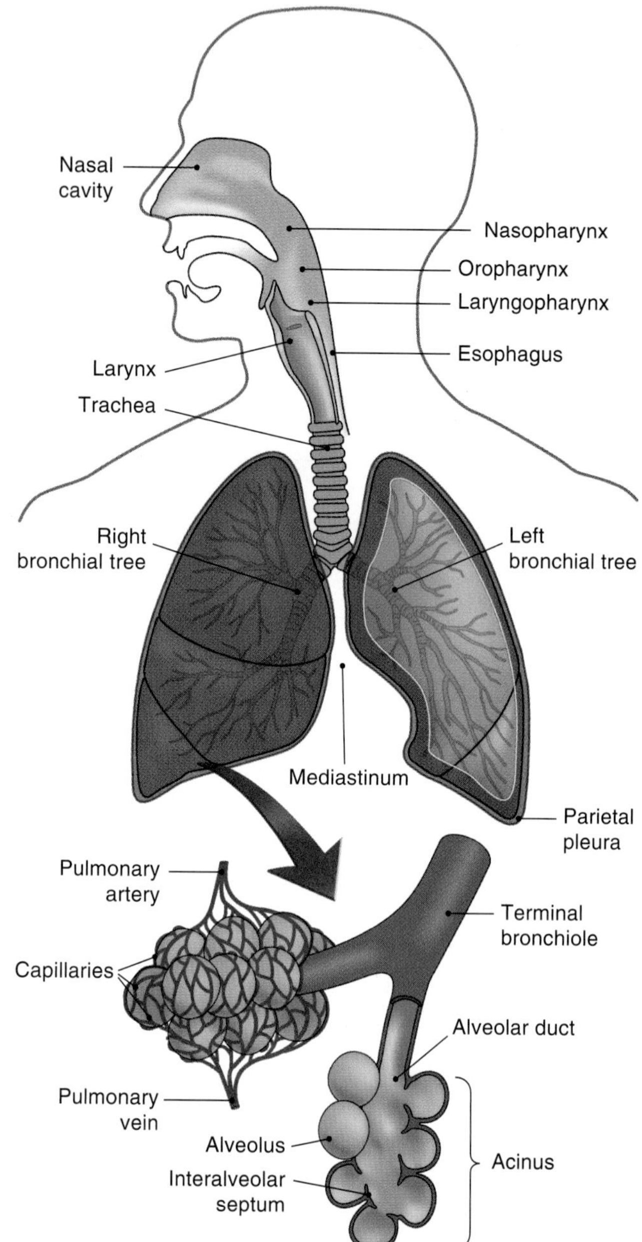

FIGURE 11–1. Structures of the respiratory system.

Structures of the Respiratory System

The respiratory system (Fig. 11–1) begins at the nose and continues as a series of airways or passages extending to the alveoli where gas exchange takes place. The nasal, oropharynx, and conducting airways are considered dead space because no exchange of gases occurs there. The nasal and oropharynx airways include the nasal cavity, pharynx, and larynx. The conducting airways include the trachea and bronchi.

The bronchioles are transitional airways where some gas exchange occurs. The alveolar ducts, sacs, and alveolus are the functional units of the lung in which exchange of gases occurs with the pulmonary capillary bed. The primary muscle of respiration is the diaphragm; the secondary muscles are called the accessory muscles. The negative lung pressure that is needed for breathing is maintained by the pleura.

Acid-Base Balance

The respiratory system plays a key role in maintaining acid-base balance by responding first to changes in blood acidity. When carbon dioxide is converted to bicarbonate or carbonic acid, the blood's pH becomes either more alkaline or more acidic. Depending on the type of acid-base problem, the respiratory system responds by changing the rate and depth of respiration.

For example, in metabolic acidosis, a metabolic imbalance characterized by excess acid retention, the rate and depth of respiration *increases* to blow off excess carbon dioxide, which reduces the amount available to make carbonic acid. This results in a decrease of hydrogen ions and subsequent movement of the pH toward its normal range. On the other hand, in metabolic alkalosis, an imbalance characterized by an excess of base, the respiratory system *decreases* the rate and depth of

Structures and Functions of the Respiratory System

STRUCTURE	DESCRIPTION/PRIMARY FUNCTION
Nasal Cavity	Warms, filters and moistens air.
Pharynx	Musculomembranous tube that acts as a passage between nose and larynx for air and between mouth and esophagus for food. Consists of three parts: the nasopharynx, oropharynx, and laryngopharynx.
Nasopharynx	Passage for air behind nasal cavities. Adenoids or pharyngeal tonsils located on posterior wall are lymphoid tissue and have a protective function. Eustachian tubes extend from middle ears and open into nasopharynx to equalize atmospheric pressure.
Oropharynx	Passage for both air and food, located behind mouth. Palatine tonsils are on lateral wall of oropharynx.
Laryngopharynx	Most inferior portion of pharynx. Opens anteriorly into larynx and posteriorly into esophagus.
Larynx	Passage between pharynx and trachea. Contains vocal cords to produce sound.
Single Cartilages	Cartilages that support larynx.
Thyroid	
Epiglottis	Prevents food from entering trachea.
Cricoid	
Paired Cartilages	Support and affect vocal cords.
Arytenoid	
Cuneiform	
Corniculate	
Trachea	Conducting airway between the larynx and bronchi, about 10 to 12 cm long. Divides into two primary bronchi midthorax at the carina.
Bronchi	Conducting airways to hilum of each lung. Each primary bronchus branches into secondary (lobar) and tertiary (segmental) bronchi.
Bronchioles	Smaller transitional airways to alveoli. Consist of bronchioles (>1 mm in diameter), terminal bronchioles (>0.5 mm) and even smaller respiratory bronchioles, in which some gas exchange occurs.
Alveolar Ducts, Sacs	Functional units of lung. Each lung has more than 350 million alveoli, in which exchange of gases between alveoli and pulmonary capillary bed occurs.
Pleura Serous	Protective linings of lungs that maintain negative pressure and aid in mechanics of breathing. Consists of parietal pleura and visceral pleura.
Parietal pleura	Line thoracic wall and superior portion of diaphragm.
Visceral pleura	Extension of parietal pleura that covers lung. Serous fluid fills and lubricates pleural cavity, preventing friction.

respiration to conserve carbon dioxide. Breathing pattern changes such as hyperventilation or hypoventilation are either compensation for an out-of-balance pH or a primary cause of acid-base imbalances. Hyperventilation can result in respiratory alkalosis; hypoventilation can result in respiratory acidosis.

Interaction with Other Body Systems

The neurological, musculoskeletal, and circulatory systems have an essential role in maintaining respiratory function. A problem in any of these systems may affect the functioning of the respiratory system.

The Neurological System

In the brain, the respiratory control centers are located in the reticular substance of the medulla oblongata and in the pons. The respiratory center within the medulla can be divided further into two opposing centers: the inspiratory center and the expiratory center. These two centers control the motor neurons to the phrenic nerve, which arises in the third, fourth, and fifth cervical nerve segments of the spinal cord and innervate the diaphragm, and the intercostal muscles, which arise in the upper thoracic segments. The inspiratory center stimulates the contractions of the respiratory muscles, at the same time

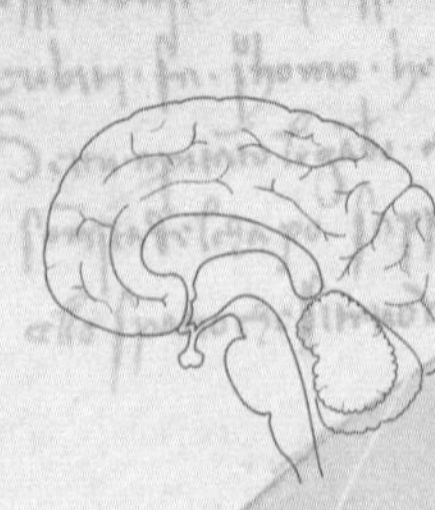

NEUROLOGICAL

Medulla is respiratory center.

Chemoreceptors respond to changes in carbon dioxide, oxygen and hydrogen ions by affecting rate and depth of respirations.

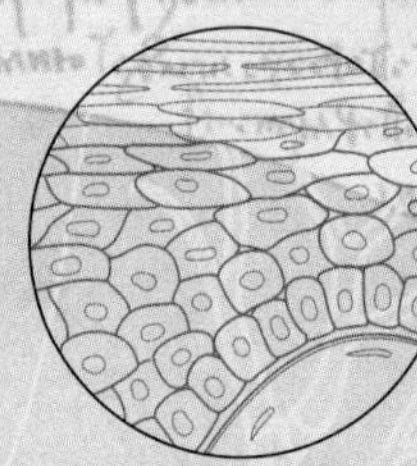
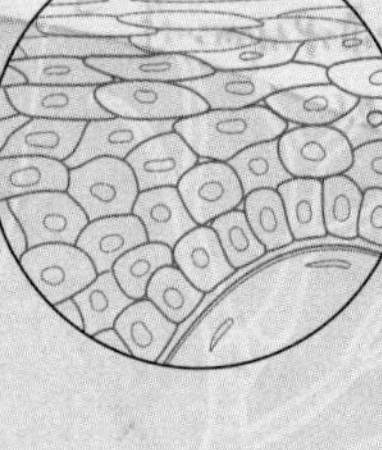

INTEGUMENTARY

Protects structures of upper respiratory tract.

Nasal hair filters air.

Skin color reflects oxygenation.

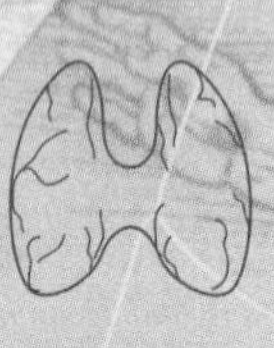

ENDOCRINE

Converting enzymes in lung convert angiotensin I to angiotensin II.

Epinephrine and norepinephrine increase respiratory rate and dilate airways.

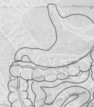

DIGESTIVE

Abdominal muscles aid with respirations.

GI tract provides nutrients to respiratory system.

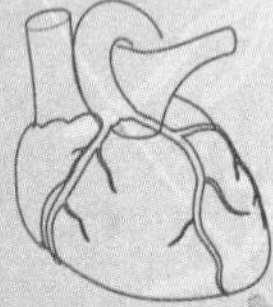

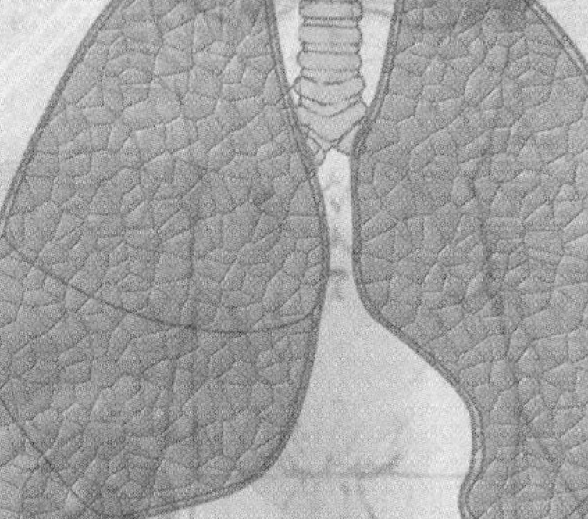

SKELETAL

Ribs provide protective framework for lungs.

CARDIOVASCULAR

Cardiovascular system transports oxygen and carbon dioxide between lungs and peripheral tissue.

Activation of angiotensin by lungs important in B/P regulation.

Peripheral chemoreceptors in aortic arch and carotid arteries respond to oxygen, carbon dioxide and hydrogen ion concentrations.

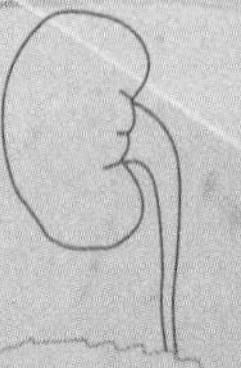
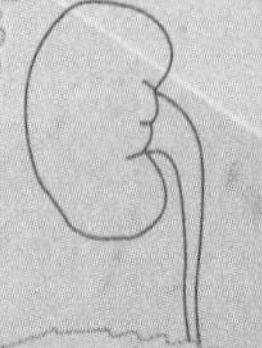

MUSCULAR

Diaphragm, chest and abdominal muscles needed for breathing.

Accessory muscles used when oxygen demands are increased, as with strenuous exercise.

URINARY

GU system works with respiratory system to eliminate wastes and maintain acid-base balance.

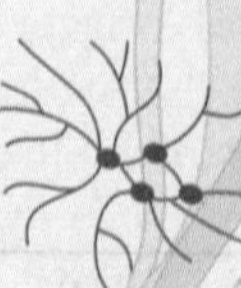

LYMPHATIC

Alveolar macrophages trap microorganisms and other foreign substances.

Foreign material removed by cilia or lymphatic system.

Tonsils and adenoids protect upper airways from infection, but also may become enlarged and obstruct breathing.

REPRODUCTIVE

Sexual activity increases oxygen demands.

Pregnancy affects oxygen demands and breathing.

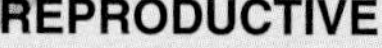

Relationship of Respiratory System to Other Systems

depressing the expiratory center. This results in inhalation. The process then reverses; as the inspiratory center is depressed, the expiratory center is stimulated, resulting in relaxation of the respiratory muscles and exhalation.

The pons also has two respiratory centers—the apneustic and the pneumotaxic—which are responsible for the rhythm of breathing. The apneustic center prolongs inspiration and the pneumotaxic center contributes to exhalation. These brainstem centers are connected to the hypothalamus and cerebral cortex, the parts of the brain that control emotions such as fear, pain, and anger. These types of emotions can affect breathing to the same extent as activities like talking or singing, which require more conscious breath control. A child who holds his or her breath during a tantrum is exhibiting conscious breath control. However, if the child loses consciousness as a result, the lower brain centers resume control again, so the child breathes automatically.

The respiratory center is sensitive to changes in carbon dioxide ($Paco_2$) levels and responds accordingly by affecting the rate and depth of respiration until homeostasis is achieved. Central chemoreceptors are found bilaterally in the medulla; peripheral chemoreceptors are located in the aortic arch and at the bifurcation of the carotid arteries. The most potent chemical affecting respiration is $Paco_2$. Even slight elevations reduce the pH of the cerebrospinal fluid, sending strong signals to the central chemoreceptors. This, in turn, stimulates the respiratory centers to increase the respiratory rate.

Changes in oxygen (Pao_2) have a weak influence on respiratory rate. Only when the peripheral chemoreceptors sense a Pao_2 less than 60 mm Hg will Pao_2 become a major stimulus to increase respiration. In general, blood oxygen levels act by increasing or decreasing the chemoreceptor's sensitivity to $Paco_2$. Homeostasis of the acid-base balance of the body is maintained by the very complex interactions between carbon dioxide, oxygen, and blood pH unless disease intervenes.

The Musculoskeletal System

The musculoskeletal system provides the bony structure (thorax) and the muscles needed for breathing. The phrenic nerve innervates the diaphragm, the primary muscle used for breathing. A dome-shaped muscle at the floor of the thorax, the diaphragm separates the thorax from the abdomen. During inspiration, the diaphragm flattens as it contracts, enlarging the chest capacity. During exhalation, the diaphragm relaxes and rises to assume a dome shape.

Accessory muscles include the sternocleidomastoid, anterior serrati, scalene, trapezius, intercostal, and rhomboid muscles. They come into play during strenuous physical activity (such as jogging) or when the body has intrapulmonary resistance to air movement. The accessory muscles enhance ventilation by increasing chest expansion and lung size during inspiration. When contracted, the external intercostal muscles pull the ribs up and out; the internal intercostal muscles pull the ribs down and inward. Contraction of these muscles decreases intrathoracic pressure, causing an inward flow of air. As the muscles relax, the lungs recoil, and exhalation occurs. The abdominal muscles also assist with rapid breathing, deep breathing, exercise, coughing, and sneezing. An intact thoracic cage is essential for normal respiratory function (Fig. 11–2).

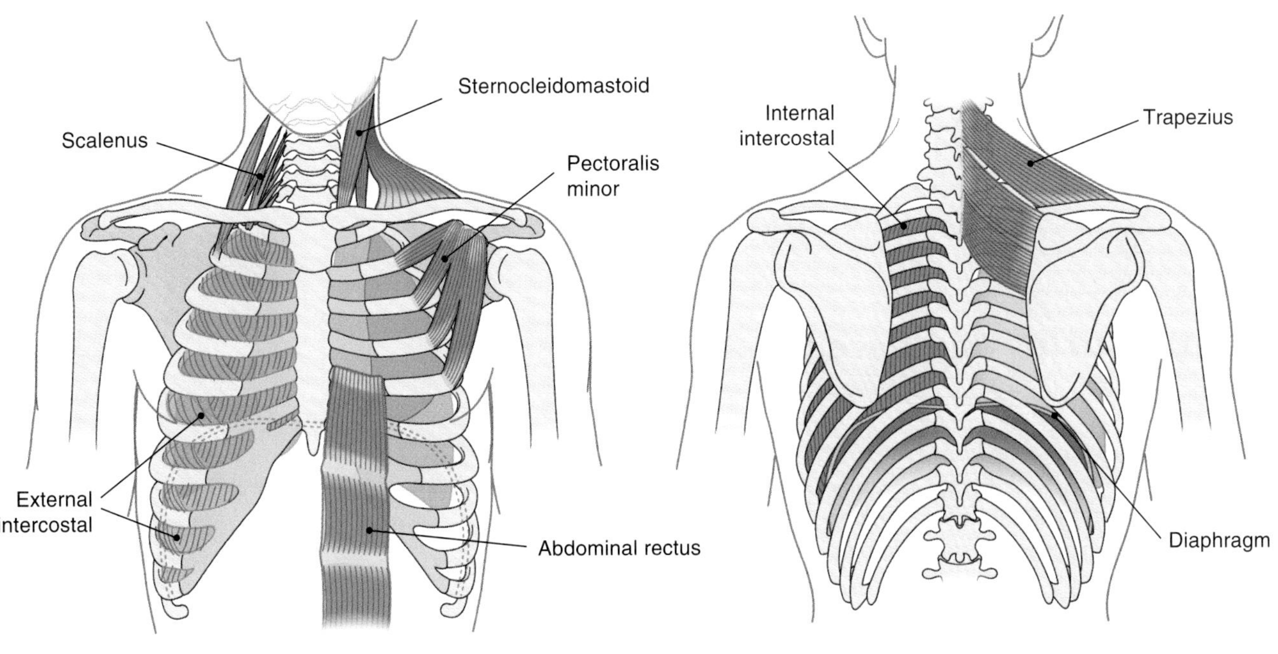

FIGURE 11–2. Muscles used for breathing.

The Circulatory System

The circulatory system of the lungs consists of the bronchial and pulmonary circulation. Bronchial circulation attends to the metabolic demands of the lung tissue. Pulmonary circulation fosters the exchange of gases between the alveoli and blood in the pulmonary capillaries. Oxygen, which diffuses from the alveoli into the pulmonary circulation, binds with hemoglobin and is transported to the cells. Similarly, carbon dioxide moves from the cells, into the pulmonary circulation, and finally into the alveoli to be exhaled from the body. Any disruption of the circulation within the lungs affects the body's ability to provide adequate oxygen to tissues or to remove enough carbon dioxide for healthy functioning.

Developmental, Cultural, and Ethnic Variations

Infants

Infants are obligatory nose breathers. Their respirations are primarily abdominal, and breath sounds are louder, harsher, and bronchovesicular. Their respiratory rhythm is often irregular, with brief periods of apnea. The shape of the chest is more round than oval, with the ribs in a horizontal position. After about age 2, the ribs become more oblique, and the breathing pattern becomes primarily intercostal.

ALERT

In infants, periods of apnea that exceed 15 seconds may indicate a cardiopulmonary or CNS disorder and need further evaluation. The infant may be at high risk for sudden infant death syndrome (SIDS).

Pregnant Women

During pregnancy, increases in tidal volume and respiratory rate allow for a 20 percent increase in oxygen consumption. Later in the pregnancy, the diaphragm rises and the costal angle widens to accommodate the enlarging uterus.

Older Adults

Alveoli usually become fibrotic with age, resulting in a decreased surface area for exchange of gases. Breathing and lung capacity decrease as a result of muscle weakness and decreased elasticity. This results in increased dead space, trapped air, and decreased vital capacity. Musculoskeletal changes that occur with aging can cause an increase in the anterior-posterior diameter from weakening of the intercostal muscles and softening of the rib cartilage. The thoracic curve may also increase, resulting in mild kyphosis, an accentuated thoracic curve. Together these changes give the appearance of a barrel chest, but without the dysfunction.

People of Different Cultures/Ethnic Groups

Chest size can vary among cultures in proportion to the person's size. For example, Chinese-Americans have smaller chests than Caucasians or African-Americans. The higher incidence of respiratory problems among certain ethnic groups relates more specifically to occupational and environmental factors than genetic ones. For example, African-Americans living in urban areas have a higher risk of respiratory disease. Appalachians have a higher risk for black lung, emphysema, and tuberculosis (TB). The Irish have a higher risk for respiratory problems related to coal mining. Navajo Indians have an increased risk for respiratory diseases because of close living quarters.

Introducing the Case Study

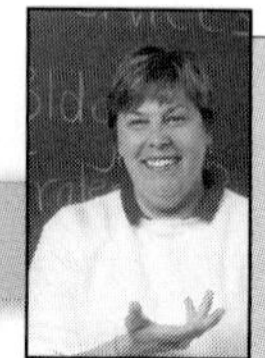

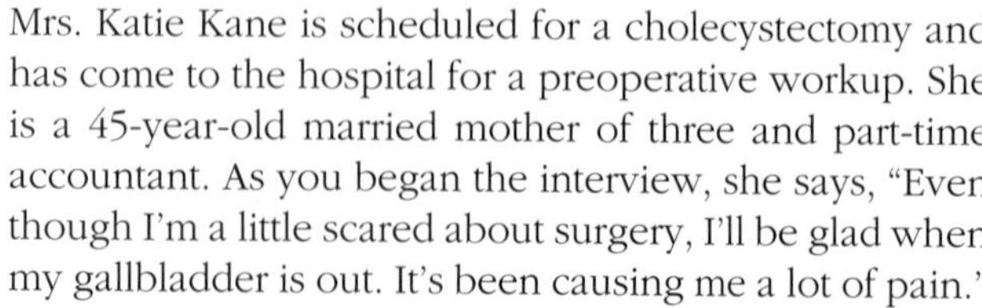

Mrs. Katie Kane is scheduled for a cholecystectomy and has come to the hospital for a preoperative workup. She is a 45-year-old married mother of three and part-time accountant. As you began the interview, she says, "Even though I'm a little scared about surgery, I'll be glad when my gallbladder is out. It's been causing me a lot of pain."

Mrs. Kane is scheduled to have general anesthesia, so a thorough respiratory assessment is necessary.

Performing the Respiratory Assessment

Assessment of the respiratory system involves a comprehensive health history and physical examination. As you perform the assessment, be alert for signs or symptoms of actual or potential respiratory problems.

Health History

The health history identifies respiratory symptoms and risk factors. It provides you with subjective data to guide your examination. As you proceed, be alert for actual or potential problems.

Biographical Data

A quick review of the biographical data may identify actual or potential problems. How old is the client? Respiratory structure and function change with age. For example, young children are more susceptible to respiratory infections because their airways are smaller, but as people age, their forced expiratory volume decreases. Residence and occupation also have an impact on the respiratory system because a person's job or environment may harbor risk factors. Chronic diseases may place financial strains on clients, so you may need to make referrals to agencies that can assist them.

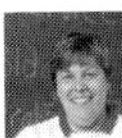

Case Study Findings

Reviewing Mrs. Kane's biographical data:

- 45-year-old white female
- Married, mother of three children, ages 15, 10, and 8
- Part-time accountant; BA degree in accounting.
- Born and raised in United States
- Catholic religion
- Healthcare insurance (HMO) through husband's work
- Referral: Preadmission workup for surgery
- Source: Self, seems reliable

Current Health Status

Begin with the client's chief complaint. Three major respiratory symptoms to watch for are dyspnea, cough, and chest pain. Perform a symptom analysis for any presenting symptom, using the PQRST format. If you notice signs of respiratory distress, such as shortness of breath (SOB), confusion, or anxiety, postpone the detailed history and focus on the acute problem. Obtain a detailed history later, when the client's condition improves, or get it from a secondary source such as a family member.

A client with chronic respiratory disease often adapts to a compromised respiratory status. Therefore compare the client's present respiratory status to his or her status at previous examinations to evaluate the impact of the disease's progression.

HELPFUL HINT

Respiratory disease makes people tire easily because most of their energy is expended on breathing. Therefore divide the history into several short interviews and ask questions that can be easily answered with few words.

Symptom Analysis

Symptom Analysis tables for all of the symptoms described in the following paragraphs are available on the Web for viewing and printing. In your Web browser, go to *http://www.fadavis.com/detail.cfm?id=0882-9* and click on Symptom Analysis Tables under Explore This Product.

Cough

Coughing is one of the most common respiratory complaints. The causes range from insignificant to life-threatening conditions. Coughing is a protective, reflexive mechanism that helps maintain a patent airway. It occurs in three phases: Deep inspiration that increases lung volume, closure of the glottis, and then muscular contraction forcing the sudden opening of the glottis, resulting in a cough. Cough receptors, located in the larynx, respiratory tree, pleura, acoustic duct, nose, sinuses, pharynx, stomach, and diaphragm respond to mechanical, inflammatory, or irritating stimuli.

Dyspnea

Dyspnea is a subjective sensation of breathing difficulty often described as shortness of breath (SOB). It may be normal with overexertion or anxiety, but it may also signal underlying cardiopulmonary or neuromuscular problems or allergic reactions.

CHRONIC OBSTRUCTIVE PULMONARY DISEASE

Chronic obstructive pulmonary disease (COPD) is a chronic, progressive disease characterized by airway obstruction and diminished lung function. It includes asthma, emphysema, and chronic bronchitis. Increasing dyspnea may correlate with the progression of the disease

CONGESTIVE HEART FAILURE

Congestive heart failure (CHF) causes the heart to pump ineffectively, resulting in volume overload. The right side, left side, or both sides of the heart can fail. Right heart failure (cor pulmonale) is frequently associated with lung disease.

Chest Pain

Chest pain may have cardiac, pulmonary, gastrointestinal, or musculoskeletal origins. However, chest pain of respiratory origin is associated with the parietal pleura, chest wall, and mediastinal structures because the lungs and visceral pleura do not have pain fibers.

Related Symptoms

Other symptoms associated with respiratory disease include edema and fatigue. Edema results from right-side congestive heart failure, a common complication of chronic obstructive lung disease. Usually edema is located in the lower extremities or abdomen. Ask your client, "Do you have swelling in your abdomen, legs, ankles, or feet?"

Hypoxia, increased energy expended for breathing, and associated cardiac involvement accompany longstanding lung disease and contribute to the development of fatigue. People adapt to fatigue by lowering their activity level, so they have more difficulty performing ADLs. Changes in rest and sleep patterns may also be seen. Ask your client, "Do you have enough energy to do your usual daily activities? Do you need to sleep or rest more than usual?"

COR PULMONALE

Cor pulmonale is right heart hypertrophy or failure resulting from disorders of the lungs or pulmonary vessels. Common causes include chronic obstructive pulmonary diseases and living at high altitudes for extended periods.

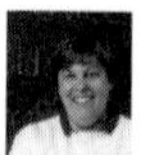

Case Study Findings

Mrs. Kane's current health status includes:

- Brief morning cough for past 5 years productive of small amount of thin, whitish-gray mucus, no odor or bad taste. Cough does not occur with activity or exercise. Positive history of smoking.
- No dyspnea or chest pain.
- No edema, loss of usual energy, change in sleeping patterns (except when gallbladder discomfort awakens her).

Past Health History

The purpose of the past health history is to compare it with the client's present respiratory status or uncover risk factors that might predispose him or her to respiratory disorders. Be sure to follow up on any unclear or

Past Health History

RISK FACTORS/ QUESTIONS TO ASK	RATIONALE/SIGNIFICANCE
Childhood Illnesses	
Did you have frequent respiratory infections, asthma, TB, or pneumonia as a child?	May indicate underlying chronic disease.
Hospitalizations/Surgeries	
Have you ever been hospitalized? What for? Have you ever had a TB test, chest x ray, or other respiratory diagnostic testing? When?	Can be used as baseline data. Also indicates disease prevention activities.
Serious Injuries/Chronic Illnesses	
Have you had fractured ribs, steering wheel injuries, or knife wounds to the chest? Have you ever had a previous respiratory illness? Do you have any other chronic medical problems, such as heart disease, renal disease, cancer, or HIV?	May explain physical findings. May have respiratory manifestations.
Immunizations	
Were you immunized as a child? Did you receive adult boosters against respiratory diseases? (e.g., pneumovax for pneumonia and bacille Calmette-Guérin [BCG] for TB?)	Identify health promotion or teaching needs; BCG explains a positive tuberculosis test (PPD).
Allergies	
Do you have any allergies (e.g., to pollens, food, drugs, environmental factors)? What type of reaction do you have?	Can cause chronic sinus or nasal congestion, trigger an asthma attack, or progress to COPD.

Past Health History

RISK FACTORS/ QUESTIONS TO ASK	RATIONALE/SIGNIFICANCE
Medications	
What prescribed and OTC drugs are you taking? For how long?	Determines compliance with treatment and therapeutic vs. toxic effects. Excessive use of medications can lead to tolerance and rebound effects. Client may be on cardiac drugs or oxygen. Corticosteroids (cortisone), which are often prescribed to relieve signs and symptoms of COPD, have serious side effects that need to be monitored. Allows evaluation of possible adverse drug interactions (e.g., beta adrenergics and antihypertensives). See box, Drugs That Adversely Affect the Respiratory System, page 322.
Recent Travel/Military Service/ Exposure to Infectious or Contagious Diseases	
Have you traveled by plane recently? Stayed in a hotel room?	Respiratory infections (e.g., upper respiratory infections or Legionnaire's disease) are more easily transmitted by the closed airflow in airplanes or faulty ventilation systems in hotels.
Have you been exposed to people with colds, flu, or cough?	Can identify contagious disorders. TB is most commonly acquired from living with infected family members.

vague answers. Rewording the question may help the client find a relevant response.

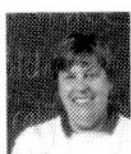

Case Study Findings

Mrs. Kane's past health history reveals:

- Frequent URIs as a child.
- No history of asthma, pneumonia, or TB.
- Never had surgery. Hospitalized only for childbirth—uncomplicated vaginal delivery of three children.
- No known exposure to people with respiratory infections.
- Denies allergies to food, drugs, or environmental factors.
- No medical problems except for gallbladder disease.
- Immunizations up to date. Last purified protein derivative (PPD) test a year ago was negative.
- Denies taking prescribed drugs. Takes acetaminophen about twice a month for headache relief.

ALERT

Side effects of oral or inhaled bronchodilators include nausea/vomiting, tremors, nervousness, insomnia, tachycardia, hypertension and oral fungus (inhaled).

Family History

The purpose of the family history is to identify any predisposing or causative factors of respiratory origin. If possible, help clients draw a family tree. This helps them remember more relevant information about family members.

Family History

RISK FACTORS QUESTIONS TO ASK	RATIONALE/SIGNIFICANCE
Genetically Linked Respiratory Disorders	
Does anyone in your family have:	
Alpha antitrypsin deficiency?	Increased risk for emphysema
Allergies or asthma?	Avoid allergens, smoking
Cystic fibrosis?	Autosomal dominant disorder
Smoking	
Are you or were you exposed to second-hand smoke in your home? If so, for how long? What type of tobacco product was used?	Second-hand smoke can cause cancer, COPD, asthma.
TB	
Does anyone in your family have TB? If so, what type and how long were you exposed?	Will need follow-up PPD or chest x ray.

Drugs That Adversely Affect the Respiratory System

Drug Class	Drug	Possible Adverse Reactions
Adrenergic agents (sympathomimetics)	epinephrine hydrochloride	Dyspnea, paradoxical bronchospasms
Adrenergic blockers (sympatholytics)	methysergide maleate	Nasal congestion; pulmonary fibrosis, resulting in dyspnea, tightness, chest pain, pleural friction rubs, effusion
Alkylating agents	busulfan	Irreversible pulmonary fibrosis (busulfan lung)
	carmustine	Pulmonary infiltrates, fibrosis
	cyclophosphamide	Pulmonary fibrosis (with high doses)
	melphalan	Pneumonitis
Antiarrhythmics	amiodarone hydrochloride	Interstitial pneumonitis, pulmonary fibrosis
Antibiotic antineoplastic agents	bleomycin sulfate	Fine crackles, dyspnea (early signs of pulmonary toxicity); interstitial pneumonitis
	mitomycin	Dyspnea, cough, hemoptysis, pulmonary infiltrates
Antihypertensives	enalapril maleate	Cough
	guanethidine sulfate	Nasal congestion
	guanabenz acetate	Nasal congestion
	reserpine	Nasal congestion
Anti-infectives	polymyxin B sulfate	Respiratory paralysis
Antimetabolites	methotrexate sodium	Pneumonitis
Beta-blockers	all beta-blockers	Bronchospasm, particularly in clients with a history of asthma; dyspnea, wheezing
Cholinergic agents	bethanecol chloride	Dyspnea, sore throat, bronchoconstriction (with subcutaneous administration)
	donepezil	
	neostigmine bromide	Increased bronchial secretions, bronchospasm
Gold salts	aurothioglucose, gold sodium thiomalate	Pulmonary infiltrates, interstitial pneumonitis, interstitial fibrosis, "gold" bronchitis
Narcotic analgesics	All types	Respiratory depression
Nonsteroidal anti-inflammatory agents	aspirin	Bronchospasm
	ibuprofen	Bronchospasm, dyspnea
	indomethacin	Bronchospasm, dyspnea
Penicillins	All types	Anaphylaxis
Sedatives and hypnotics	All types	Respiratory depression, apnea
Urinary tract antiseptics	nitrofurantoin, nitrofurantoin macrocrystals	Pulmonary sensitivity reactions, such as cough, chest pain, dyspnea, pulmonary infiltrates; interstitial pneumonitis (with prolonged use)
Miscellaneous agents	cromolyn sodium	Cough, wheezing
	levodopa	Excessive nasal discharge, hoarseness, episodic hyperventilation, bizarre breathing paterns
	thiamine hydrochloride	Tightness of throat, respiratory distress, cyanosis, pulmonary edema (with I.V. administration)

TB IN IMMIGRANTS

Because immigrants from Southeast Asia often receive the BCG vaccine before admission to the United States, they are often PPD positive without infection. They should still have a chest x ray at least every 5 to 10 years. They may need to take antituberculosis drugs if active disease is present in a family member.

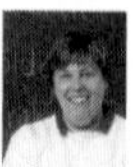

Case Study Findings

Mrs. Kane's family history reveals:

- Grandfather smoked and died of lung cancer at age 63.
- Father, age 65, recently quit after smoking a pack a day for 40 years (40 pack-years). Diagnosed with lung cancer a year ago.
- All other known relatives alive and well.

Review of Systems

Changes in the respiratory system have an impact on every other body system. In addition to helping you detect problems that directly affect the respiratory system, the review of systems (ROS) identifies changes in other systems that result from changes in the respiratory system. The ROS allows you to catch anything that you might have missed so far, and it gives meaning to the symptom by relating it to the affected system.

Review of Systems

SYSTEM/QUESTIONS TO ASK	RATIONALE/SIGNIFICANCE
General Health Survey	
Do you have fatigue or activity intolerance?	Chronic lung disease often causes fatigue and activity intolerance because so much energy is expended on breathing.
Have you had unexplained fever, night sweats, or weight loss?	May be associated with a more serious underlying disease such as tuberculosis.
Have you gained weight recently?	May correlate with fluid retention associated with right side CHF, a common complication of COPD.
Integumentary	
Have you noticed any skin color changes?	*Cyanosis:* Cardiopulmonary disease.
Do you have swollen ankles or tight shoes?	*Fluid retention:* Right-side cardiac involvement of long-standing respiratory disease.
HEENT	
Head/Neck	
Do you have any swelling, masses, or difficulty swallowing?	*Enlarged lymph nodes:* Infection or malignancy. Enlarged thyroid may compromise respiratory function.
Eyes	
Do you have excessive tearing?	Associated with allergies.
Nose/Throat	
Do you have postnasal drip, sinus pain, or sore throat?	May indicate allergies or acute/chronic URI.
Cardiovascular	
Do you have chest pain?	May indicate cardiac involvement.
Gastrointestinal	
Do you have right upper quadrant (RUQ) pain, nausea, or gastrointestinal (GI) upset?	Associated with right CHF, a common complication of COPD.
Have you experienced loss of appetite and weight loss?	Associated with chronic lung disease, TB, or lung malignancy.
Urinary	
Do you awaken during the night to urinate?	*Nocturia:* Associated with heart failure or diuretic use to treat right-side heart failure.
Reproductive	
Have you had any changes in sexual performance?	Chronic respiratory disease requires most of the client's energy for breathing.
Do you practice safe sex?	Unprotected sexual activity increases risk for HIV.
Musculoskeletal	
Have you had any weakness or muscle wasting?	Chronic lung disease.
Neurological	
Have you experienced any irritability, confusion, forgetfulness, or changes in your mental abilities? Have you had tremors?	*Change in mental status:* Early sign of hypoxia. Associated with theophylline toxicity or CO_2 narcosis.
Immune/Hematologic	
Have you had any anemia or allergies?	Directly affect respiratory system.

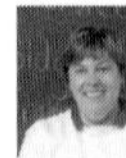

Case Study Findings

Mrs. Kane's review of systems reveals:

- General Health Survey: States that health is usually good. Has gained 15 lb in past 2 years.
- **Integumentary:** No changes in skin, hair, or nails.
- **HEENT:** ***Head/Neck:*** No swelling or masses. ***Eyes/Ears:*** Vision 20/20; hearing good. ***Nose/Throat:*** Productive morning cough with whitish-gray mucus. Has occasional cold.
- **Cardiovascular:** No chest pain.
- **Gastrointestinal:** Appetite good, no nausea or vomiting. Daily bowel movement.
- **Urinary:** No changes reported.
- **Reproductive:** Is in a monogamous relationship; satisfied with sexual performance.
- **Musculoskeletal:** No weakness or muscle wasting reported.
- **Neurological:** Memory good. No changes noted. No tremors.
- **Immune/Hematologic:** No allergies or anemia.

Psychosocial Profile

The psychosocial profile reveals lifestyle patterns that may affect the respiratory system and place the client at risk for respiratory disorders. The client's lifestyle may be affected by respiratory disease, especially when it is chronic.

Psychosocial Profile

CATEGORY/QUESTIONS TO ASK	RATIONALE/SIGNIFICANCE
Health Practices and Beliefs/ Self-Care Activities	
Do you have regular healthcare checkups; knowledge of medications, protection from environmental pollutants and allergens?	Ascertains compliance with treatment or screening for risk factors. Identifies teaching needs.
Typical Day	
What constitutes a usual day's activities? Has this changed over the last year?	Identifies whether a client is doing too much for energy level or limiting activities to compensate for loss of energy. Looks at possible disease progression. Shows ways client may be able to adapt lifestyle if needed.
Nutritional Patterns	
Have you lost weight and appetite?	Associated with lung cancer, but usually by the time weight loss is evident, metastasis has occurred.
	Dyspnea, fatigue, and decreased lung capacity from overinflation result in appetite loss and smaller amounts of food being consumed. Also evaluate ability to purchase and prepare food and effects of social isolation on eating habits.
	Weight loss is a common symptom in catabolic infections such as TB and AIDS.
Have you gained weight?	*Sudden gain:* Fluid retention from cardiac failure or secondary to medication (e.g., cortisone).
Activity and Exercise Patterns	
How would you rate your level of activity? Do you exercise regularly?	Gradual decrease or change in activity/exercise patterns seen in chronic respiratory disorders. Identifies need for physical therapy referral to improve respiratory function or for health promotion.
Pets/Hobbies	
Do you have cats, dogs, or birds in your home?	Pets and hobbies can promote health if they do not irritate respiratory function.
Do you have hobbies that require use of chemicals?	Exposure to glue, paint, sprays, silica, sawdust, or other irritants may necessitate changing hobbies.
	Allergies to pet fur or dander can trigger asthma attacks; exposure to bird droppings or feathers may cause hypersensitivity pneumonitis with eventual pulmonary fibrosis.

Psychosocial Profile

CATEGORY/QUESTIONS TO ASK	RATIONALE/SIGNIFICANCE
Sleep/Rest Patterns	
How much uninterrupted sleep do you get per night? Do you have insomnia? Do you feel rested in the morning? Do you take daytime naps?	Dyspnea, cough, pain, and medications can cause sleep pattern disturbances. Sleep apnea results in interrupted sleep and daytime fatigue.
Personal Habits	
Do you or did you ever smoke? In what form (e.g., cigarettes, cigars, marijuana)? Determine the pack-years (number of packs a day times number of years). If you quit smoking, how long ago?	Quitting smoking can improve respiratory function even if chronic respiratory problems already exist. Cigars may not be inhaled, but heat and tar can cause oral/pharyngeal/laryngeal damage. Marijuana is much more destructive to lungs than regular cigarettes, especially if smoked regularly.
Do you drink alcohol? What kind, how much, and how often?	Alcohol affects ciliary action, reducing mucus clearance and decreasing immune competence. Cough reflex may be depressed with heavy alcohol consumption, increasing risk of aspiration pneumonia.
Do you use street drugs?	IV drug abuse increases chance of HIV infection, which is associated with high incidence of opportunistic respiratory diseases such as *Pneumocystis carinii* pneumonia.
Occupational Health Patterns	
What is your occupation? Do you use protective equipment?	Looks for exposure to respiratory irritants such as chemicals and coal dust. Evaluates past employment for long-term exposure to asbestos and coal dust, which can cause cancer or black lung disease many years later. Healthcare workers may be exposed to TB and other diseases.
Is your work environment safe? Will you be able to continue in your present occupation? Do you have disability insurance?	A safe work environment provides masks, good ventilation, and freedom from second-hand smoke. Chronic respiratory disease affects job performance. Many employers allow respiratory-disabled people to work at home via computers. Explore this possibility with clients.
Environmental Health Patterns	
Where do you live?	Some respiratory diseases are more prevalent in certain areas (e.g., histoplasmosis in Mississippi River Valley, coccidioidomycosis in Southwest).
Is your home suitable for posthospital care or for person with progressive respiratory dysfunction?	Identifies discharge or home care needs, including durable medical equipment, supplies, caregivers.
Is your home environment urban or rural?	Can identify air pollutants.
Are you exposed to radon?	Radon increases risk for cancer.
What kind of heating and air conditioning do you have?	Molds and dust in heating and air conditioning systems can trigger reactive airway disease.
How many people live with you?	Multiple families in crowded conditions contribute to risk of transmitting infectious respiratory diseases.
Do you travel on freeways?	Freeway travel increases exposure to air pollutants.
Roles/Relationships/Self-Concept	
What is your role in the family? In the community? Have respiratory problems affected your family life, social life, or self-concept?	Chronic respiratory disease affects roles, relationships, and self-concept. Economic strain can occur as a result of loss of work. Limited mobility from chronic respiratory disease may lead to isolation and loss of community involvement. Be alert for signs of depression.
Cultural Influences	
Do you have any cultural influences that may affect your healthcare practices?	It is important to identify any cultural influences that may affect your client's healthcare practices.
Religious/Spiritual Influences	
Do you have any religious practices/beliefs that may influence your healthcare practices?	It is important to identify any religious practices/beliefs that may affect your client's healthcare practices.

(Continued)

Psychosocial Profile *(Continued)*

CATEGORY/QUESTIONS TO ASK	RATIONALE/SIGNIFICANCE
Sexuality Patterns	
Has your respiratory problem affected your ability to perform sexually?	Loss of energy/SOB can affect sexual performance.
Social Supports	
Are you involved in the community?	Identifies positive support systems in family and community.
Stress and Coping	
How do you manage anger, frustration, loss, and change?	Stress and coping patterns may be affected by respiratory status. Identifies and supports positive coping behaviors to decrease asthma attacks/dyspnea. For example, an action-reaction cycle occurs with stressed asthmatics: Stress triggers dyspnea; then as dyspnea worsens, person becomes more anxious. Learning appropriate coping skills to interrupt this cycle is important.

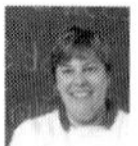

Case Study Findings

Mrs. Kane's psychosocial profile includes:

- Has a physical exam/Pap smear every 2 years. Made a special appointment when noticed RUQ colicky abdominal pain after eating high-fat meals. Scheduled surgery as soon as recommended by physician.
- Typical day consists of arising at 6 AM, having breakfast with family, and getting children off to school. Walks 5 blocks to and from work at CPA office 4 days a week. Works 8 AM to 4 PM at desk with computer. Spends evenings playing with children, helping them with homework, shopping, fixing dinner, doing housework, visiting with husband, and watching TV or reading. Showers, then goes to bed at 11 PM.
- Usually eats a healthy diet, but has gained about 15 pounds over the last 2 years. Attributes this to sedentary job, sweet tooth, and lack of exercise.
- Walks to and from work and likes to ride a bike, but doesn't have much time because of family, home, and work responsibilities.
- No pets; hobbies include reading and biking.
- Sleeps about 6 to 7 hours a night, uninterrupted, with one pillow. Denies problems falling asleep, but awakens with morning cough.
- Has smoked one pack of filtered cigarettes a day for past 10 years (10 pack-years). Lived with smokers all her life. Has tried to quit by cutting back without success. Drinks alcohol about 3 times a month at social events. Denies recreational drug use.
- Denies respiratory irritants at work.
- Lives in two-story, single-family home in suburbs with ample living space for five people; has hot water heating and air conditioning; home negative for radon gas; denies recent travel outside local community. Will stay in downstairs bedroom for the first week after surgery.
- Supportive, caring husband; good relationship with children. Concerned about father's prognosis and mother's ability to care for him. Aware of health risks of second-hand smoke for children, so tries not to smoke at home. Husband also smokes, both would like to "kick the habit." No community involvement at this time, but has several friends who will help out after surgery.
- Copes with stress by talking with husband/friends or by ignoring it; also by smoking.

FUNGAL AND BACTERIAL RESPIRATORY DISEASES

Histoplasmosis is a systemic, fungal respiratory disease whose organism is found in high organic content soil contaminated with bird droppings. Coccidioidomycosis (desert fever) is a self-limiting fungal respiratory disease that also has a more severe, progressive systemic form. Legionnaire's disease is a severe, often fatal gram-negative bacterial disease resulting in pneumonia and multisystem failure. The disease was isolated after an outbreak at an American Legion convention.

Focused Respiratory History

Your client's condition or time restraints may prohibit taking a detailed respiratory history. If so, ask questions that focus on a history of respiratory disease, the presence of respiratory symptoms, identification of risk factors, and health promotion activities. The client's response to these questions will help to direct your assessment. Key questions include the following:

- Do you have a history of respiratory disease? If so, are you taking any medications? What are they and why are you taking them?
- Do you have any other medical problems (especially cardiac problems)?
- Do you have allergies? If so, describe your reaction.
- Do you have a cough, shortness of breath, or chest pain?
- Do you use tobacco? If so, what kind, how much, and for how long?
- What is your occupation?
- Where do you live?
- When was your last PPD, and what were the results?
- Have you ever had a chest x ray? If so, what were the results?
- Have you been immunized for influenza or pneumonia?

Case Study Evaluation

Before you move on to the physical assessment, document Mrs. Kane's history findings, especially the respiratory history.

CRITICAL THINKING ACTIVITY #1

Based on the subjective information from Mrs. Kane's history, what respiratory problems do you think she might have after surgery?

CRITICAL THINKING ACTIVITY #2

What strengths have you identified that might help Mrs. Kane avoid postoperative respiratory problems?

CRITICAL THINKING ACTIVITY #3

What suggestions would you make for postoperative care?

Anatomical Landmarks

Before you begin the physical examination, you need to visualize the underlying structures and identify your landmarks to ensure an accurate and thorough assessment. Approach the respiratory assessment from anterior, lateral, and posterior views. The right lung has three lobes, and the left has two. These lobes are divided by fissures (Fig. 11–3).

Imaginary lines are used to correctly identify landmarks and document findings. When approached anteriorly, the apices of the lungs extend about 2 cm (3/4 to 1 inch) above the inner aspect of the clavicles. They then continue downward to the sixth intercostal space at the midclavicular line (MCL). Keep in mind that access to the lungs from this approach may be limited by other structures such as breast tissue or the heart (Fig. 11–4).

Laterally, the lower border of the lung is at the eighth rib at the midaxillary line. (Fig. 11–5).

The posterior approach affords the best access to the lungs because there are no underlying organs or structures to get in the way. Posteriorly, the apices of the lungs start at T1 and extend to T10 and T12 on deep inspiration. The right lung may be slightly higher because of the liver (Fig. 11–6).

HELPFUL HINTS

- Because of the anatomical position of the right middle lobe, the anterior and lateral approaches are best for assessment. The right middle lobe is not readily accessible using the posterior approach.
- An easy way to find T1 is to have the client bend his or her neck. The most prominent spinous process is C7 and the one below is T1.

CRITICAL THINKING ACTIVITY #4

The gallbladder is located in the right upper quadrant of the abdomen. How might this location affect the respiratory system?

Physical Assessment

Now that you have completed subjective data collection, begin collecting objective data by means of the physical examination. Keep key history findings in mind. These findings, along with those from the physical examination, complete your assessment picture. Now you can analyze data, formulate nursing diagnoses, and develop a plan of care.

Approach

You will use all four techniques of physical assessment to examine the respiratory system. Begin with inspection, proceed to palpation and percussion, and then perform auscultation from the anterior, lateral, and posterior approaches. The best position for the examination is with the patient sitting. For the posterior approach, ask the client to lean forward and cross his or her arms over the chest. This spreads the scapula, providing the greatest access to the lung surface. Perform all assessment techniques at each approach before changing the client's position.

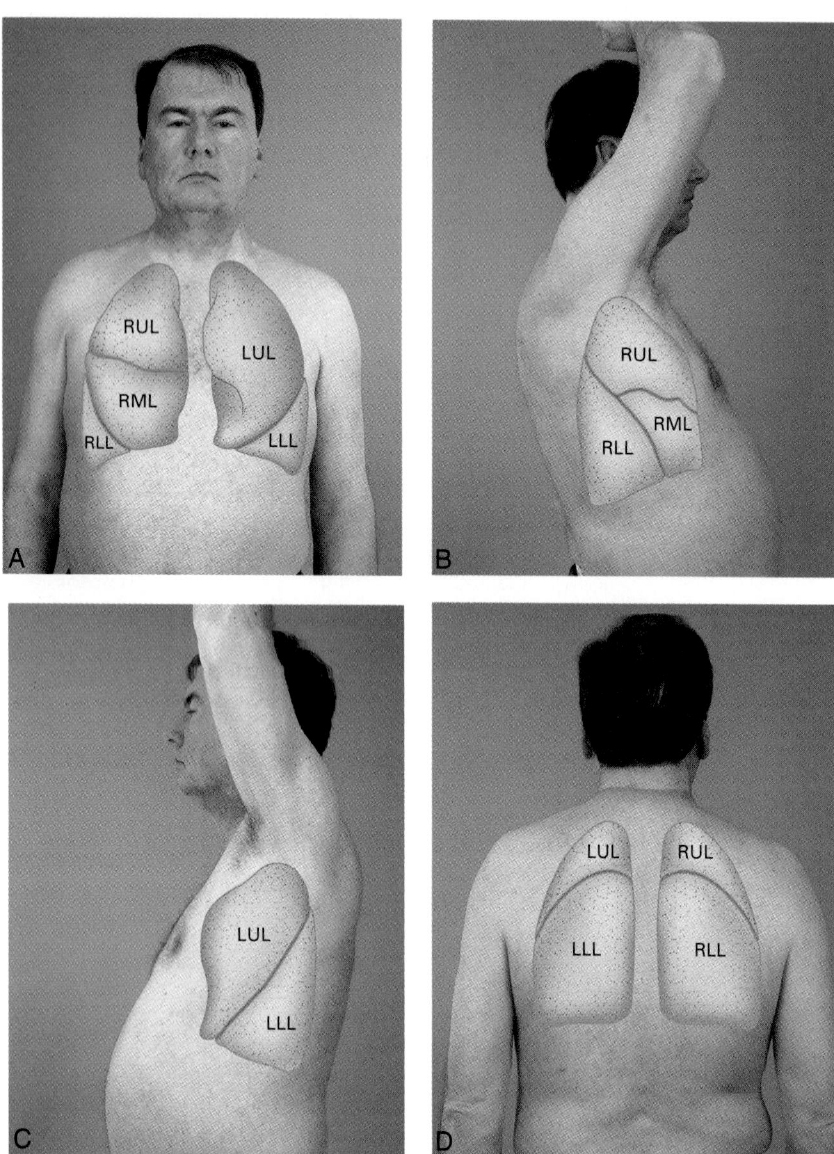

FIGURE 11-3. Lungs. (*A*) Anterior view, (*B*) Right lateral view, (*C*) Left lateral view, (*D*) Posterior view.

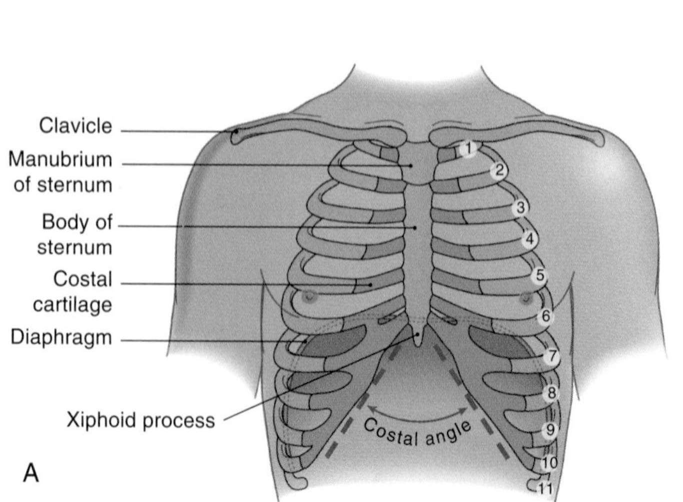

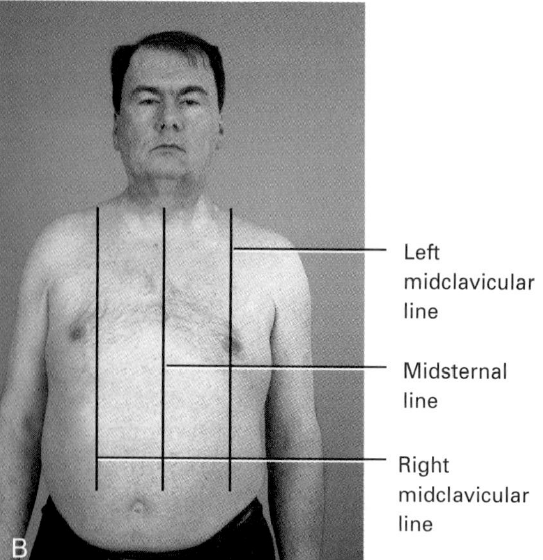

FIGURE 11-4. (*A*) and (*B*). Anterior views with landmarks.

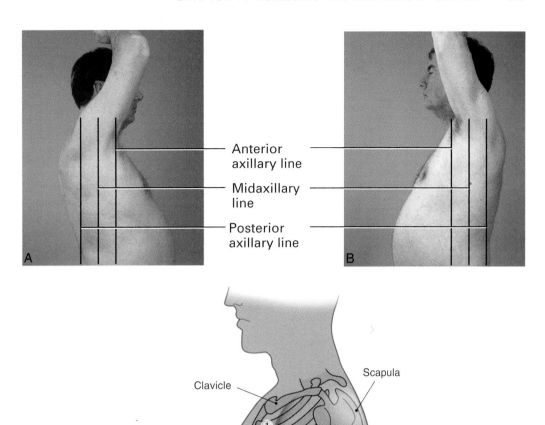

FIGURE 11–5. (*A*) Right lateral view with landmarks, (*B*) and (*C*). Left lateral views with landmarks.

If the client is unable to sit up and has to be in a supine, semi-Fowler's, or sidelying position, your findings will be distorted. Because the physical findings are more evident on the dependent side, help the client turn, and then reassess him or her from the other side.

During auscultation, have the client breathe slowly and somewhat deeply through the mouth. Be alert for dizziness and other signs of hyperventilation. To guard against this, caution the client to take slow, deep breaths and to tell you if he or she becomes dizzy.

Changes in the respiratory system can affect every other system, so you may see physical signs in many systems. Normal findings may vary from client to client, so a systematic approach is essential. Proceed from apex to base, comparing one side to the other, using the client as his or her own control. Establish a baseline that you can use to compare the client's respiratory status in subsequent assessments.

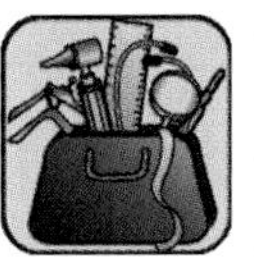

Toolbox

The tools for respiratory assessment include a stethoscope, felt-tipped marker, and metric ruler.

Also, sharpen your senses! You will use all of them during this examination.

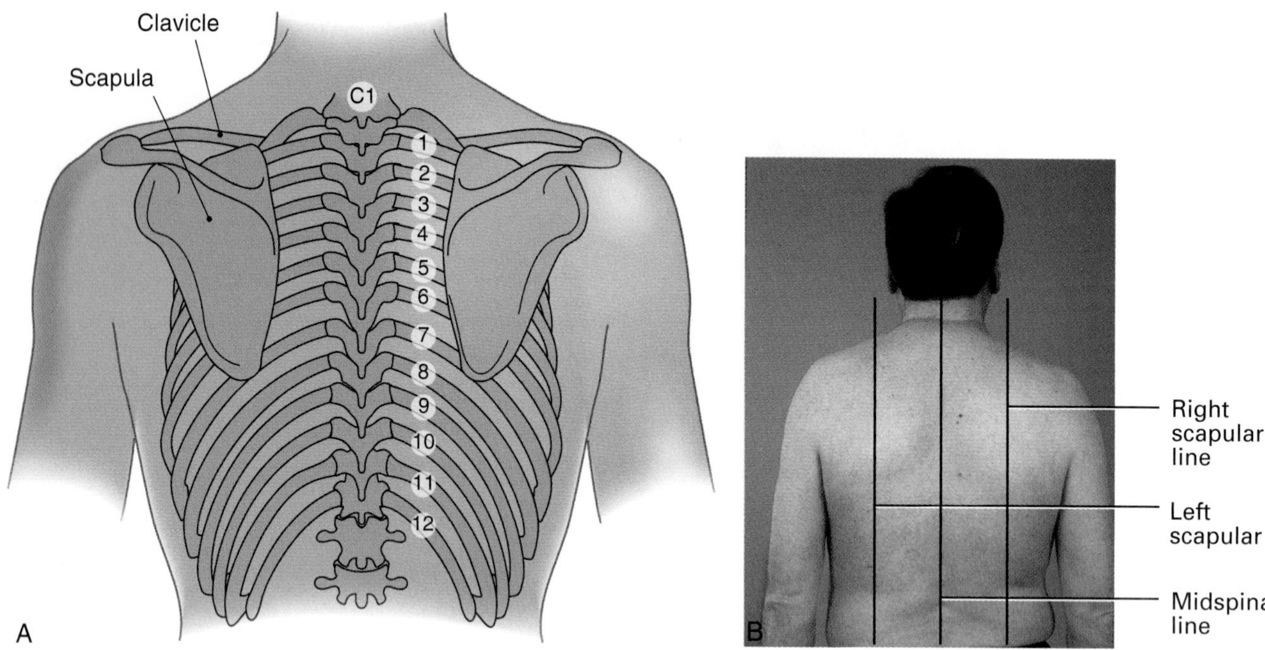

FIGURE 11–6. (*A*) and (*B*) Posterior view with landmarks.

HELPFUL HINT

Minimize position changes when examining older people or those with chronic respiratory disease. It helps conserve their energy.

Performing a General Survey

Before assessing specific areas, scan the client from head to toe, looking at general appearance and for signs of respiratory dysfunction. For example:

- Check for consistency of appearance with chronological age. Chronic illness or long-term smoking can make people appear older than they are.
- Examine weight distribution and muscle composition. Cortisone therapy can alter weight distribution and cause muscle atrophy of extremities.
- Evaluate nutritional status. People with lung cancer and chronic lung disease are frequently cachectic. Those on cortisone or with edema may appear overweight.
- Note anxiety, fear, distress, or pain. People with dyspnea or chest pain exhibit these signs.
- Consider the person's posture and assumed position. Is he or she erect and relaxed, slouched, hypererect, or leaning forward and/or using the chair arms for support (tripod position)? People with COPD or dyspnea often prefer an erect sitting or tripod position.
- Take vital signs (blood pressure, temperature, pulse, and respirations) and weigh the client. Include these results in your database. Changes in pulse and blood pressure may have a cardiopulmonary basis. Weight changes are often seen in clients with chronic respiratory disease.

Temperature

An elevated temperature may indicate a bacterial, viral, or fungal infection. Fever can also occur in noninfectious conditions such as pulmonary embolism. Remember that people who are immunosuppressed, elderly, or on corticosteroid therapy may not have a fever even with an infection.

Respirations

Eupnea refers to normal rate, depth, and rhythm of respirations. Rate varies with age. Normal adult rate is 14 to 20 breaths per minute. Depth/tidal volume for an adult is 300 to 500 mL per minute, considered moderate. Rhythm should be regular, with signs every 15 minutes at rest. Respiration should be quiet and relaxed unless the client is involved in vigorous activity.

Respiration rate, depth, and rhythm are affected by respiratory, cardiac, neurological, metabolic, and emotional disorders, as well as medications.

Rate

Tachypnea (increased rate): Can be caused by hypoxia, metabolic acidosis, anxiety, fear, pain, compromised neurological control of breathing, sepsis, fever, or increased metabolism.

Bradypnea (decreased rate): Results from excessive sedation, hypercapnea, compromised neurological control of breathing, or metabolic alkalosis.

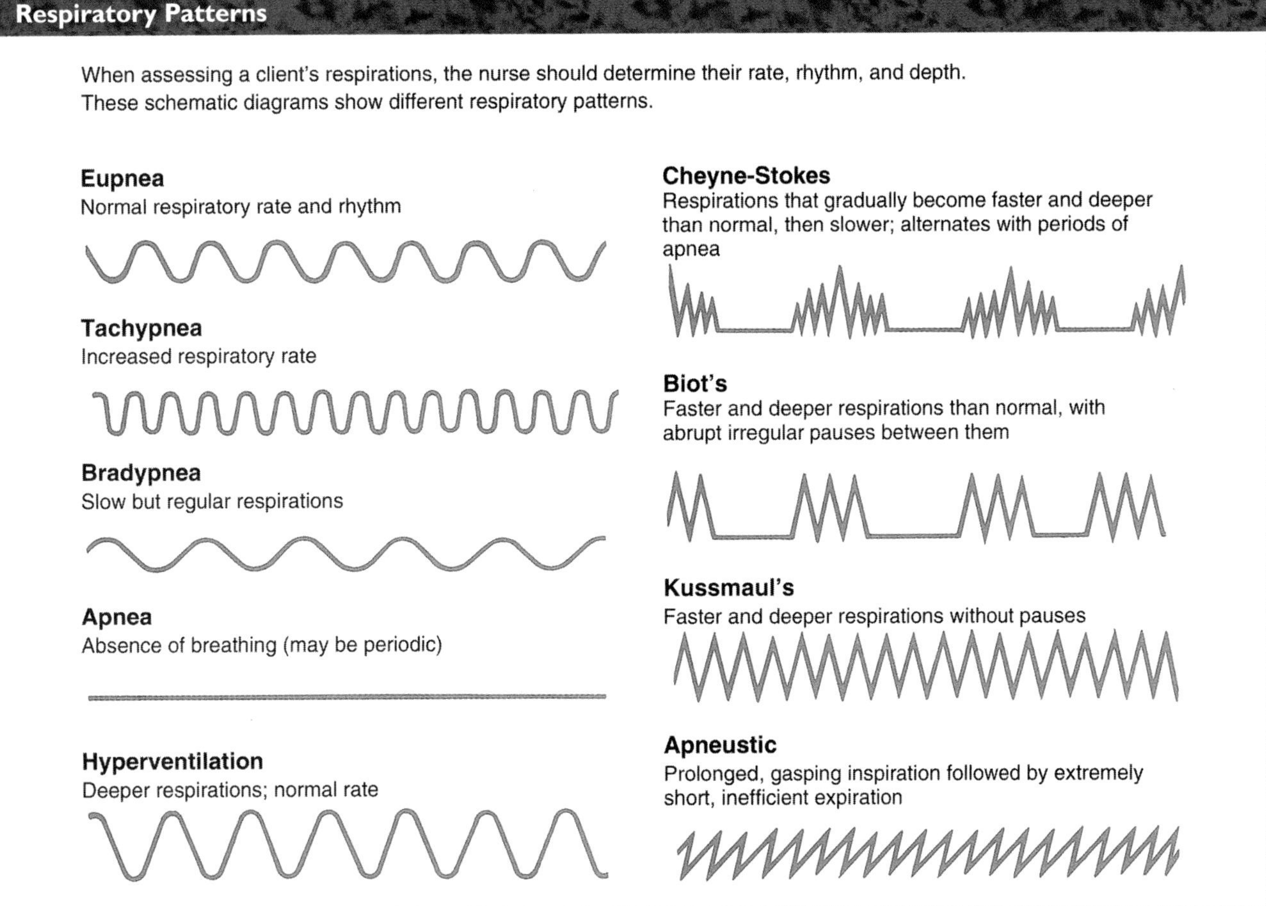

Respiratory Patterns
When assessing a client's respirations, the nurse should determine their rate, rhythm, and depth.
These schematic diagrams show different respiratory patterns.
Eupnea
Normal respiratory rate and rhythm
Tachypnea
Increased respiratory rate
Bradypnea
Slow but regular respirations
Apnea
Absence of breathing (may be periodic)
Hyperventilation
Deeper respirations; normal rate
Cheyne-Stokes
Respirations that gradually become faster and deeper than normal, then slower; alternates with periods of apnea
Biot's
Faster and deeper respirations than normal, with abrupt irregular pauses between them
Kussmaul's
Faster and deeper respirations without pauses
Apneustic
Prolonged, gasping inspiration followed by extremely short, inefficient expiration

Depth and Rhythm

Shallow respiration: Decreased depth may be a result of habit; fatigue; metabolic alkalosis; ascites; restrictive lung disease; chest, abdominal, or pleuritic pain; or neurological disorders.

Increased depth: May be related to neurological disorders, hyperventilation with anxiety, or metabolic acidosis (especially with tachypnea).

Abnormal Patterns

Kussmaul: Rapid, deep respiration associated with metabolic acidosis (body's attempt to blow off CO_2), seen in diabetic ketoacidosis or lactic acidosis.

Cheyne-Stokes: Progressively increasing rapid, deep respiration that peaks and then gradually ceases, followed by a period of apnea, after which the pattern recurs. Can be drug-induced, related to heart or renal failure, a sign of brain damage or impending death, or normal in frail elderly people during sleep.

Biot's: Ataxic breathing pattern that is irregular in rate and depth and alternates with irregular periods of apnea. Seen in respiratory depression, damage to medullary respiratory centers, or head injury.

Performing a Head-to-Toe Physical Assessment

The respiratory system affects every other system, so look for changes from head to toe in each system that might signal a respiratory problem.

Performing a Head-to-Toe Physical Assessment

SYSTEM/NORMAL FINDINGS	ABNORMAL/RATIONALE
General Health Survey	
INSPECT	
Awake, alert, oriented to time, place, person. Immediate, recent, remote memory intact. Judgment intact; compliant with treatment plan.	Early signs of hypoxia include confusion, restlessness, irritability, short attention span.

(Continued)

Performing a Head-to-Toe Physical Assessment *(Continued)*

SYSTEM/NORMAL FINDINGS	ABNORMAL/RATIONALE
General Health Survey ***(Continued)*** *INSPECT*	Short-term memory may also be affected by hypoxia. People with chronic respiratory disease may deny illness, severity of symptoms, or associated risk factors. Anxiety can trigger a respiratory problem, such as hyperventilation, or can result from a respiratory problem such as an acute asthmatic attack or pulmonary emboli. Fatigue is associated with chronic lung disease, lung cancer, and pneumonia because more energy is expended on breathing.
Integumentary/*Skin and Nails* *INSPECT*	
HELPFUL HINT When assessing for color changes in dark-skinned people, look at mucous membranes or conjunctiva. Skin color varies with racial and genetic heritage. Buccal mucosa, tongue, palates, conjunctiva and nail beds are usually pink, but may be darker pink, dark brown or even blue in people of Mediterranean or African descent.	*Pale, diaphoretic:* Sympathetic response to respiratory distress and hypoxia.
Peripheral cyanosis may be normal response to exposure to cold temperatures.	*Central cyanosis:* Dusky or blue buccal mucosa and tongue when PO_2 is less than 50. Caused by respiratory failure, shock, pulmonary edema, airway obstruction, ventilation-perfusion problems. May see cyanosis in vessels of palpebral conjunctiva in end-stage COPD. *Peripheral cyanosis:* Blue, dusky-red or purple color of lips, nail beds, tips of nose and ears, sometimes face and especially cheeks. Caused by slow or congested blood flow in peripheral vessels or disorders with compensatory polycythemia, such as COPD, CHF. *Ruddy, reddish color:* Associated with polycythemia.

Performing a Head-to-Toe Physical Assessment

SYSTEM/NORMAL FINDINGS	ABNORMAL/RATIONALE
Integumentary/*Nails* *INSPECT/PALPATE*	
No edema.	Peripheral edema frequently seen in people with chronic lung disease secondary to right-side CHF.
Positive capillary refill, nail beds pink, negative clubbing.	*Clubbing:* Long-standing lung disease. *Cyanotic or dusky nails:* Reflect peripheral cyanosis seen in vasoconstriction and slowing of peripheral blood flow. Also associated with central cyanosis. *Yellow-brown stains on nails and fingers:* Nicotine stains from long history of smoking. *Purple/dusky lower extremities:* Venous stasis, especially if PO_2 is low.
HEENT/*Head and Neck* *INSPECT/PALPATE*	
Trachea should arise out of sternal notch and be midline.	*Tracheal shifts:* Collapsed lung, tumors, pneumothorax or hemothorax.
No pursed-lip breathing, nasal flaring, neck vein distention, or use of accessory muscles unless associated with strenuous activity. Visible neck vein in older people or those with overdeveloped neck muscles. No hypertrophy of neck muscles unless occupationally related (e.g., weightlifters, singers, professional speakers). No visible/palpable lymph nodes.	Pursed-lip breathing, or physiological positive end-expiratory pressure, is a compensatory mechanism used by people with COPD to prolong expiration, help expel trapped air and keep alveoli open longer for maximum oxygenation of pulmonary blood. Nasal flaring occurs in infants and small children and indicates acute respiratory distress or cyanotic heart disease. *Neck vein distention* is a general sign of respiratory distress or air hunger. When client sits, elevating head and chest 45 degrees, neck vessels are firm and tortuous. This sign of increased venous pressure is seen in right heart failure and cor pulmonale. People with chronic lung disease may also develop hypertrophied neck muscles from increased efforts to breathe.

(Continued)

Performing a Head-to-Toe Physical Assessment *(Continued)*

SYSTEM/NORMAL FINDINGS	ABNORMAL/RATIONALE
HEENT/*Head and Neck* *INSPECT/PALPATE*	*Use of scalene, sternocleidomastoideus (SCM), and trapezius accessory muscles:* Sign of respiratory distress or COPD. *Visible/palpable lymph nodes:* Infection or malignancy.
HEENT/*Eyes* Conjunctiva pink, no excessive tearing. No papilledema.	Central cyanosis can be seen in the conjunctiva. *Excessive tearing:* Allergies. *Papilledema:* Hypercapnea or CO_2 narcosis.
HEENT/*Ears/Nose/ Throat* Oral and nasal mucous membranes pink, TM membrane pearl gray, nares patent, no drainage.	*Red mucous membranes, red TM, drainage:* UTI.
Cardiovascular *PALPATE/AUSCULTATE* Heart, regular rate and rhythm (HRRR), no extra sounds, +2 pulses, negative Homans' sign.	*Right-sided S_3 nd S_4:* Right CHF and pulmonary HTN. *Accentuated P_2:* Pulmonary HTN. *Absent/diminished pedal pulses and ankle/pedal edema:* Heart failure and cor pulmonale. Clients with polycythemia are at risk for thrombophlebitis and possibly pulmonary embolism caused by sluggish blood flow. A positive Homans' sign may indicate thrombophlebitis, but it is not conclusive.
Gastrointestinal *PALPATE/PERCUSS* No hepatomegaly or ascites.	*Enlarged liver and ascites:* Right-side CHF, a common complication of chronic lung disease.
Musculoskeletal *INSPECT/PALPATE* +5 muscle strength, no weakness or muscle wasting.	*Weakness/muscle wasting:* Long-standing respiratory disease.
Neurological *INSPECT* No tremors, +2 deep tendon reflex (DTR)	*Tremors, seizures, decreased DTRs:* Respiratory failure. *Asterixis (flapping hand tremors):* CO_2 narcosis.

CLUBBING

In people with chronic hypoxia associated with chronic lung disease, the kidneys compensate by increasing secretion of erythopoetin, a hormone that stimulates red blood cell (RBC) production. The increase in RBCs (polycythemia) results in thick, sluggish blood flow that "plugs" the capillaries of the nail folds, causing the tissue to become swollen and spongy. The result is "clubbing"—a nail plate that becomes more convex, with a rounded distal phalanx and an increased angle of attachment.

PERFUSION/VENTILATION PROBLEMS

Ventilation-perfusion problems occur when one or more areas of the lung receive adequate ventilation but inadequate blood flow (perfusion problem) or inadequate ventilation and adequate blood flow (ventilation problem). This results in increased dead space, shunting, and hypoxemia. Emphysema causes increased dead space and creates a ventilation problem. A pulmonary embolus causes inadequate blood flow and shunting and creates a perfusion problem.

Case Study Findings

Before you proceed to a focused respiratory assessment, document what you learned during Mrs. Kane's general survey and head-to-toe assessment.

Mrs. Kane's physical assessment findings include:

- **General Health Survey:** Well-developed, 45-year-old Caucasian female, appears stated age, in no acute respiratory distress. Sits upright and relaxed during interview; answers questions appropriately; affect pleasant and appropriate. Alert and responsive without complaints; oriented to time, place, situation, and person.
- **Vital Signs:** Temperature 98.6°F; pulse 64 BPM, strong and regular; respirations 16/min, unlabored; BP 120/70; height 5' 5"; weight: 165 lb.
- **Integumentary:** Skin pink and intact, no edema, nails pink, positive capillary refill, negative clubbing. Nicotine stains on nails and fingers.
- **HEENT:** Trachea midline, no palpable lymph nodes, thyroid not palpable. Oral and nasal mucosa pink, moist, and intact without lesions or discharge. TM pearl gray and intact without drainage, nares patent. Conjunctiva pink, no papilledema.
- **Cardiovascular:** HRRR, no extra sounds, +2 pulses.
- **Abdomen:** No hepatomegaly.
- **Musculoskeletal:** +5 muscle strength, no wasting.
- **Neurological:** +2 DTR, no tremors.

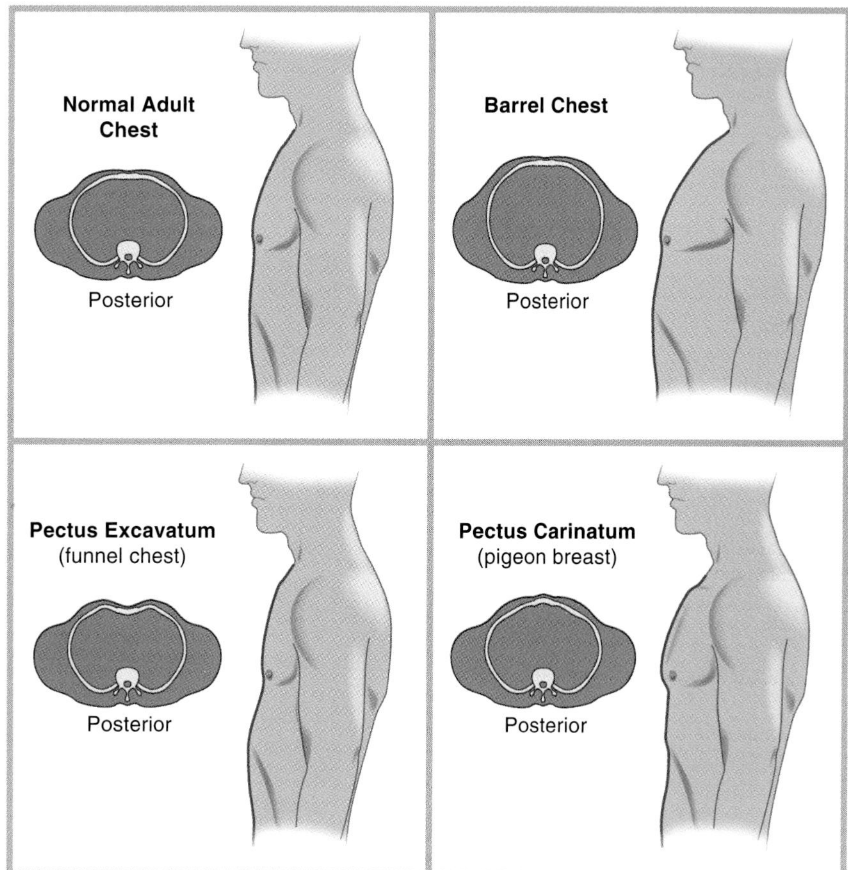

FIGURE 11-7. Chest shapes.

Performing a Focused Respiratory Assessment

Now that you have completed your general survey and head-to-toe scan, you can focus on the respiratory assessment. Begin with inspection, then palpate, percuss, and finally auscultate the lungs.

Inspection

Begin with inspection. Inspect the chest for size, shape (Fig. 11–7), symmetry, and excursion. Ask yourself: Does the chest rise equally? Are respirations quiet? What muscles are being used to breathe— chest or abdominal? Are there signs of respiratory distress, such as retractions? Inspect the skin, noting scars or color changes.

Inspecting the Chest

ASSESS/NORMAL VARIATIONS	ABNORMAL FINDINGS/RATIONALE
Anterior Chest 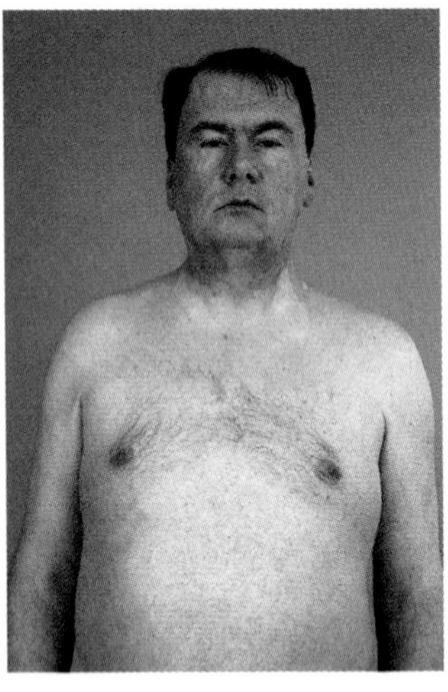 **Inspecting anterior chest** *Shape and symmetry:* Normal adult chest has anteroposterior (AP)-to-lateral ratio of approximately 1:2 and costal angle less than 90°. Ribs slope obliquely, chest symmetrical in appearance with symmetrical rise and fall when breathing. Skin intact. *Movement with breathing:* Women have more thoracic respiratory movements; men and infants have more abdominal respiratory movements. No sternal or intercostal retraction or bulging, unless associated with strenuous activity. Musculoskeletal changes associated with aging can increase the anteroposterior diameter, giving chest a barrel appearance. Anteroposterior diameter greater in infants (apple-shaped chest). *Condition of chest skin:* Skin color and hair distribution should be consistent with client's gender, ethnicity and exposure to sun. Skin intact, no scars.	*Altered chest shape:* Seen in COPD (trapped air with overinflated lungs). Anteroposterior diameter is increased, resulting in "barrel chest." Rib slope is nearly parallel, with costal angle greater than 90 degrees (see Fig. 11–7). *Altered chest symmetry:* Seen in musculoskeletal disorders of spine such as kyphosis, scoliosis, and kyphoscoliosis. Can affect respiratory function by restricting lung movement. *Altered breathing symmetry:* May be caused by rib fractures, especially at sternal border (flail chest), pneumonectomy, pneumothorax/hemothorax, and atelectasis. Affected area of chest may not move with respiration. *Sternal and intercostal retractions:* Seen in severe hypoxia or respiratory distress, especially with airway obstruction. *Altered skin color/condition:* Extreme hypoxia or cold temperature may cause blue flush on chest wall (cyanosis). Steroids may produce excessive hair in women. *Intercostal bulging:* Seen during expiratory effort of person with COPD. Scars may indicate trauma or surgery. Look for signs of lung surgery (often on lateral thorax) or 1-cm stab wounds from chest tubes.

Inspecting the Chest

ASSESS/NORMAL VARIATIONS	ABNORMAL FINDINGS/RATIONALE
Lateral Chest	Same as with anterior and posterior chest. Look for scars from pneumonectomy or lobectomy, located laterally and curving under scapula.

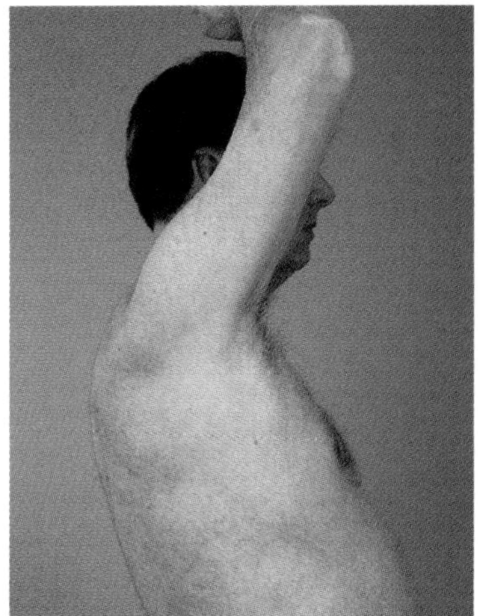

Inspecting right lateral chest

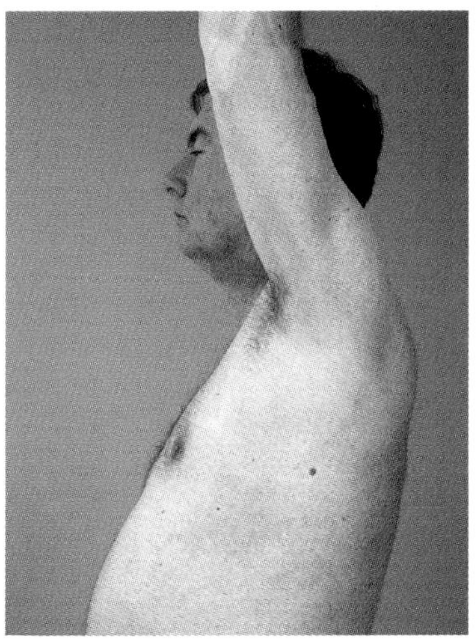

Inspecting left lateral chest

As with anterior and posterior chest, skin is intact and chest expansion equal.

ASSESS/NORMAL VARIATIONS	ABNORMAL FINDINGS/RATIONALE
Posterior Chest	Same as with anterior chest, although abnormal spinal curves are more obvious. Look for scars from pneumonectomy or lobectomy, located laterally and curving under scapula.

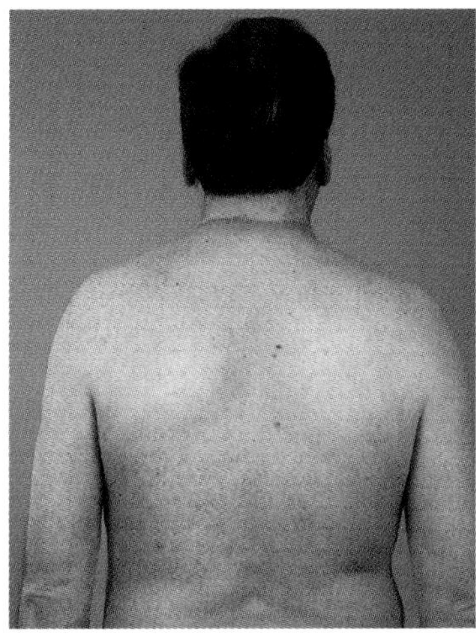

Inspecting posterior chest

Skin should be intact, chest expansion equal, and spine straight without lateral curves or deformities.

Palpation

Palpation is useful in assessing for tracheal position, tenderness and crepitus, chest excursion, and tactile fremitus. Use light palpation to assess surface characteristics of the chest, such as temperature, turgor, and moisture, as well as to identify tenderness, masses, or crepitus. Palpate from the anterior, posterior, and lateral approaches.

To assess tracheal position, place a finger on either side of the trachea. The distance between the trachea and sternocleidomastoid muscle on both sides should be equal.

Chest excursion refers to the chest's expandability. Use this technique to assess symmetrical chest expansion using both anterior and posterior approaches. Place

AREA/SYSTEM	SUBJECTIVE DATA
General	*Ask about:* Changes in energy level Activity intolerance Fatigue Weight changes
Integumentary	*Ask about:* Skin color changes Fevers, night sweats
HEENT *Head, Face, Neck, Eyes, Ears, Nose and Throat*	*Ask about:* Lumps or swelling in neck Excessive eye tearing Ear infections, sore throats, URIs, sinus problems Difficulty swallowing or breathing
Cardiovascular	*Ask about:* Chest pain Palpitations Swelling, tight shoes
Gastrointestinal	*Ask about:* Changes in appetite GI complaints RUQ pain
Genitourinary/ Reproductive	*Ask about:* Nocturia Changes in sexual activity Safe-sex practices Pregnancy
Musculoskeletal	*Ask about:* Weakness
Neurological	*Ask about:* Memory changes Morning headaches Tremors
Endocrine	*Ask about:* Thyroid disease
Lymphatic/ Hematologic	*Ask about:* Bleeding, anemia Allergies

AREA/SYSTEM	OBJECTIVE DATA
General Orthopnea	*Inspect:* Signs of acute distress, such as SOB, DOE Posture: Tripod; Position: *Measure:* Height, weight, (check for changes) Temperature, pulse, respirations, B/P (check for increases)
Integumentary	*Inspect:* Skin color changes (e.g., cyanosis, pallor, ruddiness) Central (mucous membranes) vs. peripheral cyanosis Nail clubbing *Palpate:* Skin temperature, turgor, edema Capillary refill
HEENT *Head, Face, Neck, Eyes, Ears, Nose and Throat*	*Inspect:* Facial expression (e.g., anxious) Neck vein distention, hypertrophy and use of accessory neck muscles Color of conjunctiva Ear or nose drainage, nasal flaring Color of mucous membranes, color of tonsils and enlargement *Palpate:* Sinus tenderness, lymph nodes, tracheal position, thyroid gland, patent nares, tonsilar glands *Examine:* Fundus, optic disk External ear and TM Internal nasal mucosa and structures
Cardiovascular	*Inspect:* Edema *Palpate:* Edema, Homans' sign Auscultate: Right side S4 and S3
Gastrointestinal	*Palpate:* Enlarged liver, ascites
Musculoskeletal	*Inspect:* Hypertrophy and use of accessory muscles, muscle atrophy, spinal deformities *Measure:* Muscle strength
Neurological	*Inspect:* Impaired mental status, AAO x 3 Asterixis (flapping tremors)

Assessment of Respiratory System's Relationship to Other Systems

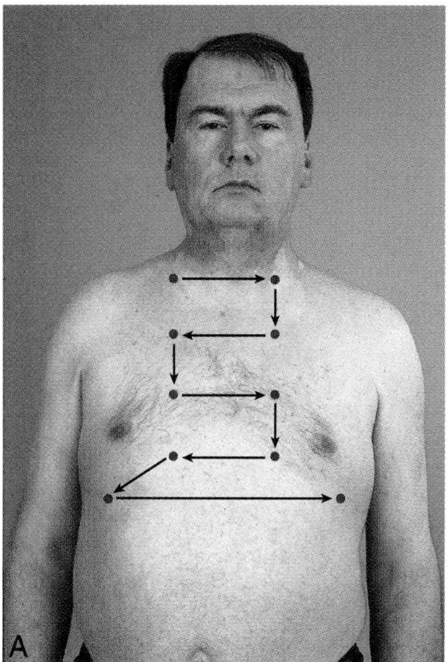

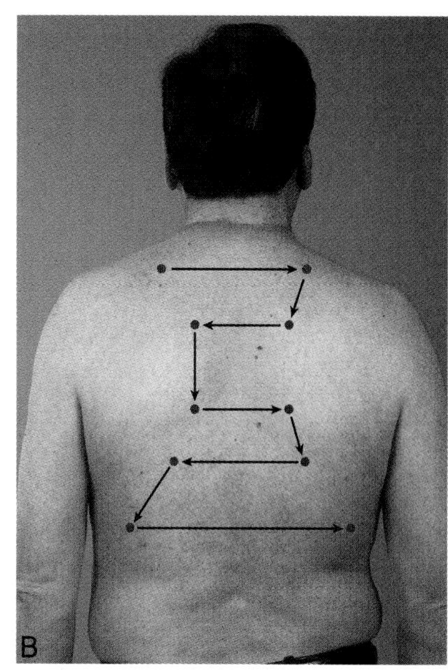

FIGURE 11–8. Palpation sequences. *(A)* Anterior, *(B)* Posterior.

your hands vertically on the client's chest, with fingers spread and thumbs at the costal margin anteriorly and at the eighth to the tenth rib posteriorly. Your palms should be firm against the skin, with thumbs touching and fingers lightly in contact with the chest wall. Gently gather a small fold of skin between your contacting thumbs. Have the client take a deep breath. You should feel equal pressure on your hands, and your thumbs should move apart evenly. If you note any abnormality, move your hands up and assess the apices of the lung.

Tactile or vocal fremitus is the palpable vibration you feel when the client speaks. Assessment of tactile fremitus is used to evaluate airflow and density of underlying tissue. Because bony prominences are best for detecting vibratory sensations, use the balls or the ulnar surfaces of your hands. Have the client say "99, 99" while you move your hands in a systematic fashion from apex to base, comparing side to side and anteriorly and posteriorly. Note the level where fremitus is palpable and where it diminishes and goes away. In the average adult, fremitus is not palpable below the third to fourth intercostal space anteriorly and at about T6 to T8 posteriorly.

Several factors besides airflow influence the quality of tactile fremitus. These include chest wall thickness, voice pitch, and airway size. Normally, the thicker the chest wall, the more diminished the fremitus; and the lower the voice pitch, the greater the fremitus. Also, fremitus is usually increased over the larger airways (Fig. 11–8).

Palpating the Chest

ASSESS NORMAL VARIATIONS	ABNORMAL FINDINGS/RATIONALE
Tracheal Position	
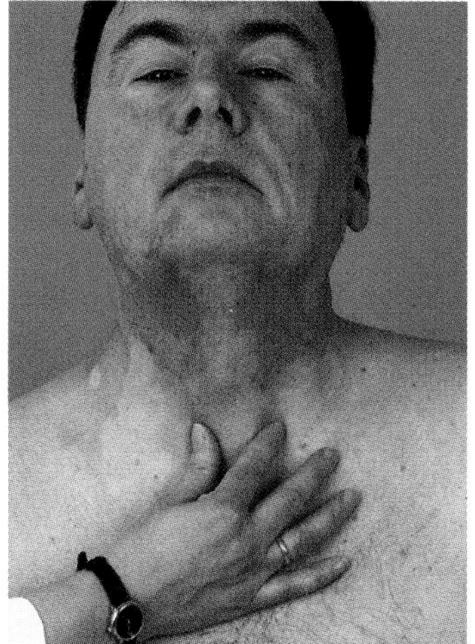 **Palpating tracheal positio** Trachea should be midline.	*Trachial deviation:* Tumor or thyroid enlargement may cause tracheal deviation. Tension pneumothorax deviates trachea *away from* affected lung. In severe atelectasis, trachea may deviate *toward* affected lung.

(Continued)

Palpating the Chest *(Continued)*

ASSESS NORMAL VARIATIONS

ABNORMAL FINDINGS/RATIONALE

Chest Tenderness and Crepitus

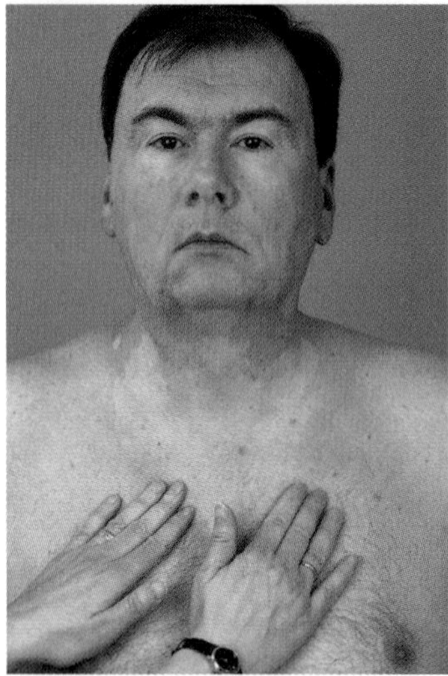

Light palpation of anterior chest

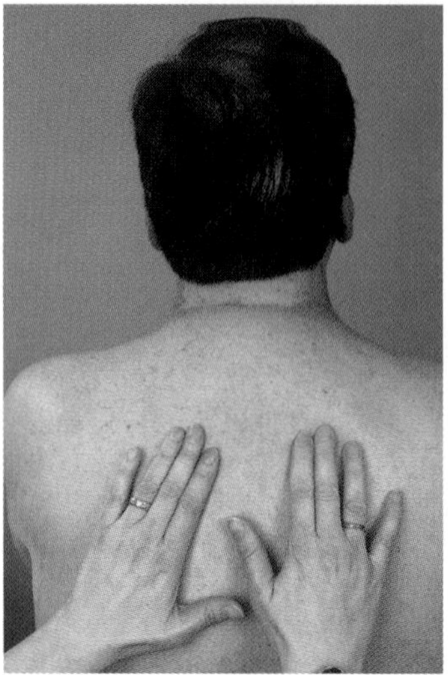

Light palpation of posterior chest

Nontender. No deformities or crepitus

Pain/tenderness at costochondral junctions/vertebral connections of ribs: Fracture. May also be present with palpation of inflamed cartilage at the rib/sternal junctions (costochondriasis).

Spontaneous pathological fractures: Corticosteroid therapy or osteomalacia.

Crepitus (subcutaneous emphysema): Results from air leaking into subcutaneous tissue. Check around wound sites, chest tubes, central lines, or tracheostomy tubes.

HELPFUL HINTS

- Chest pain that is respiratory or cardiac in origin is unaffected by palpation.
- Crepitus feels crackly, like crumpling cellophane. Although air leaking into the tissue does not hurt it, the leak must be found because that air is not going into the lungs.

Chest Excursion

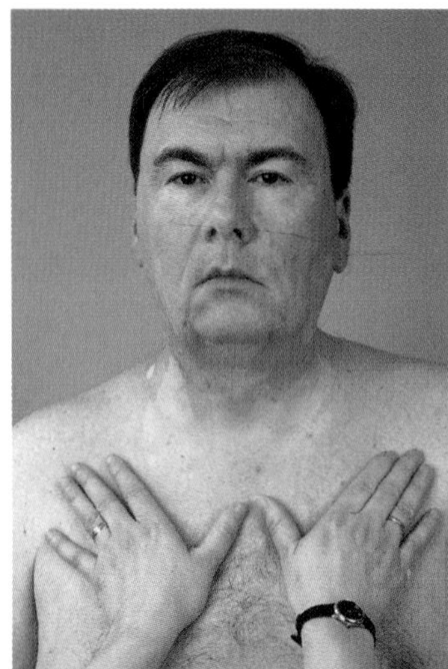

Palpating anterior chest excursion at apex

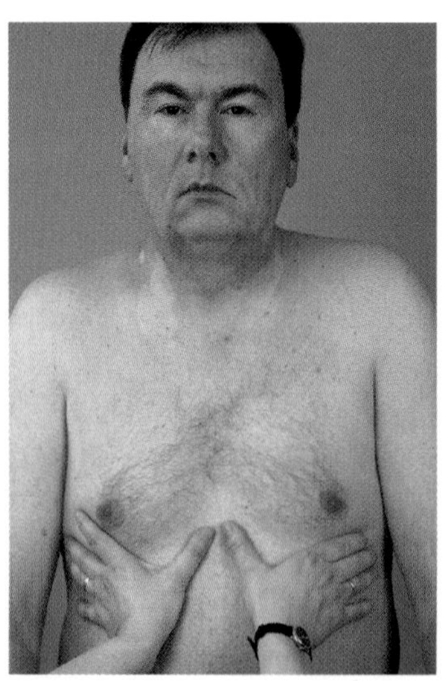

Palpating anterior chest excursion at base

Asymmetrical excursion: Associated with thoracotomy (removal of lung or lobes), complete or partial airway obstruction, pleural effusion, and pneumothorax.

Decreased excursion: May occur in clients with overinflated lungs and fixed diaphragm (COPD). May also be present with splinting because of pain of fractured ribs.

Palpating the Chest

ASSESS NORMAL VARIATIONS	ABNORMAL FINDINGS/RATIONALE

Chest Excursion *(Continued)*

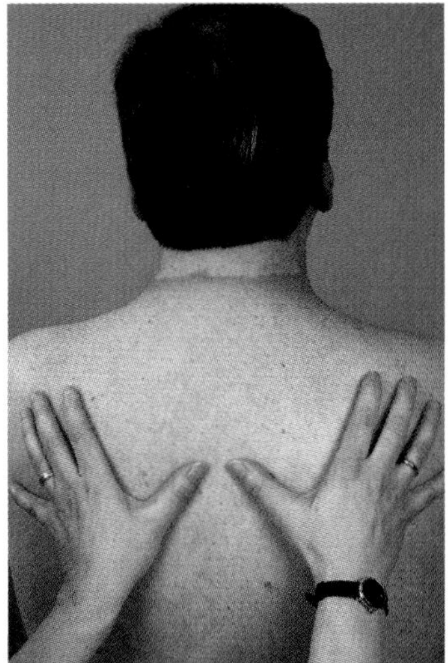

Palpating posterior chest excursion at apex

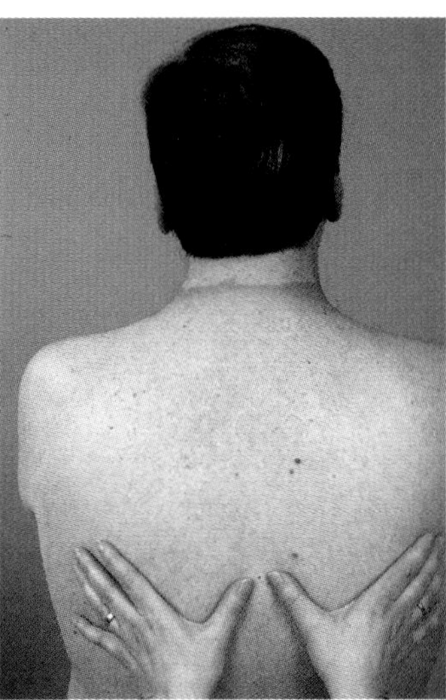

Palpating posterior chest excursion at base

Should be symmetrical without lag. Normal causes of decreased excursion are habitual shallow breathing or wearing tight, restrictive undergarments.

Tactile Fremitus

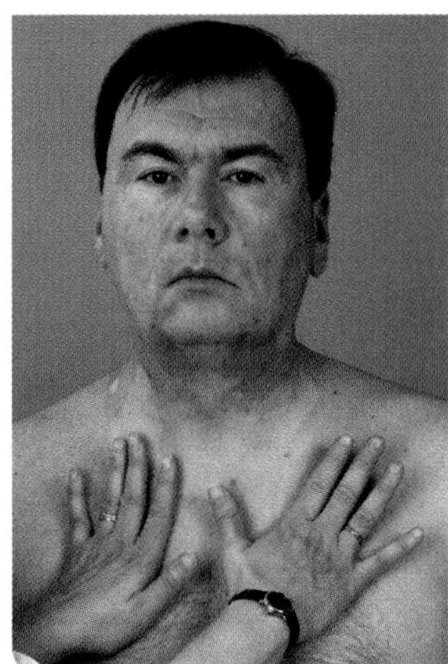

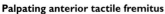

Palpating anterior tactile fremitus

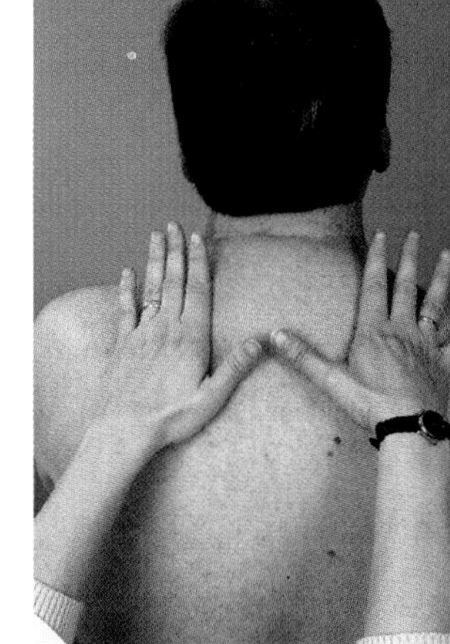

Palpating posterior tactile fremitus

Should be equal bilaterally and diminished midthorax.

Normal causes of diminished fremitus are thick chest wall or very soft voice. Young children and very thin people may have increased fremitus.

Increased fremitus: Occurs with conditions causing fluid or exudates in lungs, such as consolidating pneumonia, atelectasis, pulmonary fibrosis, pulmonary edema, or pulmonary infarction. May also occur with lung tumor, although tumor may stop vibrations, depending on its size and mobility.

Decreased or absent fremitus: Occurs where there is air trapping, solid tissue, or decreased air movement, for example, emphysema, asthma, pleural effusion, pneumothorax, or distal to airway obstruction.

Percussion

Percussion is used to assess the density of underlying lung tissue. It allows you to determine if the tissue is predominately solid or filled mainly with air or fluid. Percussion also enables you to identify the extent of the lung fields and is useful in assessing diaphragmatic excursion, the distance the diaphragm moves from expiration to inspiration. Percuss the entire anterior and posterior thorax in a systematic manner, moving from apex to base and comparing side to side. The normal percussion note over

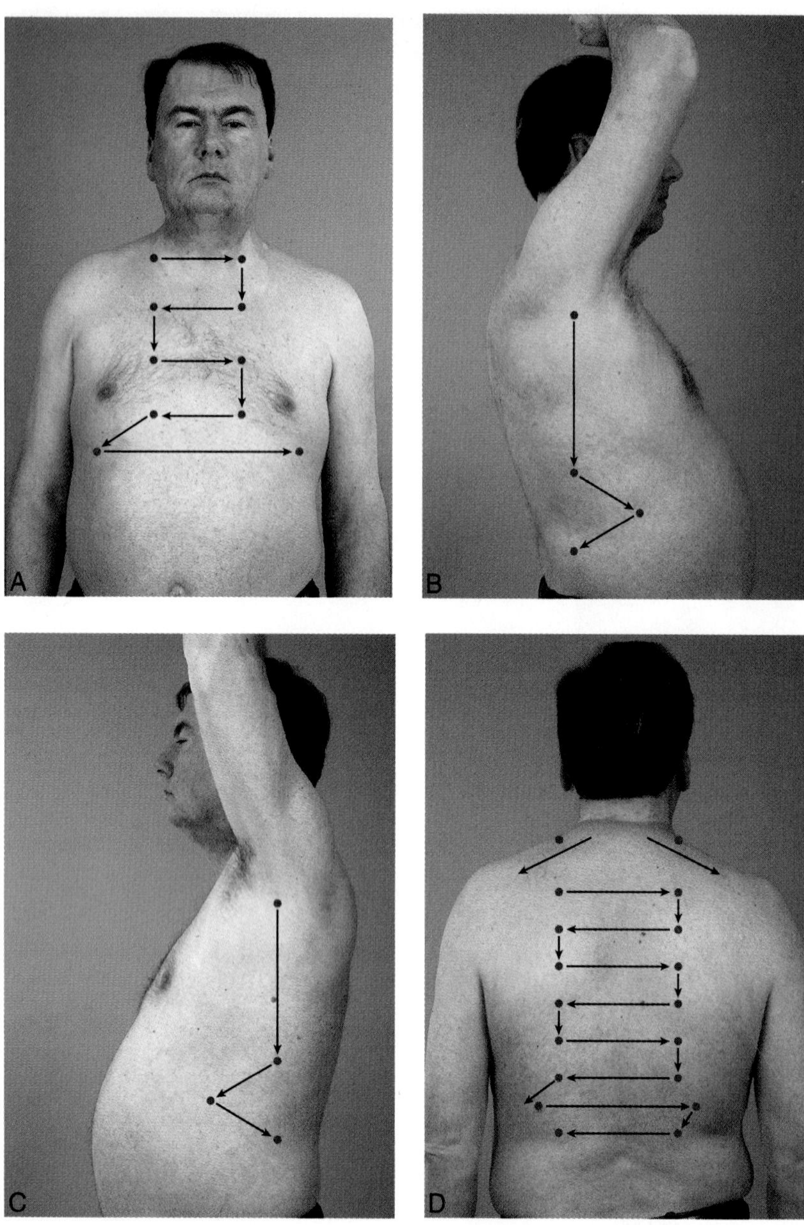

FIGURE 11–9. Percussion sequence. (*A*) Anterior, (*B*) Right lateral, (*C*) Left lateral, (*D*) Posterior.

adult lung fields is called resonance; small children will percuss more hyperresonant. It is helpful to percuss over the intercostal spaces, because percussion over bone produces a less resonant sound.

Percussion is a skill that is perfected through practice. You need to develop that skill, as well as the ability to differentiate the sounds produced by percussion. Percussion sites are the same as palpation sites anteriorly (Fig. 11–9). For more information on percussion sounds, see Chapter 3.)

Diaphragmatic Excursion

To assess diaphragmatic excursion, percuss the level of the diaphragm on full expiration and on full inspiration, noting the difference in distance in centimeters between the two. First, have the client exhale fully and then hold his or her breath as you percuss from resonance over the lung tissue to dullness over the diaphragm. Mark this area. Next, have the client take a deep breath and hold it. Continue percussing at the same location, moving from resonance to diaphragmatic dullness. Again, mark the area. Normally, the percussion that was previously dull at the diaphragm should change to resonance as the lung fills with air and the diaphragm moves downward. Measure the distance between the two marks in centimeters. Repeat the procedure on the opposite side. Normal diaphragmatic excursion is 3 to 6 cm. Remember: Work quickly to get the most accurate results and not tire the client.

Percussing the Chest

ASSESS/NORMAL VARIATIONS	ABNORMAL FINDINGS/RATIONALE

Anterior Thorax

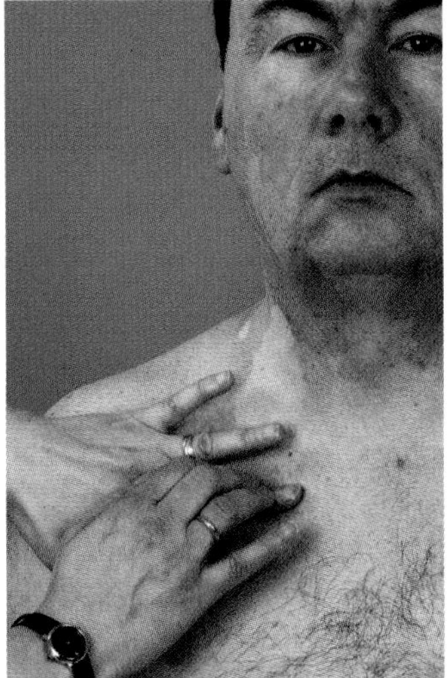

Percussing anterior chest

Resonance to 2nd intercostal space on left; slight dullness over 3rd through 5th intercostal space over heart.

Resonance to 4th intercostal space on right with dullness from approximately 5th to just above costal margin over liver. It will vary with person's size and size of liver.

Dullness: Seen with exudate, fluid, tumors, pneumonia, pulmonary edema, pleural effusion.

Hyperresonance: Noted with air trapping of emphysema.

Lateral Thorax

Resonance to 8th intercostal space.

Posterior Thorax

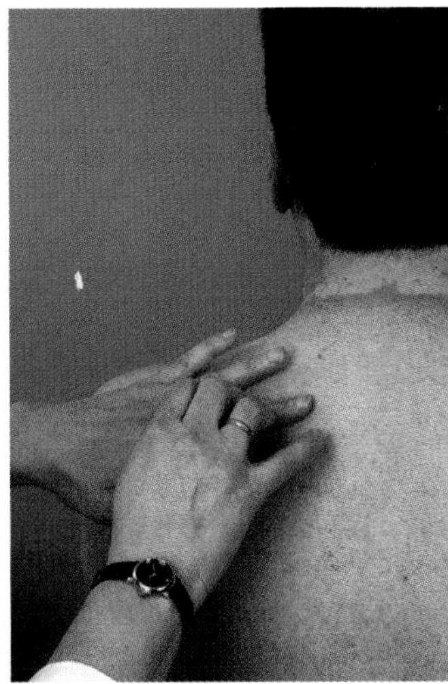

Percussing posterior chest

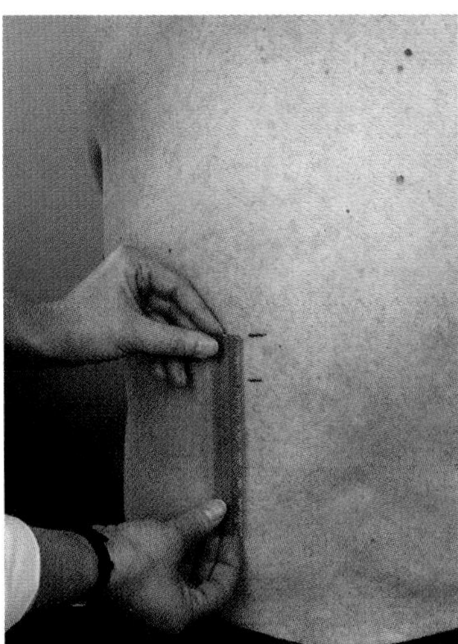

Measuring diaphragmatic excursion

Resonance to T10–T12 with deep inspiration; 3–6 cm diaphragmatic excursion.

Decreased diaphragmatic excursion unilaterally or bilaterally: Paralyzed diaphragm, atelectasis, COPD with overinflated lungs.

Hyperresonance to T12 level: Overinflated lungs.

Auscultation

Use auscultation to assess airflow through the upper airways and lungs. As you listen with the diaphragm of the stethoscope, note normal, abnormal and adventitious breath sounds, as well as abnormal vocal sounds. Be sure the room is private, warm, and quiet, and warm the diaphragm of the stethoscope between your hands before you begin. Auscultation sites are the same as for percussion.

Auscultating the Lungs

ASSESS/NORMAL VARIATIONS

Normal Breath Sounds in Appropriate Locations

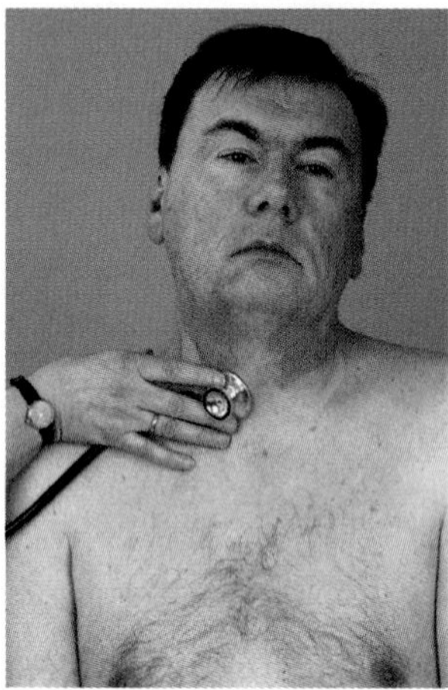

Auscultating bronchial breath sounds over trachea

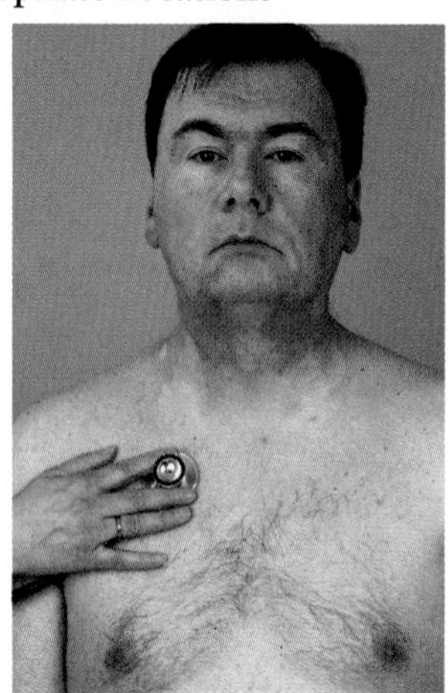

Auscultating bronchovesicular breath sounds

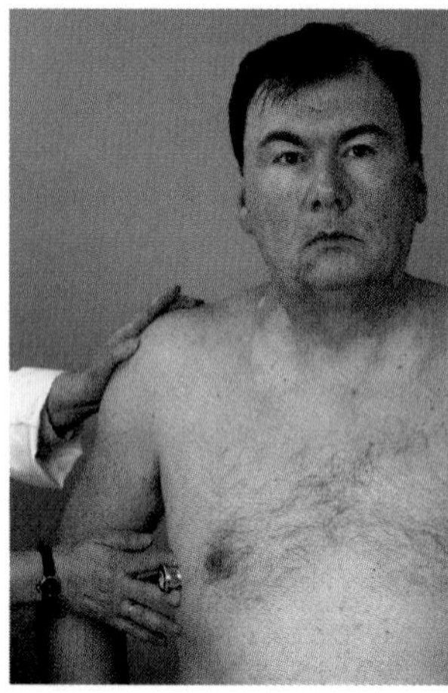

Auscultating vesicular breath sounds

Bronchial breath sounds are loud, high-pitched and hollow, with a short inspiratory phase and a long expiratory phase. They are normally heard in anterior neck and nape of neck posteriorly.

Bronchiovesicular breath sounds are moderate sounding and medium pitched, with equal inspiratory and expiratory phases. They are normally heard over 1st–2nd interspaces anteriorly and between scapula posteriorly.

Vesicular breath sounds are soft and low pitched, with a long inspiratory phase and a short expiratory phase. They are heard over most lung fields.

Adventitious Sounds

Lungs are clear to auscultation (CTA). No crackles, wheezes, or rubs.

ABNORMAL/RATIONALE

Bronchial sounds heard outside of their normal locations: Fluid or consolidated tissue, such as in pneumonia.

Diminished breath sounds: Thick, obese, or muscular chest wall, poor inspiratory effort, emphysema with air trapping, pleural effusion.

Absent breath sounds: Missing lung/lobe, airway obstruction, pneumothorax.

Crackles/rales: Pulmonary edema, pneumonia, atelectasis, and upon arising in elderly people.

Velcro rales: Pulmonary fibrosis.

High-pitched, sibilant wheezes: Bronchospasm, asthma, COPD without infection.

Low-pitched sonorous wheezes/rhonchi: Uncleared secretions, bronchitis, pneumonia, tumors.

Stridor: Laryngeal or tracheal obstruction, epiglottitis, viral croup.

Pleural friction rub: Inflammation of pleura.

HELPFUL HINTS

- If the client has a hairy chest, moisten the chest hair before auscultating to reduce interference.
- Be sure to use all of your assessment techniques, and do not rely on one finding. For example, you may hear transmitted sounds over an area with no airflow, when in fact, sounds are absent. If there is no airflow, there will be no chest movement.

Normal Breath Sounds

With the client in a sitting position, auscultate directly over the skin, exposing only the areas being assessed. Listen through at least one full respiratory cycle at each site. Be systematic in your approach, and follow the same sequence as percussion: Auscultate the anterior, lateral and posterior thorax, moving from apex to base and comparing side to side. To help differentiate breath sounds, note the relationship of inspiration to expiration (I:E) and which phase is longer, identify the pitch and intensity of the sound, and locate the area where the sound is heard best. (Fig. 11–10)

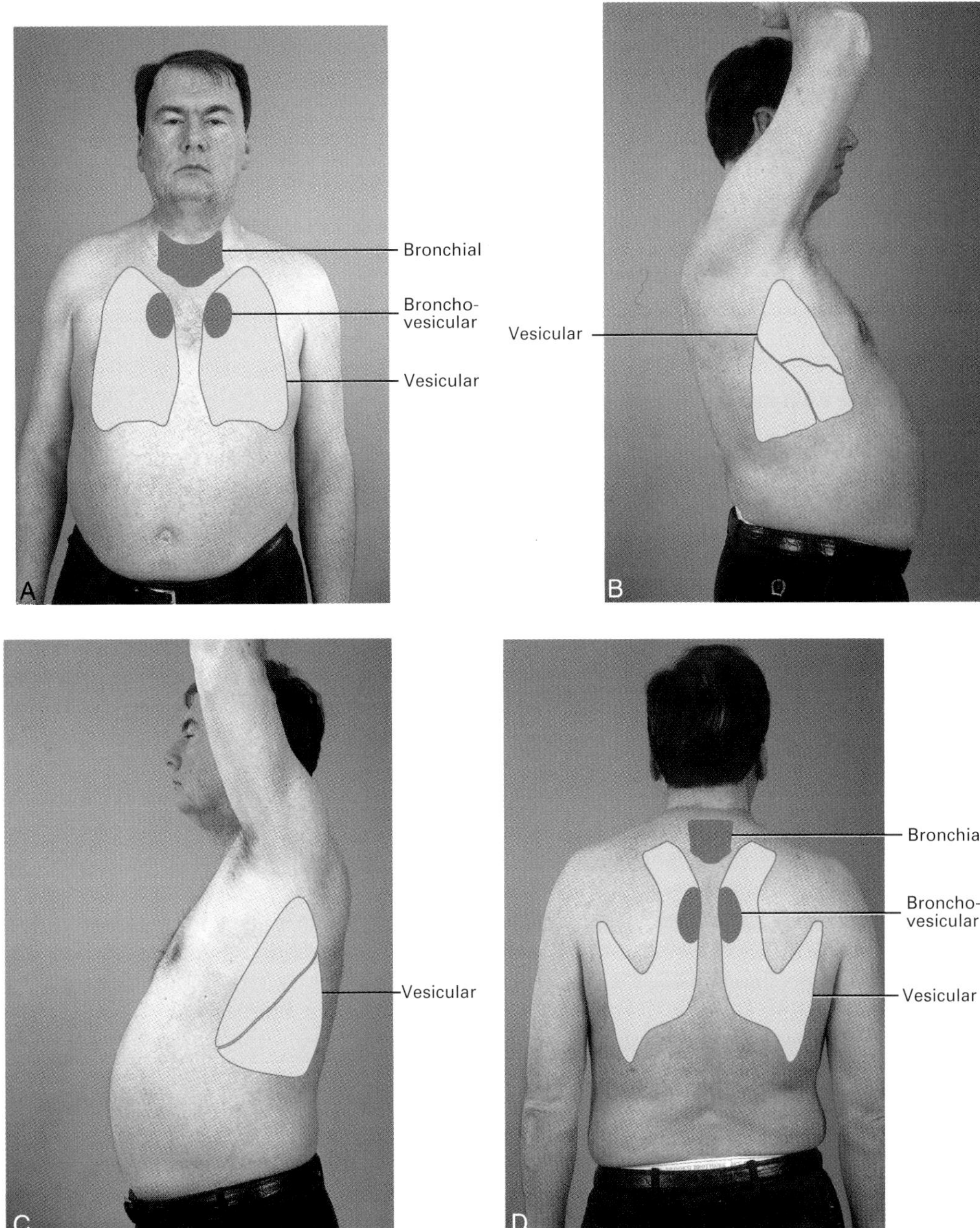

FIGURE 11–10. Normal breath sounds. (*A*) Anterior, (*B*) Right lateral, (*C*) Left lateral, (*D*) Posterior.

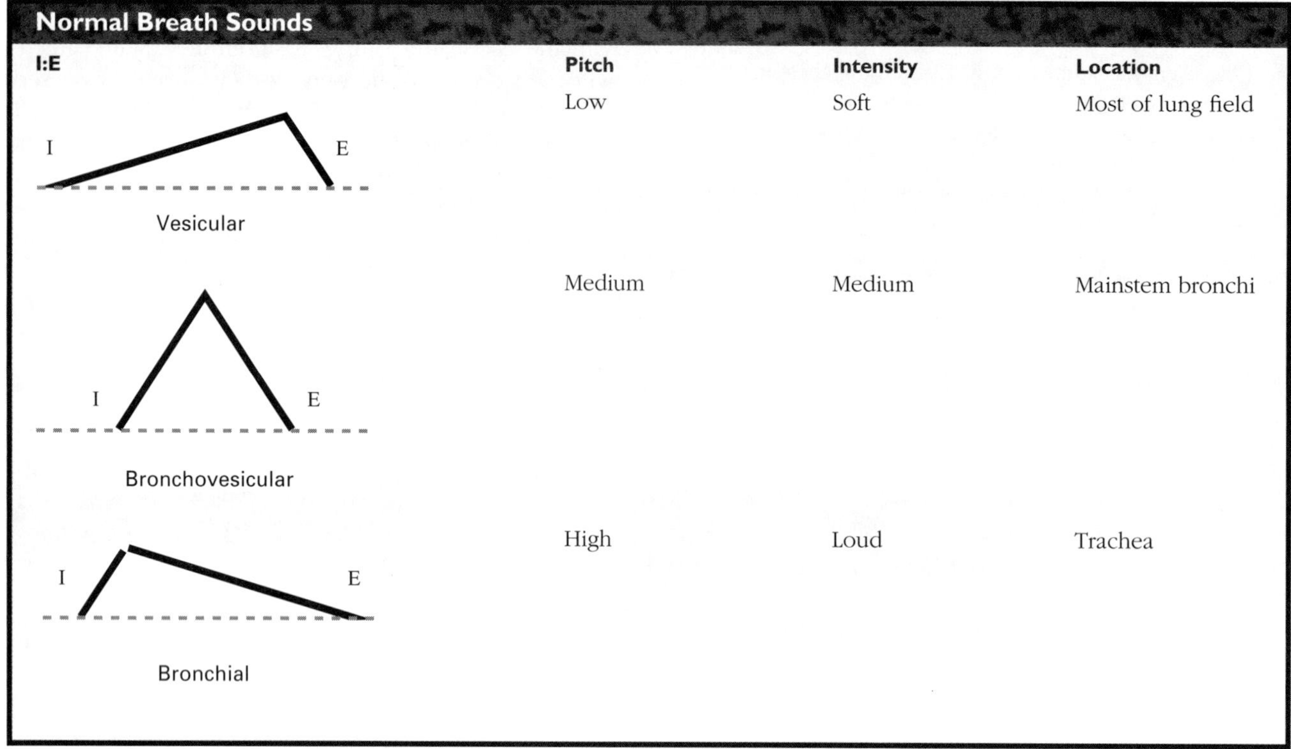

Normal Breath Sounds

I:E	Pitch	Intensity	Location
Vesicular	Low	Soft	Most of lung field
Bronchovesicular	Medium	Medium	Mainstem bronchi
Bronchial	High	Loud	Trachea

Abnormal Breath Sounds

Breath sounds that are diminished or misplaced are referred to as abnormal. Breath sounds may be decreased or diminished in a person with a thick chest wall or pleura, with shallow breathing, or with restricted/obstructed airflow. They may also be diminished in an obese or muscular person or in an older person with poor inspiratory effort.

A bronchial breath sound heard anywhere except over the trachea is a misplaced sound. For example, bronchial breath sounds are heard over areas of constriction.

Be sure to work from side to side, comparing the client to himself or herself. Examples of pathology associated with diminished breath sounds include emphysema, pleural effusion and airways blocked by mucus plugs. Remember: Do not rely on one assessment finding; evaluate the client's entire picture before coming to a decision.

HELPFUL HINT

If you hear any abnormal sounds, have the client cough, and then listen again.

Adventitious Breath Sounds

Adventitious breath sounds are additional sounds superimposed over normal breath sounds and include crackles or rales, rhonchi, wheezing, stridor, grunting and friction rubs. Unfortunately, there is no universal classification of adventitious sounds. You may hear the terms rales and crackles used interchangeably. Adventitious sounds are often classified as continuous and discontinuous. Understanding the underlying mechanism may help you to differentiate sounds. Quality, pitch, location, and timing are important characteristics that will also help you differentiate the sounds and determine their significance.

Rales/Crackles

Rales or crackles are discontinuous sounds resulting from air bubbling through moisture in the alveoli or from collapsed alveoli popping open. Crackles tend to occur at the end of inspiration, in the terminal bronchioles and alveoli. Depending on the cause, crackles may be affected by coughing—loose exudate rales may clear with cough, but the rales of pulmonary edema do not.

Rales associated with long-standing chronic lung disease or with interstitial pulmonary fibrosis are sometimes referred to as "Velcro rales" because they sound like Velcro being pulled apart. Velcro rales are louder than fluid rales and usually do not change over time. They result from air trying to force through fibrotic tissues or fibrotic tissue rubbing against the visceral pleural. Velcro rales are unaffected by coughing.

Rhonchi/Wheezes

Wheezes are continuous sounds caused by the narrowing of an airway by spasm, inflammation, mucus secre-

Adventitious Breath Sounds

Sound/Description	I:E	Conditions	Location
Crackles Popping; discontinuous; may be affected by coughing.	More prominent on inspiration	CHF, atelectasis, pneumonia, interstitial fibrosis	Periphery
Rhonchi Snore, gurgle, rattle; continuous; may be affected by coughing.	More prominent on expiration	Pneumonia	Larger airways
Mild Wheeze Musical, high pitched; continuous; may be affected by coughing. Moderate Wheeze Severe Wheeze	More prominent on expiration, but as severity increases, extends through inspiration and expiration	Asthma, cardiac asthma	Smaller airways
Friction Rub High pitched, scratching, squeaking; continuous; not affected by coughing.	Inspiratory and expiratory		Affected area

tions, or a solid tumor. Pitch is determined by the relative tightness/narrowness of the airway. For example, in asthma, tightly constricted small airways produce very high-pitched, or sibilant, wheezes. However, the loose mucus secretions in a larger airway produce lower-pitched, sonorous wheezes, often called rhonchi. These wheezes may even have a snoring or rattle-like quality.

Although rhonchi may occur in either the inspiratory or expiratory phases of breathing, they are more commonly heard during expiration when air is being forced through the obstruction or the narrowed airway. Wheezes may clear with cough if the airway narrowing is caused by secretions. So if you hear adventitious sounds, ask the client to cough, and then reassess the lung sounds.

HELPFUL HINT

The sudden absence of wheezes does not always indicate that the client's condition has improved. It may actually be a sign of a worsening condition. If the client is having difficulty speaking, he or she may be having trouble moving air.

Stridor

Stridor is a harsh, high-pitched, continuous honking sound resulting from an upper airway obstruction, a partial obstruction, or a spasm of the trachea or larynx. A person with stridor is usually in acute respiratory distress and requires immediate intervention.

Grunting

Grunting is a larger airway sound heard predominantly on expiration. It results from retention of air in the lungs, which prevents alveolar collapse.

Friction Rub

A friction rub is different from all other adventitious sounds, because it occurs between the pleural layers, not in the lung. It results from the rubbing together of the parietal and visceral layers of an inflamed pleura, which produces a high-pitched grating or squeaking sound. The rub may occur during both inspiration and expiration, but because it is not in the lung, it will never be affected by coughing. A pleural friction rub is associated with pleuritis, so people often complain of pain in the area of the rub, especially with deep inspiration.

Abnormal Vocal Sounds

Abnormal vocal sounds include bronchophony, egophony, and whispered pectoriloquy. Transmission of voice sounds through healthy lung tissue is normally muffled. Consolidated lung tissue produces clearer transmission of voice sounds over the affected area. Bronchophony is the abnormal clarity of the spoken word as heard through the stethoscope. Egophony is translated literally as "voice of the goat." Ask the client to say "eee" while you auscultate the lungs through the stethoscope at various places. Egophony is present if the sound changes from a muffled "eee" to an "ay."

To test for whispered pectoriloquy, ask the client to whisper "one, two, three" while you auscultate the lungs. Normally, you should hear "puff, puff, puff." If you hear "one-two-three" clearly through the stethoscope, whispered pectoriloquy is present.

Vocal sounds should be muffled and indistinct through stethoscope. *Bronchophony, egophony, whispered pectoriloquy:* Consolidated lung tissue, pulmonary edema, pulmonary hemorrhage.

HELPFUL HINT

Sound transmission over consolidated lung tissue is like sound transmission around an enclosed swimming pool—the sound comes across louder.

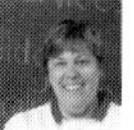

Case Study Findings

Mrs. Kane's focused respiratory assessment findings include:

- Trachea midline.
- Chest: AP:lateral 1:2, costal angle <90, equal chest excursion, normal spinal curvatures, skin intact, no use of accessory muscles, no retraction.
- Chest nontender, symmetrical chest excursion, no masses, crepitus.
- Tactile fremitus equal anterior and posterior to midthorax.
- Resonance noted throughout lung fields. Diaphragmatic excursion 4 cm bilaterally.
- Lungs CTA except for expiratory wheezing that clears with coughing; no crackles or rubs.

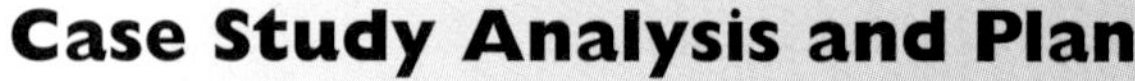

Case Study Analysis and Plan

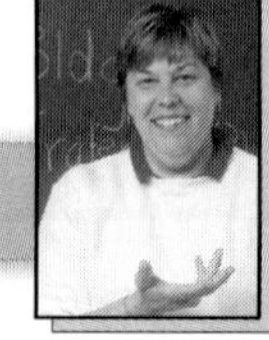

Now that you have completed your assessment of Mrs. Kane, document your key history and physical examination findings.

List key history findings and key physical examination findings that will help you formulate your nursing diagnoses.

Nursing Diagnoses

Your next step is to analyze the data from Mrs. Kane's assessment and develop nursing diagnoses. The following are possible nursing diagnoses for Mrs. Kane. Cluster the supporting data for each nursing diagnosis.

1. Anxiety, related to knowledge deficit of preoperative routine and postoperative course
2. Airway Clearance, ineffective, risk for, related to ineffective cough secondary to anesthesia, postoperative pain, and respiratory changes from smoking
3. Health Maintenance, ineffective, related to insufficient knowledge of effects of tobacco use and available self-help resources
4. Health-Seeking Behaviors
5. Health Maintenance, ineffective, risk for, related to lack of understanding of the significance of family and personal risk factors
6. Nutrition: imbalanced, more than body requirements, related to possible lack of exercise program

Identify any additional nursing diagnoses and any collaborative nursing diagnoses.

CRITICAL THINKING ACTIVITY #5

Now that you have identified some nursing diagnoses for Mrs. Kane, select one and develop a nursing care plan and a brief teaching plan for her, including learning objectives and teaching strategies.

Research Tells Us

Pulmonary complications are the leading cause of postoperative morbidity and mortality (Brooks-Brunn, 1995). Atelectasis accounts for up to 90 percent of postoperative pulmonary complications related to abdominal and cardiothoracic procedures. Smoking is a major risk factor. To minimize the risk, clients who smoke should stop at least 2 months before surgery. Teaching your client to do deep-breathing exercises is effective in improving recovery and pulmonary function. Studies show that modifying risk factors, such as smoking, doing deep-breathing exercises, ambulating early, and managing pain are effective in reducing postoperative pulmonary complications.

Health Concerns

Facts About Lung Cancer and Smoking

- Smoking is associated with 90 percent of all lung cancers in men and 79 percent of all lung cancers in women.
- Of all lung cancers, 80 to 90 percent occur in smokers.
- Heavy smokers (more than 25 cigarettes a day) have a 20 times greater chance of developing lung cancer than nonsmokers.
- Exposure to second-hand smoke may account for as many as 5 percent of all lung cancers.

Warning Signs of Lung Cancer

- Persistent cough
- Changes in respiratory pattern
- Unexplained dyspnea
- Blood-streaked sputum
- Hemoptysis
- Rust-colored or purulent sputum
- Chest, shoulder, or arm pain
- Recurring pleural effusion, pneumonia, or bronchitis

Common Abnormalities

ABNORMALITY	ASSESSMENT FINDINGS

Asthma
Reactive airway disease causing inflammation and airway obstruction because of increased reactiveness to a variety of stimuli
	• *Skin*
	  • Pallor or cyanosis caused by hypoxia
	  • Diaphoresis
	• *Position:* Sits upright and leans forward
	• *Chest*
	  • Use of accessory muscles

(Continued)

Common Abnormalities *(Continued)*

<table>
<tr><th>ABNORMALITY</th><th>ASSESSMENT FINDINGS</th></tr>
<tr><td>Asthma (Continued)</td><td>
<ul><li><ul>
<li>Intercostal and supraclavicular retraction</li>
<li>Chest tightness</li>
<li>Dyspnea, respiratory rate >30/ min</li>
<li>Increased pulse with PVCs, increased or decreased BP</li>
<li>Pulsus paradoxus >12 mm Hg</li>
<li>Crackles, rhonchi, wheezes, decreased or absent breath sounds</li>
<li>Early in disease—expiratory wheezes</li>
<li>Late in disease—inspiratory and expiratory wheezes</li>
<li>Hyperresonance</li>
<li>Decreased tactile fremitus</li>
<li>Decreased chest excursion</li>
</ul></li>
<li>Extremities: Color changes related to hypoxia</li>
</ul></td></tr>
<tr><td>Bronchitis
Excessive mucus production with recurrent, persistent cough during 3 months of the year for 2 consecutive years. Results in obstructive lung disease and hypoxic and right-side CHF.</td><td>
<ul>
<li>Body build: Average or obese</li>
<li>Head and neck
<ul>
<li>Changes in mental status related to hypoxia</li>
<li>Productive cough with copious amounts of mucus</li>
</ul></li>
<li>Skin: Cyanosis (“blue bloater”)</li>
<li>Chest</li>
<li>Increased AP diameter
<ul>
<li>Increased costal angle</li>
<li>Increased use of accessory muscles</li>
<li>Cardiac enlargement</li>
<li>Decreased excursion</li>
<li>Decreased tactile fremitus</li>
<li>Hyperresonance at bases, dullness over exudate areas</li>
<li>Crackles, rhonchi, wheezes</li>
<li>Breath sounds decreased at bases</li>
</ul></li>
</ul></td></tr>
<tr><td>Emphysema
Permanent enlargement of alveoli distal to terminal bronchioles with destruction of alveolar wall</td><td>
<ul>
<li>Body build: Thin with muscle wasting</li>
<li>Head and neck
<ul>
<li>Anxiety</li>
<li>Cough rare</li>
<li>Neck vein distention</li>
<li>Difficulty speaking because of respiratory distress</li>
<li>Pursed-lip breathing</li>
</ul></li>
<li>Skin
<ul>
<li>Pallor, ruddiness (pink puffer)</li>
<li>Decreased turgor</li>
</ul></li>
<li>Chest
<ul>
<li>Rapid, shallow respiration</li>
<li>Use of accessory muscles</li>
<li>Distant heart sounds, right-sided S_3</li>
<li>Tachycardia with arrhythmias</li>
<li>Hyperresonance at bases or in all lung fields</li>
<li>Decreased excursion</li>
<li>Decreased tactile fremitus</li>
<li>Increased AP diameter</li>
<li>Increased costal angle</li>
<li>Decreased breath sounds</li>
</ul></li>
</ul></td></tr>
</table>

Common Abnormalities

ABNORMALITY	ASSESSMENT FINDINGS
	HELPFUL HINT The disappearance of wheezes may be an ominous sign if associated with decreased breath sounds caused by decreased air movement. This may indicate severe obstruction and impending respiratory failure.

Lung Cancer
Malignant tumor of lung tissue
	• *Body build:* Thin as a result of weight loss
	• *Head and neck*
	  • Unexplained dyspnea
	  • Persistent dry or productive cough
	  • Blood-streaked, rust-colored, or purulent sputum
	  • Hemoptysis
	• *Chest*
	  • Change in respiratory pattern
	  • Wheezes
	  • Decreased breath sounds over affected lung
	  • Chest, shoulder, or arm pain

Pleural Effusion
Collection of fluid in pleural space
	• *Head and neck*
	  • Dyspnea
	  • Complaints of chest pain
	• *Chest*
	  • Decreased excursion on affected side
	  • Decreased tactile fremitus on affected side
	  • Dullness on percussion
	  • Decreased or absent breath sounds
	  • Friction rub with initial inflammation; rub disappears as fluid develops

Pneumonia
Infectious process of lung tissue. Clinical manifestations vary depending on causative agent.
	• *Head and neck*
	  • Changes in mental status related to hypoxia or fever
	  • Pharyngitis
	  • Productive cough; pink, rusty, purulent, green, yellow, or white sputum
	• *Skin*
	  • Diaphoretic or dry with poor turgor
	  • Pallor or flushing
	  • Circumoral or nailbed cyanosis
	• *Chest*
	  • Tachypnea
	  • Use of accessory muscles
	  • Asymmetrical chest movement
	  • Decreased excursion
	• *Head and neck*
	  • Changes in mental status related to hypoxia or fever
	  • Pharyngitis
	  • Productive cough; pink, rusty, purulent, green, yellow, or white sputum
	• *Skin*
	  • Diaphoretic or dry with poor turgor
	  • Pallor or flushing
	  • Circumoral or nailbed cyanosis

(Continued)

Common Abnormalities *(Continued)*

ABNORMALITY	ASSESSMENT FINDINGS
Pneumonia *(Continued)*	• *Chest* • Tachypnea • Use of accessory muscles • Asymmetrical chest movement • Decreased excursion • Increased tactile fremitus • Crackles, rhonchi • Bronchial breath sounds • Positive bronchophony • Dullness on percussion
Pneumothorax Complete or partial collapse of lung	• *Head and neck* • Shallow, rapid respiration • Dyspnea • Complaint of chest pain with or without hemoptysis • *Chest* • Asymmetrical excursion • Decreased fremitus • Hyperresonance • Absent breath sounds • If tension pneumothorax, severe respiratory distress, tachycardia, cyanosis, tracheal shift away from affected lung, and displaced point of maximal impulse occur.
Pulmonary Fibrosis ("Stiff Lung") Restrictive lung disease Chronic, nonmalignant, noninfectious inflammatory process of interstitial lung tissue	• *Head and neck* • Weakness • Fatigue • Dyspnea • Weight loss • Anorexia • *Chest* • Vesicular breath sounds, occasionally bronchovesicular • "Velcro rales" • Decreased excursion • Pulmonary hypertension occurring late; if present, prominent P wave, neck vein distention, right ventricular heave, split S_2 and accentuated pulmonic component • *Extremities:* Clubbing (late sign)
Tuberculosis Mycobacterial infection of lung	• *Head and neck:* • Fatigue • Persistent, long-term, low-grade fever • Chills and night sweats • Anorexia and weight loss • *Chest* • Dyspnea. • Productive cough with nonpurulent, blood-streaked sputum. • Hemoptysis. • Pleuritic or dull chest pain. • Chest tightness. • Apical posterior segment of upper lobes or superior segments of lower lobes usually affected. Alters normal breath sounds.

Summary

- A thorough respiratory assessment provides invaluable data about your client's overall health status.
- Before you begin the assessment, visualize the underlying structures and landmarks and review expected normal findings.
- As you work through the assessment, differentiate normal from abnormal, and work in a systematic manner from apex to base and from side to side.
- Remember, if a person has a respiratory problem, it may affect every other body system.
- Establish a baseline, using the client as his or her own control. If he or she has an acute respiratory problem, postpone the comprehensive respiratory assessment and perform a focused assessment.
- After completing the assessment, document your findings.
- The plan of care should flow from your assessment. Share your findings with the client. This provides an excellent opportunity for teaching, especially if you include the client in developing a plan of care that promotes a healthy respiratory system.

12

Assessing the Cardiovascular System

Before You Begin

INTRODUCTION TO THE CARDIOVASCULAR SYSTEM

The cardiovascular system is the lifeline of the body. Its primary function is to act as a transport system, delivering oxygen by way of the red blood cells and delivering nutrients, metabolites, and hormones to every cell in the body. At the same time, it transports metabolic wastes for detoxification and excretion. The cardiovascular system also contains white blood cells, whose main function is to fight infection.

Because cardiovascular disease is the leading health problem in the United States, accurate assessment of the cardiovascular system is essential to identify and evaluate changes in cardiovascular function and potential risk factors for cardiovascular disease. A thorough, accurate cardiovascular assessment will allow you to develop a plan of care that addresses not only treatment measures but also health promotion and disease prevention measures.

Anatomy and Physiology Review

A thorough, accurate assessment depends on a solid understanding of the cardiovascular system. You especially need to understand normal cardiovascular function before you can identify abnormal findings. Having a mental image of the underlying structures will help you to perform the assessment accurately, and an understanding of the physiology—especially of the mechanisms of heart sounds—will guide your assessment and help you interpret your findings.

Structures and Functions of the Cardiovascular System

The cardiovascular system is a closed system consisting of the heart and blood vessels.

The Heart

The heart is a muscle that pumps blood through a vast network of blood vessels extending over 60,000 miles through arteries, arterioles, capillaries, venules, and veins (Fig. 12–1).

The Circulatory System

The circulatory system has two main networks, the pulmonary circulation and the systemic circulation (Fig. 12–2. The coronary circulation is part of the systemic circulation and supplies the heart itself.

The pulmonary circulation involves blood vessels that circulate blood through the pulmonary arteries, the lungs, and the pulmonary veins. Unoxygenated blood enters the pulmonary circulation from the right and left pulmonary arteries. The unoxygenated blood then flows through the pulmonary arterioles to the lung capillaries, where the exchange of carbon dioxide and oxygen oc-

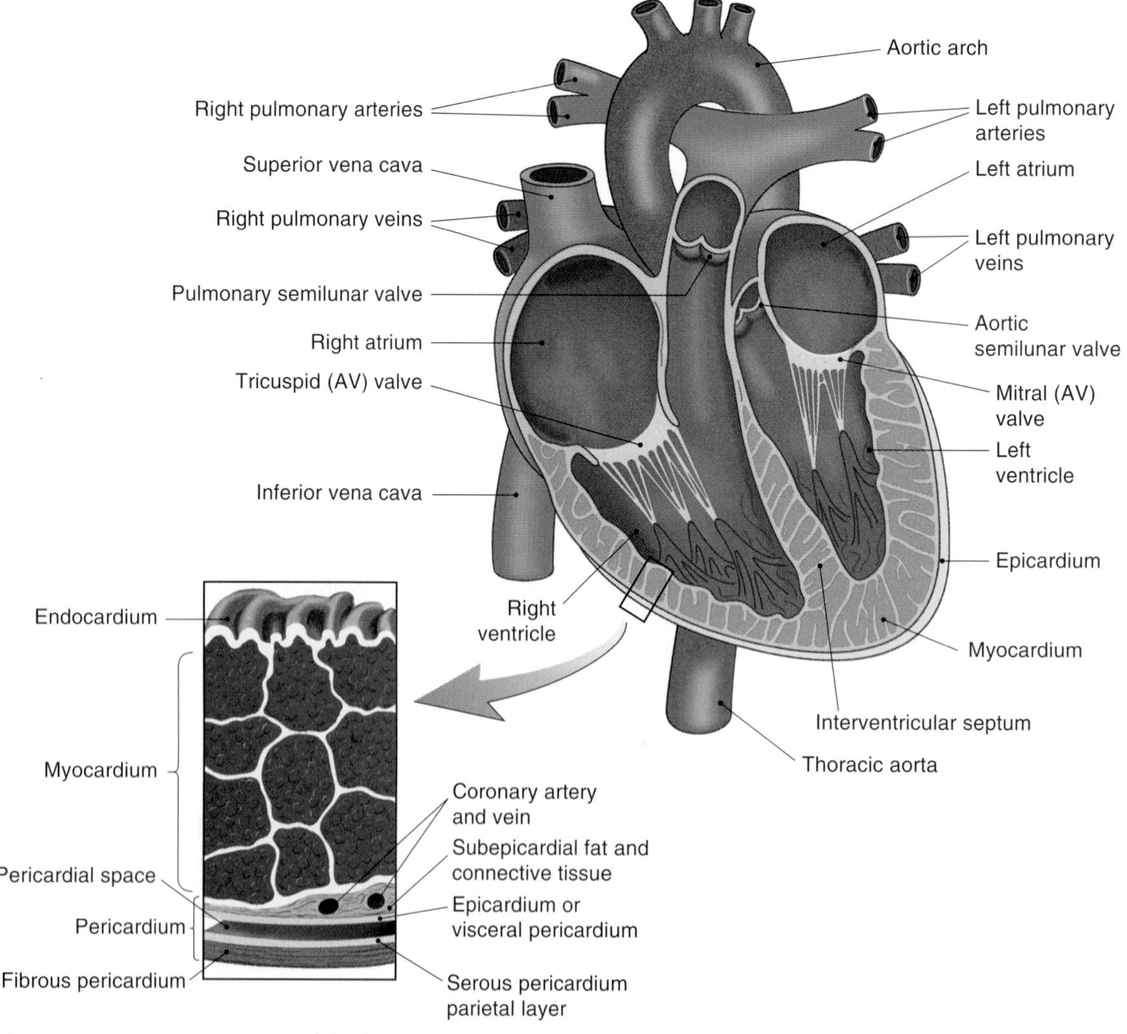

FIGURE 12–1. Structures of the heart.

Anatomy and Physiology of the Heart

STRUCTURE	DESCRIPTION/PRIMARY FUNCTION
Heart	A cone-shaped muscle with four chambers; a double pump about the size of a clenched fist (12 cm long and 9 cm wide). Weighs 250–390 g (8.8–13.8 oz) in adult males and 200–275 g (7.0–9.7 oz) in adult females Pumps blood throughout the circulatory system.
Right Side:	
Right Atrium	Upper chamber of right heart. Receives unoxygenated blood from superior and inferior vena cava.
Tricuspid Valve	Right atrioventricular valve with three cusps (tricuspid). Attached by chordae tendineae to papillary muscles, which are attached to inner heart muscle. Valve between right atrium and right ventricle.
Right Ventricle	Lower chamber of right heart. Receives blood from right atrium and pumps it into pulmonary circuit.
Pulmonary Semilunar Valve	Composed of three cusps. Valve between right ventricle and main pulmonary artery.
Main Pulmonary Artery	Artery leading from right ventricle to lungs. Divides into right and left branches supplying respective lungs. Carries unoxygenated blood from the right ventricle to the lungs.
Pulmonary Veins	Veins leading from lungs to left atrium. Carry oxygenated blood to left atrium.
Left side:	
Left Atrium	Upper chamber of left heart. Receives oxygenated blood from lungs through pulmonary veins.
Mitral Valve	Atrioventricular valve with two cusps (bicuspid) attached by chordae tendineae to papillary muscles, which are attached to inner heart muscle. Valve between left atrium and left ventricle.
Left Ventricle	Lower chamber of left half of heart. Receives blood from left atrium and pumps oxygenated blood through systemic circulation.
Aortic Valve	Composed of three cusps. Valve between left ventricle and aorta.
Interventricular Septum	Wall between left and right ventricles. Vertically separates left and right sides of heart.

Layers of the Heart

LAYER	DESCRIPTION/PRIMARY FUNCTION
Endocardium	Inner layer of the heart; a smooth, thin layer of endothelium and connective tissue. The smooth inner lining of the heart.
Myocardium	Middle and thickest layer of the heart; the heart muscle. Responsible for cardiac contraction.
Epicardium	The layer of serous pericardium on the heart's surface. Contains main coronary blood vessels.
Pericardium	Sac that surrounds the heart and roots of the great vessels. Comprised of two layers: fibrous pericardium (outer layer of fibrous connective tissue) and serous pericardium. Serous pericardium also has two layers: the outer or parietal layer that lines the fibrous layer and the visceral or inner layer that lines the heart and is also called the epicardium. The serous pericardium contains pericardial fluid (10–20 mL of serous fluid). Pericardial fluid moistens the pericardial sac between the two layers and prevents friction during systole and diastole.

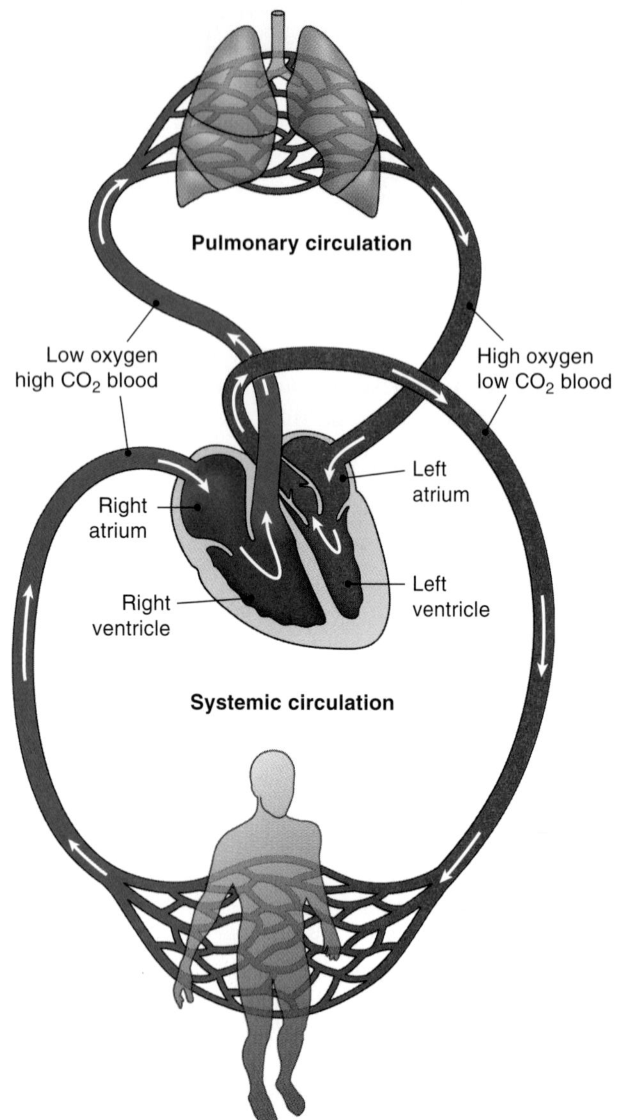

FIGURE 12–2. Systemic and pulmonary circulation.

curs. The oxygenated blood then enters the pulmonary venules that lead to the pulmonary veins. Oxygenated blood is then carried back to the left atrium through the right and left pulmonary veins.

Systemic Circulation

The systemic circulation is responsible for supplying oxygen to every cell in the body through the arterial system and then returning unoxygenated blood to the heart through the venous system. Oxygenated blood flows into the left atrium from the pulmonary circulation. The left atrium then pumps the oxygenated blood into the left ventricle, which in turn expels the oxygenated blood through the aorta into the arterial systemic circulation. From the aorta, blood then flows through smaller arterioles to the systemic capillaries. The systemic capillaries link the arterial and venous systems. At this point, exchange of oxygen, nutrients, and wastes occurs. From the capillaries, unoxygenated blood then flows through the venules, into the larger veins, and then to the superior and inferior vena cavae. Unoxygenated blood then enters the right atrium and is pumped to the right ventricle into the pulmonary circulation to continue the cycle. Layers of arteries and veins are shown in Figure 12–3.

Coronary Circulation

The heart is a muscle with the primary responsibility of circulating blood throughout the entire body. Consequently, the oxygen requirements of the heart are great, second only to those of the brain. The coronary circulation is responsible for supplying the heart with the oxygen needed to perform this task effectively. The coronary circulation consists of the right and left coronary arteries and the coronary sinus and cardiac veins. The coronary arteries are the first branches off the aorta. The cardiac veins drain into the coronary sinus, which in turn drains directly into the right atrium.

Mechanisms of Heart Sounds

To perform an accurate cardiac assessment, you need an understanding of the normal anatomy and physiology of the heart as well as knowledge of the mechanisms of heart sounds in order to interpret your findings. Heart sounds are the result of events within the heart. The movement and pressure of the blood (hemodynamics), the activity of the electrical conduction system, and the movement of the valves affect the sounds that you hear (Fig. 12–4).

The Cardiac Cycle

The cardiac cycle comprises all the physiologic events needed for the heart to beat. The valves, the hemodynamic events within the heart and the conduction system work together in the cardiac cycle. The cardiac cycle is comprised of systolic and diastolic phases. The systolic phase is the contraction or emptying phase, and the diastolic phase is the resting or filling phase. The atria and ventricles alternate through the systolic and diastolic phases; while the atria are contracting, the ventricles are relaxing, and vice versa (see Fig. 12–4).

Ventricular Diastole

Very shortly after the onset of ventricular diastole, the pressure in the ventricles descends to below that of the atria, and the mitral and tricuspid valves open to allow filling of the ventricles (the rapid filling phase of diastole). Toward the end of ventricular diastole, the atria contract to propel additional blood into the ventricles, thus completing the filling phase of the ventricles. This is referred to as the atrial kick and is responsible for

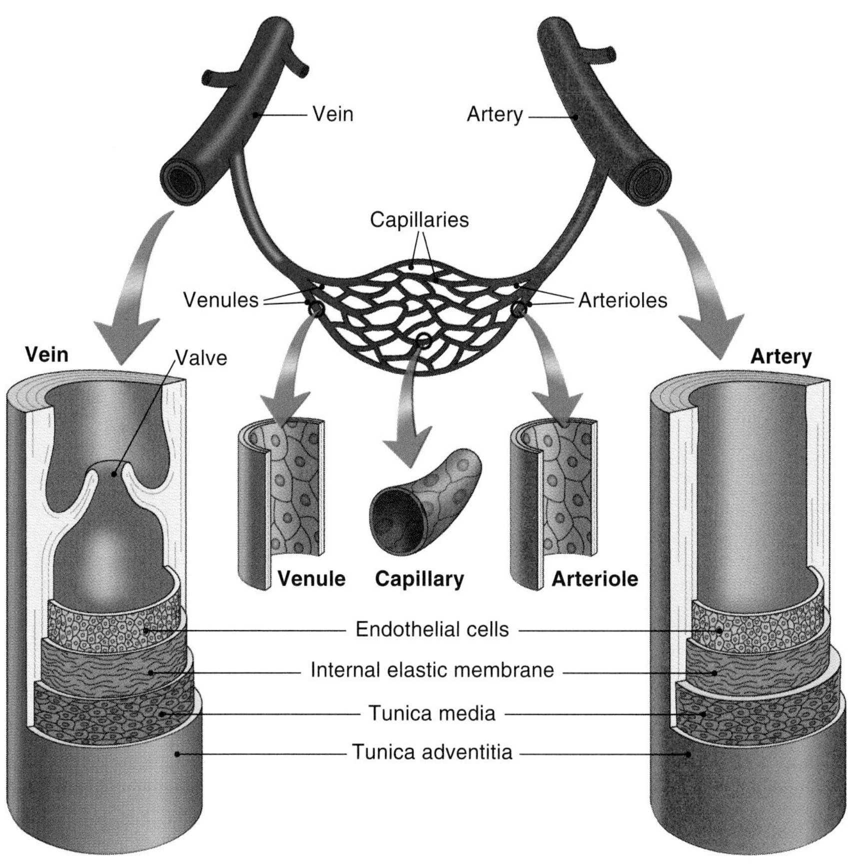

FIGURE 12–3. Layers of arteries and veins.

Layers of Arteries and Veins

STRUCTURE	DESCRIPTION/PRIMARY FUNCTION
Arteries	Blood vessels with three coats: tunica intima, tunica media, and tunica adventitia. Carry oxygenated blood away from left heart and unoxygenated blood to lungs via pulmonary arteries.
Tunica intima	Inner layer of endothelial cells containing basement membrane of fine, collagenous fibers and external elastic layer called internal elastic lamina.
Tunica media	Middle, thickest layer containing collagenous fibers, connective tissue, smooth muscle cells, and elastic fibers.
Tunica adventitia	Outer layer containing collagen and elastic fibers, nerves, lymphatic vessels.
Arterioles	Smallest arteries; contain large amount of smooth muscle cells that can dilate and constrict. Arterioles carry blood to capillaries and control blood flow to capillaries through dilation/constriction.
Capillaries	A single layer of microscopic endothelial cells. Connect arterial and venous system for exchange of gases, fluids, nutrients, and wastes.
Veins	Contain same 3 layers as arteries, but are thinner with less elastic and collagenous tissue and smooth muscle. Blood pressure in venous system is low; veins have valves to prevent backflow. Carry unoxygenated blood back to right heart, except for pulmonary veins, which carry oxygenated blood from lungs to left heart.
Venules	Smallest veins, consisting of endothelium and thin tunica adventitia. Blood from capillaries drains into venules.

Branches of the Right and Left Coronary Arteries

BRANCH	AREAS SUPPLIED
Right Coronary Artery	
Nodal branch	Sinoatrial (pacemaker) node
Right marginal branch	Ventral and dorsal surface of right ventricle
Nodal branch	Atrioventricular (AV) node
Small branches	Right AV bundle
Posterior branches	Join to anterior descending branch and circumflex artery of left coronary artery
Left Coronary Artery	
Anterior interventricular branch	Left ventricle
Small branches	Left AV bundle
Circumflex	Lateral and posterior side of heart

Branches of the Cardiac Veins

BRANCH	AREA DRAINED
Great cardiac vein	Anterior portion of heart
Middle cardiac vein and oblique vein	Posterior aspect of heart
Small cardiac vein	Drains directly into right atrium
Thebesian veins	Drain into each of heart's 4 chambers

about 25 percent of the total blood volume in the ventricles. The ventricles are now filled, marking the end of ventricular diastole. This is referred to as the end-diastolic volume.

Ventricular Systole

With ventricular contraction, the pressure in the ventricles will exceed that of the atria. This results in closure of the mitral and tricuspid valves and marks the beginning of ventricular systole. While the ventricles are contracting and blood is being propelled from them, the atria are relaxed (atrial diastole) and are filling. When pressure in the ventricles exceeds that of the aorta and pulmonary arteries, the aortic and pulmonic valves open to allow for forward flow into the systemic and pulmonic systems, respectively. While the ventricles are contracting and propelling blood into the aorta and pulmonary arteries, the pressures in the ventricles are gradually decreasing to eventually attain a level below that of the pulmonary arteries and aorta. At this point, the pulmonic and aortic valves close, marking the end of ventricular systole.

The amount of blood in the ventricles at the end of diastole is referred to as end-diastolic volume and reflects the largest volume of blood in the ventricles. The amount of blood remaining in the ventricles at the end of ventricular systole is referred to as the end-systolic volume and is indicative of the least amount of residual blood in the ventricles. The pressure of the end-diastolic volume is referred to as end-diastolic pressure; the pressure of the end-systolic volume is end-systolic pressure. The amount of blood ejected from the heart with each contraction is referred to as the stroke volume. This is the difference between the end-diastolic volume and end-systolic volume—basically the difference in volume between the beginning and end of ventricular contraction.

The Cardiac Output

The cardiac output is the amount of blood ejected per minute. Cardiac output = stroke volume × heart rate. Because so many factors can affect cardiac output, this is an important concept to understand. Although both heart rate and stroke volume affect cardiac output, the change in heart rate is the major regulator of cardiac output. The internal pacemaker of the heart controls the rate, but the autonomic nervous system also plays a major role. The heart rate also responds to various external factors, such as temperature, pain, exercise, pH, hormones, and emotions. Changes in heart rate can readily be seen in response to these factors.

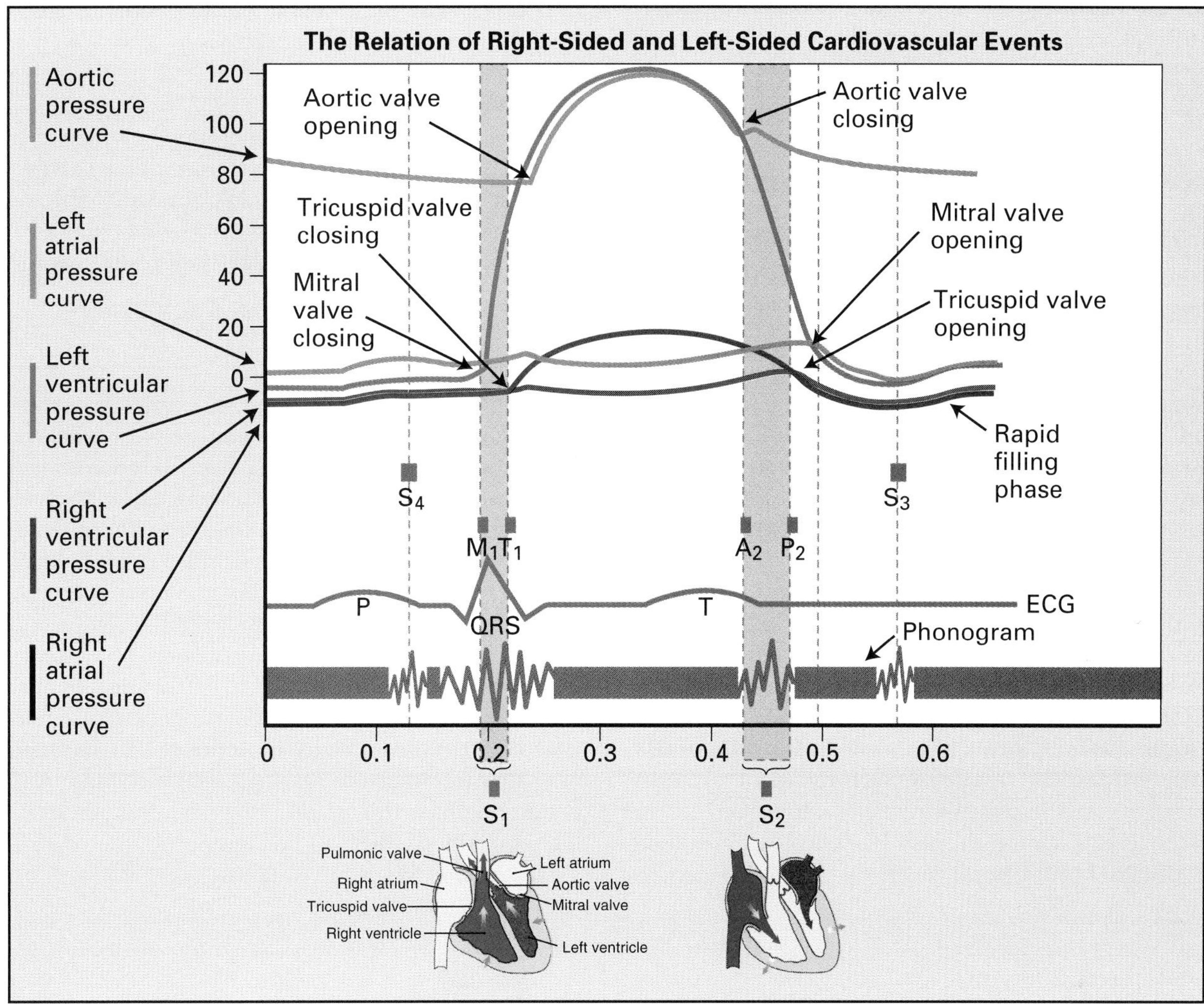

FIGURE 12–4. Mechanisms of heart sounds.

The Stroke Volume

Stroke volume is less variable and responds to changes in **preload, afterload,** and contractility of the heart. Preload refers to the volume of blood in the ventricles at the end of diastole. The greater the preload, the greater the "stretch" or contractility of the ventricles, and the greater the stroke volume. An increase in venous return to the heart will, in turn, increase preload. Factors that affect venous return include:

- Venous blood reservoirs: Distensibility of veins allows them to act as reservoirs and can either decrease or increase venous return to the heart.
- Skeletal muscle pump: Contraction of skeletal muscles pumps blood back to the heart.
- Venous tone: Sympathetic stimulation of smooth muscles in the walls of veins increases venous return to the heart.
- Respiratory pump: During inspiration, the increase in negative intrathoracic pressure increases venous return to the heart.

Afterload reflects the end-systolic volume. It is affected by the amount of resistance the ventricles have to contract against. An increase in afterload results in a decrease in stroke volume. Afterload may be affected by:

- Arterial elasticity
- Peripheral vascular resistance
- Aortic valve resistance
- Viscosity and volume of blood
- Contractility, which reflects the force of contraction
- **Positive inotropes,** increase the force of contraction.
- **Negative inotropes,** decrease the force of contraction

HELPFUL HINTS

- Remember: If contractility is increased, so are the oxygen requirements of the heart.
- In the normal heart, left-side cardiac activity occurs slightly before right-side cardiac activity.

The Heart's Electrical Conduction System

The cardiac electrical conduction system is essential for each contraction of the heart. The cardiac muscle has its own electrical system that is responsible for initiating and maintaining the rhythmic beat of the heart. The **sinoatrial (SA) node** is the normal pacemaker of the heart located in the right atrium near the superior vena cava entrance point. The SA node paces the normal adult heart at 60 to 100 beats per minute (BPM). The activation of the SA node passes through the atria and results in atrial contraction.

The electrical activity is then conducted to the **atrioventricular (AV) node.** This node is located at the base of the right atrium between the atria and the ventricles. It has the ability to pace the heart at a rate of 40 to 60 beats per minute (BPM). The electrical impulse is then transmitted from the AV node to the **bundle of His,** which divides into two branches, the right and left, which traverse the interventricular septum. Finally, the impulse is transmitted to small branches that eventuate into **the Purkinje fibers,** which stimulate the ventricles to contract. The pacer ability of the bundle of His is 20 to 40 beats per minute (Fig. 12–5).

The Valves

The most accepted theory concerning the origin of heart sounds relates primarily to the closure of the valves. The "lub-dub" sounds that are usually readily heard are referred to as $\mathbf{S_1}$ (lub) and $\mathbf{S_2}$ (dub), the first and the second heart sounds, respectively. They result from valve closure.

The First Heart Sound (S_1)

S_1 (Fig. 12–6) marks the beginning of systole and S_2 marks the end of it. S_1, the first heart sound, results from the closure of the mitral (M_1) and tricuspid (T_1) valves. M_1 and T_1 normally close within approximately 0.02 of a second or less. These valve sounds are often heard as a single sound. S_1 is best heard at the apex or left lateral sternal border with the diaphragm of the stethoscope.

The Accentuated $\mathbf{S_1}$. The intensity of S_1 may normally be increased in anemia, hyperthyroidism, and exercise. An apparent increased intensity of S_1 also may be noted with mitral or tricuspid stenosis. It is important to note that the intensity does not really change in these entities; rather, the S_1 becomes sharper (shorter and higher pitched), and consequently, is often described clinically as increased in loudness.

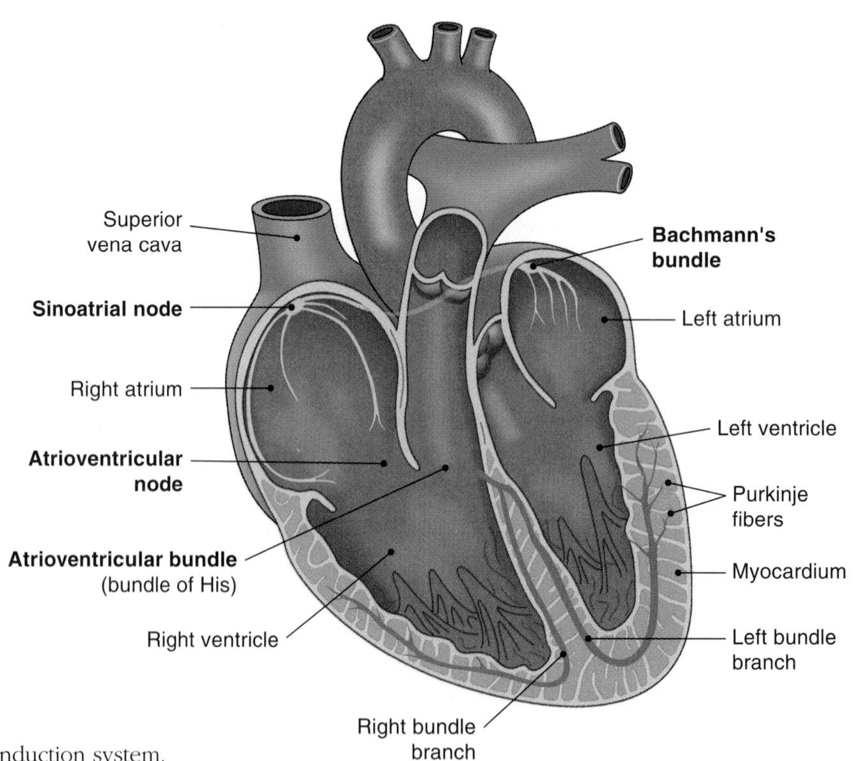

FIGURE 12–5. Electrical conduction system.

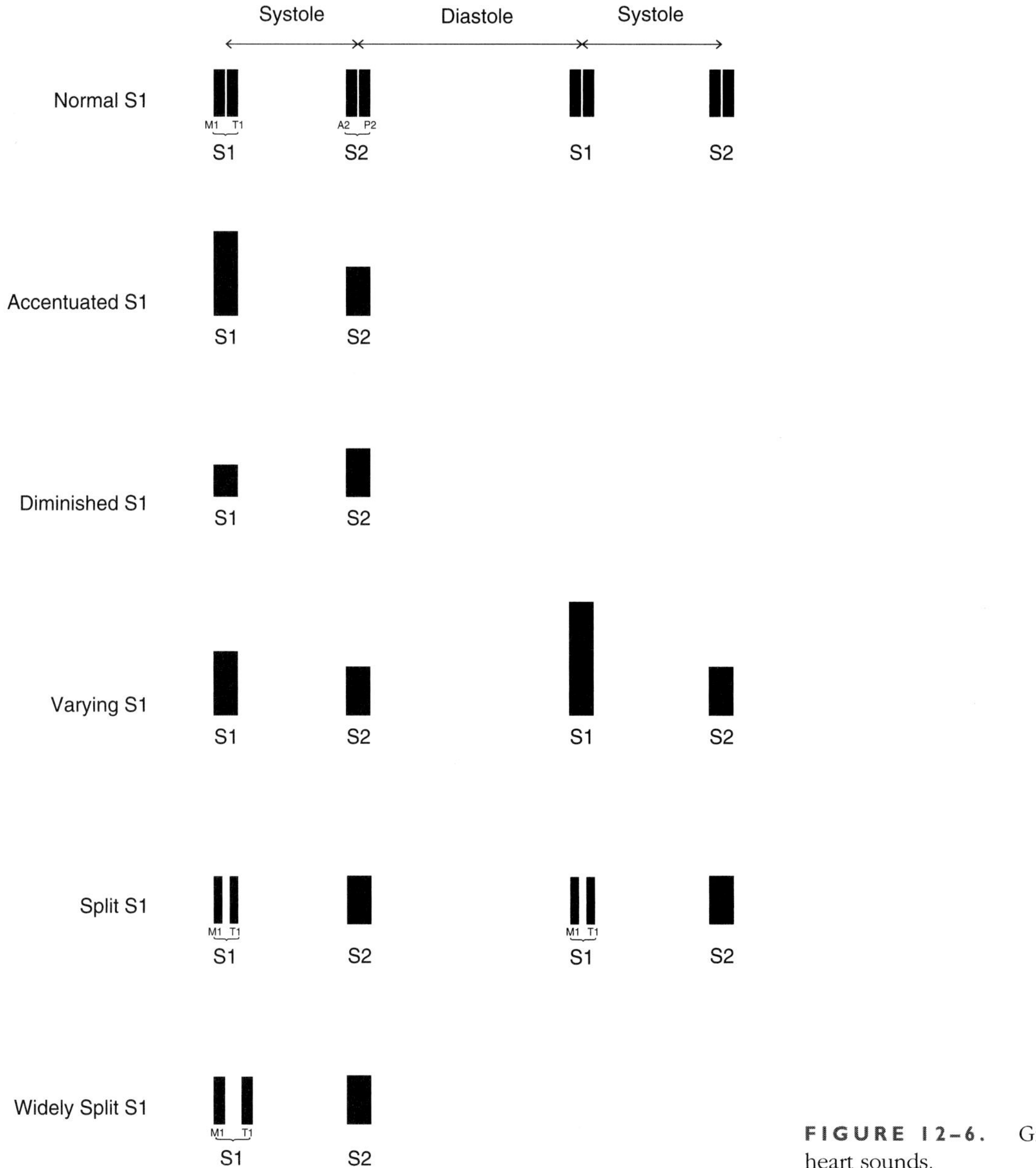

FIGURE 12–6. Graphic depiction of S_1 heart sounds.

The Diminished S_1. The intensity of S_1 may be decreased normally in patients with thick chest walls or emphysema because there is greater distance for the heart sound to traverse from the myocardium to the chest wall. S_1 may also be diminished in patients with first-degree heart block. The delay in conduction between atrial contraction and ventricular contraction allows more time for the valves to close, thus diminishing the sound's intensity.

The Varying S_1. The intensity of S_1 may vary with irregular rhythms, such as **complete heart block** or **atrial fibrillation,** a grossly irregular rhythm.

The Split S_1. In normally functioning hearts, the left side contracts before the right side; therefore the mitral valve will close before the tricuspid, and the aortic valve will close before the pulmonic. Often the closures of the mitral and tricuspid valves occur so close together that the first sound is heard as a single sound. There are times when each component (mitral and tricuspid) of the sound may be heard clearly, defining this as a normal split S_1.

If the time interval between mitral and tricuspid valve closure is greater than 0.20 of a second, each component of valve closure may be heard. If you can hear the mitral valve close and then the tricuspid valve close, this is referred to as a split S_1. The mitral component of S_1 is louder than the tricuspid component. Conduction problems such as **right bundle branch block (RBBB),**

premature ventricular contractions (PVC), and **ventricular tachycardia** may result in asynchronous closure of the mitral and triscupid valves, resulting in a widely split S1.

The Second Heart Sound (S_2)

When the systolic pressure in the ventricles decreases below that of the aorta and the pulmonary artery (toward the end of systole), the aortic (A_2) and pulmonic (P_2) valves close, producing the second heart sound (Fig. 12–7). Clinically, this sound marks the end of systole and the beginning of diastole. A_2 and P_2 normally close about 0.02 of a second from each other; consequently, they may occasionally be heard as a single sound. (See following text for an important distinction between A_2 and P_2 with respiration.)

Accentuated S_2. The intensity of S_2 also may be normally increased with high output states such as exercise, resulting also in a concomitant increased heart rate. An accentuated S_2 is also associated with pathology. A_2 may be accentuated with systemic hypertension; P_2 is likewise accentuated with pulmonary hypertension.

Diminished S_2. A thick chest wall and chronic lung disease also decreases the intensity of S_2. A_2 is also decreased characteristically in **calcific aortic stenosis,** and P_2 is diminished in **pulmonic stenosis.**

Split S_2. When the time interval between A_2 and P_2 is greater than 0.02 second, you will hear each valve component. This is referred to as a split S_2. This split differs from a split S_1 because it has a respiratory variation. During inspiration, S_2 will split, so you will hear the aortic valve close, then hear the pulmonic valve close ("blub"). Characteristically, S_2 will be heard as "blub" (A_2 followed by P_2). During expiration, the valves close as one to create a single sound ("dub").

This respiratory variation in the S_2 results from the normal physiologic changes that occur during inspiration, when an increase in negative intrathoracic pressure results in increased blood return to the right side of the heart. With more blood in the right side of the heart, the right ventricle contraction time increases, resulting in a greater time interval between A_2 and P_2, compared with the converse occurring during expiration. Thus, during inspiration you hear "lub-blub" (A_2 and P_2 as separate sounds) in comparison with "lub-dub" during expiration, when A_2 and P_2 are closer to one another and often heard as a single sound. The increased venous return to the right side of the heart that occurs during inspiration may also account for the frequent sinus variation that is noted, especially in children. During inspiration, the cardiac rate increases to accommodate the increase in venous return.

Widely abnormal split of S_2. This occurs with right bundle branch block. The delay between aortic and pulmonic valve closure will average greater than 0.03 second during expiration with further widening of the split during inspiration.

The paradoxical (reversed) split of S_2. When P_2 comes before A_2, this is defined as a paradoxical or reversed split of S_2. The mechanism relates to delayed contraction of the left ventricle, resulting from pathologic blockage or conduction through the left heart's electrical nerve conduction system. Consequently, the left heart is depolarized later by way of the electrical impulse going from the right heart and through the interventricular septum to stimulate the left ventricular muscle to contract.

Atrial septal defect. The fixed, widely split S_2 occurs in atrial septal defect. It is unaffected by respiration. In this entity and in some other congenital cardiac abnormalities, the split averages 0.04 to 0.07 second.

Extra Heart Sounds

Additional sounds that may be heard during auscultation (Fig. 12–8) include early ejection click, midsystolic ejection click, opening snap, S_3, and S_4. These sounds do not always indicate pathology.

The early ejection click. Early ejection clicks are high-pitched, short systolic sounds occurring shortly after S_1. The ejection click associated with the aortic and pulmonic valves is an early sound occurring about 0.03 to 0.08 second after S_1. The ejection click of aortic valve origin is heard at the base and better heard at the apex. The ejection click of pulmonic valve origin is best heard at the left sternal border at the second and third interspaces and rarely at the apex.

The midsystolic ejection click. This high-pitched short sound is a cardinal finding in mitral valve prolapse (MVP). The ejection click of MVP occurs at least 0.14 second after the first heart sound, but its exact placement in midsystole varies with the position of the patient (e.g, sitting, standing, lying down, squatting). It is heard best at the apex or just medial to it, but it may be widely transmitted over the precordium.

The opening snap. This is a short, high-pitched, mid-diastolic sound occurring 0.05 to 0.14 second after S_2. It is a classic finding in mitral stenosis. It is also found in tricuspid valve stenosis, a much rarer condition. It is heard best at or near the apex, with the patient in the left lateral position. It is accompanied by the other classic findings of mitral stenosis—namely, the sharp first heart sound and the midlate diastolic murmur of mitral stenosis.

The normal heart sound (S_3): The ventricles receive blood from the atria. As the blood flows torrentially from the atria into the ventricles in early diastole and forcefully impacts on the ventricular walls, it sets up vibrations that result in an audible sound—the normal S_3.

A normal finding in children and young adults, S_3 is a low-pitched, short, soft sound, occurring about 0.14 to 0.16 second after S_2. It is heard best at the apex with the patient in the left lateral position.

The S_3 gallop rhythm. **This rhythm was formerly referred to as a ventricular gallop or protodiastolic gallop, but these terms are now obsolete.** The sound of the gallop is, as its name implies, a lilt or canter similar to the sound of a galloping horse. Often, a rapid heart rate accompanies heart failure, adding to the gallop quality of the sound. The mechanism of the S_3 gallop is essentially the same as that of the normal S_3. However, it relates to hemodynamic filling of a failing, noncompliant ventricle. It is therefore a sign of congestive heart failure (CHF). The cadence of the S_3 gallop sounds like "lup-dah-dah, lup-dah-dah." It is designated as an S_3 gallop rhythm based on a constellation of other symptoms in keeping with the diagnosis of CHF associated with the characteristic lilt of canter quality present. The S_3 gallop of right-side origin is best heard at the left lateral sternal border and the S_3 of left-side origin is best heard at the apex, with the patient in the left lateral position.

The S_4 Gallop Rhythm (S_4): At the end of diastole the atria contract and expel some of the residual blood within them to complete ventricular filling. This atrial contraction at the end of diastole is referred to as the "atrial kick" and is responsible for about 25 percent of the blood entering the ventricles. The sound is not nor-

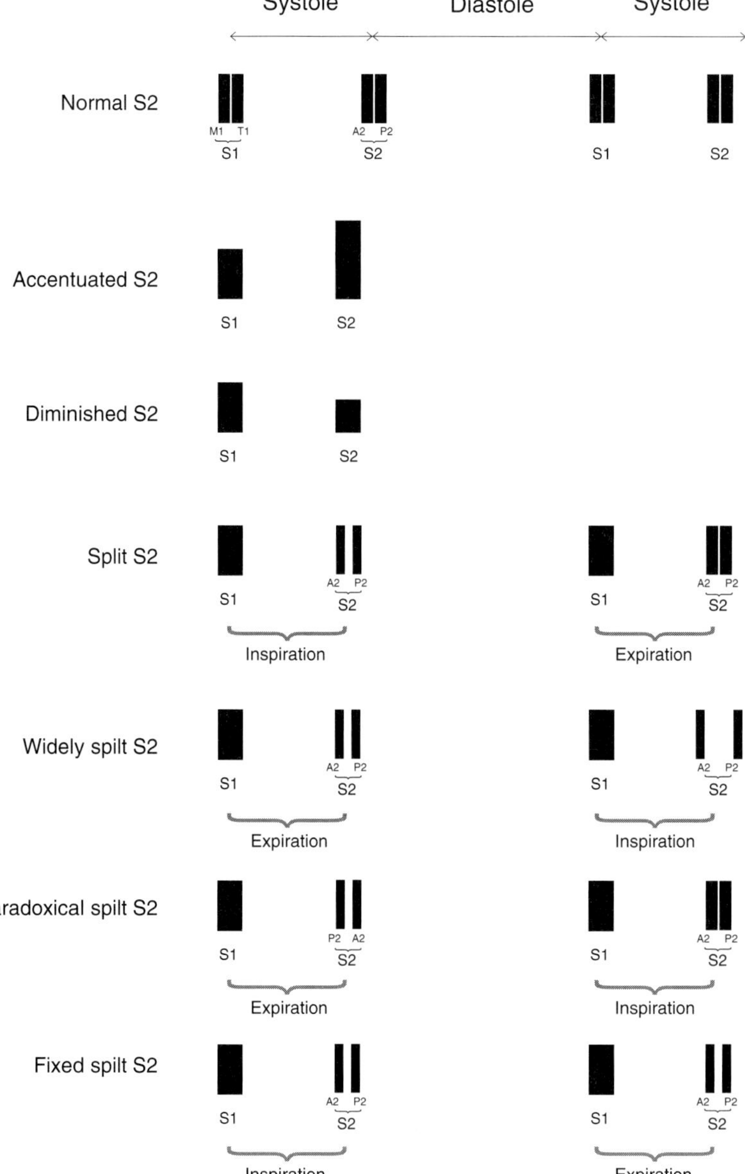

FIGURE 12–7. Graphic depiction of S_2 heart sounds.

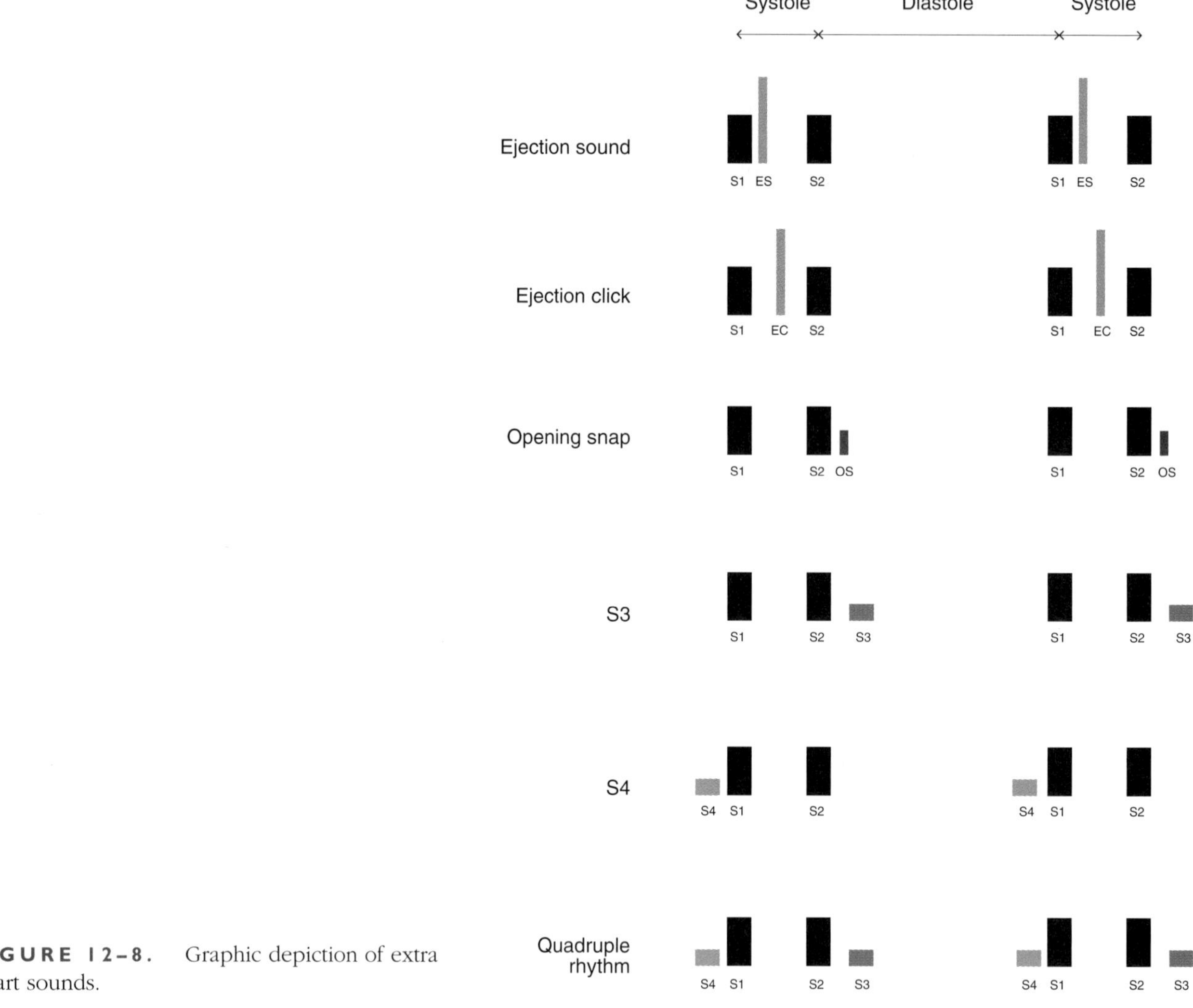

FIGURE 12–8. Graphic depiction of extra heart sounds.

mally heard. However, if the atria have to contract against ventricular resistance or decreased ventricular compliance, significant vibrations are generated, resulting in the audible S_4 sound known as an S_4 gallop rhythm. The S_4 gallop sound is a low-pitched sound occurring 0.08 to 0.20 second before S_1.

S_4 may be detected as an inaudible event on a phonocardiogram. When it is heard, it is abnormal and termed an S_4 gallop rhythm. (The terms atrial and presystolic gallop are obsolete.) The S_4 gallop may be associated with hypertension (HTN), coronary artery disease (CAD), myocardial infarction (MI), and aortic or pulmonic stenosis. The cadence of S_4 sounds like "lah-dah-dup, lah-dah-dup." The S_4 of right-side origin is best heard at the left sternal border and the S_4 of left-side origin is best heard at the apex with the patient in the left lateral position.

Murmurs

Murmurs are defined as a series of audible, prolonged sounds resulting from turbulence created within the vascular system. Causes of turbulent flow include:

- Increased flow through normal blood vessels, creating frictional, audible sounds
- Flow through constricted blood vessels (e.g., aortic stenosis)
- Flow into a dilated blood vessel from one of normal size
- Combination of the preceding causes

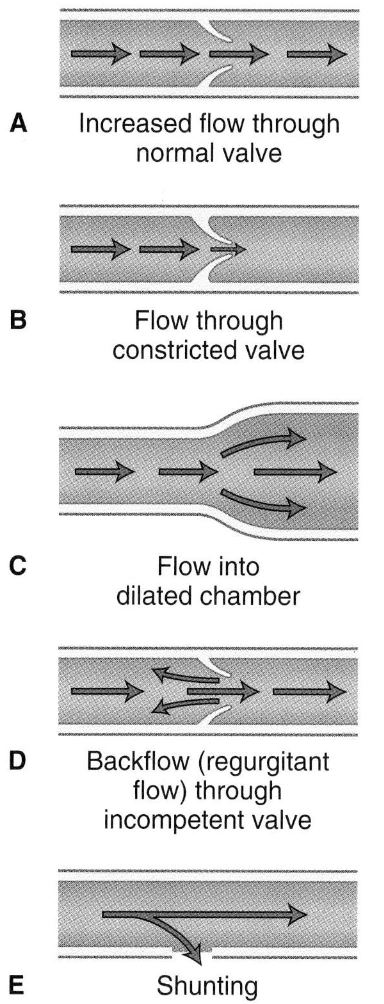

FIGURE 12–9. Graphic depiction of the causes of turbulent flow.

Figure 12–9 is a graphic depiction of the causes of turbulent flow.

Although some murmurs are "innocent," identification and thorough description of the murmur are essential in differentiating an innocent murmur from a pathological one. Murmurs are characterized in terms of their:

- Quality—blowing, rough or harsh, or musical
- Frequency—high, medium, or low
- Intensity or loudness—grades 1 through 6
- Duration—early, mid, late, holo or pan (heard throughout systole or diastole)
- Configuration—crescendo, decrescendo, or plateau
- Placement in the cardiac cycle—systole or diastole
- Location of sound
- Radiation of sound

Murmurs are also designated as: systolic, diastolic, or continuous. They may originate from either the right or the left side of the heart, and tend to radiate downstream in the direction of the jet created at their point of origin. Any changes in the quality of the murmur may indicate an acute alteration in the valve structure, such as acute valve rupture. Figure 12–10 is a graphic depiction of murmurs.

Continuous Sounds

Sounds that are heard during both systole and diastole are called continuous (Fig. 12–11). A **continuous murmur, venous hum,** and **friction rub** are continuous sounds with three different mechanisms.

Continuous Murmur. The continuous murmur is generated whenever there is uninterrupted forward flow of blood from a high pressure system into one of low pressure, as in **patent ductus arteriosus.** A continuous murmur crescendos in late systole, envelops the second sound, and decrescendos throughout diastole. This murmur is medium pitched and heard best in the infraclavicular area and in the second left interspace.

Venous hum. Turbulent flow within the venous system in the neck and superior vena cava may result in a venous hum, a continuous low-pitched sound. Venous hum may be a normal finding, especially in children. The quality of the venous hum is either blowing, rough, or musical. It is a low-pitched sound, heard best over the right internal jugular vein in the supraclavicular area, but readily disappearing when light pressure is applied to the internal jugular vein, establishing its benign nature.

Friction rub. A pericardial friction rub is a high-pitched, scratchy, leathery sound that is generated when the inflamed parietal and visceral pericardial layers rub together. A pericardial friction rub may be associated with pericarditis, pericardial effusion and acute myocardial infarction. Sharp, knifelike chest pain may accompany the rub. The pain may radiate to the left shoulder and neck, and is aggravated with deep inspiration, coughing, swallowing and position changes. The pericardial friction rub may be heard in one or all phases of the cardiac cycle. A triple component rub results from atrial contraction, ventricular contraction, and ventricular relaxation and is usually best heard at the third interspace at the left sternal border.

HELPFUL HINT

Anything that affects the valves, the hemodynamic events, or the conduction system may affect what you hear.

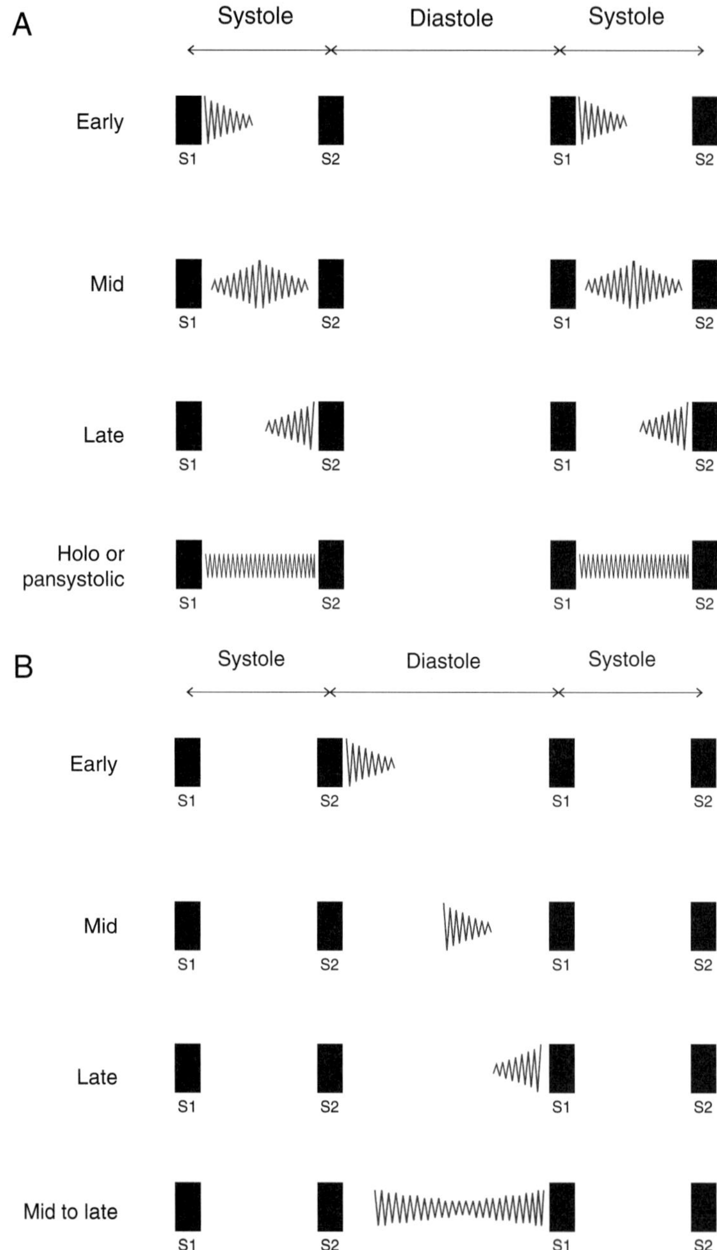

FIGURE 12–10. (*A*) Graphic depiction of systolic murmurs. (*B*) Graphic depiction of diastolic murmurs.

The Arterial System

Pressure in the arteries is much higher than in the venous system. The pressure created from the contraction of the ventricles can be converted into a waveform. The pressure creates one positive wave with a **dichrotic notch.** The positive wave represents systole. The wave has a smooth and rapid upstroke with a less acute descent. The dichrotic notch represents the closure of the aortic valve. Figure 12–12 illustrates a normal arterial pressure wave.

The Venous System

The venous system is a low-pressure system compared to the arterial system. The venous system reflects the flow of blood back to the heart. The flow of blood through the venous system is regulated by the pressure gradient for venous return, resistance to blood flow, and the venous pumps. The pressure gradient is affected by right arterial pressure and venous pressure. Resistance to blood flow also affects venous return. The venous pumps include the skeletal muscle pump and the respiratory pump.

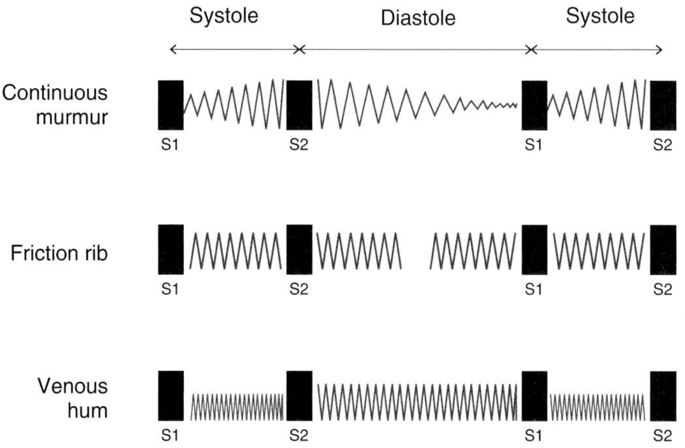

FIGURE 12–11. Graphic depiction of continuous sounds.

Assessment of venous pressure in the jugular veins is an indirect assessment of right atrial pressure. The pressure in the jugular veins can be converted into a waveform. The jugular waveform has three positive waves and two negative waves that correspond with the cardiac cycle.

Keep in mind that the atria work opposite the ventricles, so when one is contracting, the other is relaxing. So, at the end of diastole (ventricular filling), the atria contract to fill the ventricle. The force of the right atrial contraction results in the "a" wave. The ventricles are filled, diastole is completed, and the mitral and tricuspid valves close marking the beginning of systole. The "c" wave represents the force of tricuspid valve closure. As the ventricles are contracting, the atria are relaxing. The pressure in the atria at this point is low, represented by the "x" wave. The atria are now filling as the ventricles complete systole. As the atria fill, the pressure rises. The "v" wave represents right atrial filling. Once the atria are filled and the ventricles have contracted, diastole begins and the tricuspid valve opens. As the tricuspid valve opens, there is a sudden drop in right atrial pressure as the atrium empties into the ventricle, represented by the "y" wave. Figure 12–13 illustrates correlation of the jugular waveform with the cardiac cycle.

Interaction with Other Body Systems

The Respiratory System

The respiratory system works closely with the cardiovascular system to supply oxygen to and remove carbon dioxide from the body. The exchange of gases that occurs within the respiratory system could not occur without the circulatory system, which transports the gases. The respiratory system also works with the cardiovascular system to ensure that oxygen requirements are met. If the body needs more oxygen (e.g., during exercise),

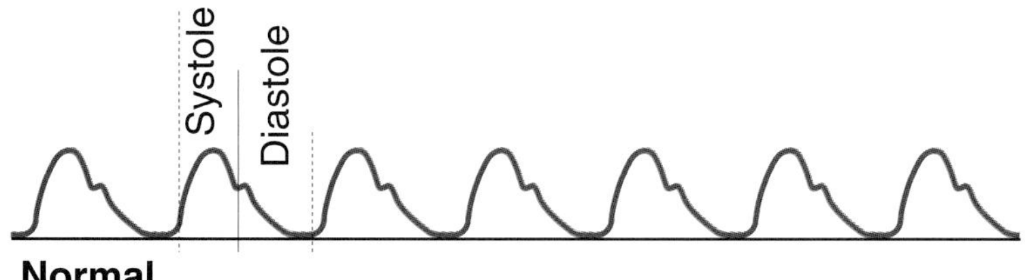

NORMAL PULSE

As shown in this illustration, a normal pulse has two components: systole and diastole. Indicated by the initial upstroke, systole signifies the arterial pressure during ventricular contraction. Diastole, the downstroke, indicates the arterial pressure during ventricular relaxation when the heart fills.

FIGURE 12–12. Normal arterial pressure wave.

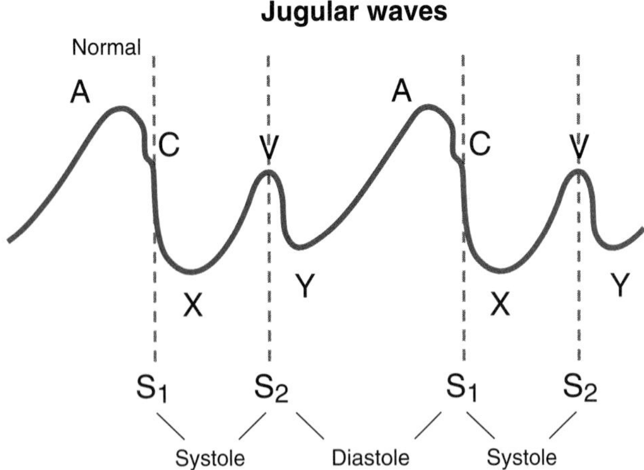

FIGURE 12–13. Correlation of jugular wave form with cardiac cycle.

the respiratory and cardiac rate will increase to meet this need. Because the two systems work so closely together, disease that affects one system eventually affects the other. For example, patients with chronic obstructive pulmonary disease (COPD) often develop right-sided CHF.

The Nervous System

The nervous system (cerebrum, hypothalamus, medulla oblongata, and autonomic nerves) has a regulatory effect on the heart. The medulla oblongata is the major control, the cardioregulatory center. In response to external factors, the cerebrum and hypothalamus send afferent information to the medulla oblongata, which then responds by changing the heart rate. The medulla oblongata also responds to afferent information from the chemoreceptors and baroreceptors in the aortic arch and carotid artery sinus. The chemoreceptors respond to changes in oxygen, carbon dioxide, and hydrogen ions. The baroreceptors respond to changes in blood pressure. The medulla oblongata responds by changing the heart rate as needed to maintain homeostasis.

The autonomic nervous system, **sympathetic** and **parasympathetic,** can affect the heart rate. The sympathetic nervous system, with the release of **norepinephrine,** accelerates the heart rate; the parasympathetic nervous system, with the release of **acetylcholine,** decreases it.

The Endocrine System

When the sympathetic nervous system is activated, the adrenal medulla responds by secreting epinephrine and norepinephrine, which both have a positive **inotropic** (contractility) and **chronotropic** (rate) effect on the heart.

Developmental, Cultural, and Ethnic Variations

Infants

Several developmental changes in the cardiovascular system occur shortly after birth. The **foramen ovale** that connected the right and left atria in fetal circulation closes after birth, allowing the heart to function as a double pump. The ductus arteriosus, a shunt between the pulmonary trunk and the aorta, also closes shortly after birth. This may result in systolic murmurs until closure occurs, usually within 48 hours after birth. The normal heart rate for the newborn is 120 to 160 BPM.

Children

Because the heart lies more horizontally in children, the apical impulse is at the fourth intercostal space until age 7, to the left of the midclavicular line till age 4, at the midclavicular line until age 6, and to the right of the midclavicular line by age 7. Sinus arrhythmia with respiratory variations is common in children. Because of the thin chest wall, heart sounds are louder, and a physiologic S_3 may be heard. Innocent murmurs are also common findings in children. These murmurs are systolic and usually of low intensity (no greater than grade 3). A venous hum is also a common benign finding in children. The heart rate gradually slows to the adult rate of 60 to 100 BPM as the child gets older.

ALERT

Although murmurs are very common in children, they need to be reported to differentiate an innocent from an abnormal murmur.

Pregnant Women

Several changes in the cardiovascular system can be seen during pregnancy. The increase in cardiac workload often results in the development of a systolic murmur. A **mammary souffle** is a murmur that develops from increased blood flow through the mammary artery

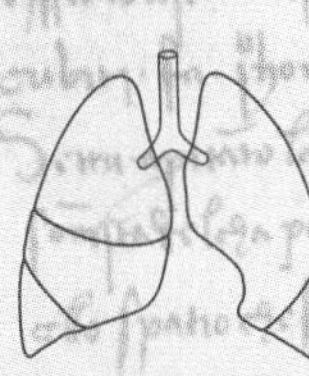

RESPIRATORY

RBCs exchange oxygen and carbon dioxide in lungs and transport it to peripheral system.

Provides oxygen to and removes wastes from cardiovascular system.

Lungs convert angiotensin I to II, which helps maintain blood pressure.

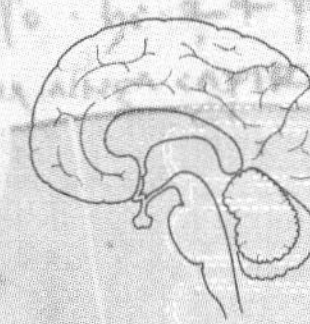

NEUROLOGICAL

Endothelial cells of brain capillaries form a semi-permeable membrane that maintains blood-brain barrier.

Controls peripheral circulation and heart rate and increases blood volume and pressure.

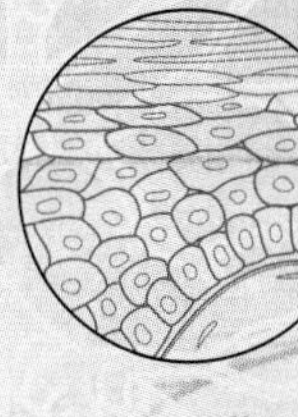

INTEGUMENTARY

Responds to skin injury or infection by delivering clotting factors and immune system response to affected area.

Stimulation of mast cells in response to injury or infection produces local changes in blood pressure and release of ADH, which helps blood flow and capillary permeability.

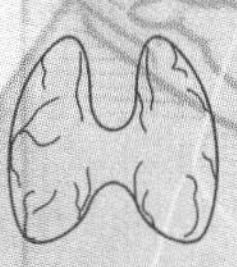

ENDOCRINE

Distributes hormones throughout body via circulatory system.

Cardiac muscle cells secrete atrial natriuretic peptide (ANP), which helps maintain fluid and electrolyte balance and lowers volume and blood pressure.

Erythropoietin regulates RBC production.

Epinephrine and norepinephrine increase heart rate and force of contraction.

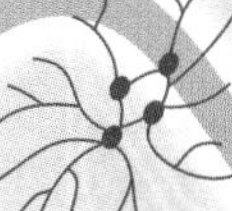

LYMPHATIC

Delivers WBCs and antibodies to fight pathogens.

Protects vascular system and heart from pathogens.

REPRODUCTIVE

Distributes reproductive hormones.

Delivers nutrients to reproductive organs.

Vascular system needed for changes that occur during sexual arousal.

Premenopausal women have lower incidence of heart disease.

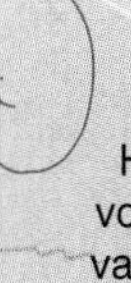

URINARY

Helps regulate volume within vascular system.

Renin/angiotensin system affects B/P.

Erythropoietin affects RBC production.

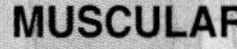

MUSCULAR

Delivers nutrients to muscles and throughout circulatory system.

Removes carbon dioxide, lactic acid and heat produced by muscle activity.

Muscles provide protection for neck vessels.

Heart is muscle responsible for pumping blood.

Muscle contraction of legs helps with venous return.

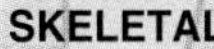

SKELETAL

Delivers calcium and minerals to bones for bone growth.

Delivers parathormone and calcitonin.

Provides calcium for normal heart muscle contraction.

Protects blood cells as they develop in bone marrow.

Skeletal framework protects heart.

DIGESTIVE

Delivers nutrients and hormones from site of absorption and transports nutrients and toxins to liver.

Supplies cardiovascular system with nutrients and absorbs water and ions that help maintain blood volume.

Relationship of Cardiovascular System to Other Systems

occurring late in pregnancy or during lactation. As the pregnancy progresses and the diaphragm rises, the heart rises and rotates, displacing the apical impulse. The blood pressure is usually lower during the first and second trimester and the heart rate is slightly higher than in the nonpregnant state.

Older Adults

Changes in blood pressure are frequently seen in older adults. **Postural (orthostatic) hypotension** results from a decrease in **baroreceptor** response, decreased elasticity of the arteries, and the increased incidence of cardiovascular disease and medications. Auscultatory gaps also frequently occur. These gaps are periods of silence after the first **Korotkoff's sound** (true systolic) and subsequent Korotkoff's sounds, and may result in inaccurate blood pressure readings.

KOROTKOFF'S SOUNDS

When you take your patient's blood pressure, you may hear five distinct phases called Korotkoff's sounds. These phases occur because the blood pressure cuff partially obstructs blood flow and disturbs the laminar flow pattern, causing turbulence. Korotkoff phases include the following:

- *Phase I:* A faint, clear, rhythmic tapping noise that gradually increases in intensity. Intraluminal pressure and cuff pressure are equal.
- *Phase II:* A swishing sound that is heard as the vessel distends with blood.
- *Phase III:* Sounds become more intense. Vessel is open in systole but not in diastole.
- *Phase IV:* Sounds begin to muffle, and pressure is closest to diastolic arterial pressure.
- *Phase V:* Sounds disappear because vessel remains open.

People of Different Cultures and Ethnic Groups

Several cultural or ethnic variations are seen in relation to the development of cardiovascular disease. These variations result from both biological and ethnic differences and lifestyles associated with the specific culture. For example:

- Japanese and Puerto Ricans have a lower incidence of hypertension and high cholesterol.
- Hispanics have a lower mortality rate from heart disease that non-Hispanics.
- Middle-aged Caucasians have the highest incidence of coronary artery disease (CAD).
- Blacks have an earlier onset and greater severity of CAD than other groups.
- Black women have a greater incidence of CAD than white women.
- Native Americans under age 35 have twice the mortality rate from heart disease as other groups.

Introducing the Case Study

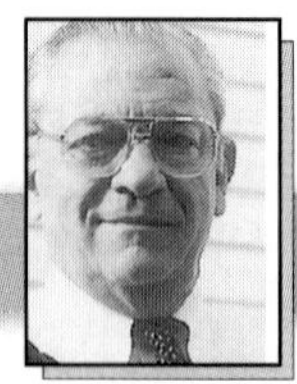

Henry Brusca is a 68-year-old, married father of 7 who was in relatively good health until 3 weeks ago. At that time, he visited the emergency room with the complaint of "just not feeling right." His blood pressure on admission was 170/118, so he was admitted to the coronary care unit with the diagnosis of uncontrolled hypertension. His blood pressure was controlled with medication, and he was discharged several days later. He is now being seen for follow-up care and management of hypertension. Because Mr. Brusca is newly diagnosed with hypertension, you will need to complete a history and thorough cardiovascular examination.

Performing the Cardiovascular Assessment

Assessment of the cardiovascular system includes a comprehensive health history and physical examination. The history will enable you to identify any cardiovascular symptoms and risk factors and the physical examination will help you evaluate the normal functioning of the heart and detect any abnormalities. As you proceed with the assessment, identify not only actual problems but also potential problems. Remember, if there is a problem with the cardiovascular system, every other system will be affected. Be alert for changes in other systems that may reflect cardiovascular problems.

Health History

During the health history, collect biographical data and ask your patient about his or her current health, past health, and family and psychosocial history. Also do a review of systems and, depending on your patient's condition, a focused cardiac history.

Biographical Data

A quick review of the patient's biographical data helps identify actual or potential problems. Begin by considering your patient's age. The risk for cardiovascular disease increases with age. Gender is also a risk factor, with men having a greater incidence of cardiovascular disease than women. On the other hand, women have a higher mortality rate within 1 year after myocardial infarction (MI) than men. CAD usually strikes women 10 years later than men. In addition, women who are having a heart attack often have different presenting symptoms than men. Besides chest pain, fatigue, and shortness of breath, they may also experience back pain, anorexia, and light-headedness.

Ethnic background is another risk factor. Certain cardiovascular diseases are more prevalent in specific races or ethnic backgrounds. For example, black men have a high incidence of hypertension. Occupation may also be a contributing factor to cardiovascular problems if the patient has a high-stress job or if progressive cardiovascular disease forces him or her to make career changes. Identify your patient's supports and financial status. Chronic cardiovascular disease may take a toll on the patient's resources, and you may need to make referrals to ensure that he or she is able to maintain the medical treatment plan.

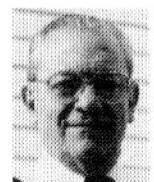

Case Study Findings

Reviewing Mr. Brusca's biographical data:

- 68-year-old white male, married, father of 7 grown children
- Self-employed entrepreneur; BS degree in engineering.
- Born and raised in the United States, Italian descent, Catholic religion.
- Blue Cross/Blue Shield medical insurance plan
- Referral: Follow-up by primary care physician
- Source: self, reliable

Current Health Status

If the patient has a cardiovascular problem, begin with his or her chief complaint. Keep in mind that the person with a cardiac problem may present with many symptoms or none at all. Identifying key symptoms may be crucial to detecting cardiac problems early and preventing complications, but interpreting these findings may be difficult. For example, symptoms that seem to be of obvious cardiac origin may actually originate in another system, whereas symptoms that seem to be from another system may actually be cardiac in origin.

If your patient presents with acute cardiac symptoms such as chest pain, defer the detailed history and focus on the acute problem. A detailed history can be obtained at a later time when the patient's condition improves, or from a secondary source, such as a family member.

Frequent cardiac symptoms include chest pain, dyspnea, cough, edema, syncope, palpitations, fatigue, and changes in the extremities such as numbness, tingling, and **intermittent claudication.** These symptoms usually do not occur in isolation, but rather in combination. One symptom may lead to another; for example, palpitations may result in **syncopal** attacks, or chest pain may be associated with dyspnea.

Symptom Analysis

Symptom Analysis tables for all of the symptoms described in the following paragraphs are available on the Web for viewing and printing. In your web browser, go to and click on Symptom Analysis Tables under Explore This Product.

Chest Pain

Chest pain is the most common presenting cardiac symptom. It may be cardiac, respiratory, gastrointestinal, musculoskeletal, or psychogenic in nature. In adults, chest pain is always treated as cardiac in origin until otherwise determined. Chest pain of cardiac nature is transmitted through the thoracic region by the five thoracic spinal nerves and may be referred to areas served by the cervical or lower thoracic segments. Also, these spinal nerves enervate the skin and the skeletal muscles. This explains the difficulty in determining the origin of chest pain and also explains the occurrence of cardiac chest pain in areas aside from the heart.

HELPFUL HINT

Chest pain that increases with position change or palpation or is described as pleuritic or sharp is probably not cardiac in origin.

ALERT

If your patient presents with chest pain, be sure to determine the time of onset because this may influence the course of treatment. Thrombolytic agents must be given within 6 hours of onset of pain to be effective.

Palpitations

A patient with palpitations has the sense that his heart is racing or skipping beats.

Syncope

Syncopal attacks (dizziness) are another symptom that may signal cardiovascular problems. These episodes can result from decreased cerebral blood flow. Keep in mind that syncopal attacks may also result from noncardiac conditions or be side effects of medications.

Edema

Edema may be seen with right-sided CHF and vascular disease. Edema may result from an increased capillary hydrostatic pressure that shifts fluid from the capillaries to the tissue.

Fatigue

Fatigue is a feeling of being tired and having no energy. Often a very subtle symptom, fatigue is associated with cardiovascular disease. However, it may not be apparent to you because patients tend to alter their activity levels to adapt to decreased energy levels.

HELPFUL HINTS

- To accurately assess fatigue, investigate changes in activities of daily living (ADLs), rest and sleep patterns.
- Visible vascular changes in the extremities may be a clue that more extensive systemic vascular changes are occurring.

Extremity Changes

Changes in the extremities may provide clues about underlying cardiovascular disease. Symptoms such as paresthesia (numbness, tingling), coolness, and intermittent claudication (pain in calves during ambulation) may be associated with vascular disease, coronary heart disease, or cerebral vascular disease.

Dyspnea and Cough

Although often associated with respiratory disorders, dyspnea may also occur with cardiac disease such as left-sided CHF. In this case, dyspnea results from pulmonary congestion or increased pulmonary venous and capillary pressure. See Chapter 11, Assessing the Respiratory System, for complete symptom analysis.

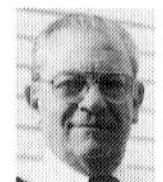

Case Study Findings

Mr. Brusca's current health status includes:

- No chest pain, dyspnea, palpitations, or edema
- Complains of fatigue, loss of energy, and occasional dizzy spells

Past Health History

The purpose of the past health history is to help you identify factors in the patient's past that may have a direct link to his or her current cardiovascular status. Or you may uncover risk factors that place your patient at risk for cardiovascular disease. This part of the assessment focuses on areas as they relate to the cardiovascular system. See table on page 375.

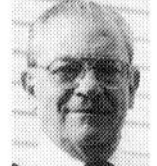

Case Study Findings

Mr. Brusca's past health history reveals:

- No rheumatic fever or heart murmurs
- No history of injuries
- Inguinal hernia repair
- Left ventricular hypertrophy revealed by EKG
- Hospitalized 3 weeks ago for hypertension
- No known food, drug, or environmental allergies
- No other previous medical problems
- Immunizations up to date
- No prescribed medications except Vasotec 5 mg bid and weekly use of antacid for indigestion

Family History

The family history will help you identify familial or genetically linked risk factors that predispose your patient to cardiovascular disease. It is important to note not only the type of problem, but also the age at which the problem occurred. See table on page 377.

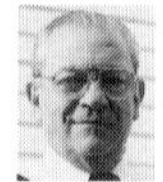

Case Study Findings

Mr. Brusca's family history reveals:

- Positive family history of HTN and CVA. Mother had HTN and died at age 78 of a CVA.
- Paternal uncle died at age 79 of MI.

Past Health History

RISK FACTORS/ QUESTIONS TO ASK	RATIONALE/SIGNIFICANCE
Childhood Illnesses	
Do you have a history of rheumatic fever or frequent streptococcal infections?	May cause rheumatic heart disease.
Do you have any congenital heart defects?	May have direct correlation to present status.
Do you have a heart murmur?	Murmurs are very common during childhood. They are often innocent but may indicate pathology.
Hospitalizations/Surgeries	
Have you ever been hospitalized for cardiovascular problems? Have you ever had an EKG?	An EKG can be used to establish baseline and comparative data and to evaluate the status of chronic cardiovascular disease.
Have you ever had surgery?	
Serious Injuries	
Have you been in an accident recently?	Blunt chest trauma or acceleration/deceleration may have caused myocardial contusion or pericardial tamponade.
Serious/Chronic Illnesses	
Do you have a history of diabetes, hypertension, or hyperlipidemia?	If controlled, these cardiac risk factors are alterable.
Do you have a history of chronic respiratory disease?	Long-standing respiratory disease often leads to cardiac involvement.
Do you have a history of renal disease or bleeding disorders?	Can affect cardiovascular system.
Immunizations	
Did you get a flu shot or Pneumovax this year?	For patients with chronic cardiovascular disease, flu or pneumonia can place added stress on an already compromised cardiac status, resulting in decompensation.
Allergies	
Do you have any allergies? (Specifically ask about allergies to iodine or shellfish.)	Allergies to foods, drugs, or environmental factors may influence treatment.
ALERT If your patient is allergic to shellfish, he or she may be allergic to the dye used for cardiac catheterization.	
Medications	
Are you on any prescribed or OTC medications, including herbal supplements?	Assess patient's compliance with treatment plan. Medications or interaction between prescribed and OTC medications, such as a side effect or toxic effect, may be a direct or contributing factor to presenting symptoms. Drugs such as digoxin, diuretics, nitrates, antihypertensives, and anticoagulants may cause a variety of symptoms, including cardiac arrhythmias, GI upset, visual disturbances, headaches, muscle cramps, dizziness, and bleeding. See box, Drugs That Adversely Affect the Cardiovascular System, on page 376.

Drugs that Adversely Affect the Cardiovascular System

Drug Class	Drug	Possible Adverse Reactions
Antidepressants	trazodone hydrochloride	Hypotension, hypertension, syncope, chest pain, tachycardia, palpitations, EKG changes
	tricyclic antidepressants	Postural hypotension, hypertension, EKG changes, dysrhythmias, syncope, thrombosis, thrombophlebitis, congestive heart failure (CHF)
Antineoplastics	daunorubicin hydrochloride, doxorubicin hydrochloride	Dose-dependent cardiomyopathy manifested by CHF, EKG changes, dysrhythmias
Antipsychotics	phenothiazines, thioridazine, mesoridizine, ziprasidone	Hypotension, postural hypotension, tachycardia, syncope, EKG changes, dysrhythmias
Anxiolytics	diazepam	Hypotension, bradycardia, cardiac arrest, dysrhythmias (with I.V. route)
	midazolam hydrochloride	Hypotension, cardiorespiratory arrest
Bronchodilators, antiasthmatic agents		
Cerebral stimulants	amphetamine sulfate	Tachycardia, palpitations, dysrrhythmias, hypertension, hypotension
	caffeine	Tachycardia
Hormones	oral contraceptives	Hypertension, fluid retention, increased risk of cerebrovascular accident, myocardial infarction, thromboembolism
	conjugated estrogens, estradiol, oral contraceptives	Hypertension, thromboembolism, thrombophlebitis
	vasopressin	Angina in clients with vascular disease; in large doses, hypertension, bradycardia, minor dysrhythmias, myocardial infarction
Narcotic agents	morphine	Hypotension
	aminophylline, theophylline	Palpitations, sinus tachycardia, extrasystoles, ventricular dysrhythmias, hypotension
Miscellaneous agents	bethanechol chloride	Hypotension, reflex tachycardia
	hydralazine hydrochloride	Tachycardia, angina pectoris, EKG changes
	levodopa-carbidopa	Orthostatic hypotension
	levothyroxine	With excessive doses, angina pectoris, dysrhythmias, tachycardia, hypertension
	phenytoin sodium	Hypotension, ventricular fibrillation (with I.V. route)

Risk Factors for CAD

Uncontrollable Factors:

Age: Risk increases with age.

Sex: Incidence is greater in men than women until women reach menopause.

Heredity: Positive family history increases the chance of heart disease.

Race: Incidence is higher for black men and women under age 45 than in white men and women in the same age group.

Controllable Factors:

Smoking: Smokers have a two to six times greater risk of developing CAD than nonsmokers.

Cholesterol: Serum cholesterol levels >200 mg/dL increase risk for CAD.

Hypertension: Uncontrolled hypertension (BP>140/90) increases risk for CAD.

Physical Inactivity: People who have a sedentary lifestyle are at greater risk for CAD.

Obesity: Obesity 30% over desired weight for height and body build increases risk for CAD and other problems, such as Type II diabetes and hypertension.

Controllable Contributing Factors:

Diabetes: Diabetes.

Stress: Stress and being a type A personality (perfectionist, hard-working, driven).

Homocystine levels: High levels of homocystine, a sulfur-containing amino acid produced by the breakdown of the essential amino acid methionine found in dietary proteins, may contribute to atherosclerosis.

Family History

RISK FACTORS/ QUESTIONS TO ASK	RATIONALE/SIGNIFICANCE
Familial/Genetically Linked CV Disorders	
Does your family have a history of:	Positive family history is an uncontrollable risk factor for CAD.
Familial hyperlipoproteinemia?	An inherited autosomal dominant trait that may increase risk for CAD at an early age.
Hypertension, CAD, or MI?	Increases risk for CAD.
Diabetes, hypertension or renal disease?	
Genetically linked cardiac disorders such as Marfan's syndrome?	An inherited autosomal-dominant trait characterized by elongation of bones that often has associated cardiovascular abnormalities.
Mitral valve prolapse?	Causes one or both leaflets to billow into the atrium during ventricular systole. Runs in families.

Review of Systems

Changes in the cardiovascular system may affect every other system of the body. The review of systems (ROS) will help you identify problems in other systems that will directly effect the cardiovascular system and also help you determine the effect and extent of cardiovascular disease on other body systems. The ROS allows you to pick up on symptoms you might have missed during your health history by jogging your patient's memory.

Review of Systems

SYSTEM/QUESTIONS TO ASK	RATIONALE/SIGNIFICANCE
General Health Survey	
Have you experienced:	
Fatigue or activity intolerance?	Chronic cardiovascular disease (chronic congestive heart failure) causes decreased cardiac output, impaired circulation, and decreased oxygen and often leads to early fatigue and difficulty performing ADLs. Increasing fatigue and activity intolerance may correlate with disease's progression.
Influenza, other recent illness, or weight gain?	Influenza or other recent illness can cause cardiomyopathy. Sudden weight gain may indicate fluid retention.
Integumentary/*Skin*	
Have you experienced:	
Changes in skin texture, color, or temperature?	Skin changes may indicate vascular insufficiency.
Sores or ulcers that won't heal?	Poor wound healing may signal diabetes, which is a risk factor for CAD.
Swelling of ankles or tight shoes?	Edema is associated with vascular disease and CHF.
Integumentary/*Nails*	
Have you experienced:	
Changes in nail shape or color?	Clubbing and cyanosis may reflect chronic cardiopulmonary problem.
HEENT/*Head*	
Have you experienced:	
Headaches?	May indicate HTN, a risk factor for CAD.
Dizzy spells?	Syncopal attacks may occur with vascular disease or cardiac arrhythmias or may be a medication side effect.

(Continued)

Review of Systems *(Continued)*

SYSTEM/QUESTIONS TO ASK	RATIONALE/SIGNIFICANCE
HEENT/*Eyes*	
Have you experienced:	
Visual problems such as blurred vision, double vision, or colored spots?	Double vision and temporary loss of vision are associated with HTN, TIA, cerebrovascular insufficiency, and digitalis toxicity. Yellow spots may signal digitalis toxicity.
HEENT/*Ears*	
Have you experienced ringing in your ears?	**Tinnitus** is associated with cerebrovascular insufficiency.
HEENT/*Nose*	
Have you experienced nosebleeds?	**Epistaxis** is associated with HTN.
HEENT/*Throat*	
Have you experienced frequent strep throats?	Beta-hemolytic streptococcal infection is associated with rheumatic heart disease.
Respiratory	
Have you experienced:	
Breathing difficulties?	Dry cough, shortness of breath (SOB), dyspnea on exertion (DOE), paroxysmal nocturnal dyspnea (PND), **orthopnea**, and cough are symptoms of left-sided CHF.
A history of COPD?	Chronic COPD can result in cardiac involvement, such as pulmonary hypertension and right-sided CHF.
Gastrointestinal	
Have you experienced right upper quadrant (RUQ) pain, nausea, GI upset?	GI upset and RUQ pain may accompany right-sided CHF. GI complaints are associated with medications such as digitalis.
Genitourinary	
Have you experienced changes in urination, such as waking up at night go to the bathroom?	CHF leads to decreased renal perfusion during the day. But at night, when patient is in a recumbent position, fluid moves from interstitial spaces back into circulatory system, increasing renal blood flow and causing diuresis **(nocturia)**.
Reproductive/*Female*	
Are you postmenopausal?	Increases CAD risk.
Do you use oral contraceptives, or are you on hormone replacement therapy (HRT)?	Oral contraceptives/estrogen supplements are associated with thrombus formation. Research on the cardiovascular value of HRT has been conflicting.
During pregnancy, did you have gestational diabetes or pregnancy-induced hypertension (PIH)?	Increased risk for developing diabetes later in life, which increases risk for CAD.
Reproductive/*Male*	
Have you experienced:	
Problems with impotence or sexual performance?	Impotence/erectile dysfunction may be caused by vascular disease, diabetes, or medication.
Chest pain during sexual activity?	Sexual activity increases the heart's workload and can precipitate an angina attack.
Musculoskeletal	
Have you experienced:	
Muscle weakness?	Chronic cardiovascular disease may result in weakness secondary to decreased use.
Leg-muscle cramps when walking?	Intermittent claudication is associated with arterial insufficiency.

Review of Systems

SYSTEM/QUESTIONS TO ASK	RATIONALE/SIGNIFICANCE
Neurological	
Have you experienced:	
Fainting episodes, loss of consciousness, or headaches?	Syncopal attacks may signal vascular problems or cardiac arrhythmias.
Behavioral changes such as confusion, decreased attention span or loss of memory?	HTN or chronic CHF may cause hypoxia and impair cerebral circulation.
Endocrine	
Do you have diabetes or thyroid disease?	Diabetes is a known risk factor for CAD. Hyperthyroid disease can lead to hypertrophic cardiomyopathy.
Lymphatic/Hematologic	
Have you experienced:	
Bleeding problems?	Anemia increases the heart's workload. **Polycythemia** increases risk for thrombus, HTN, and cardiopulmonary disease.
A recent infection?	Cardiomyopathy.

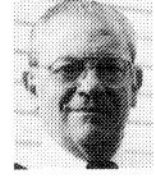

Case Study Findings

Mr. Brusca's ROS reveals:

- **General Health Survey:** Fatigue, weight gain of 60 lb over past 3 years
- **Integumentary:** Feet cold, thick nails, tight shoes
- **HEENT:** Two dizzy spells over past 6 months. ***Eyes:*** Wears glasses, no visual complaints, yearly eye examination
- **Respiratory:** "Short winded" with activity
- **Gastrointestinal:** Indigestion on weekly basis
- **Genitourinary:** Awakens at least once a night to go to bathroom
- **Reproductive:** Little sexual activity because he is "too tired"; becoming more and more difficult to have an erection
- **Musculoskeletal/Neurological:** General weakness, cramps in legs with walking
- **Lymphatic:** No reported problems
- **Endocrine:** No reported problems

Psychosocial Profile

The psychosocial profile enables you to examine your patient's lifestyle and identify risk factors for cardiovascular disease. Identifying risk factors is essential in developing an effective plan of care. Chronic cardiovascular disease can also affect your patient's lifestyle, forcing him or her to make changes to adapt to the illness.

Psychosocial Profile

CATEGORY/QUESTIONS TO ASK	RATIONALE/SIGNIFICANCE
Health Practices and Beliefs/ Self-Care Activities	
Do you get yearly physicals? Do you see a doctor or nurse regularly? What medications are you taking and why?	Determines preventive practices. Ascertains compliance with treatment program. Identifies teaching needs.
Typical Day	
What is your typical day? Has it changed over the last year? For example, are there activities you find difficult to do or are unable to do?	Activity level can correlate with energy level. Chronic heart disease decreases energy levels. Changes in ADLs may reflect patient's attempt to adapt to progression of illness.

(Continued)

Psychosocial Profile *(Continued)*

CATEGORY/QUESTIONS TO ASK	RATIONALE/SIGNIFICANCE
Nutrition/Weight Patterns	
Do you have weight problems—for example, obesity or a sudden weight increase?	Obesity is a risk factor for CAD. Sudden weight increases are usually associated with fluid retention.
What did you eat in the last 24 hours?	24-hour recall helps identify diets high in cholesterol and sodium, which may contribute to cardiovascular disease.
Do you get chest discomfort after eating?	Large, heavy meals can precipitate an angina attack in patients with CAD.
Do you have anorexia, loss of appetite, or nausea?	May indicate right-sided CHF or be a side effect or toxic effect of cardiac medications.
Activity/Exercise Patterns	
Do you exercise routinely?	A gradual decrease or change in activity or exercise patterns is seen in patients with chronic cardiovascular disease.
Do you have chest discomfort after certain types of activity or exercise?	Exercise can precipitate an angina attack in patients with CAD. May identify need for referral for cardiac rehabilitation.
Recreation/Pets/Hobbies	
Do you have any pets or hobbies? What kinds?	Pets and hobbies can be a good way to reduce stress.
Sleep/Rest Patterns	
Do you awaken during the night to go to bathroom?	Nocturia is associated with CHF.
Do you awaken with SOB?	PND is associated with CHF.
Do you awaken with chest pain?	Angina may occur during rest (nocturnal angina and **Prinzmetal's angina**). During the rapid eye movement (REM) cycle of sleep, myocardial oxygen demands increase. This may explain the high incidence of MIs in the early morning hours. **HELPFUL HINT** Prinzmetal's (variant) angina usually has no precipitating factors and occurs at rest as a result of spasms of the coronary artery. Patients with Prinzmetal's angina frequently have a history of migraine headaches and Raynaud's disease.
Do you snore?	The incidence of sudden cardiac death is higher in patients with sleep apnea.
Personal Habits	
Do you smoke cigarettes? How many packs per day and for how many years?	Smoking cigarettes is a known risk factor for CAD. Nicotine increases **catecholamine** release, which leads to vasoconstriction and increased heart rate and blood pressure. This increases the heart's workload, and increased carbon monoxide levels result in decreased oxygen supply.
Do you use street drugs such as cocaine?	*"Crack" heart:* Cocaine increases catecholamine release, which increases heart rate and the heart's workload. May result in MI, CHF, or **cardiomyopathy** (CMP).
Do you drink alcohol? How many glasses a day?	Alcohol abuse can lead to increased pulse and blood pressure, CMP, CAD, HTN, CAD, and CVA.
Occupational Health Patterns	
What is your job? Are you currently working?	Cardiac limitations may prevent patient from working.
How many hours a day do you usually work? Does your job make physical demands?	Helps establish cardiovascular workload and helps you devise an activity plan.

Psychosocial Profile

CATEGORY/QUESTIONS TO ASK	RATIONALE/SIGNIFICANCE
Occupational Health Patterns *(Continued)*	
Are you exposed to smoke, noise, extreme temperatures, or dust?	May cause CV symptoms.
Environmental Health Patterns	
Where do you live? Are there stairs?	As CAD progresses, patient may have difficulty within own environment. Referrals may be indicated. Identify discharge or home-care needs.
Roles/Relationships/Social Supports	
Do you belong to any church or community groups? What is your role in family, church, and community? What are your support systems?	Chronic cardiovascular disease may affect patient's ability to perform role tasks. Roles may change as disease progresses, and referrals may be needed. Patient may isolate self as disease progress, becoming homebound as a "cardiac cripple." Be alert for signs of depression!
Sexuality Patterns	
How has your CV problem affected your sex life?	Fear of heart damage may cause patients and spouses to avoid sex or become impotent. Antihypertensive or antianginal medications may also cause impotence.
Stress and Coping	
What do you do when you feel upset, angry, frustrated, or stressed out?	Stress increases CAD risk by increased stimulation of sympathetic nervous system. Volatile emotions such as anger also increase sympathetic nervous system response, which in turn increases the heart's workload.

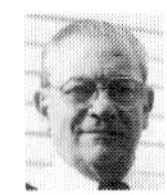

Case Study Findings

Mr. Brusca's psychosocial profile includes:

- States that he does not have time for routine checkups. "I only go to the doctor's when I'm sick." Typical day consists of arising at 7 AM, showering, having breakfast, and then going to work. Returns home by 6 PM, eats dinner, watches TV till 11:30 PM, but usually falls asleep before news is over. Usually in bed by 12 midnight.
- 24-hour recall reveals a diet high in carbohydrates and fats and lacking in fruits and vegetables. Heavy-handed with salt shaker; salts everything. Admits that he has gained weight over the years and is 60 lb overweight.
- No regular exercise program. States: "I'm too busy running my business."
- Hobbies include reading, crossword puzzles, and antique collecting.
- Sleeps about 7 hours a night, but usually feels he is not getting enough sleep. Lately is more and more tired. Wife states that he snores.
- Never smoked. Has a bottle of wine every night with dinner.
- Works at sedentary job, usually 7 days a week. No environmental hazards in workplace.
- Lives with wife of 45 years in a 2-story, single home in the suburbs with ample living space.
- Has a large, close, caring family.
- Admits that running his own business is very stressful, but feels he can handle it alone and doesn't need anyone to help him.

Focused Cardiovascular History

If your patient's condition or time prohibits a detailed cardiac history, take a history that focuses specifically on the cardiac status of your patient. The patient's response to the following questions will help direct your assessment:

- Are you having any chest discomfort? If yes, when did it start?
- What were you doing before the pain started? Did anything make it better or worse?
- Have you ever had this pain before? What does it feel like? Where does it hurt? On a scale from 1 to 10, with 10 being the worst, how severe is the pain?
- Do you have a history of cardiovascular disease? If yes, are you taking any medications? If yes, what are you taking and why?
- Do you have any other medical problems?
- Are you having any breathing difficulties?
- Do you have any allergies? If, yes, describe reaction.

CRITICAL THINKING ACTIVITY #1

From the subjective information you have obtained from Mr. Brusca's history, what are his identifiable risk factors for heart disease? Which risk factors are modifiable and which are unmodifiable?

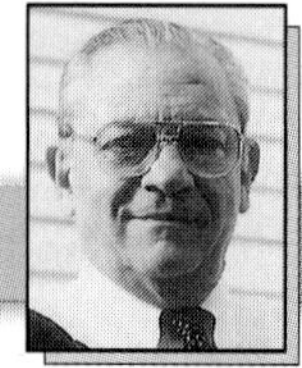

Case Study Evaluation

Before you begin the physical assessment, summarize Mr. Brusca's subjective findings obtained from his history. What key points in his history will help you plan his care? Document his cardiovascular history.

Anatomical Landmarks

Before you begin the physical assessment, visualize the underlying structures and identify cardiac landmarks to ensure an accurate and thorough assessment. The heart is situated in the chest in the third, fourth, and fifth intercostal spaces to the left of the sternum. In a normal size heart, the right side is located more anteriorly, with only the tip of the left ventricle situated anteriorly (Fig. 12–14).

Even though heart sounds may be heard anywhere on the precordium, specific sites have been identified as best for performing the cardiac assessment: right base/aortic area, left base/pulmonic area, Erb's point/third intercostal space, left lateral sternal border (tricuspid), and apex (mitral) (Fig. 12–15).

Central Artery and Jugular Veins

Before you begin assessing the central arteries and jugular veins, identify your anatomical landmarks to ensure accurate assessment. The carotid and the internal and external jugular need to be located. The sternocleidomastoid and trapezius muscles are helpful in locating these vessels. The carotid artery and the internal jugular run parallel to each other along the sternocleidomastoid muscle toward the sternal notch. The external jugular crosses the internal jugular and lies posterior to the sternocleidomastoid muscle. These neck structures are shown in Figure 12–16.

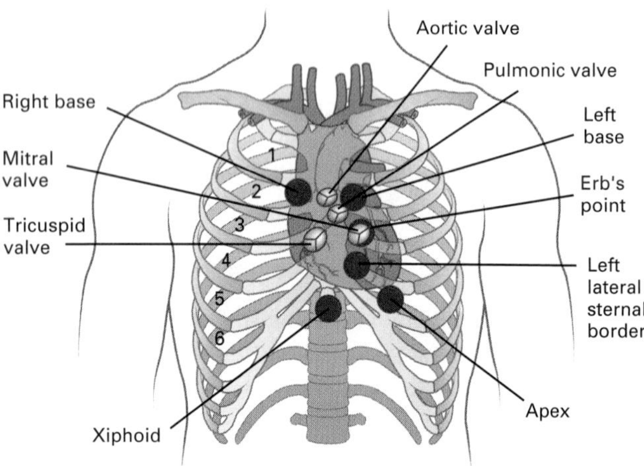

FIGURE 12–14. Anatomical site of heart.

Cardiac Auscultation Sites

Traditional Sites	Alternative Sites
Apex/Mitral area	Apex
Left lateral sternal border (LLSB)/Tricuspid area	Lower left sternal border
Erb's point	Left base
Base left/pulmonic area	Right base
Base right/aortic area	Xiphoid

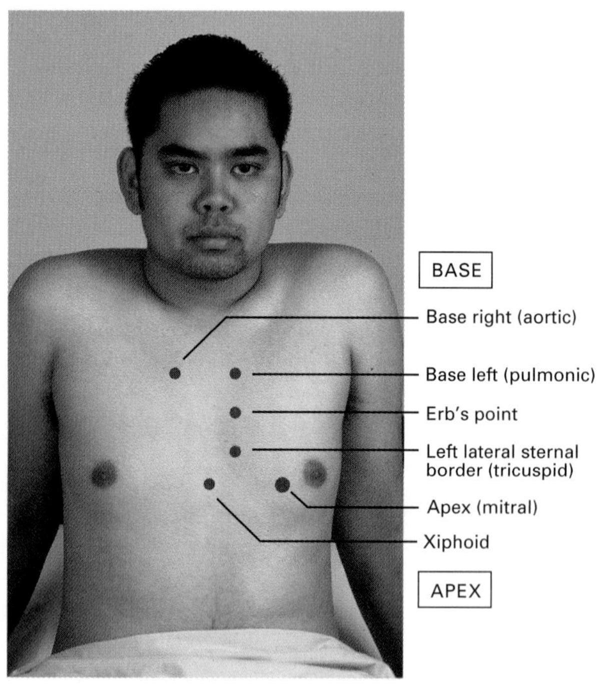

FIGURE 12–15. Sites for cardiac assessment.

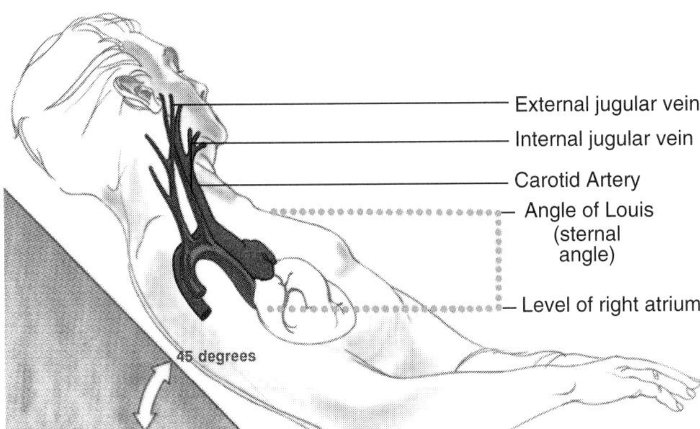

FIGURE 12–16. Neck structures.

Physical Assessment

The significant subjective data that you obtained from the health history will help to direct your physical examination. The history provides you with clues about what physical findings you can expect to find in your patient. These physical findings provide the objective database. Together, the health history and physical examination complete your assessment picture. You can then analyze the data, formulate nursing diagnoses, and develop a plan of care for your patient.

The physical examination begins with a general survey, proceeds to a head-to-toe assessment of each body system, and then ends with a focused cardiovascular assessment.

Approach

You will use all four techniques of physical assessment to assess the cardiovascular system. Because changes in this system may affect every other body system, assess for physical signs in every system. Perform the assessment in three positions: sitting, supine, and left lateral recumbent. Placing the patient in several positions facilitates the auscultation of specific heart sounds. However, keep in mind that patients with chronic cardiovascular problems may have little cardiac reserve. You may need to minimize position changes to conserve your patient's energy.

Work from the right side of your patient. This is especially helpful during auscultation because it allows you to stretch the tubing of the stethoscope and minimize interference. Allay your patient's anxiety by explaining that a cardiovascular examination always takes time. Be systematic in your approach. Your first assessment will serve as the baseline that will be used for subsequent assessments. This baseline will enable you to detect subtle changes in the patient's cardiovascular status.

Before you begin, wash your hands, assemble your equipment, and prepare a warm, quiet, private environment. Let your patient know what you will be doing. This will help to minimize his or her anxiety and maximize cooperation during the examination. Sharing your findings with your patient can help you validate them and provide an ideal opportunity for patient teaching.

Toolbox

The tools for cardiovascular assessment include a stethoscope with the ability to detect high- and low-pitched sounds, a sphygmomanometer, scale, metric ruler, thermometer, and marking pen. Sharpen your senses; you will need all of them to perform a cardiovascular assessment.

Performing a General Survey

Before assessing specific areas, perform a general survey that includes evaluating the patient's general appearance, vital signs, height, and weight. Be alert for signs of cardiovascular disease.

General Appearance

General appearance can give you important clues about the patient's cardiovascular status. Note the following:

- **Chronological age:** Is the patient's age consistent with his or her appearance? Chronic illness can "age" a person.
- **Weight distribution and muscle composition:** Look for edema that may indicate cardiovascular disease. Muscle wasting may occur from lack of use.
- **Facial expression:** Does it match the patient's behavior? If he or she presents with chest pain, his or her expression and behavior should be consistent with the complaint.
- **Posture or assumed position of comfort:** The patient's posture should be erect and midline. Variations from this may reflect fatigue associated with chronic cardiac disease. A sitting position may be the preferred position for the patient with CHF.
- **Dress and grooming:** The patient with chronic cardiovascular disease may have increasing difficulty performing ADLs, and this may be reflected in his or her dress and grooming.
- **Body stature:** Several genetic disorders have characteristic stature profiles and associated cardiac problems. Tall stature with long limbs in proportion to the trunk is seen with **Marfan's syndrome,** a genetic disorder associated with aortic dissection, aortic valve incompetence, and cardiomyopathy.

Tall stature and long extremities are also seen with **Klinefelter's syndrome,** a genetic disorder in males characterized by an extra X chromosome with possible atrial or ventricular septal defects, PDA, and tetralogy of Fallot. The short stature of patients with **Turner's syndrome** is associated with coarctation of the aorta and pulmonic stenosis.

- **Muscle wasting:** Cardiac **cachexia** and muscle wasting on the upper arms, thighs, and chest wall may be seen in patients with chronic cardiac disease. Anthropometric measurements may be made to accurately determine the degree of cachexia. The normal percentage of body fat for men is 14 to 18 percent; for women it is 20 to 25 percent. Loss of body fat and muscle mass not only reduces the body's energy stores, but also affects the immune system and healing process.
- **Abnormal movements:** Rhythmic bobbing of the head simultaneous with the heartbeat (Musset's sign) may result from high back pressure associated with aortic insufficiency or aneurysm. Squatting position is seen in patients with tetralogy of Fallot.

Vital Signs

Blood pressure, pulse, respirations, and temperature are a good reflection of how well the cardiovascular system is functioning.

Blood Pressure

Blood pressure reflects stroke volume, distensibility of arteries, peripheral vascular resistance, and volume. Blood pressure measurements greater than 140/90 may indicate hypertension; blood pressure with a systolic less than 100 may indicate hypovolemia or CHF.

HELPFUL HINT

If the patient's blood pressure is high, serial readings of elevated blood pressure will help confirm a diagnosis of hypertension.

Pulse

The quickest way to increase cardiac output is to increase heart rate. Therefore changes in heart rate are often adaptive mechanisms by the body as it attempts to maintain homeostasis. Aside from heart rate, take note of rhythm. An irregular rhythm indicates an underlying arrhythmia. Also check for a pulse deficit—a difference between the radial pulse and apical pulse—which can occur with atrial fibrillation. The strength of the pulse may reflect the vascular system; bounding pulses may be seen with hypertension, and weak pulses or **pulsus alternans** (alternating weak and strong pulse) may reflect a failing heart.

ALERT

If you get an irregular radial pulse, take an apical rate for one full minute. If the apical pulse is also irregular, report these findings to the physician.

Respiratory Rate

Patients with CHF or pulmonary edema have an increased respiratory rate, dyspnea, and orthopnea. The respiratory rate usually increases in response to hypoxia. If the patient has chest pain, you will also see changes in the respiratory rate and pattern.

Temperature

Elevated temperature may indicate an infectious disease process. Slight elevation in body temperature is often seen within the first 24 hours after an acute MI because of the inflammatory process that occurs during an MI. The elevation is usually low grade at 100.4°F, but it may rise to 102.2°F and last for one week post MI.

Acute **pericarditis** may also result in temperature elevations to 102.2°F, and even higher elevations are seen with bacterial **endocarditis.** No matter what the cause, fever increases metabolism, which in turn increases cardiac workload. The cardiac response to this increase is tachycardia.

Height and Weight

Accurate height and weight measurements are helpful in planning treatment, calculating dosages, identifying nutritional deficits, and detecting and monitoring fluid retention.

- **Height:** As mentioned previously, tall stature is linked to several genetic disorders that have associated cardiac problems, such as Marfan's syndrome, Klinefelter's syndrome, and **acromegaly.** Short stature may also have genetic links and be associated with cardiac problems. Examples are Turner's syndrome and **dwarfism.**
- **Weight:** Weighing your patient is the most accurate means of monitoring fluid status. Note any weight changes, especially sudden weight gains, which suggest fluid retention as is seen with CHF. Changes of 2 to 3 pounds in 48 hours usually reflect a change in fluid status, not body mass. A patient can gain 6 to 8 pounds before edema may be visible, so weighing your patient every day at the same time and with the same scale is the most accurate means of assessing fluid status.

Performing a Head-to-Toe Physical Assessment

The cardiovascular system can affect every other body system. Therefore, once you have done a general survey, look at the patient from head to toe, checking for changes in each body system that might signal a cardiovascular problem.

Performing a Head-to-Toe Physical Assessment

SYSTEM/NORMAL FINDINGS	ABNORMAL FINDINGS/RATIONALE
General Health Survey *INSPECT*	
Awake, alert, and oriented to time, place, and person.	*Confusion, restlessness, irritability, short attention span:* Early signs of hypoxia and impaired cerebral circulation caused by decreased cardiac output.
Immediate, recent and remote memory intact. Judgment intact, compliant with treatment plan.	*Memory loss:* Hypoxia. Patients with cardiovascular disease may deny their illness, severity of symptoms, or associated risk factors. *Fatigue:* Often accompanies chronic cardiovascular disease.
Integumentary/*Skin* *INSPECT/PALPATE*	
Normal skin color varies from patient to patient because of racial and genetic differences. Buccal mucosa pink, but may be darker (including dark brown or blue) in patients of Mediterranean or African descent.	If cyanosis is present, differentiate between central and peripheral. *Central cyanosis:* Suggests a cardiopulmonary problem, such as CHF, MI, or pulmonary edema. Look for central cyanosis in the oral mucosa.
Peripheral cyanosis can be a normal response to cold.	*Peripheral cyanosis in absence of cold:* Hypovolemia, shock, or peripheral vascular disease caused by vasoconstriction, vascular occlusion, or decreased cardiac output.
Changes from the patient's normal color should be noted.	*Ashen color:* MI. *Dependent rubor and pallor with elevation of extremities:* Arterial insufficiency. *Pallor:* Anemia and high-output failure. *Jaundice:* Hepatic congestion secondary to right CHF. *Cyanosis when dependent and brown pigmentation:* Venous insufficiency.
Skin intact, no lesions.	***Petechiae:*** Bacterial endocarditis.
Skin pink, warm and dry, +2 pedal pulses, no edema.	*Thin, shiny, hairless, cool skin with decreased or absent pulses:* Arterial insufficiency.

(Continued)

Performing a Head-to-Toe Physical Assessment *(Continued)*

SYSTEM/NORMAL FINDINGS	ABNORMAL FINDINGS/RATIONALE
Integumentary/*Skin* *(Continued)* *INSPECT/PALPATE*	*Peripheral edema, leathery skin with cyanosis and brownish discoloration:* Venous insufficiency. *Peripheral edema:* Right-sided CHF. *Cool, clammy skin:* Shock, MI, CHF, arterial insufficiency, or occlusion as a result of vasoconstriction in response to decreased cardiac output. This is a compensatory mechanism to shunt blood to vital organs.
Positive skin turgor. Poor skin turgor may be normal in older adults as a result of decreased elasticity.	*Taunt, shiny skin:* Edema caused by cardiovascular disease such as right CHF or vascular insufficiency.
No edema.	***Anasarca*** *(generalized body edema)*: Right CHF.

HELPFUL HINT

When assessing for edema, check the patient's most dependent areas such as the legs, sacrum, and scrotum.

SYSTEM/NORMAL FINDINGS	ABNORMAL FINDINGS/RATIONALE
Integumentary/*Hair* *INSPECT/PALPATE* Normal hair distribution for age and sex.	*Thinning or loss of hair on extremities:* Arterial insufficiency.
Integumentary/*Nails* *INSPECT/PALPATE* Nailbeds pink to dark brown or blue in patients of Mediterranean or African descent; positive capillary refill; angle of attachment 160 degrees; no clubbing,	*Cyanotic nailbeds with poor capillary refill and clubbing:* Cardiopulmonary disease. *Splinter hemorrhages:* Bacterial endocarditis.
HEENT/*Head and Neck* *INSPECT/PALPATE* Facial expression appropriate.	*Struggling, frightened look:* Pulmonary edema. *Apprehension:* CAD, MI.
Thyroid not palpable.	*Enlarged thyroid:* Hyperthyroid disease, which can affect the cardiac system, resulting in CHF.
HEENT/*Eyes* *INSPECT* Eyes clear and bright, no lesions or edema.	*Periorbital edema, xanthelasma, arcus senilis, sclera icterus:* Suggest cardiovascular disorders. Edema is also associated with CHF.

Performing a Head-to-Toe Physical Assessment

SYSTEM/NORMAL FINDINGS	ABNORMAL FINDINGS/RATIONALE
HEENT/*Eyes* *(Continued)*	
INSPECT	*Xanthelasma (small, yellow raised plaques on eyelids)*: Lipid deposits that may indicate **hyperlipidemia**.
Arcus senilis (thin whitish-gray ring around cornea) may be seen in older patients.	*Arcus senilis in patients under age 65:* Hyperlipidemia.
Sclera white; palpebral conjunctiva pink.	***Sclera icterus*** *(jaundiced sclera)*: Right-sided CHF (cardiac cirrhosis). *Cyanosis of palpebral conjunctiva:* CHF, MI, pulmonary edema.
No lid lag or expothalmos.	***Exophthalmos*** *and lid lag:* Hyperthyroidism, which can result in supraventricular tachycardia (SVT), **angina**, or high-output failure.
Fundoscopic examination reveals yellow to orange retina without hemorrhages or exudates. Arteriovenous (AV) crossings smooth.	HTN and diabetes are risk factors for CAD, so it is important to note fundoscopic changes. *Fundoscopic changes associated with HTN:* Papilledema, AV nicking, hard exudates, creamy yellow lesions, soft exudates, such as cotton wool (also seen with subacute bacterial endocarditis). *Fundoscopic changes associated with diabetes:* Diabetic retinopathy.
Respiratory	
INSPECT/AUSCULTATE	
Respirations 16 per minute, lungs clear on auscultation.	*Breathing difficulties, such as dyspnea, DOE, PND, and tachypnea:* Associated with CHF, pulmonary edema, MI. ***Cheyne-Stokes*** *respiratory pattern:* Severe CHF. In patients with CHF, further assessment reveals crackles and wheezes. Cardiac asthma can develop with CHF. *Barrel chest:* COPD. Chronic COPD often has right-sided cardiac involvement.
Chest AP: Lateral 1:2, negative barrel chest or spinal deformities.	***Pectus excavatum*** *(depressed sternum),* ***scoliosis*** *(lateral deviation of spine), and* ***kyphosis*** *(accentuated convex thoracic curve)*: If severe, may affect cardiac functioning by impairing chest expansion and cardiac movement.

(Continued)

Performing a Head-to-Toe Physical Assessment *(Continued)*

SYSTEM/NORMAL FINDINGS	ABNORMAL FINDINGS/RATIONALE
Respiratory *(Continued)* *INSPECT/AUSCULTATE* No retraction or use of accessory muscles	*Retraction of intercostals and use of accessory muscles:* Respiratory difficulty caused by a respiratory disorder, congenital heart defect, or CHF.
Gastrointestinal *INSPECT/PALPATE/AUSCULTATE* Positive bowel sounds; abdomen soft, nontender; no bruits or venous hums; liver not palpable; positive pulsation in epigastric area; abdominal aorta <2.5 cm.	*Ascites, hepatomegaly, RUQ tenderness, venous hum:* Right CHF. *Positive bruit or wide, diffuse pulsation in epigastric area:* Abdominal aortic aneurysm.
Musculoskeletal *INSPECT/PALPATE* Grade 4 to 5 muscle strength, no atrophy.	*Muscle weakness:* Chronic cardiac disease resulting in muscle atrophy from lack of use.
Neurological *INSPECT/PALPATE* Sensory intact in extremities. +2 DTR.	*Decreased sensation and diminished DTR:* Peripheral neuropathy associated with diabetes, which is a risk factor for CAD.

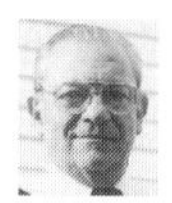

Case Study Findings

Mr. Brusca's physical assessment findings include:

- **General Health Survey:** Well-developed, well-groomed 68-year-old white male, appears younger than stated age. Sits upright and relaxed during interview, answers questions appropriately. Alert and responsive without complaint, oriented × 4 (time, place, situation and person), affect pleasant and appropriate.
- **Vital Signs:** Temperature 98°F; pulse 86 BPM , strong and regular; respirations 18 per minute, unlabored; BP 150/90; height 6′; weight 275 lb.
- **Integumentary:** Skin intact, pink, warm and dry; good turgor; mucous membranes pink and moist; nails positive capillary refill, negative clubbing.
- **HEENT:** Thyroid not palpable. Eyes: negative periorbital edema; positive arcus senilis; fundoscopic, positive AV nicking and cotton wool; negative papilledema and hemorrhages.
- **Respiratory:** Lungs CTA, AP:lateral 1:2.
- **Gastrointestinal:** Abdomen large, round, soft, nontender; positive bowel sounds; negative hepatomegaly; positive pulsation in epigastric area; negative bruits or thrills.
- **Musculoskeletal/Neurological:** Sensory intact, +2 DTR, muscle strength equal +5. Extremities: +1 pedal pulses; skin cool, pale, dry, thin, hairless and shiny; thick nails; trace edema.

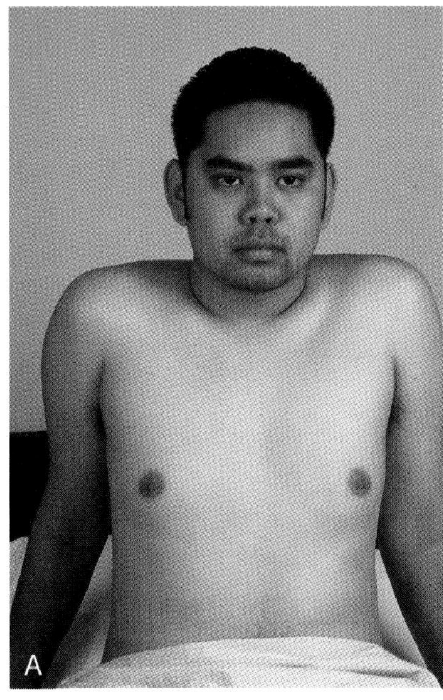

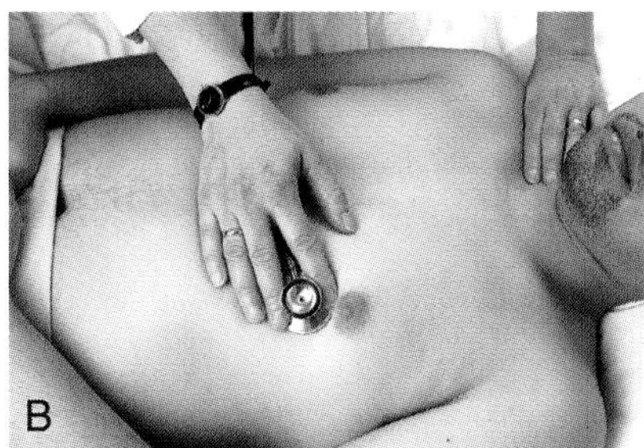

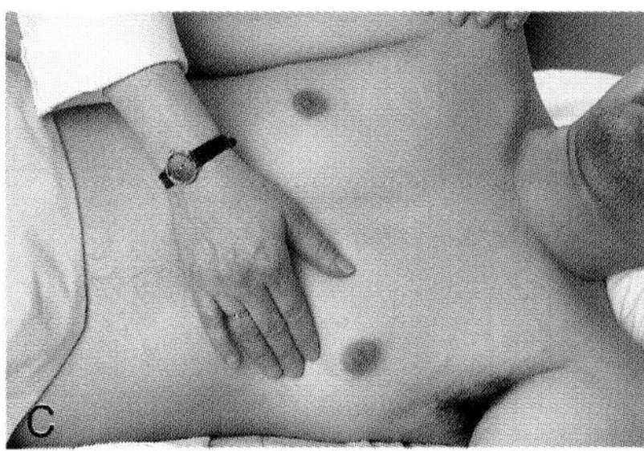

FIGURE 12–17. Positions for cardiac assessment. (*A*) Sitting position, (*B*) Supine position, (*C*) Left lateral position.

Performing a Focused Physical Assessment

Now that you have completed your general survey and head-to-toe assessment, focus your attention on assessing the cardiac system. All four techniques of physical assessment are used. Figure 12–17 shows the positions for cardiac examination.

Inspection

You will need to inspect the great vessels in the neck and the precordium for pulsations. Examining these areas from different angles and with tangential lighting will help you visualize pulsations.

Neck

With the patient in a supine position, inspect the carotid and jugular venous systems in the neck for pulsations. Remember that the carotid artery and the internal jugular vein lie parallel to the sternocleidomastoid muscle. Although the internal jugular vein is larger than the external jugular vein, the external jugular is more superficial, making visualization easier. Because the internal jugular lies deep, you will be able to see only the jugular pressure wave. To visualize external venous pulsations, look for pulsations in the supraclavicular area. To visualize internal venous pulsations, look for pulsations at the suprasternal notch. Using a penlight to cast a shadow on the neck vessels may help you visualize the pulsations.

To measure jugular venous pressure (JVP), elevate the patient's head to 30 to 45 degrees. Identify the highest point of visible internal jugular pulsation, and then place a ruler vertically at the sternal angle (angle of Louis). This is the site at which the manubrium attaches to the sternum and is used to measure jugular venous pressure because it is located 5 cm above the heart. Remember, the jugular venous system reflects right-sided heart activity. Place another ruler at the highest point of the venous wave horizontal to the ruler placed vertically. Measure the distance up from the chest wall. The normal JVP is <3 cm. A central venous pressure (CVP) can be estimated by adding 5 cm to the JVP. If venous pulsations are not visible, measure the JVP by identifying the highest point of external jugular vein distention.

Is It a Jugular Wave or a Carotid Arterial Wave?

- Carotid pulsation is normally palpable; jugular pulsation is not. Because jugular pulsation is a low-pressure wave, applying pressure can easily obliterate it.
- Carotid pulsation is not affected by position; jugular venous pulsation is.
- Carotid pulsation is unaffected by respirations; jugular venous pulsation is.
- Carotid pulsation has one positive wave; jugular venous pulsation has 3 positive waves (undulated).

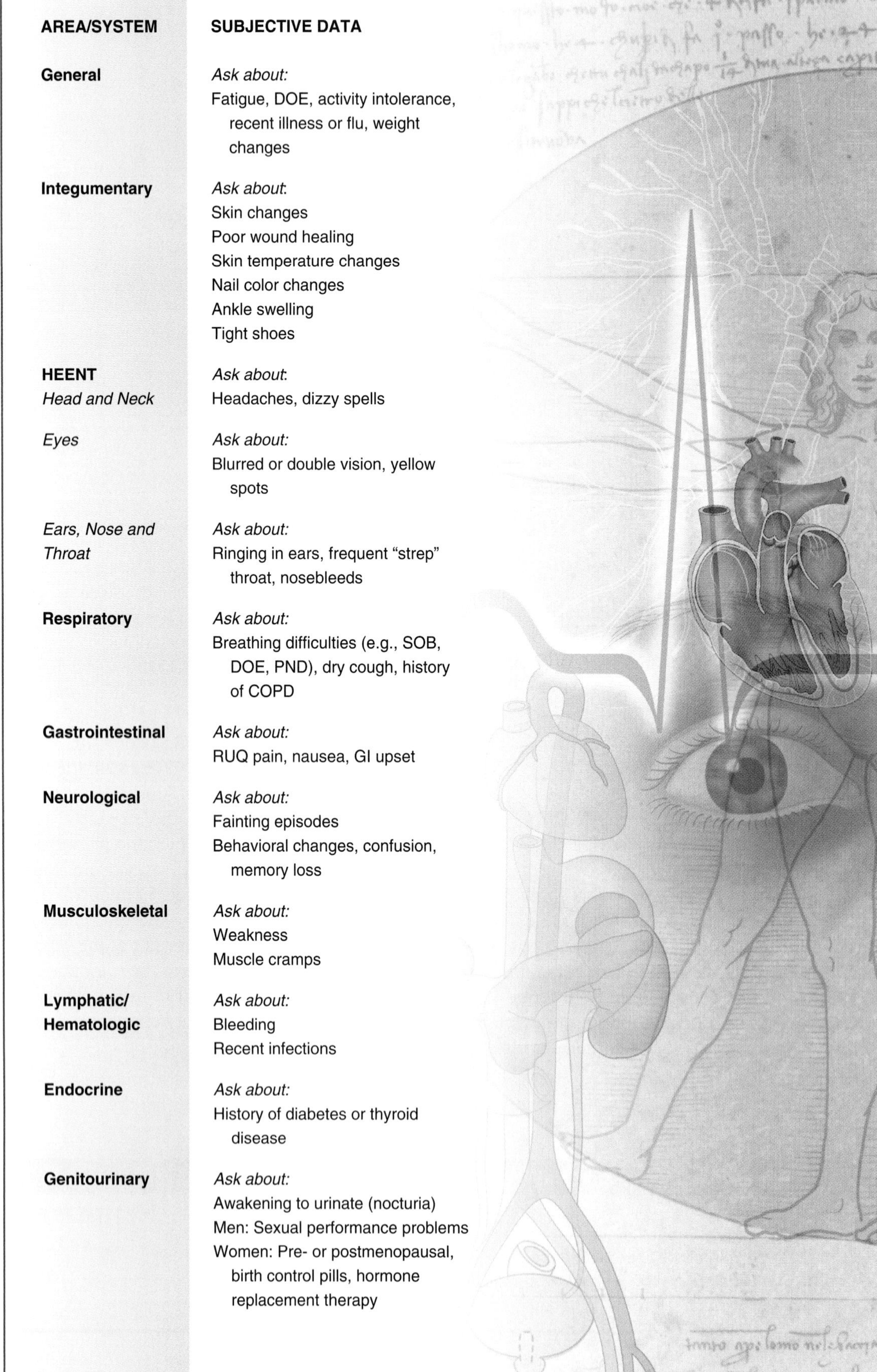

AREA/SYSTEM	SUBJECTIVE DATA
General	*Ask about:* Fatigue, DOE, activity intolerance, recent illness or flu, weight changes
Integumentary	*Ask about:* Skin changes Poor wound healing Skin temperature changes Nail color changes Ankle swelling Tight shoes
HEENT *Head and Neck*	*Ask about:* Headaches, dizzy spells
Eyes	*Ask about:* Blurred or double vision, yellow spots
Ears, Nose and Throat	*Ask about:* Ringing in ears, frequent "strep" throat, nosebleeds
Respiratory	*Ask about:* Breathing difficulties (e.g., SOB, DOE, PND), dry cough, history of COPD
Gastrointestinal	*Ask about:* RUQ pain, nausea, GI upset
Neurological	*Ask about:* Fainting episodes Behavioral changes, confusion, memory loss
Musculoskeletal	*Ask about:* Weakness Muscle cramps
Lymphatic/ Hematologic	*Ask about:* Bleeding Recent infections
Endocrine	*Ask about:* History of diabetes or thyroid disease
Genitourinary	*Ask about:* Awakening to urinate (nocturia) Men: Sexual performance problems Women: Pre- or postmenopausal, birth control pills, hormone replacement therapy

Assessment of Cardiovascular System's Relationship to Other Systems (pt.1)

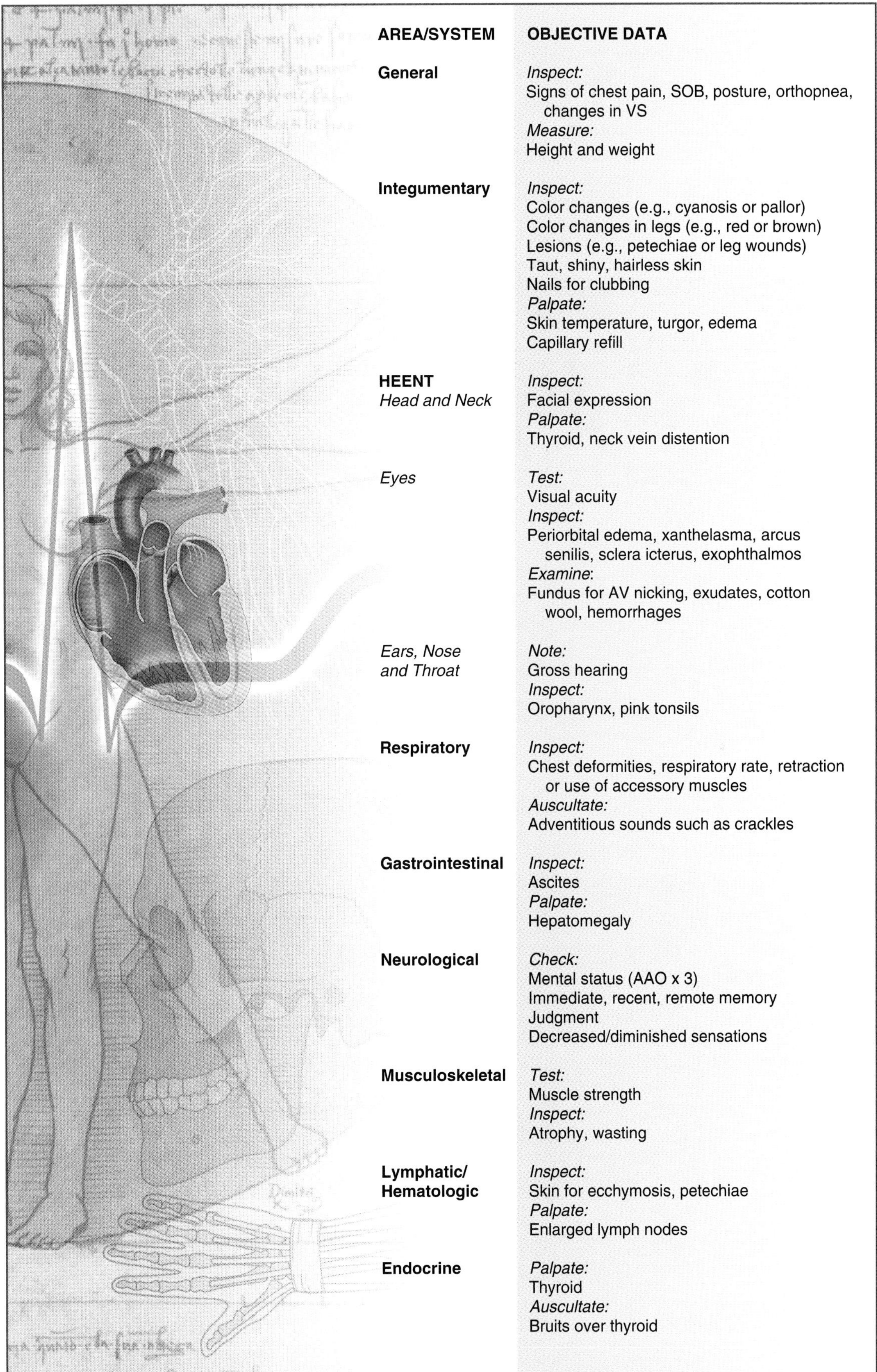

AREA/SYSTEM	OBJECTIVE DATA
General	*Inspect:* Signs of chest pain, SOB, posture, orthopnea, changes in VS *Measure:* Height and weight
Integumentary	*Inspect:* Color changes (e.g., cyanosis or pallor) Color changes in legs (e.g., red or brown) Lesions (e.g., petechiae or leg wounds) Taut, shiny, hairless skin Nails for clubbing *Palpate:* Skin temperature, turgor, edema Capillary refill
HEENT *Head and Neck*	*Inspect:* Facial expression *Palpate:* Thyroid, neck vein distention
Eyes	*Test:* Visual acuity *Inspect:* Periorbital edema, xanthelasma, arcus senilis, sclera icterus, exophthalmos *Examine*: Fundus for AV nicking, exudates, cotton wool, hemorrhages
Ears, Nose and Throat	*Note:* Gross hearing *Inspect:* Oropharynx, pink tonsils
Respiratory	*Inspect:* Chest deformities, respiratory rate, retraction or use of accessory muscles *Auscultate:* Adventitious sounds such as crackles
Gastrointestinal	*Inspect:* Ascites *Palpate:* Hepatomegaly
Neurological	*Check:* Mental status (AAO x 3) Immediate, recent, remote memory Judgment Decreased/diminished sensations
Musculoskeletal	*Test:* Muscle strength *Inspect:* Atrophy, wasting
Lymphatic/ Hematologic	*Inspect:* Skin for ecchymosis, petechiae *Palpate:* Enlarged lymph nodes
Endocrine	*Palpate:* Thyroid *Auscultate:* Bruits over thyroid

Assessment of Cardiovascular System's Relationship to Other Systems (pt.2)

Precordium

With the patient supine, inspect the precordium with tangential lighting. Check for pulsations or abnormal movements, such as lifts and heaves or thrusts. Thrills are palpable vibrations created by turbulent blood flow. Lifts or heaves are diffuse, lifting impulses. To facilitate the assessment, have the patient sit-up and lean forward or turn to the left side. This brings the apex of the heart closer to the chest wall.

HELPFUL HINT

You are more likely to see pulsations at the apex of the precordium than the base, because the apex is the more active area, whereas the base is the quiet area.

Figure 12–18 illustrates abnormal jugular venous waves.

Inspecting the Carotid Artery, Jugular Venous System, and Precordium

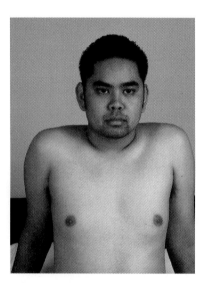

ASSESS/NORMAL VARIATIONS	ABNORMAL FINDINGS/RATIONALE
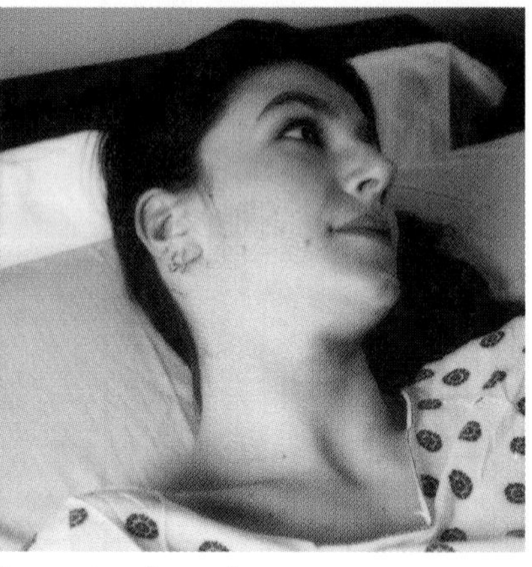 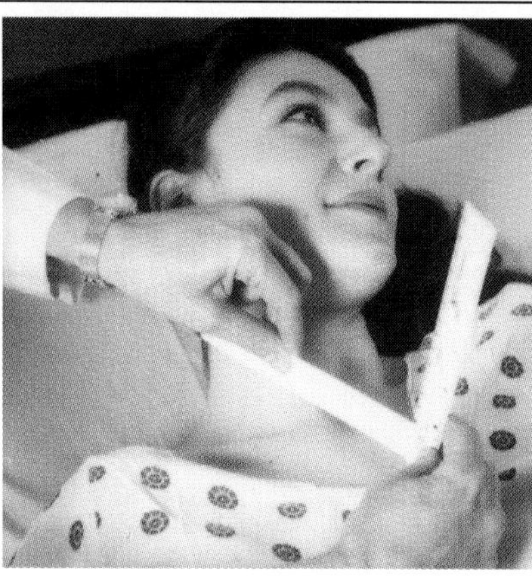 **Inspecting the neck** Neck Measuring JVP Positive carotid pulsations. JVP 2 cm at 45-degree angle. Jugular venous wave undulated, easily obliterated, varies with position change and respirations.	*Large, bounding visible pulsation in neck or at suprasternal notch:* HTN, aortic stenosis, or aneurysm. *Elevated JVP:* Right-sided CHF, constrictive pericarditis, tricuspid stenosis, or superior vena cava obstruction. *Low JVP:* Hypovolemia. *Abnormal venous waveforms:* • Giant A waves. • Tricuspid stenosis, right ventricular hypertrophy, cor pulmonale. • Absent A wave: Atrial fibrillation.
Inspecting the precordium Precordium Positive pulsation at apex. May note slight pulsations over base in thin adults and children.	*Pulsations to right of sternum or at epigastric or sternoclavicular areas:* Aortic aneurysm. *Apical pulsation displaced toward axillary line:* Left ventricular hypertrophy.

Constrictive Pericarditis

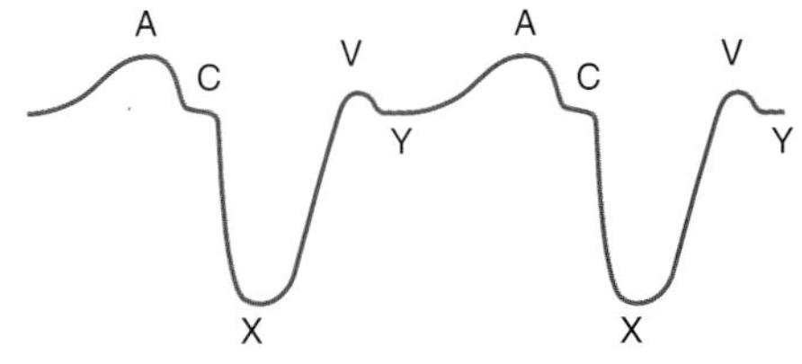

Exaggerated "x" wave

Right Ventricular Hypertrophy

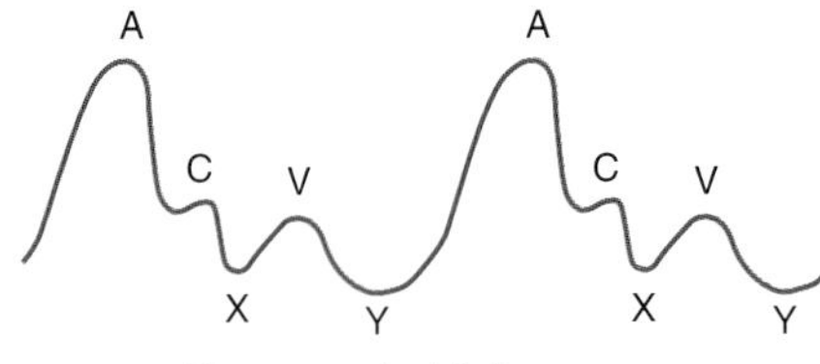

Exaggerated "a" waves

Atrial Fibrillation

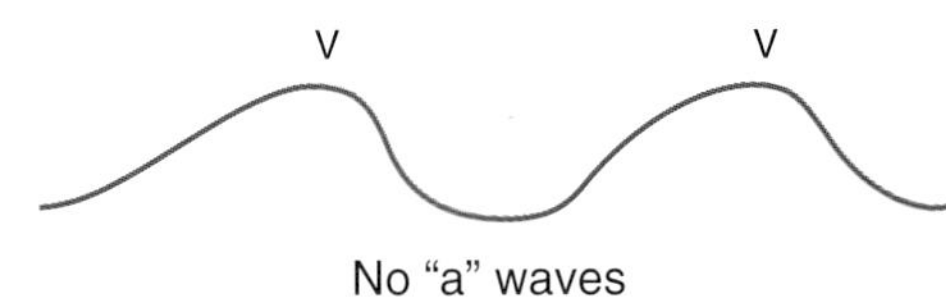

No "a" waves

Tricuspid Regurgitation

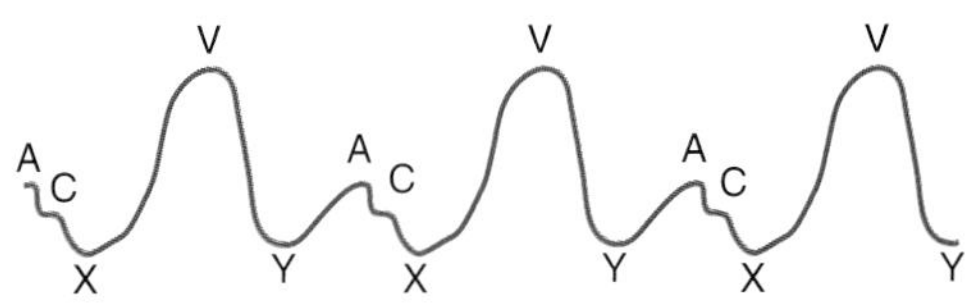

Exaggerated V waves

FIGURE 12–18. Abnormal jugular venous waves.

Palpation

Both the neck and precordium are palpated for pulsations. Palpation is also useful in detecting abnormal pulsations or movements, such as **thrills, lifts,** and **thrusts.** A thrust is a rocking movement. Light palpation with your fingerpads is best for detecting pulsations. The balls of your hand are best for detecting vibratory sensations such as thrills.

Neck

Assess the carotid artery for rate, rhythm, amplitude, contour, symmetry, elasticity and thrills.

- *Rate:* Rate is normally age dependent. Keep in mind that rates >100 BPM or <60 BPM do not always indicate pathology. Sympathetic nervous stimulation, such as fear, anxiety, and pain, may increase the rate. Vomiting or suctioning may cause vagal stimulation, which in turn may decrease the rate. Although activity and exercise often cause an increase in rate, well-trained athletes often have a slower rate with a larger stroke volume.
- *Rhythm:* Note if the rhythm is regular, fluctuating, or consistently irregular. Although a slightly irregular rhythm may occur with respirations, especially in children, irregular rhythms may also indicate an arrhythmia.
- *Amplitude:* Amplitude reflects the strength of the pulse. Amplitude is described as absent, weak, strong, or bounding or is graded on a scale of 0 to +3, with +2 as normal.
- *Contour:* Contour is the pressure wave created by the force of ventricular contraction. Both amplitude and contour are affected by the strength of ventricular contractions.
- *Symmetry:* The pulses should be equal.
- *Elasticity:* Because arteries are elastic, the carotid should be soft and pliable. Palpate the carotid medial to the trachea below the jaw angle. Do not palpate the carotids simultaneously. This can obstruct blood flow to the brain and cause a syncopal attack. Also avoid excessive carotid stimulation, which may stimulate the vagus nerve, lowering the heart rate and blood pressure and impairing cerebral circulation. If a thrill is detected, listen for a bruit.

Precordium

The thicker the chest wall, the more difficult palpating pulsations becomes. Obesity, breast tissue, and increased musculature may interfere with palpation. Also, conditions such as COPD with overinflation of the lungs increase the distance between the heart and the chest wall, making palpation more difficult. Having the patient sit brings the heart more anterior, facilitating the palpation of impulses. If the apical impulse is not palpable, turn the patient to the left lateral recumbent position and palpate again. You may also ask the patient to hold his or her breath to assist in palpation of pulsations.

Palpate the chest for pulsations, lifts, thrusts, and thrills. If you detect a thrill, listen for a murmur. Palpate the base right (aortic), base left (pulmonic), left lateral sternal border (tricuspid), and apex (mitral) areas. Be systematic in your approach. The pulsation felt at the apex originates from ventricular contraction and is referred to as the **point of maximum impulse** (PMI) or the left ventricular impulse (LVI). This is the easiest pulsation to palpate. Pulsations are least likely to be palpated at the base, the quieter area of the precordium, except in thin patients and children. Record the location, size, amplitude and duration of any pulses you palpate.

When you palpate a pulse, record the following:

- *Location:* Also note any displacement.
- *Size:* Estimate in centimeters.

- *Amplitude:* Describe as small or increased.
- *Duration:* In heart rates less than 100 BPM, duration of the apical impulse is about 1/3 of the cardiac cycle.

The apical impulse should be palpable during systole. Impulses occurring during diastole may indicate an S_3 or S_4. The location, size, amplitude, and duration of the pulsation may be affected by hyperkinetic states that results in increased preload.

HELPFUL HINT

One finger's width is about one centimeter. To determine the size of the pulsation, determine the number of finger pads you use to palpate it.

The jugulars are further assessed by evaluating for **abdominojugular reflux.** Position the patient at about a 45-degree angle or less, which allows you to easily visualize jugular venous pulsations. Place your right hand over the midabdominal area and apply 20 to 30 mm Hg of pressure for about 15 to 30 seconds. Estimate this pressure by placing a partially inflated blood pressure cuff between the abdomen and the right hand and applying sustained pressure until the desired pressure is reached. As you apply pressure, assess the jugular veins. A sustained increase in the JVP above 4 cm is considered a positive abdominojugular reflux. Valsalva's maneuver can result in false positives, so warn the patient not to hold his or her breath or bear down during this maneuver.

Abnormal pulses are shown in Figure 12–19.

Palpating the Neck and Precordium

ASSESS/NORMAL VARIATIONS

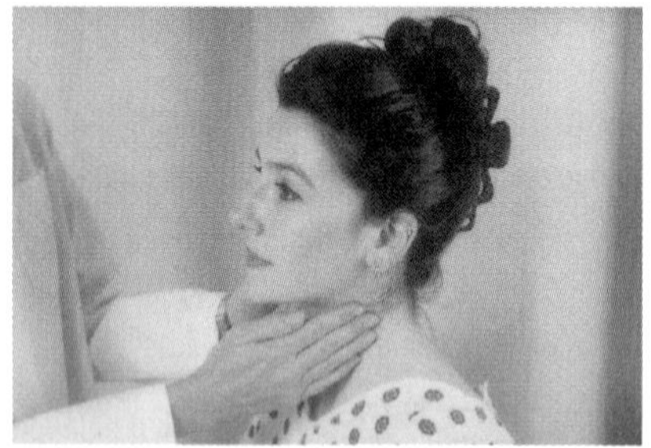

Palpating carotid artery

Neck

Carotid arteries and jugular veins

Rate: Depends on age. Rhythm: Regular

Amplitude: Strong, +2 or +3 pulses may normally be seen in high-output states such as exercise

Contour: Smooth upstroke with smooth, less acute descent

Symmetry: pulses equal

Elasticity: carotid soft and pliable

PMI 1 cm at apex; no lifts, thrills, or heaves

Slight pulsation, no diffusion

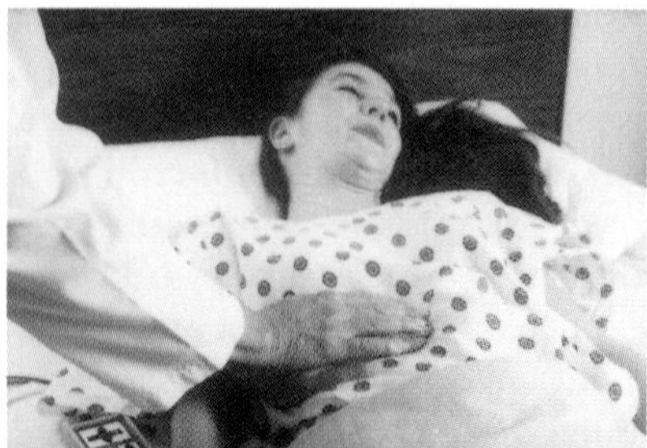

Testing hepatojugular reflux

Negative abdominojugular reflux

ABNORMAL FINDINGS/RATIONALE

Cardiac rates >100 BPM: Sinus tachycardia, SVT, PAT, uncontrolled atrial fibrillation, ventricular tachycardia. Causes include CHF; drugs, such as atropine, nitrates, epinephrine, isoproterenol, nicotine and caffeine; hypercalcemia.

Cardiac rates <60 BPM: Sinus bradycardia heart block. Causes include MI; drugs such as digoxin, quinidine, procainamide, and beta-adrenergic inhibitors; hyperkalemia.

Irregular rhythm: Arrhythmia.

Abnormal pulses: See Figure 12–19 on page 397.

Palpating the Neck and Precordium

ASSESS/NORMAL VARIATIONS

Palpating Jugulars

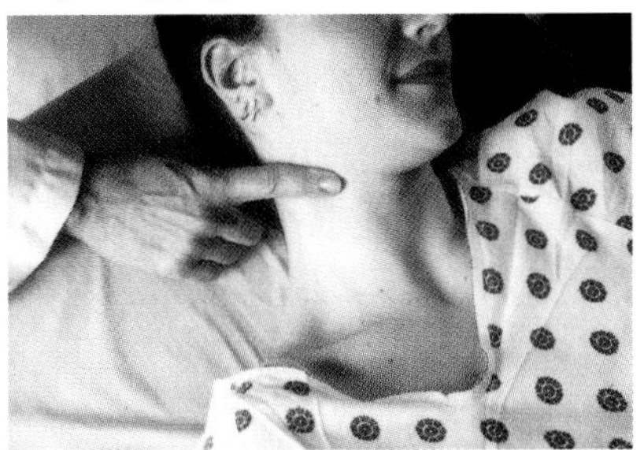

a: Assessing jugular flow. Compress jugular below jaw. Jugular vein collapses and jugular wave is more prominent at supraclavicular area.

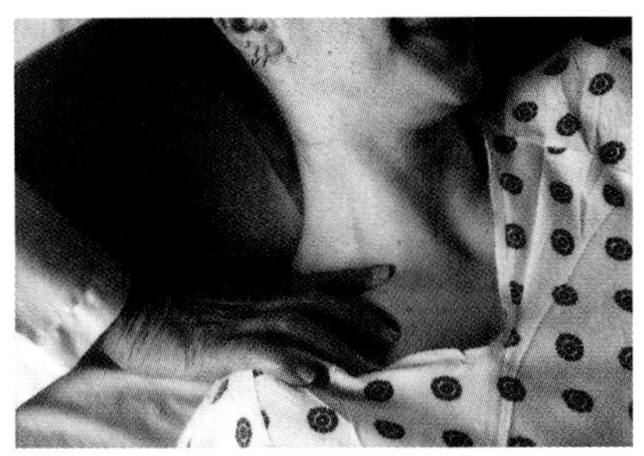

b: Checking jugular fill. Compress jugular above clavicle. Jugular distends and jugular wave disappears.

Jugulars are easily obliterated and fill appropriately.

ABNORMAL FINDINGS/RATIONALE

Unequal pulses: Obstruction or occlusion.

Stiff, cordlike arteries: Atherosclerosis

Positive abdominojugular reflux: Right-sided CHF, tricuspid regurgitation, tricuspid stenosis, constrictive pericarditis, cardiac tamponade, inferior vena cava obstruction, hypervolemia

Enlargement and displacement of PMI to left midaxillary line: Ventricular hypertrophy with dilation.

Apical impulse located on right side of precordium: Dextrocardia, a heart located on the right side, often associated with congenital heart disease.

Enlarged apical pulsation without displacement >2–2.5 cm with patient supine or >3 cm with patient in left lateral recumbent position: Ventricular enlargement, HTN, aortic stenosis.

Sustained pulsation: Hypertrophy, HTN, overload, cardiomyopathy.

Presystolic impulse: May correlate with S_4 and be seen with aortic stenosis.

Early diastolic impulse: May correlate with S_3 and be seen with CHF.

Diffuse, sustained impulse displaced downward and laterally: Congestive cardiomyopathy.

Thrills: Murmur.

Right ventricular impulse with increased amplitude and duration: Pulmonary stenosis or pulmonary hypertension.

(Continued)

Palpating the Neck and Precordium *(Continued)*

ASSESS/NORMAL VARIATIONS

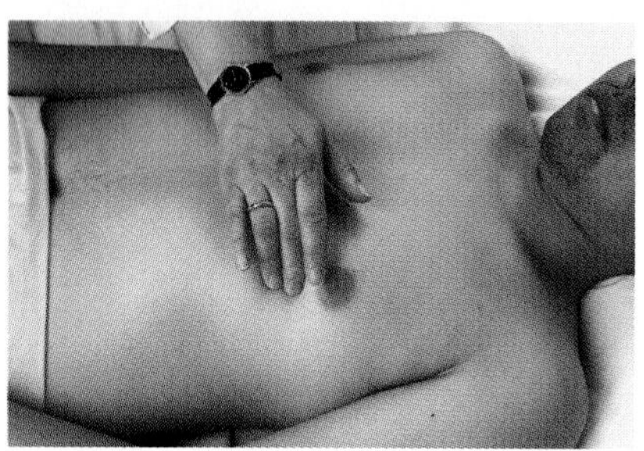

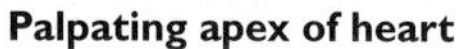

Palpating apex of heart

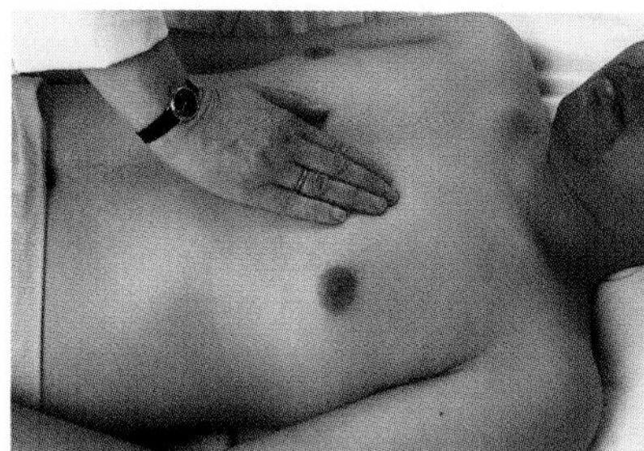

Palpating left lateral sternal border

Precordium

Apex (left ventricular area): PMI or LVI is 1–2 cm, amplitude small, duration nonsustained, systolic. Negative thrills. Amplitude may normally be increased in high-output states, such as exercise. Apical pulsation may not always be palpable. Left lateral displacement of PMI may occur during the last trimester of pregnancy.

Left lateral sternal border: May not be palpable, although small, nonsustained, systolic impulse may be palpated, especially in thin patients. Negative thrills.

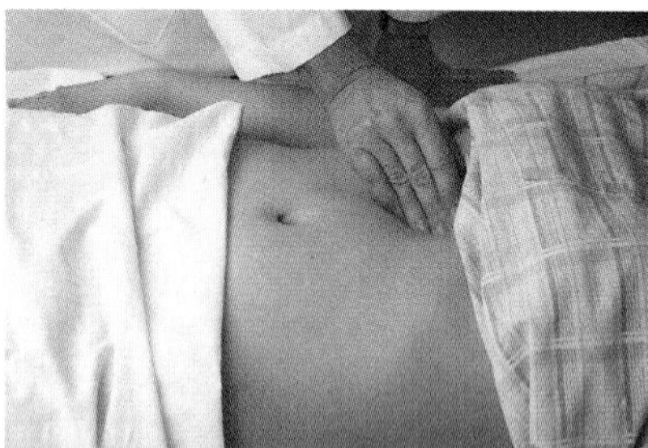

Palpating epigastric area

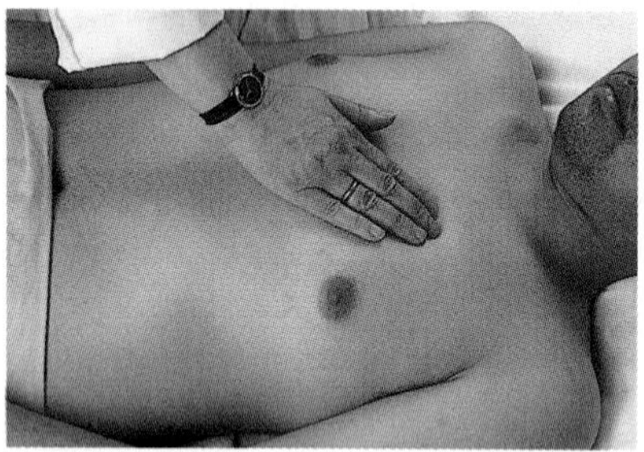

Palpating base left

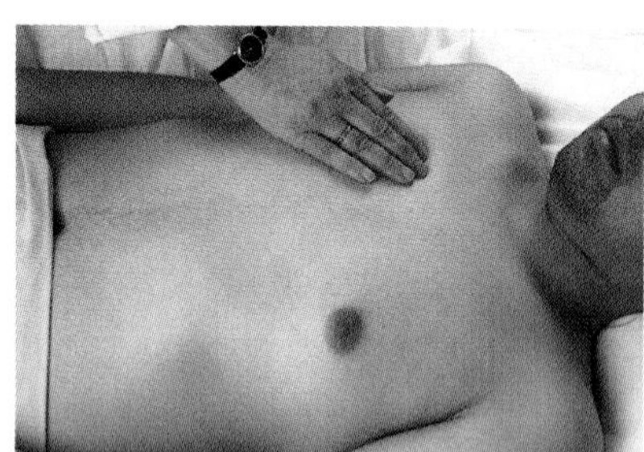

Palpating base right

Epigastric area: Positive slight pulsation may be normal. Palpations not palpable at base left, the pulmonic area, and base right, the aortic area, except in thin patients.

HELPFUL HINT

When palpating the epigastric area, pulsations originating from the abdominal aorta are felt with the fingerpads; pulsations coming from the right ventricle are felt with the fingertips.

ABNORMAL FINDINGS/RATIONALE

Palpable lifts or heaves: Right ventricular hypertrophy.

Pulsations felt on the fingertips: May come from the right ventricle, indicating right ventricular hypertrophy.

Large diffuse epigastric pulsation: Abdominal aortic aneurysm.

Accentuated pulsation in pulmonic area: Pulmonary hypertension.

Accentuated pulsation in aortic area: HTN or aneurysm.

Description	Possible Cause
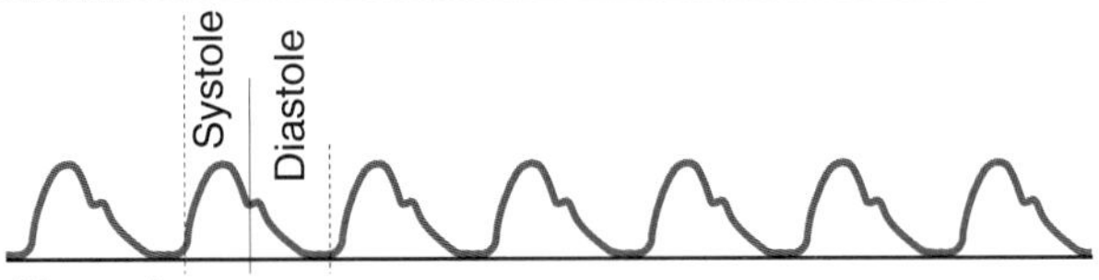 Systole Diastole **Normal**	
Small, Weak Pulse Decreased pulse pressure with a slow upstroke and prolonged peak	Increased peripheral vascular resistance such as occurs in cold weather or severe congestive heart failure; decreased stroke volume such as occurs in hypovolemia or aortic stenosis
Large, Bounding Pulse Bounding pulse in which a great surge precedes a sudden absence of force or fullness	Increased stroke volume, as in aortic regurgitation; increased stiffness of arterial walls, as in atherosclerosis or normal aging; exercise; anxiety; fever; hypertension
Corrigan's (Water-Hammer) Pulse Increased pulse pressure with a rapid upstroke and downstroke and a shortened peak	Aortic regurgitation, patent ductus arteriosus, systemic arteriosclerosis
Pulsus Alternans Regular pulse rhythm with alternation of weak and strong beats (amplitude or volume)	Left ventricular failure
Pulsus Bigeminus Irregular pulse rhythm in which premature beats alternate with sinus beats	Premature ventricular beats caused by heart failure, hypoxia, or other condition
Pulsus Bisferiens A strong upstroke, downstroke, and second upstroke during systole	Aortic insufficiency, aortic regurgitation, aortic stenosis
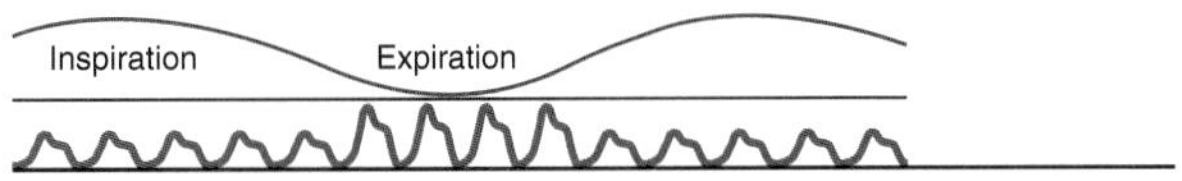 Inspiration Expiration **Pulsus Paradoxus** Pulse with a markedly decreased amplitude during Inspiration	Constrictive pericarditis, pericardial tamponade, advanced heart failure, severe lung disease

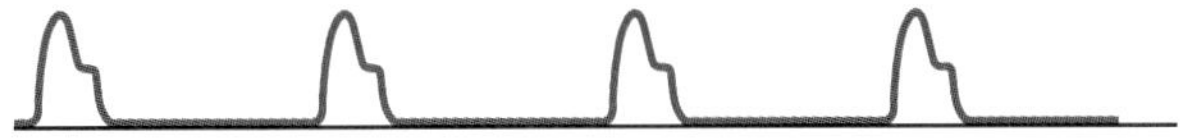

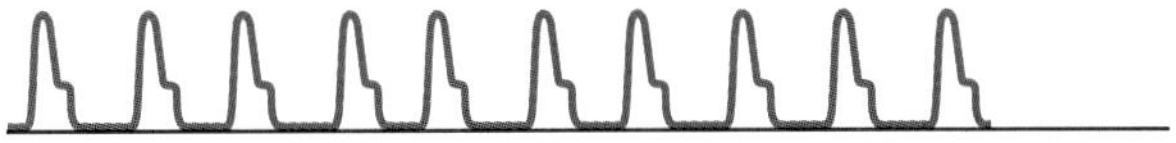

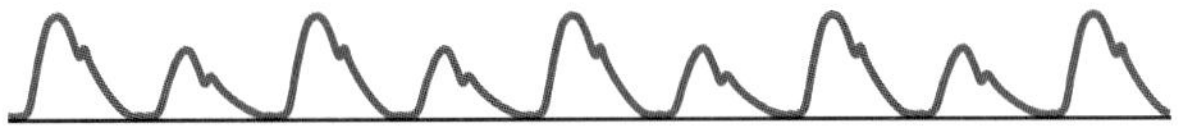

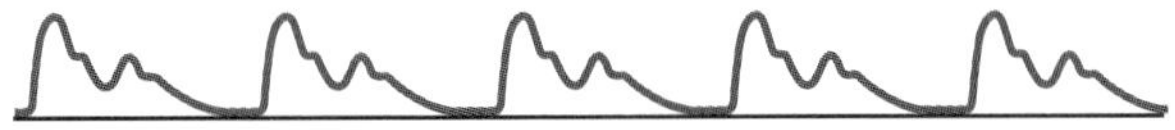

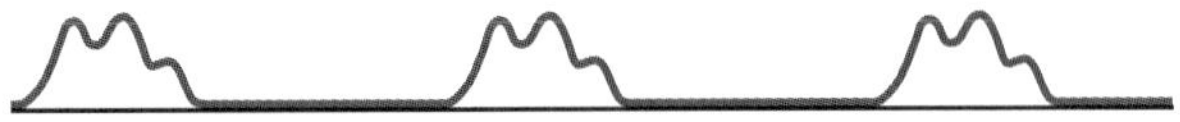

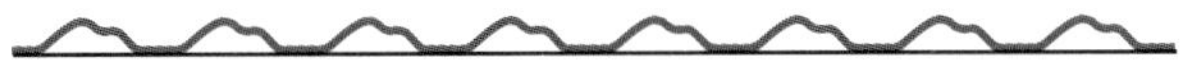

FIGURE 12–19. Abnormal pulses.

Precordial Impulses

Impulse	Normal	Increased Stroke Volume	Increased Afterload	Increased Preload
Size	Left: 2 cm Right: Slight or nonpalpable	Increased Palpable	Increased Palpable	Increased Palpable
Location	Left: Apex Right: LLSB	Apex LLSB	Apex LLSB	Displaced to left toward axilla Displaced to left toward heart
Duration	Left: Short Right: Not discernible	Short Short	Sustained Sustained	Sustained Sustained
Amplitude	Left: Small Right: Not discernible or nonpalpable	Increased Small	Increased Increased	Increased Increased
Effect			Increased pressure leads to hypertrophy	Increased volume leads to dilatation
Examples		Noncardiac conditions, such as exercise, anxiety, anemia, hyperthyroidism	Left: HTN, aortic stenosis Right: Pulmonary HTN, pulmonic stenosis	Left: Aortic or mitral regurgitation Right: Atrial septal defect

Percussion

Percussion of the precordium may be performed to determine cardiac size. However, other methods are more accurate. For example, palpation of the apical impulse, noting size and location, indirectly reflects cardiac size, and chest x ray accurately determines cardiac size. Consequently, percussion has limited value in the cardiac assessment.

If you percuss the precordium, use mediate or indirect percussion. Begin at the anterior axillary line and percuss to the sternum at the fifth intercostal space. A resonance sound will change to dullness once you reach the left border of the heart. This should normally be at the fifth intercostal space at the midclavicular line and should correspond with the PMI at the apex. Because the right border of the heart lies under the sternum, a change cannot be detected through percussion. Anteriorly, dullness is normally percussed over the third, fourth, and fifth intercostal spaces to the left of the sternum.

Auscultation

Auscultation is very useful in assessing heart sounds and vascular sounds. It is used extensively in the cardiovascular assessment to evaluate cardiac function. Auscultate the vascular structures of the neck and the precordium.

Percussing the Precordium

ASSESS/NORMAL VARIATIONS	ABNORMAL FINDINGS/RATIONALE
Precordium **Percussing precordium** Dullness at 3rd, 4th, and 5th intercostal space to the left of sternum at midclavicular line.	Left sternal border extends to midaxillary lines in an enlarged, dilated heart.

Neck

Auscultate the carotid artery and jugular veins for "flow" sounds. Assess the carotid for **bruits,** audible low-pitched sounds created by turbulent flow. Assess the jugular veins for a venous hum, a continuous low-pitched sound that reflects turbulent jugular venous flow and is often heard normally in children. These vascular sounds are low-pitched, so use the bell portion of the stethoscope.

HELPFUL HINTS

- Breath sounds over the trachea are loud, bronchial sounds, so ask your patient to hold his or her breath while you listen over the neck for vascular sounds.
- Turbulent flow in the heart is referred to as a murmur; turbulent flow outside of the heart is a bruit.

ALERT

The absence of a bruit is no guarantee that the carotid is patent. In fact, it may signal total occlusion of the artery.

Precordium

After establishing the cardiac rate and rhythm, carefully auscultate the precordium and identify normal and abnormal sounds. Listen to one sound at a time in each cardiac cycle at each auscultatory site. Closing your eyes to block out other sensory stimuli will help you focus on the sounds. When auscultating, listen for the following specific characteristics that will help you differentiate and identify sounds: location, frequency, intensity, quality, duration, and timing in the cardiac cycle. Note if the sound is affected by breathing patterns or position changes. As you listen, integrate your auscultatory findings with the hemodynamic events that they represent.

Location. Specific sites have been identified for cardiac auscultation. Ask yourself, "At what site do I hear the sound best?"

HELPFUL HINT

Use this mnemonic to help you remember auscultory sites:

All (aortic)
Patients (Pulmonary)
Take (triscuspid)
Meds (mitral)

Frequency. The frequency of a sound relates to the pitch. Heart sounds and vascular sounds may be high, medium, or low in pitch, so you need a stethoscope that can detect high- and low-pitched sounds. Ask yourself, "What part of the stethoscope allows me to hear the sound best?" The diaphragm of the stethoscope is best for detecting high-pitched sounds; the bell is best for low-pitched sounds.

HELPFUL HINT

When using the diaphragm, use firm pressure; when using the bell, use light pressure.

Intensity. Intensity relates to loudness of a sound. Ask yourself, "How loud is the sound?" Intensity can be described as soft, loud, very loud, or on a scale of 1 to 4. A +1 sound is slightly louder than normal, +2 louder than normal, +3 very loud, and +4 the loudest. A grading scale can also be used to describe intensity of murmurs. Murmurs are classified on a 1 to 6 scale:

- Grade 1: Not immediately heard. You need to "tune in" for several seconds before sound can be heard.
- Grade 2: Quiet sound, but heard immediately if you are paying attention.
- Grade 3: Loud, readily heard.
- Grade 4: Loud, with a palpable thrust or thrill.
- Grade 5: Loud with palpable thrust or thrill with stethoscope tilted slightly off chest wall.
- Grade 6: Loud with palpable thrust or thrill with stethoscope off chest wall.

Although any cardiac sound can be graded, in clinical situations, the grading scale is most frequently used to grade murmurs. If using the grading scale, document your finding as a fraction—for example, 3/6 or III/VI would represent a grade 3 sound on the 6-step scale.

Quality. Quality distinguishes one sound from another. Ask yourself, "What did it sound like?" Descriptive words such as snapping, blowing, and rumbling can be used to describe the quality of a sound.

Duration. Duration is the length of time the sound lasts. Ask yourself, "How long is the sound? Does it extend through systole, diastole, or both?" Duration is often described as short, medium, or long. Normal heart sounds are relatively short in duration as compared to murmurs, which are long-duration sounds.

Timing in the cardiac cycle. Timing in the cardiac cycle is one of the most important characteristics in distinguishing sounds. If you cannot determine where the sound is occurring in the cardiac cycle, you won't be able to distinguish one sound from another. Ask yourself, "Does the sound occur during systole or diastole or throughout the entire cardiac cycle?" Here are some ways to establish the timing of the sound in the cardiac cycle:

- **Heart rate:** The best way to identify the first and second heart sounds is to note the time interval between them. In heart rates less than 100 BPM, systole is shorter than diastole. The shorter interval between the sounds represents systole (the timing between S_1 and S_2), and the longer interval represents diastole (the timing between S_2 and the

Heart Sounds

Heart sound	Location	Pitch	Timing in Cardiac Cycle	Interpretation
S_1	Apex/mitral area	High	Systolic	Normal
S_1 split	LLSB/tricuspid area	High	Systolic	Normal RBBB
S_2	Base right/aortic area	High	Systolic	Normal
S_2 split	Base left/pulmonic area	High	Systolic	Normal RBB, ASD, VSD, PE, pulmonic stenosis
S_3 (Left ventricular origin)	Apex	Low	Diastolic	May be normal at age under 30 years Left-sided CHF
S_3 (Right ventricular origin)	LLSB	Low	Diastolic	Right-sided CHF
S_4 (Left ventricular origin)	Apex, LLSB	Low	Diastolic	May be normal in children and young adults MI, HTN, CAD
S_4 (Right ventricular origin)		low	Diastolic	Pulmonary HTN
Opening snap	Apex	High	Diastolic	Mitral stenosis
Ejection click	Base	High	Early systolic	Aortic stenosis, pulmonic stenosis
	Apex	High	Midsystolic	Mitral valve prolapse
Friction rub	LLSB	High	Systolic/diastolic	Pericarditis

next S_1). With practice and experience, you will find this method invaluable and practically infallible.

- **Location:** Different heart sounds are best heard at specific sites. For example, S_1 is best heard at the apex, and S_2 is best heard at the base. Therefore, if you are listening at the apex, the louder of the two sounds should be S_1; if you are listening at the base, it should be S_2.
- **Carotid pulsation:** The first heart sound will immediately precede the carotid pulsation.
- **Precordial movement:** Precordial apical movement is simultaneous with S_1.
- **EKG monitor:** If your patient is on a cardiac monitor, the QRS complex is simultaneous with S_1.

Auscultating Murmurs

Murmurs involving the mitral and aortic valves are the most common. They may indicate the presence of mitral regurgitation, mitral stenosis, aortic stenosis, or aortic regurgitation.

Characteristics of Murmurs

Type	Location	Pitch	Quality	Interpretation
Early systolic	LLSB	High	Blowing	VSD
Midsystolic	Base right Base left	High	Harsh	Aortic stenosis Pulmonic stenosis
Late systolic	Apex LLSB	High	Blowing	MVP Tricuspid regurgitation
Pansystolic	Apex LLSB	High		Mitral regurgitation, VSD Tricuspid regurgitation
Early diastolic	Erb's point Base left	High	Blowing	Aortic regurgitation Pulmonic regurgitation
Mid-diastolic	Apex LLSB	Low	Rumbling	Mitral stenosis Tricuspid stenosis
Late diastolic	Apex LLSB	Low	Rumbling	Mitral stenosis Tricuspid stenosis
Pandiastolic	Base left	Low	continuous	PDA

Auscultating Valvular Heart Disease

Disease | **Description/Assessment Findings**

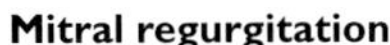

Mitral regurgitation

- Holosystolic; extends from first heart sound to second heart sound
- Loudness constant throughout systole
- Heard best at apical area
- May radiate to left lateral chest or, less commonly, to base
- Blowing, rough (harsh), or musical
- If very loud, it may mask first heart sound.

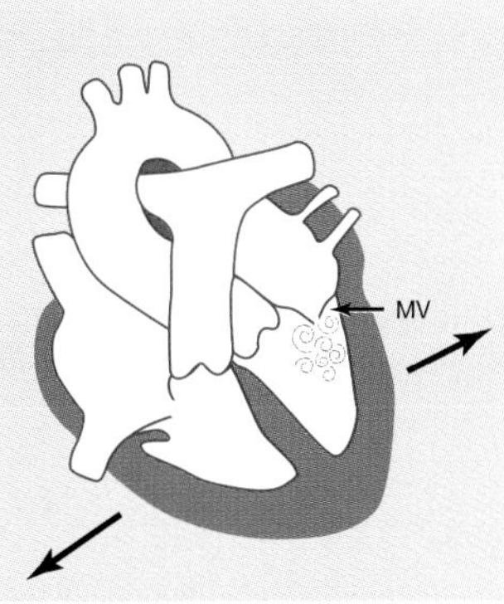

Mitral stenosis

- Occurs in diastolic phase of cardiac cycle.
- With normal sinus rhythm, characteristically a low-pitched rough or harsh murmur beginning immediately after opening snap.
- Extends to sharp first heart sound.
- Demonstrates presystolic (late diastolic) accentuation with normal sinus rhythm and just before termination.
- Presystolic accentuation of mid-late diastolic murmur disappears with atrial fibrillation.
- Best heard in apical area with patient in left lateral position and with bell portion of stethoscope.
- Localized to a very small (quarter-sized) area, so may be hard to find.

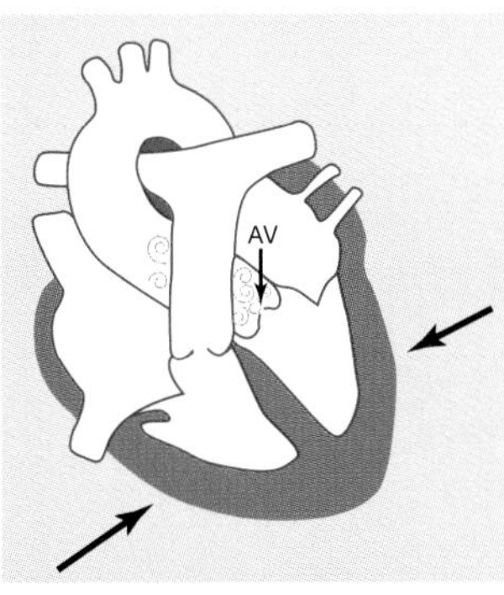

Aortic Stenosis

- Midsystolic; characterized by crescendo/decrescendo pattern.
- Begins shortly after first heart sound and ends before second sound.
- Rough (low-pitched).
- Second heart sound at base markedly diminished or absent as a result of poor movement of severely calcified valve leaflets.
- When transmitted to apex, may have musical overtone in addition to rough quality (Gallavardin effect).
- If congenital (represented by two valve leaflets instead of three), early ejection click is often heard shortly after first heart sound.
- Both acquired and congenital murmurs heard best at base in second right interspace. May also be transmitted to apex and neck.

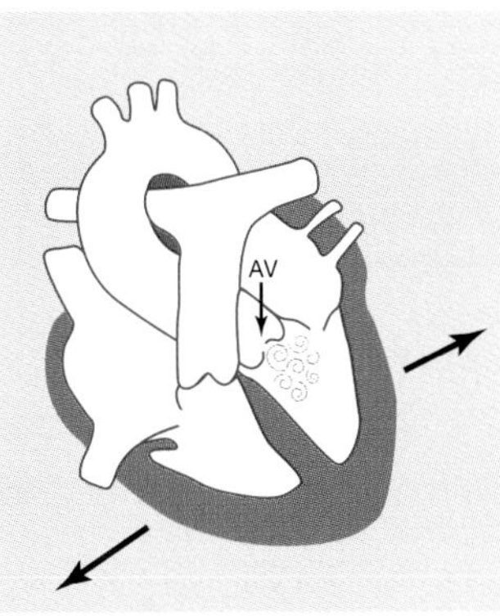

Aortic regurgitation

- Onset early in diastole.
- Decrescendo, ending before first heart sound.
- Usually blowing.
- Heard best at base of heart in third left interspace in parasternal line.
- Often transmitted toward apex, if loud enough.
- Loudness varies from Grade 1 to Grade 3 or 4.
- Often is only Grade 1 intensity. If so, to facilitate identification of murmur, have patient sit forward, exhale, and hold his or her breath while you listen in third left interspace in parasternal line.

Questions on Characteristics of Murmurs

Location: Where did you hear the murmur best? Note the area.
Pitch: Did you hear the murmur with the bell or the diaphragm? Murmurs can be high, medium, or low pitched.
Intensity: How loud was the murmur? Grade the intensity on the 1 to 6 scale.
Quality: What did the murmur sound like? Was it blowing, harsh, mechanical, or rumbling?
Timing: Where does the murmur occur in the cardiac cycle? Murmurs can be systolic, diastolic, or both.
Duration: How long is the murmur? Murmurs by their very nature are long-duration sounds. However, some murmurs are longer than others. Some occur in parts of the cardiac cycle, whereas others occur throughout the cycle.
Radiation: Do you hear the murmur in any other places? Murmurs can radiate across the chest, through the back, and to the neck.
Position: Is the murmur heard best in a particular position? Some murmurs change with position.
Respiratory Variations: Does the murmur change with breathing? Some murmurs are affected by respirations.
Shape or configuration: Does the intensity of the murmur change? Does the murmur start soft, then become louder? Start loud, then become softer? Is it consistent throughout? Describe the pattern of the intensity as crescendo, decrescendo, or crescendo-decrescendo?

Auscultating the Vascular Structures and Precordium

ASSESS/NORMAL VARIATIONS

Neck
Carotid Artery
Jugular Veins

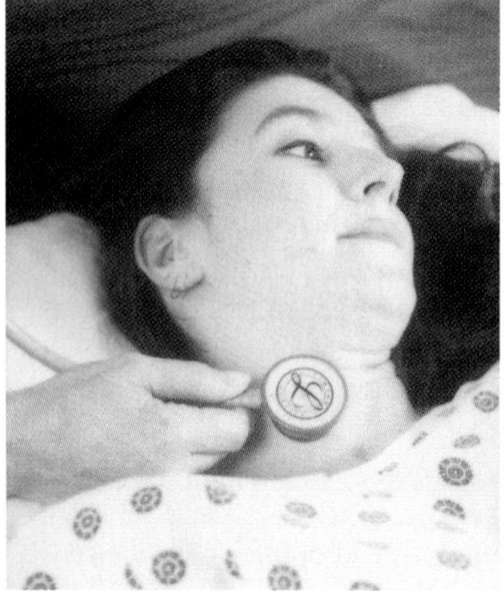

Auscultating neck

Negative bruits
Positive carotid bruit may be normal in children and is associated with high-output states.
Negative venous hum.
Positive venous hum may be normal in children.

Apex (mitral)
Rate depends on age.
Rhythm: regular; $S_1 > S_2$; high-pitched systolic, short duration. No extra sounds.

ABNORMAL FINDINGS/RATIONALE

Bruit suggests carotid stenosis. Murmurs can also radiate up to the neck from the heart, as in aortic **stenosis.**

Bradycardia rates <60 BPM or tachycardia rates >100 BPM: See variations in pulse in Palpating the Neck and Precordium, page 394.
Irregular rhythm: Arrhythmia.
Accentuated S_1: High-output states, mitral or tricuspid stenosis.
Diminished S_1: First-degree heart block, CHF, CAD.
Variable S_1: Atrial fibrillation.

ASSESS/NORMAL VARIATIONS	ABNORMAL FINDINGS/RATIONALE
Apex (mitral) *(Continued)* Physiologic S_3 and S_4 may be heard in children and young adults without heart disease.	*S_3, low-pitched, early diastolic sound:* CHF. *S_4, low-pitched late-diastolic sound:* CAD, HTN, MI. Quadruple rhythm, $S_3 + S_4$ with fast rate is called a summation gallop.
LLSB (tricuspid) $S_1 >$ or $= S_2$, + split S_1	Wide split: RBBB. *Midsystolic ejection click, a high-pitched systolic sound:* MVP. *Opening snap, a high-pitched diastolic sound:* Mitral or tricuspid stenosis, VSD, PDA. *Pericardial friction rub, a high-pitched systolic and diastolic sound:* Pericarditis or postoperative cardiac surgery.
Erb's point No aortic murmurs	Aortic murmurs
Base Base right (aortic) Base left (pulmonic) $S_1 < S_2$ + split S_2 on inspiration at pulmonic area	*Diminished S_2:* Incompetent aortic or pulmonic valves and low output states. *Ejection click, a high-pitched systolic sound:* Aortic or pulmonic stenosis. *Accentuated S_2:* Associated with HTN or pulmonary HTN. Wide split S_2 occurs with RBBB, pulmonic stenosis, ASD, VSD. *Fixed split S_2, a split with no respiratory variation:* ASD, VSD, CHF *Paradoxical split S_2, occurs during expirations:* LBBB or aortic stenosis.
Murmurs Innocent grade 2/6, systolic, blowing murmurs often heard in children. Innocent systolic murmurs may also be heard during pregnancy. The diaphragm of the stethoscope is best for detecting high-pitched sounds; the bell is best for detecting low-pitched sounds. Use firm pressure with the diaphragm and light pressure with the bell.	*Systolic and diastolic murmurs:* See box, Characteristics of Murmurs, on page 400.

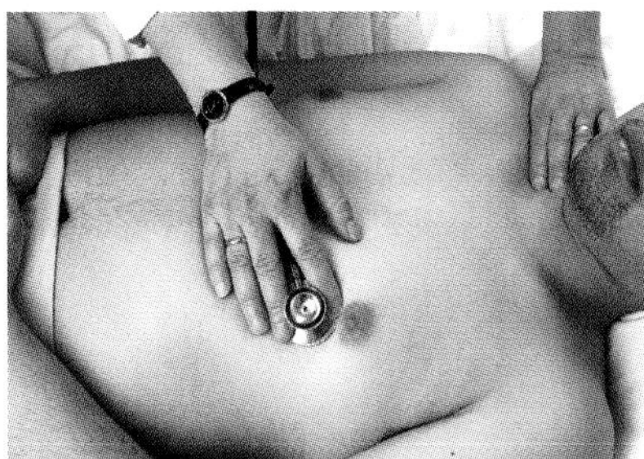

Auscultation with diaphragm of stethoscope

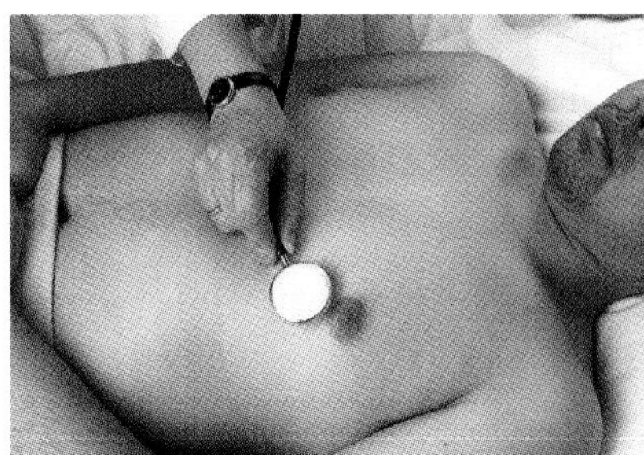

Auscultation with bell of stethoscope

Cardiac Auscultation Tips

- A quiet, warm, well-lit environment will minimize extraneous sound, facilitate cardiac inspection, and maximize patient comfort.
- Remember, you cannot auscultate heart sounds through layers of clothes. Because the patient will have to disrobe, ensure his or her privacy during the examination.
- Position changes can facilitate auscultation. The three positions for cardiac examination are supine, left lateral recumbent, and sitting. The left lateral recumbent position and sitting positions bring the apex of the heart closer to the chest wall, enhancing auscultation.
- Always work from the right side of the patient. This allows you to stretch the stethoscope across the chest wall and minimize interference from the tubing.
- Remember, a stethoscope basically transmits sound, so the better the instrument, the better your ability to hear sound.
- Be systematic in your approach. Listen with both the diaphragm and the bell. The diaphragm is best for detecting high-pitched sounds and is used by applying firm pressure. The bell is best for detecting low-pitched sounds and should be held lightly on the chest wall.
- Become a selective listener! Closing your eyes during auscultation allows you to focus your attention on listening to sound.
- Explain to your patient what you will be doing and that auscultation takes time. Teaching can be incorporated into the assessment process by sharing your findings with your patient.
- The thickness of the chest wall makes heart sounds more difficult to hear in obese and muscular patients than in patients with thin chests.
- Overinflated lungs increase the distance between the heart and the chest wall, also making auscultation more difficult. Patients with chronic obstructive pulmonary disease (COPD) often have distant heart sounds.

HELPFUL HINTS

- It can be very confusing when extra sounds are added to the normal heart sounds. To help differentiate one sound from the other, first establish the timing of the sound in the cardiac cycle.
- Diastolic murmurs are usually not considered innocent! Remember, the diastolic phase is the resting phase, and if there is turbulent flow during the resting phase, there is usually a problem.
- Murmurs above grade 3/6 are usually associated with pathology. Remember, murmurs greater than grade 3/6 are associated with a thrill. If the turbulent flow is so great that it can be felt, there is usually a problem.
- Innocent or functional murmurs are often related to increased flow through normal valves.

Figure 12–20 shows how to differentiate sounds.

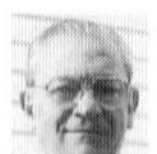

Case Study Findings

Mr. Brusca's focused physical assessment findings include:

- **Neck Vessels**
  - Positive large carotid pulsation, +3, symmetrical with smooth, sharp upstroke and rapid descent, artery stiff, negative for thrills and bruits
  - JVP at 30 degrees <3cm, negative abdominojugular reflux
- **Precordium**
  - Positive sustained pulsations displaced lateral to apex, PMI 3 cm with increased amplitude
  - Slight pulsations also appreciated at LLSB and Base, but not as pronounced
  - Negative thrills; cardiac borders percussed 3rd, 4th, and 5th intercostal space to the left of the midclavicular line
  - Heart sounds appreciated with regular rate and rhythm at apex $S_1 > S_2$ and $+S_4$, at LLSB $S_1 >$
  - S_2 negative split, at base left $S_1 < S_2$ negative split, at base right $S_1 < S_2$ with an accentuated S_2, negative for murmurs and rubs

CRITICAL THINKING ACTIVITY #2

What effect would hypertension have on Mr. Brusca's heart?

CRITICAL THINKING ACTIVITY #3

Considering the relationship of the cardiovascular system to the respiratory system, what respiratory problems might Mr. Brusca have as a result of his cardiovascular disease?

CRITICAL THINKING ACTIVITY #4

How would you explain the fact that the carotid pulse is palpable, but the jugular pulse is not?

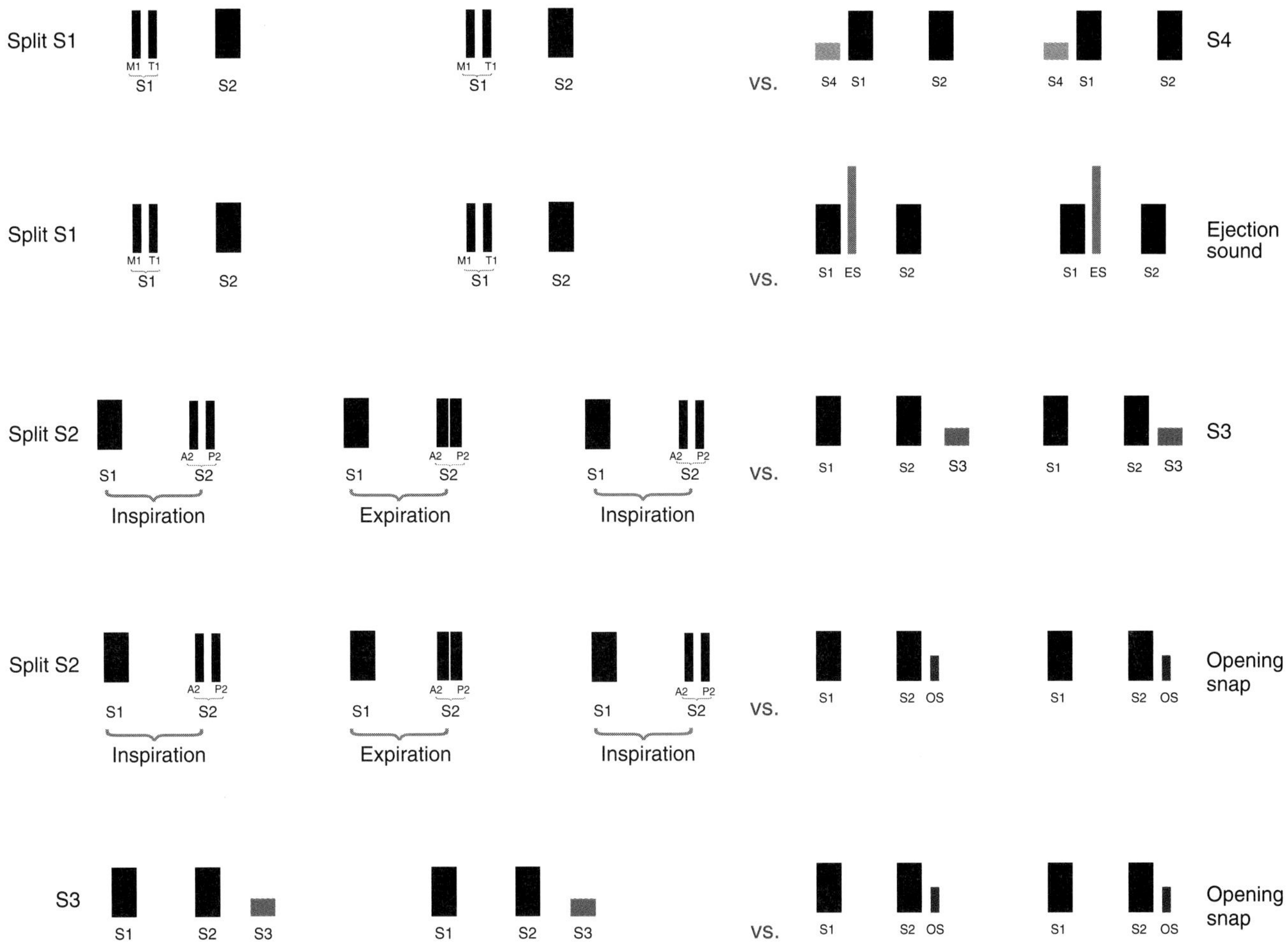

FIGURE 12–20. How to differentiate sounds.

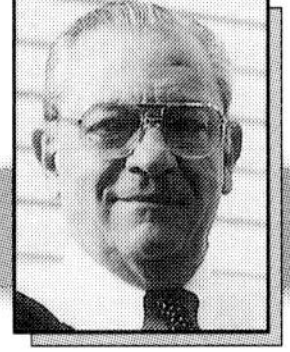

Case Study Analysis and Plan

Now that you have completed a thorough assessment of Mr. Brusca, document your key history and physical assessment findings. List key history findings and physical examination findings that will help you formulate your nursing diagnoses.

CRITICAL THINKING ACTIVITY #5

List all of the strengths and areas of concern that would affect Mr. Brusca's health status at this time.

Nursing Diagnoses

After you have completed Mr. Brusca's assessment, you need to analyze the data, cluster the data, and formulate the nursing diagnoses. Some possible nursing diagnoses for Mr. Brusca are listed below. Cluster the data that support each diagnosis.

1. **Tissue Perfusion, ineffective, related to cardiovascular disease**
2. **Nutrition: imbalanced, more than body requirements**

3. Cardiac Output, decreased, risk for
4. Health Maintenance, ineffective, related to lack of knowledge regarding pathology, complications, and management of HTN
5. Knowledge, deficient, regarding complications and management of hypertension

Identify any additional nursing diagnoses.

Collaborative Nursing Diagnoses

1. Potential Complication: Hypertensive crises
2. Potential Complication: MI, CVA
3. Potential Complication: Adverse effects from medication

CRITICAL THINKING ACTIVITY #6

Now that you have identified some nursing diagnoses for Mr. Brusca, select one and develop a nursing care plan and a brief teaching plan for him, including learning objectives and teaching strategies.

Research Tells Us

In spite of medical advances, heart disease still remains the number one killer of both men and women in the United States. The Nurse's Health Study followed 84,129 women who were free of cardiovascular disease, diabetes, and cancer in 1980 for the next 14 years. During this time, 296 women died of coronary heart disease and 832 had myocardial infarctions. The study identified lifestyle behaviors of those at low risk for developing cardiovascular disease. Diet, exercise, and abstinence from smoking were associated with a very low risk.

Source: Stampfer, M., Hu, F., Manson, J., Rimm, E., and Willet, W. (2000). Primary prevention of coronary heart disease in women through diet and lifestyle. *The New England Journal of Nursing, 343, 1:* 16–22.

Health Concerns

- In the United States, 1 million deaths annually are caused by cardiovascular disease.
- Of these deaths, 500,000 are caused by CAD, with the majority being sudden deaths.
- About 160,000 deaths occur before age 65.
- Half of all cardiovascular deaths occur in women.
- CAD is the major cause of mortality and morbidity in women in their 50s.
- Approximately 6.2 million Americans have significant CAD.
- Approximately 2/3 of sudden deaths from CAD occur within 2 hours after onset of symptoms, often before the victim ever reaches the hospital.

Source: American Heart Association, 1992.

Common Abnormalities

ABNORMALITY/AREA	ASSESSMENT FINDINGS
Angina Pectoris Chest pain resulting from myocardial ischemia.	
General	Anxiety, chest pain
Skin	Pale, diaphoretic, cool, clammy
Chest	Dyspnea, tachycardia, pulsus alternans, arrhythmias, S_4, S_3
Abdomen	Nausea, belching
Extremities	Weakness, paresthesia
Congestive Heart Failure (CHF) Failure of the heart to pump sufficiently to meet the demands of the body. CHF can be right, left, or both.	

Common Abnormalities

ABNORMALITY/AREA	ASSESSMENT FINDINGS
Right-sided failure:	
General	Fatigue, weight gain, confusion
Skin	Pale, cool
Head and Neck	NVD
Chest	Tachycardia, right ventricular heaves, murmurs, S_3, right-sided pleural effusion
Abdomen	Anorexia, bloating, RUQ tenderness, hepatomegaly, ascites
Extremities	Edema, diminished hair growth
Left-sided failure:	
General	Fatigue, confusion
Skin	Pale, dusky, cyanotic, cool
Chest	LV heaves, pulsus alternans, increased heart rate, displaced PMI, S_3, S_4, dyspnea, crackles, orthopnea, dry, hacking cough, PND
Abdomen	Nocturia
Coronary Artery Disease (CAD) A progressive narrowing of the coronary arteries. Atherosclerosis is the major cause of CAD. CAD can present as angina pectoris, acute **myocardial infarction (MI)**, or sudden cardiac death. MI is necrosis of myocardial tissue from ischemia.	
General	Anxiety, dizziness, chest pain, fatigue
Skin	Pale to ashen, cool, diaphoretic, feverish
Neck	Neck vein distention
Chest	Dyspnea, tachypnea, crackles, tachycardia or bradycardia, arrhythmias, elevated BP initially, S_3, S_4, murmur, rubs, and diminished heart sounds
Abdomen	Nausea, vomiting, low urinary output
Extremities	Cool, pale, decreased pulses
Pericarditis An inflammation of the visceral or parietal pericardium, resulting in cardiac compression, decreased ventricular filling and emptying, and cardiac failure. It often occurs 2 to 3 days after MI.	
General	Chest pain aggravated by inspiration, coughing, or movement.
Skin	Fever
Chest	Friction rub at LLSB

Summary

- A thorough cardiovascular assessment includes a health history and physical examination and provides invaluable data about the patient's overall health status.
- Before you begin, visualize the underlying structures and review expected normal findings. Understanding normal cardiovascular functioning is crucial in interpreting your findings.
- As you work through the assessment, systematically look for cardiovascular changes in every system.
- Let your patient's current health status direct your assessment. If he or she has an acute problem, perform a focused assessment.
- After you complete your assessment, document your findings. Your plan of care should flow from the assessment.
- Share your findings with your patient—this is an ideal teaching opportunity. Involving the patient in developing the plan of care allows him or her to actively participate in his or her health care and to make decisions that promote a healthy cardiovascular system.

13

Assessing the Peripheral-Vascular and Lymphatic Systems

Before You Begin

INTRODUCTION TO THE PERIPHERAL-VASCULAR AND LYMPHATIC SYSTEMS

The peripheral-vascular (PV) system is a branching network of vessels that transports oxygenated blood to all body organs and tissues and then returns it to the heart for reoxygenation in the lungs. A disruption in the PV system can cause significant pain, loss of limb, or even death. The lymphatic system helps the heart and peripheral vasculature maintain adequate circulation. The function of the lymphatic system is to collect and drain excess tissue fluid that accumulates from the cardiovascular system and return this fluid to the heart. Lymphatic dysfunction may result in reduced range of motion, permanent disfigurement, and susceptibility to infection.

When assessing these two systems, your goal is first to identify any acute changes that require immediate intervention and then to identify any unhealthy behaviors that may affect the client's health. A complete, accurate assessment is the first step in planning care, implementing therapeutic measures, and developing appropriate teaching strategies.

Anatomy and Physiology Review

Before you begin your assessment, you must understand how the PV and lymphatic systems work.

Peripheral-Vascular System

The primary function of the PV system is to deliver blood to all areas of the body. Blood flows through **arteries, veins,** and **capillaries** and is measured by pulse and pressure. Adequate perfusion to the vital organs and extremities is essential to life. Figure 13–1 and the table that follows it illustrate and describe the arterial system, and Figure 13–2 and the table that follows it illustrate and describe the venous system. (For more information on the function of arteries, veins, and capillaries, see Chapter 12, Assessing the Cardiovascular System.)

Lymphatic System

The lymphatic system complements the function of the vascular system. It is made up of lymphatic capillaries, lymph fluid, collecting ducts, and various tissues including the lymph nodes, spleen, thymus, tonsils, adenoids, and Peyer patches. The collecting ducts are thin, small, veinlike vessels that start at the capillaries and branch into their own circulation. Lymphatic vessels tend to lie near veins and drain into larger lymphatic vessels. Lymph capillaries drain the tissue spaces of lymph and tissue fluid. The lymph flows through small, oval bodies called lymph nodes before entering the bloodstream. As the lymph is returned to the central circulation, collections of lymph nodes filter large molecules and debris. The lymphatic system drains toward the center of the body. All lymphatic vessels eventually flow into two main vessels, the thoracic duct and the right lymphatic duct. The drainage point for the right upper body is a

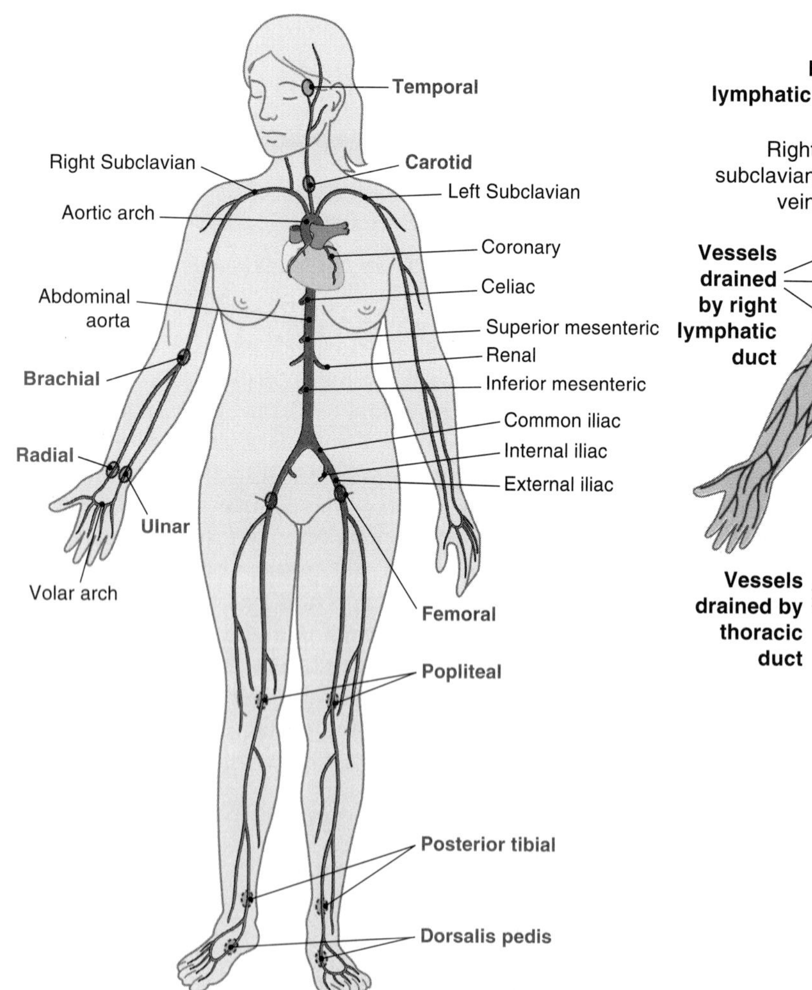

FIGURE 13–1. Peripheral arterial system. Pulse sites labeled in red.

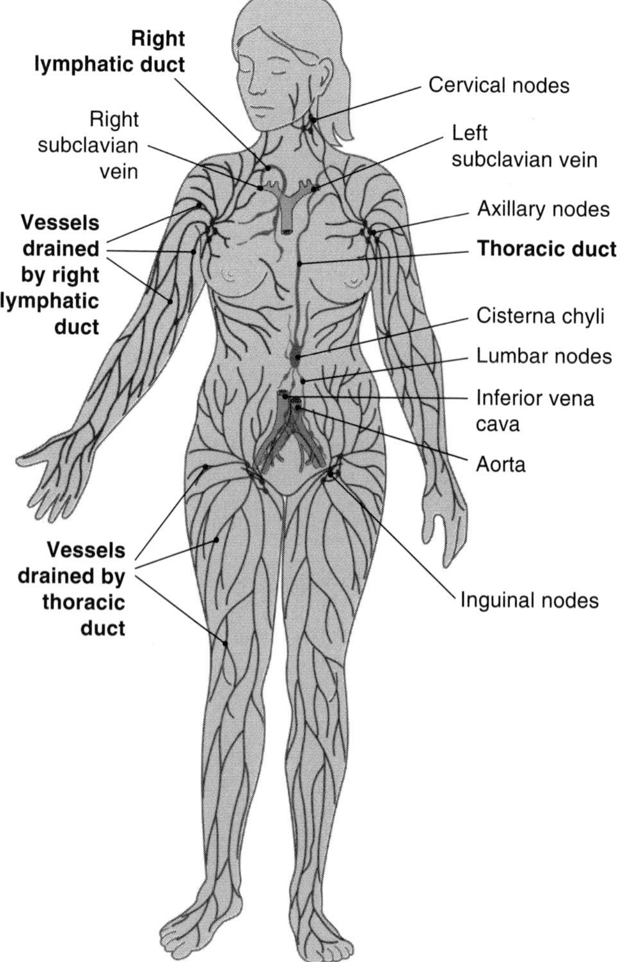

FIGURE 13–2. Peripheral venous system.

Peripheral Arterial Pulse Sites and Areas Supplied

ARTERY	AREAS SUPPLIED
Carotid	
• *Internal*	The internal carotid artery branches into the anterior and middle cerebral arteries and supplies the brain.
• *External*	The external carotid artery branches into the superior thyroid, inguinal, facial, occipital posterior auricular, superficial temporal, and maxillary arteries and supplies the thyroid, head, and mouth.
Brachial	Supplies the humerus and the muscles and skin of the upper arm.
Radial	Supplies the forearm and hand on radial side.
Ulnar	Supplies the forearm and hand on ulnar side.
Femoral	Supplies the thighs.
Popliteal	Supplies the knees; the posterior femoral, gastrocnemius, and soleus muscles; and the skin on the back of the leg.
Posterior tibialis	Supplies the back of the leg and the ankle.
Dorsalis pedis	Supplies the feet

Peripheral Venous System and Areas Drained

VEIN	AREAS DRAINED
Jugular Veins	Head, face, neck, and brain
• *Internal*	
• *External*	
Deep Veins	Arms
• *Brachial*	
• *Axillary*	
• *Subclavian*	
Superficial Veins	Elbow, forearm, and hand
• *Dorsal venous arch*	
• *Basilic*	
• *Cephalic*	
• *Medial cubital*	
Common Iliac Vein	Lower limbs, pelvis, and genitourinary structures
Inferior Vena Cava	Renal, gonadal, and hepatic veins
Portal Veins	Spleen and small and large intestines.
Azygos Vein	Chest and bronchi

lymphatic trunk that empties into the right subclavian vein. The thoracic duct, the major vessel of the lymph system, drains lymph from the rest of the body into the left subclavian vein. It returns the various fluids and proteins to the cardiovascular system, forming a closed, porous circle.

Important functions of the lymphatic system include:

- Movement of lymph fluid in a closed circuit with the cardiovascular system
- Development and maintenance of the immune system
- Reabsorption of fat and fat-soluble substances from the small intestine

Figure 13–3 and the table that follows it illustrate and describe the lymphatic system.

Interaction with Other Body Systems

The PV system has a complex mechanism to control blood flow to different parts of the body. There are three major types of control. First, local control of blood flow in each individual tissue is delivered in proportion to that tissue's need for blood perfusion. Second, nervous

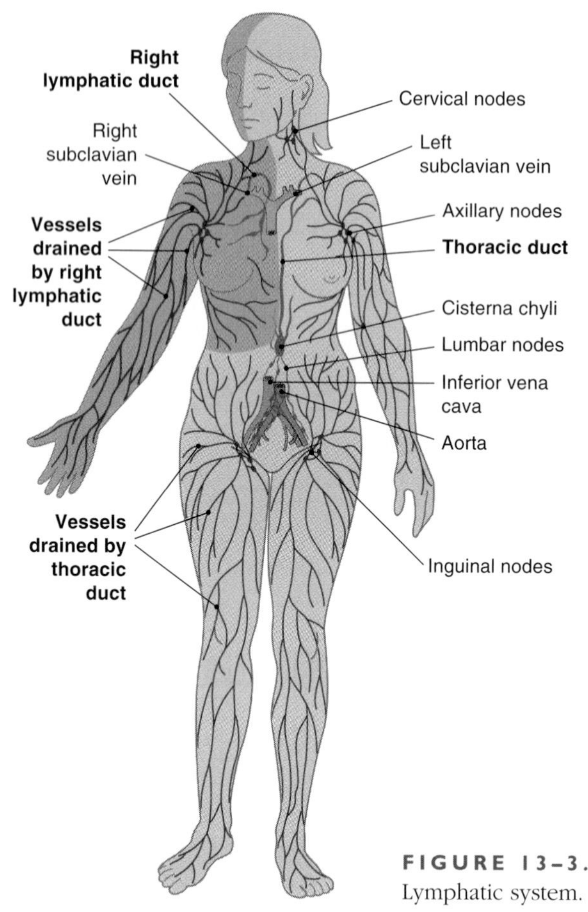

FIGURE 13–3. Lymphatic system.

system control of the blood flow affects large segments of the systemic circulation, for example, by shifting blood flow from nonmuscular vascular beds to muscular beds during exercise or by altering blood flow in the skin to control body temperature. Last, the endocrine system, through hormones, ions, and other chemicals, can cause local increases, decreases, and generalized changes in tissue flow.

The Cardiovascular System

The lymphatic system has no pumping mechanism of its own, so it depends on the cardiovascular system, contraction of smooth muscles within lymphatic vessels, and skeletal muscle contraction to pump lymph throughout the body. Like the veins, the lymphatic vessels have one-way valves to prevent backflow. As lymph volume increases, the lymph flows faster in response to an increasing capillary pressure and greater permeability of the capillary walls of the cardiovascular system. Increased metabolic activity and massage also contribute to lymph movement. Mechanical obstruction slows or stops the movement of lymph, dilating the system. If the flow of the lymphatic system is obstructed, lymph may diffuse into the vascular system or collateral channels may develop. For more information on how the PV and lymphatic systems interact with other systems, see Chapter 12, Assessing the Cardiovascular System.

Structures and Functions of the Lymphatic System

STRUCTURE	FUNCTION
Lymph	Excessive fluid from body tissue that has drained into lymphatic capillaries. Responsible for 1–3% of body weight. Contains leukocytes.
Lymphatic capillaries	Collects fluid from interstitial space and surrounding tissue.
Lymphatic vessels	Formed by merging of lymphatic capillaries. Drain lymph back to right lymphatic duct and thoracic duct.
Lymph nodes	Filter microorganisms and foreign substances from lymph.
• *Cervical*	• Drains head, face, mouth, and neck.
• *Axillary*	• Drains arms, thoracic, breast, and upper abdominal wall.
• *Supratrochlear*	• Drains hands and forearms.
• *Intestinal*	• Drains abdominal viscera.
• *Iliac*	• Drains pelvic viscera.
• *Inguinal*	• Drains legs, external genitalia, and lower abdominal wall.
• *Lumbar*	• Drains pelvic viscera.
Tonsils	Lymphatic tissue that destroys microorganisms and foreign substances at beginning of digestive and respiratory tracts.
Thymus	Lymphatic tissue in thorax that forms antibodies in newborn and developing immune system and secretes thymosin, which helps with T-cell differentiation.
Spleen	Lymphatic tissue that filters blood and produces lymphocytes and monocytes.
Peyer's Patches	Clusters of lymphoid tissue found in small intestines. Respond to antigens by producing antibodies.

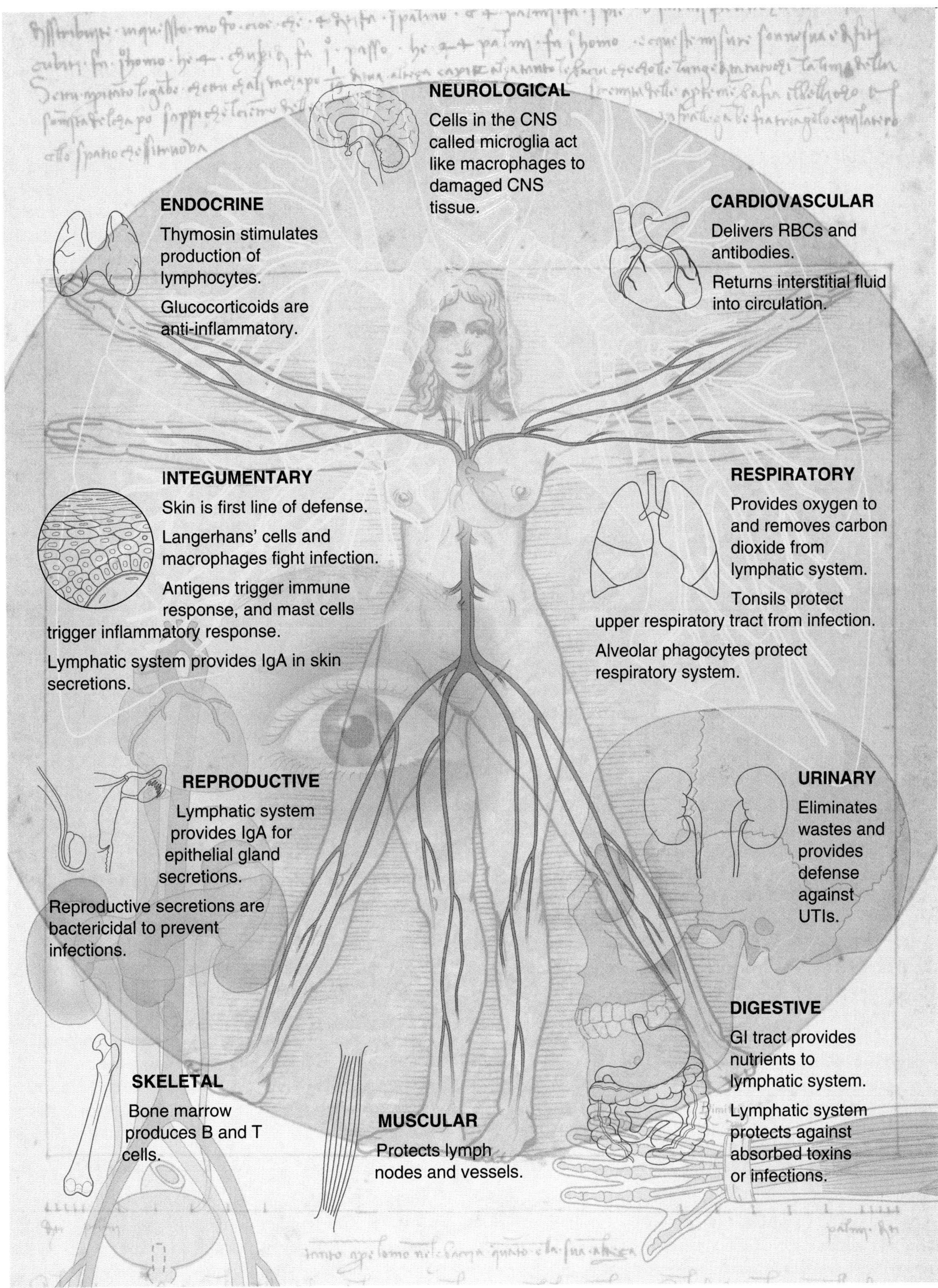

NEUROLOGICAL
Cells in the CNS called microglia act like macrophages to damaged CNS tissue.
ENDOCRINE
Thymosin stimulates production of lymphocytes.
Glucocorticoids are anti-inflammatory.
CARDIOVASCULAR
Delivers RBCs and antibodies.
Returns interstitial fluid into circulation.
INTEGUMENTARY
Skin is first line of defense.
Langerhans' cells and macrophages fight infection.
Antigens trigger immune response, and mast cells trigger inflammatory response.
Lymphatic system provides IgA in skin secretions.
RESPIRATORY
Provides oxygen to and removes carbon dioxide from lymphatic system.
Tonsils protect upper respiratory tract from infection.
Alveolar phagocytes protect respiratory system.
REPRODUCTIVE
Lymphatic system provides IgA for epithelial gland secretions.
Reproductive secretions are bactericidal to prevent infections.
URINARY
Eliminates wastes and provides defense against UTIs.
DIGESTIVE
GI tract provides nutrients to lymphatic system.
Lymphatic system protects against absorbed toxins or infections.
SKELETAL
Bone marrow produces B and T cells.
MUSCULAR
Protects lymph nodes and vessels.

Relationship of Lymphatic System to Other Systems

Developmental, Cultural, and Ethnic Variations

Infants and Children

The lymphatic system begins developing at about 20 weeks gestation. The first few months after birth, an infant's ability to produce antibodies is still immature, so he or she is more vulnerable to infection and relies on the mother's immunity. Lymphoid tissue is abundant in infants, increases especially between ages 6 and 10, and then regresses to adult levels by puberty. The thymus grows rapidly from birth to age 2, and then slows down, reaching its greatest weight at puberty. Afterward, involution begins to occur until the thymus becomes a rudimentary organ in adulthood. The palatine tonsils are larger during early childhood than after puberty. The lymph nodes have the same distribution in children as in adults.

Like the cardiovascular system, the PV system becomes very similar to an adult's early in fetal life. The fetal circulation compensates for the nonfunctional fetal lung, with the right ventricle pumping blood through the patent ductus arteriosus rather than into the lungs. In the fetus, both ventricles are equal in weight because they both pump blood into the systemic circulation.

At birth, both the ductus arteriosus and the interatrial foramen ovale close, causing pressure to rise in the left atrium. Demand on the right ventricle changes as the pulmonary circulation becomes established. Demand also changes on the left ventricle, which now assumes total responsibility for the systemic circulation. These changes increase the size of the left ventricle, and by age 1 year, the relative size of both ventricles approximates the adult ratio of 2:1. The arterial pressure on the first day after birth averages about 70/50 mm Hg, increasing slowly over the next several months to about 90/60 mm Hg. Then it rises very slowly until the adult pressure of 120/80 mm Hg is reached at adolescence.

Pregnant Women

The immunologic processes that allow a woman to tolerate the implantation and development of a fetus are not fully understood. For unknown reasons, during the first and second trimesters of pregnancy, the leukocyte count gradually increases and IgG concentrations decrease slightly. Maternal host defenses are altered because of reduced chemotaxis (the movement of neutrophils toward the infection site) and cause a delay in initial maternal responses to infection.

Systemic vascular resistance decreases with pregnancy, and peripheral vasodilatation occurs. This may lead to palmar erythema, an inflammatory redness of the palms, and to spider telangiectasis, a spiderlike image on the skin caused by a branched group of dilated capillary blood vessels. Blood pressure decreases during the second trimester and may rise thereafter to the prepregnancy level. Generally, an increase in blood pressure of more than 30 mm Hg systolic or 15 mm Hg diastolic over prepregnancy levels is cause for concern and may indicate preeclampsia, a hypertensive condition of pregnancy involving many systems and affecting primarily the vasculature, kidneys, liver, and brain.

Older Adults

The number and size of lymph nodes decrease with advancing age, and some of the lymphoid elements are lost. Typically, the nodes of older patients are more likely to be fibrotic and fatty and result in impaired ability to resist infection. Degenerative changes in the vascular system occur as part of the normal aging process. Fibrosis causes increased thickness in the intimal wall. Wall stiffness is caused by an accumulation of collagen and calcium in the intima and media. Elastic fibers of the media become thin and calcified. These changes dramatically decrease the flexibility and elasticity of the vessels and increase PV resistance. Decreased venous elasticity increases the risk of varicosities, and increased PV resistance usually elevates blood pressure. Throughout life, damage to the endothelium reduces its ability to protect the PV system and leads to the development of atherosclerotic plaques.

People of Different Cultures or Ethnic Groups

Although socioeconomic and environmental factors may play a part, certain diseases of the PV and lymphatic systems are more prevalent in certain cultural groups. For example:

- Hypertension (HTN) is the most serious health problem for African-Americans. There is also a high incidence of HTN in Puerto Ricans, Cubans, and Mexican-Americans. One-sixth of the Iranian population has HTN, with stress as a major contributing factor.
- Navajo Native Americans have a high incidence of severe combined immunodeficiency syndrome (SCIDS), failure of antibody response, and cell-mediated immunity, unrelated to AIDS.
- African-Americans account for 13 percent of the population in the United States, but they account for 30 percent of AIDS cases.

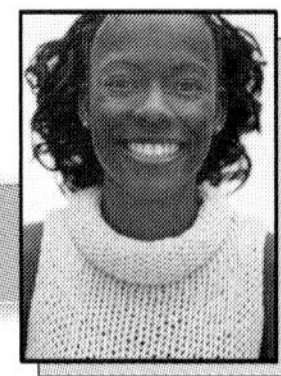

Introducing the Case Study

Tasha Jordan is a 38-year-old African-American woman who reports increasing pain and tenderness in her left leg since she delivered a premature baby 1 week ago. She describes the pain as dull and throbbing, and says that it gets worse when she stands and walks and gets better with rest and elevation. She also has noticed swelling in the leg. Aspirin has not relieved her symptoms. She has felt more tired than usual. Her past medical history is unremarkable. She is a smoker with a family history of cardiac disease. She had prolonged bed rest before delivery.

Performing the PV and Lymphatic Systems Assessment

Health History

Assessment of the PV and lymphatic systems includes a comprehensive health history that provides the framework for an accurate physical examination. If the client's medical records are available, review them before starting the interview. Medical records can help you identify areas that need further exploration, but they are never a substitute for obtaining a health history directly from the client.

Biographical Data

The incidence of PV disease increases with age. Most clients are over age 45. The incidence of hypertension also increases with age. Risk factors for vascular disease may differ according to sex and race. In men, half of all new cases occur in the fifth decade of life, but in women the disease occurs much later. By the seventh decade, prevalence is similar in both sexes. White women have a slightly higher incidence of vascular disease than African-American women. Infection in the lymphatic system can occur at any age.

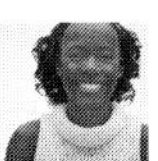

Case Study Findings

Reviewing Mrs. Jordan's biographical data:

- 38-year-old African-American female, married, one child.
- Works full-time as a secretary.
- Born and raised in the United States, Baptist religion.
- High school graduate, interested in attending community college when her baby gets older.
- Healthcare insurance, PPO, through husband's work plan.
- Husband is a firefighter.
- Referral: Private practice, internal medicine office.
- Source: Self, seems nervous but reliable.

Current Health Status

Begin your assessment by asking for the person's chief complaint. Because the assessment of the PV and lymphatic systems covers a wide range of possible symptoms, you may need to ask which symptom is the most bothersome. Major vascular symptoms to watch for are swelling, limb pain, and changes in sensation of an extremity. Always ask about fever, fatigue, and lumps when evaluating the lymphatic system.

Symptom Analysis

Symptom Analysis tables for all of the symptoms described in the following paragraphs are available on the Web for viewing and printing. In your web browser, go to http://www.fadavis.com/detail.cfm?id=802-9 and click on Symptom Analysis Tables under Explore This Product.

Swelling

Swelling (edema) can be generalized or localized, acute or chronic. It occurs when fluid accumulates in tissue because of increased cellular permeability. This results in increased capillary pressure and can be caused by venous obstruction, heart failure, renal disease, lymphatic obstruction, decreased plasma proteins, inflammatory conditions, fluid and electrolyte imbalance (especially an excess of sodium), malnutrition, bacterial toxins, venoms, caustic substances, and histamine.

Limb Pain

Limb pain associated with vascular or lymphatic problems may be associated with a chronic condition or be a signal of a more serious acute problem that requires immediate medical attention. Pain associated with venous or arterial vascular problems is often accompanied by other signs and symptoms.

Changes in Sensation

Paresthesia is a change in sensation such as numbness, tingling, pins and needles, or burning. It may be neurological in nature, but it can also be caused by vascular problems. Paresthesia can be acute or chronic, temporary or permanent.

Fatigue

Fatigue is the seventh most common complaint in primary care. Fatigue is a normal response to overexertion, but it can also be the presenting symptom of almost any disease. A thorough history and physical examination will establish the cause in about 85 percent of all patients.

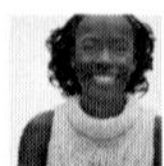

Case Study Findings

Mrs. Jordan's current health status includes:

- Six-day history of dull, aching pain and tenderness in left leg that is progressively getting worse.
- Pain is worse when standing and walking and is minimally relieved by rest and elevation.
- Aspirin has not helped.
- Denies chest pain or shortness of breath.

Past Health History

The past health history can provide direct links to your client's present health status. Look for data that may affect the PV and lymphatic systems.

Past Health History

RISK FACTORS/ QUESTIONS TO ASK	RATIONALE/SIGNIFICANCE
Childhood Illnesses	
Did you ever have Hodgkin's lymphoma, acute lymphocytic leukemia, or sarcoma?	These cancers frequently occur in children, who often receive bone marrow suppression drugs or radiation.
Surgery	
Have you ever had surgery?	May explain physical findings.
If so, when and what type?	Surgery exerts a negative effect on immune system. Splenectomy increases risk for disseminated infection. Mastectomy with lymph node removal can cause lymphedema.
Hospitalizations/Diagnostic Procedures	
Were you ever hospitalized for peripheral-vascular disease (PVD) or lymphatic disorders?	Use previous hospitalizations as a comparative.
Did you receive a blood transfusion before 1985?	Blood was not routinely screened for HIV before 1985. Transfusions can also cause other infectious disorders such as hepatitis B.
Serious Injuries	
Have you ever had trauma to your spleen?	The spleen is very vulnerable to blunt abdominal trauma and may rupture.
Serious/Chronic Illnesses	
Do you have any other medical problems, such as cardiac or renal disease, cancer, hypertension, diabetes, AIDS, or autoimmune diseases such as systemic lupus erythematosus (SLE) or rheumatoid arthritis (RA)?	All these diseases may have PV or lymphatic symptoms. *Hypertension:* Doubles risk of symptomatic peripheral artery occlusive disease. *Diabetes mellitus:* Damages blood vessels and accelerates atherogenesis. *Autoimmune diseases:* Increase risk for other diseases.
Immunizations	
What immunizations have you had? Are they up to date?	Up-to-date immunizations can prevent many communicable diseases.
Allergies	
Do you have allergies or asthma?	Allergies reflect immune system function. Asthma may indicate immunopathology.

Past Health History

RISK FACTORS/ QUESTIONS TO ASK	RATIONALE/SIGNIFICANCE
Medications	
Are you taking any medications?	*Antihypertensives, anticoagulants:* Determines compliance with treatment; therapeutic vs. toxic effects. OTC medications: May alter affects of prescribed medications. *Steroids:* Cause immunosuppression.
Are you taking birth control pills?	*Birth control pills:* Increases risk for thrombus formation.
Are you on chemotherapy?	*Chemotherapy:* May suppress the immune system and lower platelet counts. See box, Drugs That Adversely Affect the Lymphatic System, page 418.
Recent Travel/Military Service/ Exposure to Infectious or Contagious Diseases	
Have you been in the military service?	Exposure to certain chemicals or toxins may affect the immune system.

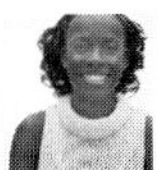

Case Study Findings

Mrs. Jordan's past health history reveals:

- Delivered premature baby 1 week ago.
- Prolonged bedrest (2 months) before delivery.
- No history of surgery. Hospitalized only for childbirth. Uncomplicated vaginal delivery; baby's gestational age is 31 weeks.
- Gained 50 lb during pregnancy.
- No history of chronic illness.
- Denies prescribed drugs.
- Has smoked 1 pack of cigarettes a day for 22 years (22 pack-years).

Family History

The family history identifies any causative factors that may lead to problems with the PV or lymphatic system. There are no known familial relationships for diseases of the lymphatic system. The cause of lymphomas, lymphosarcomas, and cancer of the lymph glands is unknown.

Family History

RISK FACTORS/ QUESTIONS TO ASK	RATIONALE/SIGNIFICANCE
Familial/Genetically Linked PV Disorders	
Does anyone in your family have heart disease, arteriosclerosis, stroke, hypertension, or hyperlipidemia?	Increases risk for PVD. Indicates need for risk factor modification.
Diabetes Mellitus	
Does anyone in your family have diabetes? If so, how old was he or she when it was diagnosed?	Diabetics are more susceptible to PVD.
Familial/Genetically Linked Lymphatic Disorders	
Is there any family history of lymphomas or leukemias?	Positive family history increases risk for malignancies.

Drugs That Adversely Affect the Lymphatic System

For information on drugs that affect the cardiovascular system, see Chapter 12, Assessing the Cardiovascular System.

Drug Class	Drug	Possible Adverse Reactions
Anticonvulsants	carbamazepine	Aplastic anemia (characterized by decreased levels of all formed elements of blood), leukopenia (decreased leukocyte levels), agranulocytosis (increased agranulocyte levels), eosinophilia (increased eosinophil levels), leukocytosis (increased leukocyte levels), thrombocytopenia (decreased thrombocyte levels)
	phenytoin	Thrombocytopenia, leukopenia, granulocytopenia (decreased granulocyte levels), pancytopenia (decreased levels of all blood cells), macrocytosis (enlarged erythrocytes), megaloblastic anemia (characterized by increased, immature, enlarged erythrocytes)
Antidiabetics	acetohexamide, chlorpropamide, glipizide, glyburide, tolbutamide	Leukopenia, thrombocytopenia, pancytopenia, agranulocytosis, aplastic anemia, hemolytic anemia (characterized by premature erythrocyte destruction)
Antihypertensives	captopril	Neutropenia (decreased neutrophil levels), agranulocytosis
	hydralazine	Positive ANA (antinuclear antibodies) titer that occurs when the immune system creates antibodies against some of the body's own cells; systemic lupus erythematosus-like syndrome
	methyldopa	Positive Coombs' test, indicating that some type of immunoglobulin coats the red blood cells
Anti-infectives	cephalosporins	Positive Coombs' test, hypothrombinemia (decreased thrombin levels), with or without bleeding
	chloramphenicol	Bone marrow depression, pancytopenia, aplastic anemia
	penicillins	Eosinophilia, hemolytic anemia, leukopenia, neutropenia, thrombocytopenia, positive Coombs' test
	pentamide isethionate	Leukopenia, thrombocytopenia
	sulfonamides	Granulocytopenia, leukopenia, eosinophilia, hemolytic anemia, aplastic anemia, thrombocytopenia, methemoglobinemia (increased levels of an oxidative compound of hemoglobin), hypoprothrombinemia (prothrombin, or Factor II, deficiency)
Antieoplastics	busulfan	Severe leukopenia, anemia, severe thrombocytopenia
	chlorambucil	Leukopenia, thrombocytopenia, anemia
	cisplatin, cyclophosphamide, doxorubicin hydorchloride	Leukopenia, granulocytopenia, thrombocytopenia, anemia
	methotrexate	Leukopenia, thrombocytopenia, anemia, hemorrhage
	mitomycin	Thrombocytopenia, leukopenia
Antipsychotic agents	chlorpromazine hydrochloride, thioridazine hydrochloride	Agranulocytosis, mild leukopenia
Cardiac agents	procainamide hydrochioride	Positive ANA titer; systemic lupus erythematosus-like syndrome
	quinidine	Thrombocytopenia, hypoprothrombinemia, acute hemolytic anemia, agranulocytosis, aplastic anemia, and leukopenia can occur as hypersensitivity reactions
Gold compounds	auranofin, gold sodium thiomalate	Leukopenia, thrombocytopenia, anemia, eosinophilia
Nonsteroidal anti-inflammatory agents	ibuprofen	Neutropenia, agranuloytosis, aplastic anemia, hemolytic anemia, thrombocytopenia, decreased hemoglobin and hematocrit
Miscellaneous agents	furosemide	Anemia, leukopenia, neutropenia, thrombocytopenia
	lithium	Leukocytosis

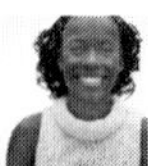

Case Study Findings

Mrs. Jordan's family history reveals:

- Mother, age 65, has HTN and is obese.
- Father, age 67, had myocardial infarction (MI) at age 50; quit smoking 17 years ago.
- All other known relatives alive and well.

Review of Systems

The review of systems (ROS) assesses the interrelationship of the PV and lymphatic systems to every other body system. Because signs and symptoms of lymphatic disorders are typically nonspecific, a complete ROS is an essential component of your assessment.

Review of Systems

SYSTEM/QUESTIONS TO ASK	RATIONALE/SIGNIFICANCE
General Health Survey	
How have you been feeling?	
Any changes in your energy level?	*Fatigue/activity intolerance:* PV changes, infection.
Fevers? Weight changes?	*Unexplained fever, night sweats, weight loss:* AIDS or cancer involving lymphatic system.
Integumentary	
Have you noticed changes in the color of your skin, hair, or nails? Hair loss?	*Color changes/hair loss:* Chronic arterial or venous insufficiency.
Ankle swelling or tight shoes?	*Ankle swelling/tight shoes:* Fluid retention associated with PV disease or **lymphadenopathy**.
HEENT	
Do you have any lumps in your neck?	*Neck swelling or masses:* Enlarged lymph nodes associated with infection or malignancy.
Sore throat?	*Sore throat/difficulty swallowing:* Bacterial or viral infection of lymphoid tissue.
Vision problems?	*Vision problems:* PV disease such as HTN.
Respiratory	
Do you have breathing problems?	*Dyspnea with sputum production:* Respiratory infection such as pneumonia. Dyspnea is also associated with CV problems.
Cardiovascular	
Do you have cardiovascular problems?	*Color changes in fingers and toes, leg pain, ankle swelling:* PVD. *Chest pain/dyspnea:* Cardiac involvement.
Gastrointestinal	
Do you have GI complaints? Bowel changes?	*Diarrhea, abdominal tenderness and pain, weight loss:* Infections occurring with immunodeficiency disorders.
Genitourinary	
Do you have to urinate frequently, especially at night?	*Nocturia:* Congestive heart failure (CHF).
Reproductive	
Do you have reproductive/sexual performance problems?	*Impotence:* PV disease.
Do you practice safe sex?	*Unprotected sexual activity:* Increased risk for HIV.
Musculoskeletal	
Do you have limb pain on activity?	*Exercise-induced limb pain:* Peripheral arterial disease.
Limb tenderness?	*Bone tenderness:* Leukemic or immunoproliferative disorder.
Neurological	
Do you have numbness or tingling anywhere in the body?	*Paresthesia:* Arterial insufficiency.
Endocrine	
Do you have a history of diabetes or thyroid disease?	Diabetes can cause vascular changes. Hypothyroidism can cause edema.

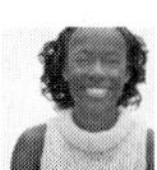

Case Study Findings

Mrs. Jordan's review of systems reveals:

- **General Health Survey:** General health good, feeling tired since delivery of baby.
- **Integumentary:** Inflammation and swelling of left calf.
- **HEENT:** Head/neck: No swelling or masses, no sore throat.
- **Respiratory:** No breathing problems.
- **Cardiovascular:** No chest pain.
- **Gastrointestinal:** No complaints, daily bowel movement.
- **Genitourinary:** No nocturia since delivery of baby.
- **Reproductive:** Has not been sexually active for about 3 months because of complications of pregnancy. No problems before this. Plans to bottle-feed baby.
- **Musculoskeletal:** Tenderness in left calf.
- **Neurological:** No numbness, tingling, or loss of sensation.
- **Endocrine:** No history of thyroid disease or diabetes

Psychosocial Profile

The psychosocial profile reveals patterns in the client's life that may affect the health of his or her PV and lymphatic systems. It may also help determine the cause of a particular health concern. Assessing the lifestyle may identify specific health maintenance educational needs.

Psychosocial Profile

CATEGORY/QUESTIONS TO ASK	RATIONALE/SIGNIFICANCE
Health Practices and Beliefs/ Self-Care Activities	
Do you have regular health checkups? Do you know the risk factors for PVD (e.g., high-fat diet, protein-deficient diet, smoking, lack of exercise)?	May identify screening for risk factors and teaching needs.
Typical Day	
Can you describe your typical day?	Fatigue and limb pain may limit ability to perform ADLs.
Nutritional Patterns	
What did you eat in the last 24 hours?	Protein-deficient diets can cause edema. High-fat diet is risk factor for PVD.
Has your weight changed recently?	Weight loss seen with cancer and AIDS; weight gain seen with edema. Obesity is risk factor for cardiovascular (CV) disease.
Activity/Exercise Patterns	
Do you exercise? What type of activity?	Exercise decreases risk for CV disease. Arterial insufficiency can cause intermittent claudication with exercise.
Pets/Hobbies	
Do you have any pets? Do any of your hobbies involve using chemicals?	Pets and hobbies can enhance mental well-being if they do not compromise immunocompetence.
Sleep/Rest Patterns	
How many hours of sleep do you get a night?	Pain can interrupt sleep.
Personal Habits	
Do you or did you ever use tobacco? If so, in what form and how much?	Smoking is a major risk factor for vascular disease.
Do you drink alcohol?	Regular consumption of three or more drinks a day increases risk of hypertension and decreases immune competence.
Do you use street drugs?	Intravenous drug use may transmit infectious diseases like hepatitis and HIV.
Occupational Health Patterns	
What type of work do you do?	Prolonged sitting or standing and exposure to temperature extremes may contribute to circulatory problems.

compare the contralateral side of the body. Also ensure your client's privacy and comfort.

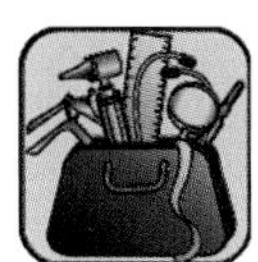

Toolbox

The tools for the PV and lymphatic systems include a stethoscope, sphygmomanometer, flashlight, ruler, and nonstretchable tape measure.

Performing a General Survey

Before examining specific areas, scan the client from head to toe, looking for general appearance and signs of PV and lymphatic system dysfunction. For example:

- Be alert for signs of an acute illness, such as grimacing, pallor, or diaphoresis, or of a chronic problem, such as wasting or listlessness.
- Check appearance against chronological age. Does the person look older than his or her stated age? Chronic autoimmune diseases can "age" a person.
- Observe for edema, which is associated with PV or lymphatic disease.
- Observe posture. Abnormal posture, gait, and movements may signal an autoimmune disease such as rheumatoid arthritis.
- Check vital signs. Elevated temperature may indicate an infection, changes in blood pressure and pulse may indicate a CV problem.

Performing a Head-to-Toe Physical Assessment

Next, look for changes in every system that might signal a PV or lymphatic system problem.

Performing a Head-to-Toe Physical Assessment

SYSTEM/NORMAL FINDINGS	ABNORMAL FINDINGS/RATIONALE
General Survey *INSPECT* Awake, alert, and oriented to time, place, and person. Affect appropriate.	Changes in mental status may indicate impaired cerebral circulation or an autoimmune disease such as SLE, which can cause mental status changes, including depression or even psychosis.
Integumentary *INSPECT/PALPATE* ***Skin*** Skin color varies with client's ethnicity. Texture smooth and skin intact with no lesions.	*Cyanosis:* Impaired circulation. *Pallor or rubor:* Vascular problems. *Thin, shiny skin:* Arterial insufficiency *Thick, leathery skin:* Venous insufficiency. *Rash:* Immune disorders such as the butterfly rash of SLE. *Poor wound healing:* Vascular insufficiency or immune deficiency.
Hair Even hair distribution.	*Alopecia and short broken hair above forehead:* SLE. *Decreased hair on extremities:* Arterial insufficiency.
HEENT *INSPECT, PALPATE* Oral and nasal mucosa pink, moist, and intact without lesions.	*Pale nasal mucosa, boggy turbinates:* Chronic allergies.

(Continued)

Performing a Head-to-Toe Physical Assessment *(Continued)*

SYSTEM/NORMAL FINDINGS	ABNORMAL FINDINGS/RATIONALE
HEENT *(Continued)* *INSPECT, PALPATE*	
Tonsils pink; gum pink and intact with no bleeding.	*Enlarged, red, inflamed tonsils with exudates:* Infection.
No masses or nodes.	*Oral lesions (e.g., lacy leukoplakia):* AIDS.
Thyroid not palpable.	*Bleeding gums:* Leukemia. *Enlarged nodes:* Infection or malignancy. *Enlarged thyroid:* Chronic thyroiditis (Hashimoto's), an autoimmune disorder.
Eye clear and bright, vision and hearing intact	*Ptosis, extraocular movement deficits:* Myasthenia gravis. *Decreased auditory function:* May occur with Hashimoto's.
Respiratory *AUSCULTATE*	
Lungs clear	Adventitious sounds such as wheezes associated with asthma or allergic responses.
Cardiovascular *AUSCULTATE*	
Regular heart rate/rhythm. PMI 1 cm at apex. No extra sounds.	Enlarged, displaced PMI associated with ventricular hypertrophy such as occurs with HTN.
Gastrointestinal *INSPECT/PALPATE/AUSCULTATE*	
Positive bowel sounds; abdomen soft, nontender, no organomegaly.	*Hyperactive bowel sounds:* Ulcerative colitis, an autoimmune disorder. *Hypoactive bowel sounds:* Scleroderma, an autoimmune disorder. *Enlarged liver:* Infection, CV problem, immune disorder, malignancy. *Enlarged spleen:* Infection or cancer.
Genitourinary *INSPECT/PALPATE*	
External genitalia pink, intact, no lesions	*Lesions:* Associated with STDs and may cause lymphadenopathy.
Musculoskeletal *INSPECT/PALPATE*	
Full ROM in joints, no deformities or tenderness, +5 muscle strength	*Joint pain, deformity, limited ROM, muscle weakness:* PVD, MS, or autoimmune disorder such as rheumatoid arthritis.
Neurological *INSPECT/PALPATE*	
	Decreased sensation: Vascular insufficiency.
Sensory intact, +2 DTR	*Decreased DTR:* Peripheral neuropathies.

AREA/SYSTEM	SUBJECTIVE DATA
General	*Ask about:* Fatigue Fevers Weight changes
Integumentary	*Ask about:* Skin lesions, rashes Hair loss Tight shoes
HEENT	*Ask about:* Mouth lesions Bleeding gums Sore throat
Respiratory	*Ask about:* History of asthma, allergies
Cardiovascular	*Ask about:* Chest pain History of murmurs
Gastrointestinal	*Ask about:* GI complaints History of abdominal trauma
Genitourinary/ Reproductive	*Ask about:* UTIs Safe sex practices STDs
Musculoskeletal	*Ask about:* Weakness Joint pain
Neurological	*Ask about:* Changes in mental status Loss of sensation

AREA/SYSTEM	OBJECTIVE DATA
General	*Inspect:* Signs of distress *Measure:* Vital signs Weight
Integumentary	*Inspect:* Skin lesions Hair distribution Edema
HEENT	*Inspect:* Oral mucosa, gums, tonsils Nasal mucosa
Respiratory	*Auscultate:* Adventitious breath sounds
Cardiovascular	*Auscultate:* Heart sounds Murmurs, rubs
Gastrointestinal	*Palpate:* Organs for enlargement
Genitourinary/ Reproductive	*Inspect:* Discharge STDs, lesions
Musculoskeletal	*Palpate:* Muscle strength Joints
Neurological	*Test:* Mental status Sensation

Assessment of the Lymphatic System's Relationship to Other Systems

Case Study Findings

Before you proceed to a focused PV and lymphatic system assessment, document what you learned during Mrs. Jordan's general survey and head-to-toe assessment.

Mrs. Jordan's physical assessment findings include:

- **General Health Survey:** Well-developed 41-year-old female, appears stated age. Posture relaxed, sitting upright. Guarding left leg. Alert, cooperative, responding appropriately.
- **Vital Signs:** Temperature 99.8°F; pulse 90 BPM, strong and regular; respirations 20/min, unlabored; BP 140/70;height 5 ft 1 in; weight 160 lb.
- **Integumentary:** Skin intact, no lesions.
- **HEENT:** Thyroid not palpable; vision and hearing intact; EOM intact; mucous membranes and tonsils pink; no lesions, palpable nodes, or masses.
- **Respiratory:** Lungs clear.
- **Cardiovascular:** Regular heart rate/rhythm, no extra sounds.
- **Gastrointestinal:** Positive bowel sounds, abdomen soft and nontender, no organomegaly.
- **Genitourinary:** No lesions on external genitalia. Small amount of pink lochia serosa.
- **Musculoskeletal:** Decreased ROM left lower extremity, calf warm and tender, positive Homans' sign.
- **Neurological:** Sensory intact, positive deep tendon reflex.

Performing a Focused Physical Assessment

Now that you have looked at the relationship of the PV and lymphatic systems to all other systems, focus on the specifics of the examination. Begin with inspection of the veins and lymph nodes, and then proceed to palpation and auscultation. The client should be sitting for most of the assessment and be supine only for palpation of the pulses of the lower extremities. Palpation of the lymph nodes and pulses is essential. For best results, use the pads of your index and middle fingers. Always palpate gently, beginning with light pressure and gradually increasing it.

Inspection

Begin with inspection. Work from head to toe, inspecting the head and neck, upper extremities, abdomen, and lower extremities. For information on inspecting the neck, see Chapter 9, Assessing the Head, Face, and Neck, and Chapter 12, Assessing the Cardiovascular System.

Inspecting the Veins and Lymph Nodes

ASSESS/NORMAL VARIATIONS	ABNORMAL FINDINGS/ATIONALE
Upper Extremities 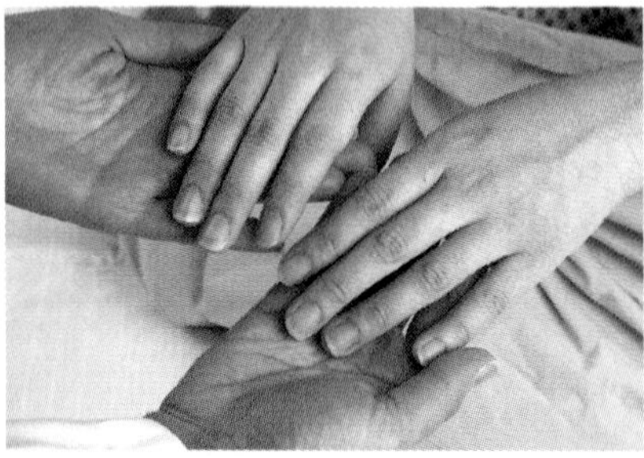 Inspecting the hands 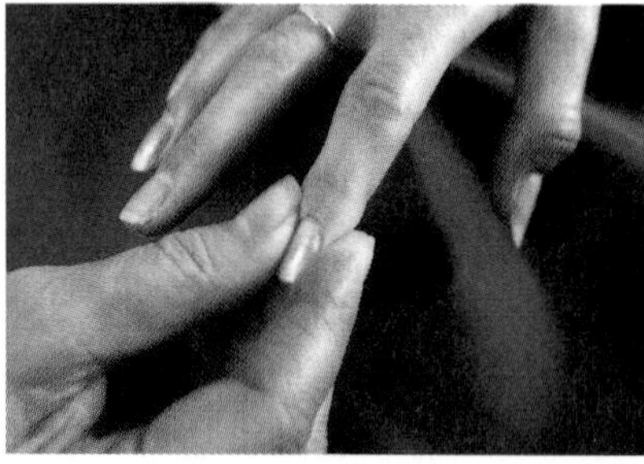 Checking capillary refill	*Delayed capillary refill time:* Arterial occlusion, hypovolemic shock, hypothermia.
Skin color uniform. Fingernails of equal thickness. Positive brisk capillary refill less than 2 to 3 seconds.	Capillary refill time may also be delayed by environmental influences such as decreased ambient temperature, suggesting a problem that may not exist.
No edema, erythema, red streaks, or skin lesions.	*Edema:* Cellulitis, lymphedema, venous obstruction (thrombophlebitis). *Intermittent pallor and cyanosis of hands and fingers:* Episodic constriction of peripheral small arteries or arterioles caused by Raynaud's phenomenon or

Inspecting the Veins and Lymph Nodes

ASSESS/NORMAL VARIATIONS	ABNORMAL FINDINGS/ATIONALE
Upper Extremities *(Continued)*	Raynaud's disease (a condition in which digital arteries respond excessively to vasospastic stimuli). Constriction causes hyperemia and rubor (redness). *Ischemic changes and gangrene of hands and fingers:* Buerger's disease (thromboangiitis obliterans). *Streaky redness, tenderness, warmth along course of a vein:* Thrombophlebitis
Abdomen 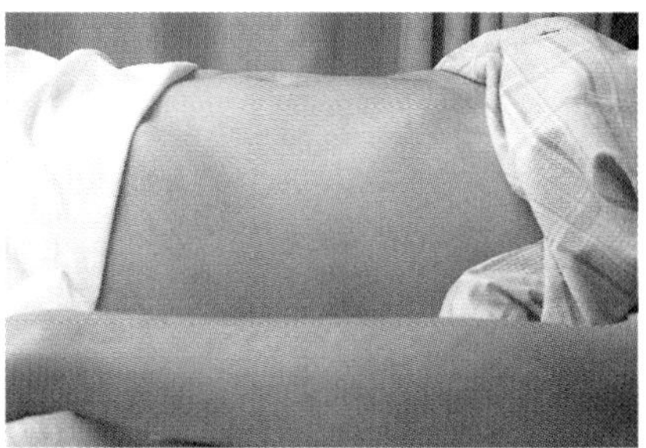 **Inspecting the abdomen**	*Tense, shiny abdominal skin:* Ascites or edema
Abdominal contour flat, concave, or round. Abdominal veins barely visible. Veins flowing upward above and downward below umbilicus. Arterial pulsations at midline over aorta in thin adults.	*Upward or centrifugal venous flow:* Inferior vena cava obstruction or portal hypertension. *Visible, large, diffuse pulsations:* Aneurysm (For more information, see Chapter 15, Assessing the Abdomen.)
Lower Extremities Leg hair distributed evenly. Older clients may have thinner, drier skin with less leg hair and altered pigmentation.	*Hair loss:* Arterial insufficiency. *Eczema, stasis dermatitis:* Chronic venous insufficiency
No varicosities or only superficial ones. 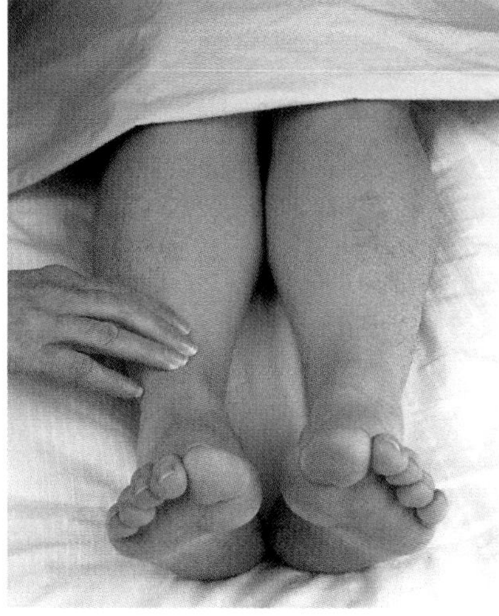 **Inspecting the legs** 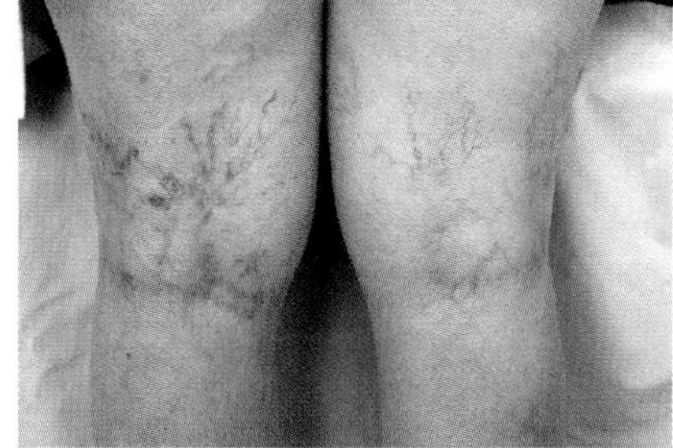 **Superficial varicosities**	*Prominent leg veins, possibly with ropelike, dilated appearance or purplish spiderlike appearance:* Chronic venous insufficiency.

(Continued)

Inspecting the Veins and Lymph Nodes *(Continued)*

ASSESS/NORMAL VARIATIONS	ABNORMAL FINDINGS/ATIONALE

Lower Extremities *(Continued)*

HELPFUL HINT

Have client stand when assessing for varicosities so that veins are more prominent.

No swelling or edema.

Edema: Injury, cellulitis, venous/lymph obstruction, thrombophlebitis, varicosities.

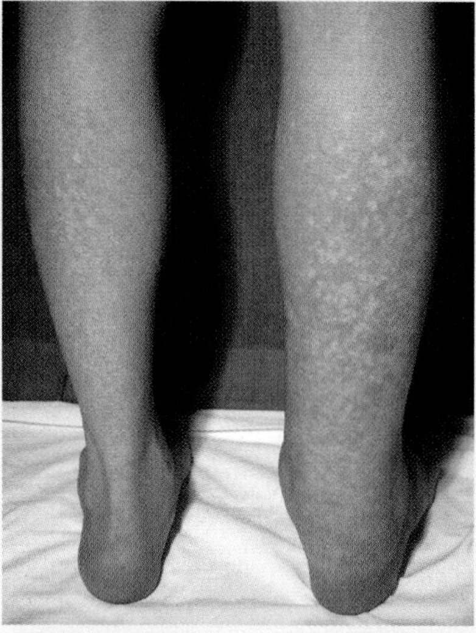

Lymphedema

No lesions or ulcers.

Skin ulcers: Trauma or venous/arterial insufficiency.

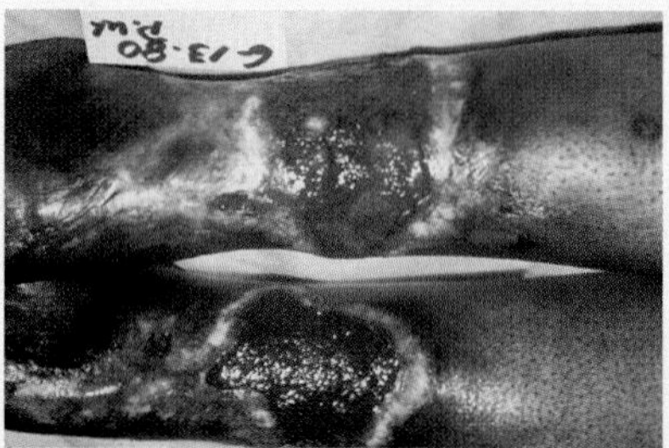

Venous stasis ulcer

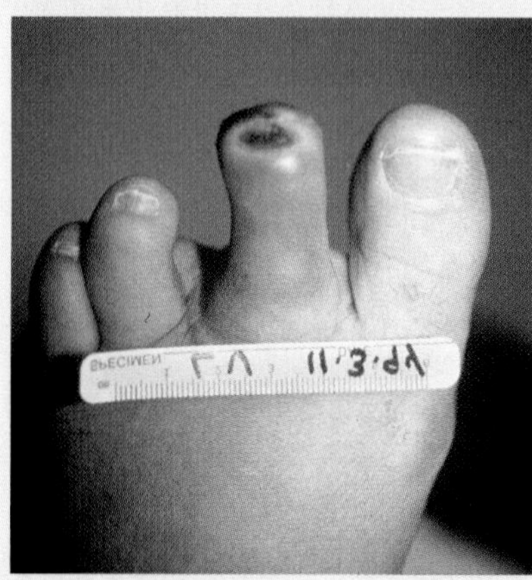

Arterial insufficiency

ASSESSING EDEMA

To assess edema, press your index finger over the bony prominence of the tibia or medial malleolus. Orthostatic (pitting) edema results in a depression that does not rapidly refill and resume its original contour. It is not usually accompanied by thickening or pigmentation of the overlying skin. The severity of edema can be graded on a scale of +1 to +4.

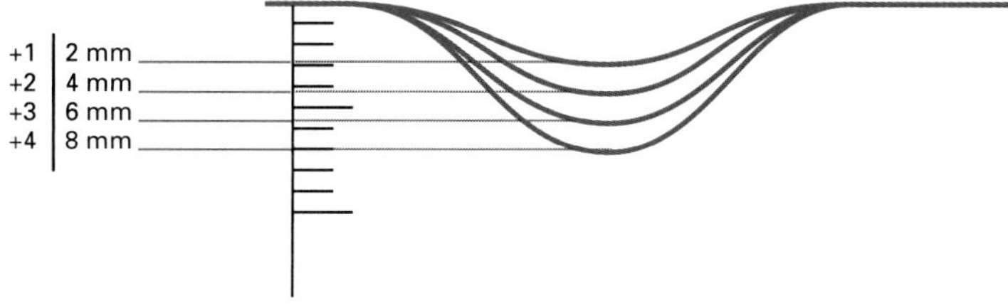

- +1: Slight pitting with about 2-mm depression that disappears rapidly. No visible distortion of extremity.
- +2: Deeper pitting with about 4-mm depression that disappears in 10 to 15 seconds. No visible distortion of extremity.
- +3: Depression of about 6 mm that lasts more than a minute. Dependent extremity looks swollen.
- +4: Very deep pitting with about 8-mm depression that lasts 2 to 3 minutes. Dependent extremity is grossly distorted.

HELPFUL HINT

- If edema is unilateral, suspect occlusion of a major vein. If edema occurs without pitting, suspect arterial disease and occlusion. Arterial insufficiency may occur without edema.
- Because arteries are elastic, if you push them into soft tissue, you will have trouble palpating the pulse. So try to palpate arteries over bone.

Palpation

Certain parts of your hands and fingers are better than others for specific types of palpation. When evaluating pulses, use the distal pads of your second and third fingers. Palpate firmly but not so hard that you occlude the artery. If you have trouble finding a pulse, vary your pressure, feeling carefully at the correct anatomical location. Be sure you are not feeling your own pulse. Assess pulses for rate, rhythm, equality, amplitude, and elasticity. Pulse amplitude should be described on a scale of 0 to 4 as follows:

- 0 = absent, not palpable
- 1 = diminished, barely palpable
- 2 = normal, expected
- 3 = full, increased
- 4 = bounding

For more information, see Chapter 12, Assessing the Cardiovascular System.

To palpate lymph nodes, use the pads of your second, third, and fourth fingers, and gently palpate for superficial nodes. Be sure to note the size, shape, symmetry, consistency, delineation, mobility, tenderness, sensation, and condition of overlying skin. In areas where the skin is more mobile, move it over the area of the nodes. Press gently at first, adding pressure gradually. If you find enlarged lymph nodes, explore adjacent areas and regions drained by those nodes for signs of possible infection or malignancy. The following section shows how to palpate the head and neck and upper and lower extremities. For more information on palpation, see Chapter 9, Assessing the Head, Face, and Neck, Chapter 14, Assessing the Breasts, and Chapter 15, Assessing the Abdomen.

Auscultation

Auscultate the pulses in the head, neck, upper extremities, and abdomen, and check blood pressure.

Palpating the Pulses and Lymph Nodes

ASSESS/NORMAL VARIATIONS

Head and Neck Pulses

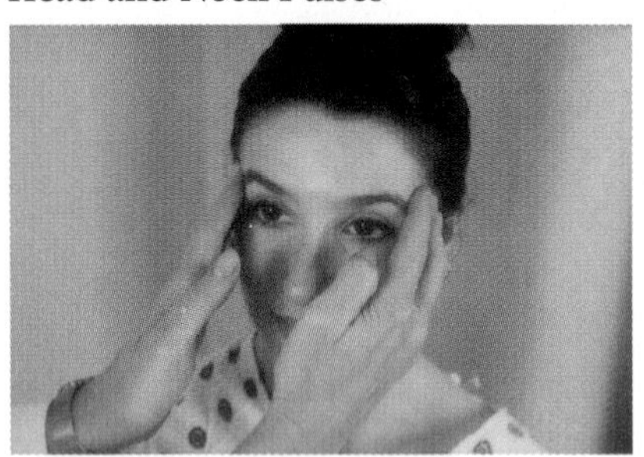

Palpating the temporal artery

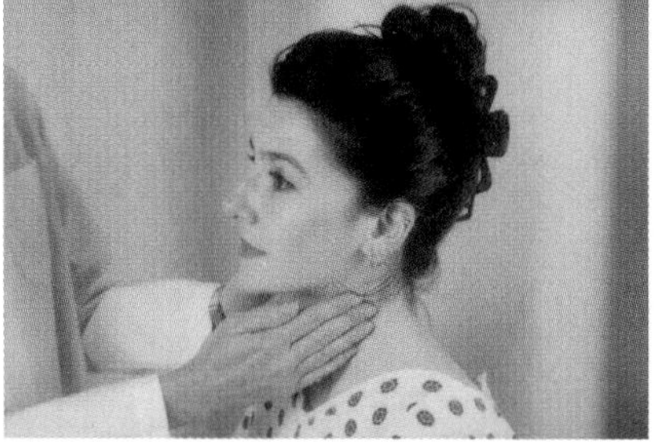

Palpating the carotid artery

Temporal and carotid arteries are regular, smooth, and +2 bilaterally.

Neck Lymph Nodes

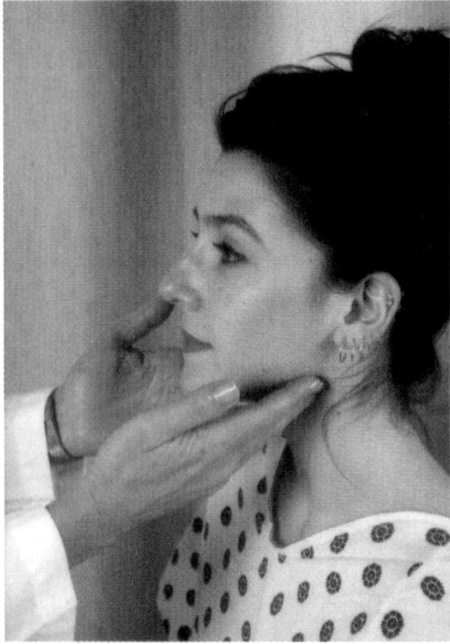

Palpating the cervical lymph nodes

Cervical nodes are nonpalpable.

Upper Extremity Pulses

Skin temperature is warm bilaterally.

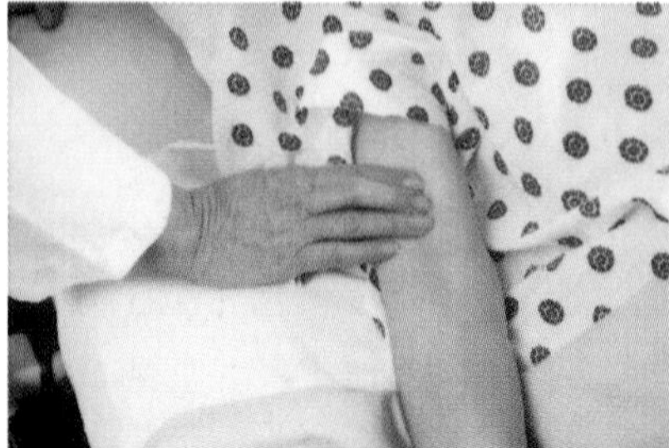

Palpating the brachial pulse

ABNORMAL FINDINGS/RATIONALE

Alterations in pulse rate/rhythm: Cardiac arrhythmia.

Absent pulse: Arterial occlusion.

Tender, palpable lymph nodes: Recent infection.

Large, well-defined nodes: Acute infection.

Less defined node borders: Chronic infection.

Firm, enlarged, nontender, immobile nodes: Malignancy.

Involvement of three or more node groups (generalized lymphadenopathy): Autoimmune disease or neoplasm.

(For more information on assessing lymph nodes in the head and neck, see Chapter 9, Assessing the Head, Face, and Neck.)

Cool extremities: Decreased circulation, vasoconstriction, Raynaud's disease, Buerger's disease, response to cold external temperature.

Absent pulse, pallor, pain, or paresthesias of distal upper extremities: Arterial occlusion.

Palpating the Pulses and Lymph Nodes

ASSESS/NORMAL VARIATIONS | **ABNORMAL FINDINGS/RATIONALE**

Upper Extremity Pulses *(Continued)*

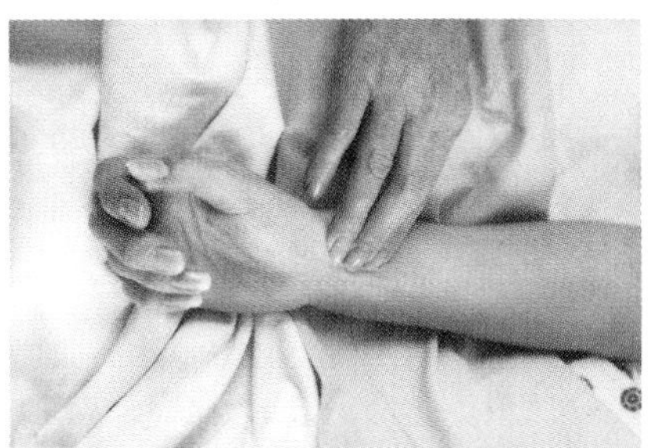

Palpating the radial pulse

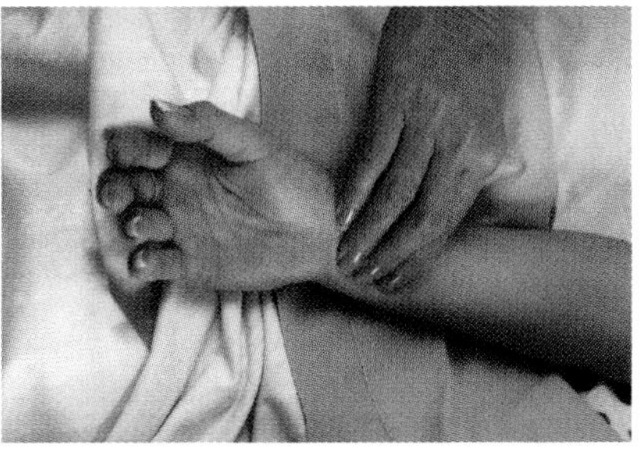

Palpating the ulnar pulse

Brachial, radial, ulnar pulses are easily palpated and equal in strength and amplitude bilaterally.

Ulnar artery may be difficult to palpate.

Unequal pulses: Arterial narrowing or obstruction on one side.

Upper Extremity Lymph Nodes

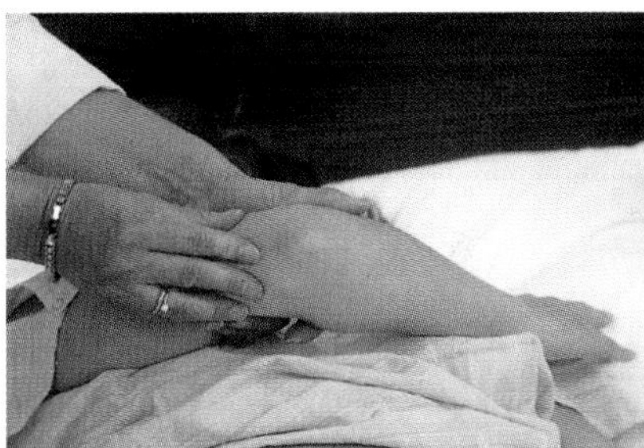

Palpating the epitrochlear nodes

Infraclavicular, axillary, and epitrochlear nodes are either nonpalpable or small, soft, mobile, and nontender. See Chapter 14, Assessing the Breasts.

Extremity swelling, along with pallor or cyanosis and dilation of superficial veins: Thrombosis of axillary or subclavian veins.

Diminished or absent pulses: Arterial spasm.

Painful reddish streaks beneath skin; tender, enlarged nodes: Inflamed lymphatic vessels caused by bacterial infection.

Lower Extremity Pulses

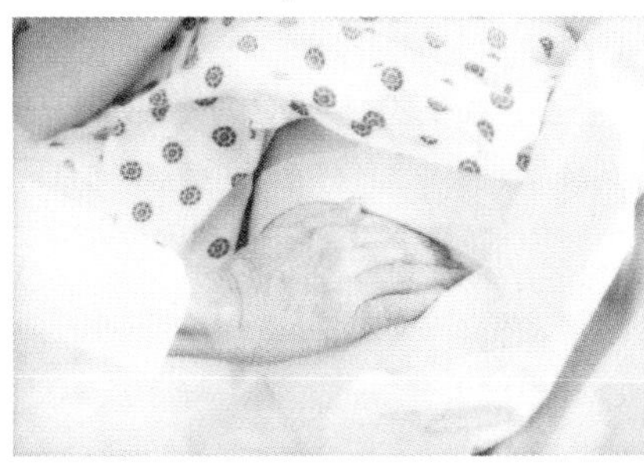

Palpating the femoral pulse

To palpate the femoral pulse, place client supine and feel below the inguinal ligament, halfway between the symphysis pubis and the anterior-superior iliac spine. Palpate in the groin crease halfway between the symphysis pubis and the anterior-superior iliac spine.

Diminished or absent pulses: Partial or complete arterial occlusion of proximal vessel, often caused by arteriosclerosis obliterans.

(Continued)

Palpating the Pulses and Lymph Nodes *(Continued)*

ASSESS/NORMAL VARIATIONS

Lower Extremity Pulses *(Continued)*

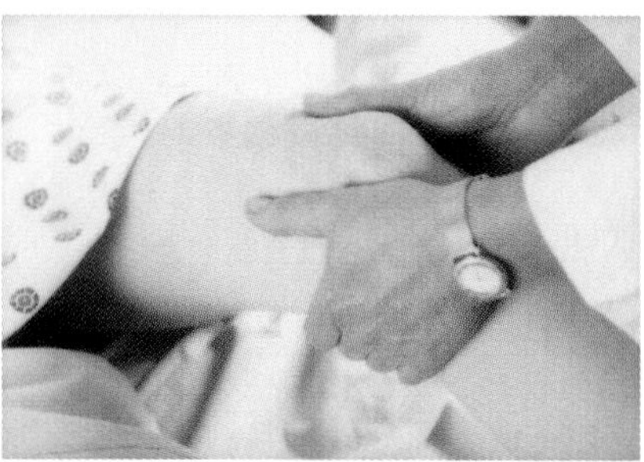

Palpating the popliteal pulse

To palpate the popliteal pulse, flex the client's knee so that his or her foot rests on the examination table. Place one hand on each side of the knee with your thumbs near the front of the patella. Curl your fingers around the knee and rest them in the popliteal fossa. If the pulse is difficult to feel, try slightly straightening the client's leg.

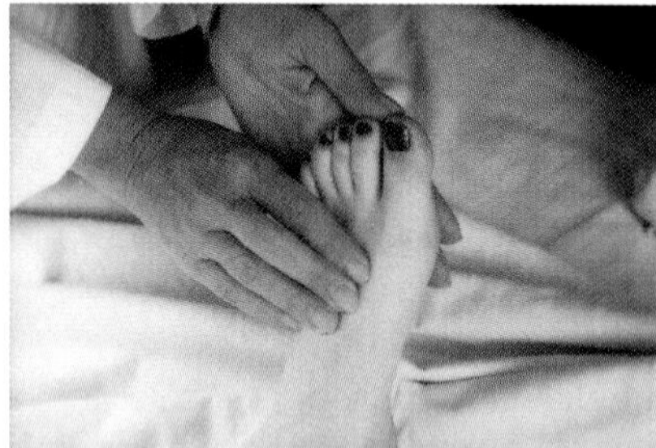

Palpating the dorsalis pedis

To palpate the dorsalis pedis pulse, place your fingers between the client's great toe and first toe and slowly move away from the toes between the extensor tendons until you feel pulse. Plantarflexing the foot may make pedal pulse easier to palpate. Pedal pulse may be congenitally absent or branch high in the ankle.

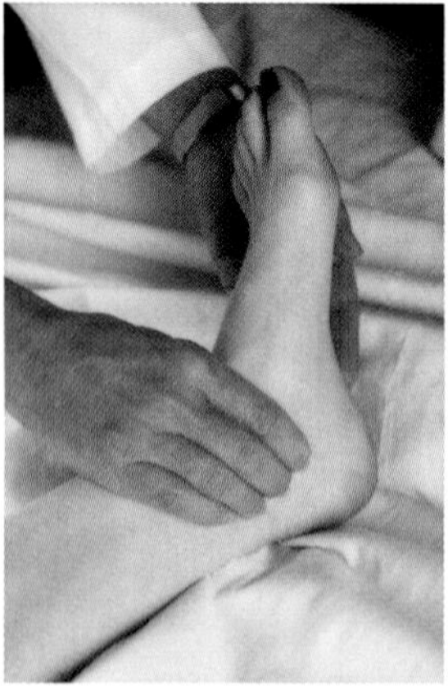

Palpating the posterior tibialis

To palpate the posterior tibial pulse, place your fingertips in the groove between the medial malleolus and the Achilles tendon, and feel for pulse. Passive dorsiflexion of the foot makes this pulse easier to palpate.

ABNORMAL FINDINGS/RATIONALE

Absent posterior tibial pulse with signs and symptoms of arterial insufficiency: Acute occlusion by thrombosis or embolus.

Increased, widened popliteal pulses: Aneurysm.

Palpating the Pulses and Lymph Nodes

ASSESS/NORMAL VARIATIONS | **ABNORMAL FINDINGS/RATIONALE**

Lower Extremity Pulses *(Continued)*

HELPFUL HINT

If you are unable to palpate a pulse, use a Doppler if available.

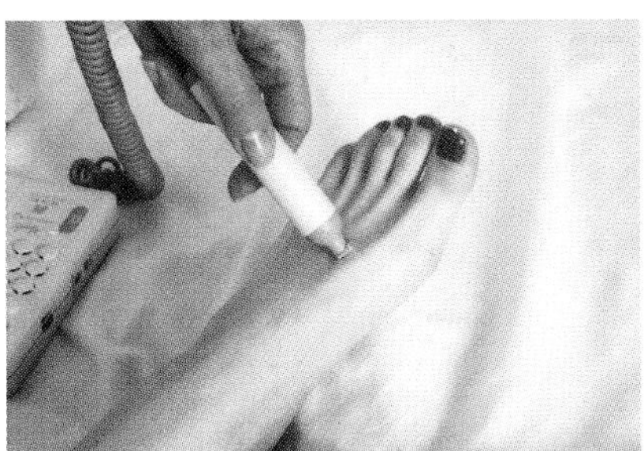

Using a Doppler

Femoral, popliteal, posterior tibial, and dorsalis pedis pulses are easily palpated and bilaterally equal in strength and amplitude. Pedal pulses may be congenitally absent.

Popliteal occlusion associated with diabetes mellitus.

Skin Temperature

ALERT

Sudden loss of peripheral pulse with cold, mottled extremity suggests arterial occlusion, a medical emergency.

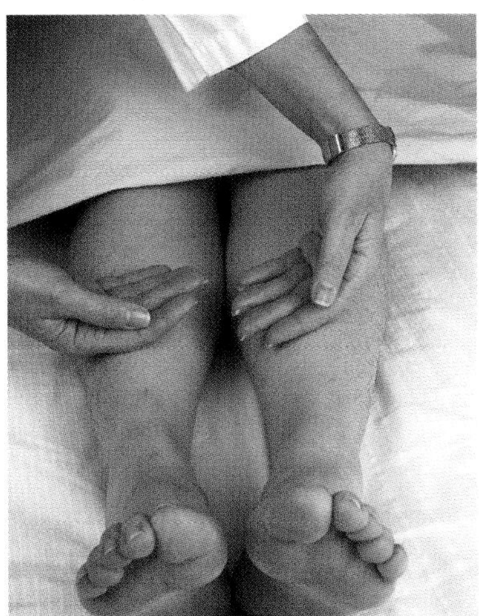

Checking skin temperature

Temperature is cool to warm.

Cold feet: Arterial insufficiency, especially if unilateral.

Calf Circumference

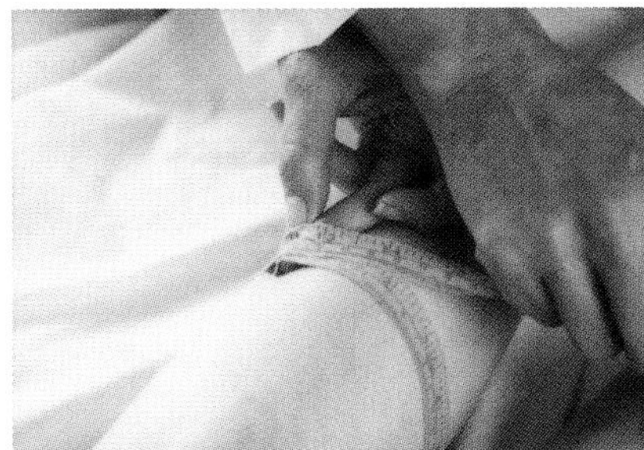

Measuring calf circumference

Leg circumferences at forefoot, above ankle, at calf, and at midthigh are equal bilaterally.

Difference in leg circumference over 1 cm above ankle or 2 cm at calf: Edema

(Continued)

Palpating the Pulses and Lymph Nodes *(Continued)*

ASSESS/NORMAL VARIATIONS	ABNORMAL FINDINGS/RATIONALE
Calf Pain 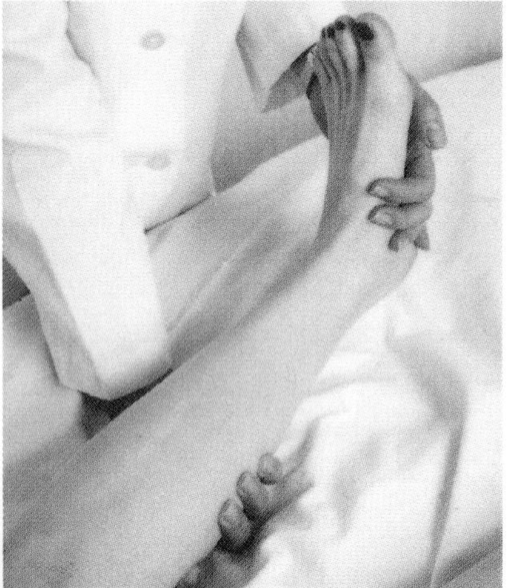 **Assessing for Homans' sign** No calf pain is present on dorsiflexion.	*Pain on dorsiflexion (Homans' sign)*: DVT (in 50% of clients). Negative sign does not rule out DVT.
Lower Extremity Lymph Nodes 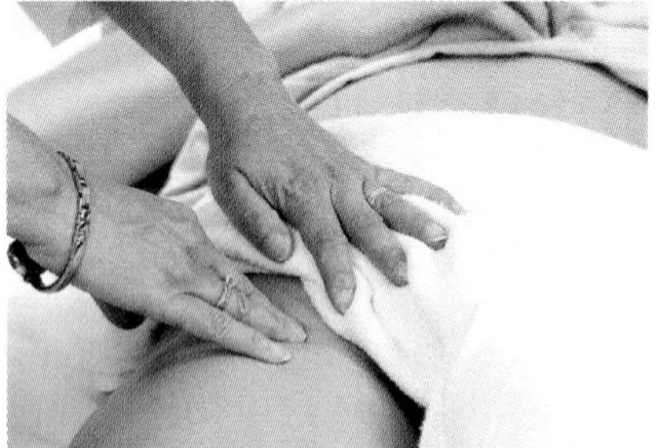 **Palpating the horizontal lymph nodes** 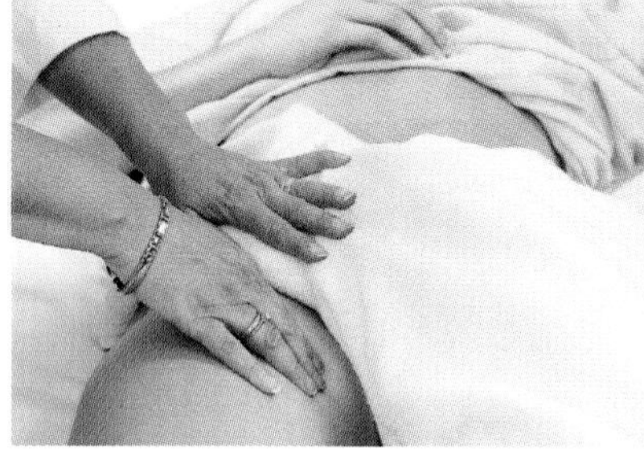 **Palpating the vertical lymph nodes** Horizontal and vertical nodes are either nonpalpable or small (0.5–1 cm), soft, mobile, and nontender.	*Enlarged or tender nodes:* Current or recent infection in abdominal or genital area. *Difference in leg circumference:* infection. *Nodes that run together (confluent)*: Chronic infection. *Unilateral discrete, nontender, firm or hard, fixed nodes:* Metastasized cancer. *Generalized lymphadenopathy (of three or more node groups)*: Autoimmune, infectious, or neoplastic disorder.

Auscultating the Pulses

ASSESS/NORMAL VARIATIONS	ABNORMAL FINDINGS/RATIONALE
Head and Neck Pulses 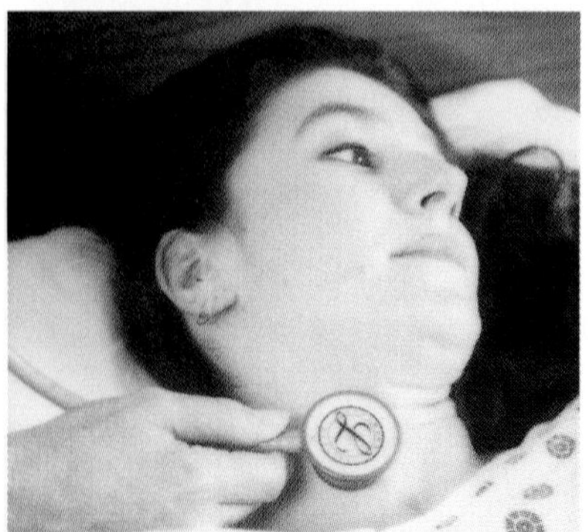 **Auscultating for bruits**	*Soft, low-pitched, rushing sound during cardiac cycle:* Bruit in temporal or carotid artery signifies narrowing of artery.

Auscultating the Pulses

ASSESS/NORMAL VARIATIONS	ABNORMAL FINDINGS/RATIONALE
Head and Neck Pulses *(Continued)* To listen to carotid arteries, place bell of stethoscope over each artery and ask client to hold his or her breath. Heart sounds should normally be heard in neck. No other audible sounds when auscultating temporal and carotid arteries.	
BP in Upper Extremities Systolic BP <140 mm Hg bilaterally in adults. Diastolic BP <90 mm Hg bilaterally in adults. Systolic BP dropping less than 20 mm Hg when client rises from sitting position. Pulse pressure (difference between systolic and diastolic pressure) 1/3 of systolic pressure. BP rises slightly with age.	*Below normal BP (hypotension)*: Heart failure, dehydration, endocrine disorders (hypothyroidism), neurogenic vena cava obstruction, cardiac tamponade. *Decrease in systolic BP of 10–15 mm Hg and drop in diastolic BP on standing accompanied by rise in pulse rate:* Orthostatic hypotension caused by antihypertensive medications, volume depletion, peripheral neurovascular disease, or bedrest. *Three consecutive BP readings above 140/90:* Hypertension. *Auscultatory gap (silent interval between systolic and diastolic BP)*: Normal variation or sign of systolic hypertension. *Korotkoff's sounds down to zero:* Cardiac valve replacement, hyperkinetic states, severe anemia, thyrotoxicosis, or following strenuous exercise. *Difference of over 10 mm Hg between arms:* Arterial compression on side of lower reading, aortic dissection, coarctation of aorta. *Widened pulse pressure with increased systolic BP:* Exercise, arteriosclerosis, severe anemia, thyrotoxicosis, increased intracranial pressure (ICP). ***Narrowed pulse pressure with decreased systolic BP:*** Shock, cardiac failure, pulmonary embolus.
Abdominal Pulses No vascular sounds heard on auscultation.	Abdominal bruits reflect turbulent blood flow associated with partial occlusion. Bruits heard over epigastrium and radiating laterally, especially with

(Continued)

Auscultating the Pulses *(Continued)*

ASSESS/NORMAL VARIATIONS	ABNORMAL FINDINGS/RATIONALE
Abdominal Pulses *(Continued)*	hypertension, suggest renal artery stenosis or aneurysm. Bruits heard in lower abdominal quadrants suggest partial occlusion of iliac arteries.

STEPS FOR OBTAINING AN ACCURATE BLOOD PRESSURE READING

- Tell client to rest for 5 minutes before you take his or her BP and to wait 30 minutes if he or she has smoked or ingested caffeine.
- Have client sit comfortably with arm resting on a flat surface at heart level.
- Palpate brachial artery. Center cuff bladder over this artery with bottom edge of cuff 1 inch above antecubital space.
- Estimate systolic BP by applying cuff and palpating radial pulse. Then inflate cuff until pulse disappears—this point is estimated systolic pressure. Deflate cuff and wait 1 minute before taking BP.
- Wrap cuff evenly and snugly around upper arm and place manometer at eye level. Place bell of stethoscope over brachial artery. Apply light pressure with good skin contact; heavy pressure may distort sounds. The bell transmits low-frequency sounds better than the diaphragm.
- Close valve of pressure bulb clockwise until tight. Rapidly and steadily inflate cuff 30 mm Hg higher than client's estimated systolic BP.
- Release valve at rate to 2 to 3 mm Hg/second.
- Note point at which first sound is heard (Phase I Korotkoff's sound). This is systolic pressure. Deflate cuff and note point at which sound disappears (Phase V Korotkoff's sound).
- In adults, Phase V is diastolic pressure.
- Listen 10 to 20 mm Hg below last sound and then deflate cuff rapidly and remove it from client's arm. Wait 2 to 3 minutes before repeating procedure.

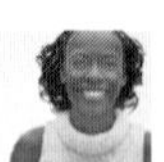

Case Study Findings

Mrs. Jordan's focused PV and lymphatic system findings include:

- Temperature 99.8°F.
- Skin moist and of uniform color throughout except for slight cyanosis of left leg.
- Capillary refill <2 seconds.
- Leg hair distributed evenly.
- No prominent leg veins or skin lesions.
- Left leg warm to touch, markedly tender on palpation, and edematous from popliteal space to ankle.
- Femoral and popliteal pulses +2 bilaterally; left posterior and pedal pulses difficult to locate.
- Calf circumference right leg 38 cm; left leg 41 cm.
- Positive Homans' sign.
- No palpable lymph nodes.

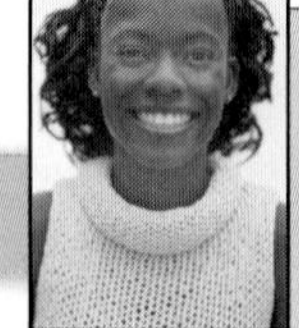

Case Study Analysis and Plan

Now that you have completed your assessment of Mrs. Jordan, list the key history and physical examination findings that will help you formulate your nursing diagnoses.

Nursing Diagnoses

Now, from the data collected, develop nursing diagnoses for Mrs. Jordan. The following are some possible nursing diagnoses. Cluster the supporting data for each.

1. Pain, chronic, related to interruption of venous blood flow and inflammation in left leg.
2. Anxiety, related to unexpected hospitalization
3. Role Performance, ineffective, related to being a new mother
4. Walking, impaired, related to pain and edema in left leg

Additional Tests to Assess PV Flow

Allen Test

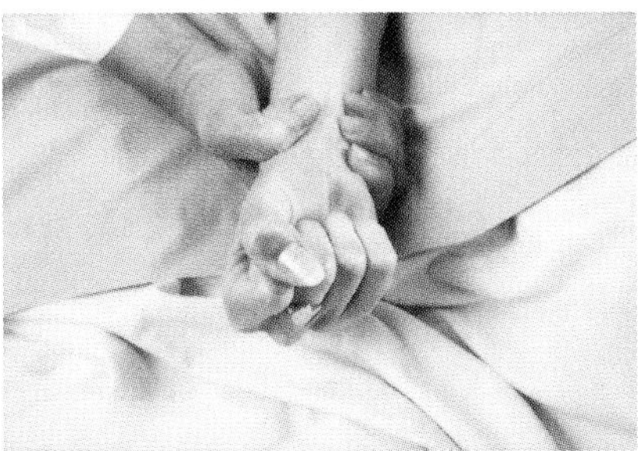

Compressing the radial and ulnar arteries

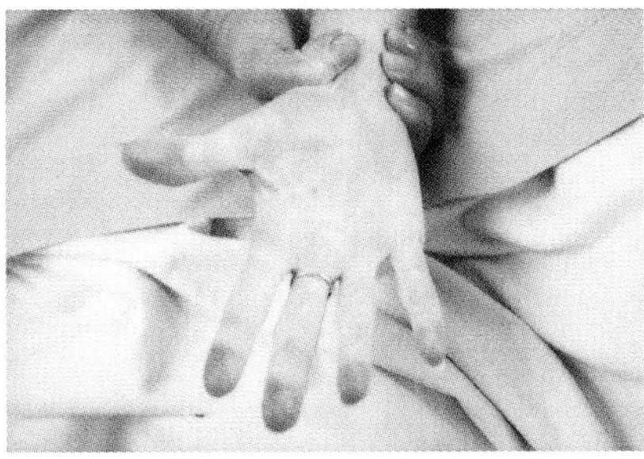

Observing for pallor

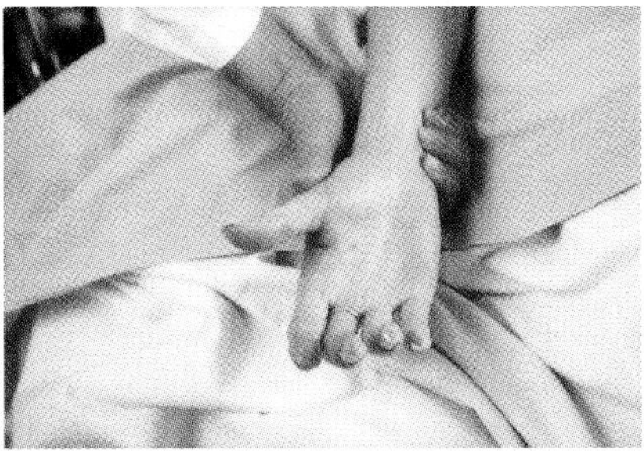

Releasing pressure and observing for return of normal color

This test assesses arterial flow in the hands. Follow these steps:

- Have client make a tight fist.
- Compress radial and ulnar arteries.
- Tell client to open hand to a slightly flexed position.
- Observe for pallor.
- Release ulnar artery and watch for return of pink color in 3 to 5 seconds.
- Repeat procedure on radial artery.

Persistent pallor with the Allen's test suggests ulnar artery occlusion. Perform this test before obtaining an arterial blood specimen from the wrist. If both ulnar and radial arteries are not patent, the site cannot be used to obtain an arterial specimen.

Ankle-Brachial Index

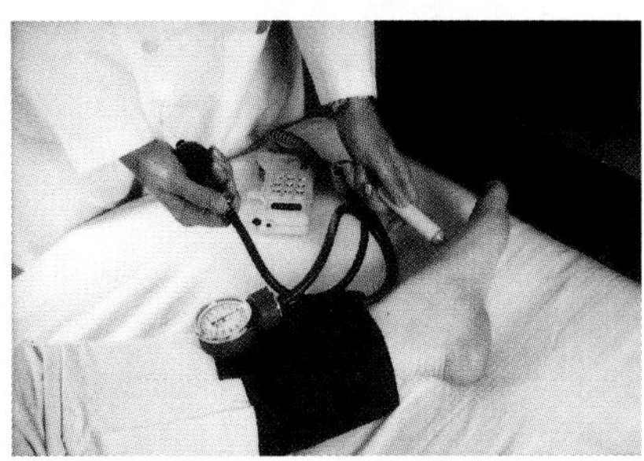

Ankle-brachial index

This test assesses circulation to the feet. Measure ankle BP using a Doppler at the posterior tibialis or dorsalis pedis pulse site; then measure brachial BP. Normally, leg pressures are equal to or slightly greater than arm pressures. This test has limited use in diabetics with vascular calcification because the findings may be falsely high.

Equate the ankle-brachial index by:

Ankle systolic pressure divided by brachial systolic pressure = ABI

For example, if ankle pressure is 140 and brachial pressure is 110, ABI is 1.25.

ABI findings:

Normal = 1 or greater
Minimal disease = 0.8–0.95
Moderate disease = 0.8–0.4
Severe disease = 0.4–0

Manual Compression Test

This test checks venous valve competence in clients with varicose veins. Have the client stand and then compress first the distal portion of the vein and then the proximal portion. Normally, no backflow should occur, and you should not feel a wave with your distal hand. If the valves are incompetent, you will feel a wave with your lower hand as a result of backflow.

Trendelenburg Test

This test also evaluates venous valve competence. With the client supine, elevate the leg to promote venous return. Then place a tourniquet around the thigh and have the client stand. The veins should fill slowly from the lower leg up. After 30 seconds, remove the tourniquet. If the veins fill rapidly from the upper leg down, the saphenous valves are incompetent.

Color Change Test

This test evaluates arterial insufficiency. With the client supine, elevate the legs to increase venous return, and then have the client sit and dangle the legs. Note color changes. Normally, color returns to the feet within 10 seconds. Elevation pallor and dependent rubor are associated with arterial insufficiency.

5. Health-Seeking Behaviors
6. Nutrition: imbalanced, more than body requirements, related to prolonged period of bedrest during pregnancy

Identify any additional nursing diagnoses and any collaborative nursing diagnoses.

CRITICAL THINKING ACTIVITY #3

Now that you have identified some nursing diagnoses for Mrs. Jordan, select one and develop a nursing care plan and a brief teaching plan for her, including learning objectives and teaching strategies.

Research Tells Us

In younger patients, inherited or acquired hypercoagulable disorders account for up to 48 percent of cases of idiopathic DVT, making them the most common cause of this disorder. Most hypercoagulable states occur as a result of a prothrombotic stimulus, such as surgery, trauma, pregnancy, or oral contraceptive use. In the general population, the most common hypercoagulable disorder is activated protein C resistance, usually from a defect in the gene for factor V. Ridker (1997) found that, up to age 50, men with the factor V Leiden mutation had a very low incidence of DVT and pulmonary embolism. After age 50, the incidence increased in proportion to age. People over age 70 had 7.83 events per 1000 person-years, compared with 1.86 in people under 50 years. Ginsberg (1996) identifies the following situations when a search for a hypercoagulable state is indicated:

- Any idiopathic DVT associated with a family history of DVT
- DVT in a client under age 50
- DVT in an unusual site (e.g., other than an extremity)
- Massive venous thrombosis
- Recurrent episodes of thrombosis
- Recurrent fetal loss

Health Concerns

Facts about Peripheral Arterial Disease and Hypertension

- The "big three" modifiable risk factors for coronary heart disease are cigarette smoking, dyslipidemia, and elevated BP.
- The prevalence of peripheral arterial disease (PAD) increases with age, and rates are higher among men than women.
- Rates of systolic BP are higher in older adults and in men.
- Other important risk factors include diabetes, obesity, and physical inactivity.
- Because each of the above risk factors is thought to influence atherosclerosis, they should be related to PAD as well as coronary heart disease (CHD).
- Cigarette smoking and diabetes appear to be the most important risk factors for PAD.

Ways to Promote Lymphatic Health

- Drink plenty of good-quality drinking water.
- Eat healthfully.
- Exercise regularly.
- Avoid exposure to the causes and sources of disease and infection.
- Avoid pollutants, toxic substances, and unhealthy environments.
- Manage stress in a manner that promotes wellness and health.

How to Manage Patients with Lymphedema

- Support and compress the affected limb, using multilayer bandaging, which gives a nonrigid outer casing of pressures up to 40 mm Hg.
- Use a combination of spiral and figure-8 bandage techniques to give an increased massage effect at rest and on exercise.
- Position wadding and foam of different densities along limb at pressure points to protect delicate areas, encourage fibrotic breakdown, and give an even compression once the entire bandage is in place.
- Change bandages daily because compression loosens with movement and bandages may slip.

Common Abnormalities

ABNORMALITY/AREA	ASSESSMENT FINDINGS
Acute Lymphangitis An inflammation of one or more lymphatic vessels. The cause is usually a bacterial infection that has spread from its initial site (e.g., skin cut) to nearby lymph glands. Area affected depends on site of inflammation.	• Chills and fever. • Swelling of lymph glands. • Red lines on arms or legs if lymphatics are inflamed, indicating concentration of inflammation along lymph channels • Inflammation may be slightly indurated and palpable to gentle touch. • Infection may occur distal to inflammation, particularly interdigitally.
Aneurysm An abnormal dilation of a blood vessel, commonly at the site of a weakness or tear in the vessel wall. The following are possible areas affected:	
Thoracic Aorta	• Pain in back, neck, and substernal areas. • Dyspnea, stridor, or cough if pressing on trachea. • Asymptomatic—first sign may be rupture. • Hoarseness and dysphagia if pressing on esophagus or laryngeal nerve.
Abdominal Aorta	• Pulsating abdominal mass. • Mild midabdominal or lumbar pain to severe abdominal and back pain. • Peripheral emboli. • Cool, cyanotic extremities if renal, iliac, or mesenteric arteries are involved. • Possible claudication, depending on which vessels are affected.
Dissecting Aorta	• Abrupt, extreme, tearing pain in area of aneurysm. • Blood pressure markedly elevated initially; then drops. • Radial pulses may be unobtainable as disorder progresses. • Syncope, hemiplegia, or paralysis of lower extremities. • Possible heart failure.
Arterial Embolism Occlusion of blood flow by a foreign object or blood clot within the vessel. Area affected varies because embolism moves.	• Sudden or insidious pain in extremity • Numbness in extremity • Coldness of extremity • Tingling in extremity • Pulselessness distal to blockage • Pallor or mottling of extremity • Muscle weakness • Muscle spasm • Paralysis • A line of demarcation, with pallor, cyanosis, and cooler skin distal to blockage
Arterial Thrombosis (Blood Clot) An aggregation of blood and other cells that adhere to the vessel wall. Area affected depends on site of blockage.	• Pain in region of affected vessel • Numbness in affected vessel • Pallor or mottling of skin in affected area • Muscle spasms • Pulselessness distal to blockage • Possible paralysis
Buerger's Disease A vasculitis confined to the intermediate and small arteries and veins of the extremities, which are the areas affected.	• Claudication. • Migrating thrombophlebitis. • Numbness, pain, and ulceration of toes.

(Continued)

Common Abnormalities *(Continued)*

ABNORMALITY/AREA	ASSESSMENT FINDINGS
Buerger's Disease ***(Continued)***	• Pain in arch of foot that may occur at rest. • Paresthesias. • Sensitivity to cold. • Diminished peripheral pulses. • Stasis dermatitis and trophic nail changes. • Ulceration and gangrene. • Nicotine use is strong risk factor.
Chronic Arterial Insufficiency Reduced blood flow to the lower extremities (area affected), usually caused by an atherosclerotic process.	• May be asymptomatic or present as intermittent claudication. • Pulses decreased or absent. • Pale color, especially when elevated; dusky red when dependent. • Temperature of extremity is cool. • Edema may be absent or mild. • Skin is thin, shiny, and atrophic. • Loss of hair is seen over foot and toes. • Nails are thickened and ridged. • Ulcers, if present, involve toes or points of trauma on feet. • Skin around ulcer has no excess pigment. • Pain is often severe unless neuropathy masks it. • Gangrene may develop.
Chronic Venous Insufficiency Stasis of blood in lower extremities (area affected), resulting from chronic lower leg edema caused by thrombophlebitis or valvular incompetence.	• Prominent leg veins, may appear ropelike and dilated or purplish and spiderlike. • Lower leg edema may extend to knee of affected extremity. • Affected leg hard and leathery to touch. • Pulses normal, but may be difficult to feel through edema. • Normal temperature. • Brownish skin pigmentation. • Gangrene does not occur. • Ulcers may occur at sides of ankles. • Skin surrounding ulcers pigmented and sometimes fibrotic. • Pain is not severe. • Eczema or stasis dermatitis.
Deep Vein Thrombosis (DVT) A thrombus formation that obstructs venous flow. Area affected may be anywhere in the body.	• Local tenderness and pain • Increased skin turgor • Swelling • Increased skin temperature • Possible positive Homans' sign
Lymphedema A blockage or dysfunction of lymph vessels or nodes. It is often associated with lymphatic disorders following surgery for breast cancer or prostate cancer. Congenital lymphedema (Meige-Milroy's disease) is chronic edema of the lower extremities, resulting in swelling and often grotesque distortion. Areas affected are extremities.	• Swelling of arms or legs. • Overlying skin eventually thickens and feels tougher than usual. • Usually painless.

Common Abnormalities

ABNORMALITY/AREA	ASSESSMENT FINDINGS
Peripheral Atherosclerotic Disease (Arteriosclerosis obliterans)	
Occlusion of the blood supply by atherosclerotic plaque. The following areas are affected:	• Weak or absent peripheral pulses. • Color changes associated with position changes (blanching when raised above heart level; rubor when dependent)
Lower Extremities	• Filling of dorsal veins • Ulceration and gangrene
Upper Extremities	• Aching, fatigue, weakness in upper arm • Unilateral coolness • Pallor • Weak or absent radial or ulnar pulses • Unilateral and focal filling abnormalities
Raynaud's Phenomenon/ Raynaud's Disease	
Involves enhanced response to cold or stress. Idiopathic, intermittent spasm of the arterioles in the digits (Raynaud's disease) occurs most frequently in young, otherwise healthy women. Raynaud's phenomenon is secondary to connective tissue diseases, neurogenic lesions, and trauma. Areas affected are hands and fingers.	• Pallor of fingertips with cold exposure, followed by cyanosis, then redness and pain with warming. • Ulceration of finger pads, progressing to autoamputation in severe, prolonged cases. • Raynaud's phenomenon is almost always bilateral. • Physical exam is normal when patient is not having symptoms. • May see pitting digital scars.
Thrombophlebitis	
Inflammation of a vein associated with thrombus formation. Area affected may be anywhere in the body.	• Redness and cyanosis of affected extremity • Warmth and tenderness to touch • Increased size of affected extremity caused by swelling • Palpable cordlike structures (if superficial) • Possible positive Homans' sign • Decreased or absent pedal pulse on affected extremity • Slowed capillary refill
Varicose Veins	
Irregular, tortuous veins with incompetent valves. Areas affected are lower extremities.	• Severe, aching pain in leg • Leg fatigue, heaviness • Itching over affected leg (stasis dermatitis) • Feelings of heat in leg • Visibly dilated veins

Summary

- The incidence of PV disease continues to rise.
- Lower-extremity edema is common and represents a variety of possible disease processes. Therefore it is essential that nurses understand the arterial, venous, and lymphatic circulatory mechanisms and the pathophysiologic alterations that accompany common diseases of these systems.
- A thorough patient history and physical examination are the mainstays of assessing for PV and lymphatic disorders and the cornerstones for further diagnostic and laboratory evaluation.
- Providing an initial and ongoing assessment to obtain a diagnosis and monitor disease progression is a key task for the nurse and enhances the preservation of function, life, and limb in clients with these disorders.

CHAPTER 14

Assessing the Breasts

Before You Begin

INTRODUCTION TO THE BREASTS

Assessment of the breasts enables you to identify abnormalities and obtain valuable data, especially information that can help in early detection of disease. Breast cancer is the second leading cause of death in women, and successful treatment depends on early diagnosis. Knowing how to perform an accurate and thorough breast examination is crucial. Because most breast masses are detected by self-examination, teaching your clients how to examine their breasts is just as critical.

Anatomy and Physiology Review

To perform the assessment accurately, you must understand the anatomy and physiology of the breast. You need to be able to identify normal structures before you can identify abnormal findings. Understanding the physiology will also guide your assessment and enable you to interpret your findings.

Structures and Functions

The breast contains the mammary gland. The primary function of the breasts in female mammals is to produce nourishment to feed their offspring. In many countries, including the United States, the breasts are also associated with female sexuality. The breast lies between the second and sixth ribs and between the sternal edge and the midaxillary line. The tail of the breast extends into the axilla. Approximately two-thirds of the breast lies over the pectoralis major muscle, and the remaining one-third is superficial to the serratus anterior muscle.

Breasts are conical in shape and often unequal in size. The primary structures of the breast include lobes, lobules, milk (lactiferous) ducts, milk (lactiferous) sinuses, acini cells, areola, nipple, ligaments, blood vessels, lymphatic tissue, and supporting muscular tissue. The breast is composed of glandular, connective, and adipose tissues, as well as smooth muscle and nerve fibers. Figure 14–1 shows external breast structures and quadrants. Figure 14–2 is a cross-section of the breast, and Figure 14–3 shows the breast lymph nodes.

Although men's breasts are different from women's, men do have a few ducts surrounded by breast and other tissue. However, men generally do not secrete the same amounts of hormones (such as estrogen) that cause breasts to develop. Although the incidence is very rare (about 10 in a million), men can develop breast cancer. Therefore you need to carefully examine male clients' breasts also.

Interaction with Other Body Systems

The breasts are not a system in and of themselves, but are a part of the reproductive system. However, the breasts have a specific relationship to other systems.

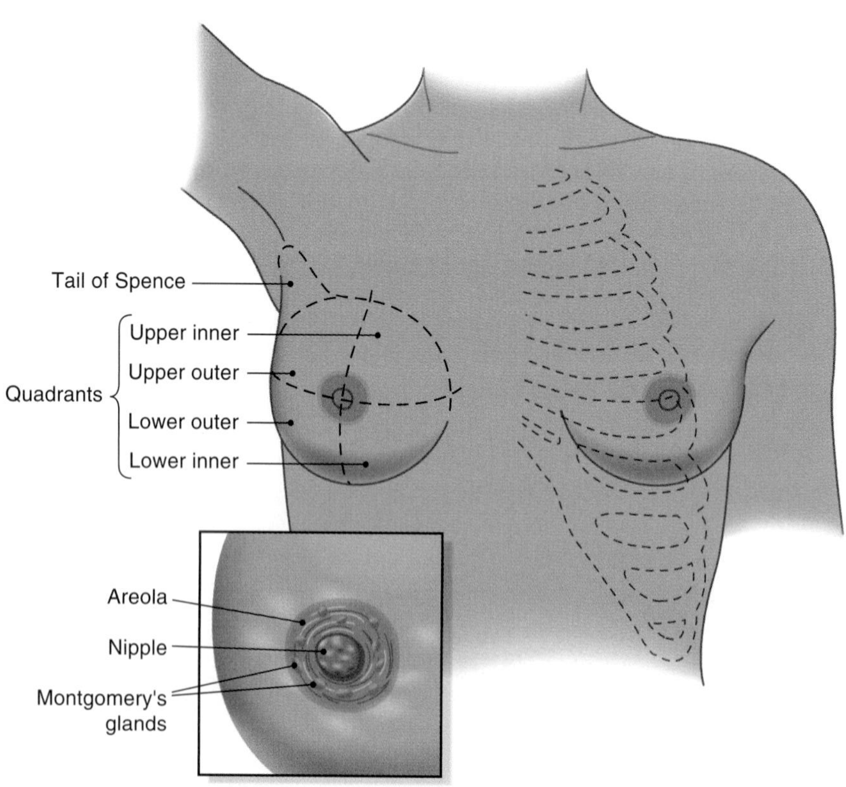

FIGURE 14–1. External breast structures and quadrants.

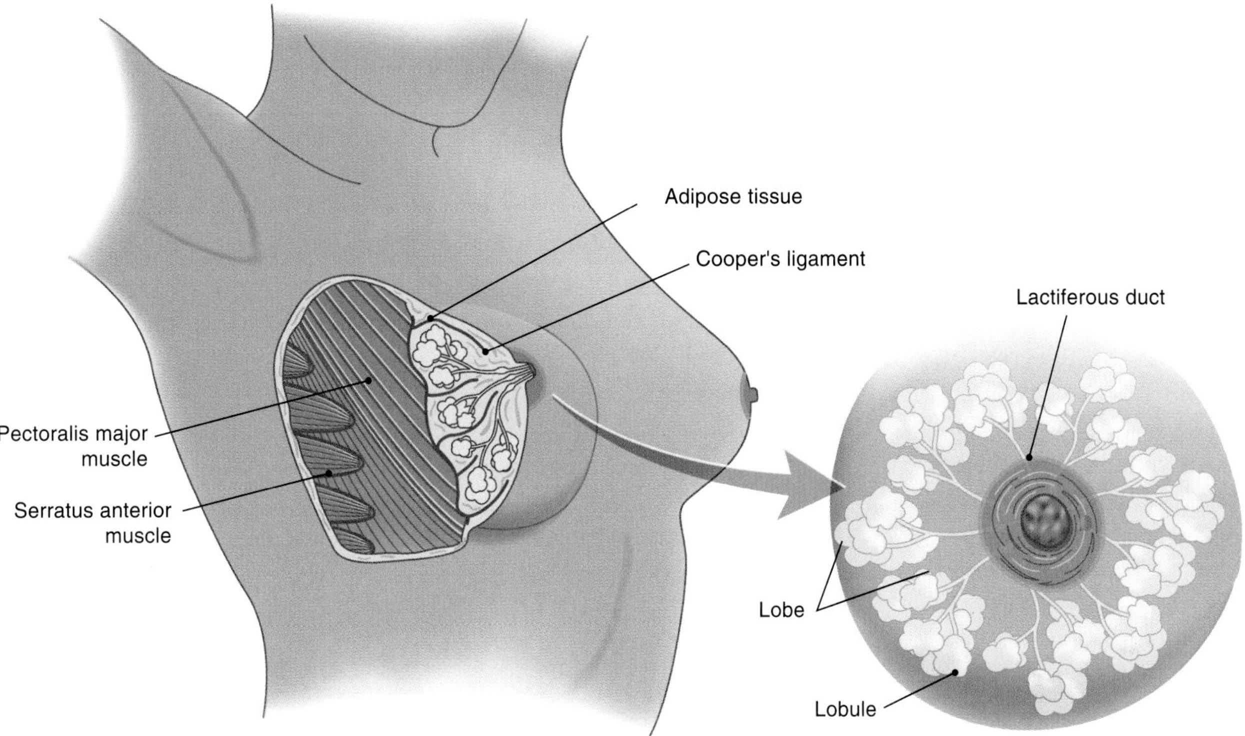

FIGURE 14–2. Cross section of breast.

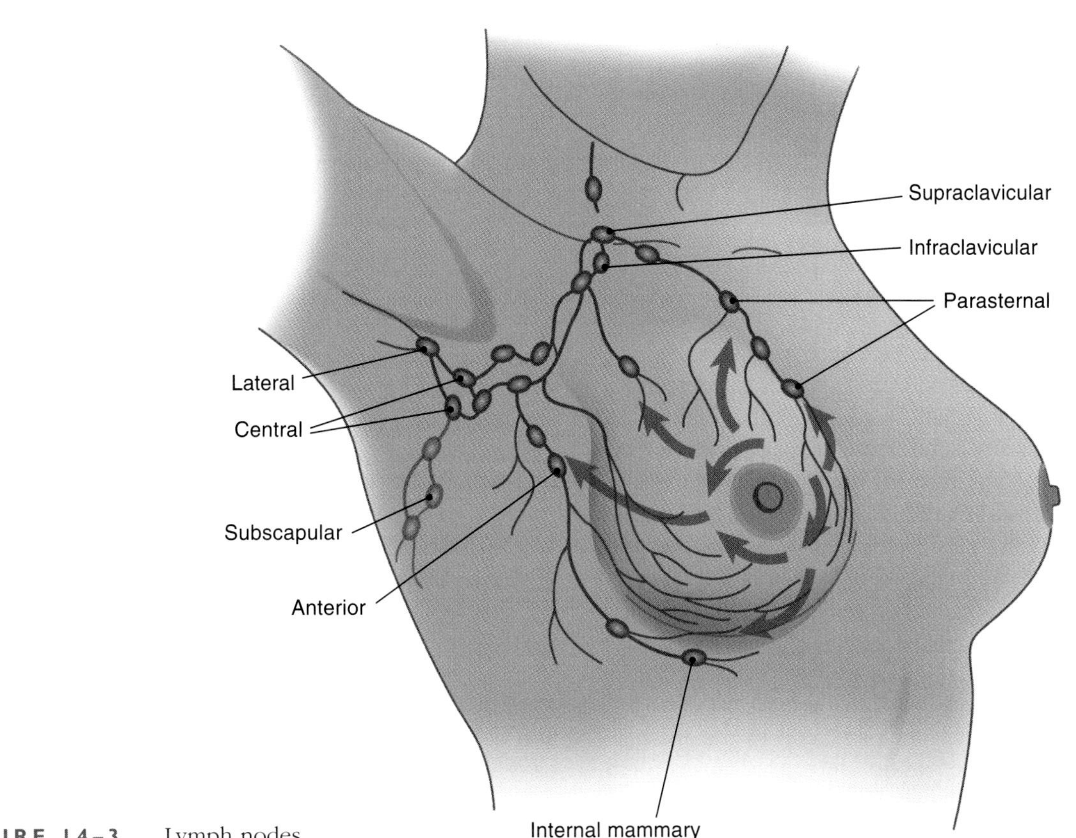

FIGURE 14–3. Lymph nodes.

Structures and Functions of the Breast

STRUCTURE	FUNCTION
Mammary Gland: Composed of 15–20 lobes. Each lobe has 50–75 lobules.	Lobules contain acini cells, which produce milk.
Lactiferous Ducts	Carry milk from glands to lactiferous sinuses.
Lactiferous Sinuses	Store milk.
Areola	Darker tissue surrounding nipple. Contains occasional hair follicles and small glands that lubricate nipple during breastfeeding.
Montgomery's Glands	Sebaceous glands.
Nipple: Composed of connective tissue, smooth muscle, blood vessels, and nerve endings	Contraction of smooth muscles makes nipple firm and erect. Sensitive nerve endings are important area for sexual stimulation.
Cooper's Ligament: Composed of bands of breast tissue fused with outer layers of superficial fascia	Suspensory ligaments attached to chest wall musculature that supports breasts.
Pectoralis Major and Serratus Anterior Muscles	Breast lies over these chest muscles.
Internal Mammary Artery	Supplies blood to breast.
Lymph Nodes of Breasts:	
Anterior (pectoral)	On lower border of pectoralis major in anterior axillary fold; drains most of breast and anterior chest wall.
Central (midaxillary)	High in axilla; pectoral, brachial, and subscapular drain into central nodes.
Lateral (brachial)	High in axilla on inner aspect of humerus; drains most of arm.
Posterior (subscapular)	High in axilla on lateral scapular border deep in posterior axillary fold; drains part of arm and posterior chest wall.
Internal Mammary	Deep in anterior chest; drains mammary glands.
Epitrochlear	In depression above and posterior to medial area of elbow; drains arm.
Supraclavicular	Above clavicle; often site for metastatic breast cancer.
Infraclavicular	Below clavicle; often site for metastatic breast cancer.

The Neuroendocrine System

Sucking stimulates impulses to the hypothalamus. The hypothalamus stimulates the production of prolactin by the anterior pituitary, which stimulates milk production. The hypothalamus also stimulates the production of oxytocin by the posterior pituitary gland, which stimulates muscle cells surrounding the glandular tissue to contract and force the milk into the excretory ducts. Estrogen and progesterone are hormones that influence breast growth.

The Reproductive System

Breast development and function depend on estrogen and progesterone, which are produced in the ovaries. Estrogen elongates the excretory ducts and causes them to create tributaries. Progesterone increases the number and size of the lobules to prepare the breasts for milk production and storage for nourishing a baby. Progesterone increases breast cell growth and dilation of blood vessels after ovulation. This engorgement is the reason why the breasts often become tender and swollen 5 to 7 days before menstruation, increasing in size, nodularity, density, and sensitivity.

Developmental, Cultural, and Ethnic Variations

Infants

At birth, the infant's nipple is elevated, and a slight secretion of milky material, "witch's milk" may occur for 5 to 7 days after birth. Palpable breast tissue is normal in infancy, but not beyond this period. Some newborns have supernumerary nipples, a normal finding.

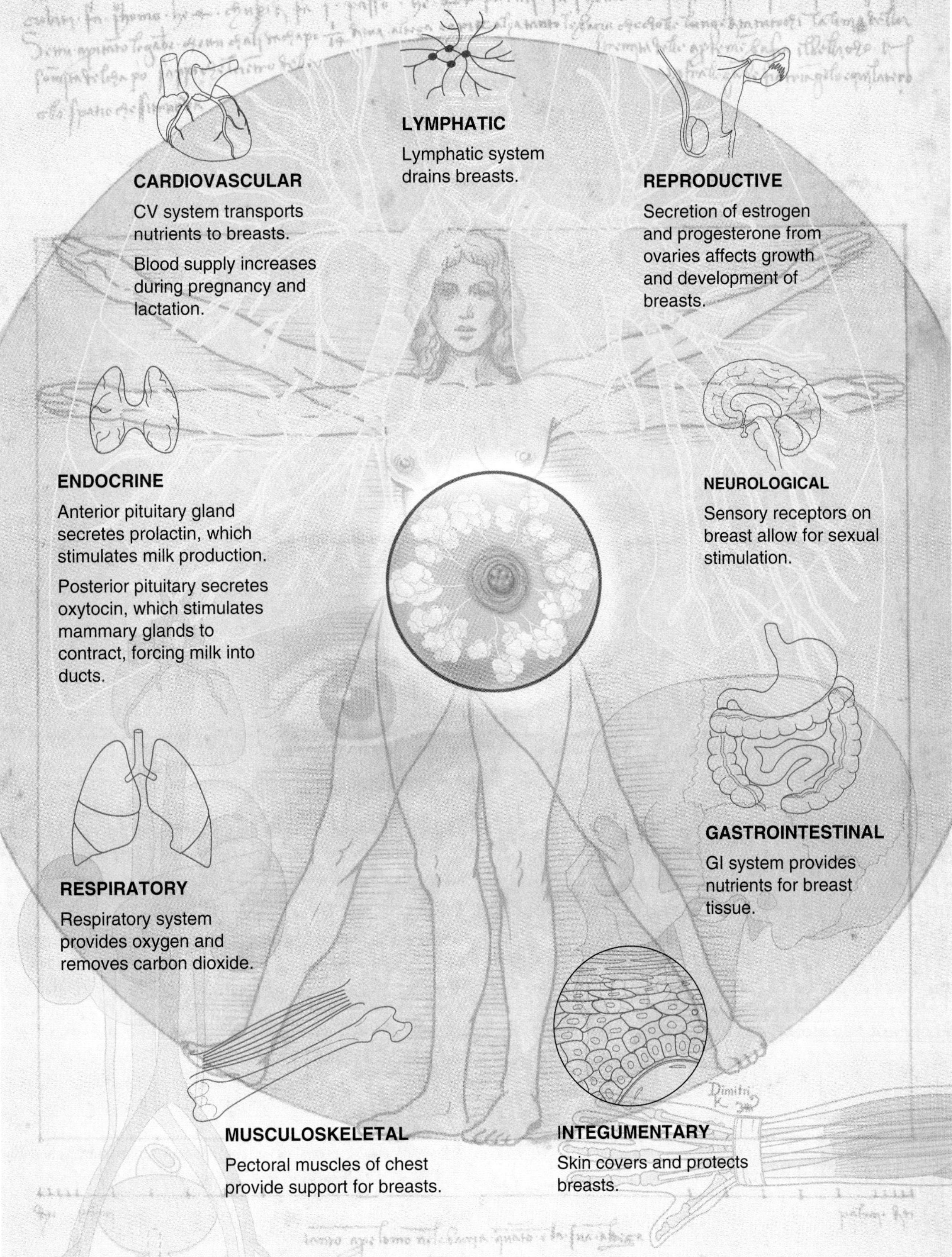

LYMPHATIC
Lymphatic system drains breasts.
CARDIOVASCULAR
CV system transports nutrients to breasts.
Blood supply increases during pregnancy and lactation.
REPRODUCTIVE
Secretion of estrogen and progesterone from ovaries affects growth and development of breasts.
ENDOCRINE
Anterior pituitary gland secretes prolactin, which stimulates milk production.
Posterior pituitary secretes oxytocin, which stimulates mammary glands to contract, forcing milk into ducts.
NEUROLOGICAL
Sensory receptors on breast allow for sexual stimulation.
GASTROINTESTINAL
GI system provides nutrients for breast tissue.
RESPIRATORY
Respiratory system provides oxygen and removes carbon dioxide.
MUSCULOSKELETAL
Pectoral muscles of chest provide support for breasts.
INTEGUMENTARY
Skin covers and protects breasts.
Dimitri K

Relationship of Breasts to Other Systems

Stages of Breast Development

Stage 1: Prepuberty
Elevation of papilla

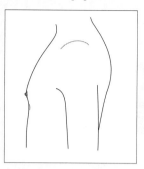

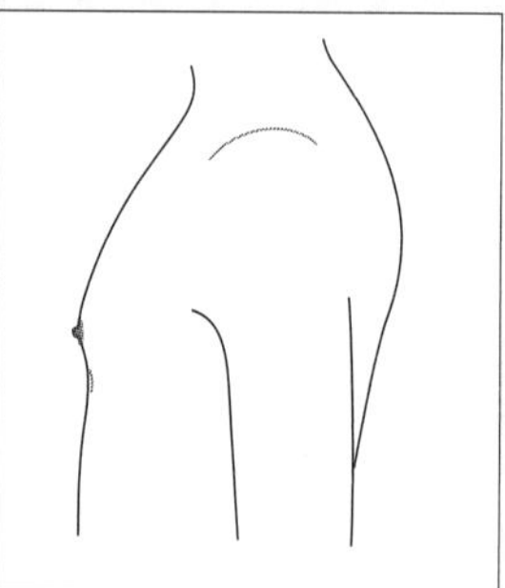

Stage 2: Breast bud
Elevation of breast and nipple and increased diameter of areola

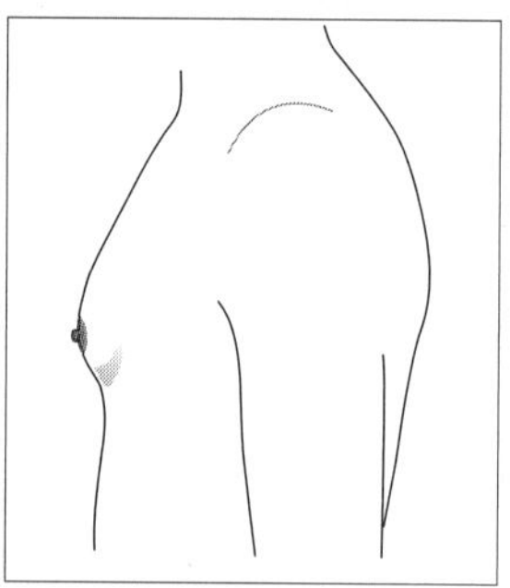

Stage 3: Areola deepens in color and enlarges further. Glandular tissue begins to develop beneath areola.

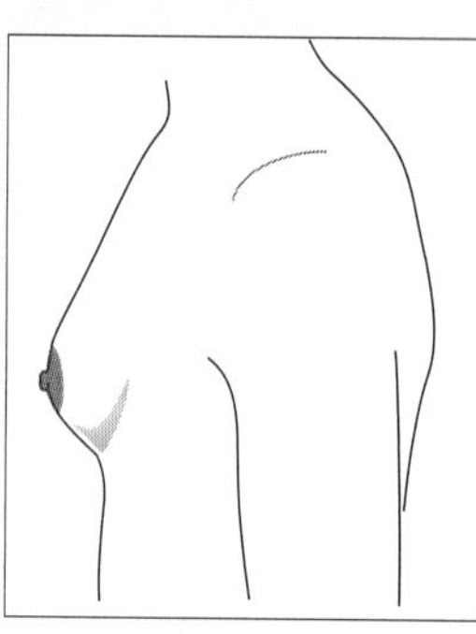

Stage 4: Areola appears as a mound; breast appears as a mound.

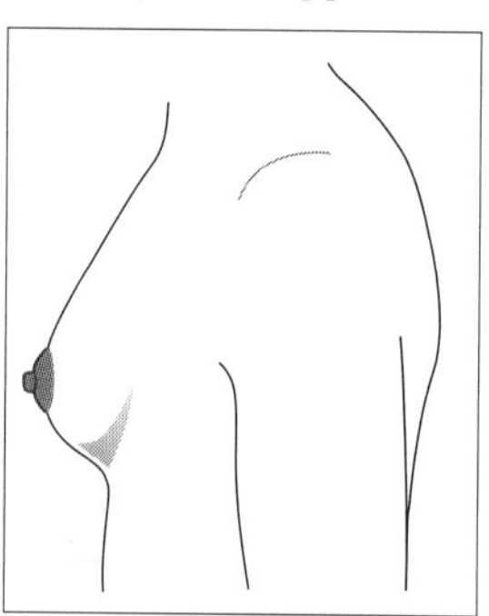

Stage 5: Mature breast
Areola recesses to general contour of breast; nipple projects forward.

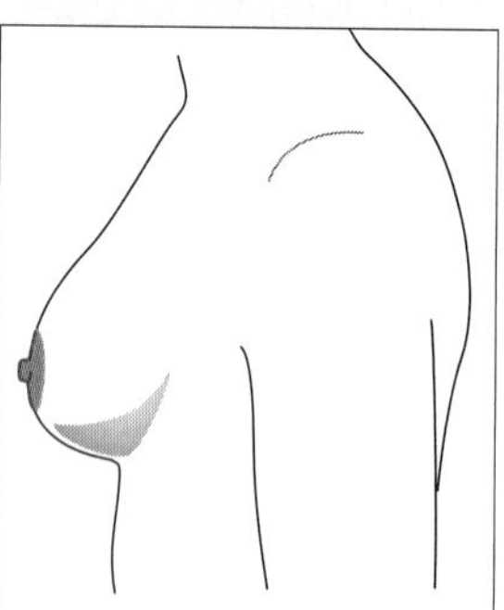

Children and Adolescents

A female child's breast is underdeveloped compared to an adult's. Growth of breast tissue generally begins in the prepubertal period. Physiologic changes occurring in the breasts are the result of growth. Tanner staging (box, Stages of Breast Development) is used to track breast development in females during puberty. (For more information, see Chapter 24, Assessing the School-Age Child and Adolescent.)

Pregnant Women

Breasts become fuller and firmer, and the areola and nipples darken and enlarge. In the third trimester, colostrum, a yellow secretion, occurs. Colostrum continues to be secreted after the birth of a baby until milk is produced. (For more information, see Chapter 21, Assessing the Mother-to Be.)

Older Adults

As women age, glandular tissue is replaced with adipose tissue and the ducts become more fibrous. These changes, along with a general reduction of muscle mass and tone, cause breasts to be less firm and more pendulous. Arthritic changes in the joints and hands make BSE a little more challenging. (For more information, see Chapter 25, Assessing the Older Adult.)

HELPFUL HINTS

- Pregnancy is not an ideal time for a woman to learn how to do breast self-examination (BSE). Getting to know what is normal for her will be difficult until pregnancy and lactation are completed.
- Older women may be reluctant to examine their breasts because they have the idea that "touching yourself" is taboo.
- Older women may have trouble assuming some positions necessary for the physical examination. Besides being sensitive to their needs, you may need to be creative!
- Advise older women to sprinkle talcum powder on their hands so that they will glide more smoothly during BSE.

People of Different Cultures and Ethnic Groups

Some health problems are culturally or racially bound. That is, diseases are either associated exclusively with a certain race or ethnic group or occur more frequently in that group. Ashkenazi Jews have a greater incidence of breast cancer than other ethnic groups because they are believed to have a gene that predisposes them to "familial breast cancer." White women have a higher incidence of breast cancer than nonwhite women, but African-American women have lower survival rates than white women. African-American men appear to be at greater risk than white men for breast cancer. In addition, some cultural practices may delay early diagnosis or treatment. For instance, African-American women in the southern United States have been known to treat breast lesions with home remedies.

Introducing the Case Study

Lynn Kobrynski is a childless 46-year-old married woman who visits her nurse practitioner for an annual physical exam. She states: "My husband thinks I have a lump in my right breast." Mrs. Kobrynski has been active and healthy and has never been pregnant. She has a family history of breast cancer. Considering her complaint and the fact that she has not had a complete physical in 5 years, a complete health history and physical examination are warranted.

Performing the Breast Assessment

A comprehensive assessment includes taking the client's health history and performing a physical examination of the breasts and axillae.

Health History

The health history involves interviewing the client regarding her perception of her health status. It includes a broad range of questions so that possible problems associated with breast cancer may be identified. Keep in mind that information collected as part of the health history may uncover problems related to systems outside the breast (e.g., metastatic disease).

Biographical Data

Biographical information can provide valuable insights about the health of your client's breasts. Begin by asking your client's age—it influences the questions you ask during the rest of the health history. Breast development varies according to the age of your client, and various breast problems are age related. For example, the risk for breast cancer increases with age; fibroid adenomas usually occur before age 30; the incidence of intraductal papilloma, a benign lesion of the lactiferous duct, peaks at age 40; fibrocystic breast changes usually occur between ages 35 and 50; and ductal ectasia occurs most commonly in perimenopausal women in their 50s.

Also ask about your client's ethnic background because it may influence the risk for breast disease. For example, the incidence of breast cancer is greater in white women than in nonwhite women, and fibroadenomas most commonly occur in African-Americans.

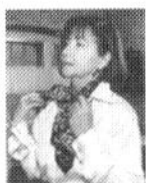

Case Study Findings

Reviewing Mrs. Kobrynski's biographical data:

- 46-year-old married woman
- No pregnancies, no children
- Caucasian, Catholic religion, Polish descent
- College graduate; employed as high school teacher
- Contact person: Husband, Edward Kobrynski, a steelworker
- Insurance from full-time work
- Source of information: Self, seems reliable

Current Health Status

If your client's chief complaint is about her breast, investigate this first; then perform a symptom analysis. Common chief complaints involving the breast include lumps or masses, breast pain or tenderness, and nipple discharge. Related complaints include changes in the venous pattern of the breast (increased vascularity), dimpling or puckering of breast skin, redness or scaliness of breast skin, and change in the direction of the nipple.

Symptom Analysis

Symptom Analysis tables for all of the symptoms described in the following paragraphs are available on the

Web for viewing and printing. In your Web browser, go to http://www.fadavis.com/detail.cfm?id=0882-9 and click on Symptom Analysis Tables under Explore This Product.

Lump or Mass

The most common complaint related to the early detection of breast cancer, a lump or mass, may be a normal physiologic nodularity or may indicate a neoplasm. Careful analysis of this symptom can provide data that will help you distinguish between normal and abnormal breast changes.

HELPFUL HINTS

- If your client is premenopausal, be sure to determine the relationship of symptoms to the menstrual cycle.
- When assessing precipitating or palliative factors, explore the client's use of culturally related health practices or remedies. Use of these remedies may delay the initiation of traditional Western treatment, which can be deleterious to the client's health.
- Give special attention to adolescent girls who are sensitive about body image. Ask about recent breast trauma.

Pain or Tenderness

Breast pain or tenderness (**mastalgia**) is usually related to the normal menstrual cycle and is generally not characteristic of a malignant lesion. However, it may be associated with extensive or metastatic disease and therefore needs to be evaluated. Pain can also be caused by a rapidly enlarging cyst, an infection or abscess, mastitis, hematoma, trauma, or fibrocystic disease. Some disorders have classic signs located in the breast that are diagnostically significant. For instance, redness and pain may indicate inflammatory breast cancer, trauma, or an abscess.

CRITICAL THINKING ACTIVITY #1

How would you explain pain or tenderness associated with the menstrual cycle?

Nipple Discharge

Nipple discharge may be normal or abnormal. Discharge may occur spontaneously or be manually expressed and may be white, milky, serous, clear, bloody, gray, brown, or green. A thorough evaluation is necessary to determine the cause. Unless the client is lactating, spontaneous discharge is usually not considered normal and warrants further investigation.

ALERT

Any spontaneous discharge from a nonpregnant woman's breast is an abnormal, potentially serious finding and must be followed up.

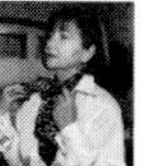

Case Study Findings

Mrs. Kobrynski's current health status includes:

- Chief complaint is that her husband thinks she has a lump.
- Does not perform monthly BSE.

CRITICAL THINKING ACTIVITY #2

What other questions would you ask Mrs. Kobrynski to further assess her chief complaint?

Past Health History

The past health history compares the client's past health and present health and uncovers risk factors that might predispose her to breast disease. The following questions will help you explore specific areas related to the breast.

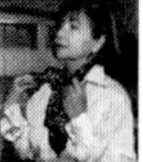

Case Study Findings

Mrs. Kobrynski's past health history includes:

- Menarche at age 12; menstrual cycles have always been regular—every 28 days and lasting 3 days.
- Had lumpectomy for benign breast lesion; otherwise negative.
- No pregnancies; no history of infertility.
- No known food, drug, perfume, or deodorant allergies.
- Does not take any medications other than occasional Tylenol for headache. No history of birth control pills (BCP) or hormone replacement therapy (HRT).
- No other medical problems. Does not examine breasts, and has never had a complete breast examination (CBE) or mammogram.

Past Health History

RISK FACTORS/ QUESTIONS TO ASK	RATIONALE/SIGNIFICANCE
Childhood Illnesses	Childhood illnesses may cause permanent effects.
Do you have a history of breast lumps as an adolescent or young adult?	Fibroadenomas usually occur between ages 15 and 25.
When did you begin menstruation?	Early menarche (< age 12) is a risk factor for breast cancer because breasts are under hormonal influence longer.
Surgery	
Have you ever had surgery or other treatments involving the breasts?	Provides information on possible reasons for symptoms (e.g., breast implants).
Hospitalizations/Diagnostic Procedures	
Have you ever been treated for a breast problem?	Helps identify potential or recurring problems, or may explain physical findings.
How often do you have a mammogram?	Identifies current health practices.
Serious Injuries	
What serious injuries have you had?	Data on past breast injuries provides baseline data for physical assessment.
What treatment did you receive?	
Do you have any residual effects from injuries or treatments?	Women who received radiation therapy for breast disorders may have redness, scaliness, and other symptoms that may appear to be a malignancy.
Serious/Chronic Illnesses	
Do you have any other medical problems? For example, cancer in any other area?	Liver disease, testicular tumors, hyperthyroidism, and adrenal and pituitary tumors can cause gynecomastia in men.
Recent infection?	Cancer from another area may have local spread involving the lymph nodes.
Have you recently stopped nursing a child?	Stopping nursing abruptly can cause breasts to become engorged, red, and hard.
Allergies	
Do you have any allergies (e.g., to perfume or deodorant)?	May cause redness, pruritus, and scaliness in breasts and axillae.
Medications	
Are you taking any prescribed or over-the-counter medications?	Data on use of HRT is conflicting.
Hormones or hormone replacement therapy?	Unopposed use of estrogen may increase risk of breast cancer.
Birth control pills?	Digoxin can cause gynecomastia in men. See box, Drugs That Adversely Affect the Breasts.

Drugs That Adversely Affect the Breasts

Drug Class	Drug	Possible Adverse Reactions
Androgens	danazol, fluoxymesterone, methyltestosterone, testosterone	*Female:* decreased breast size *Male:* gynecomastia
Antidepressants	tricyclic antidepressants	*Female:* breast engorgement and galactorrhea (spontaneous milk flow) *Male:* gynecomastia

(Continued)

Drugs that Adversely Affect the Breasts *(Continued)*

Drug Class	Drug	Possible Adverse Reactions
Antipsychotics	chlorpromazine hydrochloride, fluphenazine, haloperidol, perphenazine, prochlorperazine maleate, thioridazine, thiothixene	*Female:* galactorrhea, moderate engorgement of the breast with lactation, mastalgia (breast pain) *Male:* gynecomastia, mastalgia
Cardiac glycosides	digitoxin, digoxin	*Male:* gynecomastia
Estrogens	chlorotrianisene, conjugated estrogens, esterified estrogens, estradiol, estrone, ethinyl estradiol	*Female:* breast changes, tenderness, enlargement, secretions *Male:* breast changes, tenderness, gynecomastia
	dienestrol	*Female:* breast tenderness
	diethylstilbestrol	*Female:* breast tenderness, enlargement *Male:* breast tenderness, gynecomastia
Oral contraceptives	estrogen-progesterone combinations	*Female:* breast changes, tenderness, enlargement, secretions
Progestins	hydroxyprogesterone caproate, medroxyprogesterone acetate, norethindrone, norethindrone acetate, norgestrel, progesterone	*Female:* breast tenderness or galactorrhea
Miscellaneous agents	isoniazid	*Male:* gynecomastia
	reserpine	*Female:* breast engorgement, galactorrhea *Male:* gynecomastia
	spironolactone	*Female:* breast tenderness *Male:* painful gynecomastia
	cimetidine	*Female:* galactorrhea *Male:* gynecomastia

Family History

The family history identifies familial tendencies toward breast disease and disorders. The following questions may help you elicit this information.

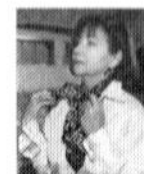

Case Study Findings

Mrs. Kobrynski's family history reveals:

- Positive for ductal breast cancer.
- Maternal grandmother deceased age 87; diagnosed with ductal breast cancer at age 85.
- Mother had benign breast lesion at age 57.
- Client has two younger sisters, both alive and well.
- One maternal aunt, alive and well.
- No other cancer history in family.

Family History

RISK FACTORS/ QUESTIONS TO ASK	RATIONALE/SIGNIFICANCE
Familial or Genetically Linked Breast Problems	
Do you have a family history of breast cancer?	Women with two or more first-line relatives (mother or sister) with breast cancer have increased risk.
If yes, what family members were afflicted? What type of breast cancer?	Number of first-line relatives with breast cancer may raise questions about genetic alterations leading to predisposition for breast cancer. Women with altered or mutated BRCA1 or BRCA2 gene have an 85% to 95% lifetime chance of developing breast cancer. Positive family history for cancer increases risk to client.
How old were they when diagnosed?	Risk of cancer increases with age. If any family member had premenopausal breast cancer, need to investigate possibility of genetic alteration.
Do you have a family history of other types of cancer? What types?	May indicate hereditary family syndromes.

Review of Systems

The review of systems enables you to relate the breast to other systems and often reveals information that your client might have been omitted earlier.

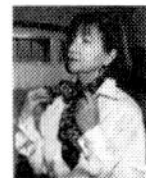

Case Study Findings

Mrs. Kobrynski's review of systems reveals:

- **General Health Survey:** Usual state of health good
- **Integumentary:** No dimpling, redness, or rashes on breasts or axillae
- **Cardiovascular:** Reports no problems or medications
- **Reproductive:** Menarche at age 12; menstrual cycle regular every 28 days, lasting 3 days; no history of BCP or HRT.

Review of Systems

SYSTEM/QUESTIONS TO ASK	RATIONALE/SIGNIFICANCE
General Health Survey	
How have you been feeling?	Provides an indicator of general overall health.
Do you have a fever?	Associated with mastitis, abscess, infection, and sometimes metastatic disease.
Have you lost weight?	Unexplained weight loss may be associated with malignancy.
Integumentary/*Skin on Breasts and Axillae*	
Do you have any dimpling, redness, rashes, lesions, or lumps?	*Dimpling:* Malignancy. *Scaly erosion of areola and nipple:* Paget's disease (breast malignancy of areola and nipple). *Redness over affected area:* Mastitis.
Respiratory	
If client has breast cancer: Any breathing difficulty?	Lung is common site for metastasis.
Cardiovascular	
Are you on any cardiovascular medications?	Some medications such as digoxin have side effect of gynecomastia.
Gastrointestinal	
If client has breast cancer: Any increase in abdominal size?	
Liver disease?	Liver is common site for metastasis. Can cause gynecomastia in men.
Reproductive	
At what age did your menstrual cycle begin?	Early menarche and late menopause are risk factors for breast cancer.
Have you ever taken BCP?	
Have you ever been pregnant? If so, at what age(s)?	Nulliparity, first pregnancy after age 30, and infertility have been linked to breast cancer.
Do you have a history of infertility?	
Did you breastfeed?	Breastfeeding decreases risk for breast cancer.
If postmenopausal: At what age did your menstrual cycles cease?	
Have you ever been on HRT? If so, what type and for how long?	HRT has been linked with increased incidence of breast cancer.
Endocrine	
Do you have a history of hyperthyroidism?	Can cause gynecomastia in men.

Psychosocial Profile

The psychosocial profile can reveal patterns in your client's life that place her at risk for breast disease. You may also identify teaching needs.

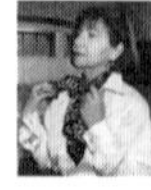

Case Study Findings

Mrs. Kobrynski's psychosocial profile includes:

- Has not had physical exam in 5 years; has never had a mammogram; does not perform BSE; has not had CBE in 5 years.
- Typical day consists of awakening at 6 AM, showering and dressing, eating breakfast with husband, and driving 30 minutes to school. Works 8 AM to 3:30 PM Monday through Friday. Returns home by 4 PM, takes a walk or relaxes, fixes dinner. After dinner, corrects papers, watches TV, or reads. Spends weekends catching up on housework, shopping and running errands, socializing with friends.
- Usually eats well, although diet premenstrually tends to be high in fats and salt. Temporarily gains 5 lb before she gets her period; otherwise, weight stable for last 10 years.
- Walks 3 miles, 3–4 times a week.
- Usually gets 8 hours sleep; no difficulty sleeping.
- Denies use of alcohol and caffeine.
- Employed full time, likes job, which does not require lifting.
- Satisfied with sex life.
- Married 15 years, husband and friends are supports.
- Goes to church weekly; religion is an important aspect of her life.

Psychosocial Profile

CATEGORY QUESTIONS TO ASK	RATIONALE/SIGNIFICANCE
Health Practices and Beliefs/ Self-Care Activities	
How do you promote breast health?	Helps identify activities that reduce breast cancer risk.
Do you get regular CBEs?	Early detection decreases morbidity and mortality.
Mammograms?	American Cancer Society (ACS) screening guidelines include:
Do you perform monthly BSEs?	• Monthly BSE beginning at age 20
	• Annual screening mammography beginning at age 40
HELPFUL HINT Ask client to demonstrate BSE. Do not rely on self-report to ascertain adequate knowledge of technique.	CBE by medical professional every 3 years from age 20–40; then yearly.
Typical Day	
Do you have trouble performing activities of daily living (ADLs)? Is your range of motion (ROM) restricted?	Helps identify if client will have trouble caring for herself and performing BSE.
Nutritional Patterns	
What did you eat in the last 24 hours?	May provide baseline information on dietary habits.
Have you recently lost or gained weight?	Weight gain may increase breast size, causing tenderness.
Does your menstrual cycle affect your appetite and the type of food you eat?	May need dietary consultation to discuss foods to decrease PMS symptoms (low sodium, low fat).
Do you have PMS?	Cancer, especially of the breast, is associated with a high-fat diet. ACS recommends <30 grams of fat/day.
Do you eat a lot of high-fat foods? Salty foods?	Diets high in sodium and methylxanthines, such as chocolate and coffee, can aggravate fibrocystic breast disease.

Psychosocial Profile

CATEGORY QUESTIONS TO ASK	RATIONALE/SIGNIFICANCE
Activity and Exercise Patterns	
Do you exercise? If so, how much and what type?	Sedentary lifestyle increases risk for cancer. Exercise is linked with decreasing cancer risks overall.
Sleep and Rest Patterns	
Do you have trouble sleeping at night?	Clients with breast swelling or pain/tenderness may have trouble finding a comfortable position for sleep.
Personal Habits	
Do you drink alcohol? If so, how much?	High intake of alcohol may be linked with cancer.
Do you drink caffeinated beverages?	Can worsen fibrocystic breast disease.
Do you use heroin or marijuana?	Can cause gynecomastia in men.
Occupational Health Patterns	
What type of work do you do? Does it involve heavy lifting?	Diagnosis or treatment of breast disorder may affect whether client can return to work at same job.
Roles/Relationships/Self-Concept	
How important are your breasts to a positive view of yourself? Do you have a difficult time discussing your problem?	Breast cancer can cause body image disturbances and have a major impact on a woman's self-image. Fear of losing breast may delay treatment.
Religious/Cultural Influences	
What are your religious practices/beliefs or cultural influences in regard to health care?	May affect client's healthcare practices.
Sexuality Patterns	
Has your breast disorder affected your sex life? How?	Breast pain or tenderness (**mastalgia**) can interfere with sexual activity. Loss of a breast to cancer can make a woman avoid sex because she feels less attractive.
Social Supports	
Who are your main sources of support? Have you seen a change in the way your support person or spouse sees you since you developed a breast problem?	Identifying client's support system is essential in planning care.

Focused Breast History

If you are unable to perform a detailed history, ask key questions that focus on a history of breast problems, presence of symptoms, identification of risk factors, and health promotion activities. The following questions focus on the warning signs of breast cancer:

- Do you have a lump or thickening in or near your breast or under your arm that persists through the menstrual cycle?
- Is the skin on your breast or nipple red, dimpled, puckered, scaly, or inflamed?
- Do you have nipple changes? For example, a change in the direction in which one nipple points, inversion, eversion, or discharge?
- Has your breast changed in size, shape, or contour?

Case Study Evaluation

Before you begin the physical examination, document the findings from your interview with Mrs. Kobrynski.

CRITICAL THINKING ACTIVITY #3

Based on the history you obtained from Mrs. Kobrynski, what breast problem is she at risk for? What are the risk factors?

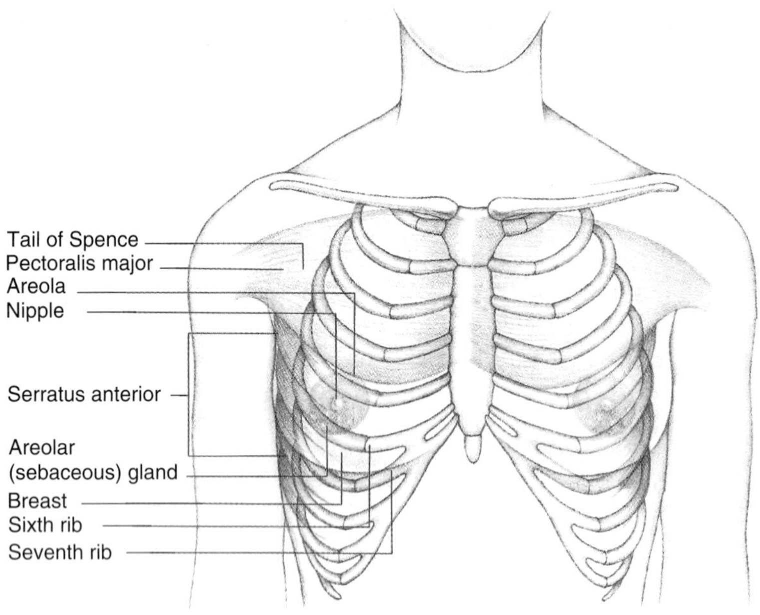

FIGURE 14–4. Anatomical landmarks.

Physical Assessment

Now that you have obtained the history, turn your attention to collecting objective data by performing the physical examination. As you assess your client's breasts, remember that this is an ideal opportunity to teach BSE.

Anatomical Landmarks

The breast examination should include the areas above the clavicle to the 6th or 7th rib, and from the sternum to the midaxillary line (Fig. 14–4).

Approach

You will use the techniques of inspection and palpation to examine the breasts. The examination is performed in several positions: sitting, arms at side; sitting, arms over head; sitting, hands on hips; sitting leaning forward; and supine with pillow under shoulder of breast being examined. The hands over head and hands pressed on hips positions are helpful in detecting dimpling or retraction of the breast tissue. The sitting, leaning forward position is helpful when assessing large, pendulous breasts. With the supine position, have the woman lie on the examination table and place a small pillow or rolled towel under the shoulder of the breast you will examine first. The pillow or towel helps spread the breast tissue over the chest wall.

Examination in Breast Reconstruction

Today many women have breast reconstruction for cancer or for cosmetic reasons. Breast examination in these women is done exactly the same way as for natural breasts and must not be omitted. If an implant was used for the reconstruction, press firmly inward at the edges of the implant to feel the ribs beneath.

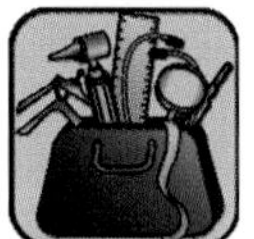

Toolbox

Assemble the following equipment for a routine breast examination: Small pillow or towel, mirror, centimeter ruler, nonsterile gloves, specimen slide, and specimen culture swab.

Performing a General Survey

Before examining specific areas, scan your client from head to toe, looking at her general appearance. Then take vital signs and document them. A temperature elevation may be associated with mastitis.

Performing a Head-to-Toe Physical Assessment

Now, look for changes in every system that may relate to the breast. Because the breasts are not a system, there may not be an obvious relationship to other systems. However, if your client has breast cancer, be alert for changes in other systems that reflect metastatic disease.

Performing a Head-to-Toe Physical Assessment

SYSTEM/NORMAL FINDINGS	ABNORMAL FINDINGS/RATIONALE
General Health Survey *INSPECT* No acute distress; AAO ×3; responses clear and appropriate; affect pleasant; well-groomed.	*If client has breast cancer:* Changes in level of consciousness (LOC), dyphasia, or hemiparesis may indicate brain metastasis. If client has breast lump, mood may be depressed or anxious.
Integumentary *INSPECT* No rashes or lesions on breasts or axillae.	*Axillary rashes:* Allergies. *Breast lesions/redness:* Malignancy or mastitis.
HEENT/*Eyes* *INSPECT* Vision intact; no papilledema.	*If client has breast cancer:* Visual changes and papilledema may indicate brain metastasis.
HEENT/*Neck* No palpable nodes.	*Enlarged lymph nodes:* Infection or metastasis.
Thyroid nonpalpable.	*Palpable thyroid:* Hyperthyroidism, which can cause gynecomastia in men.
Respiratory *AUSCULTATE* Respiratory rate 18 per minute. Lungs clear.	*If client has breast cancer:* Adventitious breath sounds, decreased chest excursion, and dullness to percussion seen with pleural effusion and may indicate metastasis to lungs.
Cardiovascular *INSPECT* No increased venous pattern on chest.	*Increased venous pattern, especially asymmetrical:* Breast cancer.
Gastrointestinal *INSPECT, PALPATE, AUSCULTATE* Swallowing intact; positive bowel sounds; abdomen soft, nontender, no hepatomegaly.	*If client has breast cancer:* Ascites and hepatomegaly may indicate metastasis to liver.
Genitourinary/Reproductive *INSPECT, PALPATE* Normal pelvic exam.	Endometrial and ovarian cancer increase risk for breast cancer.
Musculoskeletal *INSPECT* Muscle strength +5. Movements smooth and coordinated.	*If client has breast cancer:* Weakness and ataxia may

(Continued)

Performing a Head-to-Toe Physical Assessment *(Continued)*

SYSTEM/NORMAL FINDINGS	ABNORMAL FINDINGS/RATIONALE
Musculoskeletal *(Continued)* *INSPECT* Gait balanced, no ataxia.	indicate metastasis to bone and brain.
Neurological *INSPECT* No sensory loss.	*If client has breast cancer:* Unilateral sensory loss and hemiparesis may indicate metastasis.

Case Study Findings

Mrs. Kobrynski's physical assessment findings include:

- **General Health Survey:** No acute distress; AAO × 3; responses clear and appropriate; affect pleasant, but slightly anxious; well-groomed, looks younger than stated age.
- **Vital signs:** Temperature 98.4°F; pulse 72 bpm; respirations 18/min; BP 110/68; height 5′4″; weight 116 lb
- **Integumentary:** Skin intact; no rashes or lesions
- **HEENT:** No palpable lymph nodes; thyroid not palpable
- **Respiratory:** Lungs clear
- **Cardiovascular:** Heart regular
- **Gastrointestinal:** Abdomen soft, nontender; no hepatomegaly
- **Genitourinary/Reproductive:** Normal pelvic exam; day 7 of menstrual cycle
- **Musculoskeletal:** Normal findings
- **Neurological:** Normal findings

Performing a Focused Physical Assessment

Now that you have looked at the relationship of the breasts to other systems, focus on the specifics of the examination. First inspect the breasts and axillae; then palpate them.

Inspection

Inspect the breasts with the client in all five positions, as described in the Approach section. Inspect the breasts for size, shape, symmetry, skin condition, and venous pattern. Inspect the nipple and areola for nipple inversion or eversion, nipple direction, and nipple discharge.

Figure 14–5 shows milk lines, mentioned under Nipples and Areolae.

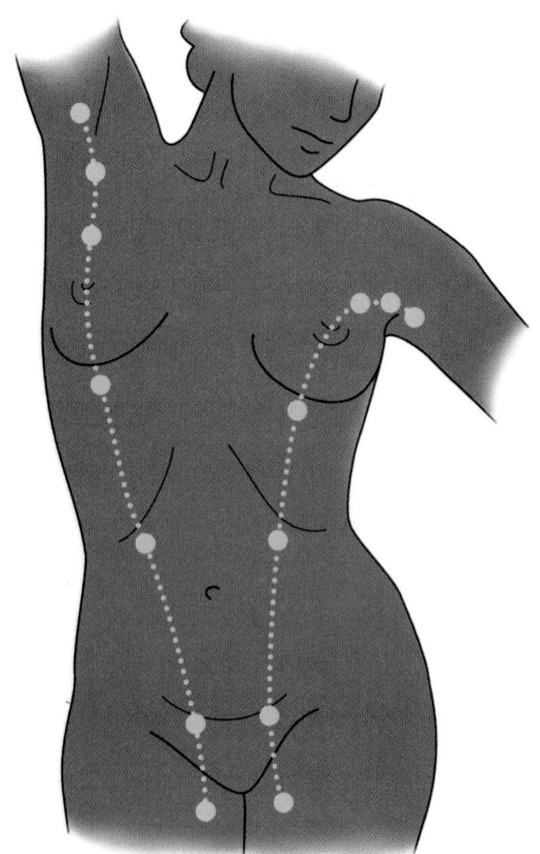

FIGURE 14–5. Milk lines.

Inspecting the Breasts

ASSESS/NORMAL VARIATIONS

Positions for breast examination

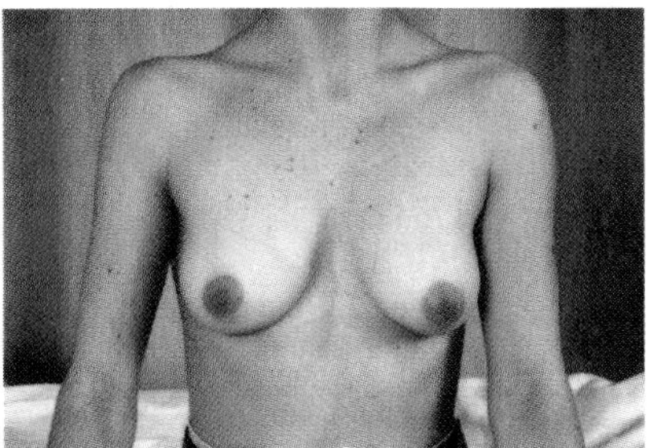
Sitting with arms at sides

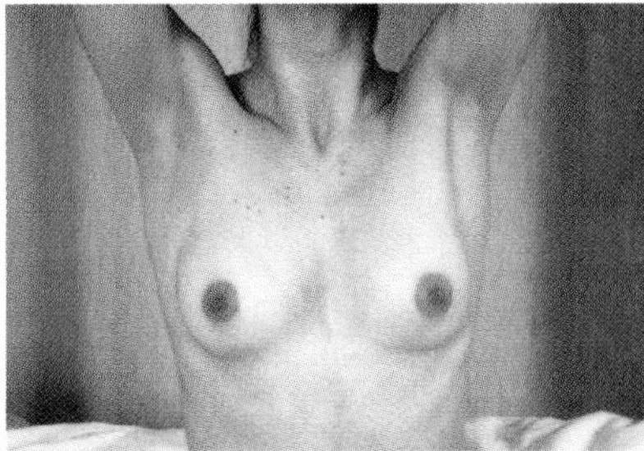
Sitting with arms above head

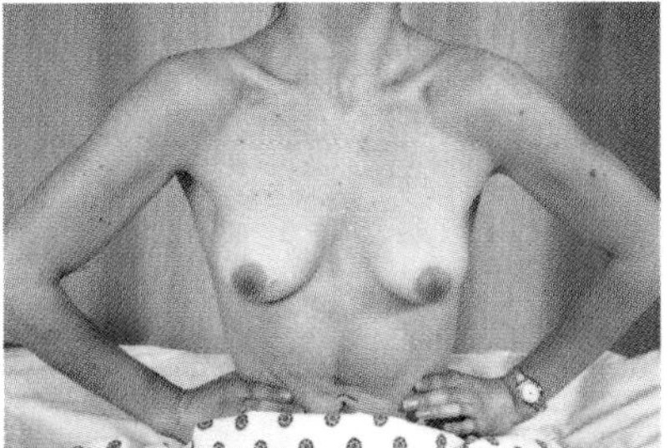
Sitting with hands on hips

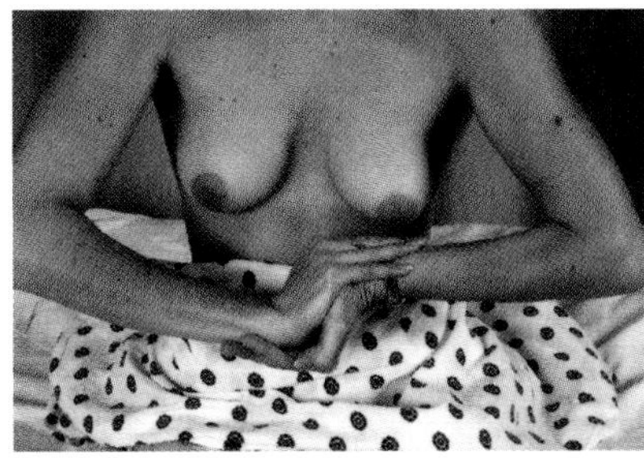
Sitting, pushing hands together

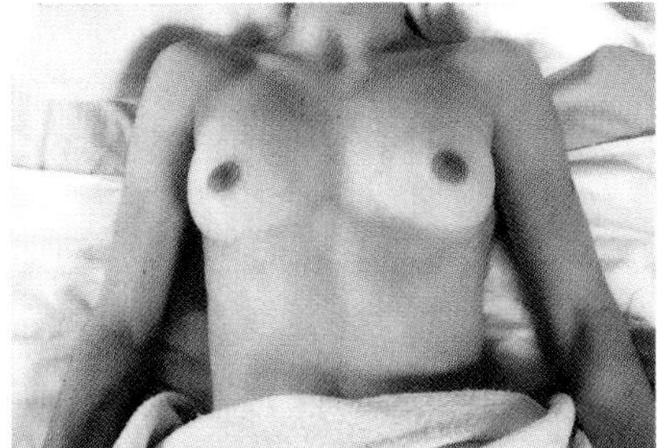
Supine

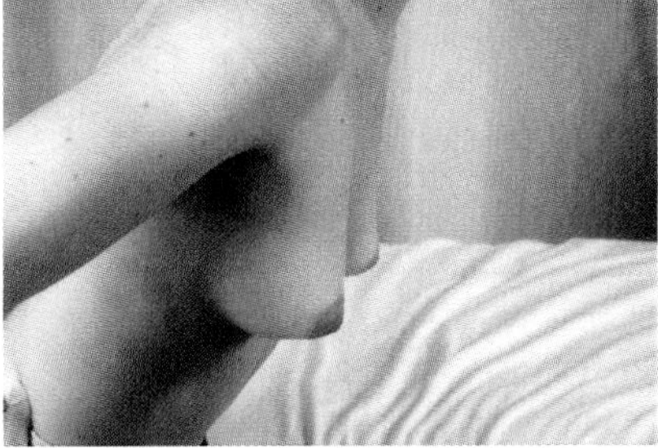
Sitting, leaning forward

HELPFUL HINT

- Large, pendulous breasts are easier to visualize if woman leans forward so they hang free..
- Note client's dominant side—it may be more developed.

Breast conical, symmetrical, or slightly asymmetrical.

Skin color lighter than in exposed areas; no lesions, redness, or edema; texture even.

Striae often seen with breast enlargement during pregnancy.

No dimpling or retraction.

No increase in venous pattern unless client is pregnant. Then symmetrical increase is normal.

ABNORMAL FINDINGS/RATIONALE

Change in symmetry warrants further investigation.

Edema and peau d'orange (orange skin appearance): May be related to lymphatic obstruction.

Erythema: Infection, abscess, or inflammatory carcinoma of breast.

Dimpling/puckering: Sign of retraction phenomena or abnormal traction on Cooper's ligaments caused by neoplasm. Attachment of tumor to fascia and pectoralis muscle pulls on skin and produces dimpling.

Lesions/asymmetrical increased venous pattern: Signs of breast cancer.

(Continued)

Inspecting the Breasts *(Continued)*

ASSESS/NORMAL VARIATIONS	ABNORMAL FINDINGS/RATIONALE
Nipples and Areolae Nipples everted, pointing in same direction, no discharge or lesions.	Inverted nipples may make breastfeeding difficult. Nipple changes—eversion to inversion or changes in direction they are pointing—may indicate an underlying mass. Flattened or inverted nipples are caused by shortening of mammary ducts.
Spontaneous discharge normal during pregnancy and lactation.	Spontaneous discharge not associated with pregnancy or breastfeeding warrants follow-up. Obtain a specimen for evaluation.
Areola and nipple darker than breast tissue. Become even darker during pregnancy. Supernumerary breasts or nipples are congenital anomalies in which small, palpable masses or nipples are present along milk lines, embryonic ridges that extend from axilla to groin. They usually atrophy during fetal development, except where the breasts develop. Cracks, redness of nipple can occur with nursing.	*Lesions/erosion/ulceration of areola and nipple:* Paget's disease. Discoloration of areola and nipple that is not associated with pregnancy warrants follow-up.
Axillae 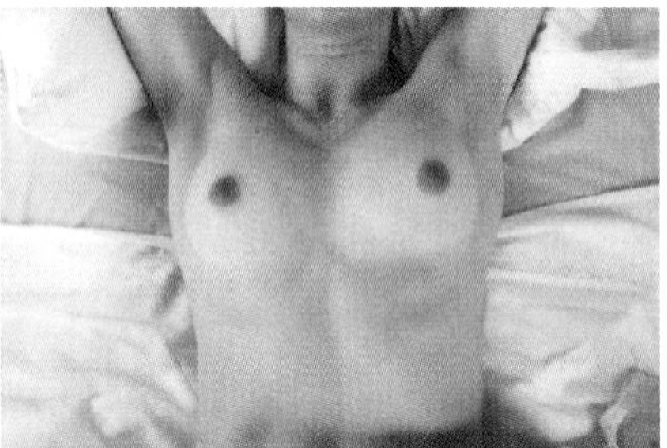 **Inspecting axillae** Skin intact. No rashes or lesions.	*Rashes/redness/unusual pigmentation:* Infection, allergy. *Dark pigmentation/velvety skin texture of axilla:* Malignant acanthosis nigricans, a rare cancer.

Palpation

Palpation enables you to feel for lumps, masses, and other abnormalities. Palpate the entire breast and axilla on both sides, making three small circles with the fingerpads of your middle three fingers. Use different pressure for each circle—light, medium, and deep. Light pressure allows you to palpate lesions beneath the skin; deep pressure allows you to palpate lesions that are deeper and near the ribs. Feel for lumps, thickening, or other changes. Because the breast extends from the midaxillary line to the sternal notch and the 2nd to 6th ribs, you must palpate all these areas. Put another way, you must palpate from the bottom of the bra line (6th or 7th intercostal space) to the collarbone (clavicle) and from the line down the middle of the breastbone (sternum) to the line down the middle of the armpit (midaxillary line), including the axilla.

HELPFUL HINTS

- Do not remove your fingerpads from the skin surface or jump from area to area.
- Most breast lesions in women are found in the upper outer quadrant. This area includes the tail of Spence and contains more breast tissue than the other quadrants.
- Although only about 1% of men get breast cancer, you still need to assess their breasts. Breast cancer in men most frequently occurs in the areola.

Palpating the Breasts

There are three techniques of breast palpation—the vertical strip method, the pie wedge method, and the concentric circle method. When demonstrating these methods for your client, stress that it doesn't matter which method she uses during BSE, as long as she uses the same

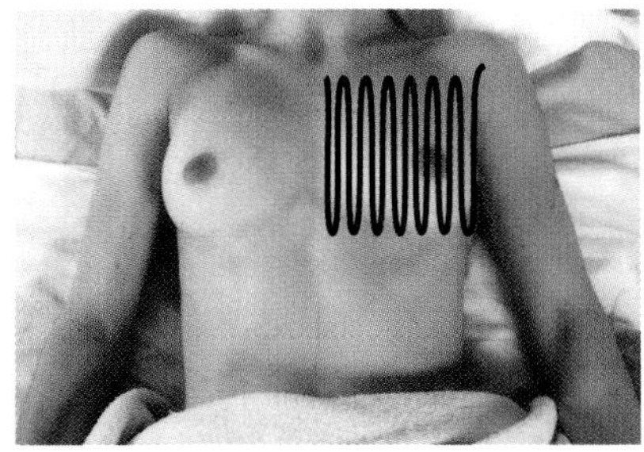
FIGURE 14–6. Vertical strip method.

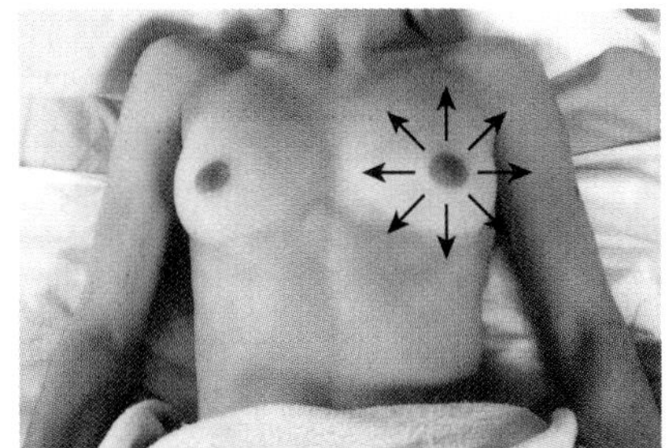
FIGURE 14–7. Pie wedge method.

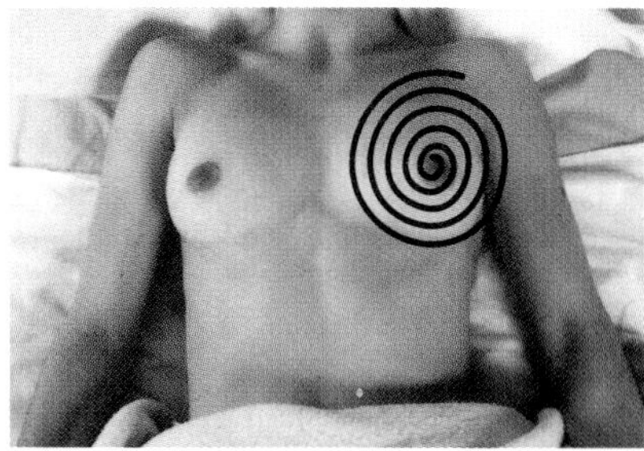
FIGURE 14–8. Concentric circles method.

method consistently and examines the entire breast area and axillae.

Vertical Strip Method

With this method (Fig. 14–6, you start at the sternal edge and palpate the breast in parallel lines until you reach the midaxillary line. This is like "mowing the grass," in which you go up one area and down the adjacent strip. Be sure to palpate the tail of Spence as well. End by examining and palpating the nipple. Note its elasticity, and squeeze it between your thumb and index finger to see if there is a discharge. Because of the possibility of discharge, be sure to wear nonsterile gloves when palpating the nipple. If the client is supine, shift the pillow or rolled towel to the opposite side and repeat the procedure with the other breast.

ALERT

If you notice an open lesion on the breast or axillae, wear nonsterile gloves to prevent contact with body fluids.

Pie Wedge Method

This method (Fig. 14–7) examines the breast in wedges or "pie slices." Once one wedge is examined, move to the adjacent wedge until you examine the entire breast and the tail of Spence. Then examine the nipple as you did in the vertical strip method. Repeat with the opposite breast.

Concentric Circles Method

This method (Fig. 14–8) uses concentric circles to examine the entire breast area. Start in the outermost area (or largest circle) at 12 o'clock; then move to 1 o'clock, 2 o'clock, and so on until the first circle is completed. When you complete the circle and return to 12 o'clock, move your fingers two fingerbreadths inward and examine another concentric circle. Repeat this procedure until you reach the nipple area. Examine the nipple in the same fashion as the previous two methods. Also examine the tail of Spence. Repeat with the other breast.

Palpating the Axillae and Lymph Nodes

Using your fingerpads, move your fingers in circular fashion to lightly palpate the axillary and clavicular nodes. Palpate the axillae with the client supine or sitting up with her arms at her sides. Palpate the supraclavicular, infraclavicular, central, lateral, anterior, posterior, and epitrochlear nodes. (For more information, see Chapter 13, Assessing the Peripheral-Vascular and Lymphatic Systems.)

HELPFUL HINT

Older women may have trouble changing positions, so examine the axillae after examining the breasts, with the client in the same position.

Documenting Your Findings

If you palpate a mass or lump, describe its size, shape, symmetry, mobility, delimitation, tenderness, consistency, temperature, and degree of redness. To document the location of breast masses, divide the breast into four quadrants by horizontal and vertical lines. Then visualize the breast as a clock face with the nipple as the center. Locate the pain or lump by the time on the clock (e.g., 2 o'clock), and measure the distance in centimeters from the nipple (Fig. 14–9).

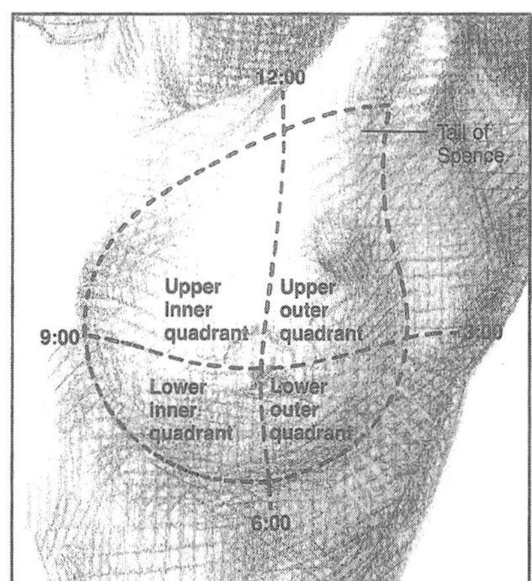

FIGURE 14–9. Describing the location of abnormalities.

Palpating the Breasts, Axillae, and Lymph Nodes

ASSESS/NORMAL VARIATIONS

Breasts

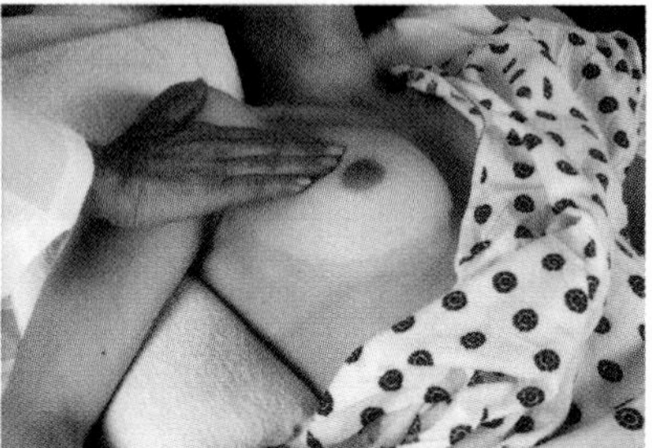

Palpating breast

Breasts soft, nontender.

Consistency is age dependent: More firm and elastic in premenopausal women; less firm and elastic with ducts that may feel stringy or cordlike in postmenopausal women.

ABNORMAL FINDINGS/RATIONALE

Benign breast lumps:

Fibroadenoma: Smooth, firm, round, movable, nontender, 1–5 cm in size.

Fibrocystic breast disease: Nodular, tender, movable, soft to firm, in postmenopausal women. multiple, fluctuate with menstrual cycle.

Malignant breast lumps:

Breast cancer: Irregular shape; irregular, poorly defined borders; nontender, immovable; increase in size as disease progresses.

Breast warm and indurated (hard): Mastitis; *Staphylococcus aureus* is most common cause.

HELPFUL HINTS

- In older adults, the inframammary ridge below the breast thickens and can be mistaken for a mass.
- In pregnancy, the breast may feel firm; during lactation, it may feel hard if engorged.

Nipples

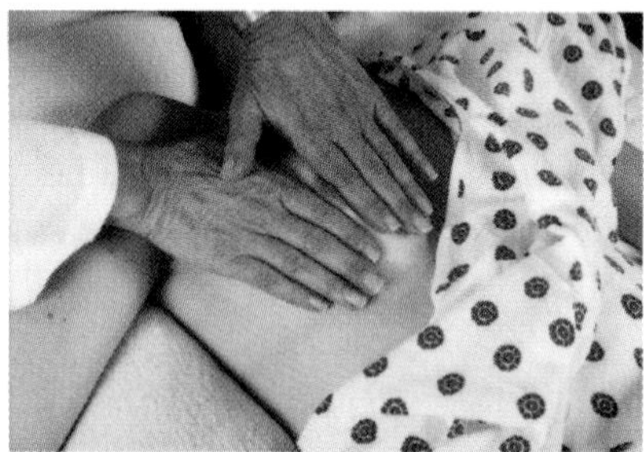

Palpating nipple

Nipples elastic, nontender. No discharge or white, sebaceous secretion.

Loss of elasticity may indicate underlying malignancy.

Bloody, purulent discharge: Infection.

Serous, serosanguinous, or bloody drainage: Intraductal papilloma.

Thick, gray drainage, fixation of nipple: Ductal ectasia.

Axilla and Clavicular Nodes

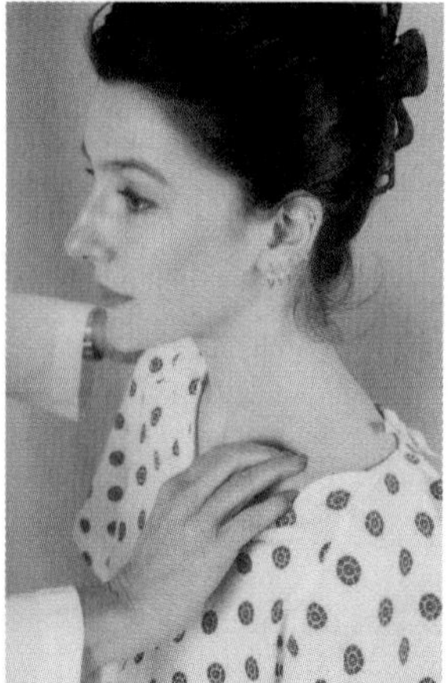

Palpating supraclavicular nodes

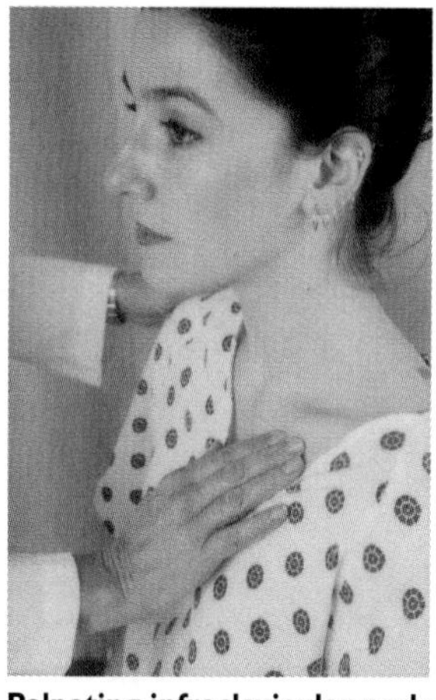

Palpating infraclavicular nodes

Palpable nodes: Infection or metastatic disease.

Enlarged lymph nodes caused by infection are usually tender; those caused by malignancy are nontender.

Palpating the Breasts, Axillae, and Lymph Nodes

ASSESS/NORMAL VARIATIONS	ABNORMAL FINDINGS/RATIONALE

Axilla and Clavicular Nodes *(Continued)*

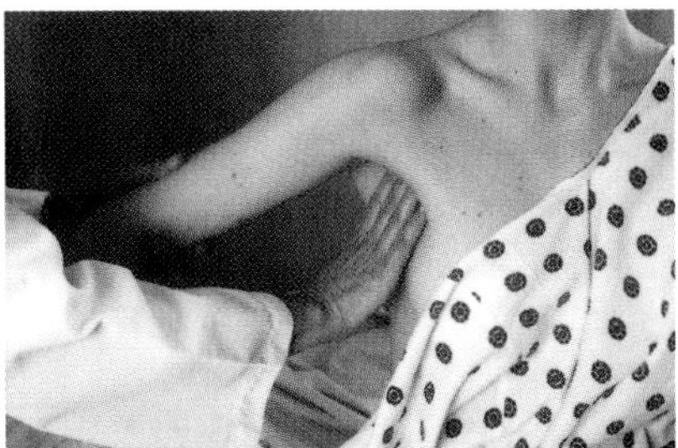

Palpating central nodes

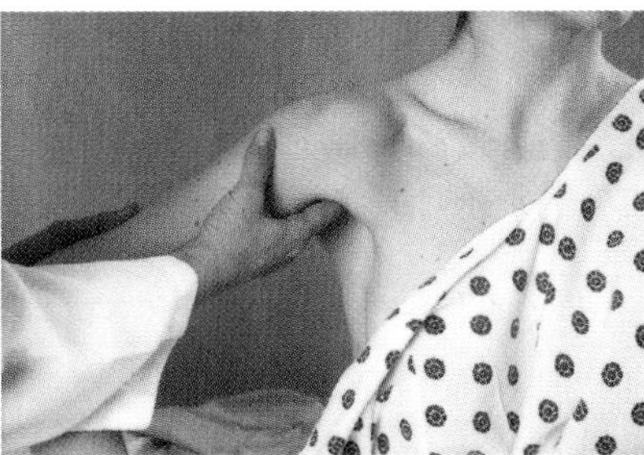

Palpating lateral nodes

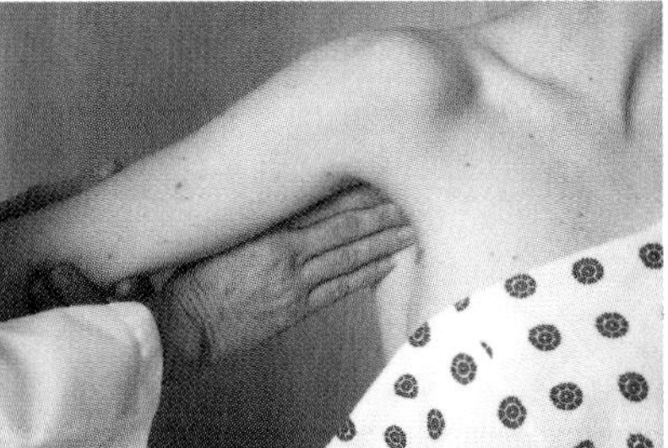

Palpating posterior nodes

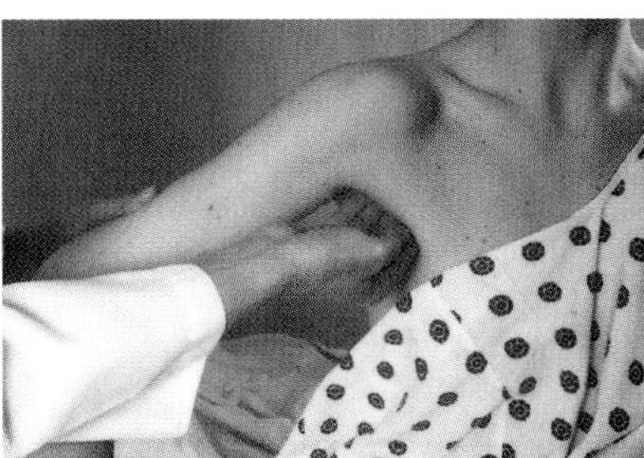

Palpating anterior nodes

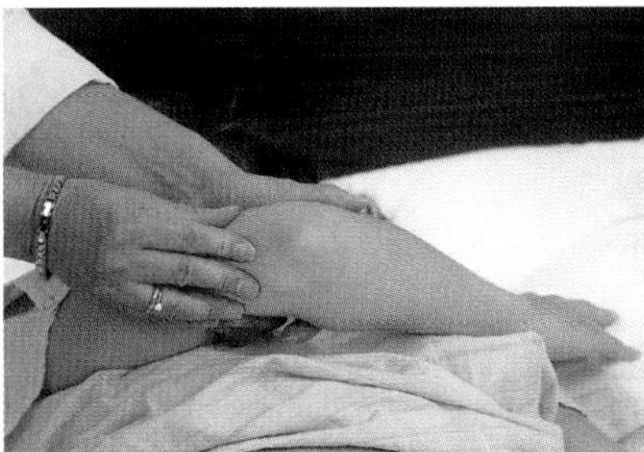
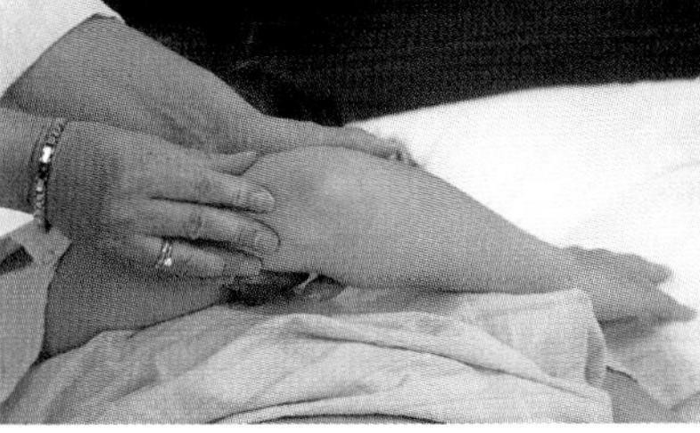

Palpating epitrochlear nodes

Nonpalpable

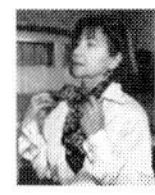

Case Study Findings

Mrs. Kobrynski's focused breast findings include:

- **Breasts:** Right breast slightly larger than left; uniform and symmetrical; ovoid in shape; no skin lesions noted; no redness or dimpling. Small, pea-sized (0.5 cm), easily movable, rubbery, smooth-edged lesion palpated in right breast at 2 o'clock; 4 cm from areola in the right upper outer quadrant; no lesions palpated in left breast.
- **Nipple:** No lesions observed or palpated; nipples erect and point in same direction; no inversion or eversion; denies discharge from nipple; unable to elicit discharge from either nipple; no specimens sent.
- **Axillae:** No lesions or thickening noted.

AREA/SYSTEM	SUBJECTIVE DATA
General	*Ask about:* General health Fever, weight changes
Integumentary	*Ask about:* Rashes Lesions Allergies
HEENT	*If patient has breast cancer, ask about:* Headaches Changes in mentation
Respiratory	*If patient has breast cancer, ask about:* SOB Cough Breathing difficulty
Cardiovascular	*Ask about:* CV medications
Gastrointestinal	*If patient has breast cancer, ask about:* Increase in size of abdominal girth.
Genitourinary/ Reproductive	*Ask about:* Last menstrual period, whether patient is pregnant, number of pregnancies, year of first pregnancy, whether patient is pre- or postmenopausal. Medications (BCP, HRT)
Musculoskeletal	*If patient has breast cancer, ask about:* Weakness Bone pain Fractures
Endocrine	*Ask about:* History of thyroid disease
Lymphatic/ Hematologic	*Ask about:* Infection or malignancy

AREA/SYSTEM	OBJECTIVE DATA
General	*Observe:* LOC Affect *Measure:* Vital signs Weight
Integumentary	*Inspect:* Rashes Lesions Color changes
HEENT	*If patient has breast cancer:* Test vision.
Respiratory	*If patient has breast cancer:* Auscultate and percuss lungs
Cardiovascular	*Inspect:* Increased vascularity of breasts
Gastrointestinal	*If patient has breast cancer:* Palpate abdomen.
Genitourinary/ Reproductive	*Inspect:* Perform pelvic exam
Musculoskeletal	*If patient has breast cancer:* Test muscle strength
Neurological	*If patient has breast cancer:* Test LOC, sensory and motor function
Endocrine	Palpate thyroid
Lymphatic/ Hematologic	Palpate lymph nodes

Assessment of the Breasts' Relationship to Other Systems

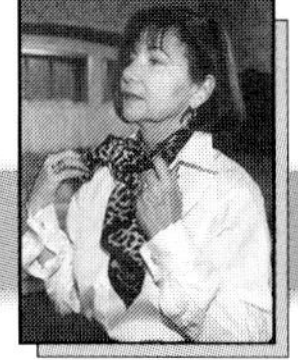

Case Study Analysis and Plan

Now that you have completed a thorough assessment of Mrs. Kobrynski, list the key history and physical examination findings that will help you formulate your nursing diagnoses.

Nursing Diagnoses

After you complete the assessment, formulate nursing diagnoses. The following are possible diagnoses. Cluster the supporting data for each.

1. Knowledge, deficient, related to BSE
2. Health Maintenance, ineffective, related to need for incorporation of preventive behaviors
3. Fear, related to presence of lump and need for mammogram/potential for life-threatening disease
4. Body Image, disturbed, potential

CRITICAL THINKING ACTIVITY #4

Now that your have identified some nursing diagnoses for Mrs. Kobrynski, select one diagnosis and develop a nursing care plan and a related teaching plan, including learning outcomes and teaching strategies.

Research Tells Us

Today, one in eight women in the United States will develop breast cancer in her lifetime. The lifetime risk (to age 85) of a woman developing breast cancer in 1940 was 5 percent, or 1 in 20; today, the risk is 12.6 percent, or 1 in 8. In women 40 to 49 years of age, there is a 1 in 66 risk of developing breast cancer; in women aged 50 to 59, the risk is 1 in 40.

Breast cancer is the second leading cause of cancer death in women and the leading cause of cancer death among women aged 35 to 54. Approximately 205,000 new cases of breast cancer will be diagnosed each year, and approximately 40,600 women will die.

Breast cancer is a major health risk, but early detection decreases morbidity and mortality and increases treatment options. Women need to take charge of their own health and learn how to examine their breasts and detect changes from month to month. The nurse's role is to teach women the importance and techniques of monthly BSE.

Molyneaux (1995) conducted a descriptive-correlational study of 289 second-semester senior baccalaureate nursing students from seven generic NLNAC approved programs and found that only 20 percent reported doing regular BSEs. Most of the students said that they learned BSE from nursing faculty in their nursing program. In addition, the study revealed that the students did not teach BSE to their clients, family, or friends. Nursing students had a presumed greater knowledge of the importance of preventive health behaviors, yet failed to incorporate them into their practice. Molyneaux recommended that adequate attention be given to preventive health practices and health teaching in nursing curricula. In addition, students should be required to teach BSE to clients so that students learn the process of teaching and are able to incorporate lifelong preventive health behaviors themselves.

Health Concerns

BSE should be performed monthly. In premenopausal women, examination should occur 5 to 7 days after the menstrual cycle begins, or 3 to 5 days after it ends. In postmenopausal women, BSE should be performed on the same day each month—such as the first day of the month, the client's birthday, or another meaningful day—so that the client will be reminded.

The purpose of BSE is to allow women to detect breast changes from month to month. At first, a woman may not know how to interpret what she feels, but she will soon become familiar with what is normal for her.

Studies show that 80% of all lumps found in breast tissue are benign, and most lumps are found by the women themselves. Mammography is the best method of early detection because it detects breast cancers before they can be felt. However, because annual screening mammography generally begins at age 40, this eliminates younger women. Women may also be without insurance or financial means to have mammograms. In addition, a small percentage of breast cancers may not show up on mammograms, so monthly BSE and regular clinical exams by a trained medical professional are necessary.

Risk Factors for Breast Cancer

- Older age
- Personal or family history of breast cancer
- Nulliparity or having a first child after age 30
- Early menarche (<12)
- Late menopause (>50)
- Unopposed estrogen stimulation of breasts by BCP or HRT.
- Being a carrier of either of two familial breast cancer genes called BRCA1 or BRCA2. Ten percent of women are carriers of these genes.

Teaching Breast Self-Examination

1 First, teach the client how to look at herself in a mirror and, with her arms at her sides, check for any visible abnormalities. She should observe for dimpling, retraction, or breast flattening as she first elevates her arms slowly, then presses her hands against her hips, and finally, bends forward.

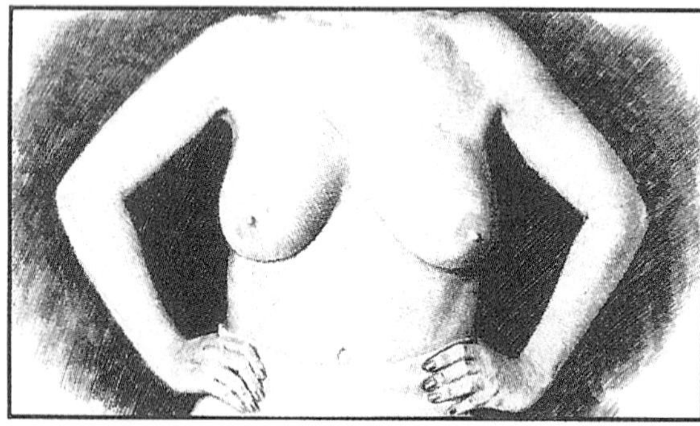

2 Next, by placing your hand over the client's, show her how to use the pads of the middle three fingers of the opposite hand to palpate the breast systematically by compressing the breast tissue against the chest wall. She should palpate all portions of the breast, areola, nipple, tail of Spence, and axilla when she is in the shower or standing before a mirror. She should repeat the procedure lying down with a pillow or folded towel under the shoulder of the side she is examining.

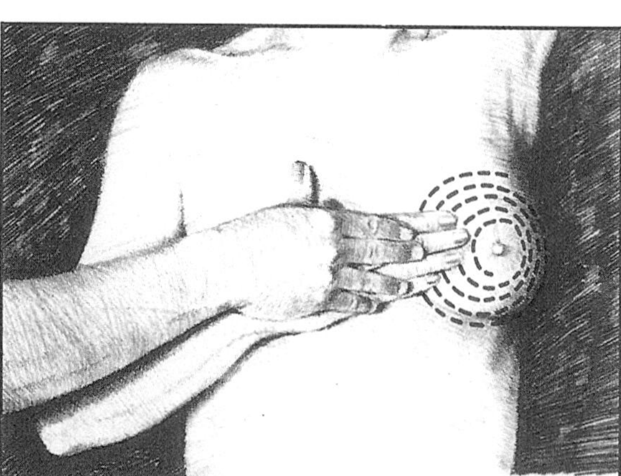

3 Next, show her how to compress the nipple gently between the thumb and index finger as she observes for any discharge.

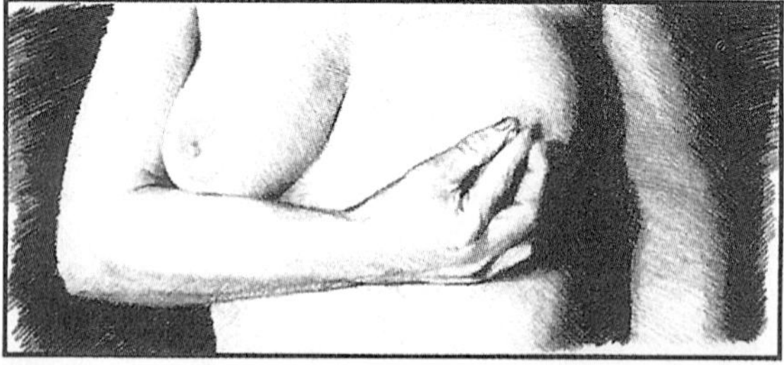

4 Finally, explain that she should report any redness or inflammation, swelling, masses, flattening, puckering, dimpling, retraction, sunken areas, asymmetrical nipple direction, discharge, bleeding, lesions, or eczematous nipple changes to her physician.

HELPFUL HINTS

- Some women do not feel comfortable touching their own breasts. Before teaching BSE, ascertain a women's comfort level regarding touching herself.
- Suggest that the client stand in front of a mirror to inspect her breasts.

Common Abnormalities

ABNORMALITY	ASSESSMENT FINDINGS
Breast Cancer	• Nipple erosion; retraction; or discharge, usually bloody. • Enlarged, shrunken, or dimpled breast with no pain. • Nontender, firm or hard lump, irregularly shaped and fixed to skin or underlying tissues. • Enlarged surrounding lymph nodes. • Usually seen in white women over 35 with family history of breast cancer; personal history of long menstrual cycles, early menarche, late menopause, or first pregnancy after 35. • Possible history of endometrial or ovarian cancer.
Fibroadenoma of Breast	• Well-defined mass or masses in breast, no pain. • Mass is round, firm, discrete, movable, 3/8″ to 2″ (1 to 5 cm) in diameter. • Usually solitary but may be multiple and bilateral. • Client usually in teens or early 20s.
Fibrocystic Disease Includes mammary dysplasia, cystic adenosis, chronic cystic disease, cystic mastitis.	• Thickened, nodular areas in breast (usually bilateral); may be slight; pain and tenderness possible, especially premenstrually. • May be single or multiple; mobile, well defined, tender; in upper outer quadrant. • Exacerbated by caffeine intake. • Cystic fluid (typically gray-green) from aspirated cysts. • Client in childbearing years.
Interductal Papilloma	• Serous or serosanguineous discharge from one nipple duct unilaterally, moderate pain. • No palpable tumor or mass, or soft mass difficult to distinguish from surrounding tissue. • Client usually aged 35 to 55.
Mammary Duct Ectasia (Dilatation)	• Nipple discharge and retraction, pain in affected areas, itching around nipple • Subareolar ducts feel like rubbery lesions filled with pastelike material • Enlarged regional lymph nodes possible. • Client usually in early-stage menopause.
Mastitis	• Pain accompanied by breast tenderness. • Firm, tender, warm, and reddened area in affected breast. • History of cracked nipples. • Breast abscess. • Painful, enlarged axillary lymph nodes. • Client usually 3rd or 4th week postpartum.

Summary

- Assessment of the breast provides invaluable information about the overall health of your client.
- A primary goal of breast assessment is to detect changes in the breast.
- Early detection of breast disease leads to early treatment.
- For breast cancer, the earlier the diagnosis and treatment, the better the prognosis.
- Assessment of the breast also provides an ideal opportunity to teach BSE to your client.

15

Assessing the Abdomen

Before You Begin

INTRODUCTION TO THE ABDOMEN

The abdominal assessment provides information about a variety of systems because every system, with the exception of the respiratory system, is found within the abdomen. The stomach, small and large intestines, liver, gallbladder, pancreas, spleen, kidneys, ureters, bladder, aortic vasculature, spine, uterus and ovaries or spermatic cord are all located in the abdomen. Assessment of the abdomen not only enables you to obtain valuable information about the functioning of the gastrointestinal, cardiovascular, reproductive, neuromuscular and genitourinary systems; it can also provide vital information about the health status of every other system.

Anatomy and Physiology Review

Before you begin your assessment, an understanding of the anatomy and physiology of abdominal structures is essential. You must be able to recognize normal structures before you can identify abnormal findings. Recognizing the structures will enable you to perform the assessment accurately, and understanding the physiology will guide your assessment and allow you to interpret your findings.

Structures and Functions

The major system assessed in the abdominal examination is the gastrointestinal (GI) or digestive system. The digestive system is responsible for the ingestion and digestion of food, absorption of nutrients, and elimination of waste products.

The primary structures of the digestive system (Fig. 15–1) include the mouth, pharynx, esophagus, stomach, small intestines (duodenum, jejunum, and ileum), large intestines (cecum, colon [ascending, transverse, descend-

Primary Digestive Organs/Structures and Functions

ORGAN/STRUCTURE	PRIMARY FUNCTION
Mouth	Mastication (chewing) of food particles and mixing them with saliva. Primarily mechanical digestion and the beginning of chemical digestion.
Pharynx	Swallowing of food particles into esophagus.
Esophagus	Propelling of food downward into stomach
Stomach	Stores food until it can be moved farther along GI tract. Parietal cells secrete hydrochloric acid to aid in digestion. Mucus cells secrete substances to coat the stomach. Chief cells secrete pepsinogen, which is converted to pepsin, which in turn digests protein. Churns food and breaks it down into small particles, then mixes them with gastric juices. Secretes gastrin, which stimulates secretion of acid and pepsinogen and increases gastric motility. Secretes intrinsic factor that protects vitamin B_{12} from stomach acids and facilitates absorption of B_{12} across the membranes of the small intestines (parietal cells) Absorbs some water, alcohol, and certain drugs. Destroys some bacteria found in foods. Site for both mechanical and chemical digestion.
Small intestine *Duodenum:* 25 cm (10 inches) long *Jejunum:* 2.5 meters (8 feet) long *Ileum:* 3.5 meters (12 feet) long	Bile and pancreatic juices facilitate absorption of nutrients in small intestines. Primary site for digestion, especially chemical digestion. Enzymes include: • Enterokinase: coverts trypsinogen to active trypsin. • Peptidases: help break down proteins. • Maltase, lactase, and sucrase: break down carbohydrates. Hormones include: • Cholecystokinin : secreted from duodenal wall; stimulates gallbladder to secrete pancreatic enzymes • Gastric inhibitory peptide: inhibits gastric motility • Secretin: secreted by duodenal wall; stimulates pancreatic secretions to neutralize gastric acid.
Appendix	Function is unknown. Narrowest part of intestines and a frequent site for bacteria and indigestible matter to become trapped leading to inflammation (appendicitis). May serve as a breeding ground for intestinal bacteria because it contains large amounts of lymphatic tissue.
Large intestine 1.5–1.8 meters (5–6 feet) long	Absorbs salt and water and excretes waste products of digestive process (feces) from the rectum (defecation). Helps synthesize vitamins B_{12} and K.

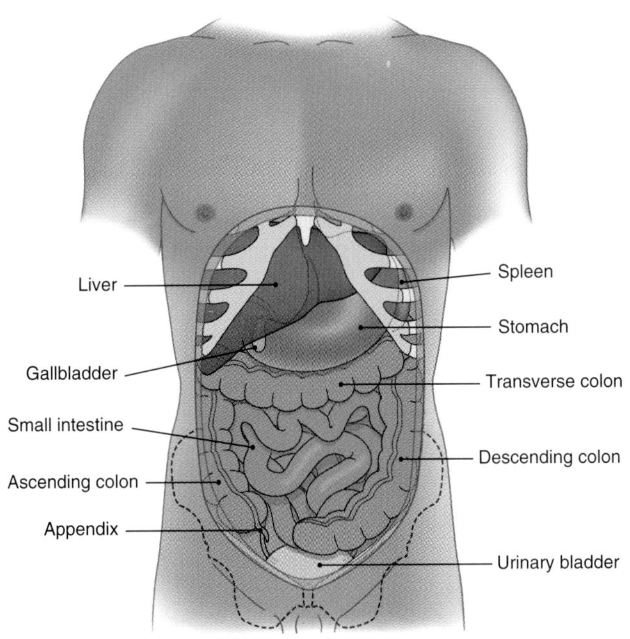

FIGURE 15–1. Abdominal organs and structures.

ing, and sigmoid]), and rectum. These main structures of the digestive system form a hollow tube that is actually outside the internal environment of the body even though it is located inside the body. This tube, referred to as the alimentary canal or the gastrointestinal tract, begins at the mouth and ends at the anus.

The digestive system also contains accessory organs that aid in the digestion of food. The accessory organs of the digestive system include the salivary glands (parotid, submandibular, sublingual), liver, gallbladder, and pancreas.

The Digestive Process

The digestive process consists of mechanical digestion, the breakdown of food through chewing, peristalsis, and churning; and chemical digestion, the breakdown of food through a series of metabolic reactions with enzymes.

The digestive process begins in the mouth, where food is taken in and masticated. The bolus of food is then

Accessory Digestive Organs/Structures and Functions

ORGAN/STRUCTURE	PRIMARY FUNCTION
Salivary glands: *Parotid, submandibular, sublingual*	Produce saliva that moistens and lubricates food Secrete amylase, which converts starches to maltose
Liver	Produces and secretes bile to emulsify fats Metabolizes protein, carbohydrates, and fats Converts glucose to glycogen where it is stored in the liver Produces clotting factors and fibrinogen Produces plasma proteins such as albumin Detoxifies a variety of substances such as drugs and alcohol Stores vitamins A, D, E, K, and B_{12} and minerals iron and copper Converts conjugated bilirubin from blood to unconjugated bilirubin
Pancreas, 12–5 cm (6–9 inches) long	As an endocrine gland, the pancreas secretes: • Beta cells, which secrete insulin to regulate blood sugar levels • Alpha cells, which secrete glucagons that store carbohydrates • Delta cells, which secret somatostatin, the hypothalamic growth inhibiting hormone that inhibits insulin and glucagon secretion • F cells, which secrete pancreatic polypeptide that regulates the release of pancreatic enzymes As an exocrine gland, the pancreas secretes the following digestive enzymes and alkaline materials: • Acinar units, which secrete digestive enzymes • Amylase, which digests starches into maltose • Lipase, which breaks down lipids into fatty acids and glycerol • Pancreatic proteolytic enzymes (trypsinogen, chymotrypsinogen and procarboxypeptidase), secreted in inactive form and activated in small intestine
Gallbladder, 7–10 cm (3–4 inches) long and 3 cm wide.	Stores and concentrates bile

swallowed into the esophagus, where is it is propelled slowly via peristaltic contraction to the stomach. In the stomach the food bolus is churned, breaking it down further into smaller particles and mixing it with digestive juices and hydrochloric acid that is produced by the stomach. The food bolus becomes chyme and progresses down into thTae first portion of the small intestine called the duodenum. In the duodenum, pancreatic juices and bile are secreted in the chyme. The food then enters the jejunum and ileum, where nutrients are absorbed into the circulatory system. Food particles that are not absorbed by the small intestines proceed into the large intestine, where they are eventually excreted as feces.

Additional Abdominal Structures

Along with the organs of the digestive system, the abdomen also contains the spleen; the urinary tract including the bladder, kidneys, and ureters; the uterus and ovaries; the aorta; and the iliac, renal, and femoral arteries. The uterus and ovaries are covered in Chapter 16. The other abdominal organs are shown in Figure 15–2.

The abdominal cavity has a serous membrane called the peritoneum, which covers the organs and holds them in place. The peritoneum contains a parietal layer that lines the walls of the abdomen and the visceral pleura, which coats the outer surface of the organs. There is a small amount of fluid between these membranes that allows them to move smoothly within the cavity.

Interaction with Other Body Systems

The GI system requires the proper functioning of the nervous, endocrine, respiratory, cardiovascular, integumentary, and musculoskeletal systems in order to function at its full capacity.

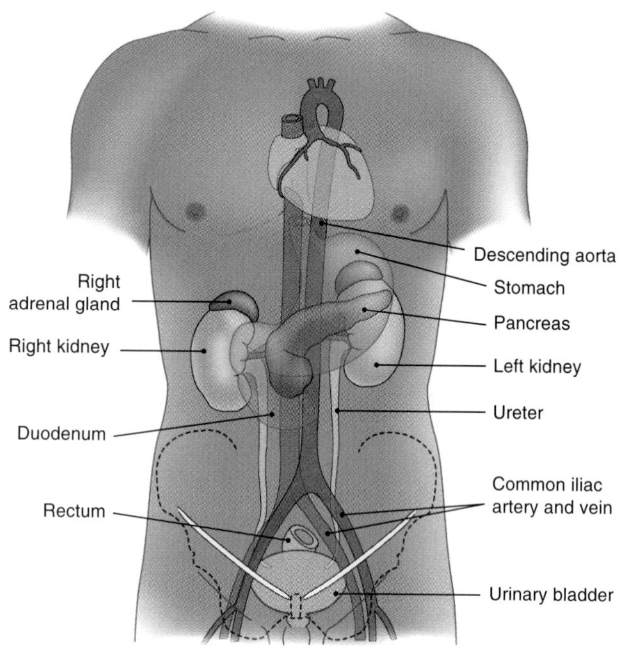

FIGURE 15–2. Other abdominal organs and structures.

The Integumentary and Musculoskeletal Systems

The digestive system is protected and supported by the musculoskeletal and integumentary systems. The musculoskeletal system also assists with ingestion, mastication, deglutition (swallowing) of food, and eventual defecation of its by-products.

Other Abdominal Organs and Structures

ORGAN/STRUCTURE	PRIMARY FUNCTION
Spleen	Stores RBCs and platelets. Produces RBCs and macrophages. Activates B and T lymphocytes.
Urinary Tract, Bladder, Kidneys	Maintain homeostasis of fluid-and-electrolyte and acid-base systems. Control blood pressure through secretion of renin. Secrete erythropoietin to stimulate RBC production. Remove waste products from body.
Spine	Supports weight of body. Protects spinal cord.
Spermatic Cord	Protects the vas deferens, blood vessels, lymph, and nerves that run from the scrotum to the penis.
Uterus and Ovaries	Ovaries produce ova and secrete estrogen and progesterone. The uterus allows the sperm to reach the uterine tubes, where it can make contact with an ovum. If conception occurs, the uterus develops an environment where the embryo can grow.
Vasculature of the Abdomen: Aorta and Inferior Vena Cava	Supplies oxygenated blood to the cells and organs in the lower half of the body.

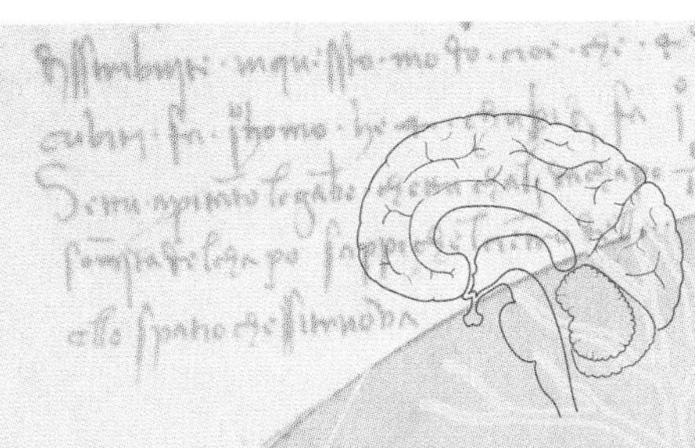

NEUROLOGICAL

Parasympathetic nervous system increases peristalsis; sympathetic nervous system decreases peristalsis.

Many cranial nerves are essential for eating.

Spinal cord problems may affect bowel and bladder control.

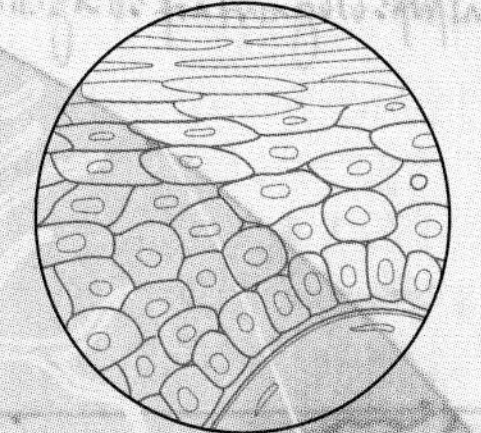

ENDOCRINE

Thyroid regulates metabolism.

Pancreas is an endocrine organ producing insulin, glucagons, and digestive enzymes.

INTEGUMENTARY

Skin-color changes such as jaundice may indicate liver disease.

Nutritional deficits or malabsorption problems can affect growth of skin, hair, and nails.

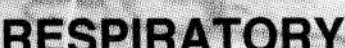

RESPIRATORY

A distended abdomen can impinge on respiratory structures.

Chronic lung disease with overinflation of lungs can push diaphragm farther into abdomen.

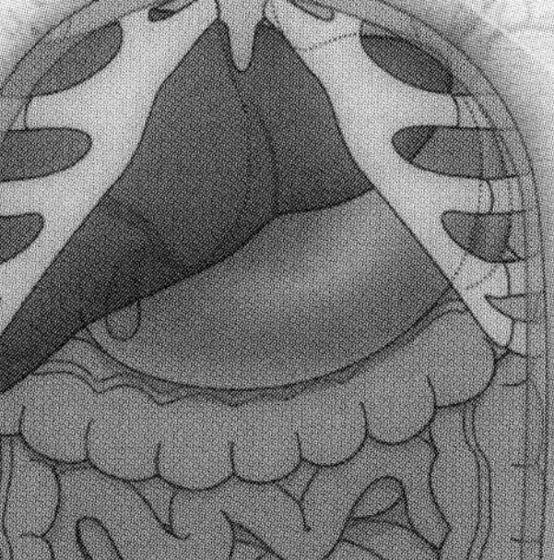

DIGESTIVE

Digestive system is found in abdominal cavity.

Problems with digestive system may affect other abdominal structures.

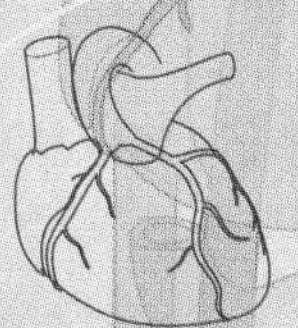

CARDIOVASCULAR

CV system transports nutrients and wastes.

Abdominal aorta is located in abdominal cavity.

Right-side heart problem can result in fluid accumulation in abdomen (ascites).

MUSCULAR

Abdominal muscles protect and support abdominal contents.

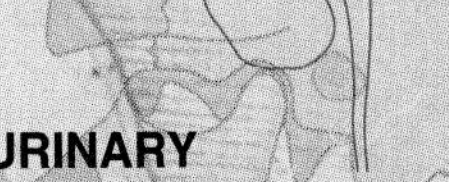

URINARY

Urinary structures are located in abdomen.

Problems with urinary system may affect other abdominal structures.

LYMPHATIC

The spleen is a lymphatic structure.

SKELETAL

Osteoporosis and arthritis are complications of ulcerative colitis.

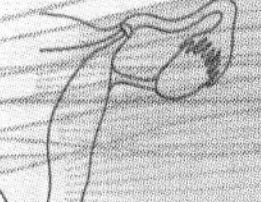

REPRODUCTIVE

Pregnancy displaces abdominal contents.

Relationship of GI System to Other Systems

The Respiratory and Cardiovascular Systems

The respiratory and cardiovascular systems provide the oxygen needed for the digestive organs to function. The respiratory system gets oxygen for the cells of the body and rids the body of carbon dioxide. All the cells in the body need oxygen to function appropriately, including the digestive system. The cardiovascular system circulates the oxygen-rich blood to all the cells in the body. Any decrease in oxygen to the cells of the digestive system affects organ function. For example, if blood flow to the bowel is disrupted, a bowel infarct can occur, causing the bowel to stop functioning.

The Neurological Systems

The neurological system plays an important role in digestion. When the body is in a parasympathetic response or the "rest and repair" phase, the neurological system releases acetylcholine, the neurotransmitter for the parasympathetic system. In relation to the digestive system, acetylcholine stimulates the secretion of digestive juices and increases peristalsis.

The opposite is true for the sympathetic response. The sympathetic system is stimulated at times of physical or psychological stress. When stimulated, a "fight or flight" response occurs, causing the release of norepinephrine, which causes a decrease in peristalsis and secretion of digestive juices. Therefore the digestive system functions to its maximum capacity when it receives parasympathetic responses from the peripheral nervous system.

The Endocrine System

The secretion of digestive juices also depends on the proper functioning of the pancreas, an organ that has both endocrine and exocrine functions. The endocrine function is to release insulin, glucagon, and gastrin into the bloodstream to assist in carbohydrate metabolism. The exocrine function is to secrete bicarbonate and pancreatic enzymes into the duodenum to aid in the digestion of proteins, fats, and carbohydrates.

Developmental, Cultural, and Ethnic Variations

Infants

Some anatomical characteristics in infants are different from those in adults. It is important to note that the newborn's bladder is located above the symphysis pubis. The liver proportionally takes up more space in the abdomen and may extend 2 cm (3/4 inch) below the rib cage. Because the infant's abdominal muscles are weak, the abdomen normally protrudes (see Chapter 22, Assessing the Newborn and Infant).

Children

A child's abdomen is proportionally larger than an adult's and has a slightly protuberant appearance because of the curvature of the back. This protuberance is most obvious in toddlers and preschoolers and diminishes to adult proportions during adolescence. Abdominal respiration is common in most children. Because the abdominal muscles are underdeveloped, the organs are more easily palpated (see Chapter 24, Assessing the Preschool and School-Age Child).

Pregnant Women

Many changes occur in the abdomen of the pregnant client. The abdominal muscles relax, allowing the uterus to protrude during a normal pregnancy. For women having multiple pregnancies or a multiple birth, the rectis abdominal muscles, which are located medially on the anterior aspect of the abdomen, may become separated (diastasis recti abdominis). As the fetus grows, it takes up even more room in the uterus, causing the stomach to rise up and impinge on the diaphragm.

Also, bowel sounds are diminished in the pregnant client because the bowels are compressed by the fetus. This decreased activity in the lower GI tract, along with the ingestion of prenatal vitamins containing large amounts of iron, contributes to constipation. Because of increased venous pressure in the lower abdomen, hemorrhoids may develop and cause further problems with elimination.

It is important to note that the location of the appendix in the pregnant woman is different from that in a nonpregnant woman. During pregnancy, the appendix is displaced upward and laterally to the right. This can complicate the diagnosis of appendicitis.

Pregnant clients have several particular alterations in their integumentary system. One characteristic skin change is the linea nigra, a darkly pigmented line that appears on the anterior abdomen from the pubis to the umbilicus in most pregnant women. Near the end of pregnancy the umbilicus may become everted and **striae** (stretch marks) may develop on the skin of the abdomen from the increased tension of the expanding uterus (see Chapter 21, Assessing the Mother-to-Be).

Older Adults

As people age, many of their body systems slow down and become less efficient. Elderly people have changes in dentition that may affect their chewing ability and digestion. Poorly fitted dentures may result in painful mastication, which causes the client to select foods that are

Culturally Related Health Problems with GI Symptoms

Cultural Group	Health Problem	GI symptoms
African-Americans	Sickle cell anemia	Splenomegaly and jaundice Sickle cell crisis: acute abdominal pain, vomiting
	Obesity	Weight >20% ideal weight
	Lactose intolerance	See symptoms above
Asian-Americans	GI cancer	Anorexia, bowel and digestion problems, pain, problems with weight loss
	Lactose intolerance	Abdominal cramping, diarrhea
Jews	Crohn's disease	Abdominal pain, diarrhea
	Ulcerative colitis	Abdominal pain, diarrhea, rectal bleeding
	Colon cancer	Changes in bowel habits, blood in stool, constipation
Mediterranean-Americans	Lactose intolerance	See symptoms above
(Greek and Italian descent)	Thalassemia, anemia	Jaundice, splenomegaly
Native Americans	Alcoholism, liver disease, pancreatitis	Jaundice, anorexia, ascites, pain, jaundice, steatorrhea
	Diabetes	Polyuria, thirst, weakness, weight loss, itching
	Gallbladder disease	Pain

easier to chew but not necessarily nutritionally balanced. In the GI tract, there is a reduction of saliva, stomach acid, gastric motility, and peristalsis that causes problems with swallowing, absorption, and digestion. These changes along with a general reduction of muscle mass and tone also contribute to constipation. Fat accumulates in the lower abdomen in women and around the waist in men, making physical assessment of the organs a little more challenging. The liver becomes smaller and liver function declines, making it harder to process medications (see Chapter 25, Assessing the Older Adult.)

HELPFUL HINTS

- Be aware that older adults have a diminished response to painful stimuli that may mask abdominal health problems.
- Older adults may have difficulty assuming some positions necessary for the physical examination, so modify positions to meet their needs.

People of Different Cultures and Ethnic Groups

Some health problems are considered culturally or racially related. This means that some diseases are seen either exclusively in a certain race or ethnic group or occur more frequently in that group. For instance, sickle cell anemia is seen almost exclusively in blacks. Ashkenazi Jews have a greater incidence of colon cancer than other groups because they are believed to have a gene linked to the development of "familial colorectal cancer."

Introducing the Case Study

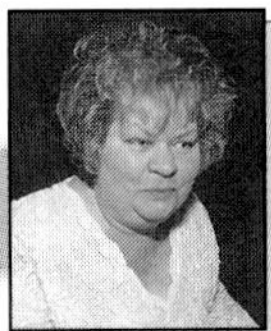

Anne Robichaud is a 56-year-old divorced mother of two grown children who came to see her nurse practitioner for an annual physical examination. She is a Roman Catholic of French-Canadian descent who speaks English and French and works in a local mill. Mrs. Robichaud states, "I'm constipated all the time." She has a family history of colon cancer. Considering her chief complaint and the fact that she has not had a complete physical for several years, a complete health history and physical examination are warranted.

Performing the Abdominal Assessment

Assessment of the abdomen involves obtaining a complete health history and performing a physical examination. As you assess the client, be watchful for signs and symptoms of actual and potential problems involving the different organs and structures in the abdomen.

Health History

The health history precedes the physical examination and involves interviewing the client about his or her perception of his or her health status. The health history interview includes a broad range of questions so that possible problems associated with each of the systems of the abdomen may be identified. Remember that information collected as part of the health history may uncover problems related to systems outside the abdomen (e.g., myocardial infarction).

Biographical Data

Gathering biographical information can provide valuable insights about the client's health status in several ways. Certain age groups are at greater risk for problems in the GI system. For example, infants and toddlers have a higher incidence of **hernias** than older children. Preschoolers are more likely to get parasitic infections, and teenagers may have abdominal symptoms as a result of pregnancy, sexually transmitted diseases, eating disorders like **anorexia nervosa** or bulimia, and infectious mononucleosis. Appendicitis occurs more frequently in children and teenagers than it does in adults. Older adults commonly develop problems with digestion, absorption, metabolism, and elimination because of changes caused by the aging process. Women aged 65 and over are commonly diagnosed with **hiatal hernia,** constipation, and diverticulosis.

Certain diseases occur more frequently in some races and cultures (see previous section). You will need to ask additional health history questions to determine whether symptoms of these diseases are present so that appropriate screening measures can performed, if necessary.

Also ask what drugs the person is taking. Many drugs have adverse effects on the GI system (see box, Drugs That Adversely Affect the GI system, on page 477).

The potential for exposure to environmental and occupational hazards can also be discovered in the biographical data. Where a person lives or works may raise questions about environmental hazards such as lead exposure in children (from inhalation of lead-based paint dust in older houses) or occupational health hazards such as chemical exposure (arsenic, benzene).

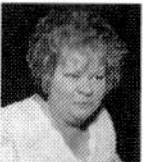

Case Study Findings

Reviewing Mrs. Robichaud's biographical data:

- 56-year-old divorced woman, mother of 2 grown children
- French-Canadian descent, speaks English and French
- Roman Catholic
- High school graduate and mill worker
- Source of information: self, reliable

Current Health Status

If your client has an abdominal complaint, investigate this first. Common chief complaints involving the body systems in the abdomen include:

- *Lymphatic:* Swelling, lymph node tenderness
- *Digestive:* Anorexia, bruising, constipation, diarrhea, distention, dysphagia, epigastric burning, gastric reflux, indigestion, jaundice, nausea, vomiting, pain, weight changes
- *Reproductive:* Cramping, nausea, pain, vomiting, weight gain
- *Neurological:* Pain
- *Cardiovascular:* Pain
- *Urinary:* Edema, pain, problems with urination (burning, frequency)

HELPFUL HINTS

- Rapid onset of symptoms usually indicates a serious problem. Note date and time pain started.
- Women of childbearing age with abdominal complaints should always be asked about the possibility of pregnancy.

The most common abdominal complaints—pain, changes in weight, changes in bowel habits (constipation, diarrhea), indigestion, nausea, and vomiting—are analyzed in the subsequent text using the PQRST format. The nature and intensity of the symptoms dictate the order and extent of questioning during the symptom analysis.

Drugs That Adversely Affect the GI System

Drug Class	Drug	Possible Adverse Reactions
Analgesics	acetaminophen	Hepatic necrosis with high (toxic) doses
	aspirin	GI disturbances, GI bleeding, ulceration
Antacids	aluminum hydroxide	Constipation
	calcium carbonate	Constipation, gastric hypersecretion, acid rebound
	magnesium hydroxide	Diarrhea
Anticholinergic agents	All anticholinergics	Nausea, vomiting, constipation, xerostomia (dry mouth), bloated feeling, paralytic ileus
Antidepressants	amitriptyline hydrochloride, nortriptyline hydrochloride	Constipation, adynamic ileus, elevated liver enzyme concentrations, jaundice, hepatitis
	Selective serotonin reuptake inhibitors	Nausea, vomiting, diarrhea, constipation
Antidiabetic agents	acetohexamide	Nausea, vomiting, diarrhea, heartburn, cholestatic jaundice
	chlorpropamide	Nausea, vomiting, diarrhea, heartburn (pyrosis), jaundice
Anti-infectives	ampicillin	Diarrhea, nausea, vomiting, pseudomembranous colitis
	ciprofloxacin	Heartburn
	clindamycin hydrochloride	Nausea, vomiting, diarrhea, tenesmus (straining at stool), pseudomembranous and nonspecific colitis
	erythromycin	Abdominal pain and cramping, nausea, vomiting, diarrhea, hepatic dysfunction, jaundice
	metronidazole	Taste disturbances, abdominal discomfort, diarrhea, nausea, vomiting
	sulfonamides	Nausea, vomiting, hepatic changes
	tetracycline hydrochloride	Nausea, vomiting, diarrhea, stomatitis
Antihypertensives	clonidine hydrochloride	Nausea, vomiting, constipation
	guanethidine sulfate	Increased frequency of bowel movements, explosive diarrhea
	methyldopa	Elevated liver function tests
Antineoplastic agents	All antineoplastics	Nausea, vomiting, stomatitis
Antituberculosis agents	isoniazid	Increased liver enzyme concentrations
	rifampin	Heartburn, nausea, vomiting, diarrhea, increased liver enzyme concentrations
Biphosphonates	alendronate	Esophagitis, heartburn
Cardiac agents	digoxin	Nausea, vomiting, diarrhea, anorexia with high (toxic) doses
	quinidine sulfate	nausea, vomiting, diarrhea, abdominal cramps, colic
Narcotic analgesics	codeine, meperidine, hydrochloride, methadone hydrochloride, morphine sulfate, oxycodone	Nausea, vomiting, constipation, biliary spasm or colic
Nonsteroidal anti-inflammatory agents	ibuprofen, indomethacin, salicylates	Nausea, vomiting, dyspepsia, GI bleeding, peptic ulcer
Phenothiazines	prochlorperazine maleate, thioridazine hydrochloride	Constipation, dyspepsia, paralytic ileus, cholestatic jaundice (hypersensitivity reaction)
	acarbose	Diarrhea, flatulence, abdominal pain
Miscellaneous agents	allopurinol	Altered liver function, nausea, vomiting, diarrhea
	aminophylline, theophylline	GI irritation, epigastric pain, nausea, vomiting, anorexia
	barium sulfate	Cramping, diarrhea
	colchicine	Diarrhea, nausea, vomiting, abdominal pain
	estrogen-progestin combinations	Nausea, vomiting, diarrhea, abdominal cramps, altered liver function tests, cholestatic jaundice
	iron preparations	Constipation, nausea, vomiting, black stools
	gold sodium thiomalate, auranofin	Changes in bowel habits, diarrhea, abdominal cramping, nausea, vomiting
	griseofulvin	Nausea, vomiting, diarrhea, flatulence
	levodopa	Nausea, vomiting, anorexia
	lithium	Nausea, vomiting, diarrhea
	phenytoin sodium	Nausea, vomiting, constipation, dysphagia
	potassium supplements	Nausea, vomiting, diarrhea, abdominal discomfort, small-bowel ulceration (with enteric-coated tablets)
	prednisone	Epigastric pain, gastric irritation, pancreatitis
	zidovudine	Nausea, vomiting, anorexia

Symptom Analysis

Symptom Analysis tables for all of the symptoms described in the following paragraphs are available on the Web for viewing and printing. In your Web browser, go to *http://www.fadavis.com/detail.cmf?id=0882-9* and click on Symptom Analysis Tables under Explore This Product.

Abdominal Pain

The most common complaint related to the abdomen, pain is often classified as visceral, parietal, or referred. Visceral pain results from distention of the intestines or stretching of the solid organs. It is often described as burning, cramping, diffuse, and poorly localized. Parietal pain results from inflammation of the parietal peritoneum. The pain is usually severe, localized, and aggravated by movement. Referred pain is felt at a site away from the site of origin. Impulses from the internal organs and structures that share nerve pathways inside the central nervous system explain the nature of referred pain.

HELPFUL HINT

When assessing severity of pain, use an accepted pain intensity rating scale consistently. Be sure to document what tool you used and the words the client uses to describe the pain's intensity.

Acute abdominal pain ("acute abdomen") may indicate a life-threatening abdominal condition that requires immediate medical intervention. In this situation, you should assess the client's vital signs to determine whether he or she is in imminent danger. Vital signs provide information about the possibility of cardiac irregularities and reveal symptoms of shock and signs of an infectious process such as peritonitis. In addition, you need to prioritize the symptom assessment questions on the Web to elicit the most essential information. The order of symptom assessment becomes RTQSP.

Pain Location

The location of the pain is often diagnostically significant. Some disorders have classic signs located in specific regions of the abdomen. For instance, pain in the umbilical region may indicate an abdominal aortic aneurysm or early appendicitis. Abdominal problems may also cause referred pain to the chest, so chest pain can indicate either an abdominal problem or a cardiac event. Clients with a **gastric ulcer** can have pain in the upper epigastric region left of midline, which is also the location for angina and myocardial infarction (MI). Clients with **gastroesophageal reflux disease (GERD)** may have chest pain that radiates to back, neck, or jaw, which also mimics an MI. Clients with a **hiatal hernia** may complain of substernal chest pain and difficulty breathing, especially after a meal. Note location of pain by quadrant or region:

- Pain in shoulder: Ruptured spleen, ectopic pregnancy, pancreatitis
- Pain in scapula: Cholelithiasis, MI, angina, biliary colic, pancreatitis
- Pain in thighs, genitals, lower back: Renal problems, ureteral colic
- Pain in lower and middle back: Abdominal aortic aneurysm

Recognizing the relationship between the location of the pain and the possible health problem has important implications for immediate nursing assessment and care of the client.

Significance of Pain by Abdominal Quadrant

Left Upper Quadrant	Right Upper Quadrant
Heart: MI/ Ischemia	*Heart:* MI/Ischemia
Lungs: Pulmonary embolism, pneumonia	*Lungs:* Pneumonia
Pancreas: Pancreatitis	*Gallbladder:* Cholelithiasis, cholecystitis
Spleen: Ruptured spleen	*Liver:* Hepatitis, cancer
Stomach: Gastric ulcer, esophagitis, GERD, hiatal hernia, varices	*Intestines:* Duodenal ulcer
	Appendicitis
Left Lower Quadrant	**Right Lower Quadrant**
Ovary/Uterus: Ectopic pregnancy, ovarian cyst, pelvic inflammatory disease (PID)	*Ovary/Uterus:* Ectopic pregnancy, ovarian cyst, PID
Intestines: Perforation, constipation, diverticulitis, hernia, ulcerative colitis	*Intestines:* Perforation, obstruction, constipation, Crohn's disease, diverticulitis, hernia, ulcerative colitis
Kidney: Nephrolithiasis (kidney stones), infection	*Kidney:* Nephrolithiasis, infection

ALERT

If a client presents with chest pain or indigestion, rule out cardiac disease first.

TERMS USED TO DESCRIBE QUALITY AND RADIATION OF PAIN

Quality:

- Aching
- Burning
- Colicky
- Dull
- Nagging
- Piercing
- Pressure
- Cramping
- Pulsing
- Sharp
- Spasms
- Squeezing
- Stabbing
- Throbbing
- Viselike
- Waves

Radiation:

- Radiating
- Shooting

HELPFUL HINTS

- Remember to assess each new complaint as it arises in the client history and physical examination.
- When assessing palliative or provocative factors, ask about the client's use of culturally related remedies. These remedies may be tried first, delaying the initiation of traditional Western treatment. For some illnesses, a delay in treatment may have serious repercussions.

CRITICAL THINKING ACTIVITY #1

How would you explain the pain associated with appendicitis, beginning first in the umbilical region, then localizing to the right lower quadrant?

HOW CLIENTS WITH EATING DISORDERS LOSE WEIGHT

Diets: Reducing calories by stopping or skipping meals
Cathartics: Abusing laxatives, enemas, suppositories, diuretics
Exercise: Excessive exercise to burn off calories
Purgatives: Using ipecac or self-induced vomiting

Weight Change

Weight change may indicate diseases in many body systems, reflect unhealthy behaviors, or even reveal a normal state such as pregnancy. Weight changes can be a sign of GI disease, cancer, congestive heart failure with fluid retention, metabolic or endocrine disorders, unhealthy lifestyles, major depressive disorder, and eating disorders. A careful analysis of this symptom provides data that allows the nurse to distinguish between medical and behavioral problems causing the weight change. Weight changes of 2 to 3 lb (1 to 1.4 kg) within 48 hours result from fluid changes. Unexplained weight loss in adult should raise suspicions of underlying malignancy.

Change in Bowel Patterns

Alterations in bowel movements are associated with a variety of GI disorders, such as malabsorption disorders, irritable bowel syndrome, cancer, infections (viral, bacterial, parasitic), food intolerance, and reactions to medications, as well as non-GI disorders. To determine whether a client is having health problems that affects bowel function, first establish a baseline by asking general questions about bowel habits, such as: "How often do you have bowel movements? Do you have any problems with your bowels, such as straining, pain, constipation, or diarrhea?" Then ask more specific questions to help identify the origin of the problem.

Bowel pattern range from two movements per day to two or three per week. Identify the color of the stool:

- Black, tarry: Upper GI bleeding
- Red, bloody: Lower GI bleeding
- Clay colored: Increased bile in obstructive jaundice

COMMON CAUSES OF CONSTIPATION

- Medications
- Lack of exercise
- Lack of dietary fiber
- Lack of response to urge to defecate
- Loss of abdominal muscle tone
- Cancer
- Depression
- Dehydration
- Impaction
- Lead poisoning
- Intestinal obstruction
- Hypothyroidism

Diarrhea (frequent loose bowel movements) can have a variety of causes: diet; medications; viral or bacterial infections; and medical problems such as ulcerative colitis, irritable bowel syndrome, and Crohn's disease.

ALERT

Never give a cathartic to a client with abdominal pain, nausea, and constipation who also has absent bowel sounds..

HELPFUL HINTS

- If your client has abdominal cramps, diarrhea, nausea, vomiting, and fever lasting 7 to 10 days, he or she probably has gastroenteritis caused by a virus.
- Diarrhea assessment tools such as the National Cancer Institute Scale of Severity of Diarrhea are helpful to use when assessing clients, especially those with ongoing episodes of diarrhea who are taking antineoplastic drugs.

ALERTS

- *Extended hospitalization, abdominal surgery, and antibiotics (especially cephalosporins) increase the client's risk for developing pseudomembranous colitis. This potentially life-threatening disorder causes abdominal cramps, fever, and watery or bloody diarrhea*
- *Prolonged diarrhea can cause loss of fluids and electrolytes such as potassium. Assess for dehydration by checking skin turgor, taking orthostatic blood pressure (BP) and pulse and observing for signs of hypokalemia, such as cardiac arrythmias and muscle weakness.*
- *If your client complains of indigestion, take his or her vital signs immediately. People having an MI commonly complain of indigestion.*

Indigestion

Indigestion—also called dyspepsia or pyrosis—is a frequent abdominal complaint that is usually described as "heartburn." This burning sensation is usually worse after eating a meal. Acid from the stomach flows into the lower esophagus causing the burning sensation. GERD has heartburn as its chief symptom, but the epigastric distress occurs more frequently, lasts longer, and has more severe symptoms than indigestion. Heartburn is also a common complaint in both gastric ulcer and duodenal ulcer disease and gallbladder disease. Indigestion that increases when the person is lying flat may indicate a hiatal hernia or GERD. Indigestion associated with belching (eructation) and flatulence suggests cholecystitis.

Nausea

Nausea is caused by stresses on the stomach wall or esophagus. Distention, alterations in peristalsis, negative olfactory stimulation, inner ear problems, or medications can also cause nausea. Many GI medical conditions have nausea as an assessment finding.

Vomiting

During vomiting, peristalsis is reversed and the esophageal sphincter opens to allow the contents of the stomach to be ejected. The involuntary emptying of stomach contents is caused by irritation of the stomach lining caused by chemicals, trauma, or distention; stimulation of the vomiting center in the brain (medulla); and head injury. Some GI conditions that cause vomiting are intestinal obstruction, peptic ulcer, viral or bacterial infection, and appendicitis. A person with repeated vomiting is always at risk for fluid and electrolyte problems.

ALERT

Projectile vomiting without nausea (unexpected vomiting) results from central stimulation of the vomiting center (medulla) and is a sign of head injury or neurological or vascular abnormalities in the brain.

HELPFUL HINT

Coffee-ground colored emesis indicates the presence of blood in the stomach.

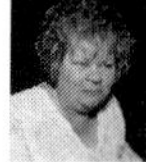

Case Study Findings

Mrs. Robichaud's current health status includes:

- No bowel movement in 4 days.
- Dull, intermittent lower abdominal pain rated 2 on a 0 to 10 scale. Walking around makes it better and nothing makes it worse.
- Denies visible red blood in stool, black stool, or symptoms in other body systems.
- Says she has had problems with constipation for the last few years.

ALERT

Foods do not have to be eaten to elicit an allergic reaction. Just smelling or touching the food is enough to produce an allergic response in some people.

Past Health History

This section of the health history involves asking questions about childhood and adult illnesses, injuries, hospitalizations, allergies; immunizations, and medications that can affect the abdominal structures. Remember to document specific dates in the client's record.

Past Health History

RISK FACTOR / QUESTIONS TO ASK	RATIONALE/SIGNIFICANCE
Childhood Illnesses	
Did you have chickenpox (varicella)?	Varicella always precedes herpes zoster or "shingles" (vesicular rash on lower aspect of rib cage in hypochondriac regions of the abdomen).
Did you have digestive problems?	May indicate a pattern of GI problems or risk for developing megacolon
Did you have malabsorption diseases?	May indicate celiac disease (impaired GI absorption related to wheat and rye ingestion)
Did you have an eating disorder?	Eating disorders often begin during adolescence and continue into adulthood.
Do you have sickle cell anemia?	Abdominal pain is associated with sickle cell crisis
Hospitalizations	
Have you ever been hospitalized for GI problems? Have you ever had any GI diagnostic tests, such as guaiac tests, colonoscopy, CT, MRI, GI series, or barium swallow?	Present symptoms may relate to previously diagnosed condition.
Surgeries	
Have you had any of the following, and if so, when?	Surgical procedures increase risk for adhesions, infections, obstructions, and faulty vitamin absorption.
Abdominal surgery, such as an appendectomy?	Rule out appendix as origin of current abdominal problem.
Blood transfusions?	Hepatitis and HIV are transmitted via blood. Increases risk for infection.
Recent insertion of GI tubes?	Assess signs and symptoms of infection
Serious Injuries	
Recent trauma, such as auto accident, workplace injury, or sports injury?	Can injure organs such as the spleen. Symptoms may develop hours or days after an accident. Hemorrhage is a danger.
Serious/Chronic Illnesses	
Have you had cancer?	Cancer in one site in the body may spread to other locations. The liver is a common site for cancer metastasis. Cancer of the stomach, intestines, colon, pancreas, spleen, ovaries, and uterus is often associated with abdominal complaints, including changes in bowel habits, abdominal pain, and weight loss.
Do you have inflammatory bowel disease (Crohn's disease)?	High risk for developing colorectal cancer.
Hypertension?	Increases risk for abdominal aortic aneurysm.
Heart disease?	Cardiac problems, including angina and MI, often present with indigestion, abdominal pain or pressure, and nausea and vomiting. Right-sided heart failure increases systemic venous pressure, which causes spleen and liver enlargement and GI complaints.
HIV or AIDS?	HIV clients are at high risk for developing Kaposi's sarcoma of the abdominal organs, infections, and multiple GI problems, such as anorexia, weight loss, and cachexia. Antiviral agents used to treat HIV have side effects that compound these problems.
Diabetes?	Diabetes can result in gastroparesis.
Immunizations	
Hepatitis A or B series	Note dates of all immunizations. Discuss need for other primary prevention activities.

(Continued)

Past Health History *(Continued)*

RISK FACTOR / QUESTIONS TO ASK	RATIONALE/SIGNIFICANCE
Allergies	
Do you have allergies to any medications or foods?	Note all allergens and responses. Milk (lactose intolerance), wheat, chocolate, peanuts, and shellfish are common food allergens. Symptoms of food allergies range from GI upset with diarrhea and vomiting to hives to life-threatening anaphylaxis.
Medications Prescribed	
List all current medication dosages and frequencies.	Many medications have GI effects. Opioids, psychiatric medications, and iron supplements cause constipation.
OTC agents	
Identify all over-the-counter preparations, including nutritional supplements, antacids, antihistamines, and laxatives.	Nonsteroidal anti-inflammatory drugs (NSAIDs) and aspirin increase the risk for GI bleeding. Overuse of laxatives may contribute to bowel problems.

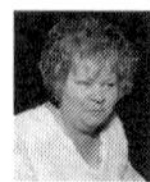

Case Study Findings

Mrs. Robichaud's past health history reveals:

- Positive for varicella and measles.
- No history of GI problems as a child.
- Cholecystectomy in 1997; appendectomy in 1953.
- Denies having any GI assessment procedures or blood transfusions
- Denies lactose intolerance or any allergies to substances, foods, or medications.
- Denies having any other health problems.
- Up to date on all immunizations; had hepatitis B series in 1997, pneumovax in 1997, tetanus in 1997, yearly flu shot last fall.
- Takes no prescribed medications.
- Takes no OTC medications now. Has used laxatives to relieve constipation over past few years.
- Uses no herbal preparations.

Family History

Questioning about diseases in the client's family enables you to identify those that the client may be at risk for because of genetic predisposition. Then you can help the client plan lifestyle changes that will help prevent those diseases and promote health.

Family History

RISK FACTORS / QUESTIONS TO ASK	RATIONALE/SIGNIFICANCE
Genetically Linked GI Conditions	
Do you have a family history of colorectal cancer?	Some colorectal conditions, such as familial adenomatous polyposis (FAP), increase the risk of colon cancer. Clients over age 35 with a family history of FAP should be screened with fecal occult blood testing and endoscopic assessment of colon. Stress high-fiber, low-fat diet to minimize risk of colorectal cancer.
Do you have a family history of cystic fibrosis?	Cystic fibrosis is a life-threatening, genetically transmitted disease that usually occurs in infancy and causes severe respiratory problems, pancreatic enzyme deficits, and reduced pancreatic functioning, leading to digestive difficulty. Tell clients about the availability of genetic testing.
Familial/Genetically Linked Disorders with Gastrointestinal Symptoms	
Do you have a family history of alcoholism?	Alcoholism has severe GI consequences.

Family History

RISK FACTORS / QUESTIONS TO ASK	RATIONALE/SIGNIFICANCE
Do you have a family history of aneurysm?	One of several factors contributing to aneurysm formation is a genetic link. Assess abdominal vasculature for signs of abdominal aneurysm.
Do you have a family history of sickle cell disease?	Sickle cell disease is an inherited autosomal recessive disorder caused by a genetic aberration in hemoglobin A. Vaso-occlusive crisis ("sickle cell crisis") may cause severe abdominal pain.
Do you have a family history of GI cancers?	Family history of GI cancer increases risk of cancer. Teach preventive activities and recommended cancer screening procedures.
Do you have a family history of colorectal cancer?	Assess colorectal cancer in family and polyps that may precede some types of colon cancer.
Absorption disorders	
Do you have a family history of celiac disease (also called nontropical sprue and gluten-sensitive enteropathy)?	Genetic susceptibility exists for this sensitivity to the protein from cereal grains (e.g., wheat, rye, oats). Results in malabsorption of nutrients in small intestine. Teach about diet free of cereal glutens and lactose.
Inflammatory bowel disorders	
Do you have a family history of Crohn's disease or ulcerative colitis?	Teach clients about increased risk for colorectal cancer with Crohn's disease and ulcerative colitis and importance of having regular cancer screening exams.
Metabolic disorders	
Do you have a family history of diabetes mellitus?	Type 1 (insulin-dependent diabetes mellitus or IDDM) is an autoimmune disorder that occurs more frequently in children whose parents have IDDM, especially the father. Type 2 (non–insulin-dependent diabetes mellitus or NIDDM) occurs even more frequently in children whose parents have the disease.
Do you have a family history of obesity?	Both genetic and environmental factors may contribute to obesity, which is an important risk factor for many serious diseases. Assess family eating and exercise patterns, explore desire for weight reduction, and teach proper nutrition and lifestyle changes to family.
Do you have a family history of porphyria?	Porphyria is a relatively rare type of anemia that causes nausea, vomiting, abdominal pain, and neurological and psychological problems.

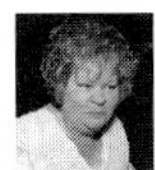

Case Study Findings

Mrs. Robichaud's family history reveals:

- Mother and brother died of colon cancer.
- Father died of congestive heart failure.
- No family history of obesity or diabetes.

Review of Systems

A disruption in the systems contained in the abdominal cavity can cause problems in many other areas of the body. The problem in another body system depends on which organ of the abdomen is involved. For example, liver problems may cause malaise, nausea and vomiting, bruising, jaundice, and fluid in the abdomen. This is one reason why taking a careful review of systems is so important.

Another reason is that the review of systems might reveal that the primary health problem does not originate in the abdomen. Instead, you may uncover medical illnesses that have abdominal symptoms. So be sure to keep an open mind about the nature of the client's health problem and not conclude that it lies in the GI system simply because he or she has abdominal complaints. Instead, assess each system methodically until you have collected all the data.

Review of Systems

SYSTEM/QUESTIONS TO ASK	RATIONALE/SIGNIFICANCE
General Health Survey	
Do you have changes in your energy level? Weakness? A general feeling of ill health?	Fatigue or weakness may reflect poor nutritional state, anemia related to blood loss in the GI tract, or vitamin B_{12} deficiency. Malaise is commonly associated with GI diseases.
Do you have fever or chills?	Fever or chills are seen with infections.
Have you been sweating?	Sweating may indicate infection, female hormonal changes, or thyroid disturbances.
Do you have pain with movement or inability to perform daily activities?	Difficulty with changing positions may indicate musculoskeletal problems, pain, or an infection in the abdomen. Inability to carry out daily activities indicates the severity of the abdominal problem.
Integumentary/*Skin*	
Do you have any rashes?	Complaints of pruritus or pain along a dermatomally distributed vesicular rash located on the lower aspects of the rib cage indicates herpes zoster (shingles). Other rashes may reflect reactions to an antibiotic, which may also cause pain, nausea, cramping, and diarrhea.
Do you have itching?	Associated with liver disease.
Have you noticed any skin color changes?	Jaundice is associated with liver disease.
Do you have any swelling (edema)?	Ascites is associated with liver disease and edema with renal disease.
HEENT/***Head/Neck***	
Have you had a recent head injury?	Can be related to projectile vomiting. Infections, such as mononucleosis, can cause spleen enlargement.
Have you noticed any neck masses, swollen nodes, or thyroid problems?	Weight loss or gain is associated with thyroid problems. History of goiter (hypothyroidism) may be related to iodine deficiency in diet.
HEENT/***Eyes/Ears***	
Have you seen any changes in the whites of your eyes?	Icteric sclera are seen with liver disease.
Do you have ear or balance problems?	Dizziness is a sign of Ménière's disease, which causes nausea.
HEENT/***Nose/Throat***	
Do you have difficulty swallowing?	May be a sign of esophageal mass, muscular or neurological problems, or benign diagnoses.
Do you have a sore throat or fever?	Infections, such as strep throat, often cause abdominal discomfort.
Respiratory	
Do you have any difficulty breathing?	Dyspnea may be caused by edema in the abdomen or large tumors of the liver, esophagus, or stomach, which impinge on respiratory structures, or may be by portal hypertension from liver congestion.
Do you have any respiratory problems?	Clients with chronic obstructive pulmonary disease (COPD) often have right-sided heart failure that may cause liver enlargement.
Cardiovascular	
Do you have cardiovascular disease such as CHF?	Cardiac disease often mimics GI complaints. CHF can cause liver enlargement and ascites.
Do you have pain and pulsations in yournavel or back?	Pain associated with a pulsating mass may indicate an abdominal aortic aneurysm.

Review of Systems

SYSTEM/QUESTIONS TO ASK	RATIONALE/SIGNIFICANCE
Genitourinary	
What color is your urine?	Dark yellow, orange, or brown urine can be caused by excessive breakdown of red blood cells or liver problems. Blood in the urine is caused by renal calculi, renal infarct, glomerulonephritis, or pyelonephritis.
Do you have burning, frequency, urgency, or blood in your urine?	Urinary tract infections can cause flank pain and costovertebral angle tenderness.
	Difficulty starting urine stream or urinary hesitancy indicates possible prostate disease in men.
Female Reproductive	
When was your last menstrual period?	Important to rule out pregnancy in women of childbearing age. After menopause, bleeding may signal a gynecological problem. Amenorrhea may indicate an eating disorder such as anorexia nervosa.
Do you have any vaginal discharge or itching?	May indicate vaginal infection that could lead to pelvic inflammatory disease (PID).
Male Reproductive	
Do you have a discharge from your penis?	Penile discharge is related to STDs.
Do you practice safe sex?	Unprotected sex increases the risk for STDs for both men and women, which in turn may affect the GI system.
Musculoskeletal	
Do you have joint pain?	Arthritis and osteoporosis are extraintestinal complications of ulcerative colitis.
Have you had any broken bones?	
Do you have rheumatoid arthritis?	Splenomegaly is associated with rheumatoid arthritis.
Neurological	
Do you drink alcohol? How much?	A deficiency of vitamin B_1 (thiamine) may present with numbness or parathesias in the extremities and is commonly seen in alcoholics and people with long-standing diarrhea.
Do you have back problems, herniated disk, numbness, or loss of bowel and bladder control?	Loss of bowel and bladder control can occur with disk problems, such as cauda equina syndrome.
Endocrine	
Do you have diabetes or thyroid disease?	Diabetes can result in gastroparesis, polyuria, and polydipsia. Thyroid disease can affect weight, appetite, and bowel patterns.
Immune/Hematologic	
Do you have food allergies?	May cause GI tract pain and changes in bowel habits.
Do you have HIV/AIDS?	Clients with AIDS have problems maintaining their weight.
Do you have mononucleosis?	Risk of an enlarged tender spleen.
Do you have sickle cell anemia?	Often causes abdominal pain.

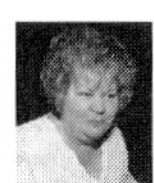

Case Study Findings

Mrs. Robichaud's review of systems reveals:

- **General Health Survey:** No changes in energy level, just feels "bloated"
- **Integumentary:** No changes
- **HEENT:** No problems with head, face, neck, eyes, ears, nose, mouth, throat; no difficulty swallowing, last dental exam 6 months ago
- **Respiratory:** No breathing difficulties
- **Cardiovascular:** No problems
- **Genitourinary:** No burning, frequency or incontinence, no history of renal disease
- **Reproductive:** Postmenopausal

- **Neurological:** No loss of sensation, bowel and bladder control intact
- **Musculoskeletal:** No changes, no history of arthritis
- **Immune/Hematologic:** No allergies
- **Endocrine:** No history of thyroid disease or diabetes

Psychosocial Profile

The psychosocial profile describes your client's lifestyle and habits. How your client eats, exercises, rests, and copes with the stresses of every day has an impact on the health of the GI system.

Psychosocial Profile

CATEGORY/QUESTIONS TO ASK	RATIONALE/SIGNIFICANCE
Health Practices and Beliefs/Self-Care Activities	
When was your last dental exam?	Good dentition is required for proper mastication and digestion of food. Regular flossing reduces the risk of infection.
Have you ever had: • Your stool tested for occult blood? • An endoscopy? • Women: When was your last gynecologic examination? • Men: Have you ever had a prostate examination or prostate-specific antigen test?	Recommended screenings include: *Men after age 40:* Digital rectal and prostate examination annually *Women:* Gynecologic/rectal examination annually *Men and women after age 50:* Baseline endoscopy, then every 5 to 10 years depending on results and history.
Typical Day	
How do you usually spend your days? Has your daily pattern changed?	Reflects energy expenditure and stressors that exacerbate GI problems, such as colitis and gastric ulcers. Pattern changes indicate how abdominal problem affects life and what adjustments client has made.
Nutritional Patterns	
What have you eaten in the past 24 hours? Are you on a special diet? Are you concerned about your weight?	Assesses usual dietary intake. Screens for eating disorders.
Have you lost your appetite?	May indicate cancer, ascites, depression.
Who prepares your meals and does the food shopping?	Improper food preparation and cooking puts client at risk for salmonella and other infections.
Have you lost weight?	Weight loss is associated with long-standing diarrhea, cancer, and eating disorders such as anorexia nervosa.
Have you gained weight?	Assesses eating patterns and nutritional knowledge, stress level, fluid retention, and ascites in abdomen.

HELPFUL HINT

Take a socioeconomic history to ascertain the client's ability to pay for food. If he or she needs financial assistance, refer him or her to the hospital social worker who can help the client access the needed resources.

CATEGORY/QUESTIONS TO ASK	RATIONALE/SIGNIFICANCE
Activity and Exercise Patterns	
Do you have any mobility problems?	Immobility contributes to constipation.
Do you exercise regularly? What do you do and how often?	Exercise expends calories and strengthens abdominal muscles, which facilitates elimination.
Recreation/Pets/Hobbies	
Do you have any pets? If so, what? Are you responsible for animal care?	Pregnant clients should avoid handling cat feces to prevent infection with toxoplasmosis.

Psychosocial Profile

CATEGORY/QUESTIONS TO ASK	RATIONALE/SIGNIFICANCE
What are your hobbies?	Hobbies may involve toxic substances. For example, inhaling model airplane glue causes kidney problems.
Sleep/Rest Patterns	
What is your usual sleep pattern?	Establishes baseline sleep schedule.
Do you ever awaken with indigestion?	Indigestion, GERD, and hiatal hernias may interfere with falling asleep. Assess whether pain or abdominal symptoms awaken client from sleep.
Personal Habits	
Do you drink alcohol? If yes, how much?	Alcohol can damage the GI tract, create vitamin deficiency states, and with chronic abuse, cause cirrhosis and esophageal varices.
Do you use tobacco?	Smoking increases risk for mouth, throat, lung, and GI cancer; chewing tobacco increases risk of mouth cancer.
Do you use street drugs or share IV needles? Do you have body piercing or tattoos?	IV drug use puts client at risk for hepatitis and HIV.
Do you wash your hands after using the bathroom or preparing food?	Careless personal hygiene increases risk for infections, such as *Escherichia coli* and hepatitis. Handwashing is most important preventive measure.
Environmental Health Patterns	
Where do you live?	Farmers may be exposed to insecticides or leaded gas (used in farm machines), which increase risk of GI problems.
Do you have public water or well water?	Wells may be infected with microbes such as *Giardia* or *Cryptosporidium,* which cause diarrhea, vomiting, and other GI symptoms. Public water may also contain chemicals that cause abdominal and neurological complaints.
How old is your home?	Older homes may contain lead-based paint, putting young children at risk for lead poisoning. Chronic lead poisoning is associated with appetite loss; acute lead poisoning has symptoms of colicky abdominal pain and constipation or diarrhea.
Are you exposed to insects or parasites?	Black widow spider bites cause abdominal pain. Tapeworms and other parasitic intestinal worms cause abdominal symptoms.
Stress and Coping	
How do you deal with anger and stress?	Explore what client perceives as stressful and identify adaptive and maladaptive coping strategies. Stress exacerbates ulcers and colitis.

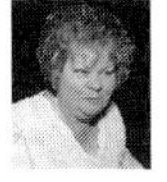

Case Study Findings

Mrs. Robichaud's psychosocial profile includes:

- Goes for yearly physical and dental examination.
- Denies having any GI assessment procedures.
- Typical day begins at 5:30 AM, when she bathes, eats breakfast, and gets ready for work at the textile mill. Works 7 AM to 3 PM. Goes grocery shopping after work, prepares supper, does housework, calls her sister, and then relaxes by watching TV. Goes to bed at 10 PM every night.
- 24-hour recall reveals that Mrs. Robichaud likes "junk food," especially high-fat dishes traditional to the French culture. Breakfast usually consists of pancakes with butter and syrup; for lunch she has a sandwich and chips; and for dinner, baked beans and brown bread. Says desserts are her weakness. She eats 1 serving of fruit; 1 serving of vegetables; 3 servings of meat; 1/2 serving of milk; 2 servings of white breads/pasta/rice/grains and at least 5 fats aday. She reports that her usual weight is 175 pounds and she is 5′3.″

- No exercise program; uses car to get to work.
- Likes to make stained glass objects in her spare time. Has no pets.
- Sleeps 7.5 hours a night, more on weekends.
- Doesn't drink alcohol or smoke cigarettes.
- Works in a textile mill, but does not know what chemicals she may be exposed to.
- Lives alone in an apartment in a part of town where she doesn't feel safe walking alone. Her apartment was built in 1985.
- Mother of two adult children, lives by herself and calls her sister every day.
- Mill where she works has been laying off employees, and she is worried that she will be next. Has been talking with her sister and other mill workers about this concern.

Focused Abdominal History

If there is little time to do a complete history, a focused history can provide a baseline of information. Identify current symptoms related to digestion and elimination as well as risk factors for GI disease by asking the following questions, using the PQRST format.

- Do you have any abdominal pain?
- Have you ever had the following: stomach ulcer, hemorrhoids, hernia, bowel disease, cancer, hepatitis, cirrhosis, or appendicitis?
- Have you had abdominal surgery? If so, when, what type, and were there any subsequent problems?
- Do you have a family history of ulcer, gallbladder disease, bowel disease, or cancer?
- Do you have any problems with swallowing, heartburn, nausea, yellowing of your skin, gas, bloating, or vomiting? (Note onset, quality, and quantity.)
- Do you have any food allergies or lactose intolerance?
- Have you noticed any recent weight changes? What is your usual weight and height?
- How is your appetite? What did you eat in the last 24 hours?
- How is your health usually?
- Are you currently being treated for a health problem? If so, what?
- How often do you usually have a bowel movement? Have you noticed any changes in your bowel movements?
- Are you having problems with diarrhea, constipation, hemorrhoids, or fecal incontinence? Have you ever noticed blood in your stool or had black, tarry stools?
- How often do you urinate? Do you have incontinence or burning when you urinate?
- When was your last menstrual period?
- Do you smoke? How many packs a day? (Calculate pack-years.)
- Do you drink alcohol? If so, how often? Do you use street drugs?
- How many cups of coffee, tea, or caffeinated soda do you drink every day?
- Have you been exposed to an infectious disease recently?
- What is your occupation?
- Have you been immunized against hepatitis B?
- Have you ever had a blood transfusion? If so, when?
- Do you take any prescribed medications? What are they?
- Do you have any allergies to medications?
- What over-the-counter medicines or herbal preparations do you use?
- Do you use antacids, laxatives, enemas, NSAIDs, or aspirin?
- What home remedies do you use?

Case Study Evaluation

Before you move on to the physical examination, review and summarize the key information from Mrs. Robichaud's health history. Document the abdominal history related to Mrs. Robichaud.

CRITICAL THINKING ACTIVITY #2

What risk factors for abdominal problems are evidenced in Mrs. Robichaud's history?

CRITICAL THINKING ACTIVITY #3

What factors may contribute to her chief complaint?

Anatomical Mapping

Anatomical mapping helps pinpoint the location of findings during the abdominal assessment. There are three ways to identify the location of these findings: anatomical landmarks, the four-quadrant method, and the nine regions of the abdomen.

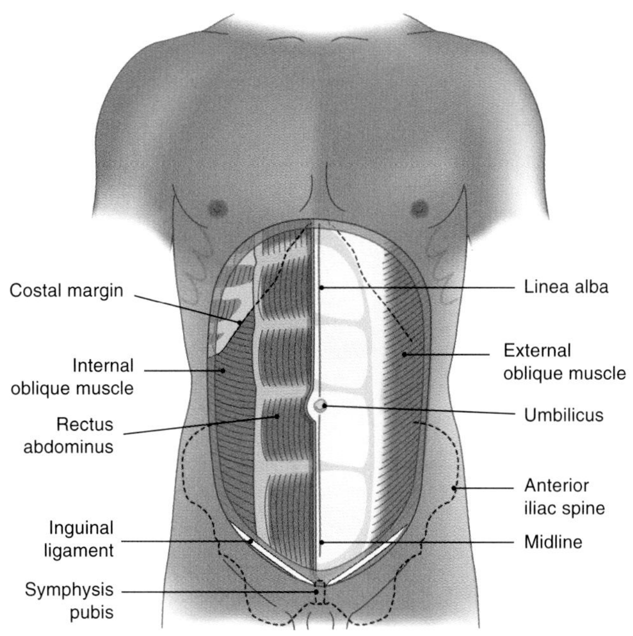

FIGURE 15–3. Anatomical landmarks (front).

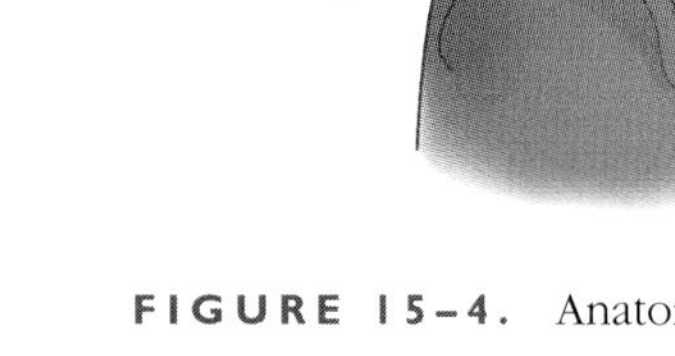

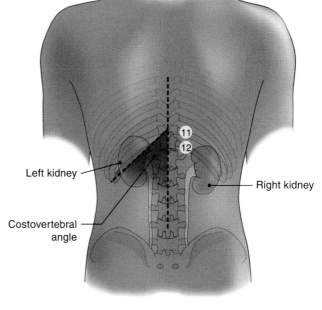

FIGURE 15–4. Anatomical landmarks (back).

Anatomical Landmarks

Anatomical structures are used as landmarks to help you describe abdominal findings. The following landmarks are used: xiphoid process of the sternum; costal margin; midline (down the center of the abdomen); umbilicus; anterosuperior iliac spine; inguinal ligament (**Poupart's**) and superior margin of the pubic bone (Figs. 15–3 and 15–4).

Four-Quadrant Method

Another way to mark the location of your findings is by the four-quadrant method. To use this method, draw imaginary lines separating the abdomen into four quadrants, with one line at the midline and the other horizontal at the umbilicus. These lines should intersect at the umbilicus. The aorta and the spine are located midline in the abdomen. The uterus and bladder, when enlarged, may be palpable midline in the abdomen (Fig. 15–5).

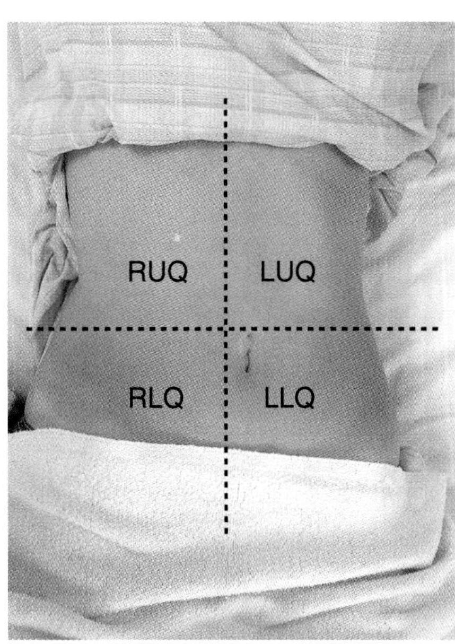

FIGURE 15–5. Four-quadrant method.

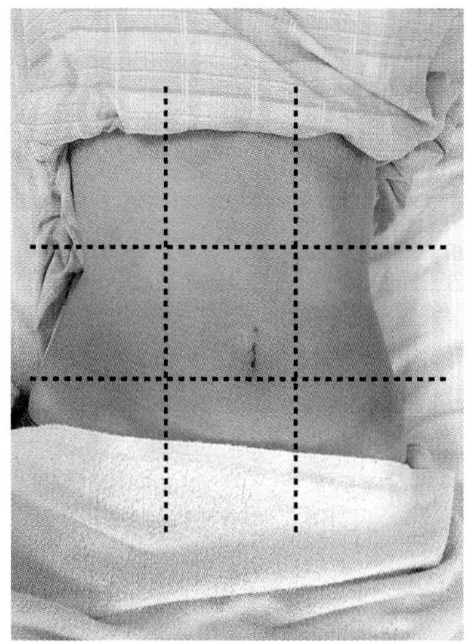

FIGURE 15–6. Nine regions of the abdomen.

Four-Quadrant Method

RIGHT UPPER QUADRANT	LEFT UPPER QUADRANT
Liver	Left lobe of liver
Gallbladder	Spleen
Pylorus	Stomach
Duodenum	Body of pancreas
Head of pancreas	Left adrenal gland
Right adrenal gland	Portion of left kidney
Portion of right kidney	Splenic flexure of colon
Hepatic flexure of colon	Portions of transverse and descending colon
Portions of ascending and transverse colon	
RIGHT LOWER QUADRANT	**LEFT LOWER QUADRANT**
Lower portion of right kidney	Lower section of left kidney
Cecum and appendix	Sigmoid colon
Portion of ascending colon	Descending colon
Bladder (if distended)	Bladder (if distended)
Ovary and salpinx	Ovary and salpinx
Uterus (if enlarged)	Uterus (if enlarged)
Right spermatic cord	Left spermatic cord
Right ureter	Left ureter

Source: Adapted from Thompson et al., p. 448.

Nine Regions of the Abdomen

The third way to document the location of your findings is to separate the abdomen into nine regions, similar to a tic-tac-toe grid. The first two lines are vertical at the right and left midclavicular lines to the middle of the inguinal ligaments. The second two lines are horizontal beginning at the lower edge of the costal margin and at the antero-superior iliac spine of the iliac bones (Fig. 15–6).

Physical Assessment

Now that you have completed the subjective part of your examination, proceed to the objective part. The purpose

Nine Regions of the Abdomen

RIGHT HYPOCHONDRIAC	EPIGASTRIC	LEFT HYPOCHONDRIAC
Right lobe of liver	Pyloris	Stomach
Gallbladder	Duodenum	Spleen
Duodenum	Head of pancreas	Pancreas tail
Hepatic flexure	Portion of liver	Splenic flexure
Portion of right kidney		Upper portion of left kidney
Suprarenal gland		Suprarenal gland
RIGHT LUMBAR	**UMBILICAL**	**LEFT LUMBAR**
Portion of right kidney	Lower duodenum	Descending colon
Hepatic flexure of colon	Jejunum and ileum	Lower half of left kidney
Ascending colon	Jejunum and ileum	
Duodenum		
Jejunum		
RIGHT INGUINAL	**HYPOGASTRIC**	**LEFT INGUINAL**
Cecum	Ileum	Sigmoid colon
Appendix	Bladder (if distended)	Left ureter
Ileum	Uterus (if enlarged)	Left spermatic cord
Right ureter		Left ovary
Right spermatic cord		
Right ovary		

Source: Adapted from Thompson et al., p. 449.

of the physical assessment is to identify normal structures and functions as well as actual and potential health problems.

Just as all the organs of the body are interrelated, so are the assessments. Assessment findings in other body areas can also indicate problems with abdominal organs. So your assessment should begin with a general survey and a head-to-toe scan to detect clues that may indicate an abdominal problem.

Approach

Perform the abdominal examination in a warm, private environment. Have your client empty his or her bladder before the examination, so that you do not mistake a full bladder for a mass. Ask the client to lie supine with his or her arms at the sides. Warm both your stethoscope and hands before proceeding with the examination, and remember to work from the right side of your client.

Once your client is comfortable, expose the abdomen from the lower thorax to the iliac crests. Other things to remember include:

- Explain what you will be doing during the examination.
- Have adequate lighting so that you can visualize the abdomen without difficulty.
- Observe the client's face for signs of discomfort.
- Perform the examination slowly and avoid quick movements.
- Make sure that your fingernails are short, to prevent injuring the client during palpation.
- Distract the client with questions or conversation.

You will use all four techniques of physical assessment to examine the abdomen. However, the sequence is inspection, auscultation, percussion, and palpation. During an abdominal examination, it is important to auscultate before percussion and palpation because the manipulation that occurs with these techniques may increase the frequency of bowel sounds.

HELPFUL HINTS

- If your client tenses his or her muscles when you are palpating the abdomen, place a pillow under his or her knees to relax the abdominal muscles.
- If your client complains of pain when you palpate an area, stop, and then palpate that area last.

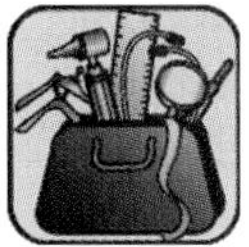

Toolbox

The equipment needed for an abdominal examination includes the following: stethoscope (bell and diaphragm), pen, metric ruler, and reflex hammer or tongue blade to assess abdominal reflexes. Remember: Always listen before palpating!

Performing a General Survey

Before physically assessing the abdomen, perform a general survey, observing the client's overall appearance. Using your inspection skills, note nutritional status, emotional status, body habitus, and any changes that might relate to the abdomen.

Begin by taking vital signs, height, and weight. Changes in vital signs may alert you to a serious medical problem. Vital sign changes and related abdominal problems include the following:

- **Hypertension:** Abdominal aortic aneurysm or dissection, renal infarction, glomerulonephritis, vasculitis, or abdominal pain.
- **Orthostatic Hypotension:** Hypovolemia (fluid or blood loss).
- **Fever:** GI infection, peritonitis, pelvic infection, cholangitis.
- **Pulse Deficit:** Aortic dissection or aneurysm.
- **Hypotension/Bradycardia:** Hypotension may indicate shock associated with ruptured abdominal aortic aneurysm. Vasovagal reaction caused by bearing down or straining with a bowel movement. Resulting decrease in pulse and BP is a result of decreased blood return to the heart and therefore decreased cardiac output.

In addition to taking vital signs, be alert for signs that may indicate underlying abdominal problems. For example, note the following:

- **Facial Expression:** Is it appropriate? If your client complains of pain, does his or her nonverbal behavior reflect this? For example, is he or she grimacing?
- **Posture:** Does your client assume a particular posture for comfort? For example, is he or she splinting a section of the abdomen, **guarding** an area of the abdomen, or drawing the knees up to his or her chest? Clients with acute appendicitis often flex their legs, because lying supine often increases the intensity of pain. Does pain seem to increase with movement?
- **Weight/Nutritional Status:** Is your client malnourished and underweight or overweight? Severely thin clients may have an eating disorder. Overweight clients may have underlying cardiovascular or renal disease as a result of fluid retention. Gross abnormalities such as abdominal distention warrant further investigation.

Performing a Head-to-Toe Physical Assessment

An abdominal assessment reflects many different systems. Therefore, next examine the client for specific changes that may indicate underlying pathology and might have an impact on the structures of the abdomen.

Performing a Head-to-Toe Physical Assessment

SYSTEM/NORMAL FINDINGS	ABNORMAL FINDINGS/RATIONALE
General Health Survey	
• Alert and oriented to time, place, and person. Remote and recent memory intact.	• *Diminished mental status:* Can occur with **hemorrhaging.** Confusion or other nervous system problems may relate to liver's inability to detoxify medications or toxins or kidneys' inability to rid body of harmful wastes.
Integumentary/*Skin* *INSPECT/PALPATE*	
• Skin color normal and appropriate for ethnic background	• *Yellow skin:* Jaundice, associated with liver disease or biliary obstruction.
• Skin warm and moist	• *Dry skin and mucous membranes/poor skin turgor with tenting:* Dehydration. GI diseases may cause dehydration with fluid and electrolyte disturbances. For example, **ulcerative colitis** causes frequent, loose diarrhea and deficits in sodium, potassium, chloride, magnesium, zinc, copper, and other minerals. **Gastroenteritis** causes severe fluid and electrolyte imbalances from vomiting and diarrhea that result in loss of water, sodium, chloride, potassium, and bicarbonate. • **Peptic ulcer disease** may cause bleeding, resulting in hematemesis and melena. Besides dehydration and fluid and electrolyte imbalances, severe blood loss (> 1 liter) may cause hypovolemic shock, with symptoms including hypotension, weak pulse, chills, palpitations, and cold, clammy skin.

HELPFUL HINT

Because diarrhea and other GI disorders may cause fluid and electrolye imbalance, be sure to monitor your client's input and output (I&O) and serum electrolytes.

SYSTEM/NORMAL FINDINGS	ABNORMAL FINDINGS/RATIONALE
• No edema	• *Lower extremity edema:* Can be caused by iliac obstruction, pelvic mass, or renal disease.
• No lesions	• *Linear lesions on one-half of the abdomen:* Shingles, an infection of herpes zoster that follows the dermatome of the nervous system.

Performing a Head-to-Toe Physical Assessment

SYSTEM/NORMAL FINDINGS	ABNORMAL FINDINGS/RATIONALE
Integumentary/*Hair/Nails*	
• Hair of normal texture. Nail shape within normal limits.	• *Cachexic appearance with dry, brittle hair, thin hair, dry skin:* **Anorexia nervosa** and/or **malnutrition.** • *Curved fingernails:* Cirrhosis or some type of bowel disease.
HEENT/*Head/Eyes/Ears/Nose*	
INSPECT/PALPATE	
• Normocephalic, even distribution of hair.	
• Sclera white, conjunctiva pink.	• *Icteric sclera:* Liver disease or biliary obstruction. • *Conjunctivitis, uveitis, episcleritis:* Extraintestinal complications of ulcerative colitis.
• No periorbital edema.	• *Periorbital edema:* Renal disease.
• No alterations in sight (CN IX).	• *Sight alterations:* Can affect food intake.
• No alterations in hearing (CN VIII).	• *Altered hearing:* Can affect food intake.
• No alterations in smell (CN VII).	• *Altered smell:* Can affect food intake.
HEENT/*Neck*	
• No masses or palpable lymph nodes	• *Neck masses:* Goiter and other masses may reflect thyroid disease and impair swallowing. • *Cervical lymphadenopathy:* May indicate a systemic infection or malignancy, such as mononucleosis or Hodgkin's disease, and cause splenomegaly.
HEENT/*Mouth/Throat*	
• Lips and mucous membranes intact, pink and moist; 32 white teeth in good repair. Positive swallow and gag reflex. Tongue pink and moist without lesions and with full mobility (CN IX, CN X, CN XII intact).	• *Dental caries/mouth lesions (aphthous ulcers)*: Affect nutritional intake. Mouth lesions associated with ulcerative colitis. • *Dry lips/mucous membranes:* Dehydration. • *Red, beefy tongue:* Pernicious anemia. • *Parotitis, dental problems, irritated pharynx:* Bulimia. • *Absence of gag/swallowing reflex:* Neurological diseases such as cerebrovascular accident (CVA) may alter nutritional status.
• No alterations in taste (CN I).	• *Taste alterations:* Can affect food intake.

(Continued)

Performing a Head-to-Toe Physical Assessment *(Continued)*

SYSTEM/NORMAL FINDINGS	ABNORMAL FINDINGS/RATIONALE
Respiratory *AUSCULTATE*	
• Respirations 16 with normal depth and regular rhythm.	• *Hypoxia:* May be caused by distended abdomen, which raises diaphragm and inhibits respiration. • *Shallow respirations:* An attempt to avoid abdominal pain caused by movement in clients with peritonitis.
Cardiovascular *PALPATE/AUSCULTATE*	
• Apical and radial pulses within normal limits.	• *Right-sided CHF:* Can cause ascites.
• S_1, S_2 present and regular with no adventitious or extra heart sounds.	
• Pulses +2/3.	
• No bruits or thrills.	• *Bruits and thrills:* Abdominal aortic aneurysm.
Reproductive	
• External genitalia pink, intact, no lesions or discharge.	• *STD:* May cause painful oral lesions that affect client's nutritional status. • *AIDS:* Associated with weight loss and viral and fungal infections that affect the GI tract, causing diarrhea, abdominal pain, stomatitis, esophagitis, and gastritis.
Musculoskeletal *INSPECT/PALPATE*	
• 5/5 strength of upper and lower extremities. No joint deformities.	• *Arthritis and osteoporosis:* Extraintestinal complications of ulcerative colitis. • *Rheumatoid arthritis:* Associated with splenomegaly. • *Muscle weakness:* Lack of protein intake or absorption problems. • *Muscle twitching:* Associated with loss of electrolytes from diarrhea.
Neurological *INSPECT/PALPATE*	
• Cranial nerves intact, positive 2 DTR	• *Numbness/parathesias in extremities:* Vitamin B_1 deficiency, commonly seen in alcoholics and people with long-standing diarrhea. • *Disc problems such as cauda equina syndrome:* Loss of bowel and bladder control.

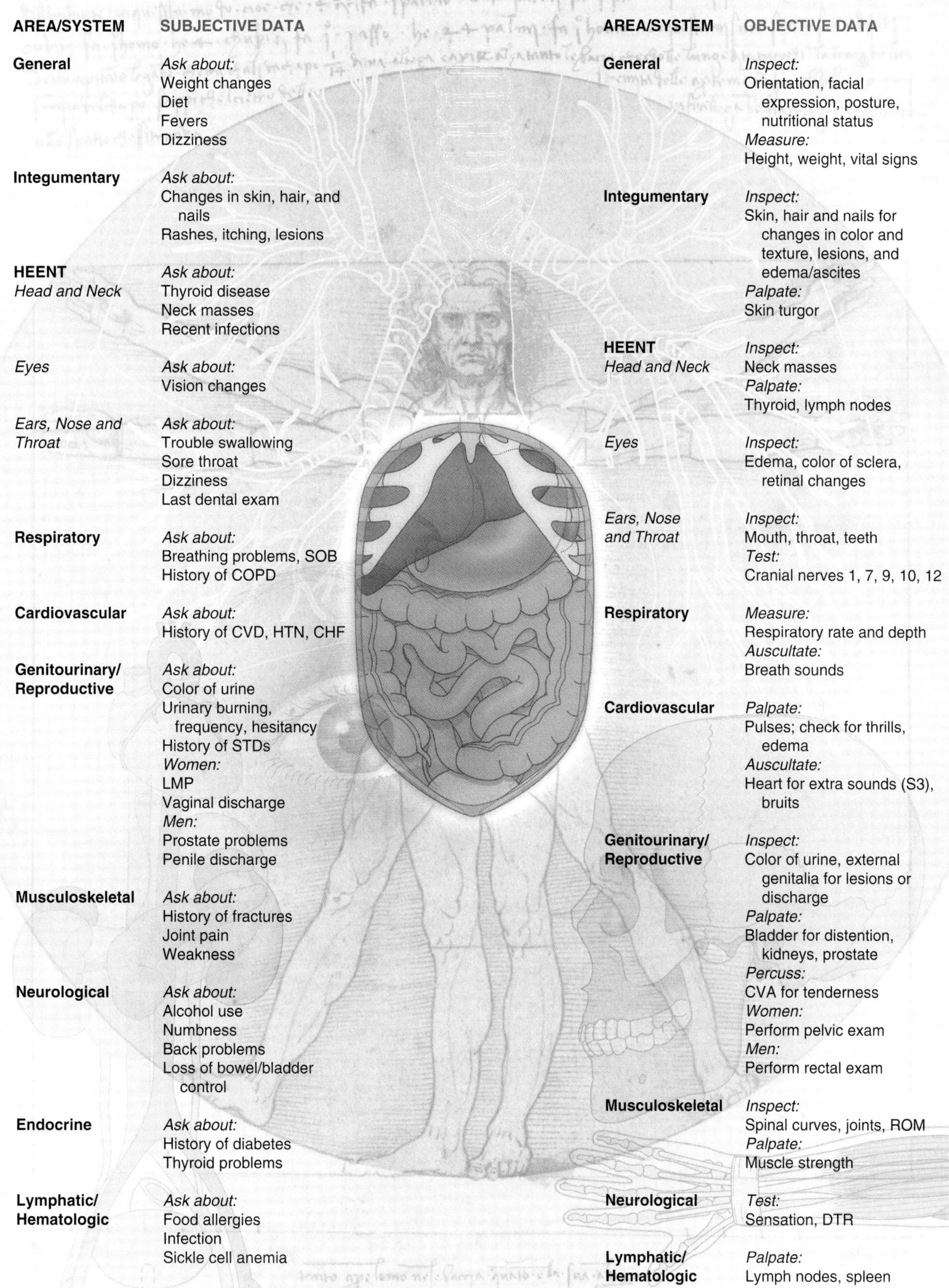

AREA/SYSTEM	SUBJECTIVE DATA
General	*Ask about:* Weight changes Diet Fevers Dizziness
Integumentary	*Ask about:* Changes in skin, hair, and nails Rashes, itching, lesions
HEENT *Head and Neck*	*Ask about:* Thyroid disease Neck masses Recent infections
Eyes	*Ask about:* Vision changes
Ears, Nose and Throat	*Ask about:* Trouble swallowing Sore throat Dizziness Last dental exam
Respiratory	*Ask about:* Breathing problems, SOB History of COPD
Cardiovascular	*Ask about:* History of CVD, HTN, CHF
Genitourinary/ Reproductive	*Ask about:* Color of urine Urinary burning, frequency, hesitancy History of STDs *Women:* LMP Vaginal discharge *Men:* Prostate problems Penile discharge
Musculoskeletal	*Ask about:* History of fractures Joint pain Weakness
Neurological	*Ask about:* Alcohol use Numbness Back problems Loss of bowel/bladder control
Endocrine	*Ask about:* History of diabetes Thyroid problems
Lymphatic/ Hematologic	*Ask about:* Food allergies Infection Sickle cell anemia

AREA/SYSTEM	OBJECTIVE DATA
General	*Inspect:* Orientation, facial expression, posture, nutritional status *Measure:* Height, weight, vital signs
Integumentary	*Inspect:* Skin, hair and nails for changes in color and texture, lesions, and edema/ascites *Palpate:* Skin turgor
HEENT *Head and Neck*	*Inspect:* Neck masses *Palpate:* Thyroid, lymph nodes
Eyes	*Inspect:* Edema, color of sclera, retinal changes
Ears, Nose and Throat	*Inspect:* Mouth, throat, teeth *Test:* Cranial nerves 1, 7, 9, 10, 12
Respiratory	*Measure:* Respiratory rate and depth *Auscultate:* Breath sounds
Cardiovascular	*Palpate:* Pulses; check for thrills, edema *Auscultate:* Heart for extra sounds (S3), bruits
Genitourinary/ Reproductive	*Inspect:* Color of urine, external genitalia for lesions or discharge *Palpate:* Bladder for distention, kidneys, prostate *Percuss:* CVA for tenderness *Women:* Perform pelvic exam *Men:* Perform rectal exam
Musculoskeletal	*Inspect:* Spinal curves, joints, ROM *Palpate:* Muscle strength
Neurological	*Test:* Sensation, DTR
Lymphatic/ Hematologic	*Palpate:* Lymph nodes, spleen

Assessment of Abdomen's Relationship to Other Systems

Case Study Findings

Before you proceed to a focused examination of the abdomen, review what you discovered during your general survey and head-to-toe assessment of Mrs. Robichaud.

Mrs. Robichaud's physical assessment findings include:

- **General Health Survey:** Well-nourished, obese 56-year-old woman who appears older than her years. Awake, alert, oriented × 3, memory intact. No distress noted. Posture erect, pleasant and cooperative, provides history with ease. In no acute distress, but mildly anxious.
- **Vital signs:** Temperature 98.8°F; pulse 86 and regular; respirations 22; BP 168/98; height 5′2″; weight 175 pounds.
- **Integumentary:** Skin warm, moist, and intact. Normal turgor, no edema.
- **HEENT:** Normocephalic; even hair distribution with no alopecia. Mucous membranes moist, 28 teeth in good repair, positive gag and swallow reflex. Tonsils pink, tongue pink and moist with full motility. Senses of taste and smell intact. No masses or palpable cervical lymph nodes, thyroid not palpable. Eyes clear, conjunctiva pink, sclera white, no periorbital edema.
- **Respiratory:** Respirations 22, lungs clear with no adventitious sounds.
- **Cardiovascular:** Heart rate and rhythm regular, no extra sounds, no thrills or bruits.
- **Rectal:** Brown stools with no evidence of blood. Negative guaiac test.
- **Reproductive:** External genitalia pink without lesions or discharge, nonpregnant uterus.
- **Musculoskeletal:** 5/5 muscle strength of upper and lower extremities, no joint deformities, full ROM.
- **Neurological:** Cranial nerves intact, sensory intact, +2 deep tendon reflexes (DTR).

Performing a Focused Abdominal Assessment

After you have completed your general survey and head-to-toe assessment, focus on the abdomen. Begin with inspection and proceed with auscultation, percussion, and palpation. Next, examine each structure separately. As you proceed with the assessment, try to visualize the underlying structures.

Inspection

Inspect the abdomen for size, shape, and symmetry. Look at it from different angles. Check color, surface characteristics, contour, and surface movements. Look for lesions, **striae,** or scars. Striae, also known as lineas albicantes or stretch marks, are streaks of light-colored skin that occur after rapid skin stretching. Observe the location of the umbilicus and note any visible veins on the abdomen. Then have the client take a deep breath and bear down to assess for bulges that may indicate a hernia or organomegaly.

Assess for distention—any unusual stretching of the abdominal wall. If present, determine if it is generalized or in one area. Fluid and gas usually result in generalized, symmetrical distention, whereas anything solid, such as a fetus, mass, tumor, or stool results in asymmetrical distention. Sometimes distention is difficult to assess, so ask the client if his or her abdomen looks or feels any different from normal. A concrete way to measure abdominal distention is to measure abdominal girth and compare measurements daily. Measurements should be taken at the umbilicus for consistency.

Also inspect the abdomen for any visible aortic pulsations, peristalsis, and respiratory pattern. Slight aortic pulsations and respiratory movements are readily seen in adult clients. Visualization of peristalic waves may be seen in infants and small children, but usually indicate a problem if seen in an adult.

Inspection of the Abdomen

ASSESS/NORMAL VARIATIONS	ABNORMAL FINDINGS/RATIONALE
Color 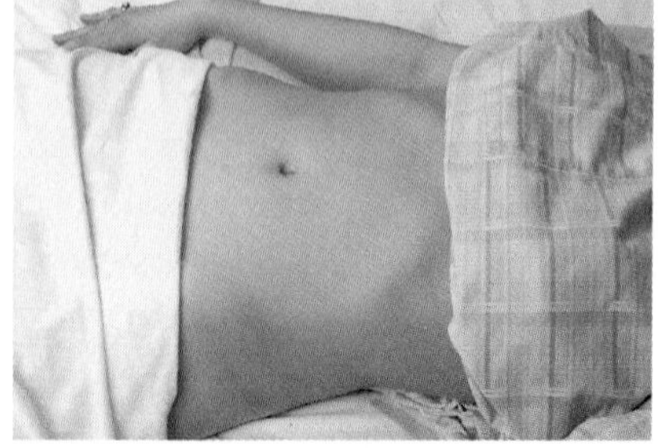 **Inspecting the abdomen** Skin color should be consistent with client's ethnicity. Color may be lighter on abdomen than on other areas of body because of lack of sun exposure. Skin color should be the same throughout the abdomen.	*Jaundice:* Liver disease *Redness:* Inflammation *Cyanosis:* Hypoxia *Bluish discoloration around umbilicus (Cullen's sign):* Hemorrhagic pancreatitis or intraperitoneal bleeding *Discoloration of lower abdominal flanks and lower back (Grey-Turner's sign):* Pancreatitis or extraperitoneal bleeding

Inspection of the Abdomen

ASSESS/NORMAL VARIATIONS	ABNORMAL FINDINGS/RATIONALE

Surface Characteristics

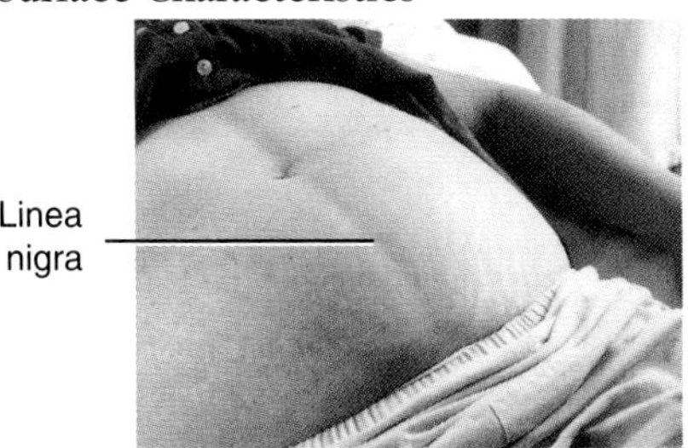

Striae

Abdominal skin intact with no lesions or masses. Striae may be present. If new, should be pink; if old, white/silver. In a pregnant client, striae and linea nigra may be present.

Bruises: Recent trauma

Pink-purple striae: Cushing's syndrome

Spider angioma: Liver failure

Caput medusa (dilated veins that extend from the umbilicus): Liver failure

Hernias (protrusion of abdominal organs through opening in abdominal wall): Caused by weakness of abdominal muscles. Seen as bulges that occur when client bears down. Occur on old surgical incisions, around umbilicus, or in inguinal area. Epigastric or linea alba hernias occur when intestine protrudes through opening in midline of abdomen above umbilicus.

Diastasis recti (separation of rectus abdominis muscle that occurs in linea alba): Occurs in pregnant women and newborns

Dermatomally distributed vesicular rash on lower rib cage in upper quadrants: Herpes zoster

Umbilicus

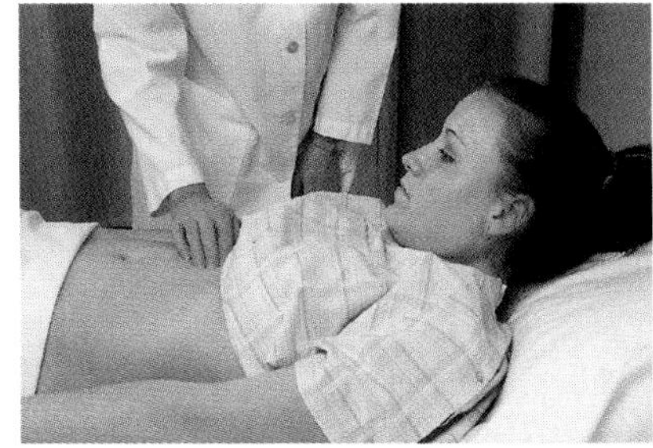

Lifting head to accentuate hernia

Umbilicus inverted and midline.

Protrusion of umbilicus: Umbilical hernia. An underlying mass may cause umbilicus to deviate from midline.

Symmetry

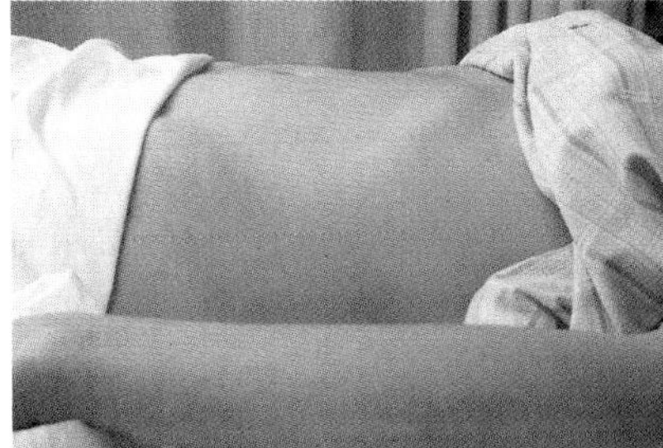

Angle 1: Looking across abdomen

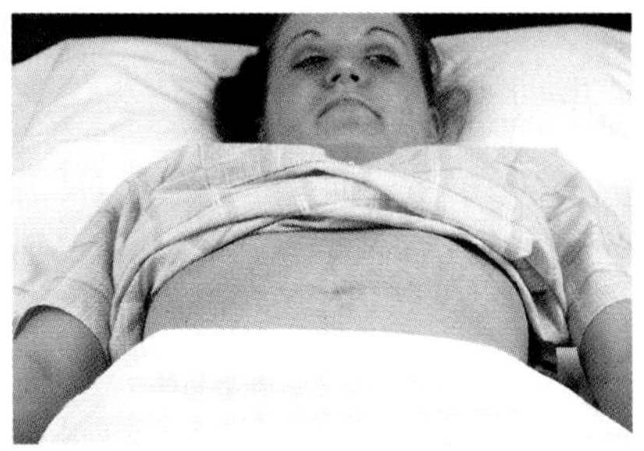

Angle 2: Looking down at abdomen

Asymmetry: Tumors, cysts, bowel obstruction, organomegaly, or scoliosis.

(Continued)

Inspection of the Abdomen *(Continued)*

ASSESS/NORMAL/VARIATIONS	ABNORMAL FINDINGS/RATIONALE
Symmetry *(Continues)* View abdomen from different angles. Abdomen should be symmetrical bilaterally from costal margin to iliac crest, with umbilicus in center.	
Contour and Distention No abdominal distention. In average adult, contour should be either flat, round, or scaphoid. A flat contour is seen in a muscular client who is physically fit. A round or convex contour is normal in infants or toddlers but indicates poor muscle tone or excessive fat deposits in adults. A scaphoid or concave contour may be seen in thin clients of all ages. 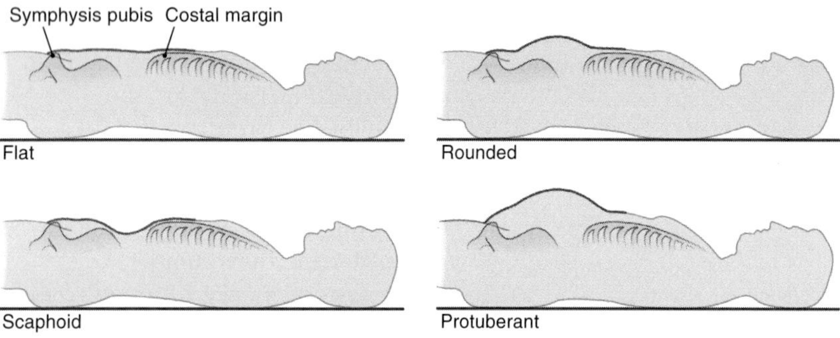 **Shapes of abdomen**	*Abdominal distention:* Causes are "Nine F's:" Fat, fluid, feces, fetus, flatus, fibroid, full bladder, false pregnancy, and fatal tumor. The area of abdomen that is distended can pinpoint cause of distention. *Right lower quadrant and left lower quadrant:* Pregnancy; ovarian or uterine tumor, bladder enlargement. *Left and right upper quadrants:* Pancreatic cyst or tumor or gastric distention. *Asymmetrical:* Tumor, hernia, cyst, bowel obstruction. *Concave abdomen:* Can also indicate malnutrition.
Surface movements On a thin client, peristalsis and aortic pulsations may be visible. Women's respirations are more thoracic, whereas men tend to use their abdominal muscles more with breathing.	*Increased peristaltic waves:* Intestinal obstruction. *Reverse peristaltic waves:* Pyloric stenosis. Abnormal respiratory movements (use of accessory muscles, grunting, restricted abdominal movements, labored respirations: *May indicate respiratory distress.* *Shallow respirations in male clients:* Abdominal pain. *Increased/diffuse pulsations:* Aortic aneurysm.

Auscultation

Begin auscultating the abdomen by placing the warmed diaphragm of the stethoscope gently in one quadrant. Proceed in an organized fashion, listening in several areas in all four quadrants. Use the diaphragm to listen for bowel sounds, which sound like high-pitched gurgles or clicks that last from one to several seconds. They are assessed to determine bowel motility. There will be 5 to 30 clicks per minute, or bowel sounds occur every 5 to15 seconds on an average adult client. If bowel sounds are hypoactive, listen over the ileocecal valve, to the right of the umbilicus.

Listen for vascular sounds with the bell of the stethoscope. These sounds include bruits, venous hums, and friction rubs. Apply the bell of the stethoscope lightly on the abdomen. Listen over the aorta in the epigastric region, over the renal, iliac, and femoral arteries. Listen for the presence of bruits, or a swishing sound, which indicates turbulent blood flow caused by constriction or dilation of a tortuous vessel. Also listen over the epigastric region and

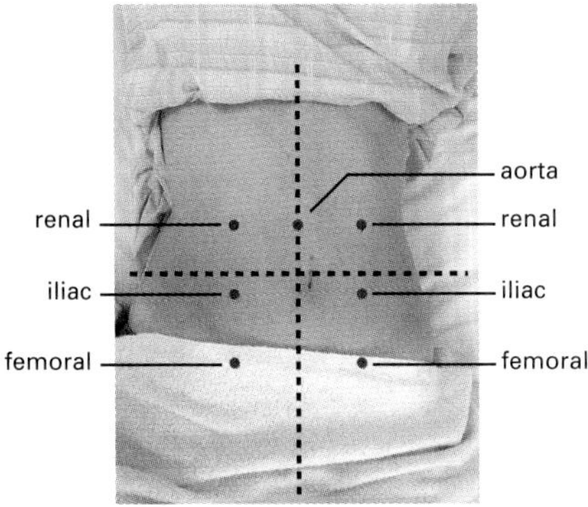

FIGURE 15–7. Auscultating sites for vascular sounds.

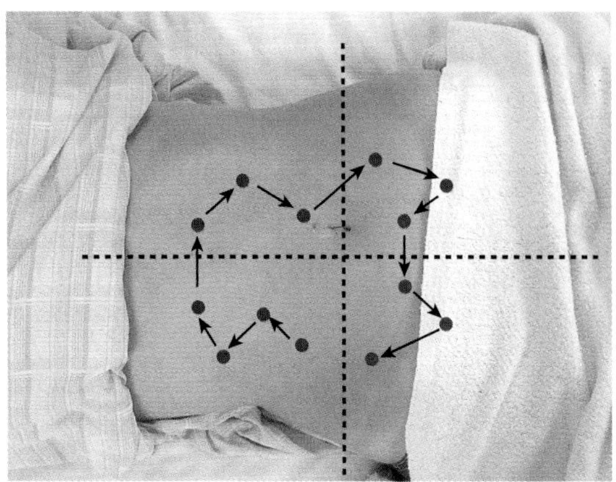

FIGURE 15–8. Percussion sites.

liver and around the umbilicus for a venous hum—a soft, low-pitched humming noise with a systolic and diastolic component. Last, listen over the liver and spleen, along the right and left costal margins, for friction rubs. These are grating sounds that increase with inspiration and indicate peritoneal irritation (Fig. 15–7).

HELPFUL HINTS

- If the client identifies an area of pain, examine that area last to minimize discomfort.
- Warm your stethoscope and hands to prevent the client from tensing the abdominal muscles.
- If the client has a nasogastric tube attached for suction, be sure to pinch the tube off or turn off the suction before you auscultate. Otherwise, you may think the client has bowel sounds, when what you are really hearing is gastric secretions being suctioned out into the tube.

Percussion

Percussion is a technique used to assess the presence of fluid, air, organs, or masses in the abdominal cavity. Indirect or mediate percussion is best for assessing the abdomen. Always ask the client if he or she has abdominal pain, and percuss painful areas last. Percuss all four quadrants, listening for tympany and dullness (Fig. 15–8). Tympany is the most common finding and indicates the presence of gas. Dullness can also be heard when percussing organs, masses, or fluid.

Percussion is also valuable for determining organ size and tenderness. The following methods are used for estimating the size of the liver, spleen, and bladder and for assessing kidney tenderness.

Assessing Liver Size

To help you locate the lower edge of the liver where it is difficult to percuss, use the **scratch test.** Place your stethoscope over the RUQ above the liver, and with one finger of your other hand, lightly scratch the abdomen starting in the RLQ and moving up toward the liver. When the scratching sound in your stethoscope becomes magnified, you have reached the liver border.

The **liver span test** gives you an estimate of the size of the liver at the midclavicular line. To assess the upper border of the liver, start at the right midclavicular line at the third intercostal space over lung tissue and percuss down until you hear resonance change to dullness over the liver (around the fifth to seventh intercostal space). Place a mark where the dullness begins. The upper border of the liver usually begins at the fifth to seventh intercostal space. To determine the lower border of the liver, start at the right midclavicular line at the level of the umbilicus and percuss upward until tympany turns to dullness (usually at the sternal border). Mark this area with a pen. Measure the distance between the two marks—this is the liver span. The normal liver span at the midclavicular line is 6 to 12 cm. If you have a liver span greater than 12 cm at the midclavicular line, you can measure the liver span at the midsternal line. The normal midsternal measurement is 4 to 8 cm.

Assessing Spleen Size

Percussion is also helpful in estimating the size of the spleen. Three methods are used. The first method is to percuss from the left midclavicular line along the costal margin to the left midaxillary line. If you hear tympany, splenomegaly is unlikely. Dullness in the area of the anterior axillary line to the midaxillary line is a sign of spleen enlargement.

A second method of assessing splenomegaly is to percuss at the lowest intercostal space at the left anterior axillary line (Fig. 15–9). Ask the client to take a deep breath and percuss again. Tympany is normal, but with splenomegaly, the tympany turns into dullness on inspiration.

The third method is to percuss from the third to the fourth intercostal space slightly posterior to the left midaxillary line, and percuss downward until dullness is heard instead of tympany or resonance. Dullness of the

Auscultation of the Abdomen

ASSESS/NORMAL VARIATIONS | **ABNORMAL FINDINGS/RATIONALE**

Bowel Sounds

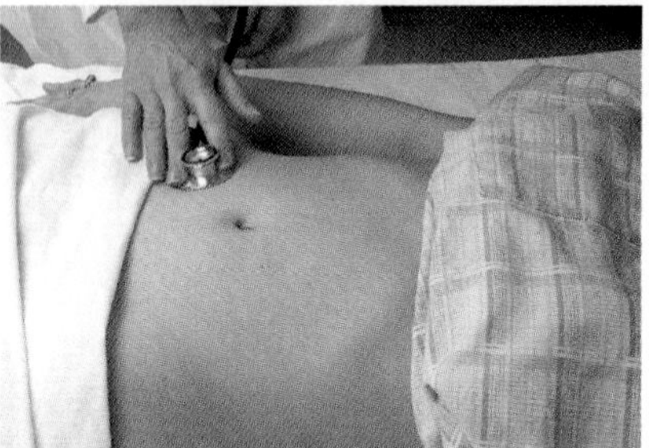

Auscultating the abdomen

In an average adult client, bowel sounds present at a rate of 5–30 clicks/bowel sounds per minute in each quadrant.

HELPFUL HINT

Listen over the ileocecal valve in the right lower quadrant to the right of the umbilicus. This is normally a very active area connecting the small intestine to the large intestine.

Bowel sounds more than 30 clicks/minute: Hyperactive bowel sounds or **hyperperistalsis.** Causes include: irritable bowel disease, bowel infection, early bowel obstruction, diarrhea, resolving paralytic ileus, or laxative use.

Types of hyperperistalsis include:

Borborygmi, which may be audible without a stethoscope and are characterized by a long stomach "gurgling."

Succussion splash, a loud sound like splashing water, often heard without a stethoscope as the client moves from side to side. It occurs when the abdomen is filled with air or fluid and indicates delayed gastric emptying from an obstruction or gastric dilatation.

Bowel sounds less than 5 clicks/minute but present: Hypoactive or hypoperistalsis. Causes include: peritonitis, medications such as opioids, bowel obstruction, or postoperative occurrence.

Absent bowel sounds are caused by late bowel obstruction, peritonitis, or paralytic ileus after surgery during which the bowel was manipulated.

HELPFUL HINT

Listen for at least 5 minutes before determining that bowel sounds are absent.

Arterial and Venous Vascular Sounds

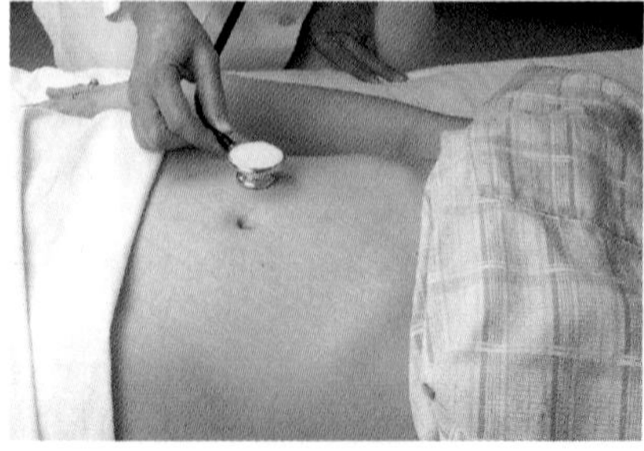

Auscultating the renal artery

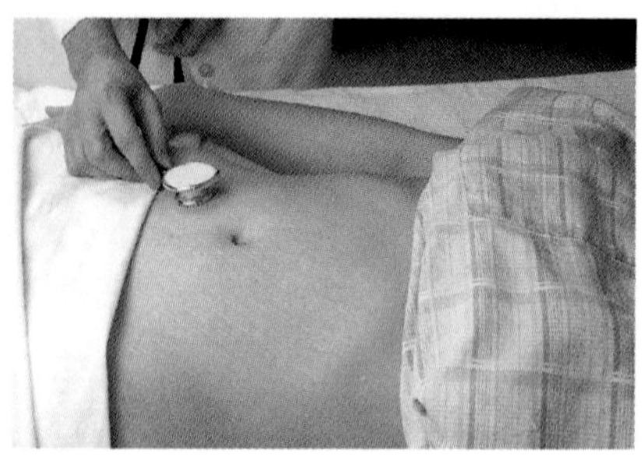

Auscultating the iliac artery

Auscultation of the Abdomen

ASSESS/NORMAL VARIATIONS | **ABNORMAL FINDINGS/RATIONALE**

Arterial and Venous Vascular Sounds *(Continued)*

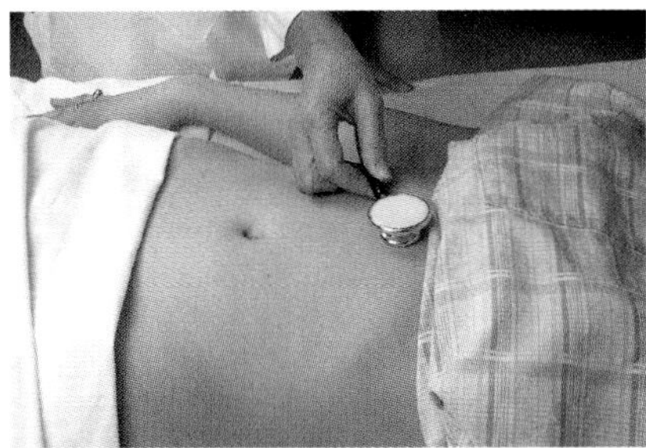

Auscultating the abdominal aorta

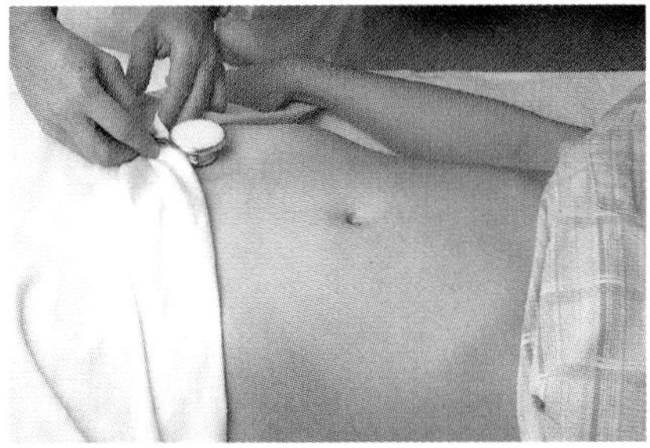

Auscultating the femoral artery

Bruits

No bruits; although bruits with only a systolic component can be a normal finding.

A bruit with a systolic and diastolic component is abnormal. The etiology of the bruit depends on the area where it is heard. The following are some possible causes of bruits in these areas:

Aortic: Aortic aneurysm

Epigastric: Renal artery stenosis

Aortic, Iliac, or Femoral: Arterial insufficiency

Venous Hums

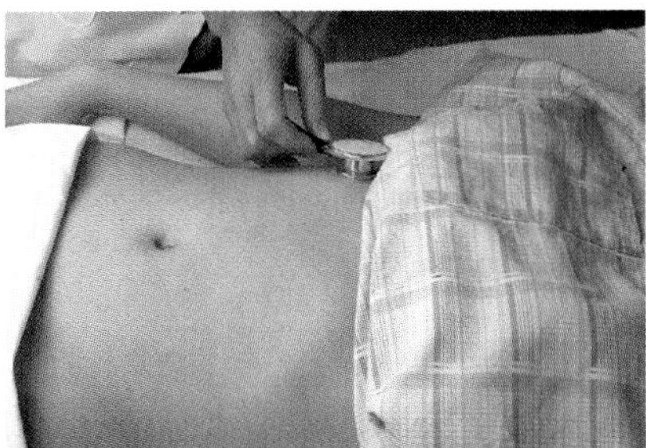

Auscultating the liver

No venous hums

Venous hums: Venous portal hypertension and liver disease.

Continuous murmur in epigastric region

(*Cruveilhier-Baumgarten murmur:* Portal hypertension.

Friction Rub

No friction rub

Friction rub: Inflammation of peritoneal surface of an organ from tumor, infection, or infarct. Liver and spleen cause friction rubs because they are in close contact with the peritoneum. Splenic friction rubs are caused by infection, abscess, infarction, or tumor and are best heard at lower rib cage in left anterior axillary line. Liver friction rubs are caused by liver cancer or abscess and can be auscultated over the lower right sternal border.

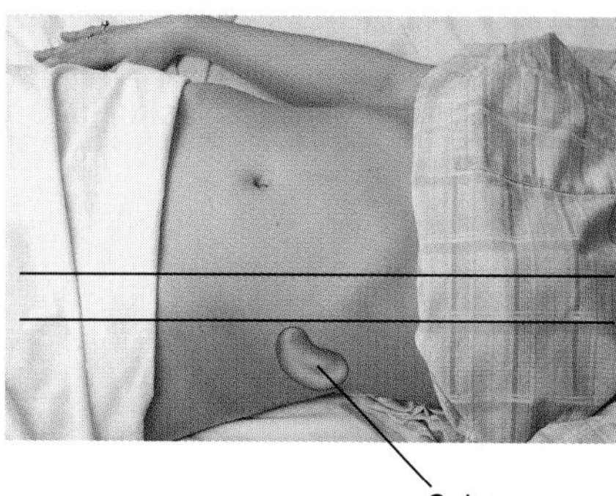

FIGURE 15–9. Percussing at lowest intercostal space at left anterior axillary line.

normal spleen will be noted around the ninth to the eleventh rib.

Assessing Bladder Size

To percuss the bladder for distention, begin at the symphysis pubis and percuss upward to the umbilicus, noting any dullness. Normally, an empty bladder does not rise above the symphysis pubis.

Assessing Kidney Tenderness

Fist or blunt percussion can be used to assess the kidneys for tenderness. Assess the kidneys at the costovertebral angle (CVA). Posteriorly, identify the CVA where the end of the rib cage meets the spine. Place the palm of your nondominant hand over the CVA, and strike that hand with the fist of your other hand. Repeat on the other side. Tenderness upon blunt percussion at the costovertebral angle is positive CVA tenderness.

Percussion of the Abdomen

ASSESS/NORMAL VARIATIONS	ABNORMAL FINDINGS/RATIONALE
Abdomen 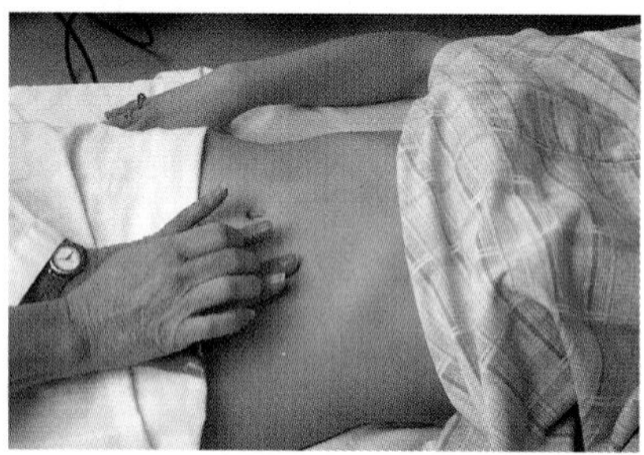 **Percussing the abdomen** Tympany to dullness, depending on abdominal contents.	*Extremely high-pitched tympanic sounds:* Distention. *Extensive dullness:* Organ enlargement or underlying mass.
Liver 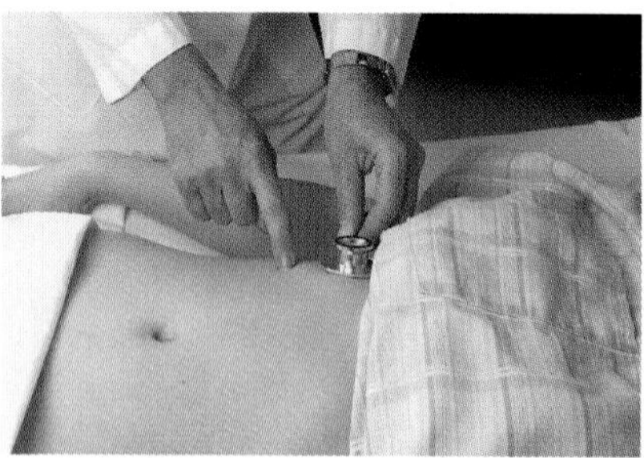 **Scratch test** Average adult liver span at midclavicular line is 6–12 cm, 4–8 cm at midsternal line. Measurements vary according to gender and height. Men have larger liver spans than women; tall clients have larger liver spans than short clients. Liver spans in children vary with age. For example, the liver span of a 6-month-old child is around 2.5 cm, whereas that of a 24-month-old is about 3.5 cm.	*Liver span greater than 12 cm:* Hepatomegaly.

Percussion of the Abdomen

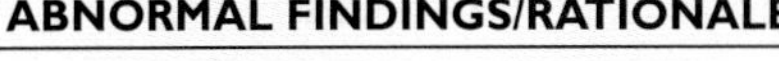

ASSESS/NORMAL VARIATIONS | **ABNORMAL FINDINGS/RATIONALE**

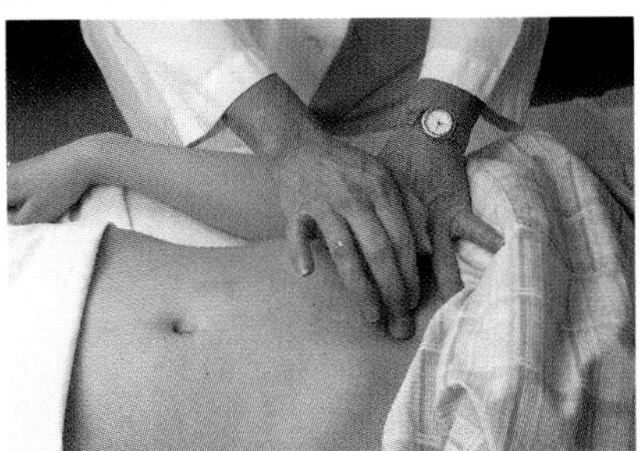

Percussing the upper liver edge

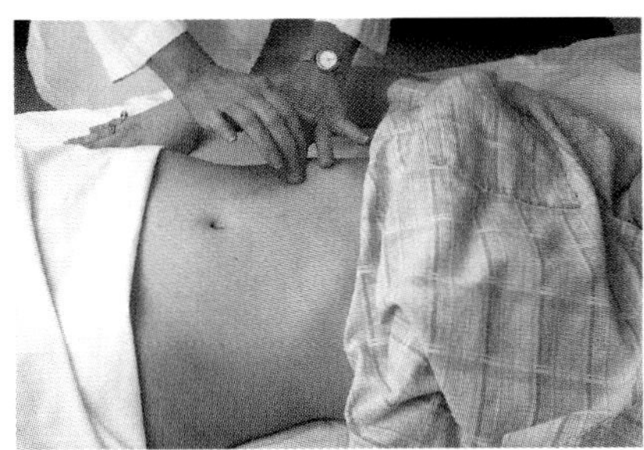

Percussing the lower liver edge

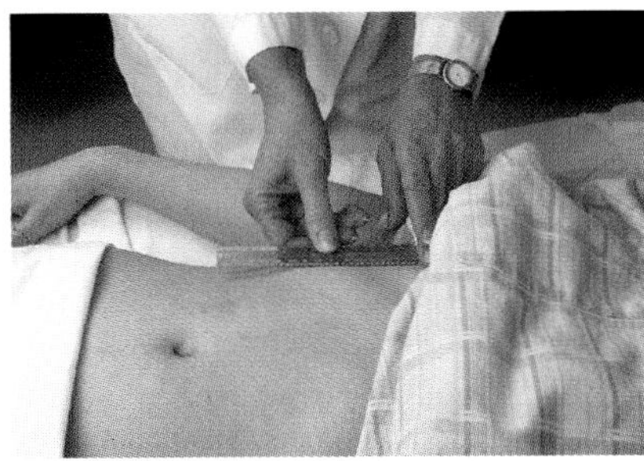

Measuring the liver

Spleen

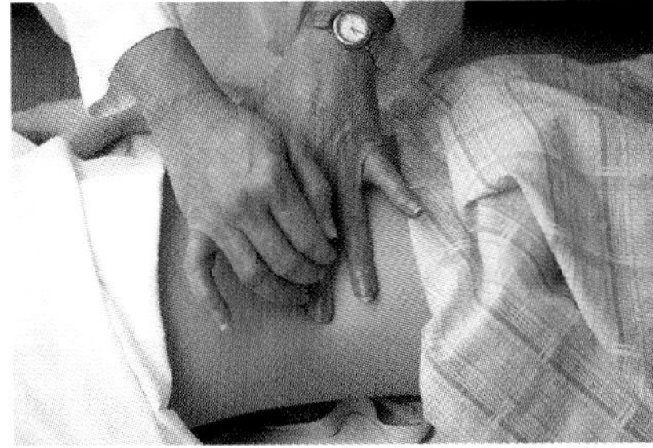

Percussing splenic dullness

The spleen may not be detected in a normal client. If detected, the upper border should be percussed 6–8 cm above the left costal margin. The body of the spleen should be percussed between the 9th and 11th ribs.

Upper border percussed beyond 8 cm above costal margin: Enlarged spleen. Causes include: Portal hypertension, thrombosis, stenosis, atresia, deformities of splenic vein, cysts, cancer, mononucleosis, trauma, and infection as long as client does not have a full stomach or intestines. (Dullness from full stomach and intestines is diffcult to differentiate from splenic dullness.)

Bladder

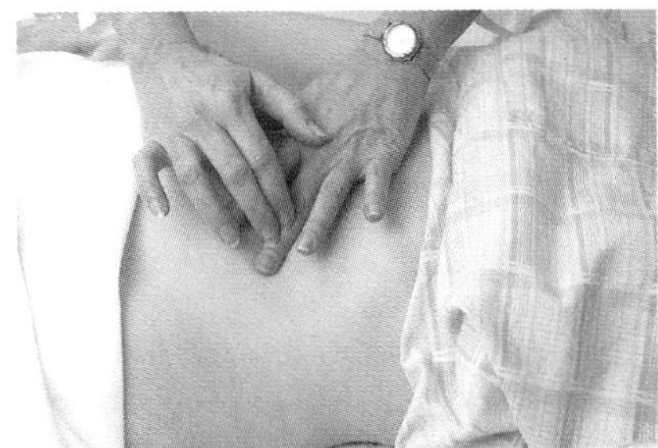

Percussing the bladder

You should not be able to percuss the bladder above the level of pubic symphysis after the client has voided.

Dullness in suprapubic area: Full bladder (for other causes, see section on abdominal contour and distention).

(Continued)

Percussion of the Abdomen *(Continued)*

ASSESS/NORMAL VARIATIONS	ABNORMAL FINDINGS/RATIONALE
Costovertebral Angle (CVA)	*Severe pain or tenderness:* Kidney infection or a musculoskeletal problem.

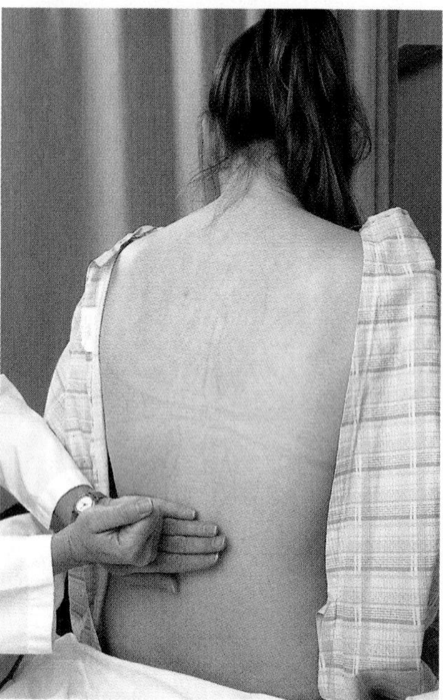

Checking for CVA tenderness

No CVA tenderness.

Palpation

You will use both light and deep palpation to assess the abdomen. Begin with light palpation to put your client at ease. Light palpation is useful in assessing surface characteristics and identifying areas of tenderness. If the client has identified an area of pain, examine that area last. Otherwise the client may tense his or her muscles, affecting the accuracy of your assessment.

Perform light palpation in all four quadrants, using your fingertips. Press down 1 to 2 cm in a rotating motion, then lift your fingers and assess the next location. Palpate as much of the abdomen as possible. Observe for nonverbal signs of pain, such as grimacing or guarding. No tenderness should be noted.

To palpate for muscle guarding, perform light palpation over the rectus muscles of the abdomen. The normal response is easy palpation of the muscle. If guarding is present, determine if it is voluntary or involuntary by placing a pillow under the client's knees and asking him or her to take several slow, deep breaths. Palpate the rectus abdominal muscles on expiration. The client cannot voluntary tense this muscle during expiration, so if involuntary guarding is present, you will feel a boardlike rigidity that indicates peritonitis.

Deep palpation is used to assess organs, masses, and tenderness. It can be done using a manual or bimanual technique. To perform single-handed deep palpation, use the distal portion of your fingertips and depress 4 to 6 cm in a dipping motion in all four quadrants, assessing for masses or areas of tenderness. To perform bimanual deep palpation, place your nondominant hand on your dominant hand, then depress your hands 4 to 6 cm. Bimanual palpation is useful when palpating a large abdomen. Tenderness may be noted in a normal adult near the xiphoid or over the cecum or sigmoid colon. If you find a mass, note its location, size, shape, consistency (soft, firm, hard), tenderness, pulsation, mobility, and movement with respiration.

HELPFUL HINTS

- If the client is ticklish, have him or her place a hand over his or her abdomen and then place yours over it and do light palpation. When the client starts to feel more relaxed, slip your hand underneath.
- If you detect a mass, have the client tighten his or her abdominal muscles. If the mass is in the abdominal wall, it will become easier to palpate. If the mass is deep in the abdomen below the muscles, it will be difficult to palpate.

Palpation of the Abdomen

ASSESS/NORMAL VARIATIONS	ABNORMAL FINDINGS/RATIONALE
Abdomen *Light palpation*	*Involuntary guarding and rigidity:* Peritonitis. *Areas of tenderness:* Indicates underlying problem. *Masses:* May indicate underlying tumor, enlarged uterus, feces-filled colon. *Enlarged liver:* May indicate cirrhosis, tumor, hepatitis. *Enlarged spleen:* May indicate malignancy, infection, trauma to spleen.

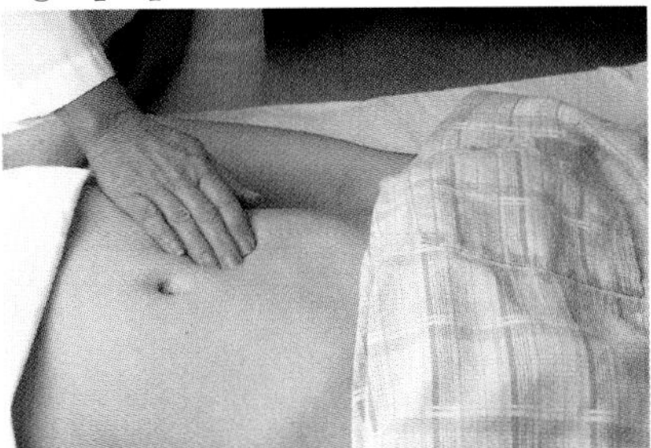

Light palpation

Light palpation using client's hands

Deep palpation

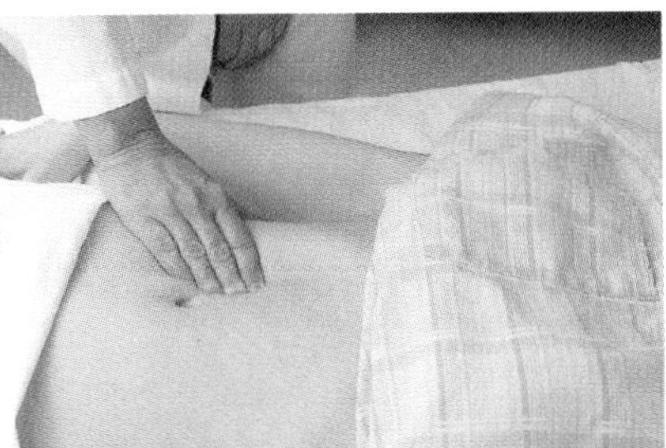

Single-handed deep palpation

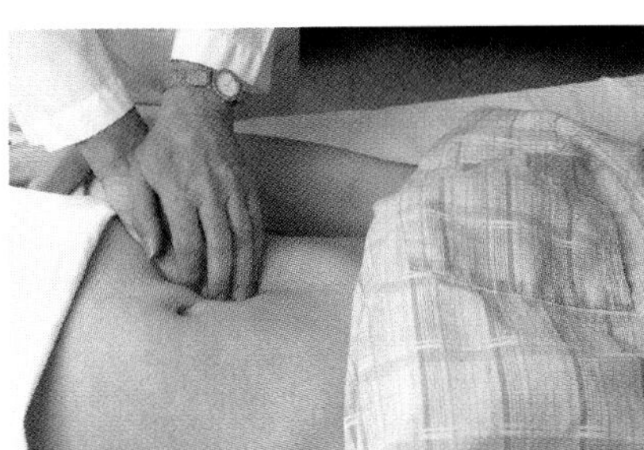

Bimanual deep palpation

Abdomen should be soft and nontender.
No organomegaly or masses, nontender.

ALERT

- *Do not palpate clients who have had an organ transplant.*
- *Do not palpate the abdomen of a child with suspected Wilm's tumor because it may cause the tumor to seed into the abdomen.*

Assessing Abdominal Structures

While assessing the abdomen, you will need to examine specific abdominal structures. The following section describes the examination of these structures and explains the difference between normal and abnormal findings.

Abdominal Aorta

To palpate the abdominal aorta, place your fingers in the epigastric portion of the abdomen and slightly toward the client's left midclavicular line. Palpate for aortic pulsations. You can also assess the width of the aorta by placing one hand on each side of the aorta.

Liver

To palpate the liver, place your right hand at the client's right midclavicular line under the costal margin. Place your left hand posteriorly on the client's right eleventh to twelfth rib and press upward to elevate the liver toward the abdominal wall. Have the client inhale and exhale deeply while you press your right hand gently but deeply in and up during inspiration.

The hooking technique is another way to palpate the liver. Place your hands over the right costal margin and hook your fingers over the edge. Have the client take a deep breath and feel for the liver's edge as it drops down on inspiration, then rises up over your fingers during expiration.

ALERT

Always percuss the spleen before palpation. Palpate gently so that you do not rupture an enlarged spleen.

Palpating the Abdominal Aorta

ASSESS/NORMAL VARIATIONS	ABNORMAL FINDINGS/RATIONALE
Aortic pulsations 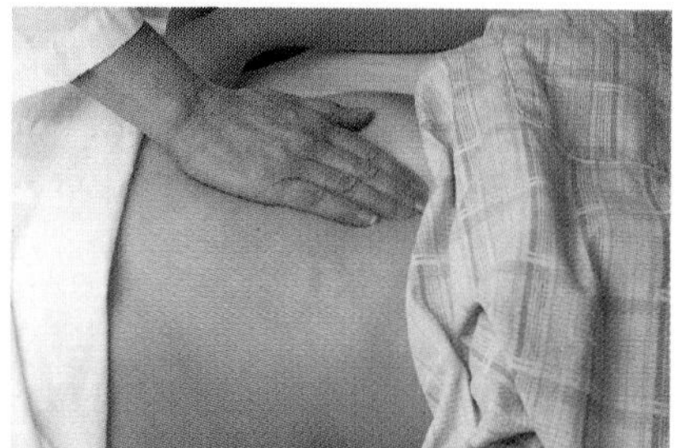 **Palpating aortic pulsations** Aorta pulsates in an anterior direction. Normal width 1.3–3 cm. **ALERT** *Do not palpate a client who has a suspected abdominal aortic aneurysm. It can cause the aneurysm to rupture, resulting in renal failure, loss of limbs, or even death.*	*Lateral diffuse pulsation:* Abdominal aortic aneurysm. *Width greater than 3 cm:* Abdominal aortic aneurysm.

Spleen

To palpate the spleen, stand on the client's right side, place your left hand under the left costovertebral angle, and pull upward to move the spleen anteriorly. Place your right hand under the left anterior costal margin and have the client take a deep breath in and out. During exhalation, press inward along the left costal margin and try to palpate the spleen.

IS IT A KIDNEY OR THE LIVER?

An enlarged liver is usually larger then an enlarged kidney. An enlarged liver extends along the right costal margin to the xiphoid, whereas an enlarged kidney does not. An enlarged liver has a sharper edge than an enlarged kidney, which is more rounded. You cannot "capture" a liver.

Kidneys

To assess the left kidney, stand on the client's right side and place your left hand in the left costovertebral angle of his or her back. Place your right hand at the left anterior costal margin. Have the client take a deep breath, then press your hands together to "capture" the kidney. As the client exhales, lift your left hand and palpate the kidney with your right hand.

To assess the right kidney, remain on the client's right side and place your right hand on the right posterior costovertebral angle and your left hand on the client's right anterior costal margin. When the client exhales, palpate the kidney.

IS IT AN ENLARGED LEFT KIDNEY OR AN ENLARGED SPLEEN?

The spleen has a palpable notch on the medial edge. Percussion of tympany in the left upper quadrant (LUQ) favors an enlarged kidney rather than an enlarged spleen.

Bladder

Palpate the bladder in the hypogastric area up to the umbilicus, using deep palpation.

Inguinal Lymph Nodes

Using the pads of your fingers, palpate just below the inguinal ligament for the superficial superior (also called the horizontal) inguinal lymph nodes and along the inner aspect of upper thigh for the superficial inferior (also called the vertical) inguinal lymph nodes. If nodes are palpable, note size, shape, mobility, consistency, and tenderness.

Palpating the Liver

ASSESS/NORMAL VARIATIONS	ABNORMAL FINDINGS/RATIONALE

Liver

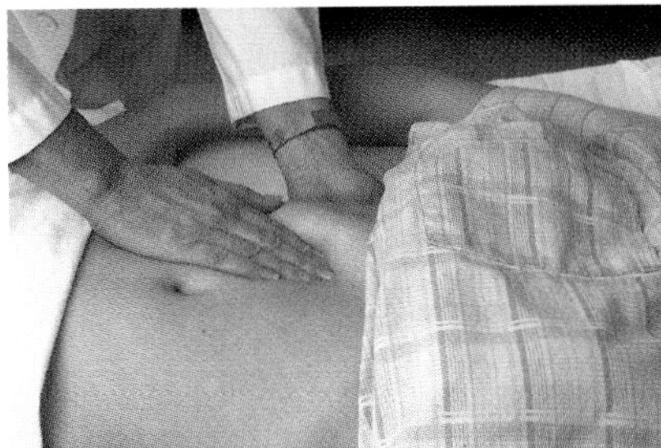

Palpating the liver

Hooking technique

The liver is normally not palpable unless the client is very thin. If it is palpable, the edge should be smooth and nontender.

Palpation below costal margin: Congestive heart failure, hepatitis, encephalopathy, cirrhosis, cysts, or cancer. If liver is enlarged, tender, firm, and nodular or has an irregular border, suspect liver cancer.

Palpating the Spleen

ASSESS/NORMAL VARIATIONS	ABNORMAL FINDINGS/RATIONALE

Spleen

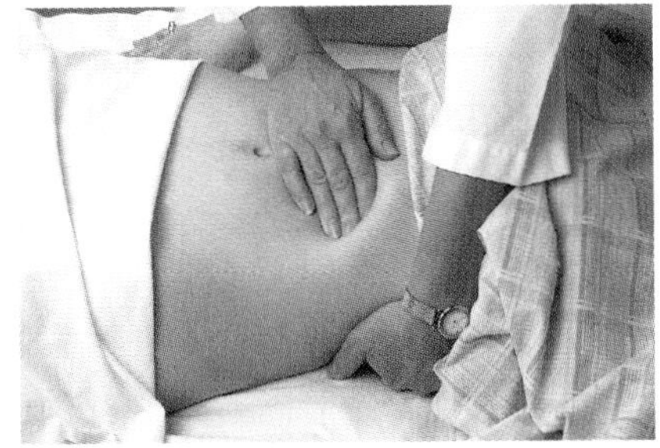

Palpating the spleen

The spleen is normally not palpable.

Splenic enlargement and tenderness: Infection, congestive heart failure, cancer, cirrhosis, or trauma.

Palpating the Kidneys

ASSESS/NORMAL VARIATIONS	ABNORMAL FINDINGS/RATIONALE

Kidneys

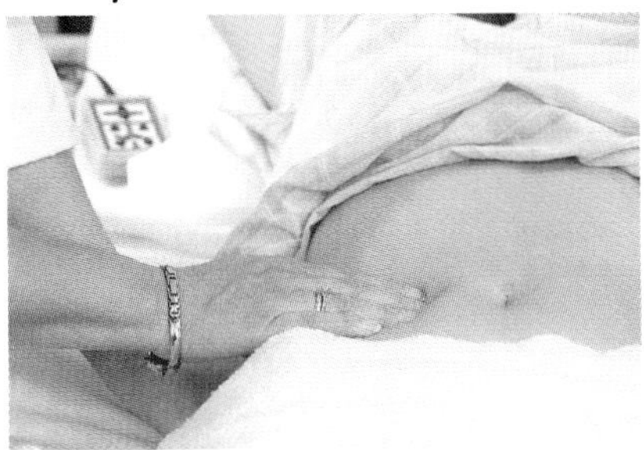

Palpating the kidneys

Kidneys are normally not palpable unless the client is very thin or elderly (owing to loss of muscle tone), and then only the right kidney is usually palpable. If kidneys are palpable, they should be smooth and nontender.

Enlarged kidneys: Hydronephrosis, neoplasm, or polycystic disease.
Kidney tenderness: Trauma or infection.

Palpating the Bladder

ASSESS/NORMAL VARIATIONS	ABNORMAL FINDINGS/RATIONALE
Bladder 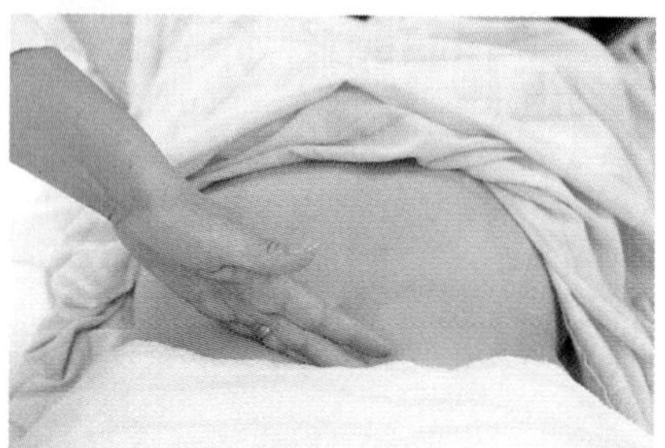 **Palpating the bladder** The bladder is usually not palpable unless it is distended with urine. If palpable, it feels like a smooth, round mass.	*Nodular or asymmetrical bladder:* May indicate malignancy.

Palpating Inguinal Lymph Nodes

ASSESS/NORMAL VARIATIONS	ABNORMAL FINDINGS/RATIONALE
Inguinal lymph nodes 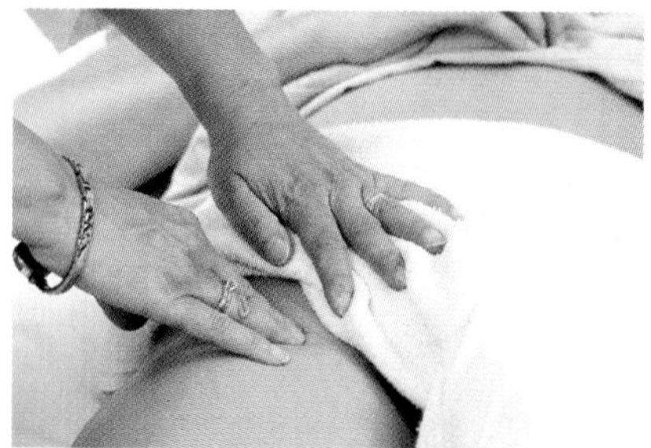 **Palpating the horizontal inguinal lymph nodes** 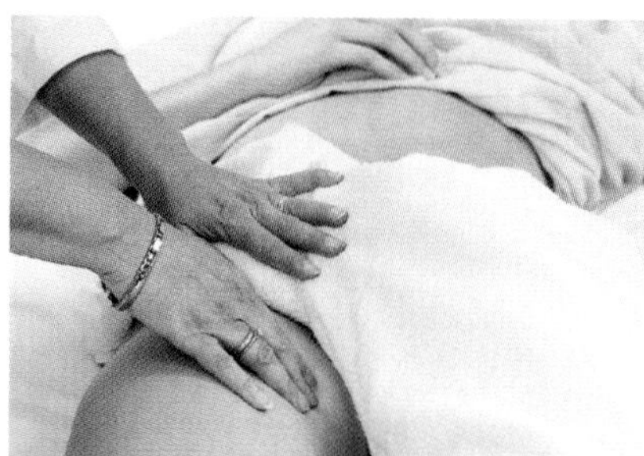 **Palpating the vertical inguinal lymph nodes** If nodes are palpable, they should be less than 1 cm, smooth, mobile, and nontender.	*Tender, unmovable nodes greater than 1 cm:* Infection, cancer, or lymphoma.

Additional Abdominal Assessment Techniques

In addition to inspection, auscultation, percussion, and palpation, several other techniques are used in assessing the abdomen. They are described in the following sections.

Assessing for Ascites

Ascites is an accumulation of fluid in the peritoneal cavity. It is usually detectable when 500 mL of fluid has accumulated. Causes of ascites include congestive heart failure, cirrhosis, nephrosis, and malignancies. There are three ways to assess for ascites: **shifting dullness, fluid wave,** and the **puddle sign.** If your client has ascites, measure abdominal girth at the umbilicus and weigh the client daily (Fig. 15–10).

- **Shifting Dullness:** Have the client lie supine and percuss the abdomen for dullness and tympany (Fig. 15–11). Normally only tympany is present. In a client with ascites, you will hear dullness laterally and tympany near the umbilical area. To further assess for ascites, have the client lie on his or her right side

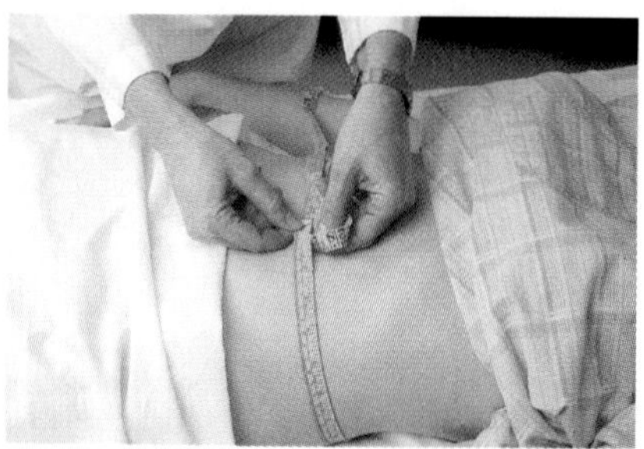

FIGURE 15–10. Assessing abdominal girth.

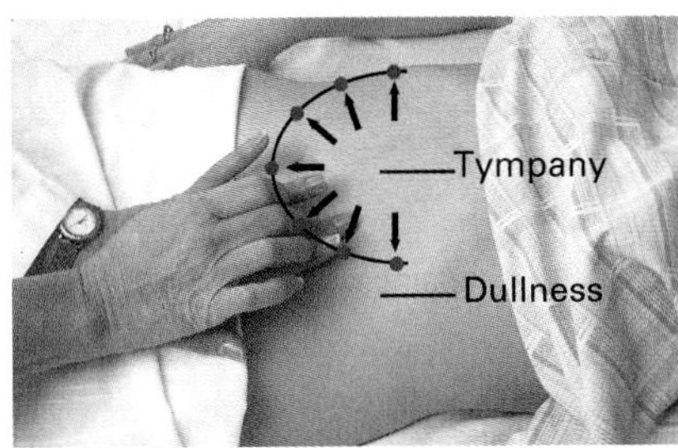

FIGURE 15–11. Percussing shifting dullness with client supine.

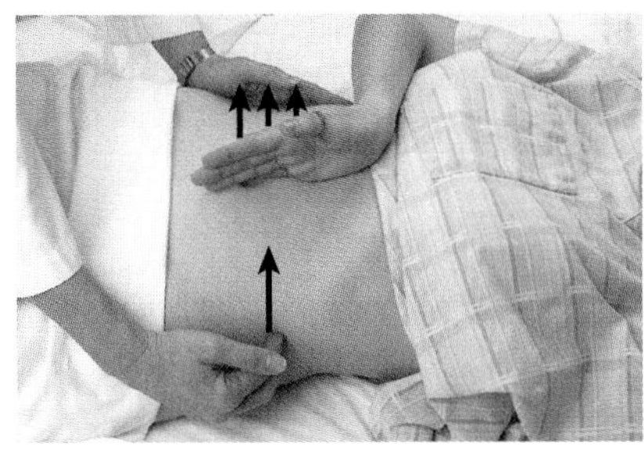

FIGURE 15–13. Fluid wave test.

and percuss again. You will note tympany on the left side of the abdomen and dullness on the right lateral aspects to the midline section. Next have the client turn on his or her left side and percuss the abdomen (Fig. 15–12). You will hear dullness from the midline to left lateral area and tympany on the right lateral area. This shifting dullness indicates ascitic fluid of greater than 500 mL.

- **Fluid Wave:** Have the client place his or her hand vertically in the middle of his or her abdomen. Place your hands on each side of the client's abdomen and tap one side while palpating the other side. If ascites is present, the tap will cause a fluid wave through the abdomen and you will feel the fluid with the other hand (Fig. 15–13).
- **Puddle Sign:** Ask the client to kneel with his or her hands on the examining table. Percussing the umbilicus normally produces tympany. If the area is dull on percussion, suspect ascites because fluid pools in the dependent areas. This is the least-popular technique to assess for fluid because it may be difficult for your client to assume the position.

Abdominal Reflexes

The abdominal reflexes are superficial reflexes. To assess them, you will need a tongue blade or a reflex hammer. The upper abdominal reflexes assess T8 through T10 and are obtained by using the end of the reflex hammer or tongue blade and stroking upward and toward the umbilicus. The lower abdominal reflexes assess T10 through T12 and are obtained by stroking downward and toward the umbilicus. The normal response is movement of the umbilicus toward the stimulation. Because this is a superficial reflex, it is either positive or negative. Absent abdominal reflexes can occur when abdominal muscles are overstretched, as in pregnancy.

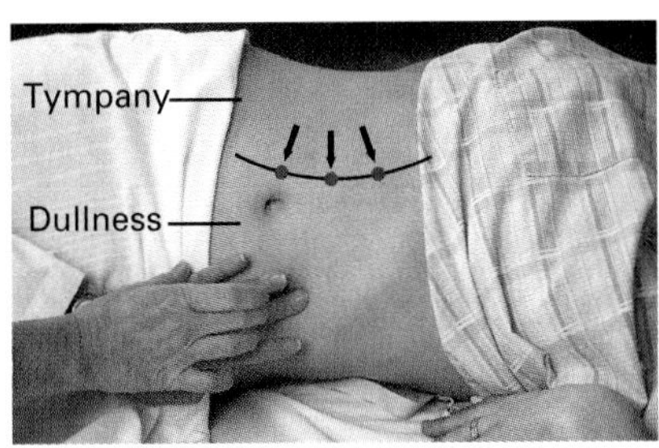

FIGURE 15–12. Percussing shifting dullness with client on side.

Ballottement

Ballottement is used to displace fluid so that a floating mass or organ can be palpated.

To perform ballottement with one hand, place your hand perpendicular to the abdomen and push in toward the mass with your fingertips. A freely movable mass will float toward your fingertips. To use the bimanual method, place one hand on the anterior abdomen and push down while the other hand is placed against the flank to push up and palpate the mass to determine the size and shape. This technique is frequently used to assess fetal position, but it may also be used to detect partially attached masses.

Kehr's Sign

Referred pain or hyperesthesia to the left shoulder is called Kehr's sign. It results from irritation to the hemidiaphragm caused by a splenic rupture with blood accumulating in the peritoneal cavity. Movement of the shoulder joint does not elicit pain, ruling out a musculoskeletal problem.

Ballance's Sign

Ballance's sign is present when dullness is percussed in the left upper quadrant. This indicates peritoneal irritation or injury to the spleen.

Murphy's Sign

Murphy's sign is used to detect an inflamed gallbladder as seen in cholecystitis. Stand at the client's right side and palpate at the right midclavicular line under the **costal angle.** When the client takes a deep breath, the

Other Physical Assessment Techniques for the Abdomen

ASSESS/NORMAL VARIATIONS	ABNORMAL FINDINGS/RATIONALE
Abdominal reflexes 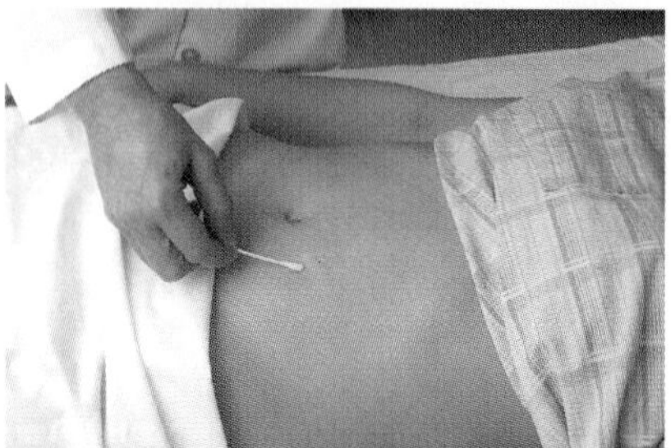 **Assessing abdominal reflexes** Positive abdominal reflexes. Diminished responses may be found in obese clients or those who have been pregnant. Abdominal reflexes may be absent in elderly clients.	*Absent abdominal reflexes:* Pyramidal tract lesion. *Absent upper abdominal reflexes:* Problems at spinal levels T8, T9 and T10. *Absent lower abdominal reflexes:* Problems at spinal levels T10, T11 and T12.
Ballottement 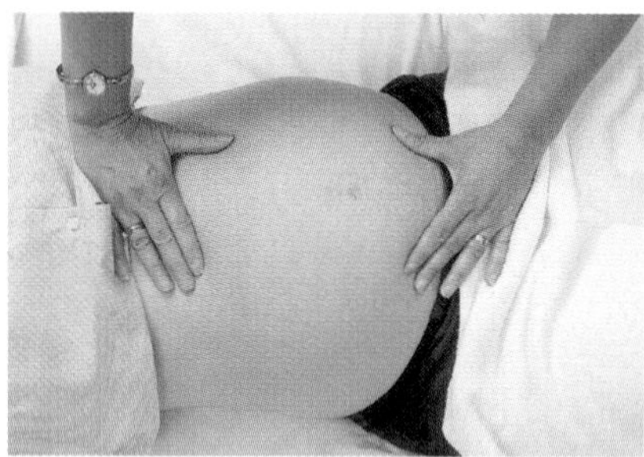 **Ballottement** In normal adults, no masses or organs should be felt. In pregnant clients, this technique is used to determine fetal position.	*Free-floating mass in abdomen:* Malignant or benign tumor.
Kehr's sign 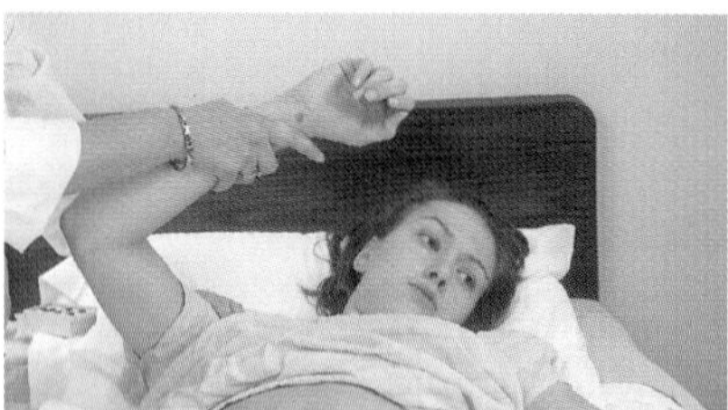 **Palpating shoulder to elicit Kehr's sign** Not normally present.	*Positive Kehr's sign:* Splenic injury, renal calculi, or ectopic pregnancy.
Ballance's sign 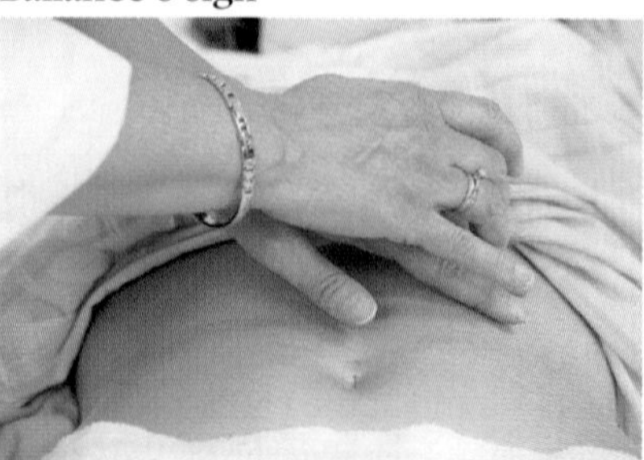 **Percussing LUQ to elicit Ballance's sign** Not normally present.	*Positive Ballance's sign:* Peritoneal irritation or injury to spleen.

Other Physical Assessment Techniques for the Abdomen

ASSESS/NORMAL VARIATIONS	ABNORMAL FINDINGS/RATIONALE
Murphy's sign 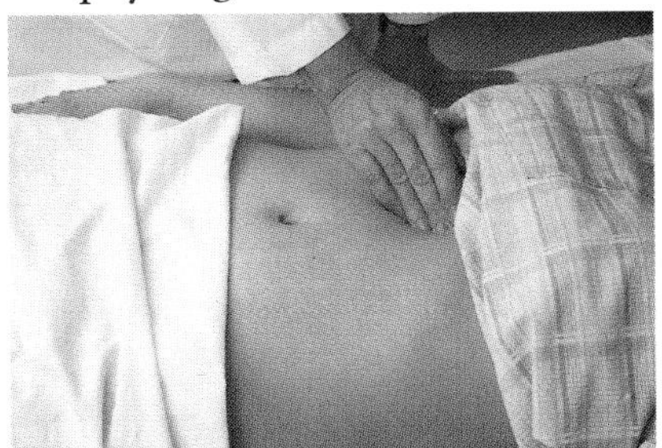 **Palpating at right midclavicular line to elicit Murphy's sign** Not normally present. Native Americans have a higher risk of gallbadder disease.	*Positive Murphy's sign:* Cholecystitis or carcinoma of the gallbladder.

gallbladder moves closer to your hand and causes pain, which stops the client from inhaling (inspiratory arrest).

The presence of pain is a positive Murphy's sign.

Assessing for Appendicitis

Various tests can be performed to assess for appendicitis. Pain during any of these tests is a positive sign.

Abdominal Signs of Appendicitis

TEST/NORMAL VARIATIONS	ABNORMAL FINDINGS/RATIONALE
McBurney's Sign 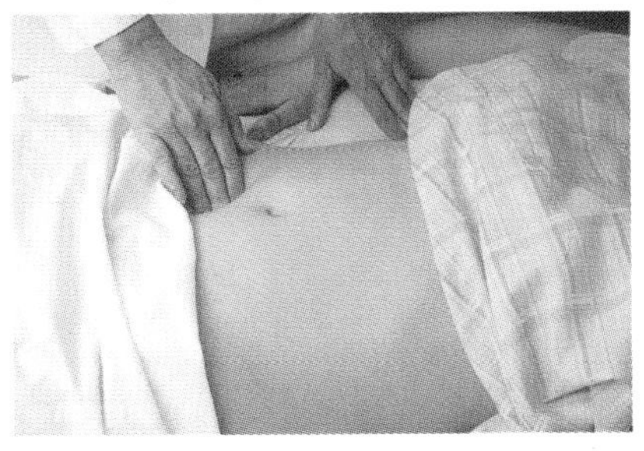 **McBurney's point** Located in RLQ, **McBurney's point** is one-third of the distance from anterior iliac crest to the umbilicus. Perform **rebound tenderness** test at this point, assessing for pain. Pain should not occur.	*Pain (positive* McBurney's sign): Appendicitis.
Obturator muscle test 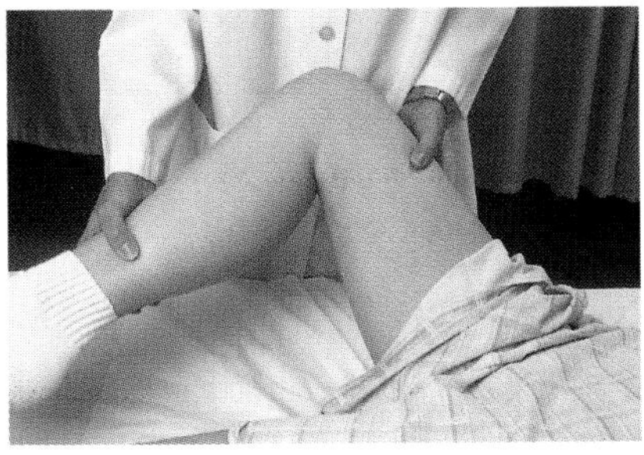 **Obturator muscle test**	*Pain (positive obturator muscle test):* Irritation of obturator muscle, which may be caused by a ruptured appendix or pelvic abscess. *(Continued)*

Abdominal Signs of Appendicitis *(Continued)*

TEST/NORMAL VARIATIONS	ABNORMAL FINDINGS/RATIONALE
Obturator muscle test *(continued)* Helps diagnose ruptured appendix or pelvic abscess. Client lies supine and flexes right leg at hip and knee. Place one hand just above client's knee and other hand at ankle, and rotate leg internally and externally. Pain should not occur in hypogastric region.	
Rovsing's sign 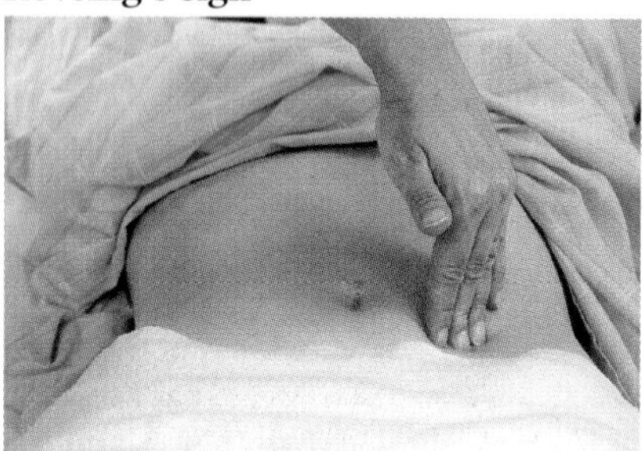 **Rovsing's sign** Assesses peritoneal inflammation caused by appendicitis. Place your hand in left lower quadrant (LLQ) and press deeply for 5 seconds. Pain should not occur.	*RLQ pain* (positive *Rovsing's sign*): Peritoneal irritation and/or appendicitis.
Cutaneous hypersensitivity 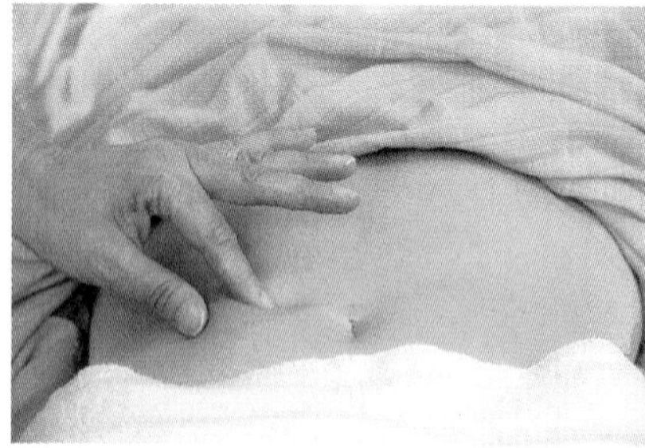 **Cutaneous hypersensitivity** Grasp a fold of skin or touch the abdominal surface with an open safety pin to assess for pain. Assess entire abdominal surface. Pain should not occur.	Cutaneous hypersensitivity: Indicates peritoneal irritation. *RLQ pain:* Appendicitis. *Pain in middle epigastric region:* Peptic ulcer.
Iliopsoas muscle test 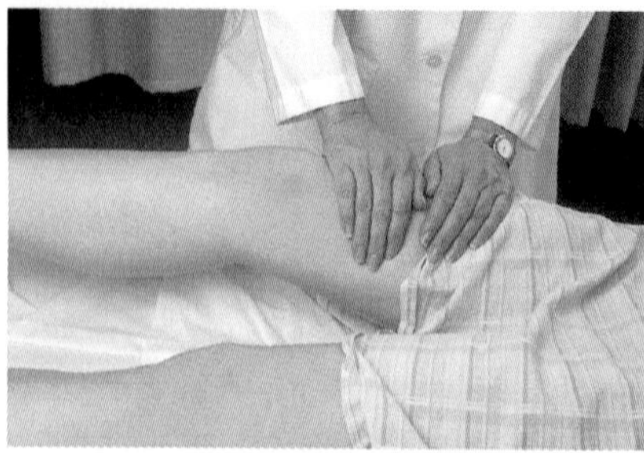 **Iliopsoas muscle test** Used when an inflamed or perforated appendix is suspected. As client lies supine, place your hand over his or her lower right thigh. Ask the client to raise his or her right leg by flexing the hip while you push downward. Assess for pain in the RLQ. Pain should not occur in RLQ.	*RLQ pain (positive Iliopsoas muscle test)*: Iliopsoas muscle irritation caused by inflamed or perforated appendix.

Abdominal Signs of Appendicitis

TEST/NORMAL VARIATIONS	ABNORMAL FINDINGS/RATIONALE
Rebound tenderness	*Rebound tenderness (pain that increases when you remove your hand)*: Peritoneal irritation. *Rebound tenderness in RLQ (McBurney's point)*: Appendicitis.

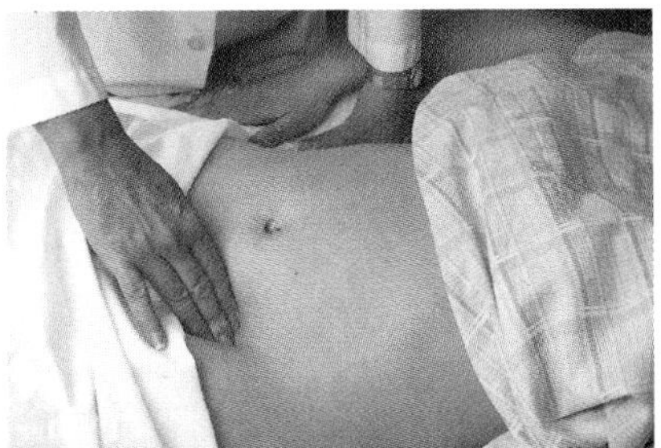

Rebound tenderness test

Place your hand perpendicular to the abdomen, press firmly and slowly, and then release quickly.

Pain should not occur.

HELPFUL HINT

Perform this test only if client complains of abdominal pain.

Assessing Drains and Tubes

If your client has an external drain, tube, or diversion (stoma), you need to evaluate how well it is functioning. Common abdominal tubes, drains, and diversions and the procedure for assessing them are as follows.

Tube/Drain/Diversion	Assess
Nasogastric (NG) Tubes Inserted into nose and advanced into stomach. Includes Levin's tubes and Salem sumps. These tubes are used to drain stomach contents or administer tube feedings.	Assess skin around insertion site for signs of drainage or breakdown. Check tube to be sure it is secured safely to nose and then more distally to client's gown. Check tube placement every shift and p.r.n. Placement can best be determined by obtaining gastric contents and testing pH and bilirubin levels. (For more information, see Research Tells Us.) Assess amount, color, and consistency of fluid if tube is used for draining secretions.
Gastrostomy and Jejunostomy Tubes (G-Tubes and J-Tubes) Inserted directly into stomach or jejunum. Used to drain GI secretions or deliver tube feedings.	Evaluate skin around tube every shift for signs of drainage or breakdown. If the client has a percutaneous endoscopic gastrostomy (PEG) tube, rotate disk every day to prevent skin breakdown. Assess amount, color, and consistency of fluid if tube is used for draining secretions. Check residual volumes every 4 hours if tube is used to administer enteral feedings.
Abdominal Cavity Drains (Biliary, Penrose, Jackson-Pratt, Hemovac, or Constavac Drains) Used to remove fluid or secretions from abdominal cavity.	Assess drain for patency. Evaluate color, consistency, amount, and odor of secretions. Note location of drains in your nurse's notes and whether they are sutured in place. Assess area surrounding drain for breakdown.
Intestinal Diversions (Colostomy or Ileostomy) Provide an alternate route for evacuation of waste products out of body. Feces are not expelled through client's rectum.	Assess stoma for color. Normal color is pink/red. Purple stoma indicates decreased circulation to stoma and needs immediate attention. Check areas surrounding stoma for skin breakdown. Note color, odor, amount, and consistency of feces excreted through ostomy. Record location of stoma in your nurse's notes.
Urinary Diversions (Ileal Conduit, Ureteral Stent, Indwelling Catheter)	Ileal conduits: Check stoma for color and skin surrounding it for areas of breakdown. Note color, odor, and amount of urine from each of these urinary diversions. Record location of diversions in your nurse's notes.

Case Study Findings

Mrs. Robichaud's focused physical assessment findings include:

- Abdomen uniformly light pink in color
- No striae, bruises, or hernias noted; umbilicus centered; scar from previous cholecystectomy
- Abdomen protuberant and slightly distended in lower half
- No aortic pulsations; peristalsis noted
- Hypoactive bowel sounds in all four quadrants
- No bruits, friction rubs, or venous hums
- Liver span 6.5 at MCL
- Unable to percuss bladder or spleen
- No CVA tenderness
- Abdomen soft and slightly tender in lower quadrants
- Liver, spleen, kidneys, bladder, and inguinal nodes not palpable
- Abdominal aorta approximately 2 cm, palpable just left of midline
- Superficial abdominal reflexes intact
- No ascites noted with shifting dullness test

Case Study Analysis and Plan

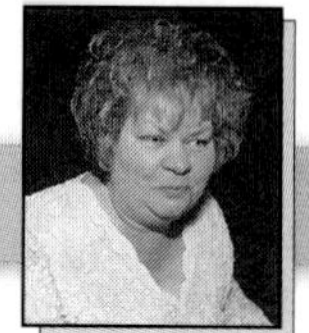

Now that you have completed Mrs. Robichaud's history and physical examination, review your key findings. List key history findings and physical examination findings that will help you formulate your nursing diagnoses:

Nursing Diagnoses

You have completed Mrs. Robichaud's physical assessment. Now you need to analyze and group the data to determine the appropriate nursing diagnoses. Below are some possible diagnoses; cluster the supporting data for each.

1. Constipation, related to decreased activity and low-fiber diet
2. Nutrition: imbalanced, more than body requirements
3. Health Maintenance, ineffective, related to dietary and exercise habits
4. Knowledge, deficient, related to high risk for colon cancer

Identify any additional nursing diagnoses.

Identify any collaborative nursing diagnoses.

 CRITICAL THINKING ACTIVITY #4

Now that you have identified some nursing diagnoses for Mrs. Robichaud, select one from above and develop a nursing care plan and a brief teaching plan for her, including learning outcomes and teaching strategies.

 CRITICAL THINKING ACTIVITY #5

What additional questions could you ask Mrs. Robichaud about her risk for constipation?

 CRITICAL THINKING ACTIVITY #6

What nursing interventions can you initiate to help her relieve her constipation?

Research Tells Us

A 1999 research study compared the pH and bilirubin levels of GI aspirates in order to check placement of feeding tubes. GI samples were obtained from 437 clients with newly inserted small-bore feeding tubes; radiographs were also done. The GI samples were tested for their pH and bilirubin level and compared to the x-ray reports of tube placement. Their results show that aspirates with a pH >5 and bilirubin value of <5 mg/dL identified feeding tubes in the lungs and a pH >5 with a bilirubin level ≥5 mg/dL correctly identified intestinal intubation.

Source: Methany, Stewart, Smith, Yan, Diebold, and Couse, 1999.

Health Concerns

The major health concern for the GI system is the prevention of colorectal cancer. Risk factors for colorectal cancer include a family history of colorectal cancer, a personal history of colorectal cancer, a personal history of polyps, a personal history of inflammatory bowel disease, aging, a diet consisting mostly of food from animal sources, and physical inactivity.

The American Cancer Society recommends taking the following measures to try to prevent colorectal cancer:

- Exercise 30 minutes on most days.
- Consume a diet rich in fiber and low in fat.
- If you are over age 50, have a yearly test for occult blood in stool with a digital rectal examination.
- If you are over age 50, have a sigmoidoscopy every 5 years or, as an alternative, a colonoscopy every 10 years or a double-contrast barium enema every 5 to 10 years.
- If you are at high risk for colorectal cancer, undergo screening more often and earlier than other people.
- The key to successful treatment of colorectal cancer is early detection and treatment.

Common Abnormalities

ABNORMALITY	ASSESSMENT FINDINGS
Abdominal Aortic Aneurysm Life-threatening outpouching of abdominal aorta, one of major blood vessels. Ruptured abdominal aortic aneurysm is a surgical emergency and must be treated immediately to prevent hemorrhages, shock, and possible death.	• Client complains of boring, tearing pain; referred pain. • Auscultation reveals bruits, exaggerated pulsations, or a mass. • Diminished or diffuse femoral pulses. • Hypotension, tachycardia, increased respirations. • Signs of shock: pale, cool, clammy skin; decreased or absent pulses; cool extremities.
Appendicitis Acute condition caused by inflammation of vermiform appendix, which may rupture, causing peritonitis.	• Abrupt onset of constant pain unrelieved by changes in body position. Pain becomes sharp and localized. • Anorexia, nausea, vomiting follow complaints of pain. • Rigid abdomen, decreased bowel sounds. • Positive rebound tenderness (Blumberg's sign), positive iliopsoas sign, positive obturator muscle response. • Increased temperature (tympanic temperature is preferred if client is nauseated).
Cancer of the Colon Occurs most frequently in descending colon, rectum, and sigmoid colon. The colon is often the primary site of cancer in the abdomen.	• Symptoms include changes in bowel habits; blood in stool; and changes in quality of stool, particularly reduction in diameter. • Pain (late sign of rectal cancer).
Cancer of the Stomach Difficult to detect on physical examination.	• Associated with epigastric distress, sense of abdominal fullness, anorexia, and weight loss. • In late stages, ascites and lymph node enlargement are seen.
Cholecystitis Inflammation of gallbladder, often accompanied by stone formation	• Positive Murphy's sign, indigestion. • May be asymptomatic.

(Continued)

Common Abnormalities *(Continued)*

ABNORMALITY	ASSESSMENT FINDINGS
Cholecystitis ***(Continued)*** (cholelithiasis). Stones may obstruct bile ducts, causing bouts of colicky, acute pain in the RUQ. Referred pain also occurs.	
Cirrhosis A degenerative disease of the liver, cirrhosis results in fibrosing and death of liver cells, which alters liver function and produces symptoms in multiple body systems. Commonly associated with alcoholism and hepatitis.	• Liver and spleen are enlarged and palpable; in advanced stages, liver is smaller and nodular. • Other symptoms: Ascites and caput medusa, changes in bowel sounds, anorexia, nausea, vomiting, dyspepsia, dull abdominal pain, hemorrhoids, jaundice, bruising, spider angiomas, portal hypertension, edema. • Encephalopathy; peripheral neuropathy with numbness and loss of sensation in extremities; asterixis (flapping hand tremor related to liver malfunction). • Amenorrhea in women; testicular atrophy, gynecomastia, and impotence in men.
Constipation Delayed movement of stool through large intestine, resulting in fewer bowel movements than usual. Because of length of time in intestine, more water is absorbed, causing stool to become dry, hard, and difficult to pass. Bowel movement may be painful. Fecal impaction, a serious condition, occurs when dry, hard feces remain in rectum or colon. Prompt intervention is needed to relieve the situation and prevent life-threatening bowel obstruction.	• Bowel sounds on auscultation • Palpation of feces in lower and possibly upper quadrants • Complaints of physical discomfort
Diverticulitis Diverticula are normal structures of the colon. When they become enlarged, they fill with fecal matter, which causes inflammation (diverticulitis) and possible infection or abscess.	• Pain or discomfort • Diminished bowel sounds with auscultation • Nausea and vomiting • Constipation
Hepatitis A liver disease caused by different viruses and transmitted by blood and bodily fluids. Different types include A, B, C, D, and E. Viral hepatitis A is the least problematic. Hepatitis B can be a lengthy illness with serious complications including death and is a necessary precursor of Hepatitis D. Hepatitis C has been associated with	• Anorexia • Malaise • Nausea and vomiting • Ascites • Enlarged liver and spleen • Jaundice • Pruritus • Amber-colored urine • Gray-colored stool

Common Abnormalities

ABNORMALITY	ASSESSMENT FINDINGS
Hepatitis *(Continued)* complications in approximately 50 percent of clients. Hepatitis D is a long-term illness. Hepatitis E is relatively uncommon and primarily occurs during disaster situations.	
Hernias ***Inguinal hernia*** Most common type of hermia. Usually occurs in men and is caused by a muscular weakness that allows the intestine to protrude through the abdominal wall, groin, or scrotum. Usually, these protrusions can be put back in place with gentle pressure.	• Discomfort worsens with prolonged standing and may diminish with rest • Pain or a feeling of fullness occurs when straining for elimination
Umbilical hernia Usually occurs in infants and children and is caused by an abdominal-wall weakness around the umbilicus that allows a portion of an internal organ to protrude.	• Protrusion becomes more prominent when an infant or child cries.
Hiatal hernia Causes the stomach to move through the esophageal hiatus (opening) and rise above the diaphragm.	• May cause esophageal constriction, acid reflux into the esophagus, and subsequent esophageal damage
Incisional hernia Occurs at site of a previous abdominal surgery. The most serious problem associated with hernias is the possibility of tissue death when circulation to a protruding intestine or abdominal organ becomes compromised (incarcerated or strangulated hernia). **ALERT** A strangulated hernia is a surgical emergency. Symptoms include severe increasing pain, vomiting, fever, and bloody stools.	
Inflammatory Bowel Diseases ***Crohn's Disease*** Common chronic inflammatory bowel disease affecting ileum and colon	• Abdominal pain • Steatorrhea

(Continued)

Common Abnormalities *(Continued)*

ABNORMALITY	ASSESSMENT FINDINGS
Crohn's Disease (Continued)	
that results in thickening of bowel and narrowing of intestinal lumen. Affects small intestine; therefore problems with vitamin absorption are common. Significantly increases risk for colon cancer and arthritis.	• Diarrhea • Vitamin deficiency states • Fatigue • Weight loss • Fever • Arthritis • Joint deformities
Ulcerative Colitis	
Inflammation of mucosa of rectum and sigmoid colon that causes cramping, diarrhea, and rectal bleeding and increases risk for colon cancer and bowel perforation. Has exacerbations and remissions.	• Watery eyes • Conjunctivitis • Mouth ulcers • Erythema nodosum • Pyoderma gangrenosum • Cramping pain in lower abdomen • Watery diarrhea • Rectal bleeding • Mucus in stool • Frequent bowel movements • Urgency • Dehydration • Fever • Weight loss
Pancreatitis	
Inflammation of pancreas that alters flow of enzymes to intestines and results in pancreatic retention of digestive enzymes. These enzymes cause breakdown of the pancreas.	• Nausea and vomiting • Weight loss • Severe "boring" pain in LUQ • Pain referred to back or shoulder • Radiating pain • Steatorrhea
Paralytic Ileus	
Lack of peristalsis, usually in the small intestine. Serious condition requiring prompt treatment. Surgery, peritonitis, or spinal injury are predisposing factors. Bowel necrosis and perforation are serious complications.	• Intermittent colicky pain • Absence of bowel sounds • Initially visible peristaltic waves • Abdominal distention • Vomiting
Peritonitis	
Inflammation of the lining of the abdominal cavity (peritoneum)	• Assessment findings include abdominal pain of varying character, cutaneous hypersensitivity • Abdominal rigidity and guarding • Diminished bowel sounds • Positive iliopsoas, Blumberg's and Rovsing's signs • Positive Murphy's sign • Fever • Nausea and vomiting
Splenic Rupture	
Serious abdominal condition resulting in hemorrhage. Usually	• Severe LUQ pain • Left shoulder pain

Common Abnormalities

ABNORMALITY	ASSESSMENT FINDINGS
Splenic Rupture *(Continued)* follows abdominal trauma, but also may be a serious sequela of infectious mononucleosis.	• Possible shock (drop in BP)
Ulcer Forms when gastric mucosa becomes permeable, when amount of protective mucus is reduced (in conditions such as gastritis) or when there is prolonged exposure to bile or other irritating substances (e.g., medications). GI ulcer sites include duodenum (duodenal ulcer) and stomach (gastric ulcer). Stress ulcers are erosions of the GI tract mucosa that arise in relation to trauma, burns, or severe illness.	• Gastric ulcer include complaints of gnawing pain, heartburn, anorexia, vomiting (hematemesis possible), eructations, and weight loss • Duodenal ulcer include intermittent RUQ pain 2 to 3 hours after meals, remissions and exacerbations; stool may be positive for guaiac.

ASSESSMENT FINDINGS IN CLIENT WITH ANOREXIA NERVOSA

Suspect anorexia nervosa if your client has a weight loss of 15 percent or more below ideal height-weight standards, says that he or she actively pursues weight loss, or expresses a distorted or almost delusional attitude about his or her body (e.g., says "I'm fat" in spite of thin appearance.) Assessment findings include starvation, decreased fluid intake, thin hair, dental erosions, dehydration, electrolyte imbalance, swollen parotid glands, decreased body temperature, dry skin, poor skin turgor, weight loss, thinness, general weakness, and constipation.

ALERT

Bulimia nervosa is harder to pinpoint than anorexia. Clients may be of normal weight or slightly over- or underweight. They binge and purge, ingesting huge amounts of food during a brief period and then inducing vomiting or diarrhea. Guilt feelings are common. Suspect bulimia nvervosa if you client exercises excessively, has eroded tooth enamel (from vomiting), and enlarged parotid glands.

Summary

- In this chapter, you learned to how take a health history related to the abdomen, perform an abdominal examination, and analyze the data to identify actual and potential health problems.
- Using this information, you made a prioritized list of nursing diagnoses and developed a plan of care with actions designed to restore and promote the client's health.

16

Assessing the Female Genitourinary System

Before You Begin

INTRODUCTION TO THE FEMALE GENITOURINARY SYSTEM

Assessment of the genitourinary (GU) system is essential to obtain a picture of a woman's overall health status. The female reproductive system undergoes cyclical changes in response to hormonal levels of estrogen and progesterone throughout the life cycle. Reproductive health issues are a concern at every stage of reproductive development. Premenarchal girls may have questions about changes that occur during adolescence and menstruation, and adolescents may be concerned about sexuality and contraception. During the childbearing years, an adult woman's concerns focus on conception and pregnancy; later in life, they focus on the changes associated with **menopause**. Identifying a woman's reproductive stage will help you identify health concerns and differentiate your findings.

Focus your assessment on identifying any acute health problems, risks for GU problems, and health promotion teaching needs. Sexually transmitted diseases (STDs) are the most common communicable diseases in the United States. If left untreated, they can have devastating, permanent effects. GU dysfunction not only has a direct impact on the reproductive and urinary systems, but it also has far-reaching effects on a woman's quality of life.

Anatomy and Physiology Review

Before you begin the assessment, you need to understand the anatomy and physiology of the female GU system. The system consists of external and internal genitalia, which develop and function according to the hormonal influences that affect fertility and childbearing. It also consists of urinary structures.

External genitalia include the mons pubis, clitoris, vestibule, labia majora, labia minora, vaginal **introitus,** hymen, Bartholin's glands, Skene's glands, and the urethral meatus. Internal genitalia include the vagina, cervix, uterus, adjacent structures **(adnexa),** ovaries, and fallopian tubes. Internal urinary structures include the ureters, bladder, and urethra (Figs. 16–1, 16–2, and 16–3).

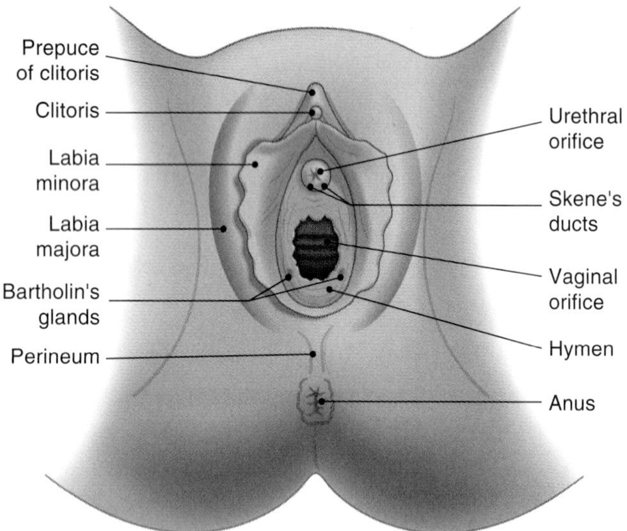

FIGURE 16–1. External female genitalia.

The functions of the female GU system are as follows:

- Manufacturing and protecting ova for fertilization.
- Transporting the fertilized ovum for implantation and embryonic/fetal development.
- Housing and nourishing the developing fetus.
- Regulating hormonal production and secretion of several sex hormones.
- Providing sexual stimulation and pleasure.
- Providing a drainage route for the excretion of urine (urinary structures).

The Process of Reproduction

Mechanical Process

The process of reproduction requires that a mature ovum be fertilized by a sperm. The ovum is viable for about 24 hours and the sperm for up to 72 hours. Fertilization must occur within 24 hours of ovulation. During male ejaculation, sperm enters the vaginal canal and travels through the uterus to the fallopian tube, where fertilization usually occurs. A fertilized ovum is called a **zygote.** Once the ovum is fertilized, embryonic devel-

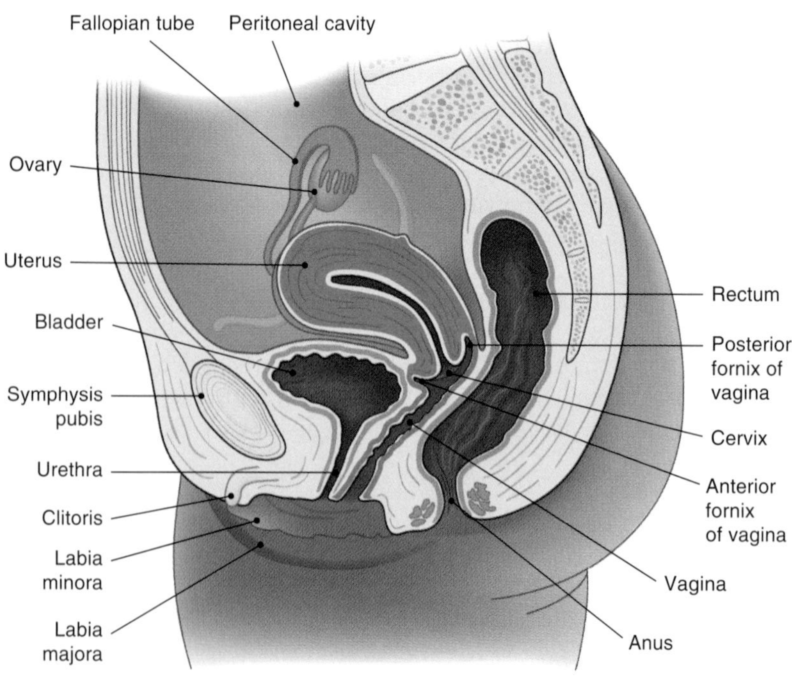

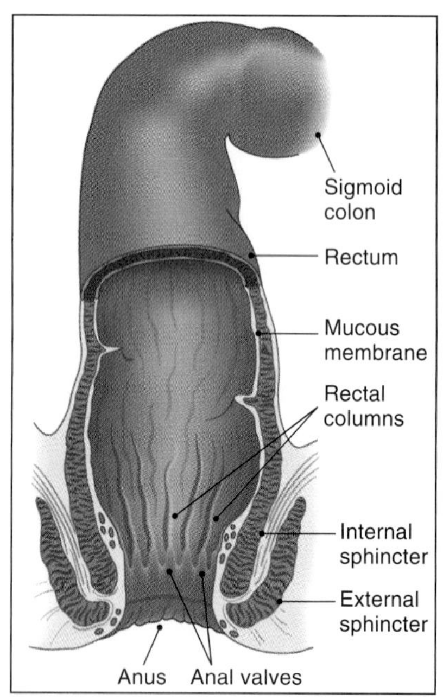

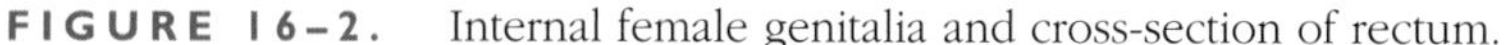

FIGURE 16–2. Internal female genitalia and cross-section of rectum.

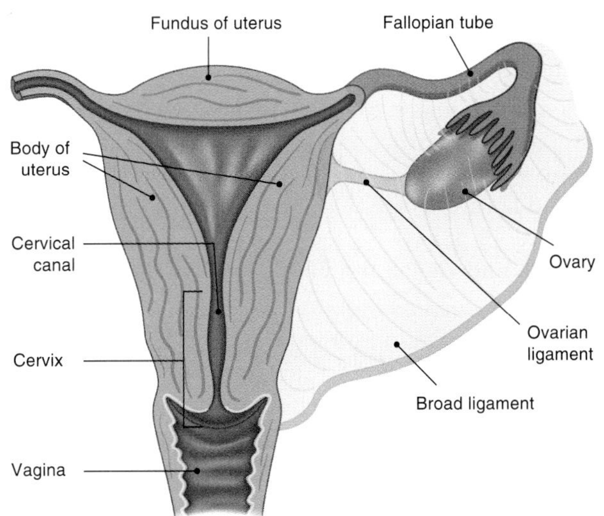

FIGURE 16–3. Internal structures of adnexa.

opment begins. The fertilized ovum travels through the fallopian tube to the uterus for implantation. Once implantation has occurred, the uterus houses, nourishes, and protects the developing fetus until the time of delivery. Hormonal influences prepare the uterus monthly for implantation of a fertilized ovum. If fertilization does not occur, the endometrium sheds and the menstrual cycle begins.

The female reproductive system consists of external and internal genitalia, which develop and function according to the hormonal influences that affect fertility and childbearing.

Physiologic Process

The hypothalamus, ovaries, and pituitary gland secrete hormones that affect the thickening and shedding of the uterine lining during the menstrual cycle. The ovarian cycle consists of two phases: the follicular phase and the luteal phase. During the **follicular phase,** the actions of the follicle-stimulating hormone (FSH) and the luteinizing hormone (LH) from the anterior pituitary stimulate the ripening of one ovarian follicle called the **graafian follicle**. The remaining follicles are suppressed by LH. Ovulation occurs when high levels of LH cause the release of the ovum from the graafian follicle. During the **luteal phase,** LH stimulates the development of the corpus luteum. The yellow pigment that fills the graafian follicle produces high levels of progesterone and low levels of estrogen. If pregnancy does not occur, the corpus luteum diminishes, hormone levels fall, and menstruation begins (Fig. 16–4).

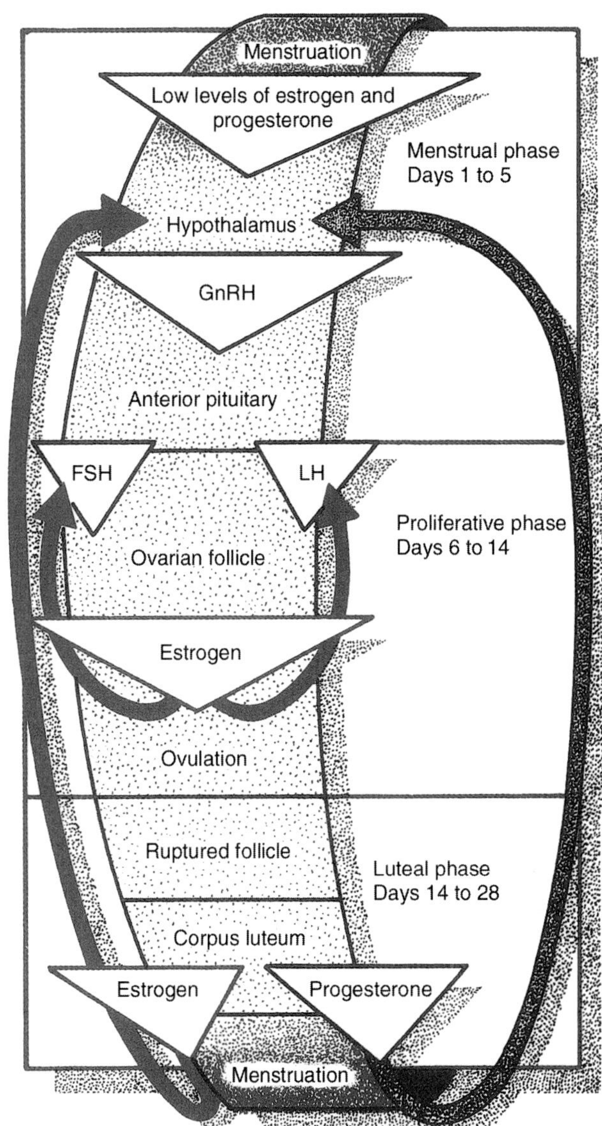

FIGURE 16–4. Menstrual cycle.

The Urinary System

The kidneys filter metabolic waste products from the blood and excrete these wastes in excessive body water. Each kidney has a single ureter connecting the renal pelvis with the urinary bladder. Each ureter then narrows on entering the posterior wall of the urinary bladder. The bladder temporarily stores the urine. As the bladder fills with urine, neuroreceptors transmit the impulse to void. Urine then flows through the urinary meatus. Any alteration in the homeostasis or structure of the urinary tract can be life threatening.

Structures and Functions of the Female Genitourinary System

STRUCTURE	DESCRIPTION/PRIMARY FUNCTION
Mons pubis	Pad of subcutaneous fatty tissue lying over anterior symphysis pubis. Protects pelvic bones during coitus.
Labia majora	Two longitudinal folds of adipose and connective tissue. Extend from clitoris anteriorly and gradually narrow to merge and form posterior commissure of perineum. Outer surface of labia majora becomes pigmented, wrinkled, and hairy at puberty. Inner surface is smoother, softer, and contains sebaceous glands. Protects vulva components that it surrounds. Protects urethra and vagina from infection.
Labia minora	Consists of two thin folds of skin that extend to form prepuce of clitoris anteriorly and a transverse fold of skin forming fourchette posteriorly. Labia minora contain sebaceous glands, erectile tissue, blood vessels, and involuntary muscle tissue. Secretions are bactericidal and aid in lubricating vulval skin and protecting it from urine. Protects urethra and vagina from infection.
Clitoris	Erectile body about 2.5 cm in length and 0.5 cm in diameter. Contains erectile tissue and has significant supply of nerve endings. Serves as primary organ of sexual stimulation.
Vestibule	Area between two folds of labia minora. A boat-shaped area containing the urethral meatus, openings of Skene's glands, hymen, openings of the Bartholin's glands and vaginal introitus.
Skene's Glands (Paraurethral Glands)	Surround urethral meatus. Provide lubrication to protect skin.
Vaginal Introitus	Entrance to vagina. Size and shape may vary.
Hymen	Avascular thin fold of connective tissue surrounding vaginal introitus in women who have not had sexual intercourse.
Bartholin's Glands	Small, pea-shaped glands deep in perineal structures. Ducts are not visible. Secrete clear, viscid, odorless, alkaline mucus that improves viability and motility of sperm along reproductive tract.
Perineum	Space between fourchette and anus. Made of muscle, elastic fibers, fascia, and connective tissue.
Vagina	Muscular tube from cervix to vulva. Located posterior to bladder and anterior to rectum. Serves as female organ of copulation, birth canal, and channel through which menstrual flow exits.
Cervix	End of uterus that projects into vagina.
Uterus	Pear-shaped, hollow, muscular organ between bladder neck and rectal wall. The mucous membrane lining is the endometrium. The muscular layer is the mesometrium. Inferior aspect is cervix and superior aspect is fundus. Major functions include serving as implantation site of fertilized ovum and as protective sac for developing embryo and fetus.
Fallopian Tubes	Two 7–10 cm long ducts on either side of fundus of uterus. Extend from uterus almost to ovaries. Normally, fertilization takes place within tubes. Major function includes serving as fertilization site and providing passageway for unfertilized and fertilized ova to travel to uterus.
Ovaries	Almond-shaped glandular structures that produce ova. Located beside fallopian tubes. Major functions include producing ova for fertilization by sperm and producing estrogen and progesterone.
Ureters	Hollow, tubelike structure connecting renal pelvis with urinary bladder.
Urinary Bladder	Muscular sac behind pubic symphysis that stores urine.
Urethra	Narrow, tubelike structure lined with mucous membrane. Opens to allow flow of urine to be excreted. It is 1 to 1 1/2 inches long and located slightly posterior to clitoris and directly anterior to vagina and rectum.

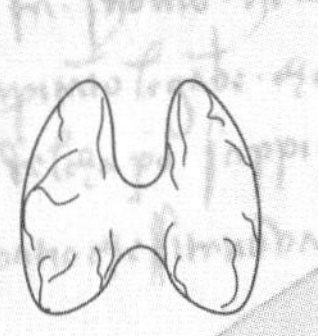

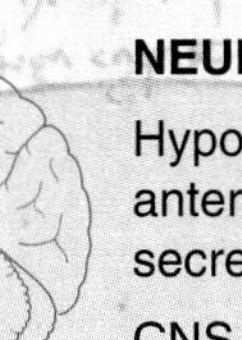

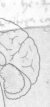

NEUROLOGICAL

Hypothalamus and anterior pituitary secrete hormones.

CNS needed for sexual pleasure.

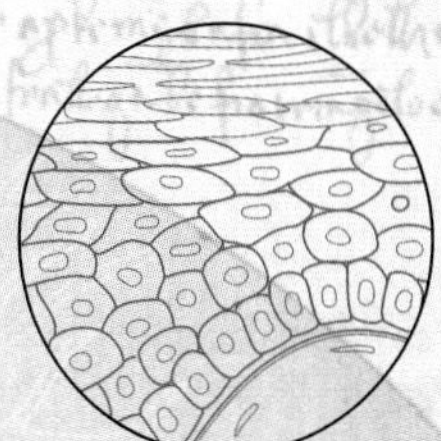

ENDOCRINE

Hypothalamus secretes GnRH.

Anterior pituitary secretes LH and FSH.

Ovaries secrete estrogen and progesterone.

INTEGUMENTARY

Female hormones influence body hair growth.

Sensory receptors on external genitalia provide sexual sensations.

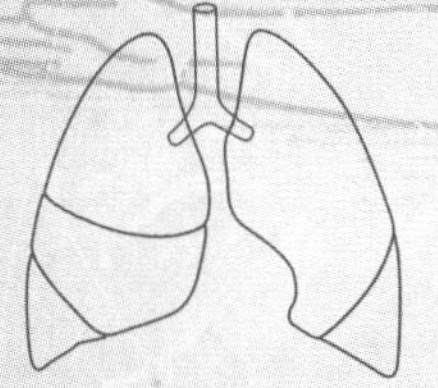

RESPIRATORY

Provides oxygen and removes carbon dioxide for reproductive system.

Respiratory system demands increase during sexual arousal and pregnancy.

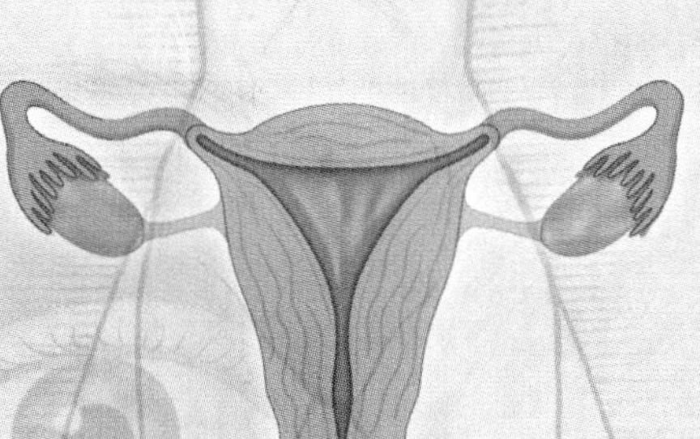

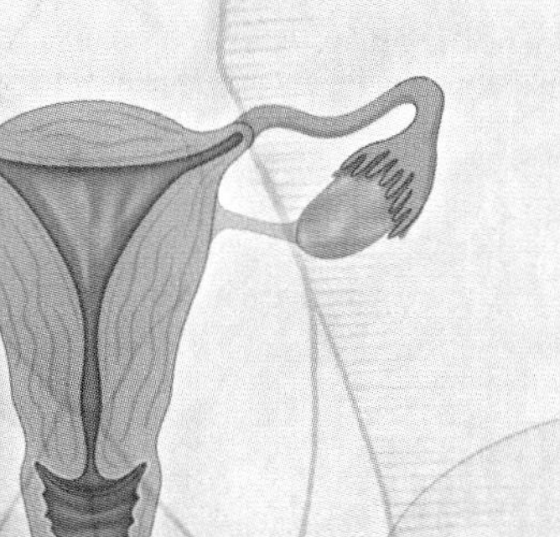

DIGESTIVE

Provides nutrients needed for genitourinary system.

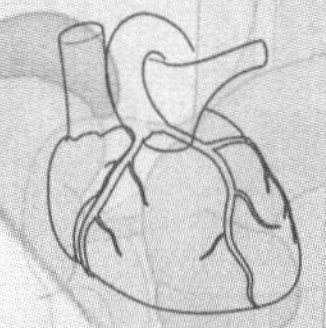

CARDIOVASCULAR

Delivers nutrients and hormones to genitourinary system.

Vascular system needed for sexual stimulation of the clitoris.

Estrogen has a protective cardiovascular effect until menopause.

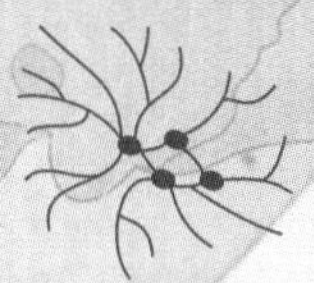

LYMPHATIC

Acidic vaginal secretions help prevent infections.

Lymphatic system defends against infection.

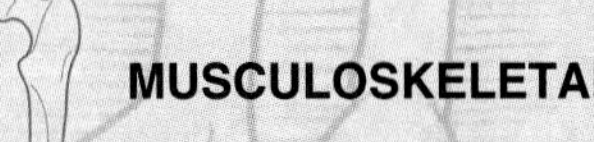

MUSCULOSKELETAL

Estrogen helps maintain bone mass and prevent osteoporosis.

Pelvis protects internal reproductive and urinary structures.

Relationship of Female GU System to Other Systems

Interaction with Other Body Systems

The Cardiovascular System

Nutrients and sex hormones are transported to the reproductive organs through the vascular system. Sexual excitement causes vasodilation of the arterioles in the clitoris. Additionally, estrogen lowers blood cholesterol levels and has positive cardiovascular effects until menopause.

The Urinary System

The close proximity of the vaginal opening to the urinary meatus increases the risk of urinary tract infections (UTIs) after frequent or vigorous sexual intercourse. Bladder continence is achieved during filling through the combination of detrusor muscle relaxation, internal sphincter muscle tone, and external sphincter contraction.

The Musculoskeletal System

The pelvic bones and pelvic floor muscles provide protection and support for some reproductive organs. Estrogen helps maintain bone mass until menopause.

The Neurological System

Neurological system impulses regulate events of the female sexual response. Hormones released by the hypothalamus of the **diencephalon** trigger the onset of the ovarian cycle.

Micturition is a reflex of parasympathetic control that stimulates detrusor muscle contraction with the simultaneous relaxation of the external sphincter and muscles of the pelvic floor. Urinary continence depends on the interaction of nerves that control the muscles for the bladder, bladder neck, urethra, and pelvic floor.

Developmental, Cultural, and Ethnic Variations

Infants

The female infant's genitals are enlarged at birth in response to maternal estrogen. The labia majora should cover the labia minora. The hormonal effect may also cause a pseudomenstruation. The urinary meatus and vaginal orifice should be visible. Androgens and progestins may cause masculine characteristics in female infants. If genitalia are ambiguous, a history is obtained to determine maternal use of sex hormones during pregnancy or a family history of adrenogenital syndrome.

Children and Adolescents

Girls begin puberty changes sometime between 8 and 13 years of age. Release of estrogen initiates the changes,

Maturation States in Females

Stage 1

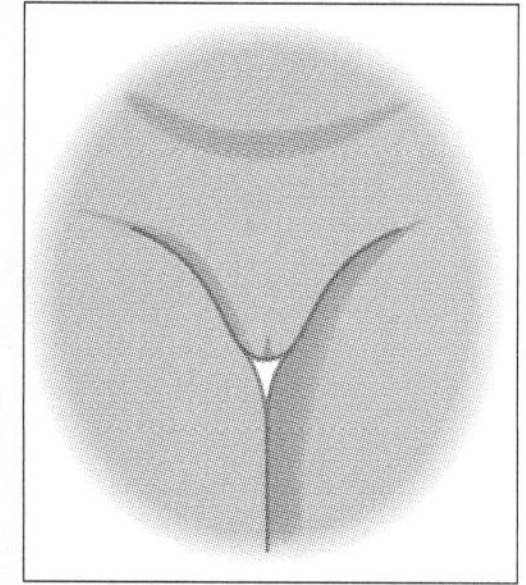

Preadolescent: No pubic hair except for fine body hair similar to hair on abdomen.

Stage 2

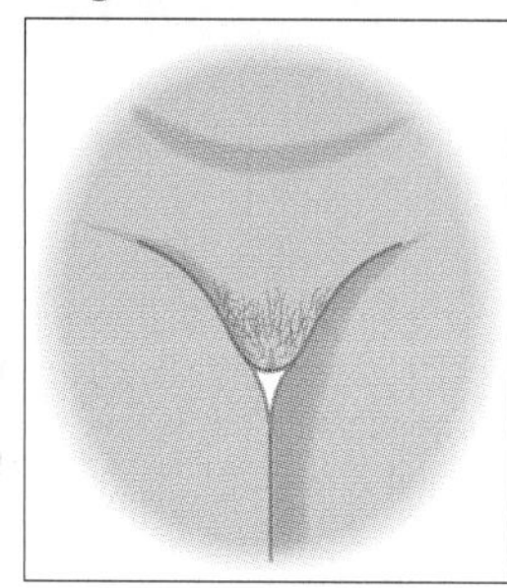

Sparse growth of long, slightly pigmented, downy hair, straight or only slightly curled, mostly along labia.

Stage 3

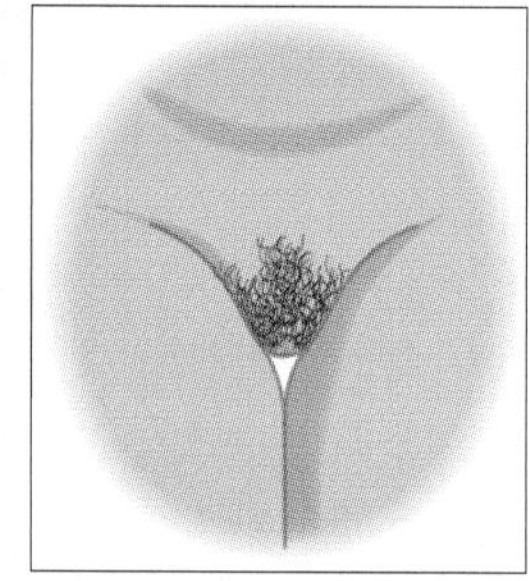

Hair becomes darker, coarser, and curlier and spreads sparsely over pubic symphysis.

Stage 4

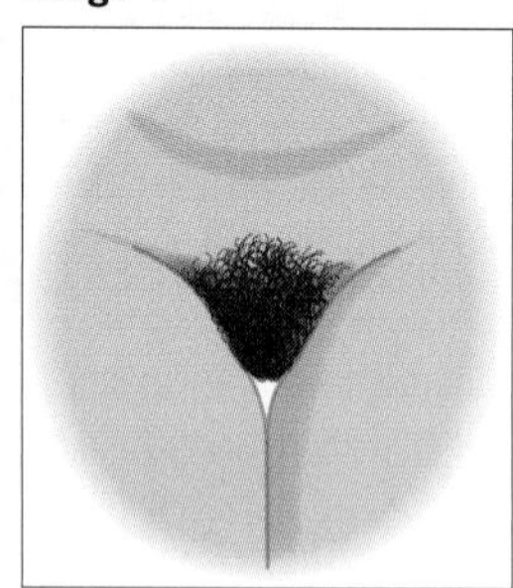

Pubic hair is coarse and curly as in adults. It covers more area than in Stage 3 but not as great as in adults.

Stage 5

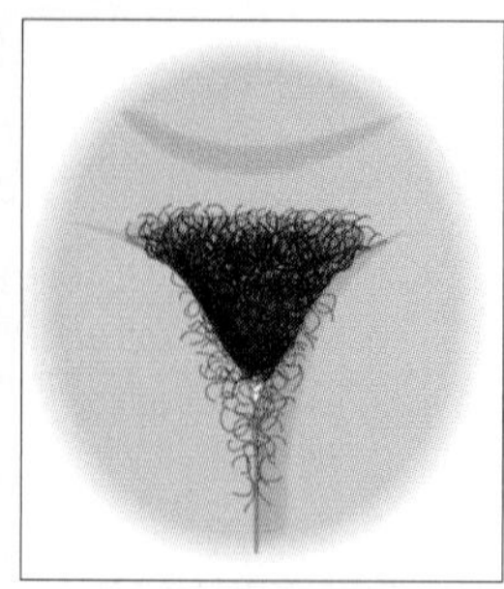

Quality and quantity are consistent with adult pubic hair distribution and spread over medial surfaces of thighs but not over abdomen.

which are first demonstrated in the development of breast buds and growth of pubic hair, followed by menstruation. The early development of sexual characteristics allows pregnancy before the child is intellectually or emotionally prepared for it. Early maturation can also lead to anemia related to menstrual bleeding. It is essential to assess for sexual molestation. Some signs include genital trauma; depression; eating disorders; and bruising, swelling, and inflammation in the vaginal, perineal, and anal areas.

Pregnant Women

Pregnancy imposes a multitude of changes to the reproductive organs. The uterus, cervix, ovaries, and vagina undergo significant structural changes related to the pregnancy and the influence of hormones. The uterus becomes hypertrophied, and its capacity increases to 500 to 1000 times its nonpregnant state. The vascularity of the cervix increases and contributes to softening of the cervix. Vascular congestion creates a blue-purple blemish or change in the cervical color (**Chadwick's sign**). Estrogen causes the glandular cervical tissue to produce a thick mucus, which builds up and forms a mucus plug at the endocervical canal.

The vagina undergoes changes similar to those of the uterus. Hypertrophy of the vaginal epithelium occurs. The vaginal wall softens and relaxes to accommodate the movement of the infant during birth.

Older Adults

Reproductive ability in women usually peaks in the late 20s. Over time, estrogen levels begin to decline and, in response, between the ages of 46 and 55, menstrual periods become shorter and less frequent until they stop entirely. Menopause is said to have occurred when the woman has not experienced a menstrual period in over a year. Sexual organs atrophy, the clitoris becomes smaller, and vaginal secretions are not as plentiful, so intercourse may become painful. These vaginal changes increase the risk for vaginal infections.

Women of Different Cultures or Ethnic Groups

Cultural and ethnic variations surrounding women often center on reproductive ability.

Cultural and Ethnic Views of Women

CULTURAL GROUP	VIEW OF WOMEN
Amish	High status associated to role of wife and mother. Responsibilities include feeding, clothing, and caring for family.
Appalachian	High status associated with motherhood. Having children associated with fulfillment. Responsible for child rearing. Older women preserve culture. Responsible for preparing herbal medicines and folk medicine.
Arab-American	Women gain status with age. Responsible for caring for and educating children and tending to husband's needs.
Chinese-American	Woman's role is to perpetuate male dominance.
Cuban-American	Women expected to stay at home and care for children.
Egyptian-American	Status and power increase with pregnancy and birthing, especially with having a son. Childbirth is expected within 1 year of marriage.
Filipino-American	Women have equal role to men in health, welfare, and family finance.
Greek-American	Pregnancy seen as a time of great respect.
Iranian-American	Prestige associated with having children.
Jewish-American	Woman runs home and is responsible for children.
Mexican-American	Woman maintains home and health of family.
Native American (Indian)	Mother is center of Indian society.
Vietnamese-American	Women expected to be dutiful and respectful of husband and to make healthcare decisions.

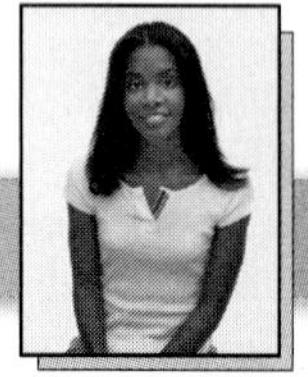

Introducing the Case Study

Mrs. Ellen James has come for her annual gynecological examination. She is 29 years old, married, and the mother of one child. She complains of scant midcycle vaginal bleeding for the last 2 months. She is not employed outside the home.

Performing the Female GU Assessment

Health History

Because assessment of the female GU system may be somewhat uncomfortable for both you and your client, begin by establishing rapport. A professional, nonthreatening approach is essential in order to collect accurate data.

Accurate data are the keys to a successful health history. When interviewing your client, keep these points in mind:

- Some cultures do not permit women to discuss sexual topics or be examined by a man.
- Reproductive system problems may adversely affect self-image, sexual functioning, and overall wellness.
- Consider the woman's age and choose your health history questions accordingly.

The history will provide you with data that will guide your physical examination.

Biographical Data

Quickly reviewing the biographical data may identify actual or potential problems. Begin with the woman's age—it influences the questions you ask. The woman's age may also help you identify risk factors such as sexually transmitted diseases (STDs), which occur more frequently in young women, and gynecological cancers, which occur more often in older adults. If your client is over age 50, you may want to ask questions related to menopause, rather than asking about the menstrual cycle.

Case Study Findings

Reviewing Mrs. James's biographical data:

- 29-year-old African-American female.
- Married, mother of a 4-year-old girl.
- American by birth; Protestant religion.
- Attended 1 year of college after high school; homemaker at present. Husband is stockbroker for investment banking company.
- Healthcare insurance with husband's company.
- Source of referral: Self, seems reliable.

Current Health Status

Reproductive health history questions relate to sexual function, fertility, sexual satisfaction, sexual practices, and self-care. Begin by asking about symptoms; leave sexuality questions to the end of the history. If the woman has a reproductive system problem, identify her chief complaint and perform a symptom analysis. Symptoms that relate to the female GU system include vaginal discharge, pain, lumps/masses, **dysmenorrhea, amenorrhea,** and urinary symptoms.

Symptom Analysis

Symptom Analysis tables for all of the symptoms described in the following paragraphs are available on the Web for viewing and printing. In your Web browser, go to *http://www.fadavis.com/detail.cfm?id=0882-9* and click on Symptom Analysis Tables under Explore This Product.

Vaginal Discharge

The only normal vaginal drainages are mucus and menstrual blood. Any other type of discharge may signal a problem. The description of the discharge may give clues to the underlying problem. Vaginal discharge is the most common presenting symptom in women with STDs. A white, curdlike discharge is seen with candidiasis; a gray or white, thin, malodorous discharge with bacterial vaginosis; and a yellow or green discharge with gonorrhea.

Lesions

Lesions may indicate a variety of problems. Vesicles, ulcers, warts, or rashes are common lesions. The morphological description of the lesion and whether or not it is painful will help you identify it. Lesions are often related to STDs, but they may also be caused by carcinoma or a systemic problem.

Vaginal Bleeding

Abnormal uterine bleeding includes excessive menstrual flow (**menorrhagia**), breakthrough bleeding (vaginal bleeding between periods), or decreased or absent menstrual bleeding (amenorrhea). Determine your client's usual menstrual cycle and flow. Changes may be associated with normal reproductive changes or signal an underlying problem, so careful assessment is needed to determine the cause.

Pain

Pain directly related to menstrual flow is called dysmenorrhea. It is the most frequent complaint of young women seeking health care. **Primary dysmenorrhea** is menstrual pain or discomfort not usually associated with a physical abnormality or pathology and can be diagnosed with a normal physical examination. **Secondary dysmenorrhea** is menstrual pain or discomfort associated with pathology, such as endometriosis, infection, IUD placement, pelvic mass, adhesions, cervical obstruction, or congenital malformations. Other causes of pelvic pain include pelvic inflammatory disease (PID) and renal and GI problems.

Pain in the lower abdomen or back can also be renal, gastrointestinal, or musculoskeletal in nature. Therefore it is important to perform a thorough symptom analysis. Perform a review of systems to identify any relevant data.

Amenorrhea

Amenorrhea is the absence of menses. **Primary amenorrhea** means that menses never occurred. In **secondary amenorrhea,** menses have ceased for 6 months if the cycle was normally regular and for 12 months if the cycle was normally irregular. Primary amenorrhea may be caused by a genetic or hormonal disorder. Secondary amenorrhea may be caused by a normal process such as pregnancy or menopause or may indicate an underlying problem. A thorough symptom analysis will help you to determine the underlying cause.

Urinary Symptoms

Urinary symptoms are often associated with female reproductive problems caused by the anatomical proximity of the systems. Urinary symptoms often cause discomfort, prompting the client to seek treatment. Dysuria, burning, frequency, change in urinary patterns, and hematuria are common problems. Because the two systems work so closely together, a problem in one often eventually affects the other. A urinary problem may cause a reproductive problem, but more frequently a reproductive problem results in a urinary problem. Urinary incontinence is a common complaint of older women, but it should not be considered a normal change associated with aging. (For more information, see Chapter 25).

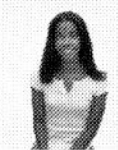

Case Study Findings

Mrs. James' current health status includes:

- Scant midcycle vaginal bleeding for the last 2 months with no other complaints at present.
- Seeking care for annual **Pap smear,** gynecological examination, and renewed prescription for oral contraceptives.

Past Health History

The various components of the past history are linked to female genitalia pathology and female genitalia-related information. You may be able to identify a direct link from the past health history to your client's current health status. The following are specific areas to explore.

Past Health History

RISK FACTORS/ QUESTIONS TO ASK	RATIONALE/SIGNIFICANCE
Childhood Illnesses	
Did you have communicable diseases transmitted at birth?	Diseases passed from mother to infant during birth include hepatitis B, herpes, HIV, chlamydia, and HPV.
Were you exposed to diethylstilbestrol (DES) before birth?	Exposure to DES in utero increases risk of cervicovaginal cancer and reproductive problems.
Hospitalizations/Surgeries	
Have you ever had gynecological surgery: hysterectomy, myomectomy, salpingectomy, oophorectomy, dilation and curettage (D & C), dilatation and evacuation, laparoscopy, vulvectomy, tubal ligation, colpotomy, cesarean section, female circumcision?	Surgical procedures affect reproductive health.

(Continued)

Past Health History *(Continued)*

RISK FACTORS/ QUESTIONS TO ASK	RATIONALE/SIGNIFICANCE
Diagnostic Procedures	
When was your last Pap test? Have any biopsies been done?	Pap test screens for cervical cancer. Biopsies detect malignancies.
Serious Injuries	
Have you ever had abdominal or vaginal trauma or injuries? Have you ever been raped or sexually abused?	May explain abnormal physical findings or sexual dysfunction.
Serious/Chronic Illnesses	
Do you have an STD, such as gonorrhea, syphilis, herpes, HIV/AIDS, hepatitis, chlamydia, condyloma (HPV)?	STDs can cause infertility. Recurrent incidence of STDs may indicate untreated sexual partner or multiple sexual partners.
Do you have any infertility problems?	Existing infertility problems may help explain physical findings. Inability to conceive after 1 year of regular coitus without contraception may indicate fertility problem and warrants referral.
Do you have diabetes mellitus, thyroid disease, incontinence, constipation, UTIs?	Diabetes mellitus increases incidence of vaginal yeast infections. There are also specific precautions for pregnant diabetics. (See Chapter 21.) A history of thyroid disease may explain menstrual irregularities. Recurrent UTIs may be a symptom of untreated vaginal infection. Voiding pattern change may be a symptom of infection or reproductive structure changes.
Are you a paraplegic or quadriplegic? Do you have a chronic neurological problem?	Disabled or handicapped clients are at increased obstetric risk depending on level of injury, tone of uterus, and competency of cervix. They are also at risk for urinary complications such as UTIs.
Immunizations	
Were you immunized against hepatitis B?	Hepatitis B can be transmitted through sexual activity and to newborns from infected mothers.
Allergies	
Do you have any allergies?	Contact dermatitis caused by condoms, nonoxynol 9, or other spermicides or latex identifies additional health promotion needs.
Medications	
Are you taking any prescribed or over-the-counter medications, including antibiotics, oral contraceptives, estrogen replacement therapy, antidepressants, antihypertensives?	Antibiotics increase incidence of *Candida* vaginosis and may lessen effectiveness of oral contraceptives. Estrogens may cause altered menstrual flow. Antidepressants and antihypertensive medications can alter libido. Antidepressants may also cause menstrual irregularities. See box, Drugs That Adversely Affect the Female Reproductive System, on page 531.
Recent Travel/Military Service/ Exposure to Infectious or Contagious Diseases	
Have you been exposed to chemicals? Do you have a history of STDs?	Increased risk for infertility. Could present an educational opportunity for disease prevention.

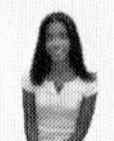

Case Study Findings

Mrs. James's past health history reveals:

- Rheumatic fever at age 7.
- Usual childhood illnesses except for measles, mumps, and rubella.
- Denies any previous surgeries or serious injuries.
- Has taken oral contraceptives since birth of child 4

years ago. No other medications except occasional aspirin.

- No history of STDs.
- **Gravida** 1, para 1, no complications with pregnancy or vaginal delivery.
- **Menarche** at age 12, LMP 21 days ago. Menses last 5 days with moderate to light flow and occurs every 21 to 23 days. Denies dysmenorrhea.
- Denies exposure to DES.

Drugs That Adversely Affect the Female Reproductive System

Drug Class	Drug	Possible Adverse Reactions
Androgens	danazol	Vaginitis with itching, dryness, burning, or bleeding; amenorrhea
	fluoxymesterone, methyltestosterone, testosterone	Amenorrhea and other menstrual irregularities; virilization, including clitoral enlargement
Antidepressants	tricyclic antidepressants	Changed libido, menstrual irregularity
	selective serotonin reuptake inhibitors	Decreased libido, anorgasmia
Antihypertensives	clonidine hydrochloride, reserpine	Decreased libido
	methyldopa	Decreased libido, amenorrhea
Antipsychotics	chlorpromazine hydrochloride, perphenazine, prochlorperazine, promazine hydrochloride, thioridazine hydrochloride, trifluoperazine hydrochloride, haloperidol	Inhibition of ovulation (chlorpromazine only) menstrual irregularities, amenorrhea, changed libido
Beta-blockers	atenolol, labetalol hydrochloride, nadolol, propranolol hydrochloride, metoprolol	Decreased libido
Cardiac glycosides	digoxin, digitoxin	Changes in cellular layer of vaginal walls in postmenopausal women
Cytotoxics	busulfan	Amenorrhea with menopausal symptoms in premenopausal women, ovarian suppression, ovarian fibrosis and atrophy
	chlorambucil	Amenorrhea
	cyclophosphamide	Gonadal suppression (possibly irreversible), amenorrhea, ovarian fibrosis
	methotrexate	Menstrual dysfunction, infertility
	tamoxifen	Vaginal discharge or bleeding, menstrual irregularities, pruritus vulvae (intense itching of the female external genitalia)
	thiotepa	Amenorrhea
Estrogens	chlorotrianisene; conjugated estrogens, esterified estrogens, estradiol, estrone, ethinyl estradiol	Altered menstrual flow, dysmenorrhea, amenorrhea cervical erosion or abnormal secretions, enlargement of uterine fibromas, vaginal candidiasis
	dienestrol	Vaginal discharge, uterine bleeding with excessive use
	diethylstilbestrol	Breakthrough bleeding, altered menstrual flow, dysmenorrhea, amenorrhea, cervical erosion, altered cervical secretions, enlargement of uterine fibromas, vaginal candidiasis, change in libido, increased risk of vaginal cancer in female offspring
Thyroid hormones	levothyroxine sodium, thyroid USP, thyrotropin, and others	Menstrual irregularities with excessive doses
Progestins	hydroxyprogesterone caproate, medroxyprogesterone acetate, norethindrone, norethindrone acetate, norgestrel, progesterone	Breakthrough bleeding, dysmenorrhea, amenorrhea, cervical erosion and abnormal secretions
Steroids	dexamethasone, hydrocortisone, prednisone	Amenorrhea and menstrual irregularities
Miscellaneous	lithium carbonate, L-tryptophan	Decreased libido
	spironolactone	Menstrual irregularities, amenorrhea, postmenopausal bleeding
	valproate	Menstrual irregularities, amenorrhea, possible polycystic ovarian syndrome

Family History

The family history can identify predisposing or causative factors of a health problem.

It not only identifies genetically linked disorders, but also familial risk factors that may predispose your client to genitourinary disease.

Family History

RISK FACTORS/ QUESTIONS TO ASK	RATIONALE/SIGNIFICANCE
Mother's Reproductive History	
Did your mother take DES while pregnant with you?	Exposure to DES in utero can cause cervicovaginal cancer and reproductive problems.
Did she transfer STDs during pregnancy or delivery, have multiple pregnancies, or have babies with congenital anomalies?	STDs can cause infertility. Spontaneous abortion, menstrual irregularities, multiple births, congenital anomalies and diseases of female genitalia may have familial tendency.
Do you have a family history of reproductive cancers?	Gynecological cancers such as ovarian and uterine have familial/genetic links.

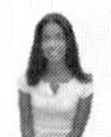

Case Study Findings

Mrs. James's family history reveals:

- No gynecological carcinomas or maternal exposure to DES.
- Parents are alive and well.
- Has two healthy female siblings, ages 33 and 35.

Review of Systems

Changes in reproductive system function have an effect on other body systems. The review of systems (ROS) can identify changes in other systems and help you identify something you might otherwise have missed.

Review of Systems

SYSTEM/QUESTIONS TO ASK	RATIONALE/SIGNIFICANCE
General Health Survey	
How have you been feeling? Have you had any changes in your energy level? Fevers? Weight changes?	Fatigue or activity intolerance is often a sign of underlying health problem. For example, fatigue from HIV/AIDS would interfere with activity tolerance; fatigue influences desire and ability to perform sexual intercourse and may also be associated with anemia.
Integumentary/*Skin/Hair/Nails*	
Have you had any rashes, lesions, or skin color changes? Any changes in hair growth?	Rashes, growths, and lumps may indicate pathology. Pruritus in hair or on labia may indicate scabies, kidney or liver problems. Estrogen and progesterone can cause changes in skin, hair and nails, such as those seen during pregnancy and menopause. Changes in hair texture, moisture, and distribution occur during pregnancy and menopause.
HEENT/*Head and Neck*	
Do you have any swollen glands or nodes?	Swelling of lymph nodes associated with infection, malignancy. Enlarged thyroid may affect sexual function.
Do you have headaches?	Headaches are a common side effect of oral contraceptives.
HEENT/*Eyes, Mouth, and Throat*	
Do you have a sore throat?	Oropharynx and eyes are sites for STDs, such as HSV II and gonorrhea. Secondary syphilis can result in oral mucous patches. Gonorrheal eye infections occur in newborns (ophthalmia neonatorum) and gonorrheal conjunctivitis in adults.

Review of Systems

SYSTEM/QUESTIONS TO ASK	RATIONALE/SIGNIFICANCE
HEENT/*Eyes, Mouth, and Throat (Continued)*	
Watery eyes? Eye drainage?	*Tearing, photophobia, eyelid edema, conjunctival edema: Chlamydia trachomatis.*
Respiratory	
Do you have any breathing problems?	Respiratory disease such as COPD may affect sexual activity.
Cardiovascular	
Do you have a heart murmur?	Some heart murmurs are associated with anemia. Cardiovascular symptoms are associated with oral contraceptive use.
Did you ever have vascular problems, thrombophlebitis, cardiovascular disease?	Chronic cardiovascular disease can affect ability to perform sexually.
Breasts	
Do you have any breast tenderness, lumps, or discharge? Where are you in your menstrual cycle?	Cyclical hormonal changes are associated with breast tenderness. Female hormones are associated with fibrocystic disease and breast cancer.
Gastrointestinal	
Do you have a history of liver disease?	Liver disease associated with gynecologic malignancy may cause ascites.
Do you have appetite or weight loss?	*Appetite or weight loss:* May indicate underlying eating disorder, malignancy, or AIDS.
Abdominal pain?	*Abdominal pain:* May indicate pathology of reproductive organs.
Reproductive/Menstrual History	
How old were you when you started to menstruate? When was your LMP? How long are your periods? How long is your cycle? Are your periods regular? Is your flow heavy, moderate, or light? Are your periods painful or extremely heavy? Do you skip periods or have you stopped getting them altogether? Do you have spotting between periods?	*Late onset of menarche (age 16–18):* Can result from inadequate nutrition caused by eating disorders, chronic diseases such as Crohn's disease, environmental stresses, intensive athletic training, hypothyroidism, or opiate or steroid use.
Reproductive/Menstrual History/ *Premenstrual Syndrome (PMS)*	
Before your period, do you have breast tenderness, bloating, moodiness; cravings for salt, sugar, or chocolate; fatigue; weight gain; headaches; or joint pain?	PMS signs and symptoms may be alleviated through stress reduction and avoidance of certain foods.
Reproductive/Menstrual History/ *Obstetrical History*	
When was your LMP? Have you ever used fertility drugs? How many pregnancies have you had? How many living children? Have you ever had an abortion, miscarriage, C-section, or other complication with pregnancy? How long were your labors? Did you have any postpartum complications?	Past obstetrical health is a predictor of future reproductive health.

(Continued)

Review of Systems *(Continued)*

SYSTEM/QUESTIONS TO ASK	RATIONALE/SIGNIFICANCE
Reproductive/Menstrual History/ *Contraceptive History*	
Do you use contraceptives? If yes, what types, how often, and have you had any problems with contraception? How do you prevent STDs? Do you or did you smoke? If yes, how much and for how long?	IUDs increase risk of PID; diaphragms may cause urinary discomfort; oral contraceptives have a variety of side effects; and some people are allergic to spermicides or latex in condoms. Oral contraceptives and smoking increase risk of cardiovascular problems. Take this opportunity to teach woman about various contraception methods.
Reproductive/Menstrual History/ *Perimenopause*	
Do you have spotting between periods, hot flashes, heart palpitations, numbness, tingling, drenching sweats, mood swings, vaginal dryness, or itching? Are you taking estrogen replacement therapy? How do you feel about menopause?	Women may have various discomforting signs and symptoms associated with menopause. Hormonal and physical changes may affect self-concept. Identifying symptoms helps you plan appropriate interventions.
Musculoskeletal	
Do you have any weakness, limitation, joint pain, swelling?	The physical act of sexual intercourse requires the musculoskeletal system to be functional.
Are you past menopause?	Postmenopausal women are at greater risk for developing **osteoporosis**.
Have you ever had a bone density test?	
Did you ever break a bone?	
Neurological	
Have you had any changes in your menstrual cycle?	Amenorrhea may result from problems with hypothalamus of diencephalon.
Have you had mood swings?	Hormonal fluctuations may affect emotional state (e.g., during pregnancy).
Have you had weakness, paralysis, tremors? Mental or personality changes?	Neurosyphilis occurs in late syphilis and can cause paresis, tremors, personality changes, and psychosis.
Endocrine	
Do you have diabetes?	Diabetes increases risk for candidal vaginal infections.
Do you have thyroid disease?	Hypothyroidism causes menorrhagia, decreased libido, and infertility. Hyperthyroidism can cause abnormal menses or amenorrhea.
Lymphatic/Hematologic	
Do you have HIV or AIDS?	AIDS affects the immune system.
Do you have a history of cancer?	Gynecological cancers can metastasize to local lymphatic tissue.
Do you have a heavy menstrual flow?	Heavy menses (menorrhagia) can lead to anemia.

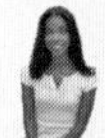

Case Study Findings

Mrs. James' review of systems reveals:

- **General Health Survey:** Usual state of health good, no changes in weight or energy level.
- **Integumentary:** No changes in skin, hair, or nails.
- **HEENT:** No sore throat, headaches, lumps, or masses in neck.
- **Respiratory:** No history of respiratory disease.
- **Cardiovascular:** No history of CV disease.
- **Gastrointestinal:** Appetite good, no GI problems.
- **Musculoskeletal:** No weakness, joint pain, or fractures.

- **Neurological:** No history of neurological problems.
- **Endocrine:** No history of diabetes or thyroid disease.
- **Lymphatic/Hematologic:** No lymphatic or hematologic disorders.

Psychosocial Profile

The psychosocial profile can provide a bridge between the health maintenance activities and female genital function.

Psychosocial Profile

CATEGORY/QUESTIONS TO ASK	RATIONALE/SIGNIFICANCE
Health Practices and Beliefs/ Self-Care Activities	
Do you get a yearly gynecological exam?	Annual exams help in early detection of problems.
When was your last Pap test? What were the results?	Pap smear can detect precancerous and cancerous cell changes in cervix and may also detect HPV. Regular Pap tests indicate client's participation in self-care. Vaginal smears are done for women who have had a hysterectomy.
What is your personal hygiene routine?	Poor personal hygiene can lead to infections of genitalia or urinary tract.
Do you douche frequently?	Excessive cleansing or frequent douching can promote rashes or genital infection. Ability to care for self indicates a high level of wellness.
Typical Day	
What is your typical day like?	May identify health teaching needs.
Nutritional Patterns	
What did you eat in the last 24 hours? What foods do you usually eat? Have you lost or gained weight recently?	Increased levels of refined sugars, salt, and caffeine enhance PMS symptoms. Extreme dieting can lead to amenorrhea.
Activity and Exercise Patterns	
Do you exercise on a routine basis? If so, how often and what type of exercise?	Exercise may diminish dysmenorrhea and menorrhagia. Excessive exercise may result in amenorrhea.
Recreation/Pets/Hobbies	
Do you have any hobbies? What do you do for recreation? Do you swim or ride horses?	Extended periods of exposure to moisture increases likelihood of *Candida* vaginosis. High incidence of genital trauma from saddle injuries.
Do you have cats?	Pregnant women can develop toxoplasmosis from touching cat litter.
Sleep/Rest Patterns	
How many hours of sleep do you average a night? Is your sleep restful or interrupted?	Lack of sleep or extreme fatigue can lead to amenorrhea.
Personal Habits/*Alcohol Use*	
Do you drink alcohol? If so, what type, how much and how often?	Significant correlation between alcohol use and date rape in college-age women. Alcohol use during pregnancy can cause fetal alcohol syndrome.
Personal Habits/*Drug Use*	
Do you use street drugs, such as cocaine, barbiturates, amphetamines, or narcotics? If so, how often and how much?	Impairs judgment, increasing risk of STD exposure. Can cause decreased libido.

(Continued)

Psychosocial Profile *(Continued)*

CATEGORY/QUESTIONS TO ASK	RATIONALE/SIGNIFICANCE
Personal Habits/*Tobacco Use*	
Do you smoke? If so, what type, how much per day and for how many years?	Smoking is a risk factor for cervical cancer. Increased incidence of strokes in smokers who use oral contraceptives.
Occupational Health Patterns	
What type of work do you do?	Exposure to some chemicals, lead, and radiation has been linked to birth defects and spontaneous abortions.
Are you exposed to arsenic, glycol ethers, lead, radiation, vinyl chloride or PCBs?	Oncology nurses exposed to antineoplastic drugs may have spontaneous abortions, fetal anomalies, and changes in menstrual cycles.
Environmental Health Patterns	
Do you live in an apartment or single home? Is sanitation adequate?	Poor sanitation may lead to numerous forms of vaginitis.
Is space adequate, or are you overcrowded?	Overcrowding can cause mite infestation.
Are you homeless?	Hygiene is a significant problem for homeless people.
Roles/Relationships/Self-Concept	
How do you see yourself?	Poor self-image and lack of self-confidence predispose a client to sexual dysfunction.
Cultural/Religious Influences	
What is your cultural and religious background?	Cultural and religious practices influence GU health. For example, abortion and contraception are prohibited in Catholic faith, and some cultures/religions have specific beliefs related to menstruation and sexual practices.
Family Roles and Relationships	
What is your present relationship status?	Grief from loss of a relationship can affect sexual desire. Abusive relationships can affect sexual functioning.
Social Supports/Stress and Coping	
Who are your supports? Do you have much stress in your life? If so, how do you deal with it?	Stress can cause amenorrhea, exacerbate genital herpes simplex, and lead to sexual dysfunction. Feelings of emotional or social isolation can increase stress.

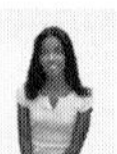

Case Study Findings

Mrs. James's psychosocial profile includes:

- Last gynecological examination and PAP smear 1 year ago with no abnormalities found. Had one cold in last year without seeking medical attention. Bathes daily and does not douche.
- Typical day includes waking at 6:00 AM, preparing family breakfast, and performing household chores. Daughter goes to day care 2 days a week while client volunteers at indigent healthcare facility.
- Eats three meals a day, drinks two cups of coffee. Does not eat at restaurants often and attempts to make healthy meals.
- Exercise/leisure activities include gardening, reading, and outside activities with family.
- Family pet is a 1-year-old beagle.
- Asleep by 10:30 PM (7 1/2 hours a night).
- Does not smoke, drinks one glass of wine occasionally with evening meals, denies recreational drug use.
- Lives in a suburban house of adequate size for a large family.
- No cultural or religious influences on health care. Family attends church most Sundays.
- Describes loving relationship with spouse, and states they intend to have three more children. Enjoys being a homemaker.
- Copes with stress by communicating with spouse.

Sexual History

Because the GU system encompasses sexuality, a more detailed sexual history may be indicated. Leaving this until the end of your history gives you time to establish rapport with the client before asking sensitive or embarrassing questions.

Asking about sexual functions and practices is important for several reasons:

- Many women have sex-related questions or problems that they want to discuss.
- Sexual practices may be directly related to the client's symptoms.
- Sexual dysfunction may be related to medications and may be reversible.
- Sexual practices are related to the client's risk for cross-contamination to other areas, STDs, hepatitis, cervical dysplasia, and cervical carcinoma. Risk for disease increases as the number of sexual partners increases.
- Changes in sexual function may indicate pain, infection, hormonal changes, disease, changes in mental status, or altered role and relationship patterns.

Depending on the individual patient, ask the following questions to assess sexual function:

- Have you ever been sexually active?
- Are you currently sexually active? That is, have you had sex with anyone in the past few months? If the answer is yes, answer the next question.
- Do you have sex with men, women, or both (heterosexual, homosexual, or bisexual)?
- What types of sexual activity do you engage in? Oral, anal, genital?
- How often do you have intercourse?
- Do you have more than one partner? How many partners have you had in the last 6 months? How many partners in your lifetime? Do you trade sexual favors for drugs or money?
- Do you use birth control? What kind? How often?
- Are you worried about the AIDS virus or other STDs?
- Do you take any precautions to avoid infections? If so, what?
- Are you able to achieve orgasm? Do you have any problems or concerns about your sexual function?
- Have you had surgery on any of your reproductive organs? If so, what kind and when?

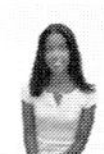

Case Study Findings

Mrs. James's sexual history findings include:

- Sexually active in a monogamous, heterosexual relationship with husband.
- Satisfied with sexual performance.
- Uses oral contraceptives.

Case Study Evaluation

Before you proceed with the physical examination of the female GU system, review the data you have obtained from Mrs. James's history. Document the GU history related to Mrs. James.

CRITICAL THINKING ACTIVITY #1

In view of the subjective data obtained from Mrs. James, what parts of the physical assessment will you be focusing on?

Physical Assessment

Once you have obtained the subjective data, focus on collecting objective data by performing the physical examination.

Approach

Instruct the client not to use vaginal sprays, douche, or have coitus for 24 to 48 hours before the examination. Doing so might affect the Pap smear and other vaginal cultures. Make sure the examination room is warm, comfortable, and private. Ideally, the foot of the examination table should point away from the door.

Many women feel anxious and fearful about having a genital assessment, so be thoroughly professional and especially sensitive to your client's needs. This will make the examination easier for both of you. Also listen for any clues that might help you uncover concerns that the woman might be reluctant to express. Having a female attendant present is also advisable. In addition, keep in mind cultural differences. For example, married Muslim women must have their husbands present during the examination. Women of some cultures will not disrobe or allow a man to perform a physical examination on them. Others will not allow a sample of their body fluids to be taken and examined by strangers.

Before you begin, ask the woman to empty her bladder. Have her completely disrobe and put on a hospital gown. She may leave on socks if the stirrups are not covered with padding. Then explain each assessment technique and its purpose, and show her the speculum and other equipment. Encourage her to express any anxieties or concerns. Reassure her that the position for the examination and the assessment techniques used may be uncomfortable at times, but they should not be painful.

Assessment of the female reproductive system consists of inspection and palpation of the abdomen, external genitalia, and internal reproductive structures. You will use the speculum to view the internal genitalia and collect specimens for laboratory analysis. Thorough palpation of the internal structures includes a bimanual examination and rectovaginal assessment.

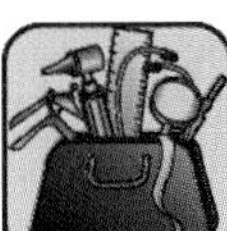

Toolbox

Assemble the following equipment for a routine examination: Large hand mirror, gooseneck lamp, disposable gloves, drape, vaginal speculum, cytological materials (Ayre spatula, cytobrush, cotton-tipped applicators, OB swabs, microscope slides), labeled

Thayer-Martin culture plate, cytology fixative spray, reagents (normal saline solution or potassium hydroxide [KOH]), Hemoccult slide and developer, acetic acid, warm water, and water-soluble lubricant.

Performing a General Survey

Before you focus on the GU assessment, perform a general survey and head-to-toe assessment, looking for clues that might suggest a GU problem. For example, obtain vital signs. Elevations in temperature may indicate an infection that might be accompanied by a GU infection.

Note the woman's emotional status. This examination can produce anxiety. Ensure privacy and expose only the area being assessed. Note the woman's posture and nonverbal behavior. Does her posture reflect pain or discomfort?

Performing a Head-to-Toe Physical Assessment

The GU system affects many different systems. So examine the client for specific changes that may affect the GU system.

Performing a Head-to-Toe Physical Assessment

SYSTEM/NORMAL FINDINGS	ABNORMAL FINDINGS/RATIONALE
General Health Survey *INSPECT* Well developed physically No acute distress	
Awake, alert, oriented. Memory intact.	Personality changes and mental deterioration can accompany late-stage syphilis.
Affect appropriate.	Depression can affect sexual functioning. Loss of height may be seen in postmenopausal women with osteoporosis.
Weight stable, no loss of height.	Weight loss resulting from anorexia can cause amenorrhea. Weight gain is associated with pregnancy. Unexplained weight loss may be associated with malignancy.
Integumentary/*Skin* *INSPECT* Intact, no lesions	Rashes and skin lesions are associated with many STDs. *Systemic rash:* Secondary syphilis *Vesicles:* Herpes simplex types 1 and 2. *Increased skin pigmentation:* Increased hormones during pregnancy.
Integumentary/*Hair* Even distribution of hair	*Alopecia:* Secondary syphilis. Abnormal increase in body hair (hirsutism): Decrease in female hormones.
HEENT/*Head and Neck* *INSPECT/PALPATE* No palpable lymph nodes	*Palpable lymph nodes:* May indicate systemic infection or malignancy.
Thyroid not palpable	*Enlarged thyroid (hypo- or hyperthyroidism):* May affect reproductive and sexual functioning.

Performing a Head-to-Toe Physical Assessment

SYSTEM/NORMAL FINDINGS	ABNORMAL FINDINGS/RATIONALE
HEENT/*Eyes, Mouth, and Throat*	
Conjunctiva pink, no drainage	Conjunctivitis: Can be caused by gonorrhea.
Oral mucous membranes pink, moist, and intact.	*Oral lesions:* Associated with STDs.
Respiratory	
INSPECT/AUSCULTATE	
Lungs clear; no shortness of breath (SOB)	Chronic lung disease may impair sexual functioning.
Cardiovascular	
INSPECT/PALPATE/AUSCULTATE	
Regular heart rate and rhythm, no extra sounds	Anemia can cause tachycardia and a systolic flow murmur.
Positive pedal pulses, negative Homans' sign, no edema	Oral contraceptives associated with increased risk of thrombus formation.
Breasts	
INSPECT/PALPATE	
Nontender, no discharge (unless lactating), no lesions	Cyclical hormonal changes may cause breast fullness and tenderness.
Abdomen	
INSPECT/PALPATE/AUSCULTATE	
Positive bowel sounds; abdomen soft, nontender, no masses	*Palpable abdominal masses:* May be a fetus or fibroid tumor.
No organomegaly	*Enlarged liver and ascites:* Associated with metastasis of gynecological cancers.
Musculoskeletal	
INSPECT	
+5 muscle strength, full range of motion, no joint deformities	Weakness or joint pain may limit sexual functioning. *Weakness/paralysis:* Neurosyphilis. *Charcot joints:* Late syphilis. *Unexplained fractures or spinal changes (dowager's hump):* Osteoporosis in postmenopausal women.
Neurological	
INSPECT	
No weakness, paralysis	*Weakness and paralysis:* Neurosyphilis
Awake, alert and oriented X 3, memory intact	*Changes in mental status/, psychosis:* Late syphilis.
Affect appropriate	Depression may affect sexual functioning.
Lymphatic/Hematologic	
INSPECT/PALPATE	
No palpable lymph nodes	*Palpable lymph nodes:* May indicate infection. *Inguinal lymph nodes:* Associated with metastatic disease

AREA/SYSTEM	SUBJECTIVE DATA
General	*Ask about:* Changes in energy level Weight changes Fevers
Integumentary	*Ask about:* Changes in hair growth Rashes, lesions
HEENT *Head and Neck*	*Ask about:* Headaches Swollen glands, nodes
Eyes, Mouth, Throat	*Ask about:* Eye drainage Oral lesions Sore throat
Respiratory	*Ask about:* History of respiratory disease
Cardiovascular	*Ask about:* History of cardiovascular disease, HTN, thrombophlebitis, heart murmurs
Gastrointestinal	*Ask about:* History of liver disease Loss of appetite Abdominal pain
Neurological	*Ask about:* History of neurological problems Paralysis Tremors Personality changes Depression
Musculoskeletal	*Ask about:* Weakness/limitations Joint pain, swelling Unexplained fracture
Endocrine	*Ask about:* History of diabetes and thyroid disease
Lymphatic/ Hematologic	*Ask about:* History of malignancies, HIV, AIDS Abnormal menses

AREA/SYSTEM	OBJECTIVE DATA
General	*Measure:* Height and weight Vital signs, checking for temperature elevations, HTN *Inspect:* Signs of discomfort Affect
Integumentary	*Inspect:* Skin lesions Hair distribution
HEENT *Head and Neck*	*Palpate:* Lymph node enlargement Thyroid enlargement
Eyes and Mouth	*Inspect:* Oral mucosa for redness and lesions Conjunctiva for drainage
Respiratory	*Inspect:* Signs of respiratory distress *Auscultate:* Abnormal breath sounds
Cardiovascular	*Inspect:* Signs of impaired circulation Skin changes *Palpate:* Pulses, edema, Homan's sign *Auscultate:* Extra heart sounds
Gastrointestinal	*Inspect:* Ascites *Palpate/percuss:* Liver enlargement Masses
Musculoskeletal	*Test:* Muscle strength *Inspect:* Joint swelling and deformity Spinal deformities
Neurological	*Test:* Changes in mental status and affect Sensory deficits
Endocrine	*Palpate:* Thyroid
Lymphatic/ Hematologic	*Palpate:* Lymph nodes

Assessment of Female GU System's Relationship to Other Systems

Case Study Findings

Before you proceed to a focused GU assessment, document what you learned from your general survey and head-to-toe assessment of Mrs. James.

Mrs. James's physical assessment findings include:

- **General Health Survey:** Well-developed 29-year-old African-American female in no acute distress.
- **Vital Signs:** Temperature 98.8°F; Pulse 80 BPM, strong and regular; Respirations 12/min, regular and unlabored; BP 122/76; Height 5'5"; Weight 122 lb.
- **Integumentary:** No skin color changes or lesions. Hair evenly distributed with no hirsutism.
- **HEENT:** Mouth: Mucous membranes pink with no lesions. Eyes: Conjunctiva pink with no pallor. Neck: Thyroid nonpalpable.
- **Respiratory:** Lungs clear.
- **Cardiovascular:** Heart regular rate and rhythm, no murmurs.
- **Breasts:** No lumps, masses, or discharge.
- **Gastrointestinal:** Abdomen soft and nontender, no hepatomegaly, no ascites.
- **Musculoskeletal:** Full ROM, no joint deformities, normal spinal curves, no loss of height.
- **Neurological:** Affect appropriate, no neurological deficits.
- **Lymphatic/Hematologic:** No palpable lymph nodes.

Positioning the Woman

Unfortunately, the GU assessment requires uncomfortable positioning for the client. The lithotomy position is preferred, but if a woman is unable to assume this position, it can be modified or a sidelying Sims' position can be used instead. Before performing the assessment, do the following:

- Drape the woman's torso and thighs while she is sitting.
- Help her into the lithotomy position with her heels in the stirrups. This abducts the legs and flexes the hips.
- Help her move her buttocks down to the end of the examination table until they are flush with the edge of the table.
- Readjust the drape to cover her as much as possible.
- Adjust the stirrups until she feels comfortable.
- Sit on a stool at the foot of the examination table facing the woman's external genitalia.
- Adjust the lighting source.
- Touch the inside of the woman's thigh before you touch her vulva. This helps her get used to your touch.

ALERT

Change gloves as needed during the examination to prevent cross-contamination.

HELPFUL HINT

Culture any abnormal discharge.

Performing a Focused Physical Assessment

Assessment of the female GU system consists of inspection and palpation, first of the external genitalia and then of the internal genitalia.

Assessing the External Genitalia

Inspection

Take note of hair pattern and distribution. With gloved hand, separate the pubic hair, checking for skin condition and the presence of lesions, discharge, or parasites. If discharge is present, obtain a specimen for culture. Sometimes a complete examination is not needed. In this case, if you are caring for a client in the home or hospital, examine her external genitals while you bathe her.

The color and odor of the discharge may suggest a specific organism. For example, frothy, malodorous, watery, green or gray discharge is associated with *Trichomonas* or ***Haemophilus*** organisms; purulent green-yellow discharge may indicate gonorrhea; heavy gray-white discharge is a sign of ***Chlamydia trachomatis***; and a cheesy discharge signals candidiasis.

Inspecting the External Genitalia

AREA/NORMAL VARIATIONS	ABNORMAL FINDINGS/RATIONALE
Hair Distribution	
Shaped like inverse triangle. May be some growth on abdomen and upper inner thighs. A diamond-shaped pattern from the umbilicus may be caused by cultural or familial differences.	Diamond-shaped pattern not associated with cultural or familial differences is abnormal and may be hirsutism, which indicates endocrine disorder.

(Continued)

Inspecting the External Genitalia *(Continued)*

AREA/NORMAL VARIATIONS

Hair Distribution *(Continued)*

No parasites should be present.

ABNORMAL FINDINGS/RATIONALE

Pubic lice, nits, or flecks of residual blood on skin is abnormal. Pediculosis pubis (pubic lice) is an infestation of hairy regions of body. It usually occurs in the pubic area, but may involve hair on the abdomen, chest, and axillae. Nits are minute white louse eggs that attach close to the pubic hair shaft.

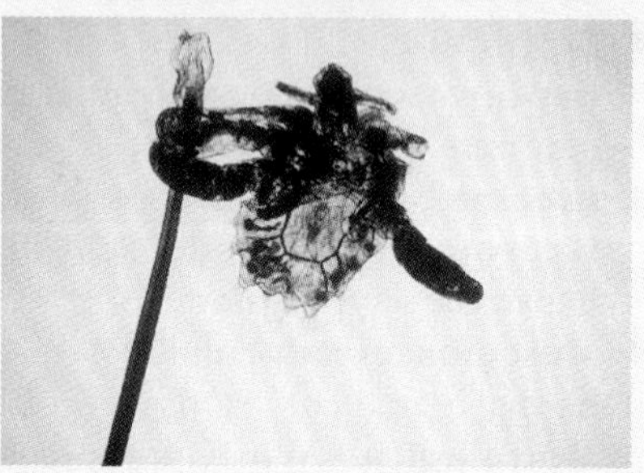

Pubic lice

Skin

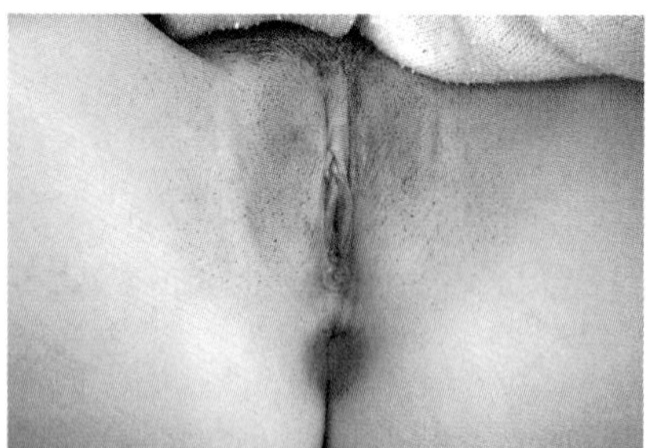

Inspecting skin

Skin over mons pubis is clear except for nevi and normal hair distribution. Labia majora and minora are symmetrical with smooth to moderately wrinkled, slightly pigmented skin without ecchymosis, excoriation, nodules, edema, rash, or lesions.

Ecchymosis: May be caused by blunt trauma.

Labial varicosities: Pregnancy or uterine tumor.

Edema: Hematoma formation, obstruction of lymphatic system, or Bartholin's cyst.

Broken areas of skin: Ulcerations or abrasions caused by infection or trauma.

Rash over mons pubis and labia is abnormal.

Chancre: Primary syphilis. Painless, reddish, round ulcer with depressed center and indurated edges. Lasts for 4 weeks and then disappears without leaving a scar.

Condylomata acuminatum (venereal warts): Caused by human papilloma virus (HPV). White, dry, painless growths with narrow bases.

Herpes simplex: Small, red, painful vesicles that progress to ulcer stage. Pruritus may be present.

Inspecting the External Genitalia

AREA/NORMAL VARIATIONS	ABNORMAL FINDINGS/RATIONALE

Skin *(Continued)*

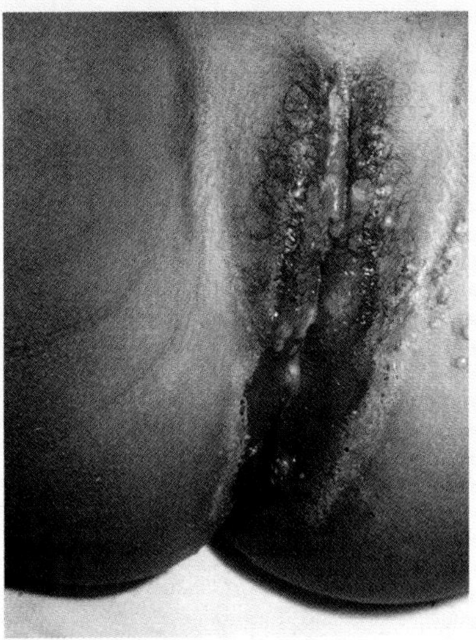

Herpes vulvovaginitis

Clitoris

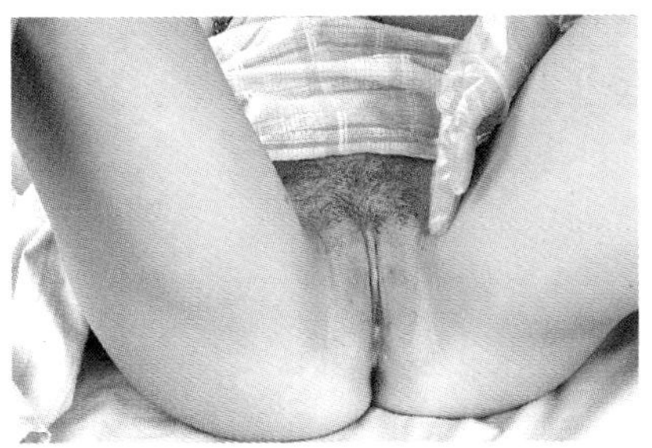

Touching inside of thigh

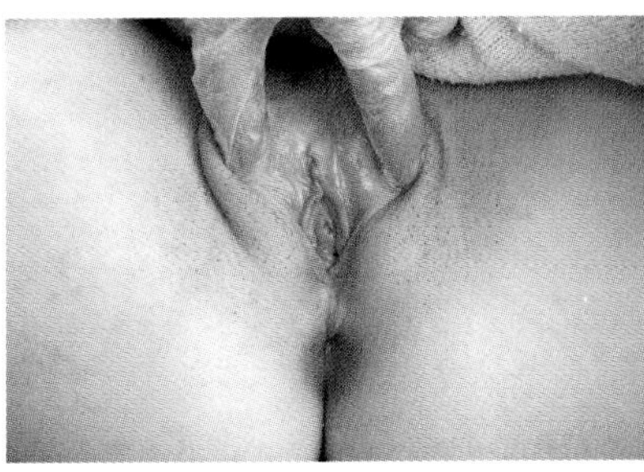

Using thumb and index finger to separate labia minora and expose clitoris

Clitoris should be about 2 cm long and 0.5 cm in diameter.

No redness or lesions.

Hypertrophy of clitoris: May indicate female pseudo-hermaphroditism caused by androgen excess.

Chancroid: Painful ulcer with rough floor and purulent yellow exudate, heals leaving a scar.

Female circumcision is removal of all or part of the clitoris, labia minora, and labia majora, usually in early childhood or early adolescence. This practice is widespread in many African countries and among some Muslim groups.

Urethral Meatus

Use thumb on dominant hand to separate labia minora to expose urethral meatus, which is very sensitive to touch. Observe shape, color and size. Urethral opening should be slitlike, midline, and free of discharge, swelling, redness, or lesions.

Discharge of any color from meatus: May indicate UTI. *Swelling or redness around meatus:* Possible infection of Skene's glands, urethral caruncle, urethral carcinoma, or prolapse of urethral mucosa.

Vaginal Introitus

With labia minora retracted, ask woman to bear down while you observe for patency or bulging.

Introitus mucosa should be pink and moist. Normal vaginal discharge is clear to white and free of foul odors. Some white clumps may be seen that are mass numbers of epithelial cells. Introitus is patent, and there is no bulging or tenderness.

Pale color, dryness: Possible atrophy from topical steroids and aging.

(Continued)

Inspecting the External Genitalia *(Continued)*

AREA/NORMAL VARIATIONS	ABNORMAL FINDINGS/RATIONALE
Vaginal Introitus *(Continued)*	Foul-smelling discharge that is not clear to slightly pale white is abnormal. Gonorrhea, chlamydia, *Candida, Trichomonas,* bacterial vaginosis, atrophic vaginitis, or cervicitis are possible infection processes that produce an abnormal vaginal discharge. *External tear:* May indicate trauma from sexual activity or abuse. *Fissure:* May indicate congenital malformation or childbirth trauma. **Cystocele** is bulging of bladder into anterior vaginal wall. **Cystourethrocele** is bulging of anterior vaginal wall, bladder and urethra into vaginal introitus. **Rectocele** is bulging of rectal wall into posterior vaginal wall.
Perineum and Anus 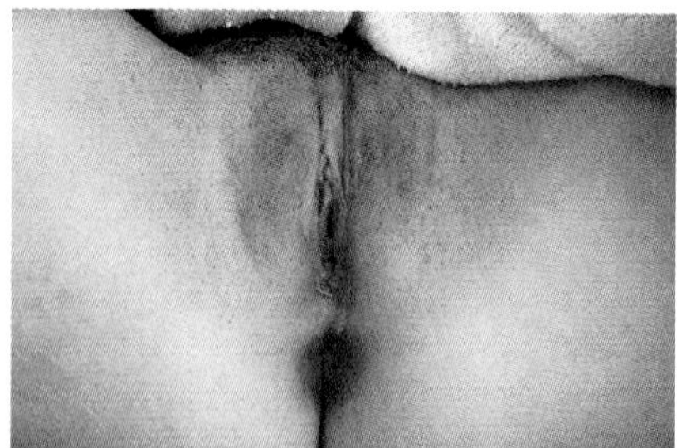 **Inspecting perineum and anus** Perineum is smooth and slightly darkened. A well-healed episiotomy scar is normal after vaginal delivery. Anus is dark pink to brown and puckered. Skin tags are common around anal area.	*Fissure or tear of perineum:* May be caused by trauma, abscess, or unhealed episiotomy. *Venous prominences in anal area:* May indicate external hemorrhoids.

Palpation

Gently palpate the external genitalia, noting any masses, nodules, discharge, or areas of tenderness. Be alert for vertical and horizontal lymph node enlargement that may indicate an infection, malignancy, or other systemic problem.

Assessing the Internal Genitalia

Next, perform the internal examination. It includes the speculum examination and specimen collection and bimanual palpation of the internal structures.

Inspection

Select the appropriate size speculum. You should have several sizes and types of sterilized, metal specula on hand. The two most commonly used types are the Graves and the Penderson. The Graves speculum is available in 3 1/2" to 5 1/2" lengths and 3/4" to 1 1/2" widths. It has a spoon-shaped flare at the distal blade ends, which helps you view the cervix and examine multiparous women. The narrow, flat Penderson speculum is used for children, women who have never been sexually active, nulliparous women, and some postmenopausal women.

Different-sized plastic specula are also available. Some of them make a loud clicking noise when the blades are opened, so be sure to warn your client before the examination. Plastic specula may be more difficult to insert into the vagina. Be very careful with insertion. Surface tension factors and rough edges on some low-cost brands may also tear the vaginal mucous membrane lining.

Palpating the External Genitalia

AREA/NORMAL VARIATIONS	ABNORMAL FINDINGS/RATIONALE
Labia 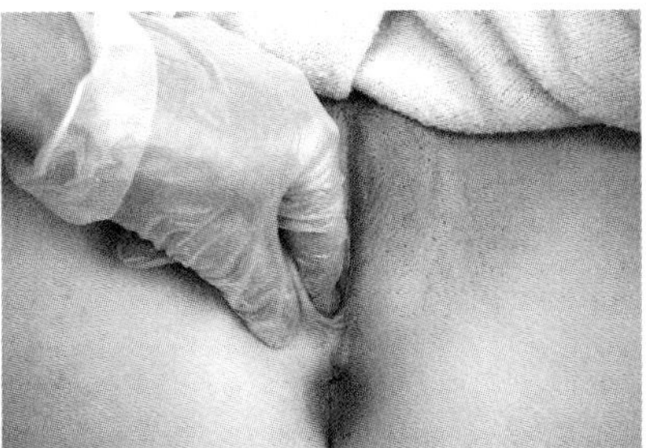 **Palpating Bartholin's glands** Palpate each labium between thumb and index finger of your dominant hand. Labia should be soft and uniform in structure with no swelling, pain, induration, or purulent discharge.	*Swelling, redness, induration, or purulent discharge from labial folds with hot, tender areas:* May indicate Bartholin's gland infection caused by gonococci or *Chlamydia trachomatis*
Urethral Meatus and Skene's Glands 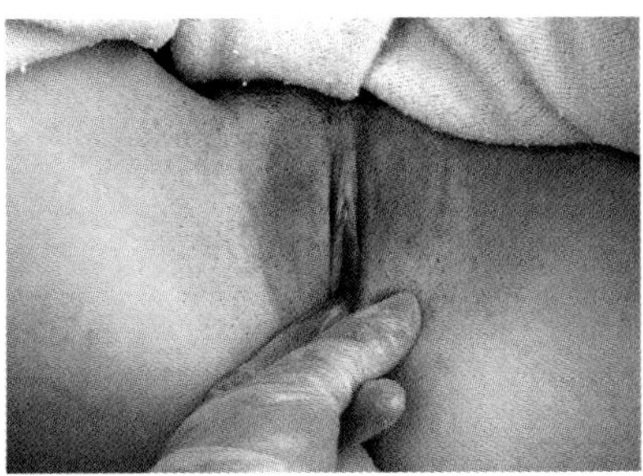 **Palpating Skene's glands and milking urethra** Insert index finger of your dominant hand into vagina and apply pressure to anterior aspect of vaginal wall to milk urethra. Swab any discharge with cotton-tipped applicator for microscopic exam. Milking urethra should not cause pain or result in any urethral discharge.	*Pain and discharge:* May indicate Skene's gland infection or UTI.
Vaginal Introitus Keep your finger in the vagina and ask the woman to squeeze the vaginal muscles around it. Vaginal muscle tone should be tight and strong in nulliparous women and diminished in parous women.	*Significantly diminished/absent muscle tone:* May result from injury, age, childbirth, or medication. *Bulging from vagina:* Cystocele, rectocele, or uterine prolapse.
Perineum Partially remove your finger from the introitus until it is posterior to the perineum, with your thumb anterior to the perineum. Assess tone and texture. Perineum should be smooth, firm, and homogenous in nulliparous women and thinner in parous women.	*Thin perineum, fissures, tears:* May indicate atrophy, trauma or an unhealed episiotomy.

ALERT

Before insertion, lubricate the speculum with warm water. Commercial lubricants may interfere with the accuracy of the cytological samples and cultures.

To perform the examination, hold the speculum in your dominant hand with the blades closed. Rest your index finger at the proximal end of the superior blade. Wrap your other fingers around the handle with your thumb over the thumbscrew. Insert your dominant index and middle fingers ventral sides down just inside the vagina and apply pressure to the posterior vaginal wall to help the perineal muscles relax. If the woman is tense, instruct her to take deep breaths. When you feel the muscles relax, insert the speculum at an oblique angle. After withdrawing your finger, gently rotate the speculum to a horizontal angle and advance it at a 45-degree downward angle against the posterior vaginal wall. Using your dominant thumb, depress the lever to open the blades and visualize the cervix. If you cannot see the cervix, close the blades and pull the speculum back 2 to 3 cm and reinsert it at a different angle. Once the cervix is visualized, lock the speculum blades into place. Adjust the light source. If any discharge obstructs the cervix, use an OB swab to clear the cervix. Inspect the cervix and os for color, position, size, surface, discharge and shape.

HELPFUL HINTS

- Avoid pinching the labia or pulling the woman's pubic hair while inserting the speculum. If insertion causes undue pain, stop and evaluate your speculum position.
- If the woman seems tense or anxious, suggest that she take deep breaths during the examination.

Collecting Specimens

Collect specimens (smears and cultures) after inspecting the cervix and cervical os. Collect the Pap smear first, using three different slides or one slide for all three smears.

Speculum Examination of the Internal Genitalia

AREA/NORMAL VARIATIONS	ABNORMAL FINDINGS/RATIONALE
Cervix 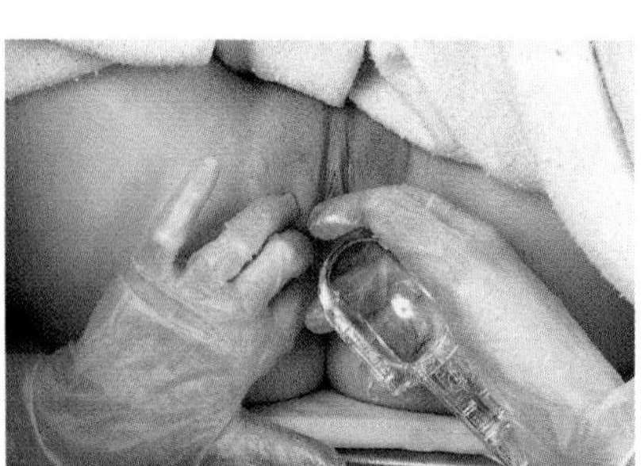 **Inserting speculum** 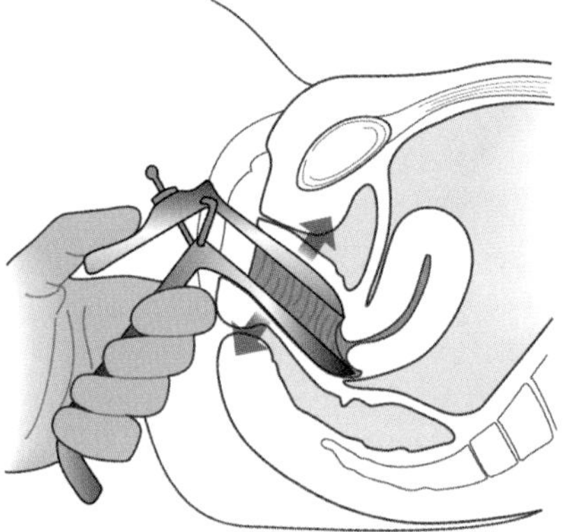 **Proper position of speculum in vagina** 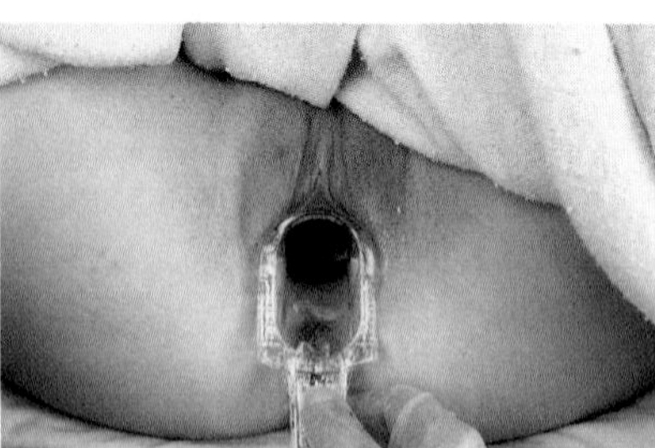 **Opening speculum** 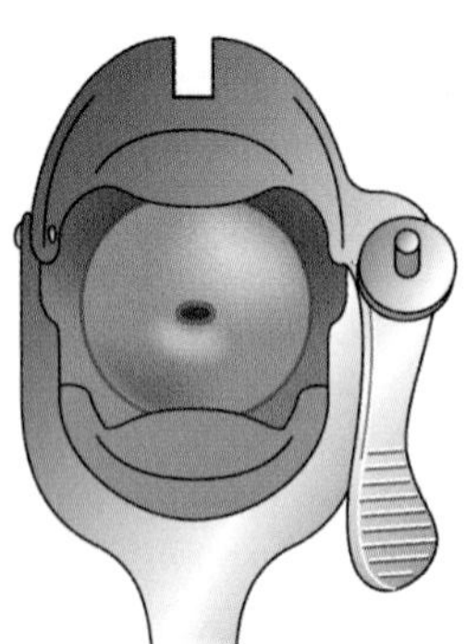 **View through speculum** Cervix is glistening pink; may be pale pink after menopause or blue (Chadwick's sign) during pregnancy.	*Cyanosis without pregnancy:* Venous congestion or systemic hypoxia as in CHF. *Redness or friable appearance:* Infection and inflammation, such as in chlamydia or gonorrhea. *Lateral positioning of cervix:* Tumor or adhesions. *Projection of cervix into vaginal vault greater than 2.5 cm:* Uterine prolapse. *Cervical size greater than 4 cm:* Hypertrophy caused by inflammation or tumor. Reddish circle around os may be abnormal. *Ectropion or eversion:* Occurs when squamocolumnar junction appears on ectocervix. Can result from lacerations during childbirth or be congenital variation. ***Nabothian cysts:*** Small, round, yellow, benign lesions from obstruction of cervical glands. ***Polyps:*** Bright-red, soft protrusions through cervical os. *Hemorrhages over cervical surface (strawberry spots):* Associated with trichomonal infection. *Unilateral transverse, bilateral transverse, stellate, or irregular*

Speculum Examination of the Internal Genitalia

AREA/NORMAL VARIATIONS	ABNORMAL FINDINGS/RATIONALE
Cervix *(Continued)*	*cervical os:* Caused by cervical tears occurring during rapid, second-stage childbirth delivery or forceps delivery, or from trauma.
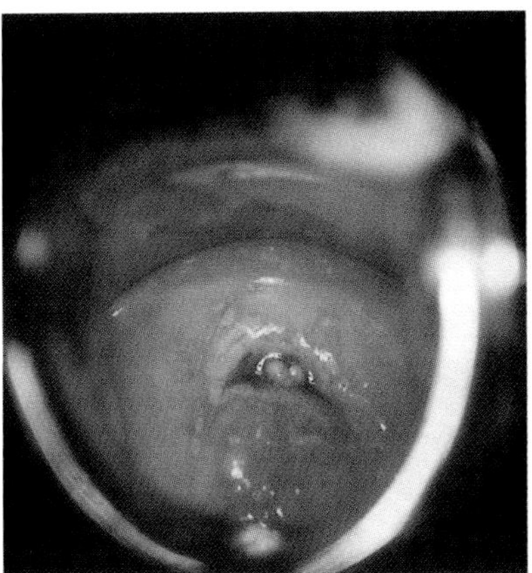 **Chadwick's sign**	*Greenish-yellow, mucopurulent discharge that adheres to vaginal walls, pus in os:* Gonococcal infection. *White, cottage cheeselike discharge that adheres to vaginal walls, with patches on os: Candida* infection. *Red spots on cervix; grayish-yellow, purulent, often bubbly discharge that smells fishy and often pools in fornix: Trichomonas.*
No lesions. Located midline in vagina with anterior or posterior position relative to vaginal vault. Size is about 2.5 cm. Normal discharge is white. No odor.	
Nulliparous woman has small round or oval os. In parous woman, os is a horizontal slit.	

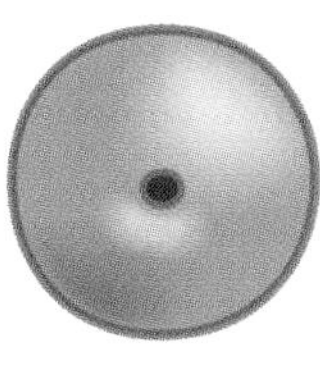

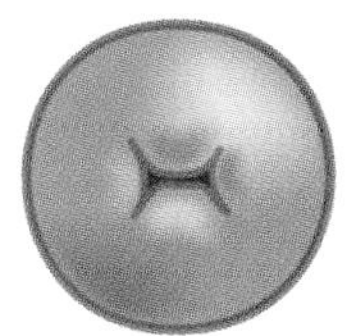

A B

a. Nulliparous cervical os; b: Parous cervical os

The Pap smear is a collection of three specimens taken from the endocervix, the cervix, and the vaginal pool. The purpose is to evaluate cervicovaginal cells for pathology that might indicate cancer. All women over age 18 or any woman who is sexually active should have an annual Pap screening.

Endocervical Smear

Using your dominant hand, insert a cotton-tipped swab, cytobrush, or the longer, serrated end of an Ayre spatula through the speculum into the cervical os about 1 cm. Rotate the instrument between your index finger and thumb, first 360 degrees clockwise and then counterclockwise. Keep the instrument in contact with the cervical tissue. If you use a swab, leave it in the cervical os for 30 seconds to ensure saturation. Remove the instrument and spread the cells in a rolling motion on the slide. If you are putting all three smears on one slide, spread the cells on one-third of the slide only. (Some cells are marked *E* to show you where to spread the cells.) Do not press down hard or wipe the instrument back and forth because this will destroy the cells. Discard the instrument after use.

Cervical Smear

Insert the bifurcated end of the Ayre spatula through the speculum base. Place the longer end of the spatula into the cervical os and put the shorter part snug against the cervix. Rotate the spatula 360 degrees one time only. Remove the spatula and gently spread the specimen on

Collecting Specimens for Culture

TEST/NORMAL VARIATIONS	ABNORMAL FINDINGS/RATIONALE
Pap Smear *Endocervical Smear* *Cervical Smear* *Vaginal Pool Smear* 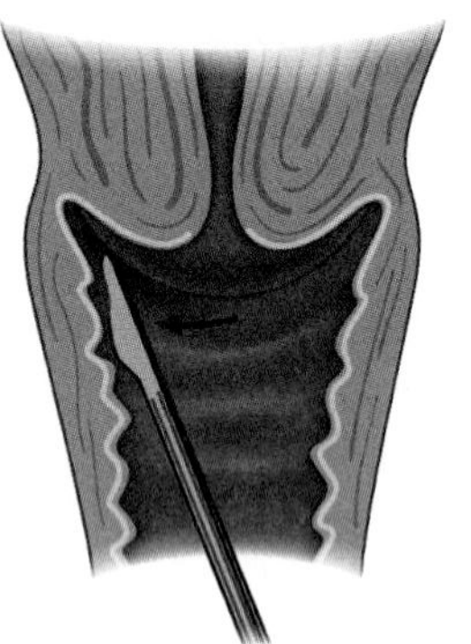 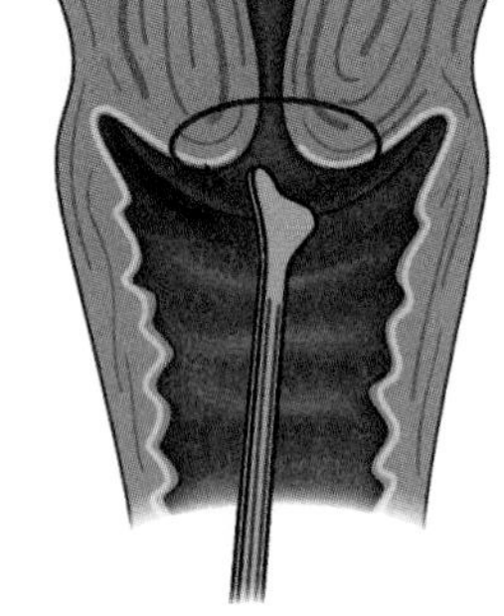 **Taking an endocervical smear** **Taking a cervical smear** Cytology report says "within normal limits" using Bethesda system. This denotes a lack of pathogenesis.	*"Benign cellular changes" on report:* May be caused by fungal, bacterial, protozoan, or viral infections. *"Atypical squamous cells" on report:* Causes include inflammatory or infectious processes, a preliminary lesion, or an unknown cause. *Epithelial cell abnormalities on report:* May indicate squamous intraepithelial lesion, squamous cell carcinoma or glandular cell abnormalities often seen in postmenopausal women not on hormone replacement therapy.
Gonococcal Smear Cervicovaginal tissues are normally free of *Neisseria gonorrhoeae.*	It is abnormal to have a large number of gram-negative diplococci present.
Saline Mount (Wet Prep) Fewer than 10 WBCs per field. No protozoa or other organisms.	*Large number of WBCs (inflammatory response): Chlamydia* or a bacterial infection. Protozoa are indicative of trichomoniasis.
KOH Prep Cervicovaginal tissues are free of *Candida albicans.*	*Presence of yeast or pseudohyphae (chains of budding yeast):* Indicates *Candida* infection.
Acetic Acid Wash No change in appearance of cervix.	*Rapid acetowhitening or blanching:* May indicate presence of human papillomavirus (HPV), causative agent of genital warts.
Anal Culture Anal tissues are free of *Neisseria gonorrhoeae.*	*Large number of gram-negative diplococci:* Indicates *Neisseria gonorrhoeae.*

another slide or on the second third of the same slide (may be marked *C*).

Vaginal Pool Smear

Reverse the Ayre spatula and place the rounded end into the posterior vaginal fornix. Gently scrape the area. You may also use a cotton-tipped applicator. Remove and gently spread the specimen on a separate slide or on the last one-third of the slide (may be marked *V*). Dispose of the spatula. Spray the entire slide (or slides) with cytological fixative within 1 minute and send to the laboratory. Slides and fixatives are not needed if you use the Thin Prep Pap Test.

Other Smears

Next, collect other smears, if needed:

- *Gonococcal Smear:* Insert a sterile cotton swab 1 cm into the cervical os. Hold the applicator in place 20 to 30 seconds. Remove the swab and roll it on a Thayer-Martin culture plate in a Z pattern. Rotate the swab as you roll it to ensure that all of the specimen is used.
- *Saline Mount (Wet Prep):* Spread a sample of the cervical or vaginal pool specimen onto a microscope slide, add one drop of normal saline solution, and apply a cover slip.
- *KOH Prep* (rapid test for *Candida*): Spread a sample of the cervical or vaginal pool specimen onto a microscope slide, add one drop of potassium hydroxide (KOH), and apply cover slip.
- *Acetic Acid Wash:* After all other specimens have been collected, swab the cervix with a 5% acetic acid solution.
- *Anal Culture:* Insert a sterile cotton swab 1 cm into the anal canal and hold in place for 20 to 30 seconds. Remove the swab. Discard the applicator if fecal material is collected and restart. Roll the swab in a Z pattern on a Thayer-Martin culture plate. Dispose of the swab.

Inspecting the Vaginal Wall

Once you have obtained the specimens, inspect the vaginal wall for color, texture, and lesions as you withdraw the speculum. To remove the speculum, disengage the locking device and slowly withdraw the speculum without closing the blades. Rotate the speculum into an oblique position as you remove it.

Palpation

Bimanual technique is used to assess the internal genitalia. Explain the assessment to the woman. As you perform the examination, observe her face for signs of discomfort. Apply a water-soluble lubricant to the first two fingertips of your dominant hand. As you stand between the woman's legs, place your nondominant hand on her abdomen below the umbilicus. Insert your dominant index and middle fingers into the vagina with your palm up. Advance slowly while palpating the vaginal walls. Keep your thumb abducted and away from the urethral meatus and clitoris. Rotate your wrist so you can palpate all surfaces in the vagina.

Next, keeping your dominant hand in the same position, with your palm up, assess the cervix for consistency, position, shape and tenderness. Move the cervix from side to side to assess mobility. Palpate the fornices with your fingertips, noting nodules or irregularities.

Now, reach under and behind the cervix and lift the uterus toward the abdomen and your external hand as you apply pressure toward the internal fingers. Keep your

Inspecting the Vaginal Wall

AREA/NORMAL VARIATIONS	ABNORMAL FINDINGS/RATIONALE
Vaginal Wall Vaginal wall is pink, moist, deeply rugated, and without lesions or redness. In postmenopausal women, walls may be smooth, shiny, and transparent.	*White spots on vaginal wall:* May be leukoplakia from *Candida albicans*. Repeated occurrences may indicate HIV infection. *Pallor of vaginal walls:* Anemia or menopause. *Redness of vaginal walls:* Inflammation, hyperemia, or trauma from tampon insertion or removal. *Vaginal lesions or masses:* Carcinoma, tumors, and DES exposure.

Bimanual Palpation of the Internal Genitalia

AREA/NORMAL VARIATIONS	ABNORMAL FINDINGS/RATIONALE
Vaginal Wall 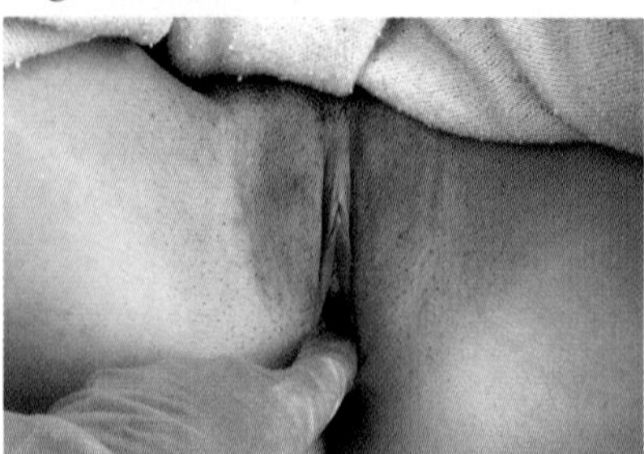 Inserting fingers into the vagina. Nontender, with smooth or rugated surface with no lesions, masses, or cysts.	*Lesions, masses, scarring, or cysts:* May be benign, such as inclusion cysts, myomas, or fibromas; or may be malignant. Most common site for vaginal malignancies is upper one-third of posterior wall
Cervix The cervix is mobile, nontender, smooth and firm, symmetrically round, and in midline, movable 1–2 cm in each direction without discomfort. Softening of cervix (**Goodell's sign**) is seen at fifth to sixth week of pregnancy.	*Pain on palpation or to assess mobility (positive **Chandleier's sign** or cervical motion tenderness):* PID or ectopic pregnancy. Irregular surface, immobility, or nodular surface of cervix is abnormal. Causes may include malignancy, nabothian cysts, or polyps.
Fornices Walls are smooth and without nodules.	*Nodules or irregularities:* Malignancy, polyps, herniations.
Uterus 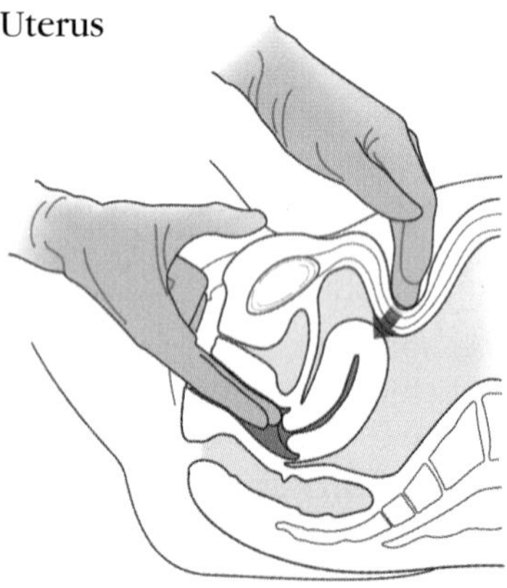 Palpating the uterus. Size varies according to **parity**. Pear shaped in nongravid woman and more rounded in parous woman. Smooth, firm, mobile, nontender and without masses.	*Enlargement/changes in shape:* Enlargement may indicate intrauterine pregnancy or tumor. *Nodules:* May be myomas—tumors containing muscle tissue.
Adnexa 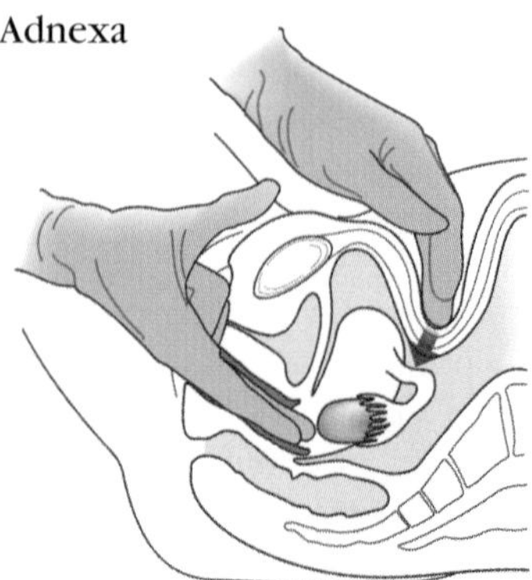 Palpating the ovaries. Ovaries are almond shaped, firm, smooth and mobile without tenderness. Nonpalpable in postmenopausal women.	*Enlarged, irregular, nodular, painful, immobile ovaries:* Ectopic pregnancy, ovarian cyst, PID, malignancy.

wrist straight. Try to grasp the uterus between your hands. Evaluate the uterus for size, shape, consistency, mobility, tenderness, masses, and position. (Note: A retroverted, retroflexed uterus can be assessed only rectovaginally.)

After assessing the uterus, palpate the fallopian tubes and ovaries. Move your intravaginal hand to the right lateral fornix, and move your external hand to the right lower quadrant of the abdomen. Push your external hand inward and downward while pushing your intravaginal hand inward and upward. Palpate for size, shape, consistency, and mobility. Repeat on the left side.

Fallopian tubes are rarely palpable. Palpation of the ovaries depends on the woman's age and size. The ovaries may be tender during palpation if the woman is in the luteal phase of the menstrual cycle.

Rectovaginal Examination

After completing the bimanual internal genitalia examination, remove your dominant hand from the vagina and change gloves. Apply lubricant to the fingertips of your dominant hand. Explain the procedure to the woman. Ask her to strain downward while you assess anal sphincter tone. To do this, insert your dominant index finger back into the vagina, and insert your middle finger into the rectum. Advance the rectal finger forward as you depress the abdomen with your nondominant hand. Assess the cervix, uterus, and rectovaginal septum for patency. Withdraw your fingers. If there is stool on your glove, you may test it for occult blood at this time.

Rectovaginal Examination

AREA/NORMAL VARIATIONS

Rectum, Anal Sphincter, Rectovaginal Septum

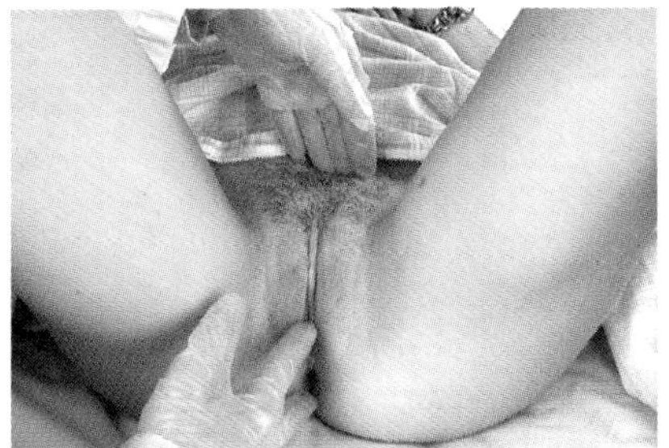

Performing rectovaginal exam

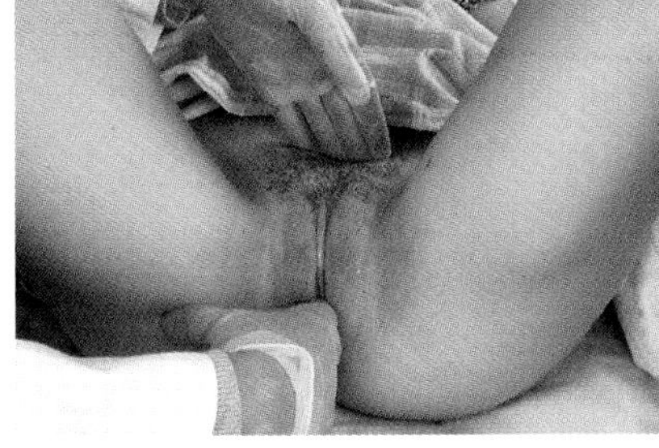

Inserting fingers for rectovaginal exam

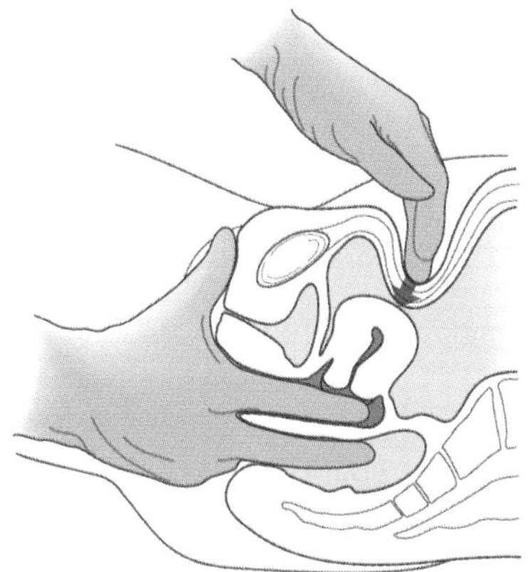

Proper position of hands

Rectal walls are smooth and free of lesions. Rectovaginal septum is patent. Rectal pouch is rugated and free of masses.

Anal sphincter tone is strong. Cervix and uterus are smooth.

Test any stool for occult blood. Test should be negative.

ABNORMAL FINDINGS/RATIONALE

Masses or lesions: Consider malignancy or internal hemorrhoids.

Anal sphincter tone is strong. Cervix and uterus are smooth.

Lax sphincter tone: Perineal trauma from childbirth, anal intercourse, or neurological disorders.

Stool test positive for occult blood: Warrants further investigation.

Case Study Findings

Mrs. James's focused physical assessment findings include:

- Appropriate pubic hair distribution for age.
- External genitalia pink and moist with no varicosities, lesions, organisms, edema, or abnormal discharge.
- Small amount of white, odorless discharge.
- No swelling, tenderness, or discharge on palpation of Bartholin's glands and Skene's glands.
- No masses, lesions, or anatomical deviations of vulva and perineum. Skin intact, smooth.
- Cervix smooth, moist, shiny pink, 2 to 3 cm in diameter at midline, firm, nontender, and midplane.
- No lesions, nodules, masses, discharge, or bleeding. Vaginal walls are pink, moist, rugose, and without lesions, swelling, or masses.
- Concentric rugae around vaginal wall, no nodules or tenderness.
- Uterus is appropriate size for age and condition. Firm, pear shaped, symmetrical, slightly mobile, and anteverted. No masses or tenderness.
- Ovaries and fallopian tubes are nonpalpable, nontender.
- No hemorrhoids, painful areas, masses or nodules in rectum.

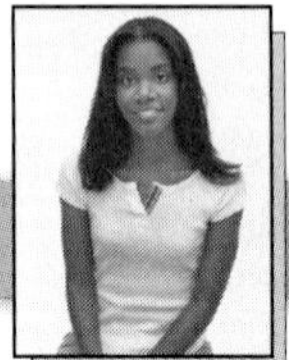

Case Study Analysis and Plan

Now that your examination of Mrs. James is complete, document your key history and key physical examination findings. List key history findings and key physical assessment findings that will help you formulate your nursing diagnoses.

 CRITICAL THINKING ACTIVITY #2

Consider the subjective information that you have obtained from Mrs. James. What other historical information should you focus on?

Nursing Diagnoses

Consider all of the data you have collected during your assessment of Mrs. James, then use this information to identify appropriate nursing diagnoses. Here are some possible ones. Cluster the supporting data.

1. **Knowledge, deficient, related to adverse effects of oral contraceptives**
2. **Potential disturbance in reproductive health related to abnormal vaginal bleeding**

Identify any additional nursing diagnoses.
Identify any collaborative nursing diagnoses.

 CRITICAL THINKING ACTIVITY #3:

Develop a nursing care plan and a brief teaching plan for Mrs. James including learning outcomes and teaching strategies, using one of these nursing diagnoses.

Research Tells Us

Deaths attributed to uterine and cervical cancers have declined by more than 50 percent since the 1960s. The decline in morbidity and mortality rates is attributed to the development of the Papanicolaou (Pap) test and increased public knowledge of routine screening techniques. Early detection is also a factor. Invasive cancer is still diagnosed in 16,000 women annually and kills 5000 each year. The importance of regular cancer screenings and client teaching cannot be overemphasized. Almost 80 percent of cervical cancers show evidence of HPV, although not all cases of HPV develop into cervical cancer (Harlan, 1991). According to the Centers for Disease Control and Prevention, HPV is one of the most prevalent STDs in the United States, infecting 5.5 million annually (MMWR, 1998). National Cancer Institute statistics show endometrial cancer constituting 13 percent of all cancers in women, with 35,000 new cases diagnosed annually. Ovarian cancer is the most prevalent cancer in women aged 40 to 70 years. It is diagnosed in 26,000 women annually in the United States and kills 14,000 each year.

Health Concerns

Risk Factors for Female Genital Cancers:

- ***Cervical Cancer***
  - Early age at first intercourse
  - Multiple sex partners
  - Previous history of HPV
  - Tobacco use
  - Positive family history
- ***Endometrial Cancer***
  - History of infertility
  - Failure to ovulate
  - Unopposed estrogen therapy
  - Use of tamoxifen
  - Obesity
  - Positive family history
- ***Ovarian Cancer***
  - Advanced age
  - Nulliparity
  - History of breast cancer
  - Positive family history
- ***Vaginal Cancer***
  - Mother who took DES during pregnancy

Warning Signs of Reproductive Organ Cancer:

- Abnormal vaginal bleeding and vaginal discharge
- Persistent aching pelvic or lower back pain
- Postmenopausal bleeding
- Abdominal pain
- Abnormal Pap smear

Risk Factors for AIDS:

- Sex with partner who engaged in homosexual activity
- History of multiple sex partners or having a partner with a history of multiple partners, especially without using condoms
- Intravenous drug use, sharing needles
- Male partner who had contacts with prostitutes, especially without using condoms
- Frequent or multiple blood transfusions

Risk Factors for Major STDs:

- Being young and sexually active (age 15 to 30)
- History of multiple sexual partners
- Early onset of sexual activity
- Previous STD
- Urban dweller
- Low income
- Unmarried

Common Abnormalities

ABNORMALITY	ASSESSMENT FINDINGS
Bacterial Vaginosis Inflammation of the vagina caused by one or more bacteria or bacteria-like organisms	• Minimal vulvar pruritus. • Yellowish-white vaginal discharge. • Occasional foul odor to discharge. • Wet mount shows WBCs and/or clue cells.
Chlamydia A sexually transmitted bacterial infection that can compromise reproductive health	• Women are often asymptomatic. • Genital symptoms: Increase in clear to white vaginal discharge, dysuria, and postcoital bleeding. • Abdominal symptoms: Increase in menstrual cramping and pelvic pain. • Dysmenorrhea **(menstrual cramping)** • Cramping or aching in lower abdomen midline • Aching in lower back • Mild tenderness on pelvic and abdominal examination bilaterally • No fever • Past history of dysmenorrhea
Endometrial Cancer Malignancy or the endometrium	• Menopausal age • History of previous estrogen therapy, nulliparity, obesity, possible diabetes or hypertension • Previous curettage, sterility, or poor fertility

(Continued)

Common Abnormalities *(Continued)*

ABNORMALITY	ASSESSMENT FINDINGS
Endometrial Cancer *(Continued)*	• Red or brown vaginal discharge or abnormal uterine bleeding, spotting for days to months • Uterine or adnexal mass, usually nontender, detected on palpation • Cervical lesion • Pain in later invasive stage
Endometriosis Inflammation of the endometrium	• Age 25 to 45 • Excessive, prolonged uterine bleeding • Menstrual pain referred to rectum and lower sacrum • Pain on defecation • Dysuria • Constipation • History of menstrual disturbances • Multiple tender nodules palpable along the uterosacral ligaments or in the rectovaginal septum • Pain on palpation of uterus
Functional Ovarian Cysts May be follicle cysts or corpus luteum cysts	• Age 20 to 40 • Mild pelvic discomfort, low back pain, or dyspareunia • Localized pain and tenderness • Abnormal uterine bleeding • Menstrual irregularities • Delayed menstruation followed by persistent bleeding • Cysts detected on bimanual palpation
Genital Herpes Viral STD	• Age teens or early 30s • Watery discharge with lesions or sores and blisters on external genitalia • Mild itching and pain • Recent urinary tract or gynecologic examination • Frequent intercourse without male partner using condom • Fever • Enlarged inguinal lymph nodes • Yellow-gray film on cervix
Monilial vaginitis (yeast infection) Fungal infection causing vaginal inflammatory process associated with the *Candida* organism	• Intense vulvar itching and/or burning. • Vulvar swelling and excoriation. • No vaginal bleeding. • Cheesy or curdlike vaginal discharge often present in labial folds. • Monilial rash may spread to upper thighs. • Wet mount shows yeast or pseudohyphae (chains of budding yeast).
Ovarian Carcinoma Malignancy of ovaries	• Early-stage menopause or postmenopause • History of urinary frequency and constipation • Abdominal pain in later stage • Lower abdominal mass • Possible ascites • Irregular postmenopausal bleeding (possible but infrequent) • Displaced cervix • Solid, bilateral ovarian mass on bimanual palpation
Urinary Tract Infection Inflammation of bladder, urethra, ureters, or kidneys.	• Suprapubic tenderness on palpation. • Low back discomfort occasionally.

Common Abnormalities

ABNORMALITY	ASSESSMENT FINDINGS
Urinary Tract Infection *(Continued)*	
Most common invading organism is *Escherichia coli.*	• Possible costovertebral angle tenderness.
Sexual intercourse may contaminate urethra with bacteria.	• No vaginal or urethral discharge.
Afebrile or low-grade temperature below 101°F.	• Bladder symptoms: Dysuria, hematuria, nocturia, and urinary frequency.

Summary

- The female reproductive system is an area where you can have a major impact on your client's health through routine screening and education.
- A thorough assessment relies on health history data, physical assessment findings, and laboratory results. It requires an understanding of normal anatomy and physiology for various age groups, good interviewing and communication skills, skill in inspecting and palpating, and expertise in the use of equipment such as the vaginal speculum.
- The assessment also requires sensitivity in responding to the woman's need for privacy and in respecting her personal boundaries.

17

Assessing The Male Genitourinary System

Before You Begin

INTRODUCTION TO THE MALE GENITOURINARY SYSTEM

Assessing the genitourinary (GU) system is essential to obtain a picture of your male client's overall health status. Assessment includes both the male reproductive system and the urinary system. The male reproductive system is anatomically divided into external and internal genital organs. The penis and scrotum are external organs and are easily inspected and palpated, whereas the internal structures have limited accessibility.

The kidneys, ureters, bladder, and urethra make up the urinary system. Because these structures are distributed among the retroperitoneal space, abdomen and genitals, examination of the urinary system is also incorporated into other areas of a total physical assessment. For example, you examine the kidneys during your assessment of the posterior thorax, back, and abdomen.

Your assessment should focus on detecting acute health problems, identifying risks for genitourinary problems, and pinpointing health promotion teaching needs. Be alert for sexual and reproductive problems. Sexually transmitted diseases (STDs) are the most common communicable diseases in the United States. Early detection is critical because untreated STDs can have permanent, devastating effects. Likewise, structural or functional problems in the urinary system can be devastating. Because this system is vital in waste removal and acid-base balance, malfunctions can affect homeostasis and even be life-threatening.

As you read this chapter, remember that the GU system affects and is affected by every other body system, having far-reaching effects on the client's quality of life.

Anatomy and Physiology Review

Before beginning your assessment, you need a clear understanding of the male GU system. Knowing normal functions and structures will enable you to detect those that are abnormal.

Functions of the male genitourinary system include the following:

- Manufacturing and protecting sperm for fertilization
- Transporting sperm
- Regulating hormonal production and secretion of male sex hormones
- Providing sexual pleasure
- Excreting urine

Structures and Functions

The male genitourinary system (Fig. 17–1) includes both internal and external structures. The penis and scrotum are the external genitalia. The internal genitalia includes the **testes, epididymis,** two vas deferens (also called ductus

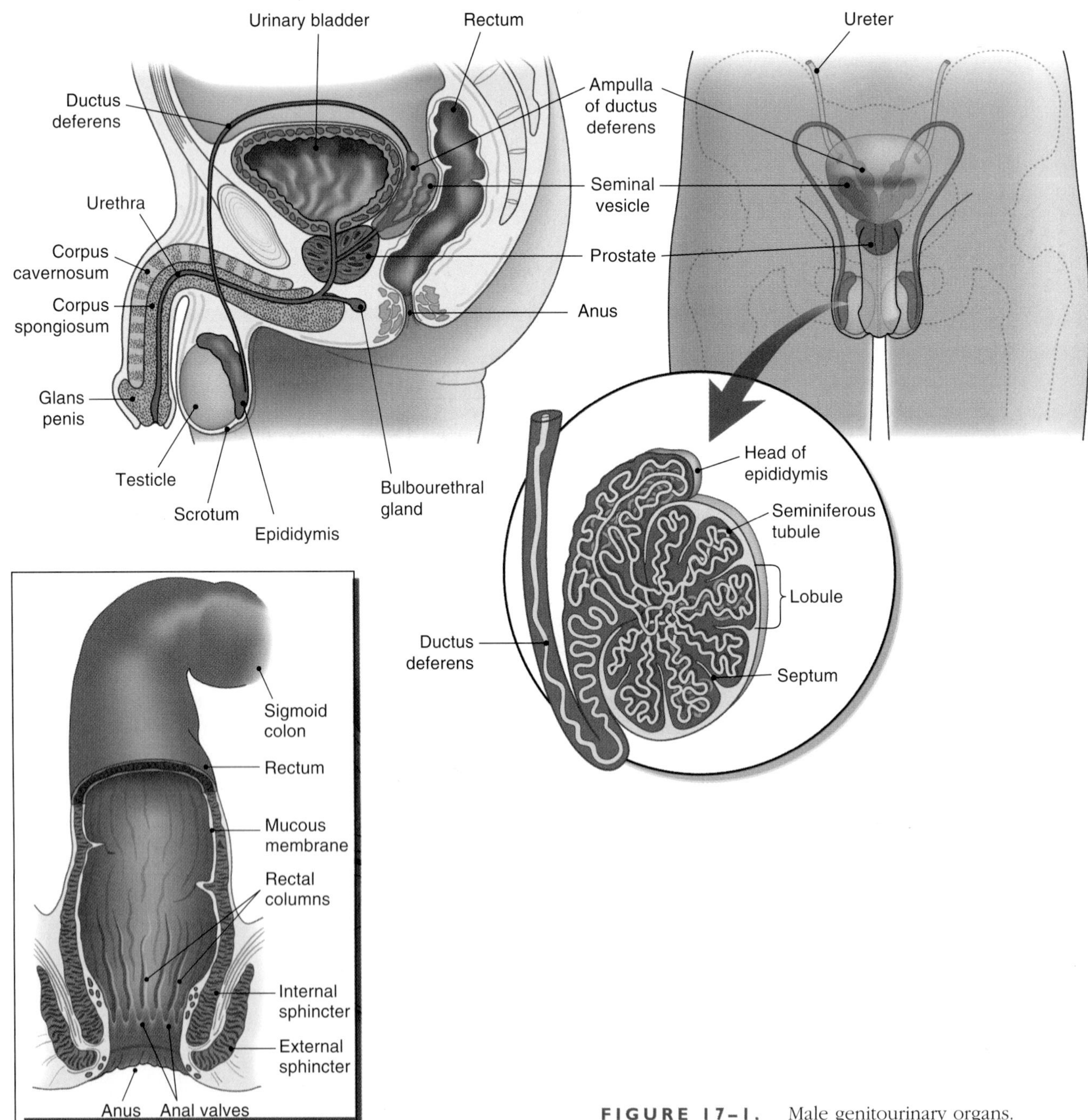

FIGURE 17–1. Male genitourinary organs.

Structures and Functions of the Male Genitourinary System

STRUCTURE	DESCRIPTION/PRIMARY FUNCTION
Scrotum	Loosely hanging pouch behind penis. Has two sacs that contain testes. Protects testes, epididymides, and part of spermatic cord. Also protects sperm production and viability by maintaining an appropriate surface temperature.
Testes	Two essential organs located in scrotum, each approximately 5 cm long by 2.5 cm wide. Each contains tightly coiled seminiferous tubules. Testes are attached to spermatic cord, which allows them to hang vertically in scrotum. Tubules are main component of testes, and they produce sperm by spermatogenesis. Testes secrete some testosterone.
Spermatic Cord	Fibrous connective tissue that forms a protective sheath around vas deferens, nerves, blood vessels, lymphatic structures, and muscle fibers associated with the scrotum.
Seminal Vesicles	Two pouches that are accessory organs, lying posteriorly to and at the base of the bladder. They contribute about 70% of the volume of semen. The fluid is alkaline and rich in fructose, water, and vitamin C and helps provide a source of energy for sperm metabolism. Vesicles also produce prostaglandins, which contribute to sperm motility and viability. The alkaline pH acts to protect the sperm by neutralizing vaginal acidity.
Bulbourethral Glands	Two accessory organs located just below the prostate. Also called Cowper's glands, they secrete an alkaline substance that protects sperm by neutralizing the acidic environment of the vagina. These glands also provide lubrication within the urethra to facilitate ejaculation and at the end of the penis during sexual intercourse.
Prostate Gland	An accessory gland that borders the urethra near the lower part of the bladder. The prostate produces a milky, alkaline solution that flows into the urethra during sexual intercourse. The liquid aids sperm transport and neutralization of the acidic vaginal secretions. The prostate also produces about 20% of all semen.
Epididymis	Tightly coiled tube located on the top and behind the testis inside the scrotum. The primary function of the epididymis is to store sperm till maturity. Sperm mature and develop as they pass through the epididymis to the vas deferens.
Vas Deferens (ductus deferens)	Muscular, tubular structure that stretches from the end of the epididymis to the ejaculatory duct. Mature sperm remain in ampulla, a wide portion of the vas deferens, before ejaculation. Smooth muscle contraction of the vas deferens propels sperm forward into the ejaculatory duct.
Urethra	The terminal end of the urethra transports both urine and semen to the outside of the body. About 6–8 inches long, the urethra passes through the prostate, the wall of the pelvic floor, and the length of the penis.
Urethral Meatus	External meatus of the urethra. Slitlike orifice located on ventral surface just millimeters from the tip of the glans.
Ureters	Hollow tubelike structures connecting the renal pelvis of each kidney with the urinary bladder. They lie within the retroperitoneal space. Ureters propel urine from the renal pelvis into the urinary bladder. Each kidney has a single ureter.
Urinary Bladder	Muscular sac that temporarily stores urine. Located anterior to rectum, directly behind the pubic symphysis.
Penis	Male sex organ that serves as passageway for sperm to exit and be deposited into the vagina during sexual intercourse. Also serves as an exit for urine.
Glans Penis	Tip of penis with many nerve endings. Very sensitive and important in sexual arousal.
Inguinal Canal	Encases vas deferens as it passes from the scrotum through the abdominal muscles into the pelvis. The external inguinal ring, located above and lateral to pubic tubercle, is the opening as the spermatic cord travels through the inguinal canal and exits from the scrotum. The spermatic cord enters the abdomen through the internal ring, located about 1 cm above the midpoint of the inguinal ligament. The inguinal ligament is located midway between the anterior superior iliac spine and the pubic tubercle of the

(Continued)

Structures and Functions of the Male Genitourinary System *(Continued)*

STRUCTURE	DESCRIPTION/PRIMARY FUNCTION
	symphysis pubis. The inguinal canal is located between the two rings. It runs parallel and above the inguinal ligament (Poupart's ligament), which connects the pubic tubercle to anterior superior iliac spine. The femoral canal runs parallel and below the inguinal ligament. Lymph nodes from the penis, scrotal surface, and anus drain into the inguinal lymph nodes. Lymph nodes from the testes drain into perivenacaval nodes in abdomen.

deferens), two seminal vesicles, the ejaculatory duct, the **prostate gland,** and two **bulbourethral (Cowper) glands**. Because of the anatomic location of the prostate gland, access to the prostate for assessment is through digital rectal examination. The urethra (about 8 inches or 20 cm long) serves as a passageway for both urine and ejaculated semen, extending from the urinary bladder to the **urethral meatus** at the tip of the penis.

These structures are further classified as accessory ducts and glands. The vas deferens, ejaculatory duct, and urethra are accessory ducts and the seminal vesicles, prostate gland, and bulbourethral gland are accessory glands. These glands are responsible for producing a secretion that combines with sperm to create **semen**.

The Process of Reproduction

Mechanical Process

Male sexual function consists of four stages: erection, lubrication, emission, and ejaculation. Erection of the penis is achieved through physical and psychogenic stimulation of sensory nerves in the genital area. Parasympathetic impulses from the sacral area of the spinal cord result in vascular dilatation of the arterioles, causing 20 to 50 mL of blood to fill the corpora cavernosa (erectile tissue), thus expanding the penis. The veins from the tissue compress to occlude venous outflow. At the same time, parasympathetic impulses cause the bulbourethral glands to secrete mucus, which provides lubrication during intercourse. Once the sexual stimulus reaches a critical intensity, the reflex centers of the spinal cord send sympathetic impulses to the genital organs, and orgasm occurs. It begins with contraction of the epididymis and the vas deferens, causing expulsion of sperm through the ejaculatory duct and prostate and into the internal urethra. During emission, the bladder neck closes to prevent the flow of semen into the bladder. Ejaculation follows, with contractions of the penile urethra expelling semen from the urethra producing a pleasurable sensation known as an orgasm. Once sexual stimulation ceases and ejaculation occurs, the penile arteries constrict and the penis returns to its flaccid state, called **detumescence.**

Spermatogenesis

Spermatogenesis is the process by which the testes produce sperm. This process begins during puberty, at around age 13, and continues throughout life. Cells in the seminiferous tubules, called interstitial cells of Leydig, secrete the male hormone **testosterone.** Testosterone is responsible for the development of secondary sexual characteristics and reproductive capacity. It is also responsible for male sexual sensation and performance as well as muscle development. Sperm is stored in the epididymis and vas deferens for about 1 month. If it is not ejaculated within that time, the sperm degenerates and is reabsorbed. The normal sperm count is 300 to 500 million sperm with each ejaculation. A man with a sperm count of less than 20 to 30 million per ejaculation is considered infertile, and a man who is unable to produce viable sperm is considered sterile.

Interaction with Other Body Systems

The cardiovascular, urinary, musculoskeletal, neurological, and endocrine systems contribute to maintaining the male reproductive system.

The Cardiovascular System

Nutrients and sex hormones are transported to the reproductive organs through the vascular system. Sexual excitement causes vasodilatation of the arterioles in the penis, resulting in erection.

The Urinary System

The male ejaculates through the urethra, which also carries urine from the bladder to the outside of the body. Hypertrophy of the prostate gland compresses the urethra, making urination difficult and increasing the risk of urinary tract infections (UTIs) and urinary retention.

The Musculoskeletal System

The bones of the pelvis and muscles of the pelvic floor provide protection and support for some reproductive organs. Androgens (male reproductive hormones) in-

Understanding Spermatogenesis

Spermatogenesis—the formation of mature sperm within the seminiferous tubules—occurs in several stages:

- Spermatogonia, the primary germinal epithelial cells, grow and develop into primary spermatocytes. Both spermatogonia and primary spermatocytes contain 46 chromosomes, consisting of 44 autosomes and the two sex chromosomes, X and Y.
- Primary spermatocytes divide to form secondary spermatocytes. No new chromosomes are formed in this stage—the pairs only divide. Each secondary spermatocyte contains half the number of autosomes, 22—one secondary spermatocyte contains an X chromosome; the other, a Y chromosome.
- Each secondary spermatocyte then divides again to form spermatids.
- Finally, the spermatids undergo a series of structural changes that transform them into mature spermatozoa, or sperm. Each spermatozoan is composed of a head, neck, body, and tail. The head contains the nucleus; the tail, a large amount of adenosine triphosphate (ATP), which provides energy for sperm motility.

Spermatogonia (44 autosomes plus X and Y)

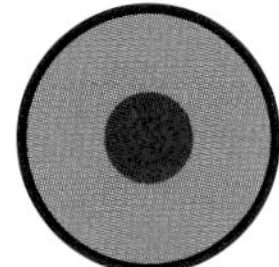

Primary spermatocytes (44 autosomes plus X and Y)

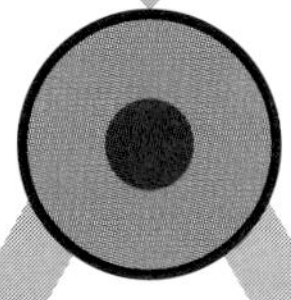

Secondary spermatocytes (22 autosomes plus X or Y)

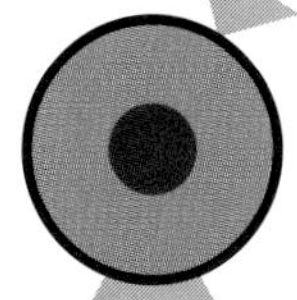

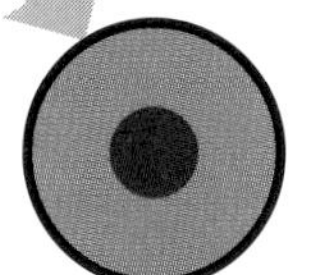

Spermatids (22 autosomes plus X or Y)

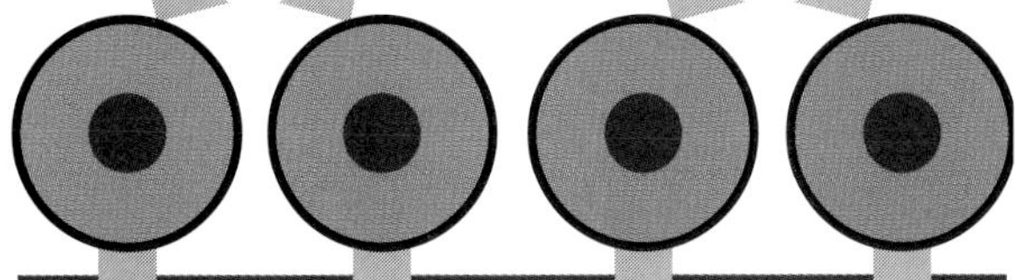

Spermatozoa (22 autosomes plus X or Y)

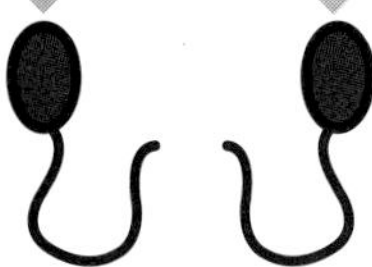

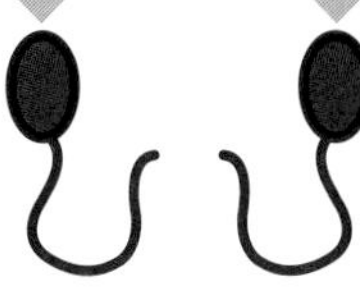

crease bone density. Bladder continence is achieved with an intact detrusor muscle, internal sphincter muscle tone, and external sphincter contraction. Structural and functional integrity of the muscles of the bladder, urethra, and pelvic floor are crucial.

The Neurological System

Parasympathetic nervous system impulses regulate events of the male and female sexual response, including the vasodilation that results in erection of the penis. Micturition is a reflex of the parasympathetic control that stimulates detrusor muscle contraction with the simultaneous relaxation of the external sphincter and pelvic floor muscles.

The Endocrine System

Gonadatropin-releasing hormone (GnRH), which is released by the hypothalamus, and luteinizing hormone (LH) and follicle stimulating hormone (FSH), which are produced by the anterior pituitary gland, trigger testosterone secretion and spermatogenesis.

Developmental, Cultural, and Ethnic Variations

Infants

Characteristics of male genitalia are used to help determine gestational age at birth. Premature infants may have undescended testes and few rugae. Breech-delivered infants may have scrotal edema and ecchymoses. Male infants should be assessed for **hypospadias** (urethral meatus opening ventrally on the glans) and **epispadias** (urethral meatus opening dorsally on the glans). **Hydroceles** and hernias are common findings in boys under age 2.

Children

You need to address specific areas when assessing a male child's GU system. Here are some questions to ask the parent or caregiver:

- Have you noticed any redness, swelling, discharge, or foul-smelling odors in the child's genital area? (Helps identify an infection.)
- Have you noticed asymmetry, lumps, or masses in the genitals? If so, where are they? Are they movable? Hard or soft? Painful to the touch? (Suggests hernia or lymphadenopathy, which may reveal an underlying problem.)
- Does the child cry and hold his genitalia as if something were hurting? (Pain may be caused by an

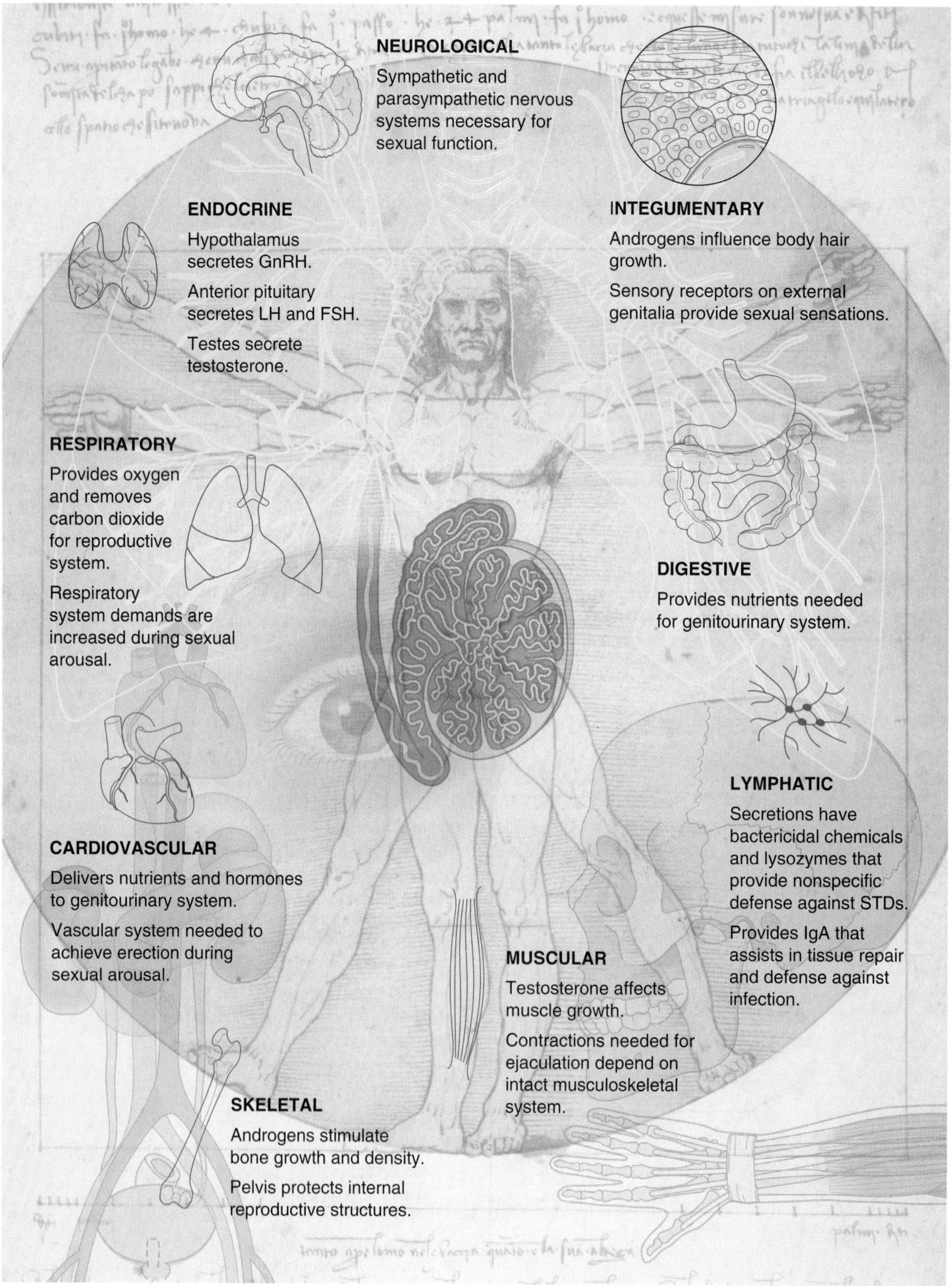

NEUROLOGICAL

Sympathetic and parasympathetic nervous systems necessary for sexual function.

ENDOCRINE

Hypothalamus secretes GnRH.

Anterior pituitary secretes LH and FSH.

Testes secrete testosterone.

INTEGUMENTARY

Androgens influence body hair growth.

Sensory receptors on external genitalia provide sexual sensations.

RESPIRATORY

Provides oxygen and removes carbon dioxide for reproductive system.

Respiratory system demands are increased during sexual arousal.

DIGESTIVE

Provides nutrients needed for genitourinary system.

LYMPHATIC

Secretions have bactericidal chemicals and lysozymes that provide nonspecific defense against STDs.

Provides IgA that assists in tissue repair and defense against infection.

CARDIOVASCULAR

Delivers nutrients and hormones to genitourinary system.

Vascular system needed to achieve erection during sexual arousal.

MUSCULAR

Testosterone affects muscle growth.

Contractions needed for ejaculation depend on intact musculoskeletal system.

SKELETAL

Androgens stimulate bone growth and density.

Pelvis protects internal reproductive structures.

Relationship of Male GU System to Other Systems

acute problem such as a strangulated hernia, but it may also suggest sexual abuse and warrants further investigation. See Appendix C for more information on assessing sexual abuse.)

- Have you ever been told that the child has a hydrocele or hernia?
- Has there been trauma to the child's genitalia, either through injury or during play?
- Is the child toilet trained (usually begins by age 2)? Are you having any toilet training problems? Does your child wet the bed (enuresis)? (Helps you assess developmental progress.)
- Does the child have any problem urinating, and is the urine stream straight? (May identify epispadias or hypospadias.)

Adolescents

Many of the questions you ask adolescents are similar to those you ask adults. But when assessing adolescent males, tailor your questions to younger and older boys. Identifying the client's understanding of sexuality and sexual practices is important because it provides an opportunity to clarify any misinformation and provide education. Above all, be nonjudgmental. A judgmental approach will almost certainly limit the amount of data you collect.

Identify any areas of concern that your client has regarding the sexual developmental changes occurring in his body. Often, adolescents need to know that these changes are normal. Also determine if he is sexually active, and if so, whether he practices safe sex. Ask if he has any concerns regarding sexual practices and whether he ever had sex education classes in school.

Tanner staging (box, page 564) is used to track the sexual maturation of males during puberty by characterizing pubic hair distribution and penile and testicular size. Assessment techniques are similar for clients of all ages, but your observations and the clients' histories are unique.

Older Adults

Normal physiological changes occur in the male reproductive system with aging. Pubic hair grays and becomes thinner; the penis appears somewhat atrophic; and the testicles may appear smaller and feel slightly softer than in a younger man. The prostate may feel larger than in youth. The scrotal sac loses its elasticity, and testosterone levels usually decrease by age 50. Although normal spermatogenesis continues, sperm output gradually decreases with age. Although the physiologic response to sexual stimulation does not change, the time required to achieve erection increases and ejaculation may be less intense, with decreased seminal fluid and rapid detumescence.

Some chronic health problems and a variety of other disease processes may have a direct effect on penile function. For example, renal failure and hypothyroidism or hyperthyroidism can alter hormonal release and metabolism at various levels. Erectile dysfunction (impotence) seems to increase with age, but it is not a normal part of aging. The most common cause of impotence in older men is vascular disease. Other causes include diabetes mellitus, hypogonadal states, medications such as antihypertensives and antidepressants, and psychological problems such as depression.

People of Different Cultures or Ethnic Groups

Cultural and ethnic variations often influence the decision regarding **circumcision**. The United States has always had a high rate of circumcision, and until recently, it was recommended for its medical benefits. However, The American Academy of Pediatrics now states that the medical benefits are not significant enough to endorse circumcision as a routine procedure. This opinion is also held in Canada, England, and Sweden, where circumcision is considered unnecessary. However, circumcision is a religious practice for Jews and Muslims.

Introducing the Case Study

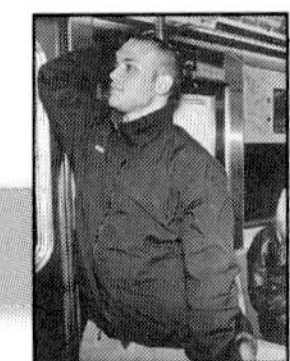

Sam Richards, age 35, works for the telephone company as a lineman. He is complaining about burning on urination for the past 3 days. He requests a "VD test" and appears anxious. He states that he has not slept for 2 nights because he is worried.

Performing the Male Genitourinary Assessment

Assessment of the male GU system consists of taking a complete health history and performing a physical exam-

Tanner Staging

Stage	Pubic Hair	Penis	Testes and Scrotum
Stage 1: Preadolescent 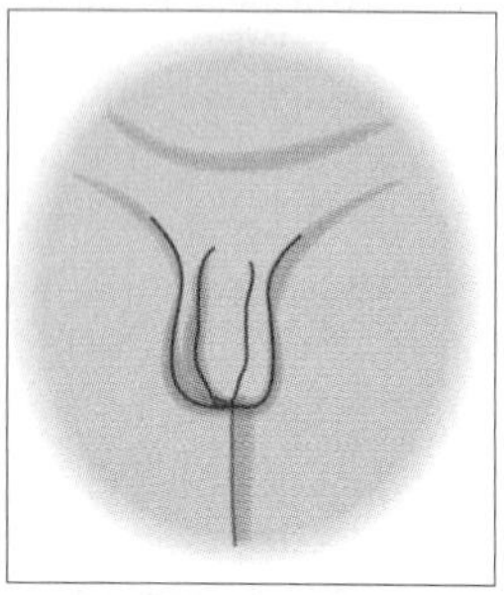	No pubic hair except for fine body hair similar to that on abdomen.	Same size and proportions as in childhood.	Same size and proportions as in childhood.
Stage 2 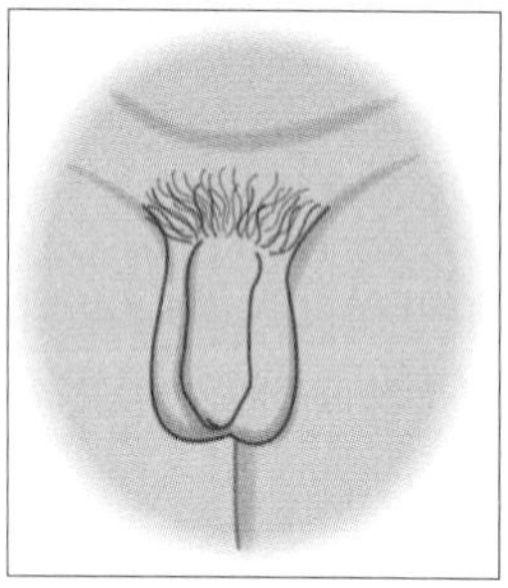	Sparse growth of long, slightly pigmented, downy hair, straight or only slightly curled, chiefly at base of penis.	Slight or no enlargement.	Testes larger; scrotum larger, somewhat reddened and altered in texture.
Stage 3 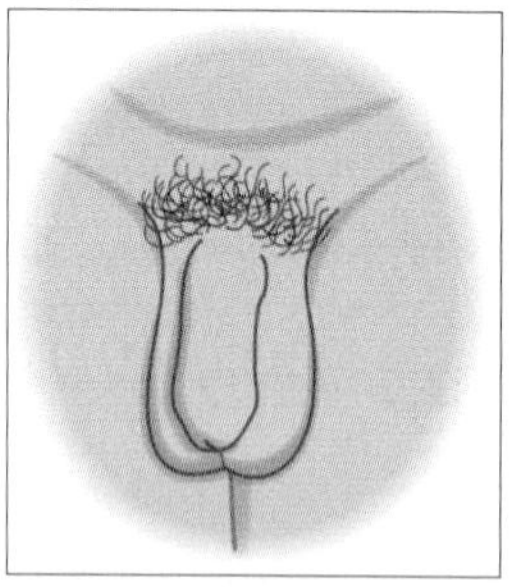	Darker, coarser, curlier hair spreading sparsely over pubic symphysis.	Larger, especially in length	Further enlarged
Stage 4 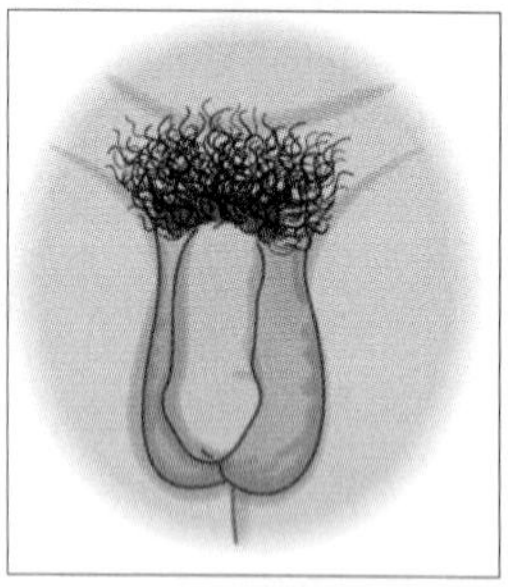	Coarse and curly hair, as in adult; area covered greater than in stage 3 but not as great as in adult.	Further enlarged in length and breadth, with development of glans.	Further enlarged; scrotal skin darkened.
Stage 5 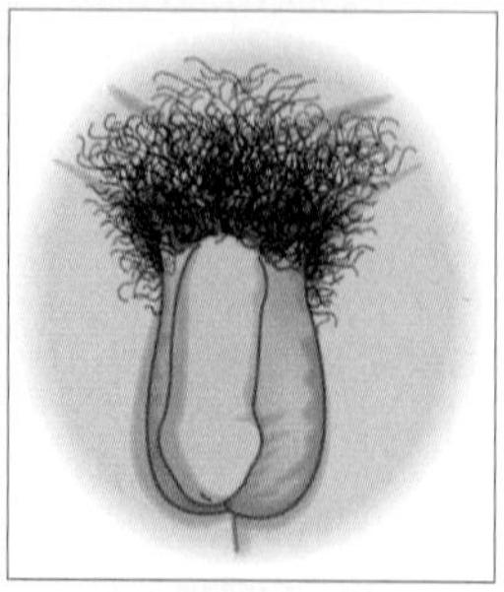	Hair same as adult in quantity and quality, spreading to medial surfaces of thighs but not up over abdomen.	Adult in size and shape.	Adult in size and shape.

ination. As you perform your assessment, be alert for signs and symptoms of actual and potential problems involving the various organs and structures in the GU system.

Health History

The purpose of the history is to identify potential or existing problems and risk factors. The history will provide you with subjective data that will guide your physical examination.

Begin by establishing rapport with your client. Assessing the male GU system may be somewhat uncomfortable for you and your client, but the more professional you are, the easier the examination will be for both of you. A nonthreatening, nonjudgmental approach is also essential. Remember to collect data about the urinary system as well as the reproductive system.

Questions about sexuality may be embarrassing for the client, or he may feel threatened. Sexual performance is often associated with a man's sense of masculinity and youth. If your client is having sexual function problems, he may be reluctant to share this information with you. Being sensitive and in tune to your client's nonverbal clues may help you uncover concerns that he is reluctant to volunteer.

Your assessment should focus on detection of any acute health problems and risks for GU problems, as well as identifying any health promotion teaching needs, especially STD prevention. STDs are the most common communicable diseases in the United States, and if left untreated, they can have devastating, permanent effects.

Biographical Data

Review the client's biographical data for clues that relate to the genitourinary system.

Begin by looking at his age—it influences the questions you ask during the health history. Because of changes in sexual development, the focus of the adolescent history will be slightly different than that of the older adult history. The age of your client may also identify risk factors. For example, testicular cancer, epididymitis, and **testicular torsion** most frequently affect young men, whereas benign prostatic hypertrophy and prostate cancer are more prevalent in older men.

Your client's occupation may put him at risk for genitourinary problems if he is exposed to chemicals or radiation that may cause infertility or increase the risk for testicular cancer. Even religion has an impact on the GU system because different cultures or ethnic groups have different circumcision practices.

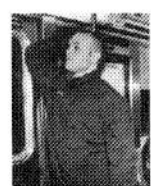

Case Study Findings

Reviewing Mr. Richards' biographical data:

- 35-year-old white male
- American by birth; Protestant religion
- Recently divorced, has a 10-year-old daughter
- Employed as telephone lineman for 10 years; healthcare insurance through work
- High-school education
- Source of referral: self, seems reliable

Current Health Status

The current health status focuses on the client's chief complaint. Common complaints include pain, lesions, swelling, discharge, urinary problems, and erectile dysfunction. Explore these complaints using the PQRST format. Begin by asking questions about genitourinary symptoms; leave questions about sexual performance until the end.

Symptom Analysis

Symptom Analysis tables for all of the symptoms described in the following paragraphs are available on the Web for viewing and printing. In your Web browser, go to *http://www.fadavis.com/detail.cfm?id=0882-9* and click on Symptom Analysis Tables under Explore This Product.

Genital Pain

Pain in the genital area usually has an acute onset and often follows trauma or infection. STDs and UTIs can cause epididymitis. Testicular torsion, a surgical emergency, causes excruciating pain and is not accompanied by urinary symptoms, fever, or elevated white blood cell (WBC) count. Prostatitis can cause perineal pain and may be bacterial or nonbacterial in origin.

Genital Lesions

Genital lesions such as vesicles, ulcers, warts, or rashes may indicate a variety of problems. The morphological description of the lesion will help with identification. Whether or not the lesion is painful is also important in differentiating lesions.

Lesions are often symptoms of STDs, but they may also be caused by carcinoma or a systemic problem.

STDS

Diseases and infections transmitted through sexual activity include chlamydia, cytomegalovirus, hepatitis B, herpes simplex, HIV/AIDS, human papillomavirus, molluscum contagiosum virus, gonorrhea, and syphilis. They may cause local or systemic effects and be long lasting or even fatal. Risk factors include:

- Multiple sex partners or having a partner with multiple partners
- IV drug use and sharing contaminated needles

- Unprotected sex
- Contacts with prostitutes, especially without using condoms
- Frequent multiple blood transfusions

Genital Swelling

Genital swelling or edema may result from local trauma or infection, but it may also be associated with systemic problems such as CHF. Swelling in the inguinal area may signal the presence of a hernia.

Penile Discharge

The only normal drainage from the penis is seminal fluid and urine. Any other discharge may signal a problem. The client's description of the discharge may give clues to the underlying problem. Copious amounts of thick, yellow discharge are associated with gonorrhea. Yellow discharge is also seen with chlamydia. Thin, watery discharge is associated with prostatitis. Bloody discharge may occur with trauma, infection, or cancer. Discharge of infectious origin is usually accompanied by pain.

Urinary Problems

Urinary problems are often associated with male reproductive problems because the penis serves as both a reproductive and a urinary structure. Urinary problems often cause discomfort, prompting the client to seek treatment. Dysuria, burning, frequency, change in urinary patterns, and **hematuria** are common complaints.

Because the two systems work so closely together, eventually a problem in one system often affects the other. However, reproductive problems more often cause urinary problems than vice versa.

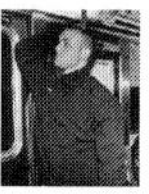

Case Study Findings

Mr. Richards' current health status includes:

- Onset of dysuria 3 days ago
- Clear urethral discharge occasionally at end of urine stream
- Denies low back pain, blood in urine, or recent trauma
- Denies suprapubic discomfort
- Had two different sex partners within the last 6 months
- Uses condoms "sometimes"

Past Health History

When taking your client's past health history, think about what information is related to male genitalia pathology. You may be able to identify a direct link between the past health history and your client's current health status. Remember to save questions about sexual performance until the end.

Past Health History

RISK FACTORS/QUESTIONS TO ASK	RATIONALE/SIGNIFICANCE
Childhood Illnesses	
Did you ever have mumps (parotitis), undescended testicles, or an **inguinal hernia** as a child?	*Mumps:* May cause infertility as a result of orchitis. *Undescended testicles (cryptorchidism):* Risk factor for testicular cancer. *Inguinal hernia as a child:* Risk factor for testicular cancer.
Hospitalizations/Surgeries	
Have you ever had a prostatectomy, transurethral prostatectomy, circumcision, orchiectomy, vasectomy,lesion or nodule removal, hernia repair, epispadias or hypospadias repair?	May explain patient complaints or physical findings.
Diagnostic Procedures	
Have you ever had a prostate-specific antigen (PSA) test? Have you ever had a rectal exam? When?	PSA is a screening test for prostate cancer. Rectal exams for prostate evaluation should be done yearly for men over age 40.
Injuries	
Have you ever had trauma to the genital area?	May explain physical findings.

Past Health History

RISK FACTORS/QUESTIONS TO ASK	RATIONALE/SIGNIFICANCE
Serious/Chronic Illnesses	
Do you have a history of STD, prostatitis, UTI, kidney stones, genital area trauma, cancer, congenital or acquired genital deformity, or infertility?	History of STDs indicates a lifestyle that predisposes client to subsequent infections. Other problems may explain physical problems. May also be used as baseline information.
Do you have a history of diabetes or vascular disease?	Can cause GU problems such as erectile dysfunction.
Immunizations	
Were you immunized for the mumps?	Mumps during adolescence may cause sterility.
Allergies	
Do you have contact dermatitis? Are you allergic to condoms, nonoxynol 9 or other spermicides, or latex?	Further identifies health promotion needs.
Medications	
Are you on any medications, such as antibiotics, hormone replacements, alpha blockers, 5-alpha-reductase inhibitors or antidepressants?	Certain medications can contribute to sexual dysfunction. See box, Drugs That Adversely Affect Male Sexual Function, below and on page 568.
Recent Travel/Military Service/ Exposure to Infectious or Contagious Diseases	
Have you been exposed to chemicals? Do you have a history of HSV, HPV, molluscum contagiosum, condyloma acuminata, syphilis, penile lesion, chlamydia, or gonorrhea?	Increased risk for infertility. Could present an educational opportunity for disease prevention.

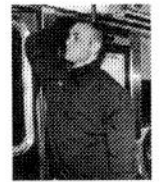

Case Study Findings

Mr. Richards' past health history reveals:

- Usual childhood illnesses except for measles, mumps, and rubella
- Tonsillectomy in 1967, no other surgeries or hospitalizations
- Had chlamydia approximately a year ago and received antibiotics
- No history of renal calculi
- Immunizations current
- Denies taking any prescription drugs; admits using aspirin occasionally for aches and pains

Drugs That Adversely Affect Male Sexual Function

Classification	Medication	Effect
Antiandrogen	finasteride	Impotence
Antianxiety/Sedative	benzodiazepines, chlordiazepoxide	Changes in libido
Anticholinergic	atropine	Impotence
Antidepressants	tricyclic antidepressants such as amitriptyline	Increased/decreased libido and impotence
	trazodone	Decreased libido, impotence, priapism, retrograde ejaculation
	selective serotonin reuptake inhibitors (SSRIs) such as fluoxetine	Decreased libido, delayed orgasm, anorgasmia, ejaculatory dysfunction

(Continued)

Drugs That Adversely Affect Male Sexual Function *(Continued)*

Classification	Medication	Effect
Antiepileptic	primidone	Impotence
Antihypertensive	methyldopa	Ejaculatory failure
	prazosin	Impotence, priapism
	clonidine	Impotence, decreased sexual activity, decreased libido
Antihypertensive/Antianginal	beta blockers, atenolol, labetalol, propranolol, nadolol	Impotence, decreased libido
Antihyperlipidemics	simvastatin	Impotence
Antipsychotics	all antipsychotics	Priapism, impotence, ejaculatory inhibition
Diuretics	chlorothiazide, spironolactone	Impotence
Estrogen	conjugated estrogen	Impotence, testicular atrophy
Tranquilizers	diazepam, alprazolam	Changes in libido

Family History

The family history can identify factors that might cause a health problem or predispose the client to one. It identifies genetically linked disorders as well as familial risk factors that put your client at risk for genitourinary disease.

Family History

RISK FACTORS/QUESTIONS TO ASK	RATIONALE/SIGNIFICANCE
Genetically Linked Diseases of Male Genitalia	
Do you have a family history of varicocele, testicular cancer, or infertility?	Increased risk for cancer and infertility. May indicate congenital deformities.
Did your mother take diethylstilbestrol (DES) during her pregnancy?	Increased risk for testicular cancer.
Familial/Genetically Linked Disorders with GU Symptoms	
Do you have a family history of diabetes or vascular disease?	Can affect sexual function.

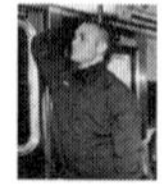

Case Study Findings

Mr. Richards' family history reveals:

- Father died at age 52 of heart attack.
- Mother, age 62, alive and well.
- Three siblings are healthy.

Review of Systems

The review of systems (ROS) allows you to assess the interrelationship of the GU system to every other system. You can determine how the GU system affects or is affected by every other system. During the ROS, you often uncover important facts that your clients failed to mention earlier.

Review of Systems

SYSTEM/QUESTIONS TO ASK	RATIONALE/SIGNIFICANCE
General Health Survey	
Have you had any changes in your energy level? Fevers? Weight changes?	Fatigue, activity intolerance, fever, and weight loss are often signs of underlying health problems, such as HIV/AIDS or prostatitis. Scrotal abnormalities may cause discomfort and affect activity tolerance. Fatigue influences desire and ability to perform sexual intercourse.
Integumentary/*Skin*	
Have you had any rashes or lesions?	May be associated with STDs, but not restricted to genitalia. Primary syphilis chancre found on lip as well as penis. Bilateral, symmetrical rash of secondary syphilis usually occurs on palms and soles.

Review of Systems

SYSTEM/QUESTIONS TO ASK	RATIONALE/SIGNIFICANCE
Integumentary/*Hair*	
Have you had any hair loss?	Male hormones affect body hair growth. Secondary syphilis can cause alopecia.
HEENT/***Head and neck***	
Do you have swollen glands or nodes?	*Swelling of lymph nodes:* Associated with infection and malignancy. *Enlarged thyroid:* May affect sexual function.
HEENT/*Eyes, Nose, and Throat*	
Do you have a sore throat? Watery eyes? Drainage from your eyes?	STDs can be found in the oropharynx and are often not assessed in client complaining of sore throat. Secondary syphilis can result in oral mucous patches. Gonorrheal eye infections occur in newborns (ophthalmia neonatorum) and adults (gonorrheal conjunctivitis). Tearing, photophobia, edema of eyelids, and conjunctival edema are symptoms of *Chlamydia trachomatis* infection.
Respiratory	
Do you have any breathing problems?	Respiratory disease such as COPD may affect sexual activity.
Cardiovascular	
Do you have cardiovascular disease, such as hypertension (HTN) or congestive heart failure (CHF)?	May compromise sexual activity. Vascular problems and HTN medications may cause erectile dysfunction. Scrotal edema may accompany CHF.
Gastrointestinal	
Do you have a history of liver disease?	Liver disease associated with ascites may cause scrotal edema.
Have you had a loss of appetite or weight loss?	Weight/appetite loss may be associated with malignancy or AIDS.
Musculoskeletal	
Do you have weakness, limitation, joint pain, or swelling?	Physical act of sexual intercourse requires functional musculoskeletal system. Late-stage syphilis damages joints (Charcot's joint).
Neurological	
Do you have any neurological problems?	May affect sexual function.
Weakness, paralysis, or tremors? Mental or personality changes or depression?	Neurosyphilis occurs in late syphilis and can cause paresis, tremors, personality changes, and psychosis. Depression is a risk factor for erectile dysfunction.
Endocrine	
Do you have diabetes or thyroid disease?	Diabetic neuropathy can cause impotence. Hypothyroidism causes decreased libido and infertility. Hyperthyroidism can cause impotence and gynecomastia.
Immune/Hematologic	
Do you have HIV or AIDS?	AIDS, an STD, affects the immune system.
Sickle cell anemia?	Sickle cell anemia can cause priapism (painful, sustained erection without sexual desire).

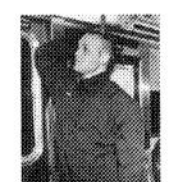

Case Study Findings

Mr. Richards' review of systems reveals:

- **General Health Survey:** Usual state of health good
- **Integumentary:** No changes in skin, hair, and nails; no lesions
- **HEENT:** No swollen glands/nodes; denies sore throat; no eye drainage
- **Respiratory:** No history of COPD
- **Cardiovascular:** No history of hypertension or cardiovascular disease
- **Gastrointestinal:** No history of liver disease
- **Musculoskeletal:** Denies joint pain or swelling

- **Neurological:** No neurological problems, weakness, or paralysis; denies personality changes or depression
- **Endocrine:** No history of thyroid disease or diabetes
- **Immune/Hematologic:** Has never been tested for HIV; no history of sickle cell anemia

Psychosocial Profile

The psychosocial profile can reveal patterns in the client's life that may affect his reproductive health and also assist in determining the cause of a health concern such as erectile dysfunction. Evaluating lifestyle may also identify specific areas where health maintenance education is needed.

Psychosocial Profile

CATEGORY/QUESTIONS TO ASK	RATIONALE/SIGNIFICANCE
Health Practices and Beliefs/ Self-Care Activities	
Do you do testicular self-exams?	Monthly testicular self-exam is recommended as well as an annual exam.
Have you had your prostate checked?	Annual prostate exam starting at age 40.
Do you use condoms and practice "safe sex"?	Use of condoms minimizes the risk for STDs.
How often do you bathe?	Poor hygiene can lead to infections of genitalia or urinary tract.
Typical Day	
What is your typical day like?	Performing ADLs indicates level of wellness. Fatigue associated with AIDS.
Nutritional Patterns	
What did you eat in the last 24 hours? What foods do you usually eat?	*High-saturated-fat, high-cholesterol diet:* Associated with arteriosclerosis, which indirectly contributes to erectile dysfunction.
Have you lost weight recently?	*Weight loss:* Associated with cancer, AIDS, and anorexia.
Activity and Exercise Patterns	
Do you exercise? How often? What type of exercise? Do you participate in sports or activities that require heavy lifting or that may cause genital injury?	May indicate reproductive health and self-esteem. Trauma to testicle may cause a hydrocele. Heavy lifting can result in hernias.
Do you wear protective equipment while participating in sports?	Use of protective equipment, such as a jockstrap or cup, decreases risk of genital trauma.
Recreation/Hobbies	
What do you do in your leisure time?	Some hobbies can expose people to carcinogens.
Sleep/Rest Patterns	
How many hours of sleep do you average a night?	Fatigue can cause sexual dysfunction.
Do you wake up to urinate? How often?	*Nocturia:* May be underlying symptom of urethritis.
Personal Habits/*Drug Use*	
Do you use street drugs, such as cocaine, barbiturates, amphetamines, or narcotics? If so, how often and how much?	May impair judgment, increasing risk of STD exposure. Street drugs may cause priapism, impotence, increased sexual excitability, increased libido, and delayed orgasm.
Personal Habits/*Alcohol Use*	
Do you drink alcohol? What type, how much, and how often?	Impairs gonadotropin release and accelerates testosterone metabolism, causing impotence and loss of libido. Large doses can acutely depress sexual reflexes. Chronic alcoholism causes high levels of circulating estrogens, which decrease libido. Alcohol intoxication may impair judgment, decreasing incidence of safe sex practices and increasing risk of exposure to STDs.

Psychosocial Profile

CATEGORY/QUESTIONS TO ASK	RATIONALE/SIGNIFICANCE
Personal Habits/*Tobacco Use*	
Do you use tobacco? What type, how much per day, and for how many years?	Cigarette smoking increases risk of atherosclerotic disease, which may decrease penile blood flow.
Occupational Health Patterns	
Does your work involve the use of heavy equipment? Does it expose you to radiation or toxic chemicals?	*Radiation/toxic chemicals:* Linked to cancer of male genitalia and infertility. *Work with heavy machinery:* Increases risk for hernias and injury to genitalia.
Environmental Health Patterns	
Do you live in an apartment or single home? What type of heating do you have? Is the plumbing adequate?	Poor sanitation may indicate poor hygiene, which can cause infections of genitalia or urinary tract.
Roles/Relationships/Self Concept	
How do you see yourself? Would you say you have a positive self-image?	Poor self-image and lack of self-confidence can predispose client to sexual dysfunction.
Cultural/Religious Influences	
Do you have any cultural or religious beliefs that affect your sexual health?	Circumcision is a religious ceremony for Jewish faith. Abortion and contraception are prohibited for members of Catholic faith.
Family Roles and Relationships	
Have GU problems affected your marriage or family life?	Premature ejaculation, impotence, and other sexual problems may affect relationships. Stress within a relationship may cause sexual dysfunction.
Social Supports/Stress and Coping	
Who are your supports? How do you deal with stress?	Stress can cause sexual dysfunction. Emotional or social isolation can increase stress.

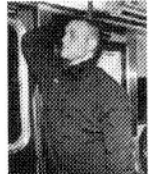

Case Study Findings

Mr. Richards' psychosocial profile includes:

- Cannot remember when he last had a physical or went to a doctor for illness.
- Does not perform testicular self-examination (TSE).
- Typical day: Awakens at 6:30 AM, has only coffee for breakfast, gets to work at 7:30 AM. Work is very physical and includes climbing up telephone poles and onto roofs of houses and crawling under houses. Usually arrives home by 5:30 PM. Spends evenings watching television or dating. Spends time with child every other weekend. Usually in bed about 10 PM on workdays. Skips breakfast, drinks 4 cups of coffee daily, eats out a lot, snacks on junk food, rarely has a nutritious meal.
- Besides work, hikes about every other weekend, plays tennis occasionally, does yard work.
- Sleeps about 7 hours a night on workdays, less on nights he has dates. Naps on weekends to "catch up" on sleep.
- Has smoked a pack of cigarettes daily for the last 15 years. Drinks beer about three times per week and about 6 to 10 beers on weekends. Denies recreational drug use.
- Job is physically taxing and potentially dangerous because of climbing.
- Has good relationship with his one child and with his mother, who cleans, irons, and occasionally cooks for him.
- No community involvement, does not attend church. Lives alone since divorce 1 year ago, in single-family home with more space than he needs.
- Copes with stress by ignoring it.

Sexual History

Because the GU system encompasses sexuality, a more detailed sexual history may be warranted. Wait until the end of the history before asking sensitive or embarrassing questions. This gives you time to establish rapport with your client. Asking about sexual functions and practices is important for several reasons:

- Many clients have sex-related questions or problems that they want to discuss.
- Sexual practices may be directly related to the client's symptoms.
- Sexual dysfunction may be a consequence of medications and may be reversible.
- Sexual practices are related to the client's risk for STDs.

Questions that are helpful in assessing sexual function include the following:

- Have you ever been sexually active?
- Are you currently sexually active? That is, have you had sex with anyone in the past few months? How often? If yes, do you have sex with men, women, or both (heterosexual, homosexual, or bisexual)?
- What types of sexual activity do you engage in? Oral, anal, genital?
- Do you have more than one partner? How many partners have you had in the last 6 months?
- Do you use birth control? What kind? How often?
- Are you worried about the AIDS virus or other STDs?
- Do you take any precautions to avoid infections? If so, what?
- Do you have any problems or concerns about your sexual function?
- Have you had surgery on any of your reproductive organs? If so, what and when?
- Have you been taught to examine your testicles?

Erectile Dysfunction

Erectile dysfunction is the inability to achieve satisfactory sexual performance. It includes the inability to achieve erection, achieve complete erection, maintain erection, or ejaculate. A specific description of the dysfunction is essential to identify the most appropriate therapy. Remember: Take a look at your client's medical history because diabetes, vascular problems, and certain medications are risk factors for erectile dysfunction. Additional questions that address erectile dysfunction include the following:

- Are you still interested in sex?
- Are you able to achieve and maintain an erection?
- Do you have morning erections?
- Were there any changes in your relationship with your partner or in your life situation when the problem began?
- How long does intercourse last?
- Do you sometimes feel that you cannot ejaculate?
- Are you satisfied with your sex life as it is now?

HELPFUL HINT

If your client can achieve a morning erection, the cause of erectile dysfunction is usually not organic.

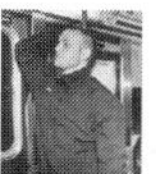

Case Study Findings

Mr. Richards' sexual history findings include:

- Currently sexually active
- Heterosexual
- Two sexual partners within last 6 months
- Inconsistent use of condoms
- Satisfied with sexual performance
- No problems achieving erection or ejaculation
- Does not perform testicular self-examination

Case Study Evaluation

Before you proceed with the physical examination of the male GU system, review and document the data you have obtained from Mr. Richards' history.

CRITICAL THINKING ACTIVITY #1

Based on your history findings, what teaching needs can you identify for Mr. Richards?

Physical Assessment

Once you have obtained the subjective data, focus on collecting the objective data by performing the physical examination.

Approach

Ensure that the examination room is warm and comfortable and that the light in the room is sufficient to adequately observe the client. Instruct him to empty his bladder and to undress to expose the groin area. Drape him appropriately for privacy. Because reproductive system assessment involves exposing and handling the genitals, the client may feel anxious and embarrassed. To help minimize discomfort, explain each assessment step before performing it and expose only the necessary areas. Keeping a professional demeanor will help you feel more at ease, too.

During the examination, the client can lie on the table in the supine position with his legs spread slightly or stand in front of you while you are sitting eye level to the genitalia. A rectal examination is used to assess the prostate gland. Your client can either assume a sidelying (Sims') position or lean over the examination table.

You will use the techniques of inspection, palpation, and auscultation to assess this client.

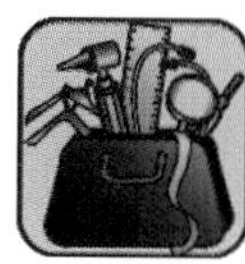

Toolbox

Assemble the following equipment for a routine examination: Nonsterile gloves, water-soluble lubricant, penlight, and stethoscope. To obtain a urethral specimen and perform a culture, you will also need cotton swabs or 1 1/2" to 2" gauze wrap, urogenital alginate swabs, and a Thayer-Martin plate (gonorrhea culture).

Performing a General Survey

Before you begin your physical examination, perform a general survey, looking for clues that suggest a GU problem. For example:

- Obtain the patient's vital signs. Elevations in temperature may indicate an infection that might be accompanied by a GU infection. HTN may affect sexual functioning.
- Because the examination can produce anxiety, take note of your client's emotional status.
- Take note of your client's posture and nonverbal behavior. Does his posturing reflect pain or discomfort?

Performing a Head-to-Toe Physical Assessment

The GU system affects many different systems. Therefore, examine the client for specific changes that may affect the GU system.

Performing a Head-to-Toe Physical Assessment

SYSTEM/NORMAL FINDINGS	ABNORMAL FINDINGS/RATIONALE
General Health Survey	
Well developed physically. No acute distress. Awake, alert, oriented. Memory intact. Affect appropriate.	Personality changes and mental deterioration can accompany late-stage syphilis. Depression can affect sexual function.
Integumentary/Skin	
Intact, no lesions	Rashes and skin lesions are associated with many STDs. *Systemic rash:* Secondary syphilis. *Vesicles:* Herpes simplex types 1 and 2.
Integumentary/Hair	
Even distribution of hair.	*Alopecia:* Associated with secondary syphilis. *Decrease in body hair:* Possible decease in male hormones.
HEENT/*Head and Neck*	
No palpable lymph nodes	*Palpable lymph nodes:* May indicate systemic infection or malignancy.
Thyroid not palpable	*Enlarged thyroid (hypo- or hyperthyroidism):* May affect sexual functioning.
HEENT/*Eyes, Mouth, and Throat*	
Conjunctiva pink, no drainage	*Conjunctivitis:* Can be caused by gonorrhea.
Oral mucous membranes pink, moist and intact.	*Oral lesions:* Associated with STDs.
Respiratory	
Lungs clear; no SOB	Chronic lung disease may impair sexual functioning.
Cardiovascular	
Regular heart rate and rhythm, no extra sounds.	HTN and CHF may impair sexual function.

(Continued)

Performing a Head-to-Toe Physical Assessment *(Continued)*

SYSTEM/NORMAL FINDINGS	ABNORMAL FINDINGS/RATIONALE
Cardiovascular *(Continued)*	
+2 pulses, extremities warm bilaterally, no edema.	CHF may cause scrotal edema. Vascular disease is risk factor for erectile dysfunction.
Breasts	
No enlargement	*Gynecomastia:* Associated with decreased male hormones.
Gastrointestinal	
Abdomen flat, positive bowel sounds, no organomegaly.	Liver disease associated with ascites may also cause scrotal edema.
No palpable lymph nodes.	*Palpable inguinal lymph nodes:* Possible infection or malignancy.
Musculoskeletal	
>+5 muscle strength, full ROM	Weakness or joint pain may limit sexual functioning. *Weakness and paralysis:* Associated with neurosyphilis.
No joint deformities	*Charcot's joints:* Associated with late syphilis.
Neurological	
No weakness or paralysis	*Weakness and paralysis:* Associated with neurosyphilis.
Awake, alert, and oriented X3, memory intact, affect appropriate	*Changes in mental status/psychosis:* Late syphilis. *Depression:* Risk factor for psychogenic erectile dysfunction.

Case Study Findings

Before you proceed to a focused GU assessment, document what you learned during your general survey and head-to-toe assessment of Mr. Richards.

Mr. Richards' physical assessment findings include:

- **General Health Survey:** 35-year-old, well-developed white male in no acute distress
- **Vital Signs:** Temperature 97.9°F; pulse 88 BPM, strong and regular; respirations 14/min; BP 128/76; height 5'11"; weight 182 lb
- **Integumentary:** Skin intact with no lesions; hair evenly distributed with no alopecia
- **HEENT:** Head and neck: no palpable nodes, nonpalpable thyroid
- **Eyes:** Conjunctiva pink and moist, no drainage
- **Mouth and Throat:** Oral mucosa pink and moist, no lesions
- **Respiratory:** Lungs clear
- **Cardiovascular:** No extra heart sounds; +2 pulses, extremities warm, no edema
- **Breasts:** No gynecomastia
- **Gastrointestinal:** Abdomen slightly rounded, positive bowel sounds, no organomegaly, positive tenderness in suprapubic area, several palpable inguinal nodes noted and tender
- **Musculoskeletal:** +5 muscle strength, full ROM, no joint deformities
- **Neurological:** No weakness, positive sensation, no paralysis

Performing a Focused Physical Assessment

Assessment of the male GU system includes inspection, palpation, and auscultation.

Inspection

Begin with inspection of the genitalia. The client should be lying on the table in a supine position with his legs slightly spread. Or he can stand in front of you and you can sit so that the genital area is at your eye level. Remember to put on gloves After inspecting the genitalia, inspect the rectal area. Have the client move to a sidelying position or stand and bend over the examination table.

AREA/SYSTEM	SUBJECTIVE DATA
General	*Ask about:* Changes in energy level, weight Fevers
Integumentary	*Ask about:* Changes in hair growth Rashes, lesions
HEENT *Head, Neck, Eyes, Mouth and Throat*	*Ask about:* Swollen glands/nodes Eye drainage Sore throat Oral lesions
Respiratory	*Ask about:* History of respiratory disease
Cardiovascular	*Ask about:* History of CVD, HTN, CHF
Gastrointestinal	*Ask about:* History of liver disease Loss of appetite
Musculoskeletal	*Ask about:* Weakness, limitations Joint pain, swelling
Neurological	*Ask about:* History of neurological problems Paralysis Tremors Personality changes Depression
Endocrine	*Ask about:* History of thyroid disease and diabetes
Lymphatic/ Hematologic	*Ask about:* History of HIV, AIDS, sickle cell anemia

AREA/SYSTEM	OBJECTIVE DATA
General	*Take:* Vital signs, checking for temperature elevations, HTN *Note:* Signs of discomfort Affect
Integumentary	*Inspect:* Skin lesions Hair distribution Areas of alopecia
HEENT *Head, Neck, Eyes, Mouth and Throat*	*Palpate:* Lymph node enlargement Thyroid enlargement *Inspect:* Conjunctiva for drainage Oral mucosa for redness and lesions
Respiratory	*Inspect:* Signs of respiratory distress *Auscultate:* Abnormal breath sounds
Cardiovascular	Inspect: Signs of impaired circulation Skin changes *Palpate:* Pulses, edema *Auscultate:* Extra heart sounds
Gastrointestinal	*Inspect:* Ascites *Palpate/Percuss:* Liver enlargement
Breasts	*Inspect:* Gynecomastia
Musculoskeletal	*Test:* Muscle strength *Inspect:* Joint swelling and deformity
Neurological	*Test for:* Changes in mental status, affect Sensory deficits

Assessment of Male GU Systems' Relationship to Other Systems

Inspecting the Genitalia

AREA/NORMAL VARIATIONS	ABNORMAL FINDINGS/RATIONALE

Hair Distribution

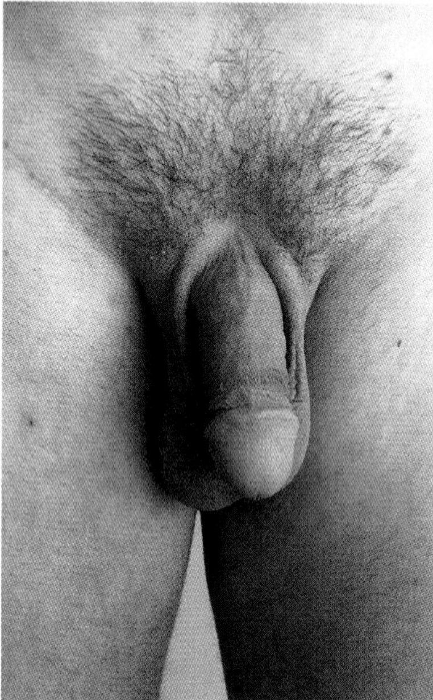

Inspecting hair distribution

Pubic hair distribution should be triangular, sparsely distributed on scrotum and inner thigh and absent on penis. Genital hair is coarser than scalp hair. No nits or lice.

Sparse or absent hair (alopecia): May result from genetic factors (developmental defects and hereditary disorders), aging or local or systemic disease. Diseases include infection, neoplasms, endocrine diseases, and nutritional or metabolic deficiencies. Other causes are physical or chemical agents and destruction or damage to hair follicles.

Penis

Skin should be free of lesions and inflammation. Shaft skin is loose and wrinkled without erection. Glans is smooth and free of lesions, swelling or inflammation. No penile discharge. Dorsal vein is sometimes visible. If client is uncircumcised, loose skin on the penis shaft folds to cover glans forming the **foreskin**. Foreskin retracts easily.

Chancre: Signals primary syphilis. Painless, ulcerated, exudative, papular lesion with an erythematous halo, surrounding edema and a friable base.

Chancroid: Caused by *Haemophilus* through small breaks in epidermal tissue. Pinhead papules to cauliflower-like groupings of painful, filiform, skin-colored, pink, or red lesions.

Condyloma acuminatum (genital warts): Caused by HPV infection. Multifocal, wartlike, maculopapular lesions that are tan, brown, pink, violet, or white.

Inspecting the Genitalia

AREA/NORMAL VARIATIONS | **ABNORMAL FINDINGS/RATIONALE**

Penis *(Continued)*

Genital Abnormalities: Inspection

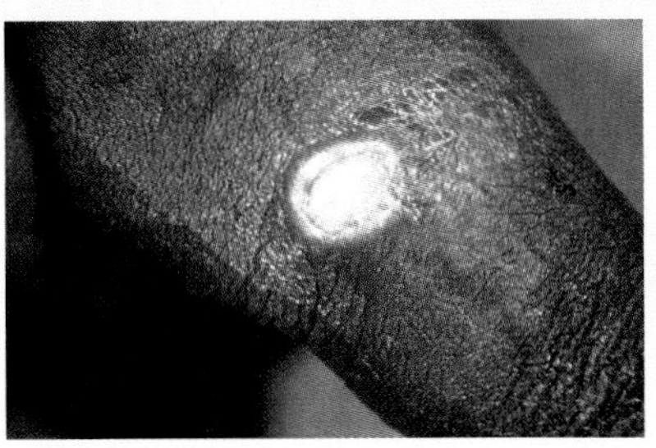

Chancre

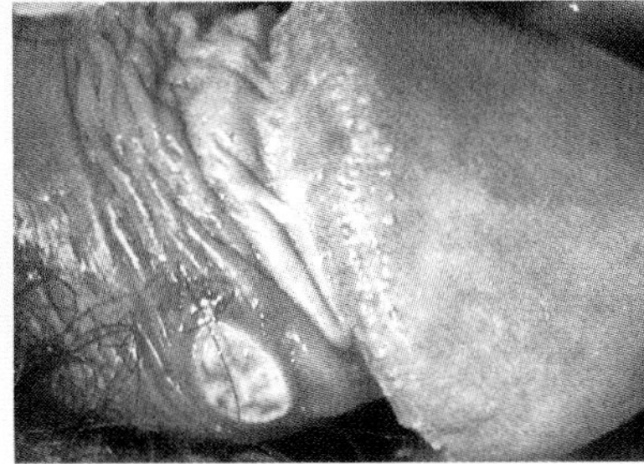

Chancroid

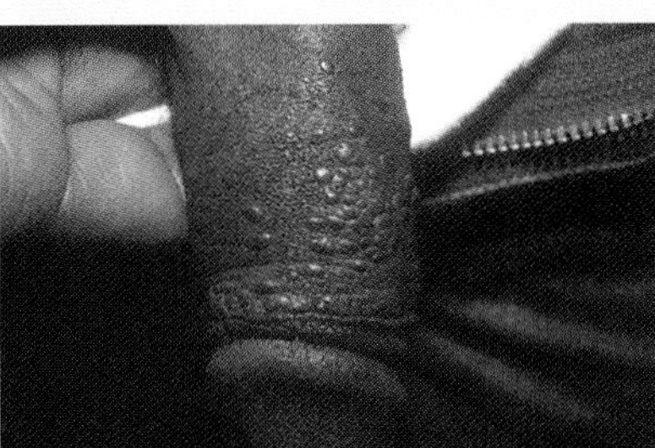

Genital warts on penis

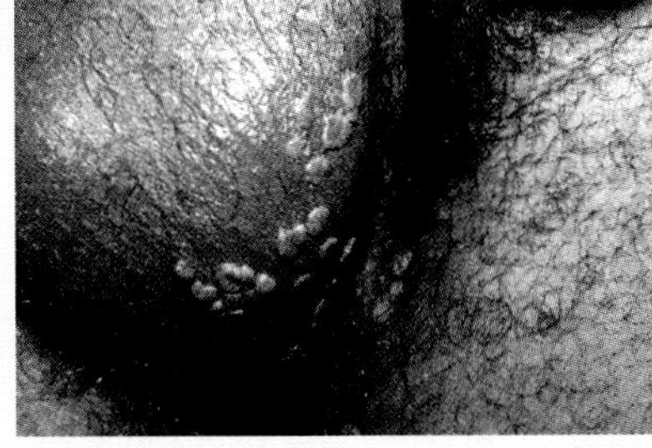

Genital warts on scrotum

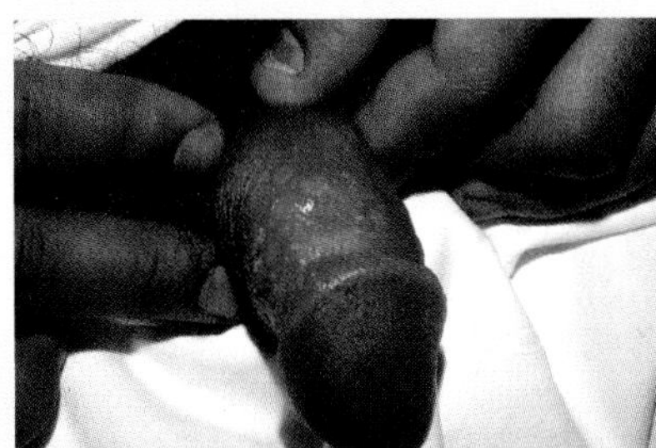

Genital herpes

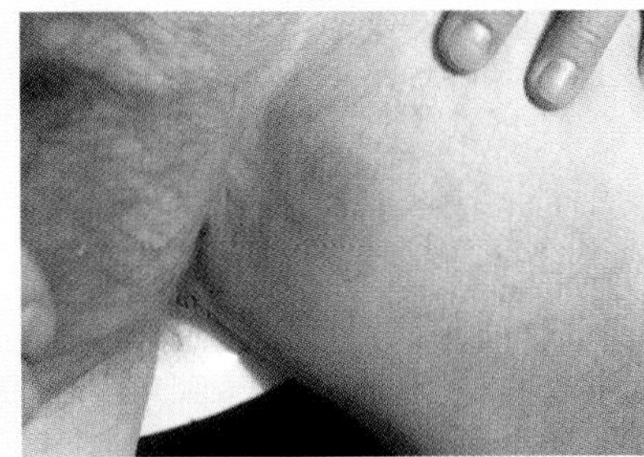

Tinea cruris

Candida: Superficial mycotic infection of moist cutaneous sites. Erythematous plaques with scaling, papular lesions with sharp margins and occasionally clear centers and pustules.

Herpetic lesion: Herpes simplex virus I and II cause painful eruptions of pustules and vesicles that rupture. Fever, headache, dysuria, dyspareunia, and urinary retention may occur.

Tinea Cruris: Fungal infection of the groin often referred to as "jock itch."

Phimosis: Occurs in uncircumcised males. Foreskin is unable to retract and may become swollen.

Priapism: Often associated with leukemia, metastatic carcinoma, or sickling hemoglobinopathies.

Chordee: Ventral or dorsal curvature of penis. Ventral chordee seen mostly with epispadias.

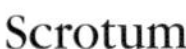

Scrotum

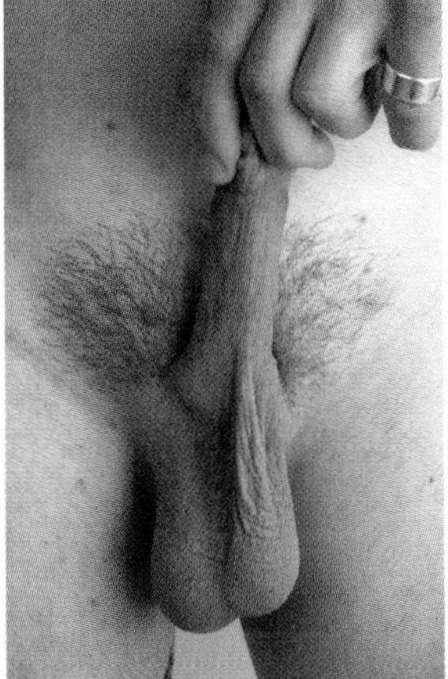

Inspecting scrotum

Masses: Can arise from benign or malignant conditions.

Scrotal swelling: Seen with inguinal hernia, hydrocele, varicocele, spermatocele, tumor, and edema.

Hydrocele: Nontender accumulation of fluid between two layers of tunica vaginalis in scrotum. May be idiopathic or a result of trauma, inguinal surgery, epididymitis, or tumor. Mass transilluminates.

Spermatocele: Nontender, well-defined cystic mass on superior testis or epididymis

(Continued)

Inspecting the Genitalia *(Continued)*

AREA/NORMAL VARIATIONS	ABNORMAL FINDINGS/RATIONALE
Scrotum *(Continued)* Scrotal skin appears rugated, thin, and more deeply pigmented than body color. Skin is firmer in young men and elongates with flaccidity in older men. Skin should be free of lesions, nodules, swelling, inflammation, and erythema. Scrotal size and shape vary greatly. Left scrotal sac is lower than right.	caused by blockage of efferent ductules of rete testis. *Varicocele:* Varicose veins of spermatic cord that feel like a "bag of worms" and slowly collapse when scrotum is elevated. Caused by dilated veins in pampiniform plexus of spermatic cord. Right-sided may indicate obstruction at vena cava. *Sebaceous cyst:* Round, firm, nontender cutaneous cyst confined to scrotal skin. May result from decrease in localized circulation and closure of sebaceous glands or ducts.
Urethral Meatus Located centrally on glans. Pink in white males and darker pink in darker-skinned males. No discharge.	*Epispadias:* Urethral meatus opens on dorsal (upper) side of penis. *Hypospadias:* Urethral meatus opens on ventral (under) side of penis.
Inguinal Area Should be free of swelling or bulges. Lymph nodes nonpalpable.	*Bulge:* May indicate a hernia or enlarged lymph node.

Inguinal Abnormalities: Inspection

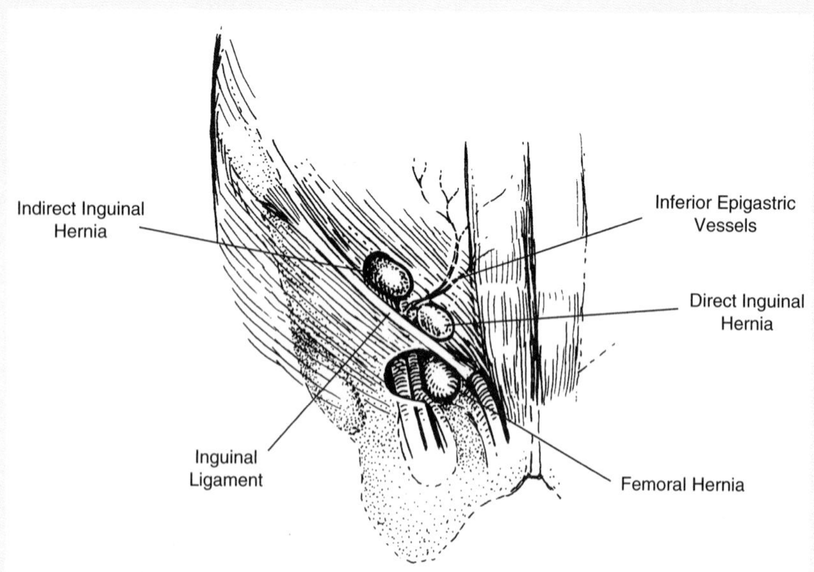

Location of indirect and direct femoral and inguinal hernias

AREA/NORMAL VARIATIONS	ABNORMAL FINDINGS/RATIONALE
Rectal Area Skin intact with slightly darker pigmentation around anus. Anus intact; no lesions, hemorrhoids, fissures, bleeding, or rectal prolapse.	STD lesions, warts, hemorrhoids, fissures, bleeding, rectal prolapse.

Obtaining a Urethral Specimen

Gonorrhea and chlamydia are classically associated with a urethral discharge. To obtain a specimen, have the client either lie supine or stand. Put on gloves and hold the penis with your nondominant hand. Use your dominant hand to clean the urethral meatus with sterile gauze or a cotton swab. Then insert a thin urogenital alginate swab 1 to 2 cm into the urethra and rotate the swab from side to side. Leave it in place for several seconds. A Thayer-Martin medium is used when collecting urethral discharge specimens for gonorrhea. A Gram stain can be done to diagnose gonorrhea, but it should be followed by a culture. A variety of tests for chlamydia are available, but the collection technique remains the same. Some laboratories can perform both tests with one swab and some will require two specimens. Chlamydia tests can also be done on urine.

HELPFUL HINT

Change gloves as needed during the exam to prevent cross contamination.

Palpation

Next, palpate the penis and scrotum for tenderness and abnormalities. Palpate the inguinal and femoral areas for hernias and enlarged lymph nodes. And palpate the rectum for masses or nodules, and note the tone of the anal sphincter. Also check the prostate and bulbourethral glands for tenderness, masses, or swelling. Remember to wear gloves!

Penis

To palpate, stand in front of the client's genital area. Palpate the entire length of the penis between your thumb and first two fingers. Note any pulsations, tenderness, masses, or plaques. If your client is not circumcised, retract the foreskin. As you retract, you may normally find white, cheesy material called **smegma.** Gently squeeze the glans of the penis to expose the meatus between your thumb and forefinger. If discharge is present or the client complains of discharge, take a culture.

Scrotum

Next, gently palpate a testicle between your thumb and first two fingers. Note the size, shape, consistency, and presence of masses. Palpate the spermatic cord from the epididymis to the external ring. Note the consistency and presence of tenderness or masses. Repeat on the opposite side. This is also a good time to teach testicular self-examination (TSE). If you detect a scrotal mass or enlargement, use transillumination to visualize it. Darken the room, apply a light source to the unaffected side behind the scrotum, and direct it forward. Repeat with the affected side.

Femoral and Inguinal Hernias

Now palpate the skin overlying the inguinal and femoral areas for lymph nodes, noting size, consistency, tenderness, and mobility. To palpate for inguinal hernias, ask the client to bear down while you palpate the inguinal area. Place your dominant index finger in the client's scrotal sac above the testicle and **invaginate** the scrotal

Teaching Testicular Self-Examination

Teach TSE to your client during the scrotal examination. Follow these steps:

- First, explain the rationale for the exam. Monthly testicular exams permit earlier detection of testicular cancer, which occurs most often in 16- to 35-year-olds. Suggest that he perform the exam on the same day each month.
- Tell him that the scrotum is easier to examine after taking a warm bath or shower.
- Now show him how to perform the exam: With one hand, lift the penis and check the scrotum for any changes in shape, size, or color. The left side of the scrotum normally hangs slightly lower than the right.
- Next, check the testes for lumps and masses. Locate the epididymis, the crescent-shaped structure at the back of each testis. It should feel soft.
- Use the thumb and first two fingers of your left hand to squeeze the left spermatic cord gently. The cord extends upward from the epididymis, just above the testis. Repeat on the right side using your right hand. Check for lumps and masses.
- Finally, examine each testis. Place your fingers on the underside and your thumb on the top and gently roll the testis between your thumb and fingers. The testis should be egg-shaped, movable, and feel rubbery, smooth and firm, with no lumps. Both testes should be the same size.
- Tell the client that if he finds any lumps, masses, or other changes, he should call his doctor.

Palpating for Inguinal and Femoral Hernias

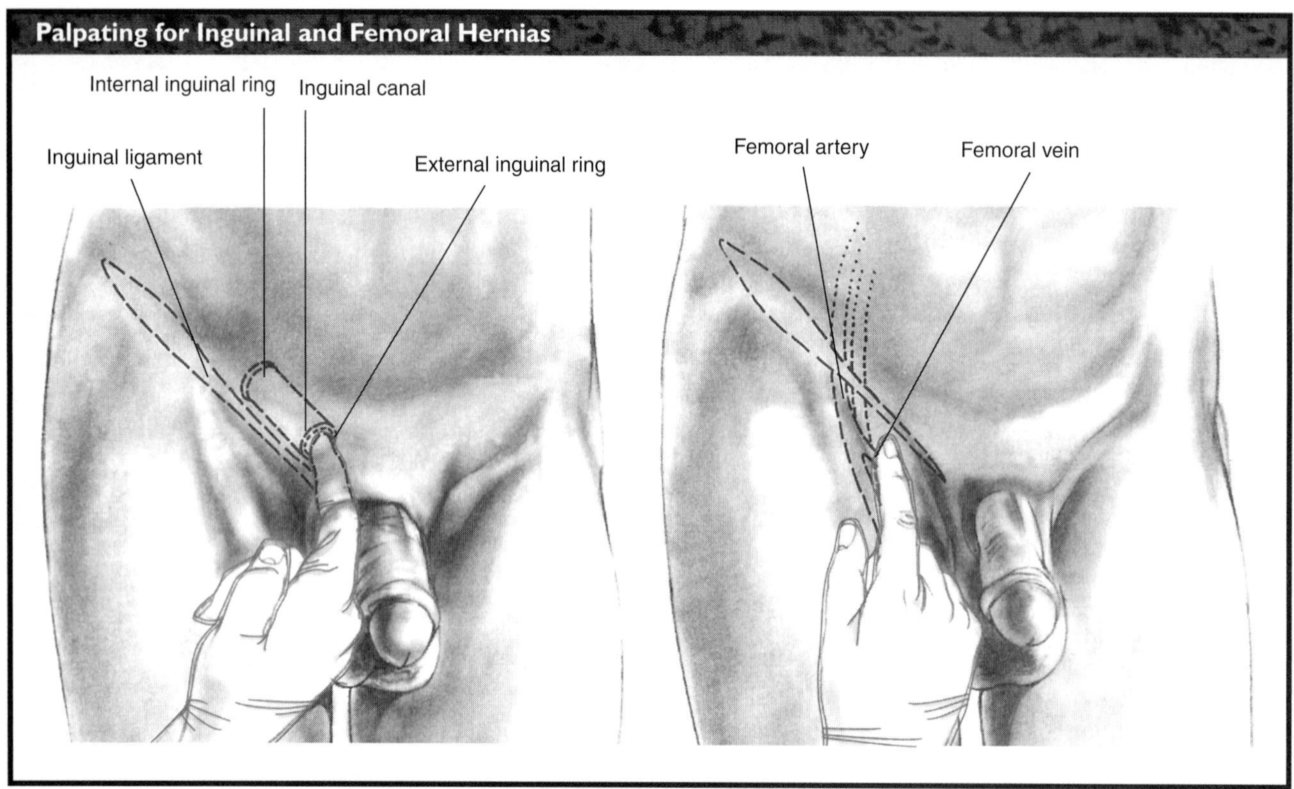

skin. Follow the spermatic cord until you reach a triangular, slitlike opening (**Hesselbach's triangle),** which is the external inguinal ring. The nail of your examining finger should be facing inward and your finger pad outward. If possible, continue to advance your finger along the inguinal canal and ask the client to cough or bear down. Note any masses. Repeat the procedure on the opposite side. To assess for femoral hernias, palpate the femoral canal, which is located below the femoral artery, and have the client bear down or cough.

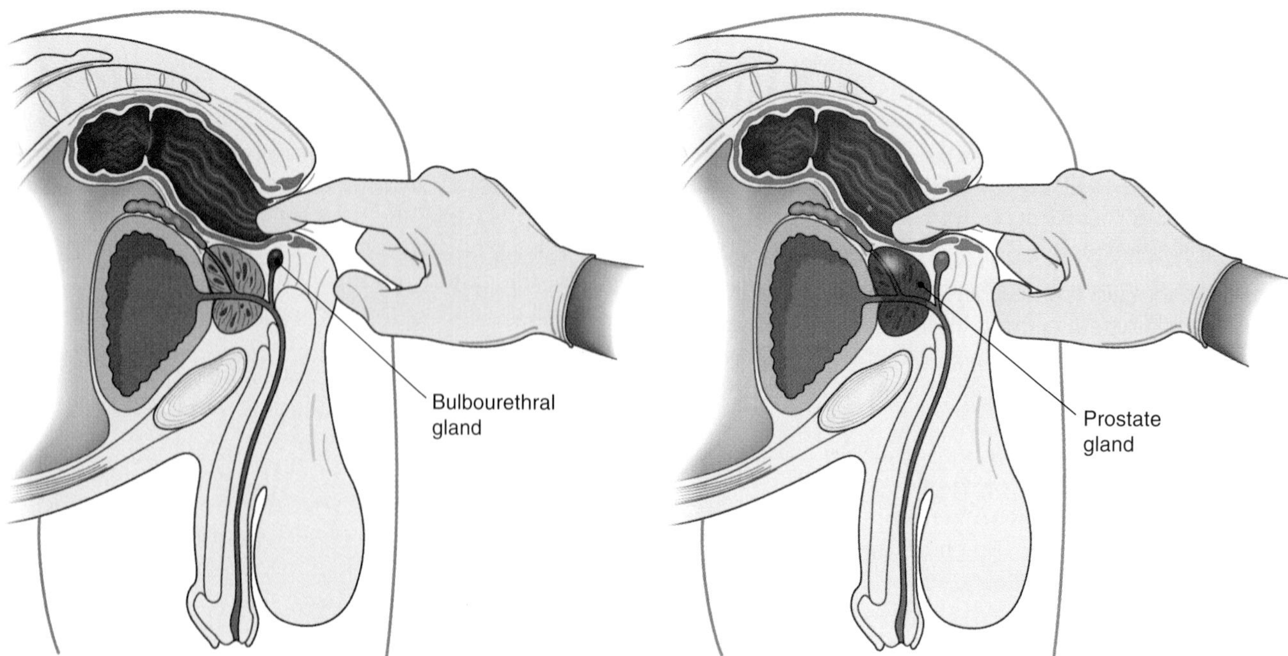

FIGURE 17–2. Palpating the prostate and bulbourethral glands.

Rectum, Prostate Gland, and Bulbourethral Gland

To examine the rectum and prostate, have the client stand and bend over the examination table. Place your lubricated, gloved index finger at the anal orifice and instruct the client to bear down. Then gently insert your finger into the anal sphincter, with the tip flexed toward the anterior rectal wall. Palpate the anterior and posterior rectal walls. They should be smooth and nontender, with good anal sphincter tone. Next, palpate the posterior surface of the prostate gland, noting size, shape, consistency, sensitivity, and mobility. Slowly withdraw your finger. If your glove contains fecal matter, perform an occult blood test. If the prostate is enlarged, determine the size and grade. Next, perform a bidigital examination of the bulbourethral gland by pressing your thumb into the perianal tissue while pressing your index finger toward it. Assess for tenderness, masses, or swelling. Release your thumb and advance your index finger (Fig. 17–2.)

Palpating the Genitalia

AREA/NORMAL VARIATIONS | **ABNORMAL FINDINGS/RATIONALE**

Penis

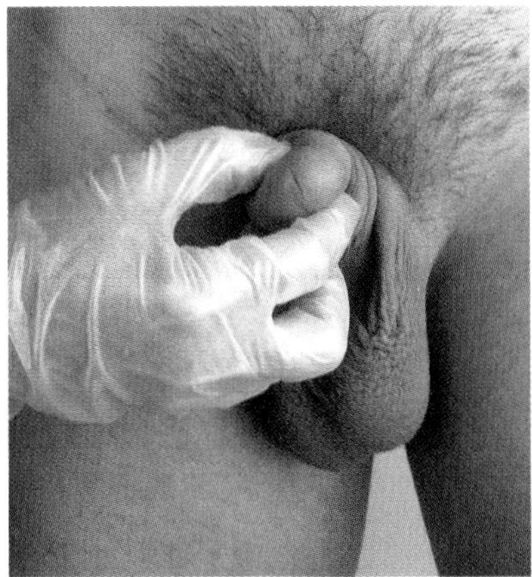

Palpating penis

Pulsations present on dorsal sides. Normally nontender. No masses or firm plaques.

Diminished/absent palpable pulse: Possible vascular insufficiency.

Normal blood flow may be affected by systemic disease, localized trauma, or localized disease.

Priapism is associated with spinal cord lesions or sickle cell anemia.

Penis should not be enlarged in nonerect state.

Phimosis and *paraphimosis* (foreskin retracts but does not return) are abnormal.

ALERT

Seek immediate assistance if foreskin cannot be retracted. Prolonged constriction of vessels can decrease blood flow and lead to necrosis.

Urethral Meatus

Should be free of discharge and drainage.

Purulent discharge or mucus shreds: Bacterial infection of GU tract. Color, consistency, and amount may vary.

Bacterial infection causes inflammation with leukocytes, shedding tissue cells, and bacteria.

(Continued)

Palpating the Genitalia *(Continued)*

AREA/NORMAL VARIATIONS	ABNORMAL FINDINGS/RATIONALE
Scrotum	A unilateral mass palpated within or about the testicle is abnormal. Intratesticular masses are nodular and painless and should be considered malignant until proven otherwise. (See section on inspecting the genitalia for description of spermatocele, hydrocele, and varicocele.)

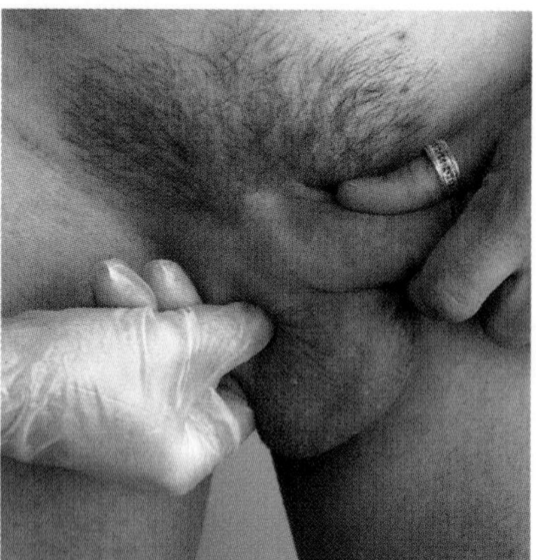

Palpating scrotum and testicles

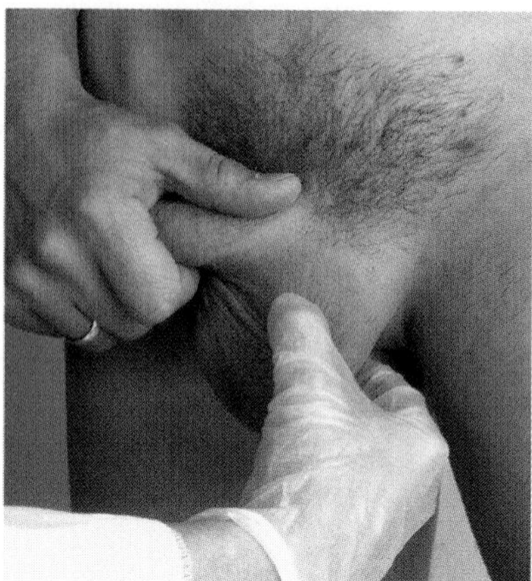

Palpating epididymis

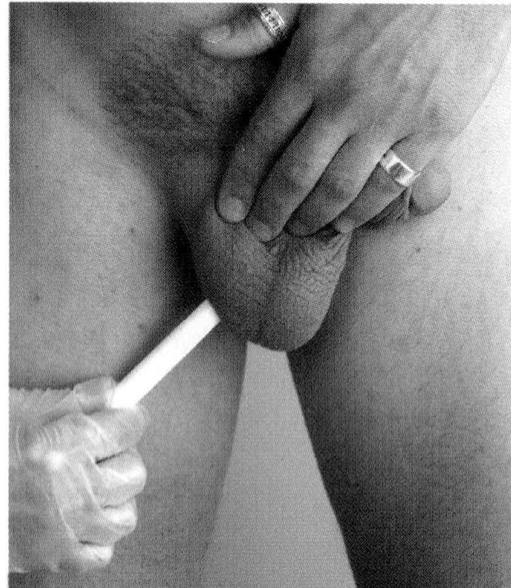

Transilluminating scrotum

ALERT

Do not squeeze or pinch any mass, lesion, or other structure that is palpated.

AREA/NORMAL VARIATIONS	ABNORMAL FINDINGS/RATIONALE
Scrotum contains a testicle and epididymis on each side. Testicles should be firm but not hard, oval, smooth, equal in size, and sensitive to pressure but not tender.	*Testicle that is enlarged, retracted, in a lateral position, and extremely sensitive:* Testicular torsion.
Epididymis is comma shaped, distinguishable from testicle, and insensitive to pressure. Spermatic cord is smooth and round.	Indurated, swollen, tender epididymis is abnormal. Undescended testes is abnormal.

Palpating the Genitalia

AREA/NORMAL VARIATIONS	ABNORMAL FINDINGS/RATIONALE

Inguinal Area

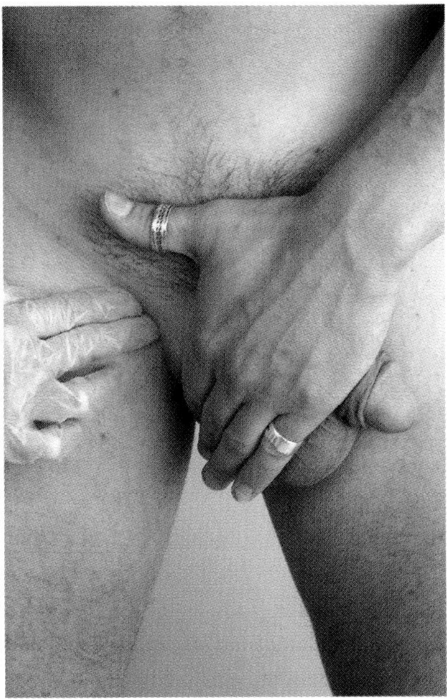

Palpating horizontal lymph nodes

Palpating vertical lymph nodes

Cryptorchidism (absence of testes and epididymis in scrotal sac): Related to testicular failure, deficient gonadotrophic stimulation, mechanical obstruction, or gubernacular defects. The undescended testes have a histologic change by age 6, so refer client as early as possible.

Orchitis is acute, painful swelling of testicle and warm scrotal skin. Client may feel heaviness in scrotum.

Atrophic testicle and scrotal edema are abnormal.

No red glow on transillumination.

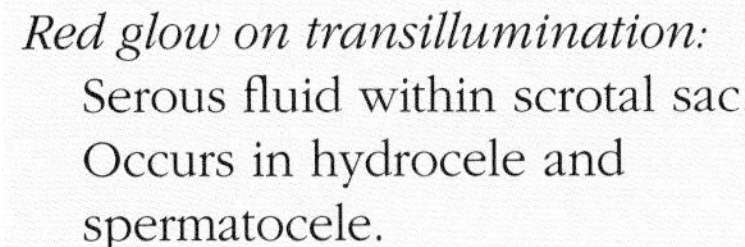

Red glow on transillumination: Serous fluid within scrotal sac. Occurs in hydrocele and spermatocele.

Unilateral or bilateral enlargement of inguinal lymph nodes: May indicate bacterial infection. Nodes may be tender or painless. Lymph node enlargement may also be associated with metastatic disease.

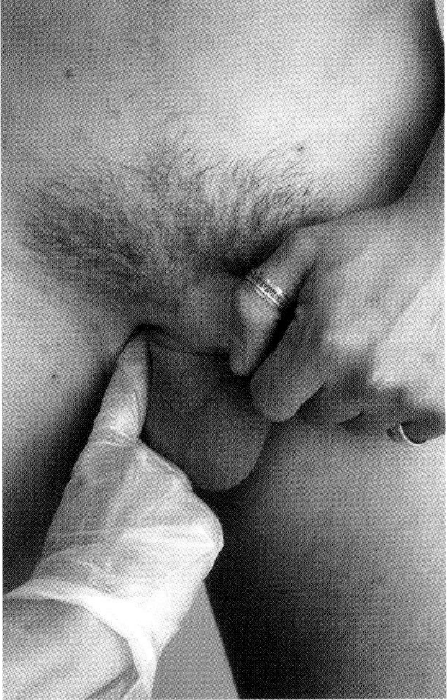

Palpating hernias

Indirect inguinal hernia comes down inguinal canal and is palpated at inguinal ring or in scrotum

Direct inguinal hernia is a mass that enlarges with coughing.

Femoral hernia is palpated medial to femoral vessels and inferior to inguinal ligament.

ALERT

A strangulated hernia is a surgical emergency.

Nodes should be less than 1 cm and freely mobile. No bulges present in inguinal area. No palpable masses in inguinal canal. No portions of the bowel enter the scrotum. No palpable masses at femoral canal.

Palpable mass or nodule: Polyp or internal hemorrhoid.

Hard mass: Possible rectal cancer.

(Continued)

Palpating the Genitalia *(Continued)*

AREA/NORMAL VARIATIONS | **ABNORMAL FINDINGS/RATIONALE**

ALERT

Do not have hypertensive patients bear down during exam. Observe for discomfort and lightheadedness. Some clients cannot tolerate bearing down for more than a few seconds.

HELPFUL HINTS

- Instruct client to inform you of any pain or discomfort during palpation. This a sensitive, ticklish area. Use firm and deliberate movements.
- If you cannot insert your finger into the inguinal canal with gentle pressure, stop. Never force it into the opening.

Rectum/Prostate

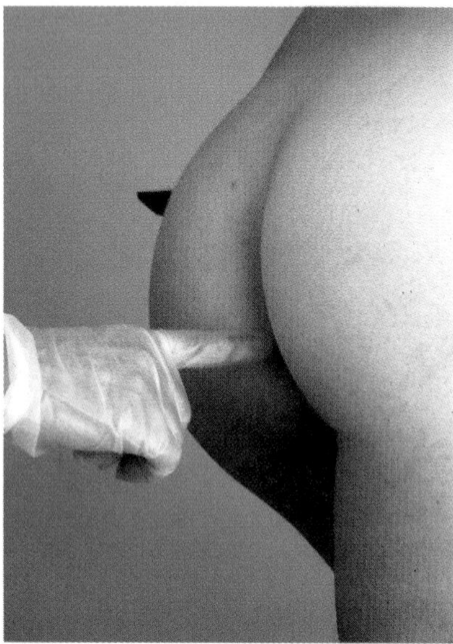

Palpating prostate

Rectum should be smooth and nontender with good anal sphincter tone.
Prostate should be small, smooth, mobile, and nontender.
Medial sulcus should be palpable.
Test stool for occult blood. Test should be negative.

Soft, nontender, enlarged prostate: Benign prostatic hypertrophy. Related to aging and presence of dihydroxy-testosterone.

Firm, tender, or fluctuant mass on prostate: Acute bacterial prostatitis. UTIs commonly occur concurrently. Increased risk for prostatic abscess.

Firm, hard, or indurated single or multiple nodules: Possible prostate cancer.

Extremely tender, warm prostate: May indicate bacterial prostatitis. Do not palpate vigorously. This would be painful and might cause bacteremia.

Positive occult blood test warrants further evaluation.

PROSTATE GLAND GRADING

Grade I: *<1 cm protrusion into rectum*
Grade II: *1 to 2 cm protrusion into rectum*
Grade III: *2 to 3 cm protrusion into rectum*
Grade IV: *>3 cm protrusion into rectum*

Auscultation

If you detect a scrotal mass on inspection and palpation, auscultate the scrotum. Ask the client to lie in a supine position, then stand at his side next to the genital area. Place your stethoscope over the scrotal mass to listen for bowel sounds. The presence of bowel sounds suggests a hernia.

Auscultation

AREA/NORMAL VARIATIONS	ABNORMAL FINDINGS/RATIONALE
No bowel sounds	*Bowel sounds in scrotum:* Indirect inguinal hernia.

Case Study Findings

Mr. Richards' focused physical assessment findings include:

- Triangular distribution of pubic hair, no nits or lice.
- Erythema at urethral meatus, skin free of lesions and inflammation, rounded glans penis, no penile curvature, circumcised
- Pulsations present on dorsal aspect of penis, no masses or firm plaques
- Scrotum rugated, no testicular swelling, no erythema, no masses or nodules, left testis slightly lower than right
- Testicles palpated bilaterally without masses or tenderness, epididymis not enlarged and nontender, no swelling or tenderness, spermatic cords intact without nodules bilaterally
- Urethral meatus centrally located
- Clear to white thin discharge expressed from urethral meatus
- No inguinal bulges, right inguinal lymph nodes slightly elevated (1.3 cm) and tender, no inguinal masses

Case Study Analysis and Plan

Now that your examination of Mr. Richards is complete, document your key history and physical examination findings. List key history findings and key physical examination findings that will help you formulate your nursing diagnoses

Nursing Diagnoses

Consider all of the data you have collected during your assessment of Mr. Richards, then use this information to identify appropriate nursing diagnoses. Here are some possible ones. Cluster the supporting data.

1. **Anxiety, related to dysuria**
2. **Fear, related to infectious process in reproductive system**
3. **Pain**
4. **Health Maintenance, ineffective, related to insufficient knowledge of safe sex practices**
5. **Health Maintenance, ineffective, related to insufficient knowledge of self-care**

Identify any additional nursing diagnoses and any collaborative nursing diagnoses.

CRITICAL THINKING ACTIVITY #2

Develop a nursing care plan and a brief teaching plan for Mr. Richards using one of the nursing diagnoses from above. Include learning outcomes and teaching strategies.

Research Tells Us

A healthy reproductive system is essential for the client's overall well-being. Research tells us that the most common sexual complaint in men is erectile dysfunction (Walsh, 1994). An estimated 30 million men in the United States have erectile dysfunction, but fewer than 5 percent are treated. Testicular cancer has an incidence of 2.8 out of 100,000 men. It is the most common form of cancer in men aged 20 to 35 (Bates, 1999). Early detection has a direct impact on prognosis. Every year more than 15 million cases of STDs are reported in the United States, yet they remain among the most underrecognized health threats (MMWR, 1998). Because infection with STDs greatly increases a person's risk of both acquiring and spreading HIV infection, do not miss the opportunity to educate your client during the physical examination.

Health Concerns

Risk Factors for Testicular Cancer:

- Cryptorchidism
- Age 20–40
- Family history of testicular cancer
- Mumps orchitis
- Inguinal hernia during childhood
- Maternal exposure to DES
- Testicular cancer in other testicle

Signs of Testicular Cancer:

- Hard, fixed, nontender mass or nodules on testicle that are not visible with transillumination
- Scrotal swelling
- Scrotal heaviness

Risk Factors for Prostatic Cancer:

- Family history of prostatic cancer
- Advanced age
- African-American ethnicity

Signs of Prostate Cancer:

- Urinary symptoms: Dysuria, frequency, nocturia, hesitancy, dribbling, hematuria, and retention
- Enlarged, hard, fixed prostate
- Back pain (may indicate metastasis)

Screening Tests:

In addition to monthly TSE, the American Cancer Society recommends an annual digital rectal exam (DRE) for all men over age 40. Serum prostate-specific antigen (PSA) is a glycoprotein exclusive to the prostate epithelium that is elevated in prostate cancer because of the accelerated metabolic rate and catabolism of the tumor. A serum PSA along with DRE increases the chance of early detection. Transrectal ultrasound may also be used to visualize the outer lobes of the prostate and localize possible cancerous sites.

Common Abnormalities

ABNORMALITY	ASSESSMENT FINDINGS
Benign Prostatic hypertrophy (BPH) Benign enlargement of prostate	• Age over 50 • Changes in urination pattern such as hesitancy, incontinence with dribbling, reduced caliber and force of urine stream, and possibly retention • Enlarged, firm, slightly elastic, smooth, possibly tender prostate • Burning on urination if accompanied by UTI
Chancroid Caused by *Haemophilus* through small breaks in epidermal tissue	• Pinhead papules to cauliflower-like groupings of filiform, skin-colored, pink or red painful lesions on genitalia heals leaving a scar
Chlamydia Caused by *Chlamydia trachomatis*	• Dysuria and clear or white penile discharge
Condyloma acuminatum Genital warts caused by the human papillomavirus	• Soft, pink papillomatous or raised warty lesions on genitalia • Blanching of areas on penis with 5% acetic acid wash
Cryptorchidism Undescended testicles	• Undeveloped scrotum (undescended testicle) • Increases risk of testicular cancer • Only one testis or epididymis palpable in scrotal sac • Testicular atrophy

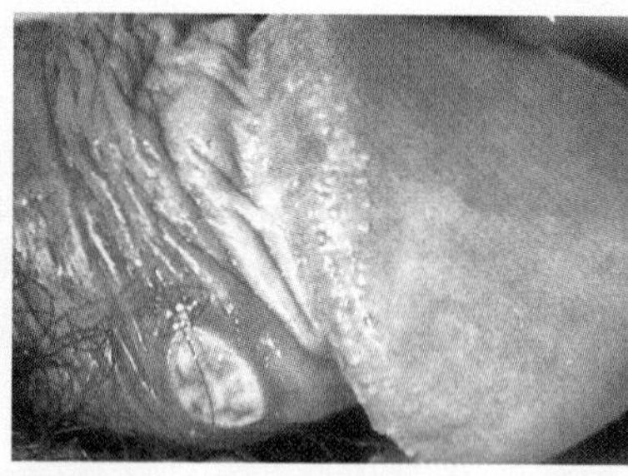

Chancroid

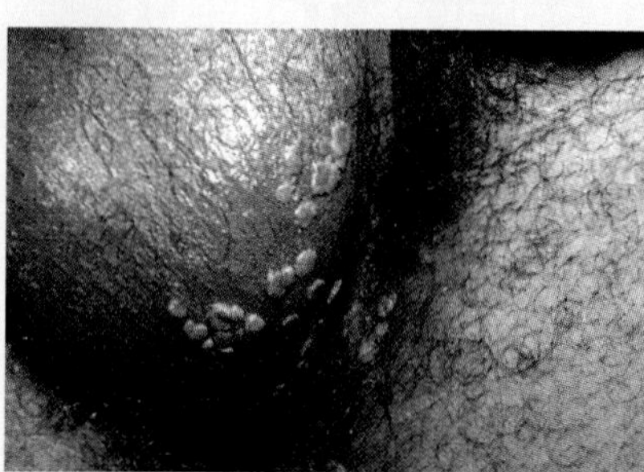

Genital warts

Common Abnormalities

ABNORMALITY	ASSESSMENT FINDINGS
Epididymitis Acutely inflamed epididymis	• Occurs chiefly in adults and may coexist with a UTI or prostatitis • Causes scrotal pain, reddened scrotum, inflamed vas deferens, and UTI symptoms
Epispadias	• Urinary meatus on dorsal side of penis
Genital Herpes Viral STD that is treatable but not curable	• Fever, malaise, arthralgia, inguinal lymphadenopathy • Multiple small vesicles on penis followed by ulcers on red bases • Pain • Possible dysuria, pruritus, urethral discharge • Recurrent infection
Gonorrhea • Caused by *Neisseria gonorrhoeae*	• Urinary symptoms • Urethral discharge
Hydrocele • Lymphatic fluid-filled tunica vaginalis around testis	• Causes enlarged, nontender scrotum • Can be transilluminated
Hypospadias	• Urinary meatus on ventral side of the penis
Indirect Inguinal Hernia • Protrusion of hernial sac containing intestine at inguinal opening	• Sac protrudes through internal inguinal ring into inguinal canal and may descend into scrotum. • Causes bulging in right or left inguinal area with heavy lifting or coughing. • Examination reveals mass in inguinal canal or scrotum. • May or may not cause tenderness or pain.
Orchitis Inflammation of the testis	• Scrotal or inguinal mass • Unilateral or bilateral scrotal swelling with pain or tenderness • Fever • Possible nausea and vomiting • Recent infection, especially epididymitis or mumps • Impotence • Possible infertility
Paraphimosis • Inability to return foreskin over penis because of edema	• Inflammation • Yeast or bacterial infection under foreskin
Phimosis Inflammation of foreskin around penis	• Causes constriction
Priapism Painful, sustained erection of penis without sexual desire	• Erect penis • History of sickle cell anemia • History of spinal cord lesion

Genital herpes

(Continued)

Common Abnormalities *(Continued)*

ABNORMALITY	ASSESSMENT FINDINGS
Prostate Cancer Malignancy of prostate	• Symptoms same as BPH • Prostate enlarged, hard, fixed, irregular on rectal exam • Lumbosacral pain radiating to hips or legs (may be seen with metastasis)
Prostatitis Inflammation of prostate gland	• Changes in urination pattern such as frequency, urgency, hesitancy, and nocturia • Dysuria and lower back pain • Penile discharge and thin, watery, possibly blood-tinged semen • Enlarged, tender, boggy prostate (firm in chronic cases) • Fever and chills • Diminished libido, impotence • Recent urinary tract infection • Possible infertility
Spermatocele Sperm-filled cyst of epididymis	• Nontender palpable cyst in scrotum • Can be transilluminated
Syphilis Caused by *Treponema pallidum* Primary, secondary, and tertiary forms	• Primary: Genital chancre, heals without leaving a scar • Secondary: Alopecia, rash, malaise, headache, arthralgia • Tertiary: Gummas, aortic valve insufficiency, thoracic aneurysm, personality changes, ataxia, paresthesia, Charcot's joints 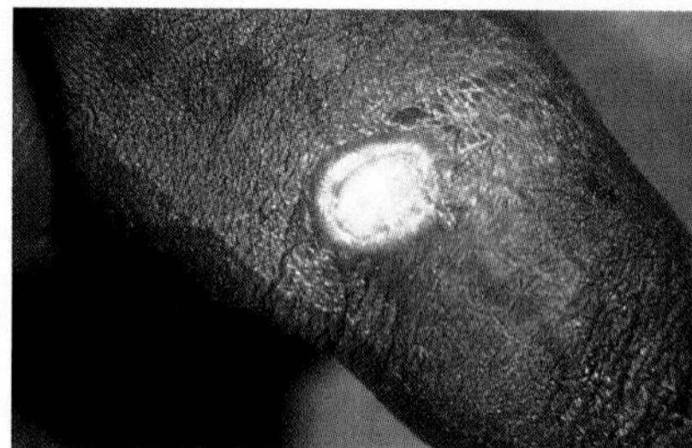 **Chancre**
Testicular Torsion Twisting of spermatic cord Surgical emergency	• Pain and swelling in testes • Nausea and vomiting 
Varicocele Varicose veins of spermatic cord	• Associated with infertility • Scrotum is purplish and soft • Scrotum feels like a "bag of worms" and collapses when it is elevated in supine position • Dull ache along spermatic cord • Slight dragging sensation in scrotum

Summary

- Assessing the male reproductive system requires knowledge of the anatomy and physiology of the male reproductive organs. These include the scrotum, testes, spermatic cord, duct system, accessory glands, lymphatic system, penis, and prostate.
- The physical assessment of the male reproductive system requires the examiner to be sensitive in responding to the client's needs for privacy.

18

Assessing the Motor-Musculoskeletal System

Before You Begin

INTRODUCTION TO THE MUSCULOSKELETAL SYSTEM

The musculoskeletal system provides shape and support to the body, allows movement, protects the internal organs, produces red blood cells in the bone marrow (hematopoiesis), and stores calcium and phosphorus in the bones. Although examining this system is usually only a small part of the overall physical assessment, everything we do depends on an intact musculoskeletal system. How extensive an assessment you perform depends largely on each patient's problems and needs.

Perform a comprehensive musculoskeletal assessment if you detect a musculoskeletal abnormality or uncover a symptom that suggests musculoskeletal involvement. Musculoskeletal problems are common in all age groups. Primary problems may result from congenital, developmental, infectious, neoplastic, traumatic, or degenerative disorders of the system itself. Secondary problems can result from disorders of other body systems.

The goal of a complete musculoskeletal assessment is to detect risk factors, potential problems, or musculoskeletal dysfunction early, and then to plan appropriate interventions, including teaching health promotion and disease prevention and implementing treatment measures. By doing so, you can play a significant role in preventing pain and dysfunction in your patients.

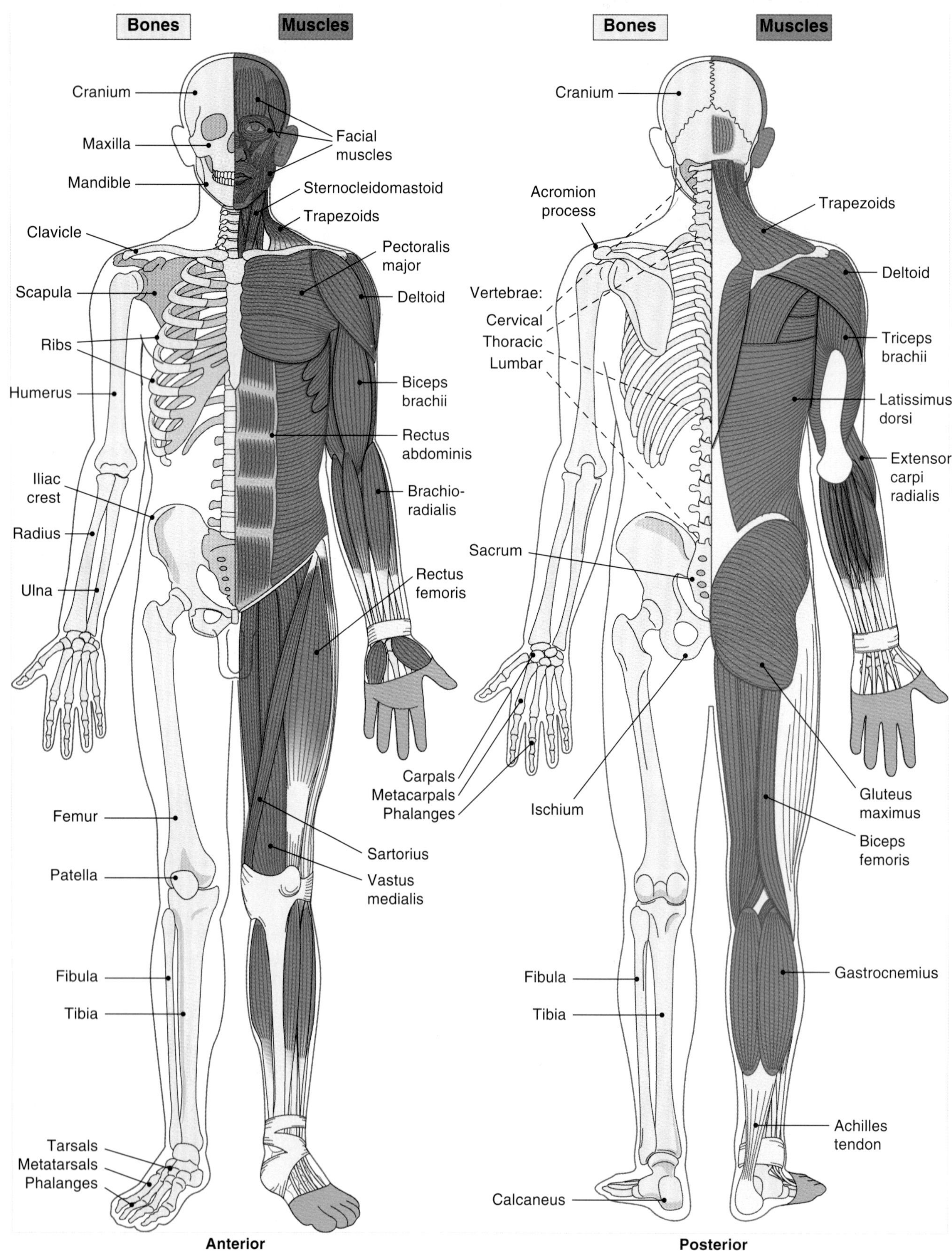

FIGURE 18–1. Cross-section of musculoskeletal system.

Anatomy and Physiology Review

Before beginning your assessment, you need to understand how the musculoskeletal system works. It consists of three major components: bones, muscles, and joints. Tendons, ligaments, cartilage, and bursae serve as connecting structures and complete the system. Figure 18–1 illustrates the musculoskeletal system, anterior and posterior views.

Bones

Composed of osseous tissue, bones are divided into two types: compact bone, which is hard and dense and makes up the shaft and outer layers, and spongy bone, which contains numerous spaces and makes up the ends and centers of the bones. Osteoblasts and osteoclasts are the cells responsible for the continuous process of creating and destroying bone. Osteoblasts form new bone tissue and osteoclasts break down bone tissue. Bones also contain red marrow, which produces blood cells, and yellow marrow, which is composed mostly of fat. The outer covering of bone is called the periosteum and contains osteoblasts and blood vessels that promote nourishment and formation of new bone tissue.

Bones vary in shape and include long bones (Fig. 18–2), such as the humerus and femur; short, flat bones, such as the sternum and ribs; and bones with irregular shapes, such as the hips and vertebrae.

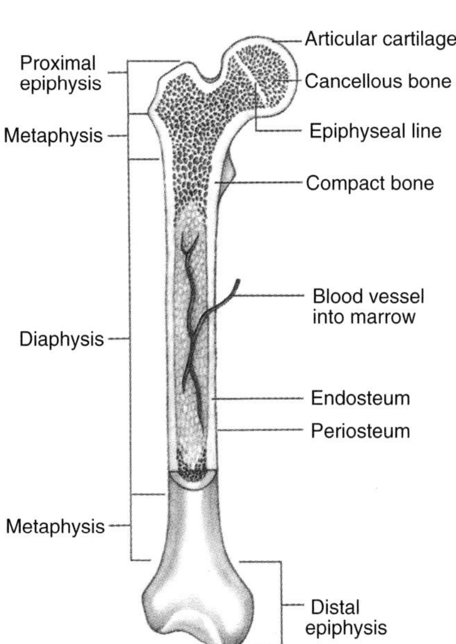

FIGURE 18–2. Cross-section of long bone.

Muscles

The body is composed of skeletal, smooth, and cardiac muscle. Made up of fasciculi (long muscle fibers) that are arranged in bundles and joined by connective tissue, skeletal muscles attach to bones by way of strong, fibrous cords called tendons. Ligaments are dense, flexible, strong bands of fibrous connective tissue that tie bones to other bones.

Cartilage is dense connective tissue consisting of fibers embedded in a strong, gel-like substance. Cartilage lacks nerve innervation, blood vessels, and lymph vessels, so it is insensitive to pain and regenerates slowly and minimally after injury. Regeneration occurs primarily at sites where the articular cartilage meets the synovial membrane. Cartilage may be fibrous, hyaline, or elastic. Fibrous cartilage forms the symphysis pubis and the intervertebral discs. Hyaline cartilage covers the articular bone surfaces (where bones meet at a joint), connects the ribs to the sternum, and is found in the trachea, bronchi, and nasal septum. Elastic cartilage is located in the auditory canal, the external ear, and the epiglottis.

Joints

The joint or articulation is the place where two or more bones meet. Joints provide range of motion (ROM) for

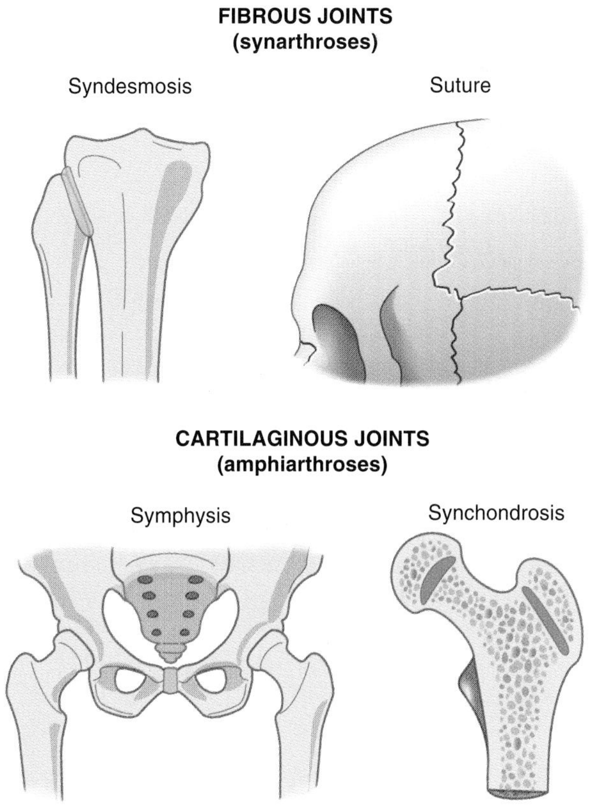

FIBROUS JOINTS (synarthroses)

Syndesmosis

Suture

CARTILAGINOUS JOINTS (amphiarthroses)

Symphysis

Synchondrosis

FIGURE 18–3. Fibrous and cartilaginous joints.

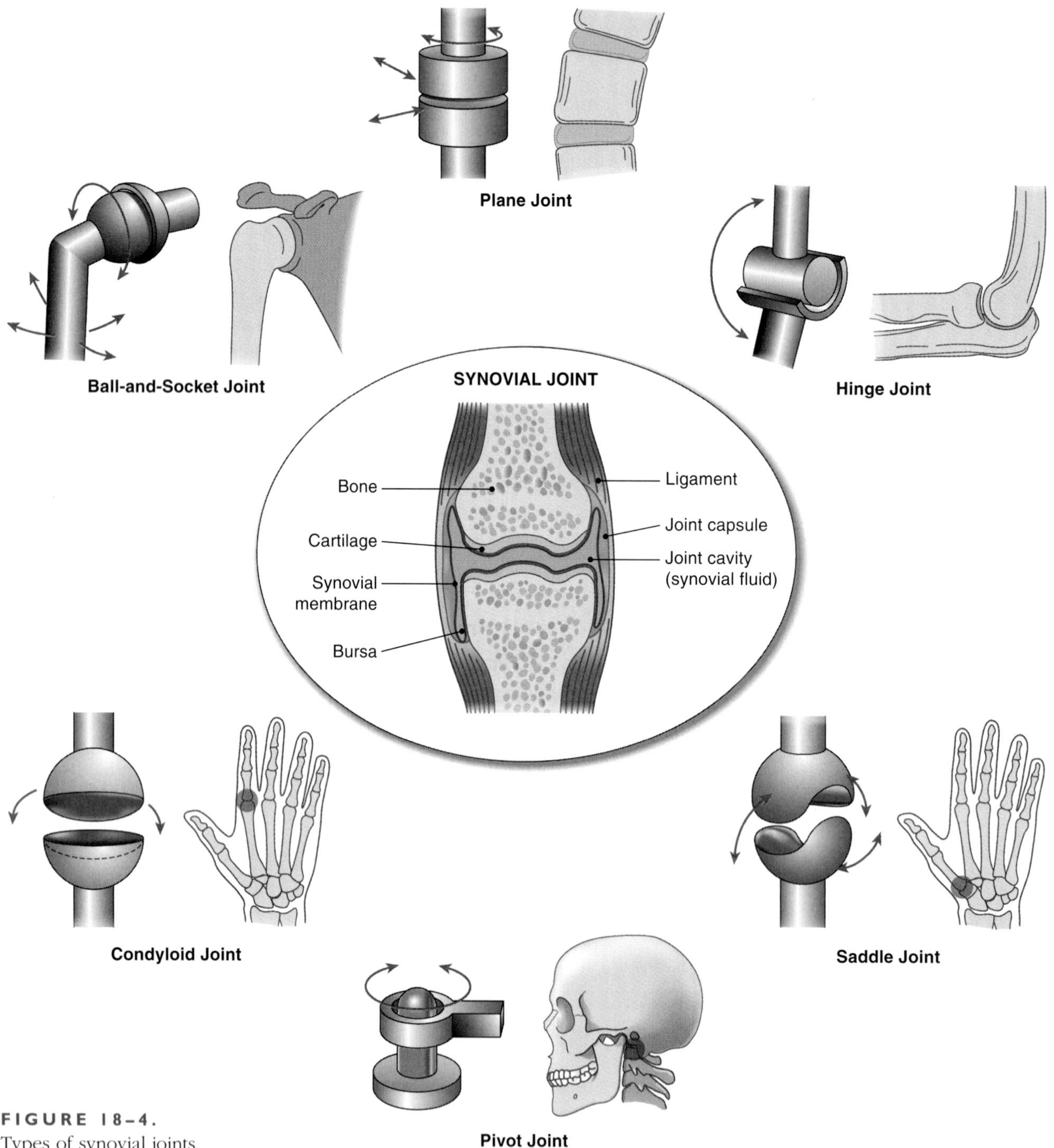

FIGURE 18–4.
Types of synovial joints.

the body parts and are classified three ways: by the degree of movement they permit, by the connecting tissues that hold them together, and by the type of motion the structure permits. Figure 18–3 illustrates the fibrous and cartilaginous joints and Figure 18–4 the synovial joints.

Bursae

Bursae are small, disc-shaped synovial fluid sacs located at points of friction around joints. They act as cushions, thereby reducing the stress to adjacent structures, and facilitate movement. Two examples of bursae are the prepatellar bursa (in the knee) and the subacromial bursa (in the shoulder).

Interaction with Other Body Systems

The neurological and respiratory systems contribute to maintaining musculoskeletal functioning. A problem in any of these systems may affect the functioning of the musculoskeletal system.

Structures and Functions of the Musculoskeletal System

STRUCTURE	FUNCTION
Bones	
206 bones make up the axial skeleton (head and trunk) and appendicular skeleton (extremities, shoulders, and hips).	Provide structure and protection, serve as levers, produce blood cells, and store calcium.
Muscles	
650 skeletal (voluntary) muscles under conscious control	Allow the body to move, stand erect, and produce body heat.
Joints (articulations)	

The place where two adjacent bones or cartilage meet	Provide range of motion for body parts
	Classification based on movement they permit:
	• *Synarthrosis:* Immovable (e.g., sutures of skull)
	• *Amphiarthrosis:* Limited movement (e.g., symphysis pubis)
	• *Diarthrosis:* Freely movable (e.g., hip)
	Classification based on connecting tissues that hold them together:
	• *Fibrous joints:* No joint cavity; fibrous connective tissue joins bones; usually allow no movement. Types include:
	  • *Sutures:* Bones fused together (e.g., skull)
	  • *Syndesmoses:* Bones very close together; held together by ligament that gives strength and support to joint and also limits movement (e.g., tibiofibular joint)
	  • *Gomphoses:* Peg and socket (e.g., root of tooth)
	• *Cartilaginous joints:* Bones joined by hyaline cartilage or fibrocartilaginous disc; allows slight movement. Types include:
	  • *Synchondrosis (primary cartilaginous joint)*: Allows for growth, but not movement (e.g., epiphyseal plate joins diaphysis and epiphysis of long bones and allows growth. Once growth is complete, joint becomes synostosic (sealed).
	  • *Symphyses (secondary cartilaginous joint)*: Articulating bones covered with hylaine cartilage; fibrocartilagenous discs that act as shock absorbers; allows for some movement (e.g., symphysis pubis moves during pregnancy to allow for fetal growth).
	• *Synovial:* Most movable and complex. Has cavity filled with lubricating (synovial) fluid to help ends of bones slide. Enclosed by fibrous capsule of connective tissue and connected to periosteum of bone. Contain free-floating synovial cells and various leukocytes that phagocytose joint debris and microorganisms. Some contain bursae. Synovial joints may be:
	  • Uniaxial: Movement limited to one axis (e.g., elbow)
	  • Biaxial: Movement on two axes (e.g., hand)
	  • Multiaxial or triaxial: Movement on three axes (e.g., shoulder)

Connecting structures	
Tendons	Connect muscles to bone. They enable bones to move when skeletal muscles contract.
Ligaments	Strong, dense bands of tissue that connect the joint (articular) ends of bones, either facilitating movement or providing stability or limiting movement.
Cartilage	Supports and shapes various structures (e.g., auditory canal), and cushions and absorbs shock that otherwise would be transmitted directly to bone (e.g., intervertebral discs).

(Continued)

Structures and Functions of the Musculoskeletal System *(Continued)*

STRUCTURE	FUNCTION
Bursae	Small, disc-shaped, flattened sacs filled with synovial fluid located at points of friction around joints. Act as cushions, reducing stress to adjacent structures and facilitating movement. Examples are prepatellar bursa in knee and subacromial bursa in shoulder.

Types of Synovial Joints

JOINT	DESCRIPTION	EXAMPLE/MOVEMENT
Pivot	Permits rotation in one axis. Axis is longitudinal with bone moving around a central axis without any displacement from that axis.	Proximal radioulnar joint **Supinates, pronates**, and rotates
Hinge	Allows movement in only one axis, namely **flexion** or **extension**, with axis situated transversely.	Elbow, knee Flexion and extension
Condyloid	Permits movement in two axes. Described as an "egg-in-spoon joint," with long diameter of oval serving as one axis, and short diameter of oval serving as other axis.	Wrist Flexion, extension, **abduction, adduction**, and **circumduction**
Saddle	Has two axis like condyloid joint. Articular surfaces are saddle shaped and move in similar fashion to condyloid joint.	Thumb Abduction, adduction, opposition, and reposition
Ball and socket	Moves across many possible axes. Articular surfaces are reciprocal segments of a sphere.	Shoulder and hip Flexion, extension, internal rotation, external rotation, abduction, adduction, and circumduction
Plane/Gliding	Moves across many axes. Articular surfaces are flat, and one bone rides over the other in many directions. Limited movement in many directions.	Patellofemoral and acromioclavicular joints, some carpal and tarsal bones, and articular vertebral processes

Neurological System

The neurological system is responsible for coordinating the functions of the skeleton and muscles. If your patient has neurological complaints, combine the musculoskeletal and neurological assessments because the spinal cord and nerves originate from the spine and innervate the musculoskeletal structures of the back and the extremities. A dysfunction in the neurological system is often reflected as pain, abnormal movement, or paresthesias in the extremities and/or back. The patient's gait may provide information on muscular weakness or neurological disease.

Back pain is a major source of disability in the United States. A large proportion of the population complains of back pain at one time or another, with the most common complaint being low back pain radiating into the hip and down the leg. This pain is usually of neurological origin and emanates from the sciatic nerve. Pain may also be caused by arthritic disease of the spine or hip or muscle spasm of the lower back. Understanding the anatomy of the back and spinal nerve tracks will help you determine the pain's origin.

Respiratory System

The respiratory system depends on the thorax, bony structures, and muscles of the chest to protect the lungs and assist with breathing. The accessory muscles, which include the sternocleidomastoid, anterior serrati, scalene, trapezius, intercostal, and rhomboid muscles, come into play when a person is involved in aerobic activities or when the body has intrapulmonary resistance to air movement (e.g., chronic pulmonary lung disease).

ENDOCRINE

MS system provides protection to endocrine structures.

Growth and sex hormones affect growth of MS system.

Thyroid/parathyroid control calcium and calcitonin.

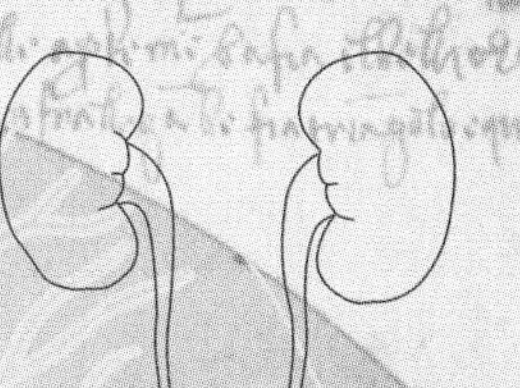

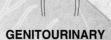

LYMPHATIC/ HEMATOLOGIC

Bone marrow produces blood cells and lymphocytes.

Lymphatic system responds as a defense for MS system.

GENITOURINARY

MS system protects renal structures.

Kidneys reabsorb calcium and phosphorus as needed.

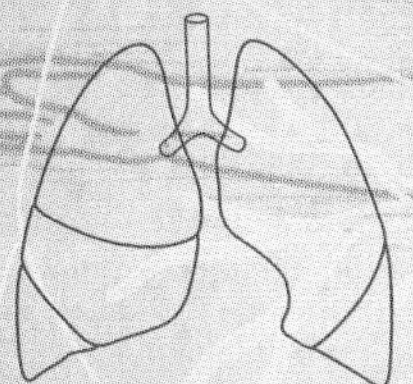

RESPIRATORY

Chest muscles and bones protect lungs.

Muscles are essential for breathing.

Respiratory system provides oxygen and removes carbon dioxide.

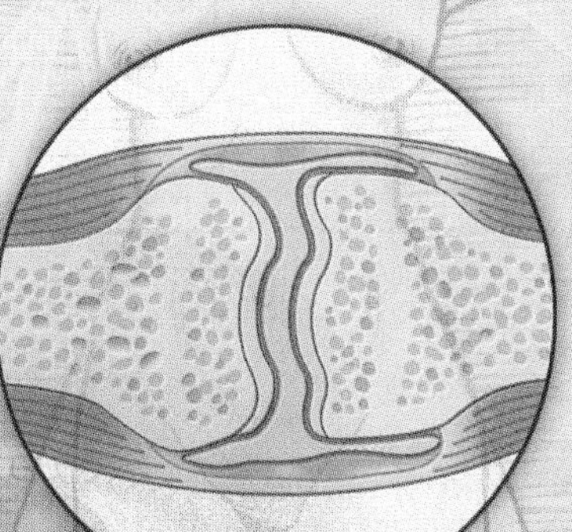

GASTROINTESTINAL

Provides nutrients to MS system, especially calcium and phosphorus.

Abdominal muscles protect abdominal structures and organs.

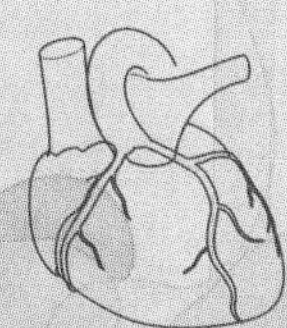

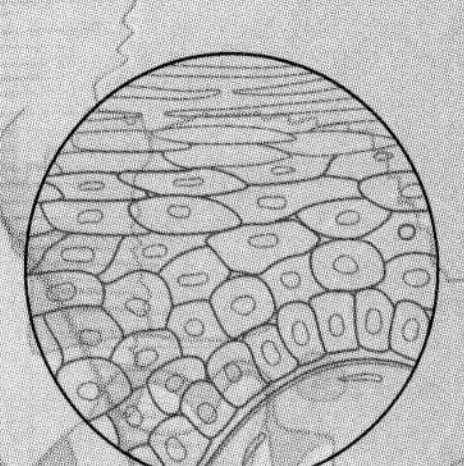

CARDIOVASCULAR

Delivers nutrients to MS system and removes wastes.

MS system provides calcium if needed for cardiac contraction.

Contraction of muscles assists with venous return.

INTEGUMENTARY

Skin provides protective covering for muscles and joints.

Skin provides vitamin D synthesis needed for calcium and phosphorus bone growth.

REPRODUCTIVE

MS system protects reproductive organs.

Sex hormones affect growth.

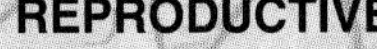

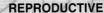

Relationship of Musculoskeletal System to Other Systems

These accessory muscles enhance ventilation by increasing chest expansion and lung size during inspiration. Intercostal muscles also coordinate rib movement; external intercostal muscles pull the ribs up and out and internal intercostals pull the ribs down and inward. Contraction of these muscles facilitates air movement into the lungs by decreasing intrathoracic pressure. As these muscles relax, exhalation occurs as the lung recoils. Abdominal muscles can also assist with deep breathing, tachypnea (rapid breathing), exercise, coughing, and sneezing. An intact thoracic cage and normal accessory and abdominal muscles are necessary for respiratory function. A musculoskeletal injury or problem in these areas can result in altered respiratory functioning.

Developmental, Cultural, and Ethnic Considerations

Infants and Children

Before birth, a skeleton forms in the fetus that is first composed of cartilage and then later ossifies into true growing bone. After birth, bone growth continues rapidly during infancy and then steadily during the childhood years. Another growth spurt occurs for both boys and girls during adolescence.

Long bones increase in diameter by depositing new bone tissue around the shafts. Lengthening occurs at the epiphyses, which are specialized growth centers (growth plates) located at the ends of long bones. Any injury or infection at these growth plates puts the growing child at risk for bone deformity. Longitudinal growth of the bones continues until closure of the epiphyses, which occurs at age 20.

Skeletal contour changes are also apparent in infants and children. At birth, the spine has a single C-shaped curve. At 3 to 4 months of age, an infant is able to raise his or her head from the prone position, allowing the development of the anterior curve in the cervical neck region. As development progresses and the infant is able to stand and walk, the anterior curve develops in the lumbar region. This occurs between 12 and 18 months of age. A toddler stands with feet wide apart to provide balance as he or she learns to walk.

The school-age child usually stands with the normal adult curvature, which should continue until old age. Throughout childhood, the skeleton continues to grow linearly; muscles and fat are responsible for significant weight increases. Individual muscle fibers continue to grow as the child grows, with a marked growth period noted during adolescence. At this time, muscles are responding to increased growth hormone, adrenal androgens, and testosterone in boys. Muscles vary in growth rate, size, and strength, depending on genetic factors, nutritional status, and amount of exercise.

Common knee deviations in children include **genu valgum** (knock knees) and **genu varum** (bowlegs). When genu valgum is present in a child, the knees touch and the medial malleoli are 2 to 3 cm or more apart when the child is standing. This variation is common during the first year when the child walks. In a child with genu varum, the knees are more than 2.5 cm apart and the medial malleoli touch when the child stands. These deviations are considered normal for a child aged 2 to 3 1/2 years and may persist until age 6.

Toddlers often have "potbellies" and **lordosis** (anterior curvature of the spine). This posture is normal and helps the child adjust to the change in the center of gravity. It should disappear as the child grows. Spinal deformities in children may be structural, but more commonly are caused by poor posture. **Scoliosis** (lateral curvature) may become apparent during adolescence, with girls at a higher risk than boys. The spine does not grow straight, and the shoulders and iliac crests are not the same height. Assessing for scoliosis is an important component when working with adolescents.

Additional history questions for parents of infants and children include:

- Was there a normal labor and delivery without trauma to the infant? (Trauma increases the risk for fractures of the humerus and clavicle.)
- Did the infant need to be resuscitated? (Anoxia may result in **hypotonia** of muscles.)
- Did the infant develop as expected?
- Has the child ever had a broken bone or dislocation? If so, how were these injuries treated?
- Have you noticed any bone deformity, spinal curvature, or unusual shape of the legs, toes, or feet?

Additional history questions for adolescents include:

- Are you involved in any sports? How often do you play or practice?
- Do you use protective or special equipment?
- Do you warm up before participating in an athletic activity?

These questions help assess the safety of the sport for the height and weight of the adolescent and gauge the risk of injuries.

Pregnant Women

Progressive lordosis is the most characteristic change in posture in pregnant women. It compensates for the enlarging fetus by shifting the center of gravity and moving the weight of the enlarging fetus back on the lower extremities. This shift in balance may create strain on the low back muscles, which may be felt as low back pain during late pregnancy. Anterior cervical flexion during the third trimester, **kyphosis** (humpback), and slumped shoulders are other postural changes that compensate for lordosis. Upper back changes may put pressure on the ulnar and median nerves, creating aching, numbness, and weakness in the upper extremities of some pregnant women. Increased mobility in the sacroiliac, sacrococcygeal, and symphysis pubis joints in the pelvis occurs in preparation for delivery, which also contributes to the characteristic waddling gait.

Older Adults

With aging, bone density decreases because loss of bone tissue occurs more rapidly than formation of new bone tissue. This results in **osteoporosis,** with women at a higher risk than men and whites more often affected than blacks.

Kyphosis with a backward head tilt to compensate and slight flexion of the hips and knees are postural changes that occur with aging. Decreased height is the most noticeable postural change. It occurs as a result of shortening of the vertebral column secondary to the loss of water content and thinning of the intervertebral discs. Both men and women can expect a decrease in height beginning in their 40s and continuing until age 60. After this age, height decreases occur secondary to osteoporotic changes in the height of individual vertebrae. This collapse of vertebrae results in a shortening of the trunk and comparatively long extremities.

Contour changes also occur as a result of the distribution of subcutaneous fat. Most men and women gain weight in their fourth and fifth decades, losing fat in the face and depositing it in the abdomen and hips. This distribution pattern continues into later years, but fat continues to decrease in the periphery, especially the forearms. The loss of subcutaneous fat in certain parts of the body contributes to marked bony prominences. The tips of the vertebrae, ribs, and iliac crests may become very noticeable and the body hollows (e.g., cheeks and axillae) become deeper. There is loss of muscle mass, a decrease in muscle size, and some muscle **atrophy,** which contributes to generalized weakness. These muscle changes can cause decreased agility; an abnormal gait with uneven rhythm and short steps; and a wide base of support. Other complicating factors include fear of falling, osteoporosis, painful arthritic joints, poor vision, and peripheral neuropathy.

Lifestyle can affect the musculoskeletal changes that occur with aging. A sedentary lifestyle leads to decreased muscle mass and strength and increased muscle atrophy. Decreased speed and strength, resistance to fatigue, reaction time, and coordination are changes that can be prevented by physical exercise. Physical activity also prevents or delays bone loss in aging adults.

Additional history questions for the aging adult should elicit information about loss of function, self-care deficits, or safety risks that may occur as a result of aging, injury, or illness. Ask the following questions:

- Have you broken any bones recently? If so, how?
- Have you noticed any weakness over the past months?
- Have you had any increase in stumbling or falls?
- Do you use mobility aids like a cane or walker to help you get around?

People of Different Cultures/Ethnic Groups

When assessing the musculoskeletal system, you need to consider your patient's ethnicity because it can affect musculoskeletal anthropomorphic and physical characteristics.

Culturally Bound Musculoskeletal Health Problems

CULTURAL GROUP	HEALTH PROBLEM
African-Americans	Tendency toward **hyperplasia** (overgrowth) of connective tissue accounts for increased incidence of systemic lupus erythematosus (SLE). Greater bone density than Europeans, Asians, and Hispanics accounts for decreased incidence of osteoporosis.
Amish	Dwarfism syndrome found in nearly all Amish communities.
Chinese-Americans	Generally shorter than Westerners. Bone structure also differs from that of Westerners: • Ulna longer than radius • Hip measurements smaller (females 4.14 cm smaller; males 7.6 cm smaller) • Bone length shorter • Bone density less
Egyptian-Americans	Relatively short in stature. Average adult height for males 5′ 10″; for females 5′4″.

(Continued)

Culturally Bound Musculoskeletal Health Problems *(Continued)*

CULTURAL GROUP	HEALTH PROBLEM
Filipino-Americans	Short in stature. Average adult height ranges from 5′ to average American size.
Irish-Americans	Taller and broader than average European-American and Asian. Hip width greater. Bone density less than that of African-Americans.
Navajo Native Americans	Taller and thinner than other Native American tribes. Noted for being good runners.
Vietnamese-Americans	Small in stature. Average adult height 5′ for women with men being a few inches taller.

Source: Adapted from Purnell and Paulanka, 1998.

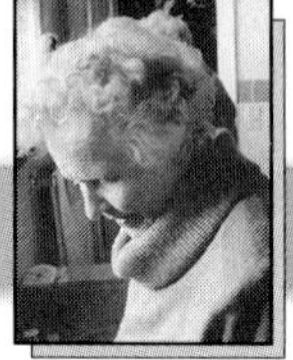

Introducing the Case Study

Maria O'Malley, age 68, is concerned with osteoporosis because she is postmenopausal and feels as though she is "shrinking." Before her routine physical examination, Mrs. O'Malley begins to ask questions about how osteoporosis occurs, what can be done to treat it, and what complications can occur from having it.

Performing the Musculoskeletal Assessment

Health History

Obtaining a thorough and accurate health history is crucial to your assessment of the musculoskeletal system. As the health history interview progresses, clarify exactly what the patient means by certain subjective complaints, including the location, character, and onset of any symptoms. Only the patient can give you data regarding pain, stiffness, ability to move, and how daily activities have been affected. The history provides the subjective data that will direct the physical examination.

Biographical Data

A review of the biographical data may identify patients who are at risk for musculoskeletal problems. Consider the patient's age, sex, marital status, race, ethnic origin, and occupation as possible risk factors. For example, women are at a higher risk than men for osteoporosis and rheumatoid arthritis (RA); an occupation that requires heavy lifting increases the risk for injury to muscles, joints, and supporting structures; and the risk for degenerative joint disease (osteoarthritis) increases with age. Even a patient's address may have significance. For example, Lyme disease, which has musculoskeletal repercussions, is endemic on the northeast coast from Massachusetts to Maryland, in the midwest states of Wisconsin and Minnesota, and on the west coast from northern California to Oregon.

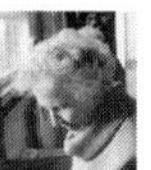

Case Study Findings

Reviewing Mrs. O'Malley's biographical data:

- 68-year-old Caucasian female, widow
- Works as housekeeper for parish priest
- Born and raised in the United States, Polish descent, Catholic religion
- Current health insurance: Medicare parts A and B, supplemented with Medicaid
- Source: Self, seems reliable

Current Health Status

Begin your assessment with questions about the patient's current health status, because he or she is most interested in this. The major symptoms to watch for, in order of importance, are pain, weakness, and stiffness.

Symptom Analysis

Symptom Analysis tables for all of the symptoms described in the following paragraphs are available on the Web for viewing and printing. In your web browser, go to *http://www.fadavis.com/detail.cfm?id=0882-9* and click on Symptom Analysis Tables under Explore This Product.

Pain

Pain can result from bone, muscle, or joint problems. Bone pain is not usually associated with movement unless there is a fracture, but muscle pain is. Current or recent illness can cause muscle aches. Bone pain is deep, dull, and throbbing; muscle pain takes the form of cramping or soreness. In rheumatoid arthritis, joint pain and stiffness are worse in the morning. In osteoarthritis, the joints are stiff after rest and pain is worse at the end of the day.

Weakness

Muscle weakness associated with certain diseases migrates from muscle to muscle or to groups of muscles. Knowing the symptom patterns and when they occur can help identify the disease process responsible for weakness. Identifying the weakness related to proximal or distal muscle groups is also helpful. Proximal weakness is usually a myopathy; distal weakness is usually a neuropathy.

Be sure to ask the patient if the weakness interferes with his or her ability to perform everyday activities. For example, proximal weakness of the upper extremities often presents itself as difficulty lifting objects or combing hair. Proximal weakness of the lower extremities presents as difficulty with walking and crossing the knees. Patients with polymyalgia rheumatica have proximal muscle weakness. A distal weakness of the upper extremities is manifested by difficulty in dressing or turning a doorknob. Patients with myasthenia gravis have difficulty with diplopia, swallowing, and chewing along with generalized muscle weakness.

Stiffness

Stiffness is a common musculoskeletal complaint. It is important to ascertain if the stiffness is worse at any particular time of the day. For example, patients with RA are stiff on arising because of the period of joint rest that occurs during sleep.

Balance and Coordination Problems

Problems with balance and coordination often indicate a neurological problem. These problems often manifest as gait problems or difficulty in performing activities of daily living (ADLs). The patient may complain of falling or losing balance or may have **ataxia**—irregular and uncoordinated voluntary movements. Gait problems are associated with cerebellar disorders, Parkinson's disease, MS, herniated disc, cerebrovascular accident (CVA), Huntington's chorea, brain tumor, inner ear problems, medications, and exposure to chemical toxins.

Other Related Symptoms

Certain musculoskeletal diseases may produce multiple symptoms. For example, acute rheumatic fever, gout, and autoimmune inflammatory diseases may cause fever and joint pain. A woman with back pain and vaginal discharge may have a gynecological disease. Lower back pain and weight loss suggest tuberculosis of the spine. Bowel and bladder dysfunction suggest a herniated disc. Therefore, also ask the patient: "Do you have a sore throat, fever, joint pain, rash, weight loss, diarrhea, numbness, tingling, or swelling?"

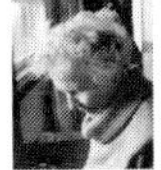

Case Study Findings

Mrs. O'Malley's current health status includes:

- "Several-year" history of aching joints in the evening after working all day.
- Discomfort first occurred in back and neck.
- Takes over-the-counter analgesic for pain with some relief.

Past Health History

After taking the past health history, compare it with the patient's present musculoskeletal status or uncover risk factors that might predispose the patient to musculoskeletal disorders.

Past Health History

RISK FACTORS/ QUESTIONS TO ASK	RATIONALE/SIGNIFICANCE
Childhood Illnesses	
Do you have a history of juvenile RA (JRA)?	Thirty percent of children with JRA have symptoms as adults. Residual deformities from JRA may be seen in adults.
Do you have cerebral palsy? Muscular dystrophy?	History of childhood musculoskeletal problems may account for current physical findings.
Surgery	
Have you ever had surgery or other treatment involving bones, muscles, joints, or other supporting structures?	Provides baseline information for physical assessment and explains physical findings.

(Continued)

Past Health History *(Continued)*

RISK FACTORS/ QUESTIONS TO ASK	RATIONALE/SIGNIFICANCE
Diagnostic Procedures	
Postmenopausal women: Have you ever had a dexa scan?	Perimenopausal and postmenopausal women should be screened for osteoporosis.
Serious Injuries	
Have you had any past problems or injuries to your joints, muscles, or bones? If so, what? What treatment was given?	Data on past injuries or problems provide baseline data for physical assessment.
Do you have any residual effects from the injury or problem?	Past trauma may affect ROM.
Serious/Chronic Illnesses	
Do you have any other medical problems?	SLE can cause arthritis, synovitis, and myositis.
Have you had a recent infection?	HIV increases risk for infectious arthritis, osteomyelitis, and polymyositis. RA and SLE may improve with HIV. Lyme disease can cause migratory joint and muscle pain; if untreated, can lead to arthritis. TB can affect bones and joints. Neuropathies associated with diabetes can lead to muscle atrophy and neuropathic arthropathy (Charcot's joint). Tertiary syphilis can also cause Charcot's joints. Recent infections such as Epstein-Barr virus may trigger RA.
Immunizations	
What immunizations have you had and when? Have you been immunized against tetanus and polio?	Tetanus and polio have symptoms that mimic other musculoskeletal disorders. Immunization information can aid in differential diagnoses.
Allergies	
Are you allergic to dairy products? Do you have lactose intolerance?	Allergies to dairy products or lactose intolerance may lead to inadequate calcium intake. Patients who are immobile or who have a reduced intake of calcium and vitamin D are especially prone to osteoporosis.
Medications	
Are you taking any prescribed or over-the-counter medications?	Certain medications can affect the musculoskeletal system. See box, Drugs That Adversely Affect the Musculoskeletal System, on p. 601.
Middle-aged women: Are you menopausal? Are you receiving estrogen replacement therapy?	Women who begin menopause early are at greater risk for osteoporosis because of decreased estrogen levels, which tend to decrease bone mass density.
Recent Travel/Military Service/ Exposure to Infectious or Contagious Diseases	
Have you been hiking or camping recently?	Lyme disease is endemic in certain areas of the country.
Were you ever in the military?	Exposure to chemicals during military service may manifest in MS symptoms.

Drugs That Adversely Affect the Musculoskeletal System

Drug Name	Drug	Possible Adverse Reactions
Adrenocorticosteroids	prednisone	Muscle weakness, muscle wasting, osteoporosis, vertebral compression fractures, aseptic necrosis of humeral or femoral heads
Adrenocorticotropic hormone (ACTH)	corticotropin	Muscle weakness, muscle wasting, osteoporosis, vertebral compression fractures, aseptic necrosis of humeral or femoral heads
Anticoagulants	heparin sodium	Bleeding into joints with high dosages
Anticonvulsants	phenytoin sodium	Ataxia, osteomalacia (softening of the bones), rickets
Antidepressants	trazadone hydrochloride	Musculoskeletal aches and pains
Antigout agents	colchicine	Myopathy with prolonged administration
Antilipemic agents	clofibrate	Acute flulike muscular syndrome characterized by myalgia (muscle pain) or myositis with symptoms of muscle cramps, weakness, and arthralgia
Benzodiazepines	diazepam	Ataxia
Central nervous system stimulants	amphetamine sulfate	Increased motor activity
Diuretics	bumetanide, furosemide	Muscle cramps
Phenothiazines	chlorpromazine hydrochloride	Extrapyramidal symptoms (dystonic reactions, motor restlessness, and Parkinsonian signs and symptoms)
Miscellaneous skin agents	isotretinoin	Bone or joint pain, general muscle aches

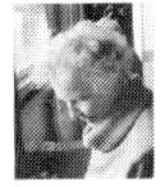

Case Study Findings

Mrs. O'Malley's past health history reveals:

- History of hypertension (HTN).
- Wrist fracture at age 65, caused by a fall on the ice. No pinning was performed.
- Cholestectomy at age 52, appendectomy at age 8, hysterectomy at age 35.
- Vaginal deliveries of 2 children with no complications.
- Denies allergies to food, drugs, or environmental factors.
- Medications include Zestril 10 mg once daily for hypertension and Alleve once daily for arthritic pain.

Family History

The purpose of the family history is to identify predisposing or causative factors for musculoskeletal problems. After assessing the current and past musculoskeletal health status, investigate possible familial tendencies toward problems.

Family History

RISK FACTORS/ QUESTIONS TO ASK	RATIONALE/SIGNIFICANCE
Familial Musculoskeletal Problems Do you have a family history of gout, arthritis, or osteoporosis?	Positive family history for these diseases increases risk to patient.

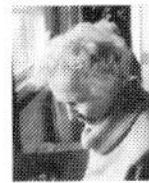

Case Study Findings

Mrs. O'Malley's family history reveals:

- Positive history of osteoporosis and HTN.
- Mother had osteoporosis and HTN; died of cardiac problems at age 82.
- Father had HTN and died of heart attack at age 65.
- Sister, age 72, positive for osteoporosis and HTN.
- One daughter and one son, alive and well.
- All other known relatives alive and well.

Review of Systems

The review of systems (ROS) allows you to assess the interrelationship of the musculoskeletal system to every other system. Often you may uncover important facts that your patient failed to mention earlier.

Review of Systems

SYSTEM/QUESTIONS TO ASK	RATIONALE/SIGNIFICANCE
General Health Survey	
How have you been feeling?	*Fatigue/activity intolerance:* RA, SLE, and Lyme disease.
Have you had any changes in weight or height?	Obesity is risk factor for DJD, osteoarthritis, and low back pain. *Anorexia/weight loss:* RA. *Loss of height:* Osteoporosis.
Have you had a fever?	RA, Lyme disease.
Integumentary	
Have you had any rashes or lesions?	*Bull's-eye rash:* Lyme disease. *Ulcers and subcutaneous rheumatoid nodules on forearm and elbow:* RA. *Butterfly facial rash:* SLE.
Have you had a change in hair growth or hair loss?	*Patchy alopecia and short broken hair above forehead:* SLE.
HEENT/*Head and Neck*	
Do you have any swollen glands or nodes?	*Enlarged lymph nodes:* Systemic infection. *Lymphadenopathy:* RA. Enlarged thyroid can affect musculoskeletal system.
HEENT/Eyes, Ears, Nose, and Throat	
Do you have dry eyes or mouth?	Sjögren's syndrome causes dry mouth and eyes and is associated with RA.
Do you have red eyes?	*Episcleritis and keratoconjunctivitis:* RA.
Respiratory	
Do you have any breathing problems?	*Interstitial fibrosis and pleuritis:* RA. *Pneumonitis and pleural effusion:* SLE.
Cardiovascular	
Do you have any cardiovascular problems?	Rheumatoid heart disease associated with RA.
Have you had changes in the color of your hands in response to cold?	*Pericarditis, myocarditis, Raynaud's disease:* RA and SLE.
Gastrointestinal	
Do you have abdominal pain, diarrhea, nausea, vomiting, or difficulty swallowing?	*GI complaints:* SLE.
Do you have any bowel problems or incontinence?	*Bowel problems, incontinence, loss of bowel function:* Cauda equina syndrome caused by compression of sacral nerve, as can occur with a herniated disc or spinal stenosis.
Genitourinary	
Do you have blood in your urine?	*Hematuria:* SLE.
Reproductive	
Do you have a history of sexually transmitted diseases (STDs)?	Tertiary syphilis can cause ataxia and Charcot's joints.
Women: Are you menopausal? If yes, are you on hormone replacement therapy (HRT)?	Postmenopausal women at greater risk for osteoporosis.
Do you have menstrual irregularities?	Menstrual irregularities are associated with SLE.
Do you have any gynecological disorders or vaginal discharge?	Gynecological disorders such as PID or ovarian cancer may cause back pain.
Neurological	
Do you have any loss of sensation, numbness, or tingling?	*Loss of sensation:* Herniated disc. *Neuropathies:* RA, SLE.

Review of Systems

SYSTEM/QUESTIONS TO ASK	RATIONALE/SIGNIFICANCE
Paralysis?	Paralysis can lead to muscle atrophy from disuse. Tertiary Syphilis can cause ataxia and Charcot's joints.
Endocrine	
Do you have diabetes mellitus?	Diabetes can cause neuropathies and muscle wasting.
Do you have thyroid disease?	Hypothyroidism can cause weakness, muscle aches, pain and arthralgia. Hyperthyroidism can cause osteoporosis.
Immune/Hematologic	
Do you have sickle cell anemia?	Can cause joint pain.
Do you bruise easily?	SLE can cause thrombocytopenia.

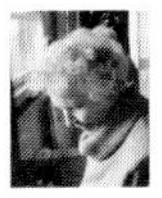

Case Study Findings

Mrs. O'Malley's review of systems reveals:

- **General Health Survey:** Describes usual state of health as "fair."
- **Integumentary:** Reports no changes in skin, hair, or nails.
- **HEENT:** Complains of pain and stiffness in neck; no swollen glands.
- **Respiratory:** No respiratory problems.
- **Cardiovascular:** Positive history of HTN, controlled with medication.
- **Gastrointestinal:** No abdominal problems.
- **Genitourinary:** No problems.
- **Reproductive:** Postmenopausal since age 35.
- **Neurological:** No changes in sensations.
- **Endocrine:** No history of diabetes or thyroid disease.
- **Immune/Hematological:** No infections or bleeding.

Psychosocial Profile

The psychosocial profile can reveal patterns in the patient's life that may affect the musculoskeletal system and put him or her at risk for musculoskeletal disorders.

Psychosocial History

CATEGORY/QUESTIONS TO ASK	RATIONALE/SIGNIFICANCE
Health Practices and Beliefs/ Self-Care Activities	
What do you do to promote the health of your musculoskeletal system?	Helps identify health promotion and preventive activities.
Do you get an annual physical exam?	
Do you wear protective equipment when playing sports?	
Do you understand proper body mechanics?	
Typical Day	
How would you describe your typical day?	MS problems, such as arthritis, may affect ability to perform ADLs. Sedentary lifestyle increases risk of osteoporosis. Prolonged immobility leads to muscle wasting. Impairment of musculoskeletal system may impair ability to perform normal activities. Assess for correct use of assistive devices.
Nutritional Patterns	
What did you eat in the last 24 hours?	Assess diet for adequate vitamin/mineral intake:
Do you drink milk?	Calcium deficiency increases risk of osteoporosis. Adequate protein promotes healthy muscle tone and bone growth.

(Continued)

Psychosocial History *(Continued)*

CATEGORY/QUESTIONS TO ASK	RATIONALE/SIGNIFICANCE
Nutritional Patterns *(Continued)*	
	Diet high in purines (organ meats and sardines) can trigger gouty arthritis. Obesity is risk factor for osteoarthritis and low back problems.
Have you lost or gained weight recently? If so, how much?	Weight loss associated with RA.
Activity/Exercise Patterns	
Do you exercise? How much and what type?	Exercise is important to a healthy musculoskeletal system. Moderate exercise builds up and maintains bone mass. Strenuous exercise increases risk for injury. Regular exercise promotes strength and flexibility and can help slow musculoskeletal changes associated with aging.
Recreation/Hobbies	
Do you participate in sports or activities that require heavy lifting?	Recreational activities may increase risk for injury.
Do you wear protective equipment?	Use of protective equipment decreases risk of trauma.
Do you participate in outdoor activities, such as hiking or camping?	Lyme disease is caused by deer ticks.
Sleep/Rest Patterns	
How many hours of sleep do you get per night?	Musculoskeletal pain may interfere with sleep. Patients with herniated discs may have trouble finding comfortable sleeping position.
Personal Habits	
Do you smoke?	Cigarette smoking increases risk of osteoporosis.
Do you drink alcohol or caffeinated beverages?	Alcohol and caffeine are risk factors for osteoporosis and gout.
Do you use drugs?	Drug use increases risk of HIV, which is associated with inflammatory arthritis.
Occupational Health Patterns	
What type of work do you do? Does it involve lifting or repetitive movements?	Occupations that require physical labor increase risk for musculoskeletal problems. Repetitive motion increases risk for carpal tunnel syndrome.
How would you describe your usual posture?	Poor body posture and body mechanics can lead to back problems.
What kind of shoes do you wear to work?	High-heeled shoes can lead to contracture of the Achilles tendon.
Have you ever lost work time because of a musculoskeletal problem?	Musculoskeletal problems may prevent patient from returning to previous work.
Are you exposured to toxic chemicals at work?	Arsenic and mercury can cause ataxia.
Environmental Health Patterns	
Where do you live?	Helps determine discharge planning needs.
How many stairs do you have to climb?	
Roles/Relationships/Self-Concept	
How did you view yourself before you had this problem, and how do you view yourself now?	Musculoskeletal deformities or disabling or crippling problems may affect patient's self-image and cause low self-esteem.

Psychosocial History

CATEGORY/QUESTIONS TO ASK	RATIONALE/SIGNIFICANCE
Roles/Relationships/Self-Concept *(Continued)*	
Have musculoskeletal problems interfered with your ability to interact with others?	Chronic musculoskeletal problems can disable the patient and impair socialization and independence.
Cultural Influences	
What is your ethnic background?	Osteoporosis has a higher incidence among Caucasians. Asians and African-Americans have 10% more bone density than whites.
Sexuality Patterns	
Have musculoskeletal problems interfered with your usual sexual activity?	Back problems, joint pain, and stiffness may interfere with sexual activities.
Social Supports	
Who are your supports?	Identifying supports is helpful in planning care.
Stress and Coping	
How do you deal with stress?	Stress can exacerbate SLE and precipitate RA.

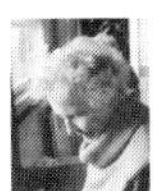

Case Study Findings

Mrs. O'Malley's psychosocial profile includes:

- Has a yearly exam because of HTN. Has not seen a gynecologist since her hysterectomy. Visits family physician every 3 months for HTN check.
- Arises at 6 AM. Does chores around own home and dresses for work. Workday is 9 AM to 5 PM. Typical day consists of daily chores around employer's home, including cooking, cleaning, and running errands. After work, she relaxes and watches the news and some television shows before going to bed at 9 PM.
- Admits she is a "tea and toast lady." Lives alone, so if she cooks, it is something quick, unless she goes out to eat with friends or family. Drinks two to four cups of caffeinated coffee a day. Has never been overweight.
- Activities include housecleaning and running errands uptown. No formal exercise program.
- Has no pets. Knits for a hobby while watching TV. Occasionally has dinner out or sees a movie with friends or family.
- Sleeps 4 to 5 hours uninterrupted, but often gets up at night to void.
- Denies smoking, alcohol use, or illicit drug use.
- Job requires some lifting (e.g., carrying vacuum cleaner upstairs) as well as bending.
- Says her self-esteem is "pretty good." Says she feels proud she can still earn a living. Admits she worries about living alone and developing health problems as she gets older, especially those that limit her mobility.
- Lives alone in a ranch home in suburbs; no steps. Is not afraid to be alone because of good neighbors.
- Has lunch or dinner once a week with daughter or son. Talks on phone to sister several times a week. Has friends in neighborhood, including younger neighbors who check on her.
- Copes with stress by talking with children or priest.

Focused Musculoskeletal History

If your patient's condition or time restraints prohibit a detailed musculoskeletal history, take a focused history instead. The patient's response to the questions below will help direct your assessment:

- Do you have a history of musculoskeletal problems, pain, or disease? If yes, are you taking any medications or undergoing any treatments?
- Do you have any other medical problems?
- Have any accidents or trauma ever affected your bones or joints?
- Do your joint, muscle, or bone problems limit your usual activities?
- Do you have any occupational hazards that could affect your muscles and joints?
- Have you been immunized for tetanus and polio?
- Do you smoke or consume alcohol or caffeine? If yes, how much and how often?

Case Study Evaluation

Before you move on to the physical examination, consider what you have learned from your interview with Mrs. O'Malley and document her musculoskeletal history:

CRITICAL THINKING ACTIVITY #1

Based on her health history, what musculoskeletal problem do you think Mrs. O'Malley is at risk for? What are the risk factors?

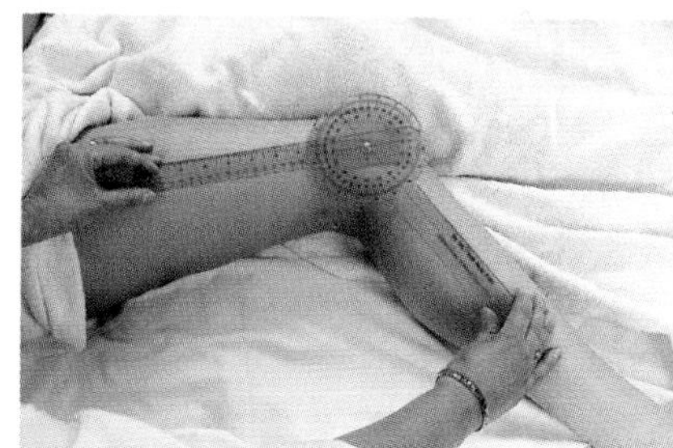

FIGURE 18–5. Using a goniometer.

Physical Assessment

Now that you have collected the subjective data, begin collecting the objective data by means of the physical examination. Keep all pertinent history findings in mind as you proceed. These findings, along with those from the physical examination, will complete the assessment picture. Then you can analyze the data, formulate nursing diagnoses, and develop a plan of a care. Because a musculoskeletal problem might be present, you will need to know normal musculoskeletal function before you can determine abnormal findings. The anatomy will direct your assessment.

Approach

Physical assessment of the musculoskeletal system provides data on the patient's posture, gait, cerebellar function and bone structure, muscle strength, joint mobility, and ability to perform ADLs. You will use inspection, palpation, and percussion to assess the musculoskeletal system. Be systematic in your approach, working from head to toe and comparing one side to the other. Inspect and palpate each joint and muscle; then assess ROM and test muscle strength. Perform inspection and palpation simultaneously during this assessment.

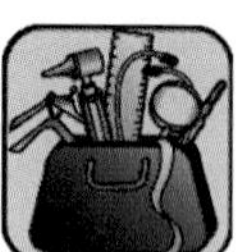

Toolbox

You will use a tape measure and a goniometer. Use the tape measure to measure limb lengths and circumferences. Use the goniometer to measure joint ROM (Fig. 18–5). To obtain a goniometer reading, match the angle of the joint being measured to the arms of the goniometer; then describe the limited motion of the joint in degrees.

Performing a General Survey

Before examining specific areas, scan the patient from head to toe, looking for general appearance and signs of musculoskeletal problems. For example:

- Obtain the patient's vital signs. Elevations in temperature are associated with Lyme disease, RA, and infections such as osteomyelitis.
- Be alert for signs of pain or discomfort as your patient performs ROM. If signs or symptoms of pain are present with movement, never force a joint.

Performing a Head-to-Toe Physical Assessment

Now look for changes in every system that might signal a musculoskeletal problem.

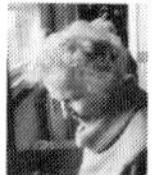

Case Study Findings

Mrs. O'Malley's physical assessment findings include:

- **General Health Survey:** Well-developed 68-year-old white female in no acute distress
- **Vital Signs:** Temperature 98.7°F; pulse 78 BPM, strong and regular; respirations 18/min., unlabored; BP 148/68; height 5′ 5″; weight 125 lb (1 1/2″ height loss since onset of menopause)
- **Integumentary:** Skin intact, no lesions; hair evenly distributed, no alopecia
- **HEENT:** No palpable nodes, nonpalpable thyroid; eyes clear and bright, no redness or drainage
- **Respiratory:** Lungs clear
- **Cardiovascular:** Heart rate, 80 with regular rhythm, +S4; +2 pulses, extremities warm, no edema
- **Gastrointestinal:** Abdomen slightly rounded, positive bowel sounds, no organomegaly
- **Genitourinary/Reproductive:** No lesions
- **Neurological:** No weakness or paralysis; positive sensation

Performing a Focused Physical Assessment

Now that you have looked at the relationship of the musculoskeletal system to all other systems, focus on the specifics of the examination. Proceed in this order:

- Assess posture, gait, and cerebellar function.
- Measure limbs.
- Assess joints and test joint movement.
- Assess muscle strength and ROM.
- Perform additional tests to assess for wrist, spine, hip, and knee problems, if necessary.

Performing a Head-to-Toe Physical Assessment

SYSTEM/NORMAL FINDINGS	ABNORMAL/RATIONALE
General Health Survey *INSPECT* Well-developed; no acute distress.	Obesity associated with osteoarthritis.
Integumentary *INSPECT* No rashes or lesions; hair evenly distributed; no alopecia.	*Bull's-eye rash:* Lyme disease. *Butterfly rash, patchy alopecia:* SLE.
HEENT/*Head,Face, Neck* *INSPECT/PALPATE* Facial expression appropriate; thyroid and nodes not palpable.	*Masklike facial expression:* Parkinson's disease. *Enlarged lymph nodes:* Infection, RA. *Weakness, pain with weight bearing, osteoporosis, decreased muscle tone:* Hyperthyroidism. *Muscle weakness and cramps, difficulty walking:* Hypothyroidism.
HEENT/*Eyes* Eyes clear and bright.	*Red eye (episcleritis)*: RA.
Respiratory *PALPATE/AUSCULTATE* Respiratory rate 18 breaths per minute. Lungs clear.	*Interstial fibrosis:* RA. *Pleural effusion, pneumonitis:* SLE.
Cardiovascular *AUSCULTATE* Regular heart rate and rhythm.	*Pericarditis, myocarditis, Raynaud's disease:* RA and SLE.
Gastrointestinal *INSPECT/PALPATE/AUSCULTATE* Positive bowel sounds; abdomen soft, nontender.	*GI complaints:* SLE.
Genitourinary/Reproductive *INSPECT* No lesions.	STDs, such as syphilis, can cause tabes dorsalis, ataxia, areflexia, and damaged joints (Charcot's joint).
Neurological *INSPECT* Sensory intact; no numbness, paralysis, or parasthesia.	Decreased sensations and numbness associated with neuropathies. Paralysis can result in muscle atrophy.

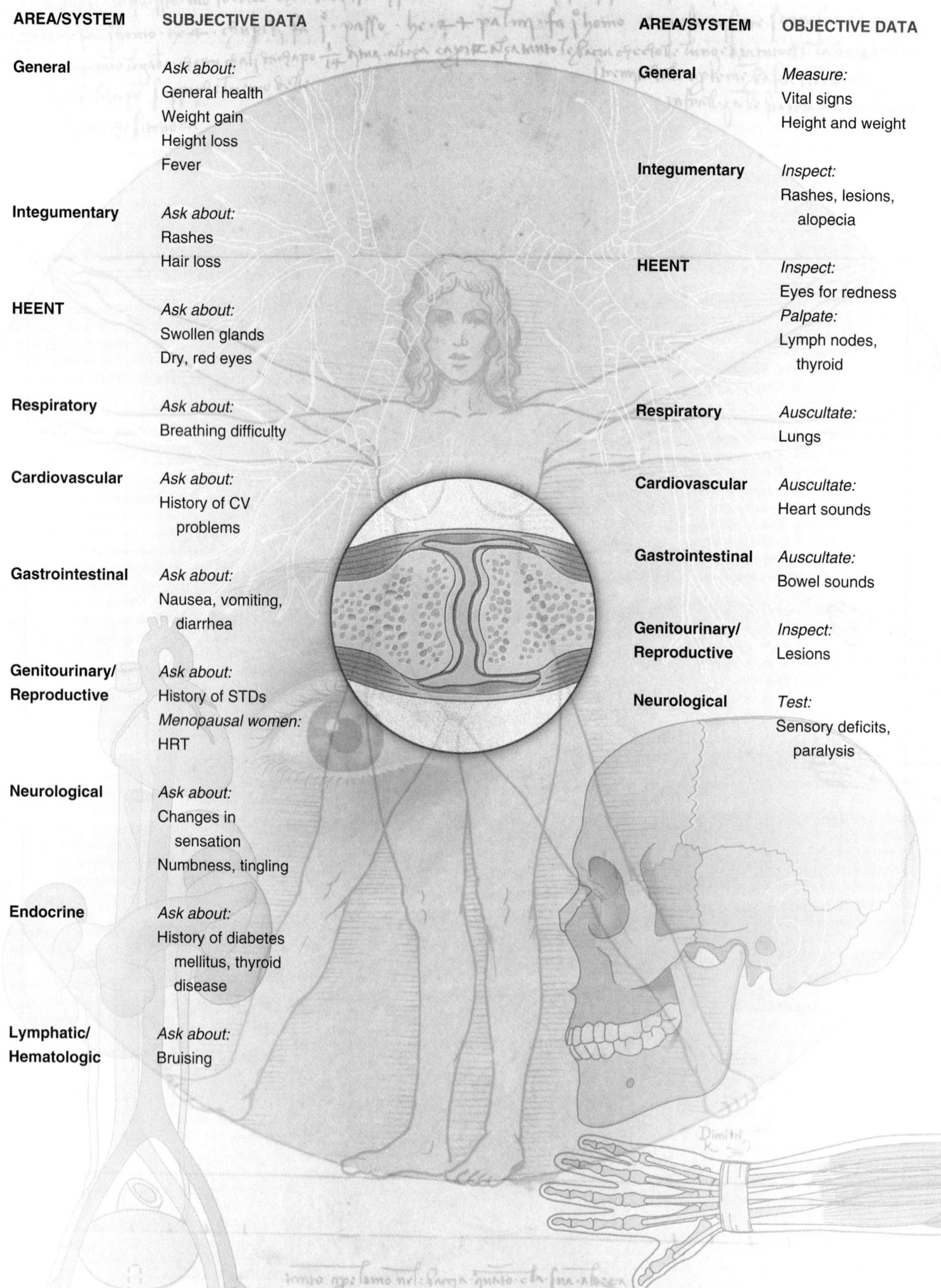

AREA/SYSTEM
SUBJECTIVE DATA
General
Ask about:
General health
Weight gain
Height loss
Fever
Integumentary
Ask about:
Rashes
Hair loss
HEENT
Ask about:
Swollen glands
Dry, red eyes
Respiratory
Ask about:
Breathing difficulty
Cardiovascular
Ask about:
History of CV problems
Gastrointestinal
Ask about:
Nausea, vomiting, diarrhea
Genitourinary/ Reproductive
Ask about:
History of STDs
Menopausal women:
HRT
Neurological
Ask about:
Changes in sensation
Numbness, tingling
Endocrine
Ask about:
History of diabetes mellitus, thyroid disease
Lymphatic/ Hematologic
Ask about:
Bruising
AREA/SYSTEM
OBJECTIVE DATA
General
Measure:
Vital signs
Height and weight
Integumentary
Inspect:
Rashes, lesions, alopecia
HEENT
Inspect:
Eyes for redness
Palpate:
Lymph nodes, thyroid
Respiratory
Auscultate:
Lungs
Cardiovascular
Auscultate:
Heart sounds
Gastrointestinal
Auscultate:
Bowel sounds
Genitourinary/ Reproductive
Inspect:
Lesions
Neurological
Test:
Sensory deficits, paralysis

Assessments of Musculoskeletal System,s Relationship to Other Systems

Assessing Posture, Gait, and Cerebellar Function

Posture

Begin by assessing your patient's posture, or his or her position in relation to the external environment. Posture should be erect, with the head midline. The spine is best assessed with the patient standing. Inspect from the front, back, and side, looking for alignment and noting symmetry of shoulders, scapula, and iliac crests. Adults have four normal curvatures. The cervical and lumbar curves are concave and the thoracic and sacral curves are convex. When assessing for spinal curvature deformities, it is important to determine if the deformity is structural or functional (postural) in nature.

To assess for kyphosis and scoliosis, have the patient bend forward from the waist with his or her arms relaxed and dangling. Then stand behind the patient to check for curvatures. The curvatures disappear in functional kyphosis and scoliosis but remain in the structural form. To assess for lordosis, have the patient stand against a wall and flatten his or her back against it. If you can freely slide your hand through the lumbar curve, the patient has structural lordosis. An alternative method is to have the patient lie supine with the knees slightly flexed and attempt to flatten his or her lumbar curve. If he or she can, the lordosis is functional.

Next, have your patient stand erect with the feet together and note the position of the knees. Are the knees midline? Draw an imaginary line from the anterior superior iliac crest to the feet. Normally, this line should transect the patella. Note if the patella deviates away from the midline. Normally, the knees should be less than 2.5 cm (1″) apart and the medial malleoli (ankle bones) less than 3 cm (1 1/8″) apart.

Gait

Next, assess your patient's gait. Pay particular attention to the base of support (distance between the feet) and stride length (distance between each step). Is there a wide base of support? The average base of support for an adult is about 2 to 4 inches. The average stride length for an adult is about 12 to 14 inches. Stride length depends in part on leg length, so the longer the legs, the greater the stride length.

HELPFUL HINT

A wide base of support and shortened stride length often reflect a balance problem.

Also pay attention to the phases of the gait—stance and swing. The stance phase has four components: heel strike, foot flat, midstance, and push-off. During midstance, the weight shifts to bearing the full body weight. The swing phase has three components: accelerate, swing-through, and decelerate. Figure 18–6 illustrates the

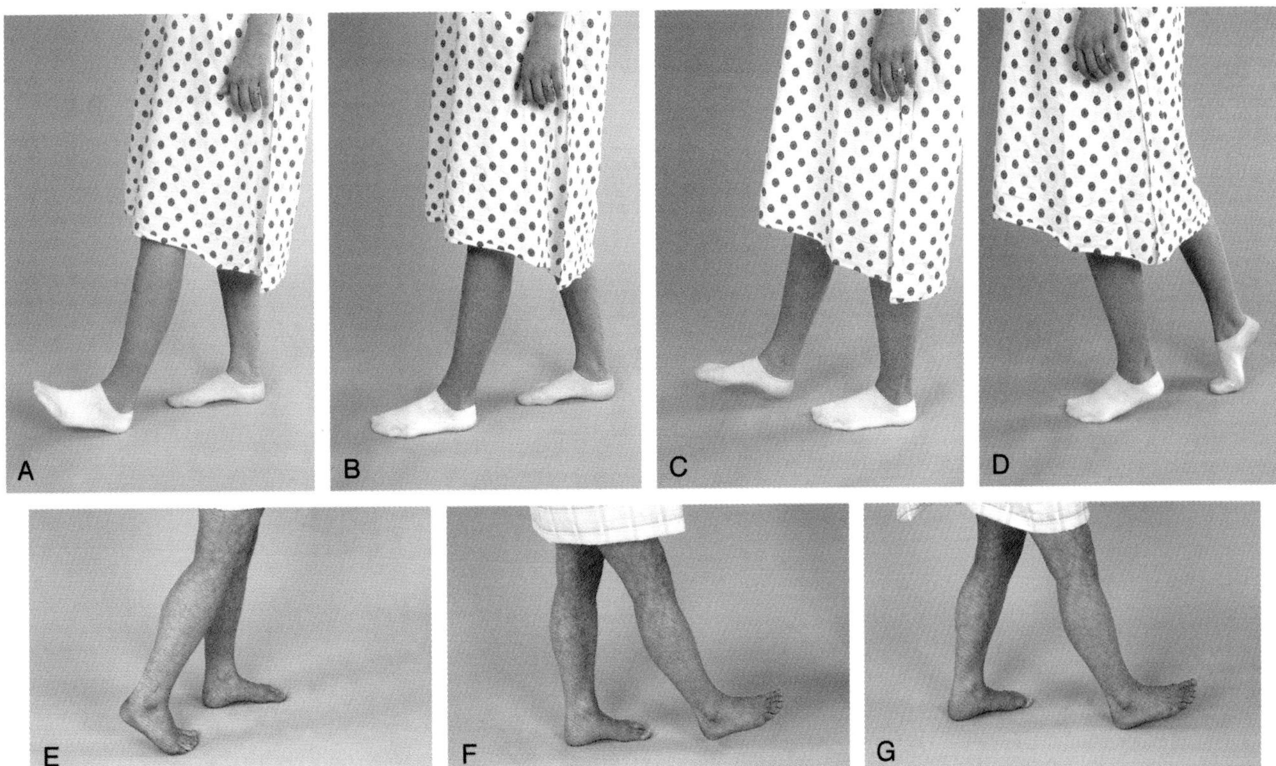

FIGURE 18–6. Stance phase: (*A*) Heel strike. (*B*) Foot flat. (*C*) Midstance. (*D*) Push-off. Swing phase: (*E*) Accelerate. (*F*) Swing-through. (*G*) Decelerate.

two phases and their components. If you do not detect a gait problem, chart "phases conform." If you do detect a problem, try to identify the specific portion of the gait that is abnormal. For example, someone with left-sided weakness from a cerebrovascular accident (CVA) may have problems with the acceleration portion of the swing phase and the midstance portion of the stance phase. Continue to observe your patient's gait, taking note of posture and cadence as he or she walks. Ask yourself: Do the arms swing in opposition? Is there toeing in or out? Are movements smooth and coordinated?

HELPFUL HINT

- Inspect the soles of your patient's shoes. How they wear is a good indicator of gait problems.
- When performing the Romberg test, stand nearby in case the patient loses his or her balance.

Cerebellar Function

Now, assess cerebellar function, including balance, coordination, and accuracy of movements.

Balance

To assess balance, look at your patient's gait. If he or she has a gait problem, you will be unable to proceed further. If there are no gait problems, have the patient tandem (heel-to-toe) walk, heel-and-toe walk, hop in place, do a deep knee bend, and perform the Romberg test. To perform the Romberg test, have the patient stand with feet together and eyes open; then have him or her close the eyes. If cerebellar function is intact, he or she will be able to maintain balance with minimal swaying with eyes closed (negative Romberg test). Keep in mind that balance problems may also occur with inner ear disorders.

Coordination

Next, assess coordination. Note the patient's dominant side. Usually this side is more coordinated. To test upper extremity coordination, have the patient perform rapid alternating movements (RAMs) by patting his or her thigh with one hand, alternating between the supinate and pronate hand position. Have him or her perform finger-thumb opposition to further test hand coordination. To test lower extremity coordination, have the patient perform rhythmic toe tapping and then run the heel of one foot down the shin of the opposite leg. Remember to test each side separately and compare findings.

Accuracy of Movements

Point-to-point localization is used to assess accuracy of movements. Have the patient touch his or her finger to the nose with the eyes open, then closed. Or have him or her touch your finger at various positions.

Assessing Posture, Gait, and Cerebellar Function

ASSESS/NORMAL VARIATIONS	ABNORMAL FINDINGS/RATIONALE
Posture	*Spinal deformities include:* *Kyphosis:* Accentuated thoracic curve. *Scoliosis:* Lateral "S" spinal deviation.

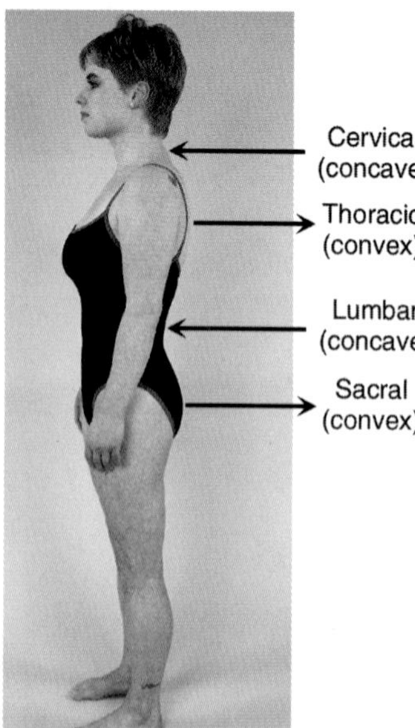

Assessing for normal curves

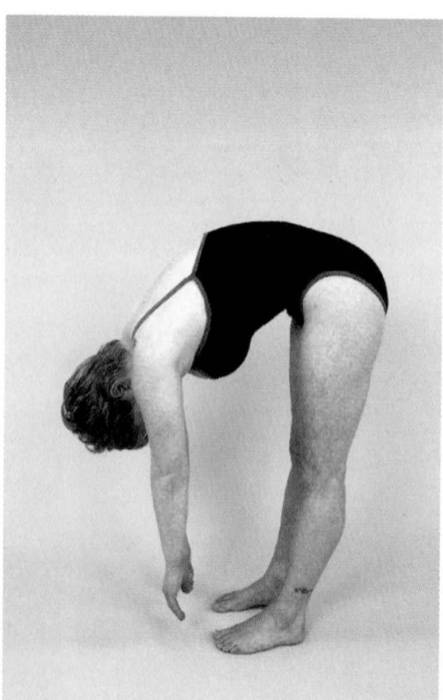

Assessing for kyphosis and scoliosis

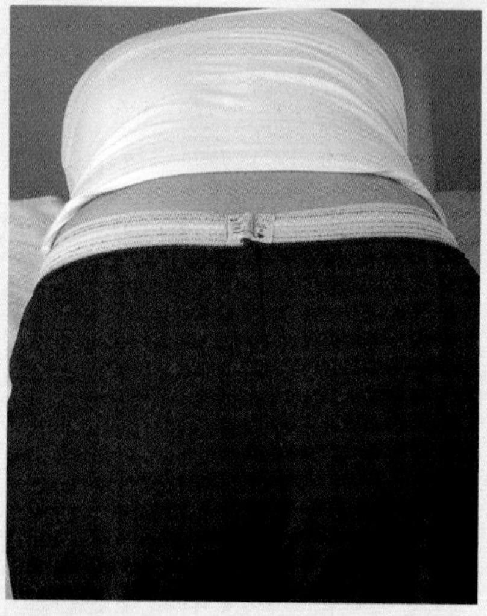

Scoliosis

Assessing Posture, Gait, and Cerebellar Function

ASSESS/NORMAL VARIATIONS

Posture *(Continued)*

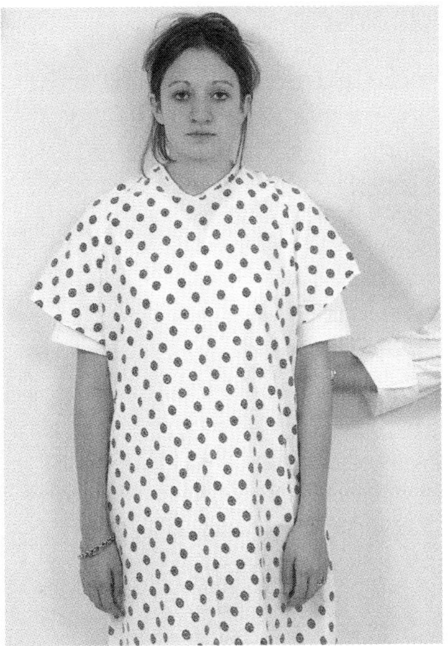

Assessing for lordosis

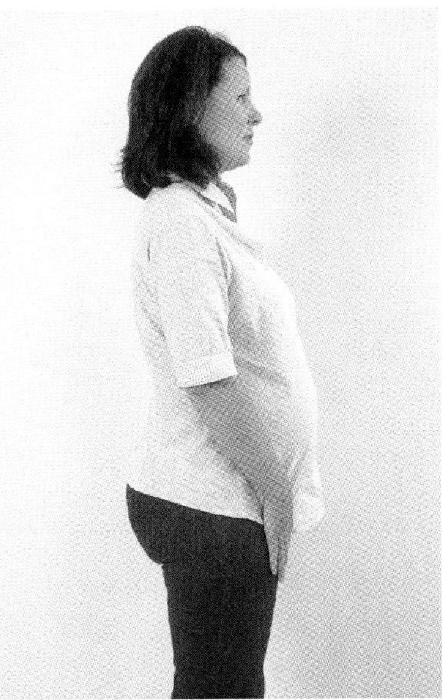

Pregnancy lordosis

Posture erect, head midline, four normal spinal curves.

In pregnancy, accentuated lumbar curve (lordosis) with a compensatory cervical flexion is normal to compensate for change in center of gravity.

In newborns, C-shaped spine without cervical curve is normal. Cervical curve develops once infant begins to hold head upright.

In toddlers, lordosis is normal as they learn to walk.

Senile kyphosis may occur in older patients.

Some African-Americans have accentuated lumbar curves.

Knees midline.

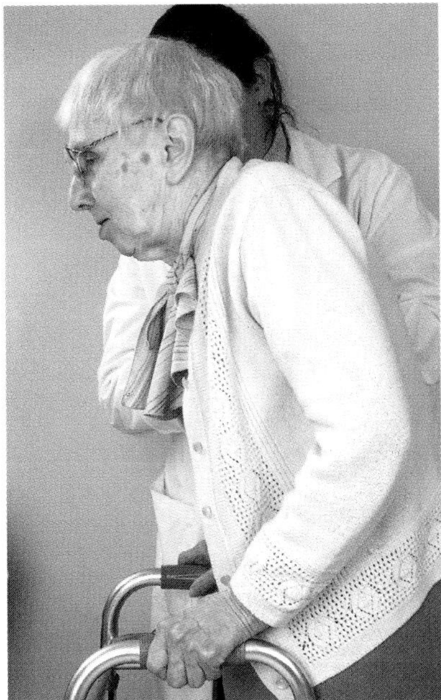

Senile kyphosis

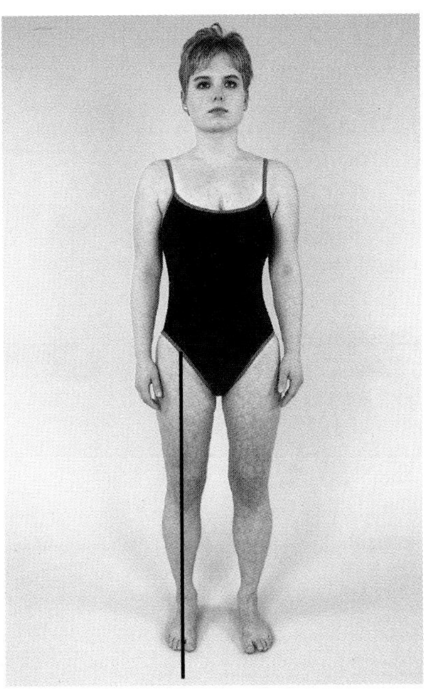

Assessing for deviation of knees

ABNORMAL FINDINGS/RATIONALE

HELPFUL HINT

To differentiate structural from functional scoliosis, have patient bend at waist. In true structural scoliosis, deviation is apparent. In functional scoliosis, deviation disappears.

Lordosis: Accentuated lumbar curve.

(Continued)

Assessing Posture, Gait, and Cerebellar Function *(Continued)*

ASSESS/NORMAL VARIATIONS	ABNORMAL FINDINGS/RATIONALE

Posture *(Continued)*

Genu valgum and genu varum often seen in toddlers and preschoolers, but should not persist beyond age 6.

Genu valgum: Knees touch and medial malleoli are 2 to 3 cm or more apart.

Genu varum: Knees are greater than 2.5 cm (1 inch) apart and medial malleoli touch.

Gait

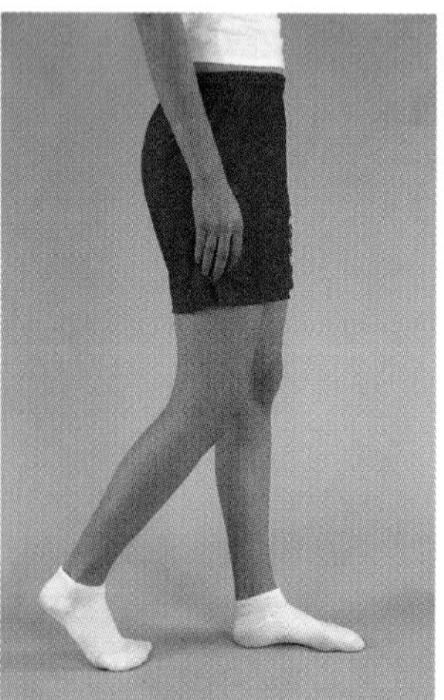

Observing gait

HELPFUL HINT

To inspect gait, observe patient as he or she walks into the examination room.

Posture erect, head midline, phases conform, weight evenly distributed, both feet point straight ahead, no toeing in or out, all movements coordinated and rhythmic, arms swing in opposition, stride length appropriate.

In pregnancy, with older patients, and in toddlers learning to walk, wider base of support gives greater stability and is normal.

Uneven weight bearing: Associated with joint pain.

Gait disorders such as wide base of support: Associated with cerebellar dysfunction.

Ataxia *(impaired coordinated movement with erratic muscular activity),* ***spasticity*** *(increased tone or contractions of muscles causing stiff, awkward movements), and tremors:* Parkinson's disease, MS, CP.

Scissors gait (legs cross over): Disorders of motor cortex or corticospinal tracts, such as bilateral spastic paresis.

Spastic movements: Upper motor neuron disorders.

Flaccidity (defective or absent muscle tone): Lower motor neuron disorders.

Flaccidity and ***foot drop*** *(affected leg drags and is unable to clear during swing phase):* Peripheral nerve disorders.

Cerebellar Function

Balance

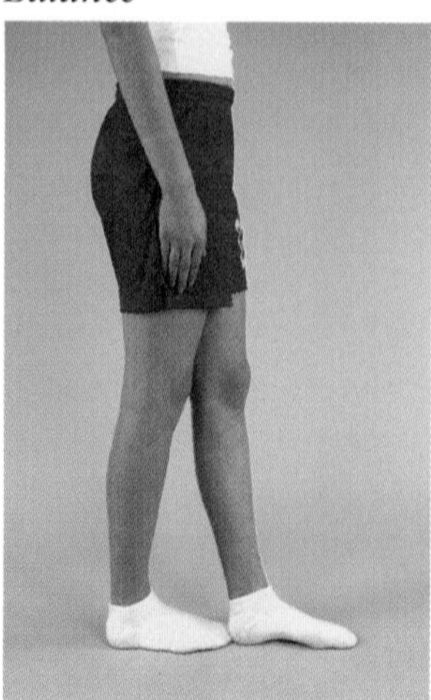

Tandem walking

Balance problems: Cerebellar disorder.

Positive Romberg Test: Cerebellar disorder if patient has difficulty maintaining balance with eyes open or closed. If the patient loses balance only when eyes are closed, there may be damage to the dorsal column.

Assessing Posture, Gait, and Cerebellar Function

ASSESS/NORMAL VARIATIONS	ABNORMAL FINDINGS/RATIONALE

Cerebellar Function *(Continued)*

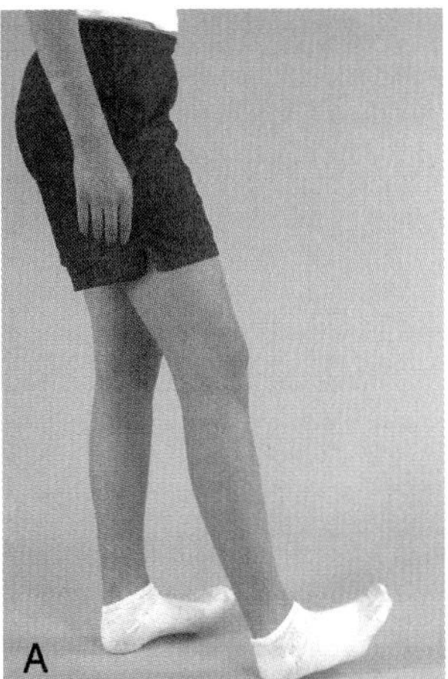

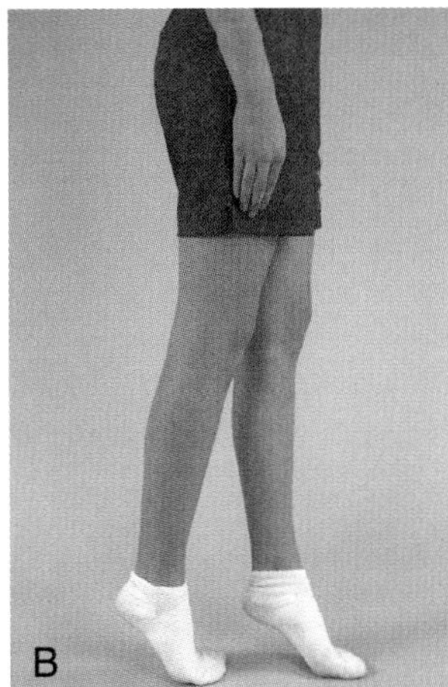

Heel-and-toe walking. A. Walking on heels, B. Walking on toes

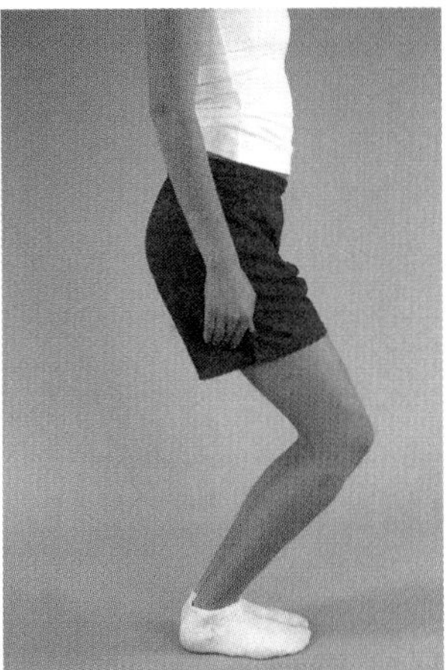
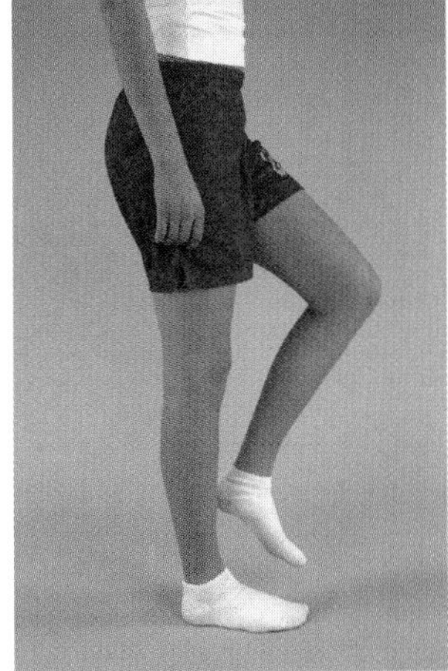

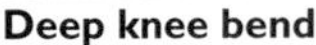
Deep knee bend

Hopping in place

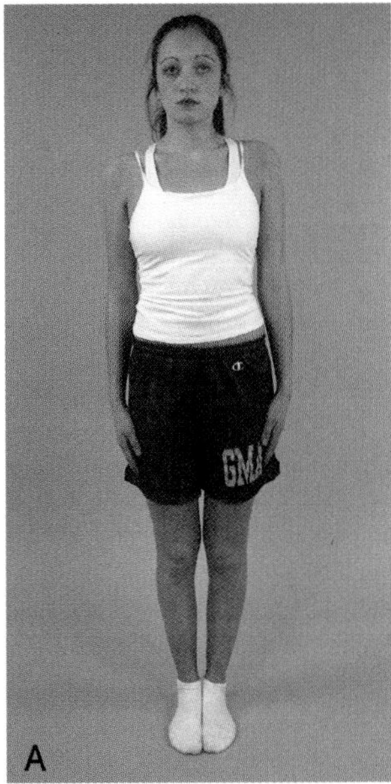

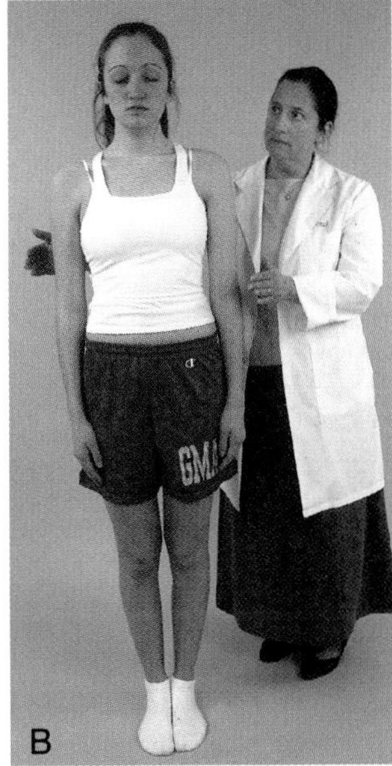

Romberg test. A. Eyes open, B. Eyes closed

(Continued)

Assessing Posture, Gait, and Cerebellar Function *(Continued)*

ASSESS/NORMAL VARIATIONS

Cerebellar Function *(Continued)*

Balance intact. Patient can tandem walk, heel-and-toe walk, perform deep knee bend, and hop in place. Negative Romberg test.

Cerebellar function cannot be tested on infants under 3 months. Instead, observe sucking, swallowing, and kicking movements to estimate cerebellar function.

Cerebellar function cannot be tested on toddlers because of their immature neuromuscular system.

Coordination

Upper extremities:

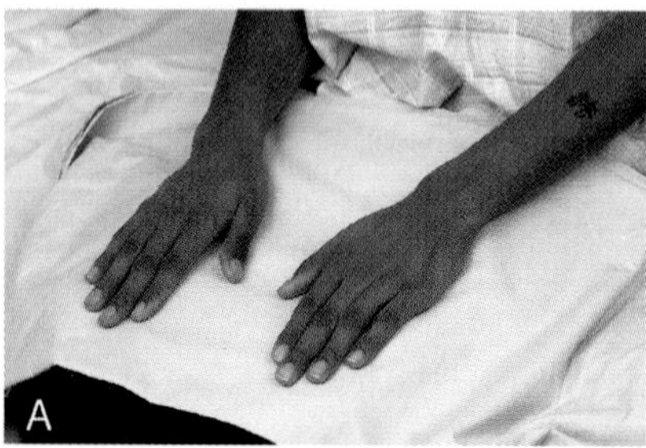

RAMs. A. Pronate position,

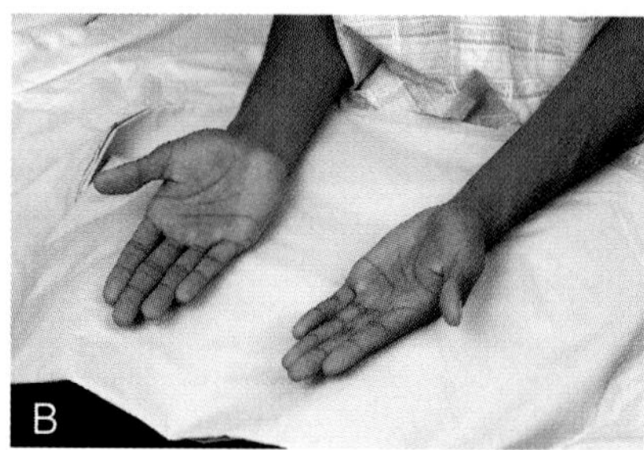

B. Supinate position

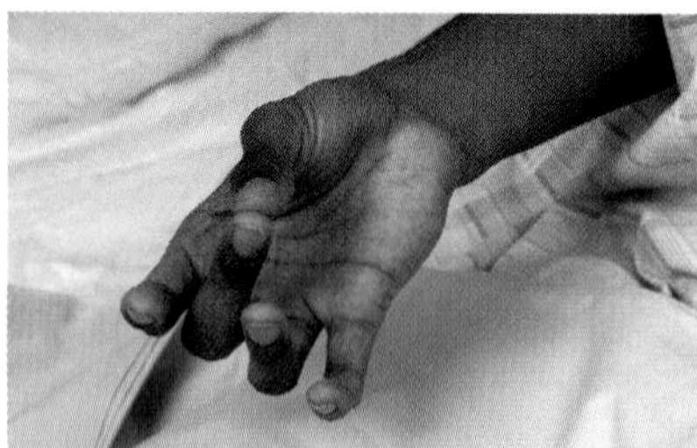

Finger-thumb opposition

Lower Extremities:

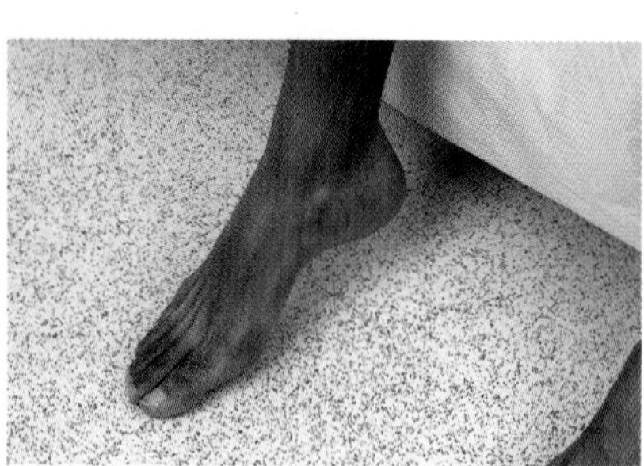

Toe tapping

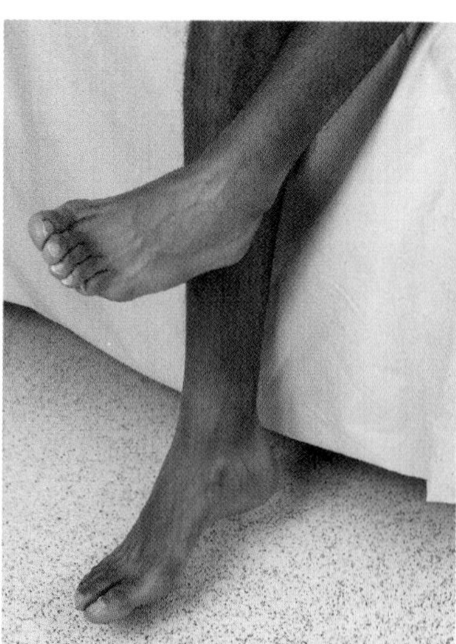

Running heel down shin

ABNORMAL FINDINGS/RATIONALE

Slowness and awkwardness in performing movements: Cerebellar disorder or motor weakness associated with extrapyramidal disease.

Assessing Posture, Gait, and Cerebellar Function

ASSESS/NORMAL VARIATIONS	ABNORMAL FINDINGS/RATIONALE
Cerebellar Function *(Continued)* Upper and lower extremity movements coordinated. Right side dominant and slightly more coordinated. Positive RAM. Positive finger-thumb opposition, toe tapping, and heel down shin.	
Accuracy of movement	*Inaccurate movements:* Cerebellar disorder.

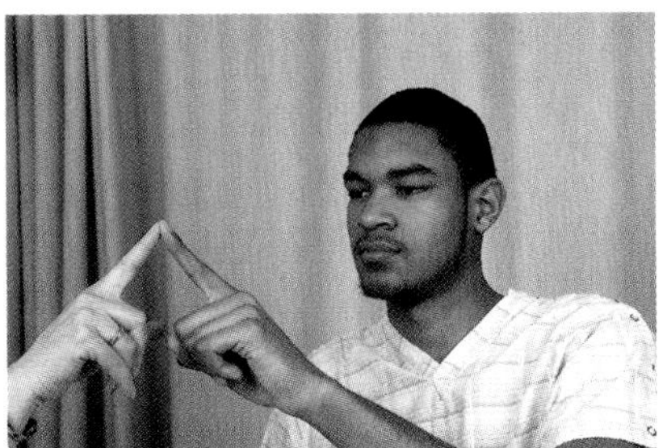

Finger to finger

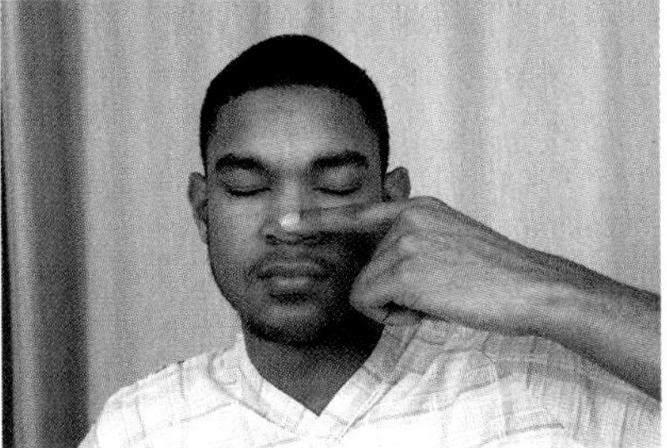

Finger to nose

Movements accurate.

Abnormal Gaits

Type of Gait	Description/Cause	Type of Gait	Description/Cause
Propulsive gait	Rigid, stooped posture with head leaning forward and arms, knees, and hips stiffly flexed. Rapid, short, shuffling steps. *Causes:* Parkinson's disease (classic gait).	**Scissors gait**	Bilateral spastic paresis of legs; arms not involved. Legs flexed at hip and knees. Knees adduct and meet or cross like scissors. Short steps, foot plantarflexed, walks on toes. *Causes:* CP, MS, spinal cord tumors.

(Continued)

Abnormal Gaits *(Continued)*

Type of Gait	Description/Cause	Type of Gait	Description/Cause
Spastic gait (hemiplegic)	Unilaterally stiff, dragging leg from leg, muscle **hypertonicity.** *Causes:* CVA, MS, brain tumor.	**Steppage gait (equine, prancing, paretic, or weak)**	Foot drop with external rotation of hip and hip and knee flexion. Foot slaps when it hits ground. *Causes:* MS, herniated lumbar disc, Guillain-Barré syndrome, perineal muscle atrophy, or nerve damage.
Waddling gait	Ducklike walk with wide base of support, chest thrown back, exaggerated lumbar curve (lordosis), and protruding abdomen. Normal in toddlers and late stages of pregnancy. Weak pelvic girdlle muscles (gluteus medius, hip flexors, and extensors). *Causes:* MS, hip dislocation.		

Taking Limb Measurements

Limb measurements include both length and circumference. Measure arm lengths from the acromion process to the tip of the middle finger. Measure leg lengths from the anterior superior iliac crest crossing over the knee to the medial malleolus. This is referred to as true leg length. An apparent leg length measurement is measured from a fixed point, the umbilicus, to the medial malleolus. Discrepancies between right and left should not exceed more than 1 cm. Obviously, a leg length discrepancy usually results in clinical problems such as gait disorders or hip or back pain.

Limb circumference reflects actual muscle size or muscle mass. Measure circumference on forearms, upper arms, thighs, and calves. Take note of the patient's dominant side, which may normally be up to 1 cm larger than his or her nondominant side. To ensure accurate circumference measurement, determine the midpoint of the extremity being assessed. For example, if you are measuring upper arm circumference, measure the distance from the acromion process to the olecranon process, and use the midpoint to determine circumference; then do the same for the opposite arm.

Taking Limb Measurements

ASSESS/NORMAL VARIATIONS	ABNORMAL FINDINGS/RATIONALE
Length *Arms:*	

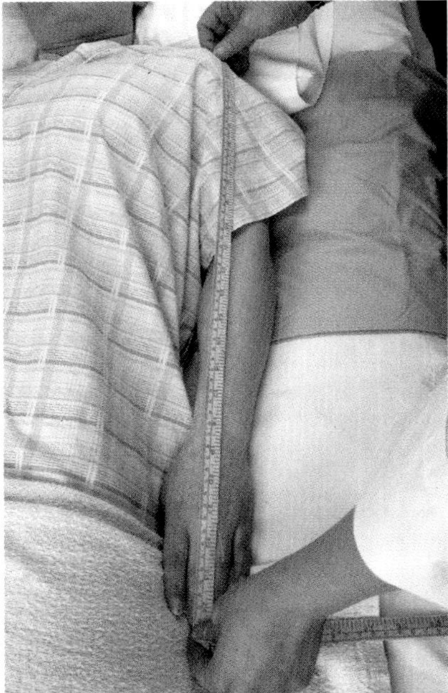

Measuring arm length

Legs:

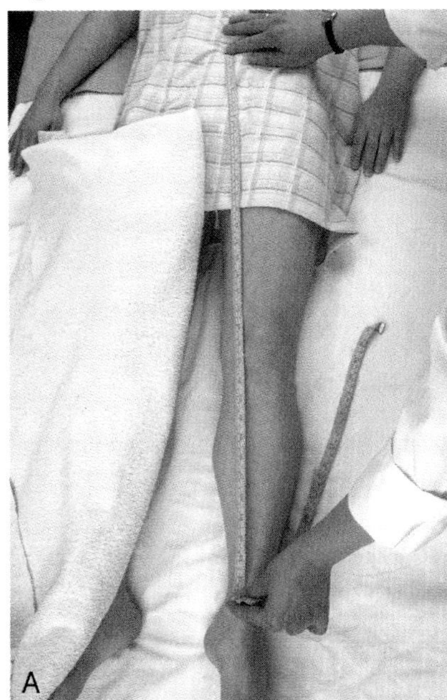

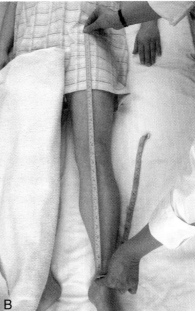

Measuring leg length. A. Apparent, B. True

Arm and leg lengths equal or < 1 cm difference between right and left.

Leg length discrepancies can cause back and hip pain, gait problems, and pseudoscoliosis, or apparent scoliosis.

Equal true leg lengths but unequal apparent leg lengths are seen with hip and pelvic area abnormalities.

(Continued)

Taking Limb Measurements *(Continued)*

ASSESS/NORMAL VARIATIONS	ABNORMAL FINDINGS/RATIONALE
Circumference *Arms:*	Circumference differences >1 cm may reflect muscular atrophy or **hypertrophy**.

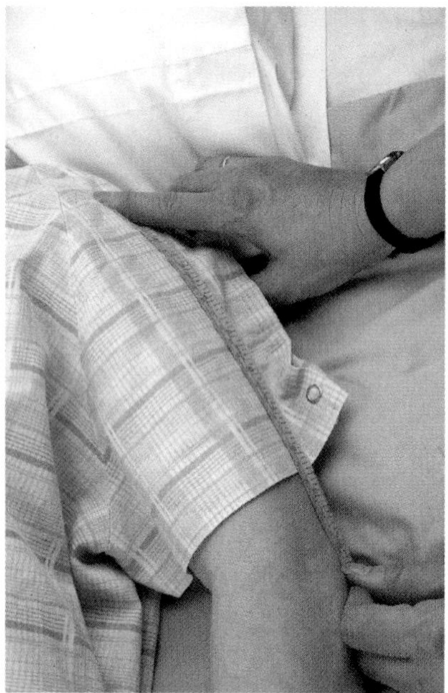

Measuring midpoint of arm

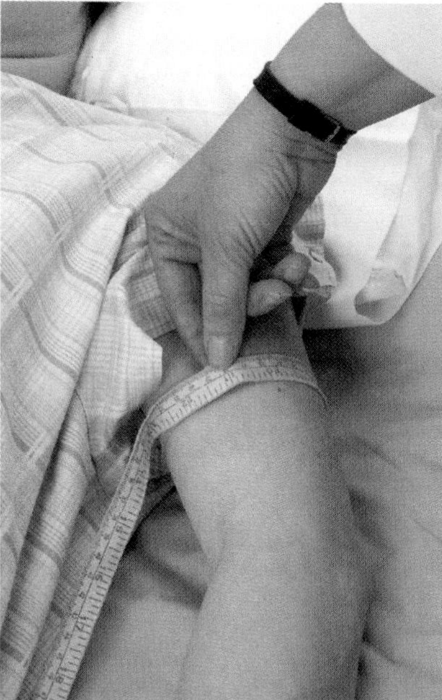

Measuring arm circumference

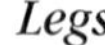

Legs

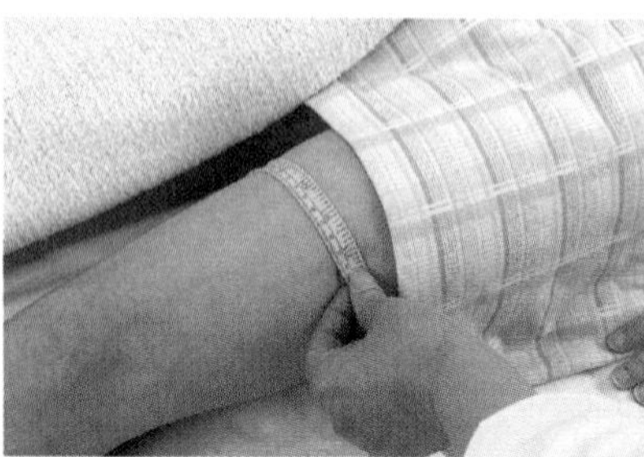

Measuring thigh circumference

Arm and leg circumferences equal to or <1 cm difference between right and left.

Assessing Joints and Muscles

Inspect the size, shape, color, and symmetry of each joint, noting masses, deformities, and muscle atrophy. Compare muscle and joint findings bilaterally and palpate for edema, heat, tenderness, pain, nodules, crepitus, and stability. Test active ROM (in which the patient performs the movement) and passive ROM (in which you put the joint through the ROM) of the joint (Fig. 18–7). Changes in articular cartilage, scarring of the joint capsule, and muscle contractures all limit motion. It is important to determine the types of motion the patient can no longer perform, especially the ADLs.

ALERT

Never force a joint!

Joint clicking or **crepitus** may occur normally sometimes or may be associated with dislocations of the humerus, temporomandibular joint (TMJ) problems, displacement of the biceps tendon from its groove, damaged knees, or DJD.

Joint deformity may result from a congenital malformation or a chronic condition. In any patient with a deformity, ask the following questions:

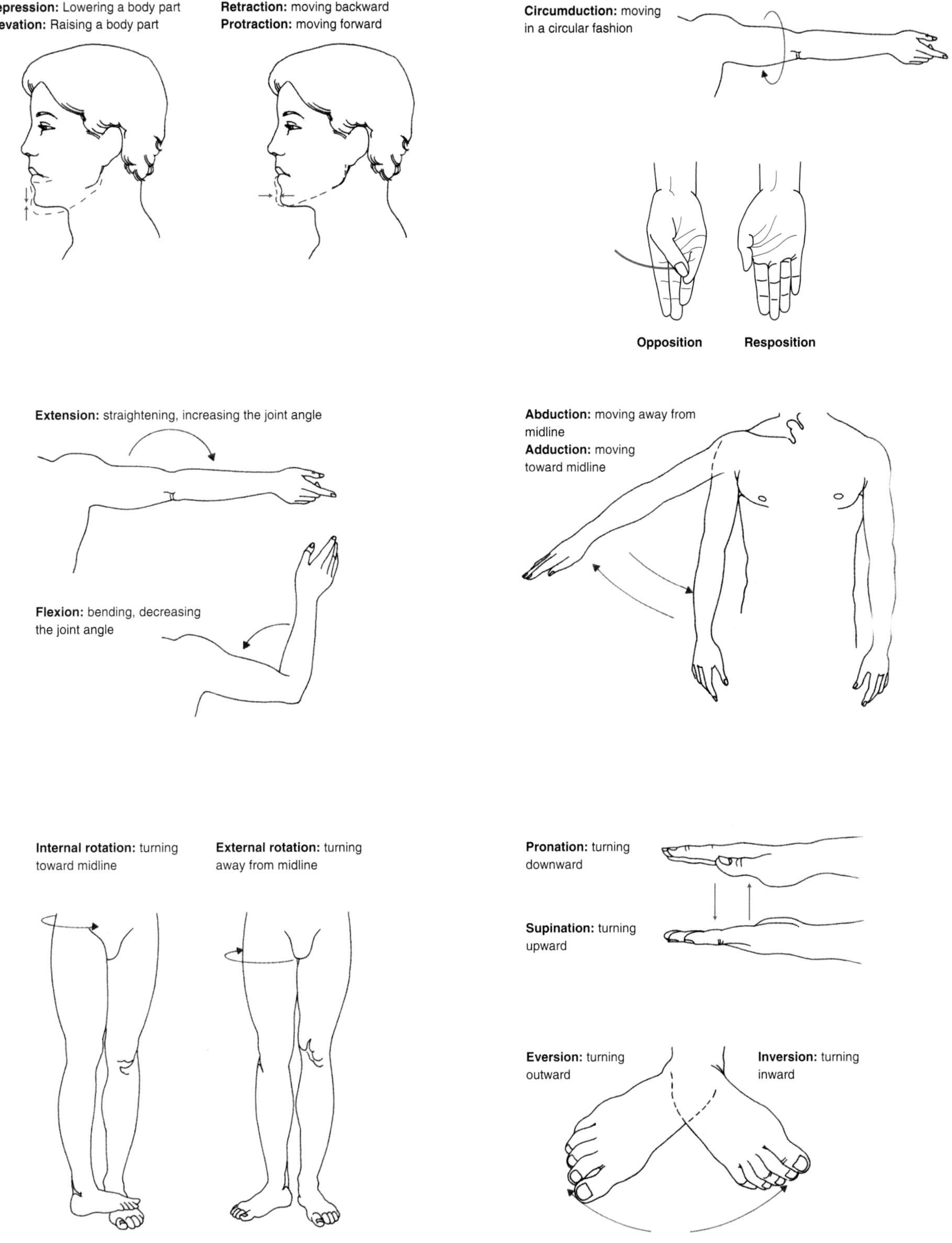

FIGURE 18–7. Body movement.

- When did you first notice the deformity?
- Did the deformity occur suddenly?
- Did it occur as the result of trauma?
- Has the deformity changed over time?
- Has it affected your range of motion?

Test muscle strength by asking the patient to put each joint through ROM while you apply resistance to the part being moved. If the patient is unable to move the part against resistance, then ask him or her to perform the ROM against gravity. If this cannot be performed, attempt

Joint Movements

Movement	Description
Extension	Straightening or increasing the angle of a joint
Flexion	Bending or decreasing the angle of a joint
Hyperextension	Straightening beyond the normal angle of a joint
Abduction	Moving away from the midline
Adduction	Moving toward the midline
Circumduction	Moving in a circular fashion
Internal rotation	Turning inward toward the midline
External rotation	Turning outward away from the midline
Pronation	Turning down
Supination	Turning up
Inversion	Turning inward (medially)
Eversion	Turning outward (laterally)
Retraction	Moving backward
Protraction	Moving forward
Opposition	Movement of thumb toward fingerpad
Reposition	Movement of thumb back to anatomical position
Depression	Movement by lowering body part
Elevation	Movement by raising body part
Ulnar deviation	Movement of hand toward ulnar side
Radial deviation	Movement of hand toward radial side

to passively put the muscle through ROM. If this is not possible (because of contraction), palpate the muscle while the patient attempts to move it. Document muscle strength as shown in the box entitled Rating Scale for Muscle Strength.

Begin your assessment by inspecting and palpating the muscles of the upper and lower extremities. Assess muscle tone and mass in both relaxed and contracted state, and then assess each joint and test muscle strength as the patient performs ROM.

Rating Scale for Muscle Strength

Rating Scale	Explanation	Classification
5	Active motion against full resistance	Normal
4	Active motion against some resistance	Slight weakness
3	Active motion against gravity	Average weakness
2	Passive ROM (gravity removed and assisted by examiner)	Poor ROM
1	Slight flicker of contraction	Severe weakness
0	No muscular contraction	Paralysis

Assessing Joints and Muscles

ASSESS/NORMAL VARIATIONS

Upper and Lower Extremities

INSPECT/PALPATE for muscle mass and tone in relaxed and contracted state

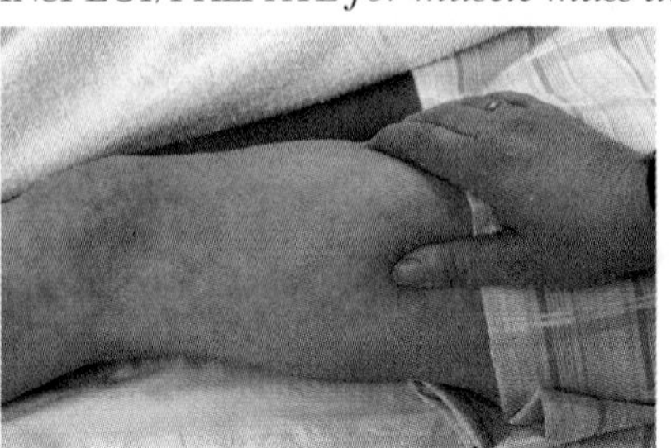

Palpating muscle tone in lower extremities

ABNORMAL FINDINGS/RATIONALE

Atrophy (muscle wasting), unexplained hypertrophy (excessive muscle size), flaccidity (**atony**), weakness (hypotonicity), **fasiculations** (involuntary twitching of muscle fibers), or tremors (involuntary contracton of muscles).

Assessing Joints and Muscles

ASSESS/NORMAL VARIATIONS	ABNORMAL FINDINGS/RATIONALE
Upper and Lower Extremities *(Continued)* Muscles soft, pliable, and nontender in relaxed state; firm and nontender in contracted state. No abnormal movements.	
Temporomandibular Joint (TMJ) (Hinge Joint and Gliding Joint) *INSPECT/PALPATE, test ROM and muscle strength* 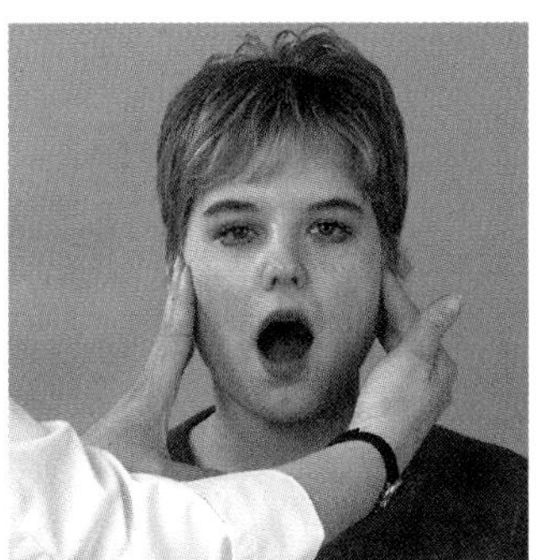 **Assessing the TMJ**	*Decreased ROM, tenderness, swelling, crepitus:* Arthritis. *Pain, swelling, popping, clicking,or grating sounds:* TMJ dysfunction. **ALERT** TMJ dysfunction may present as ear pain and headache.
Assess flexion (depression), extension (elevation), side-to-side movement, protrusion (pushing out), and retraction (pulling in) of jaw. Palpate strength of masseter and temporalis muscles as patient clenches teeth. Ask patient to laterally move the jaw left and right and then open the mouth against resistance. Feel for contraction of temporal and masseter muscles to test integrity of cranial nerve V (trigeminal). Normal ROM: • Normal opening 1–2 cm with ease. • Lateral movement 1–2 cm. Snapping and clicking are normal. • +5 muscle strength, no pain or spasms on contraction.	*Decreased muscle strength:* Muscle and joint disease. *Pain and spasms:* Myofacial pain syndrome. *Less-than-full contraction:* Lesion of cranial nerve V.
Sternoclavicular Joint (Gliding Joint) *INSPECT/PALPATE for location to midline, color, swelling, pain, and masses with patient sitting* Joint midline with no visible bony overgrowth, swelling, or redness; nontender.	*Swelling,, redness, enlargement, tenderness:* Inflammation.
Cervical, Thoracic, and Lumbar Spine (Gliding Joint for Vertebrae, Pivotal Joint for Atlantoaxial Joint) *INSPECT/PALPATE spinous processes and paravertebral muscles for tenderness or pain, test ROM* *Cervical Spine* 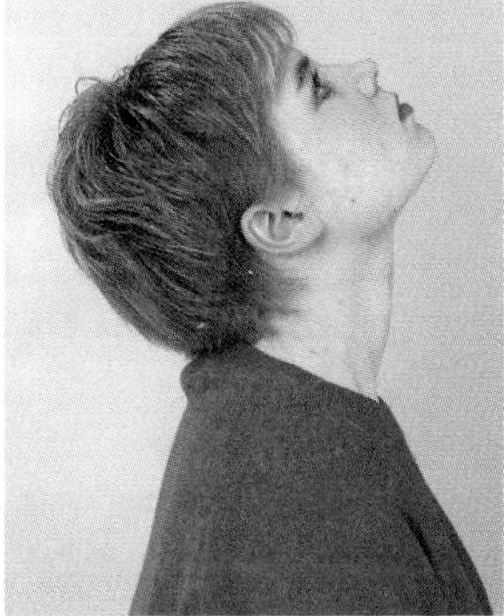 **Testing ROM and muscle strength of neck** Test ROM by having patient flex (touch chin to chest);extend (put head	A neck that is not straight and erect is abnormal. *Inability to perform ROM because of pain:* Cervical disc degenerative disease, spinal cord tumor. Pain may radiate to back, shoulder, or arms. *Neck pain associated with weakness/ loss of sensation in legs:* Cervical spinal cord compression. *Inability to perform ROM against resistance:* Muscle and joint disease. *(Continued)*

Assessing Joints and Muscles *(Continued)*

ASSESS/NORMAL VARIATIONS | **ABNORMAL FINDINGS/RATIONALE**

Cervical Spine (Continued)

in neutral position), hyperextend (look up), bend laterally, put ear to shoulder and rotate, and turn head side to side. To test muscle strength, repeat against resistance.

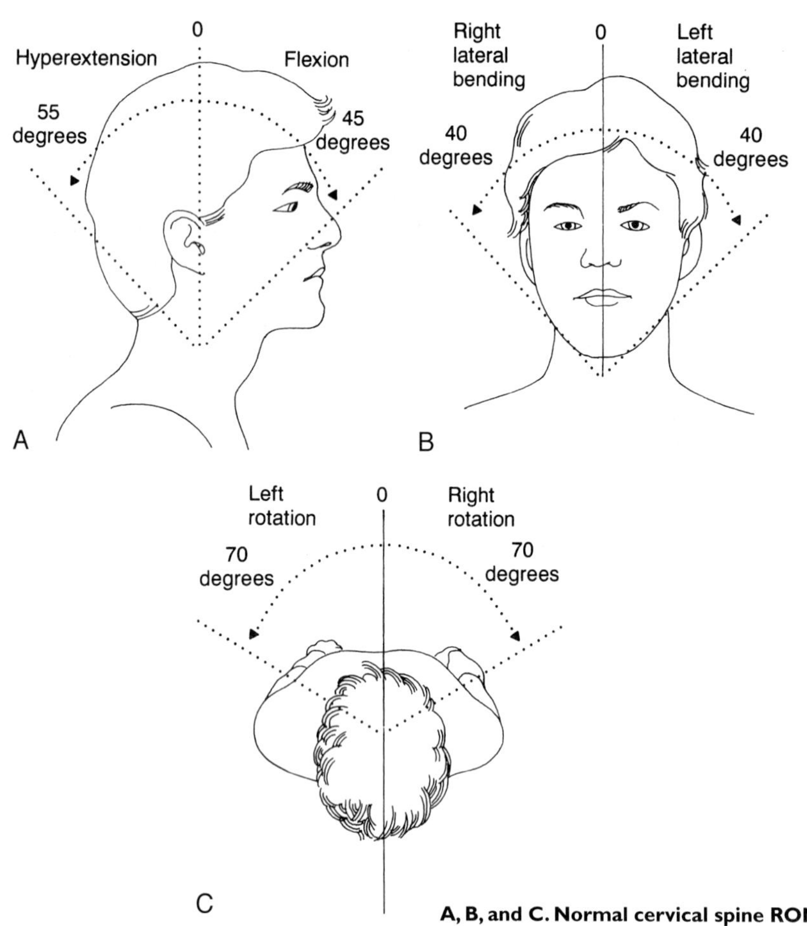

A, B, and C. Normal cervical spine ROM

Joints midline with no visible bony overgrowth, swelling, or redness; nontender.

Nontender spinous processes; paravertebral muscles well developed, smooth, firm, and nontender. Normal ROM:

- 55 degrees of hyperextension
- 45 degrees of flexion
- 40 degrees of right and left lateral bending
- 70 degrees of left and right rotation.
- +5 muscle strength

Thoracic and Lumbar Spine:

Test ROM by having patient flex (bend at waist), extend (stand upright), hyperextend (bend backward), bend laterally (side to side), and rotate (turn upper body side to side). To test muscle strength, repeat against resistance.

HELPFUL HINT

Stand behind patient and stabilize his or her pelvis with your hands as he or she performs ROM of thoracic and lumbar spine.

Assessing Joints and Muscles

ASSESS/NORMAL VARIATIONS | **ABNORMAL FINDINGS/RATIONALE**

Thoracic and Lumbar Spine: (Continued)

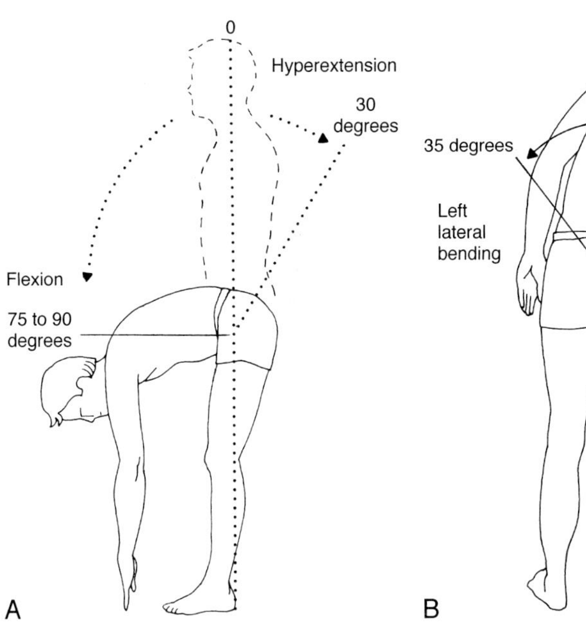

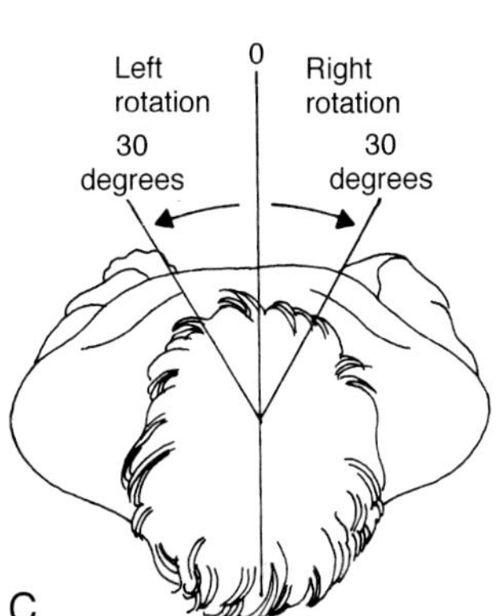

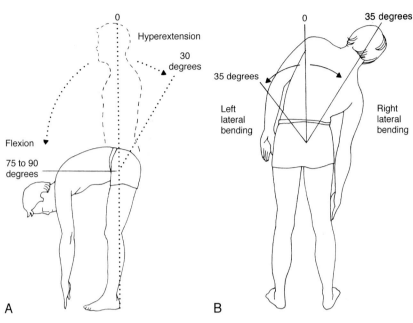

A, B, and C. Normal thoracic and lumbar spine ROM

Normal ROM:

- 75 to 90 degrees of flexion, smooth movement
- 30 degrees of hyperextension
- 35 degrees of left and right lateral bending
- 30 degrees of left and right rotation

Shoulders (Ball and Socket Joint)

INSPECT for symmetry, swelling, color, and masses; PALPATE for tenderness; test ROM

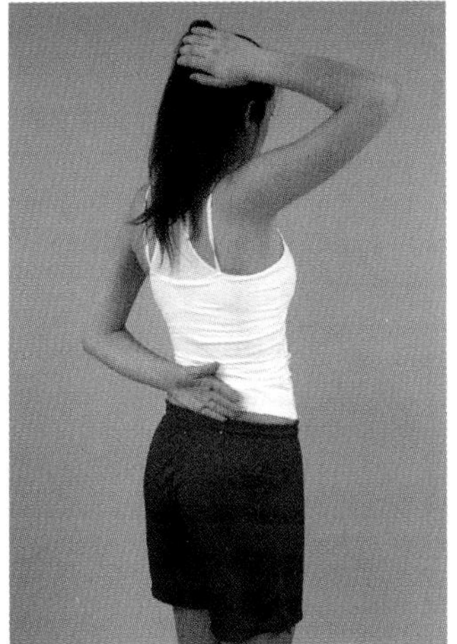

Testing ROM of shoulder

Weakness and limited ROM: Torn rotator cuff.

(Continued)

Assessing Joints and Muscles *(Continued)*

ASSESS/NORMAL VARIATIONS | **ABNORMAL FINDINGS/RATIONALE**

Shoulders (Ball and Socket Joint) *(Continued)*

Test ROM by having patient flex (move arms forward), extend (move arms backward with elbows straight), abduct (bring both hands together over head with elbows straight), and adduct (bring both hands in front of body past midline with elbows straight). Also have patient perform external rotation (with elbows flexed, bring hands behind head) and internal rotation (with elbows flexed, bring arms behind back).

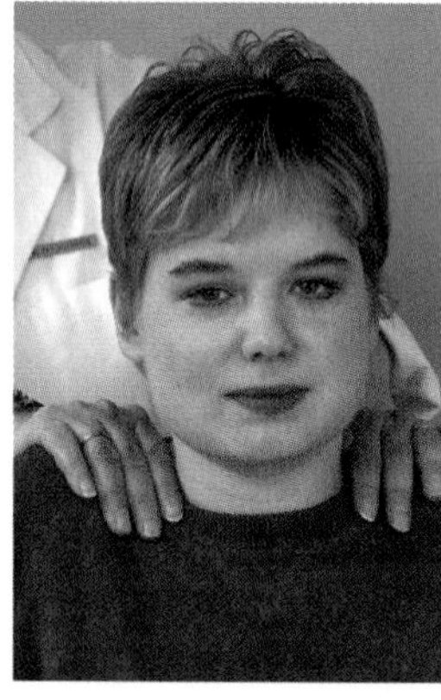

Testing muscle strength of shoulder

Test muscle strength of shoulder by performing ROM against resistance.

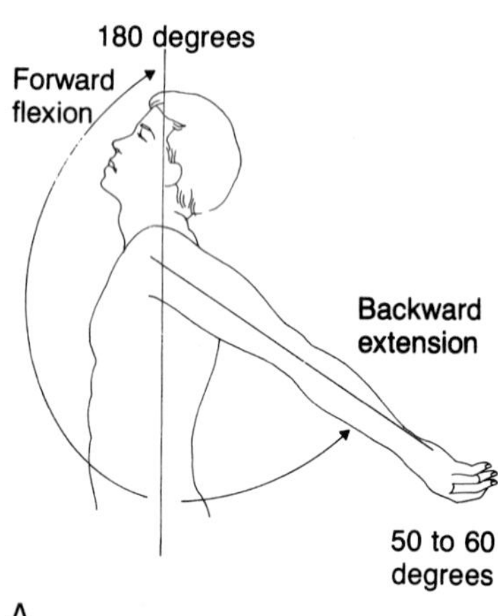

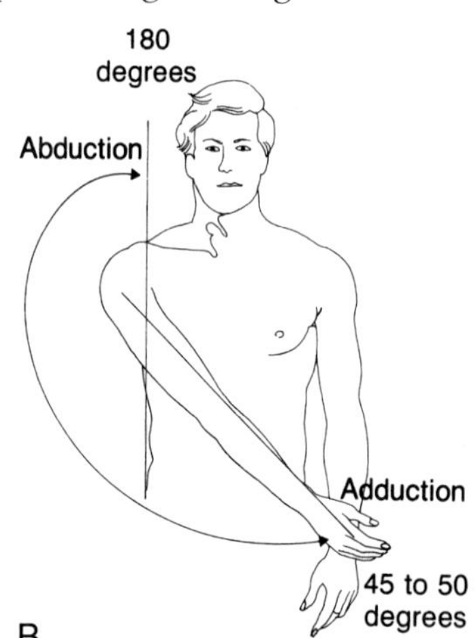

A, B, and C. Normal shoulder ROM

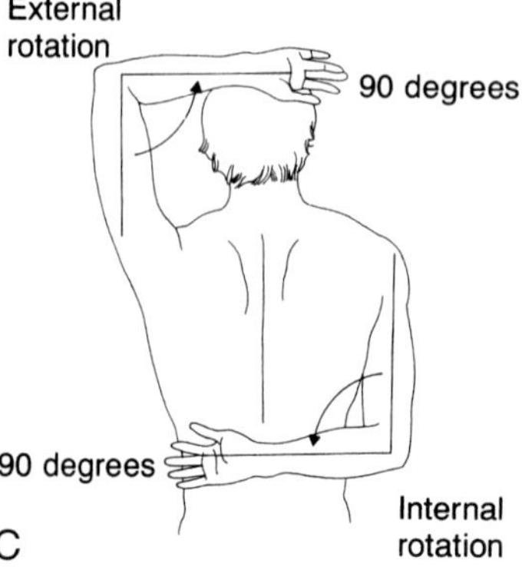

Symmetrically round; no swelling, redness, or deformity. Muscles fully developed. Clavicles and scapulae even and symmetrical. No tenderness, swelling, or heat. Flexion, extension, abduction, adduction, rotation, and shrug of shoulders should be performed without difficulty. Normal ROM:

- 180 degrees of forward flexion
- 50 to 60 degrees of backward extension

Assessing Joints and Muscles

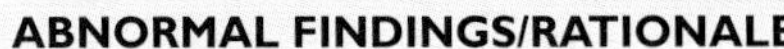

ASSESS/NORMAL VARIATIONS

Shoulders (Ball and Socket Joint) *(Continued)*

- 180 degrees of abduction
- 45 to 50 degrees of adduction
- 90 degrees of external rotation
- 90 degrees of internal rotation
- +5 muscle strength

Upper Arm and Elbow (Hinge Joint)

INSPECT for symmetry, swelling, color, and masses; PALPATE for tenderness; test ROM

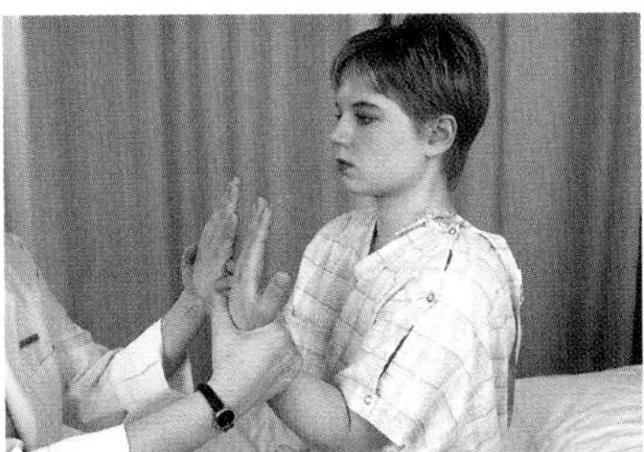

Testing ROM and muscle strength of upper arm and elbow

Test ROM by having patient flex (bend arm at elbow); extend (straighten arm at elbow); supinate (with elbow flexed, turn arm with palm up); pronate (with elbow flexed, turn arm with palm down). To test muscle strength of upper arms and elbow, repeat against resistance.

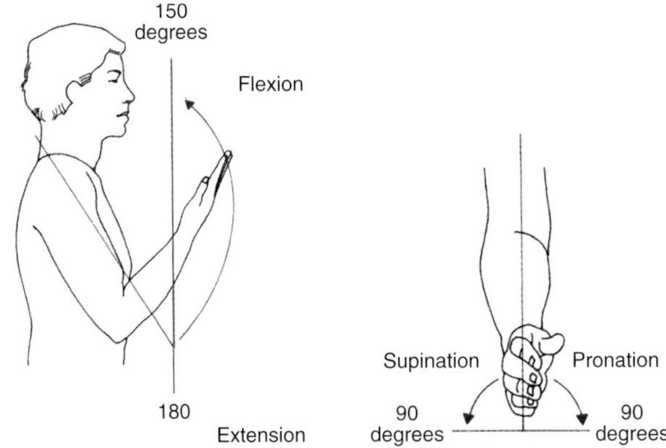

Normal upper arm and elbow ROM

Symmetrical; no redness or swelling; nontender without nodules. Normal ROM:

- 150 degrees of flexion
- 80 degrees of extension
- 90 degrees of supination and pronation
- +5 muscle strength

ABNORMAL FINDINGS/RATIONALE

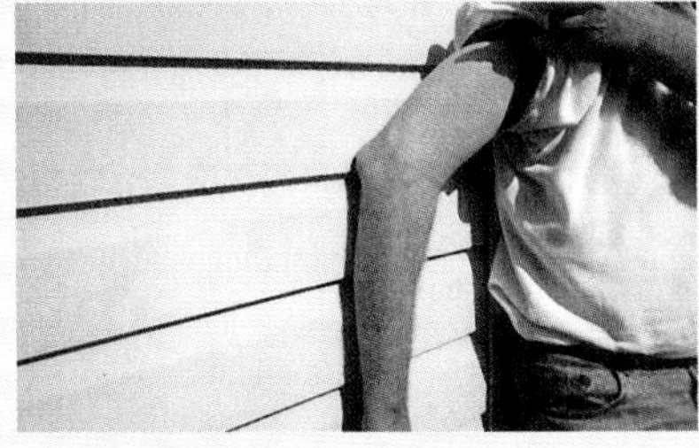

Bursitis of elbow

Redness, swelling, and tenderness at elbow (olecranon process): Bursitis.

Tennis elbow (lateral epicondylitis) is inflammation of forearm extensors or supinator muscles of fingers and wrist, and/or tendon attachment to lateral epicondyle or lateral collateral ligament caused by repetitive supination of forearm against resistance.

Golf elbow (medial epicondylitis) is same as tennis elbow, except flexor and pronator muscles and tendons are affected.

(Continued)

Assessing Joints and Muscles *(Continued)*

ASSESS/NORMAL VARIATIONS

ABNORMAL FINDINGS/RATIONALE

Wrist (Condyloid Joint)

INSPECT/PALPATE for tenderness and nodules; test ROM

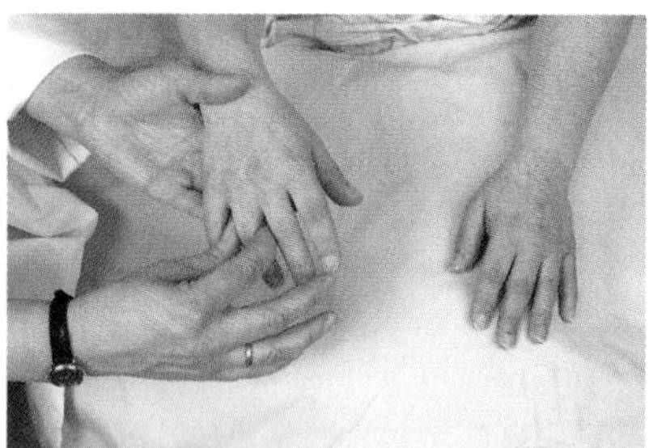

Palpating wrist joints

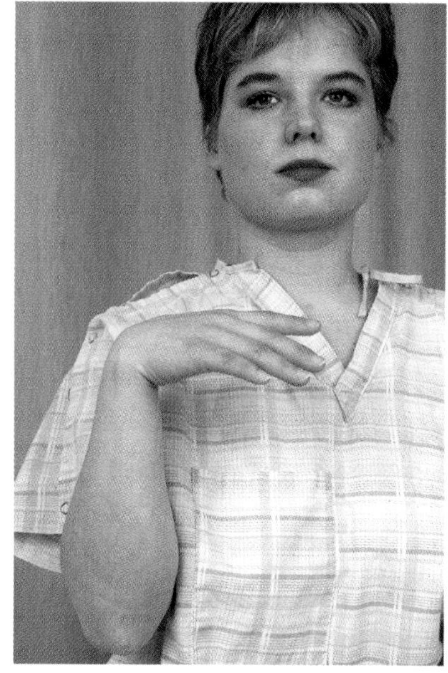

Testing ROM and muscle strength of wrist

Test ROM by having patient flex (bend wrist down), extend (straighten wrist), hyperextend (bend wrist back), perform ulnar deviation (move hand towards ulnar side), and perform radial deviation (move hand towards radial side). Test muscle strength by repeating against resistance.

Swelling, tenderness, nodules, ulnar deviation, limited ROM: RA.

Nontender, round, enlarged, swollen, fluid-filled cysts on wrists: Ganglion cyst.

Pain with movement: Tendonitis

Pain on extension of wrist against resistance: Epicondylitis.

Flexion of wrist against resistance: Medial epicondylitis.

Decreased muscle strength: Muscle and joint disease.

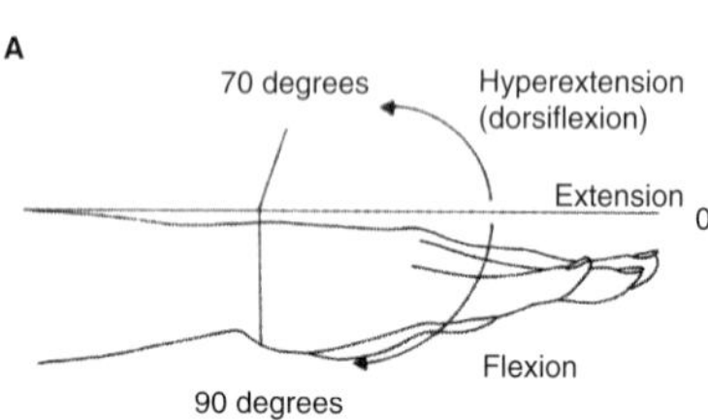

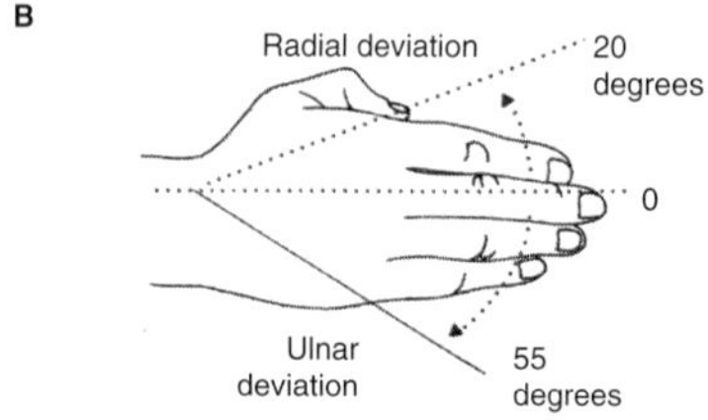

A and B. Normal wrist ROM

Symmetrical; no redness or swelling; nontender without nodules. Normal ROM:

- 90 degrees of flexion
- 70 degrees of hyperextension
- 55 degrees of ulnar deviation
- 20 degrees of radial deviation
- Full ROM against resistance
- +5 muscle strength

Hands and Fingers (Hinge, Saddle, and Condyloid Joints)

INSPECT for size, shape, symmetry, swelling, and color; PALPATE for nodules and tenderness; test ROM.

Test ROM by having patient abduct (spread fingers apart), adduct (bring fingers together), flex (make a fist), extend (open fist), hyperextend (bend fingers back), perform palmar adduction (bring thumb to index finger), perform palmar abduction (move thumb away from index finger).

Assessing Joints and Muscles

ASSESS/NORMAL VARIATIONS

Hands and Fingers (Hinge, Saddle, and Condyloid Joints) *(Continued)*

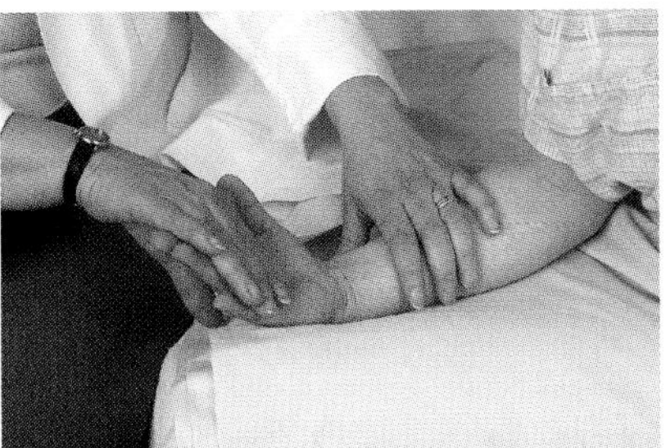

Testing ROM of hands and fingers

Test ROM by having patient abduct (spread fingers apart), adduct (bring fingers together), flex (make a fist), extend (open fist), hyperextend (bend fingers back), perform palmar adduction (bring thumb to index finger), perform palmar abduction (move thumb away from index finger).

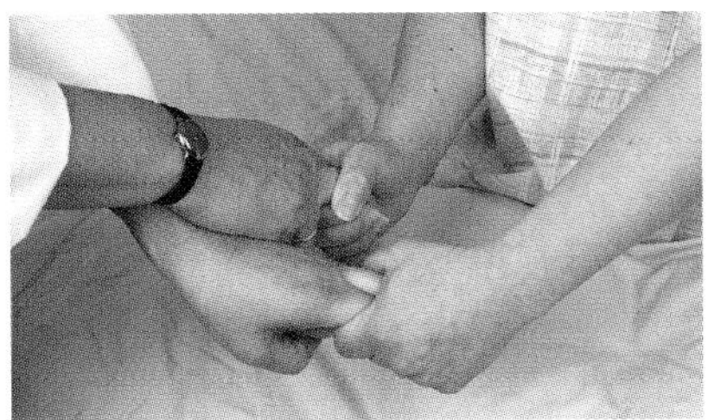

Testing muscle strength of hands and fingers

Test muscle strength by repeating movements against resistance and hand grip.

HELPFUL HINT

When testing hand grip, cross your index and middle fingers and then have patient squeeze your crossed fingers.

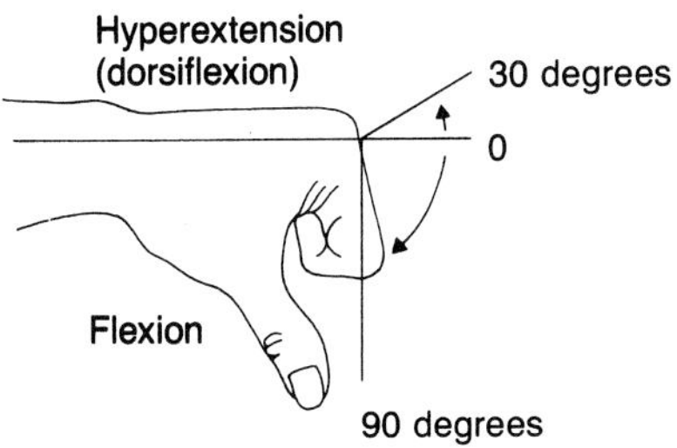

Normal hand and finger ROM

Symmetrical fingers and hands; fingers lie straight; no swelling or deformities; nontender and without nodules. Normal ROM:

- 20 degrees of abduction
- Adduction of fingers
- 90 degrees of flexion
- 30 degrees of hyperextension
- Easily moves away from other fingers, palmar abduction
- 50 degrees of flexion, palmar adduction
- Full ROM against resistance
- +5 muscle strength

ABNORMAL FINDINGS/RATIONALE

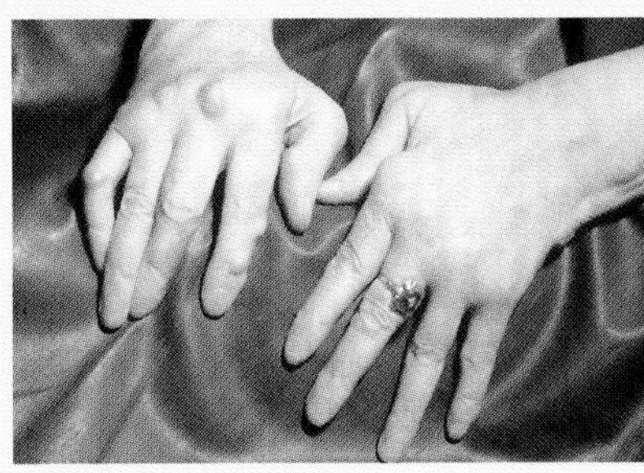

Rheumatoid arthritis

Swollen, stiff, tender finger joints: Acute RA.

Boutonnière deformity (flexion of proximal interphalangeal joint and hyperextension of distal interphalangeal joint) and swan-neck deformity (hyperextension of proximal interphalangeal joint with flexion of distal interphalangeal joint) can both be seen in long-term RA.

Atrophy of thenar prominence: Carpal tunnel syndrome.

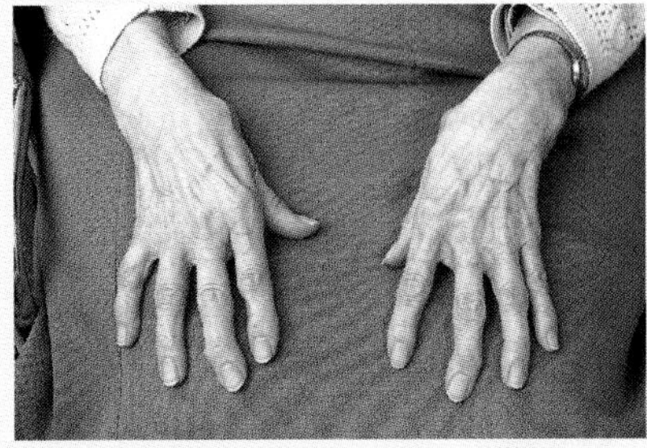

Heberden's nodes

Heberden's nodes are hard, painless nodules over the distal interphalangeal joints.

Bouchard's nodes are hard painless nodules over proximal interphalangeal joints.

Both types of nodes are seen in osteoarthritis and RA.

(Continued)

Assessing Joints and Muscles *(Continued)*

ASSESS/NORMAL VARIATIONS | **ABNORMAL FINDINGS/RATIONALE**

Hands and Fingers (Hinge, Saddle, and Condyloid Joints) *(Continued)*

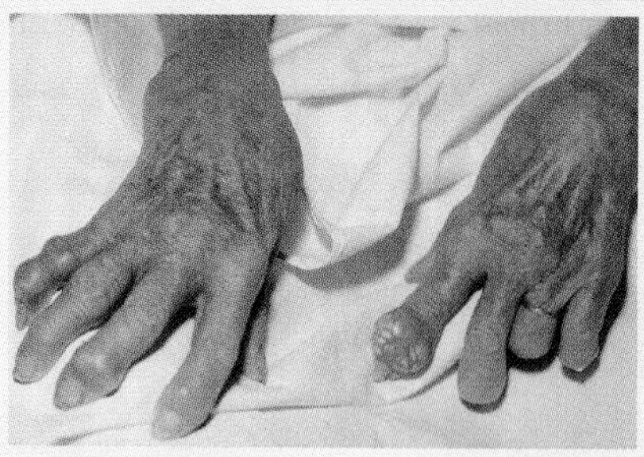

Gouty arthritis

Gouty arthritis can cause deformities and nodules of the hands.

Pain on extension of a finger: Tenosynovitis (infection of the tendon sheath)

Inability to extend ring finger: Dupuytren's contracture.

Decreased muscle strength: Muscle and joint disease may present.

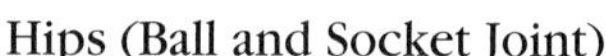

Hips (Ball and Socket Joint)

INSPECT for symmetry and shape with patient standing, PALPATE for stability, tenderness, and crepitus, test for ROM

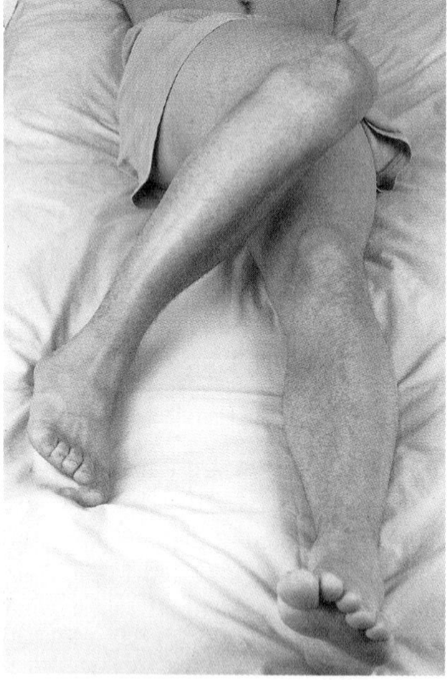

Testing ROM of hips

Test ROM by having patient extend (patient supine or standing, leg straight), flexion (raise extended leg and flex knee to chest while keeping other leg extended), abduct (move extended leg away from midline of body as far as possible), adduct (move extended leg toward midline of body as far as possible), perform internal rotation (bend knee and turn leg inward) and external rotation (bend knee and turn leg outward), hyperextend (lie prone and lift extended leg off table), and stand and swing extended leg backward.

Unequal gluteal folds: dislocated hip.

Inability to abduct hip: Common sign of hip disease.

Decrease in internal hip rotation: Early sign of hip disease.

Decreased muscle strength against resistance: Muscle and joint disease.

Assessing Joints and Muscles

ASSESS/NORMAL VARIATIONS | **ABNORMAL FINDINGS/RATIONALE**

Hips (Ball and Socket Joint) *(Continued)*

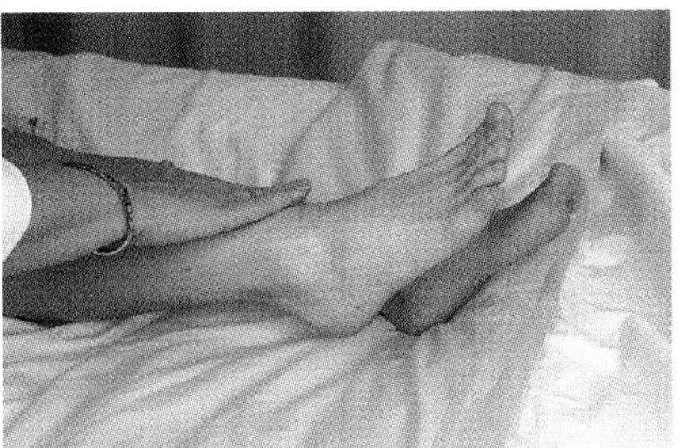

Testing muscle strength of hip

Test muscle strengtle strength by repeating ROM against resistance.

ALERT

Do not adduct, internally rotate, or flex more than 90 degrees on patients with hip replacements. Doing so may cause hip displacement!

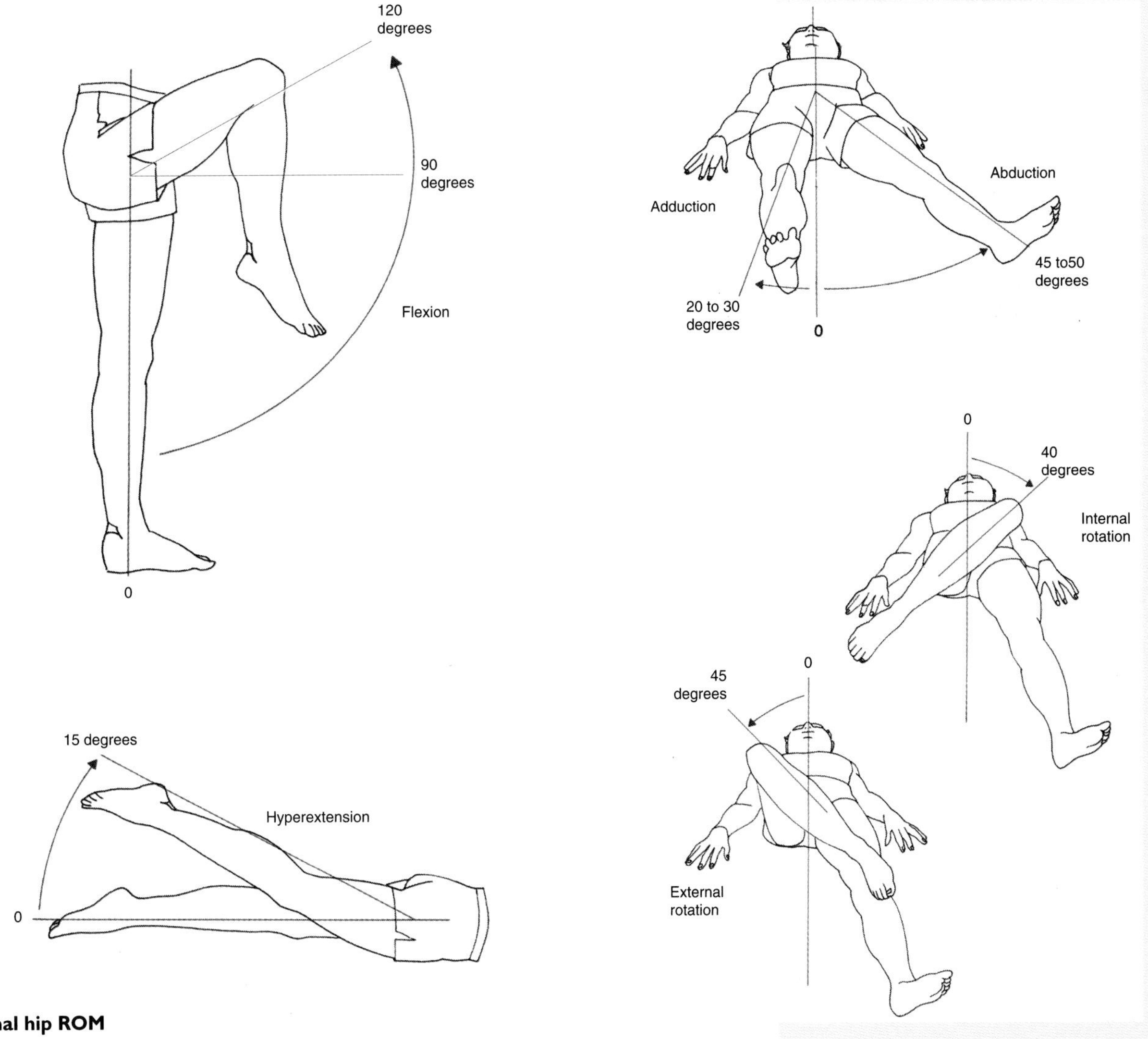

120 degrees
90 degrees
Flexion
0
Adduction
Abduction
45 to50 degrees
20 to 30 degrees
0
0
40 degrees
Internal rotation
0
45 degrees
External rotation
15 degrees
Hyperextension
0

Normal hip ROM

(Continued)

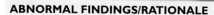

Assessing Joints and Muscles *(Continued)*

ASSESS/NORMAL VARIATIONS

Hips (Ball and Socket Joint) *(Continued)*

Buttocks equal in size; iliac crests symmetric in height; nontender, stable, and without crepitus. Normal ROM:

- 0 degrees of extension
- 90 degrees of flexion
- 120 degrees of flexion with other leg remaining straight
- 45 to 50 degrees of abduction
- 20 to 30 degrees of adduction
- 40 degrees of internal hip rotation
- 45 degrees of external hip rotation
- 15 degrees of hip hyperextension
- Full ROM against resistance
- +5 muscle strength

Knees (Hinge Joint)

INSPECT knees for size, shape, symmetry, deformities, and swelling in both supine and sitting positions with knees dangling. PALPATE for tenderness, warmth, consistency, and nodules, beginning approximately 10 cm above knee and moving downward over patella.

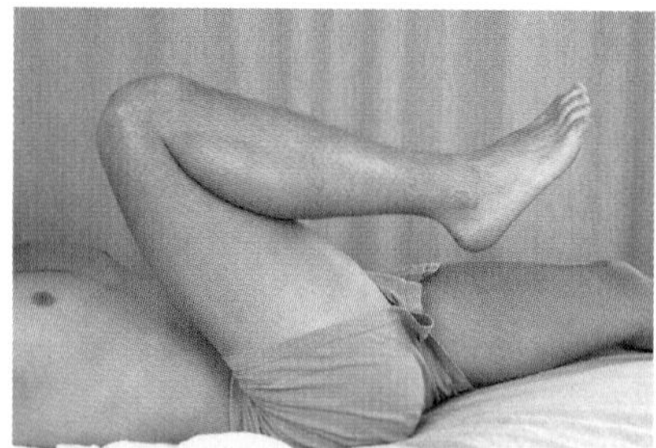

Testing ROM and muscle strength of knee

Test ROM by having patient flex (bend each knee up to chest) and extend (straighten knee). Test muscle strength by repeating ROM against resistance.

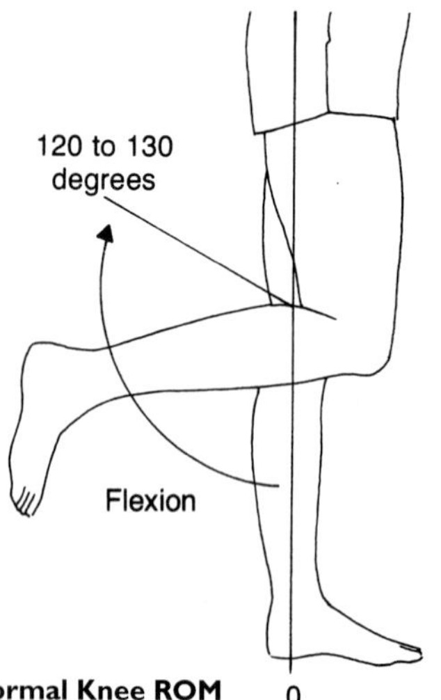

Normal Knee ROM

Symmetrical; hollow in appearance on both sides of patella; no swelling or deformities; lower leg in alignment with upper leg; nontender and cool; muscles firm and no nodules apparent. Normal ROM:

- 120 to 130 degrees of flexion
- 0 degrees of extension
- ROM not restricted against resistance
- +5 muscle strength

ABNORMAL FINDINGS/RATIONALE

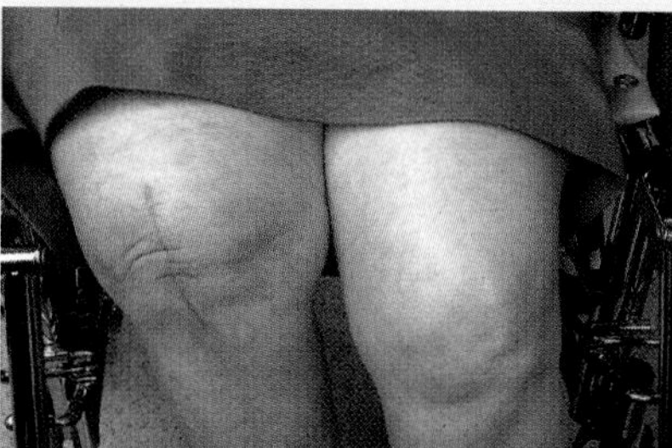

Degenerative joint disease of knees

Tenderness, warmth, boggy consistency: Synovitis.

Crepitation: Osteoarthritis.

Decreased ROM: Synovial thickening.

Inability to extend knee fully: Flexion contracture of knee.

Decreased muscle strength against resistance: Muscle and joint disease.

Assessing Joints and Muscles

ASSESS/NORMAL VARIATIONS | **ABNORMAL FINDINGS/RATIONALE**

Ankles and Feet (Hinge, Gliding, and Condyloid)

INSPECT position, alignment, shape, and skin while patient is sitting, standing and walking; PALPATE for heat, swelling, tenderness, or nodules; test ROM.

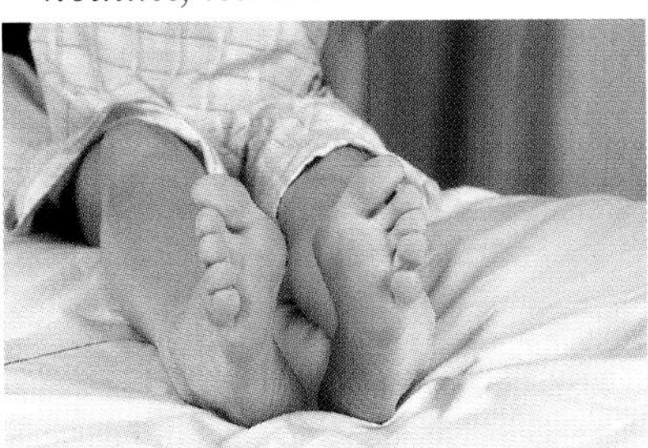

Testing ROM of ankles and feet

Test ROM by having patient dorsiflex (point toes upward), plantar flex (point toes downward), evert (turn soles outward), invert (turn soles inward), abduct (rotate foot outward), and adduct (rotate foot inward).

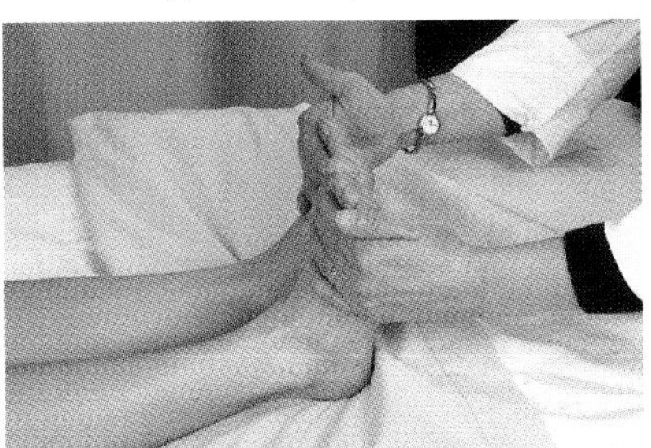

Testing muscle strength of ankles and feet

Test muscle strength by repeating ROM against resistance.

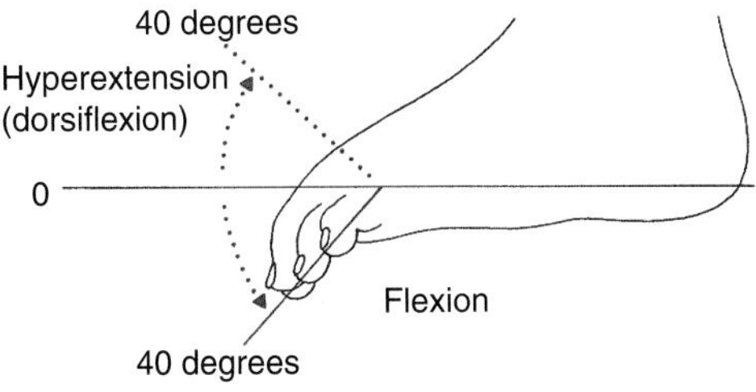

A, B, and C. Normal ankle and foot ROM

Toes and feet in alignment with lower leg; toes pointing forward and lying flat (may point in [pes varus] or out [pes valgus]; skin intact, smooth, and free of corns or calluses; longitudinal arch; weight bearing on foot midline; no heat, pain, nodules, or swelling. Normal ROM:

- 20 degrees of **dorsiflexion**
- 45 degrees of plantarflexion
- 20 degrees of eversion
- 30 degrees of inversion
- 10 degrees of abduction
- 20 degrees of adduction
- Full ROM against resistance
- +5 muscle strength

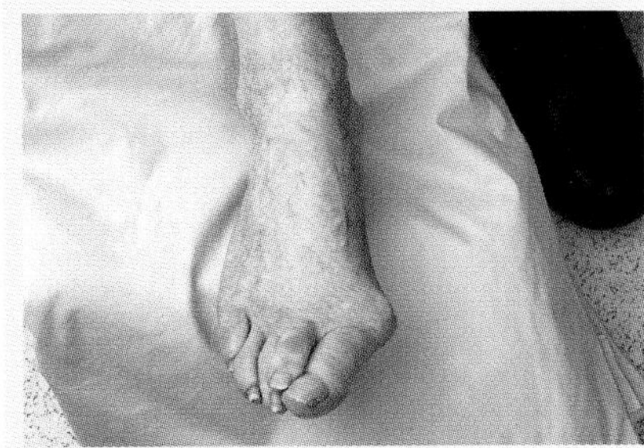

Hallux valgus, bunion, and hammer toe

Hallux valgus, often on medial side, may present with laterally deviated great toe with overlapping of second toe. A bunion is an enlarged, painful, inflamed bursa that often occurs with hammer toe, which is hyperextension of metatarsophalangeal joint and flexion of proximal interphalangeal joint.

Flat feet (pes planus) have no arches or high arches (pes cavus).

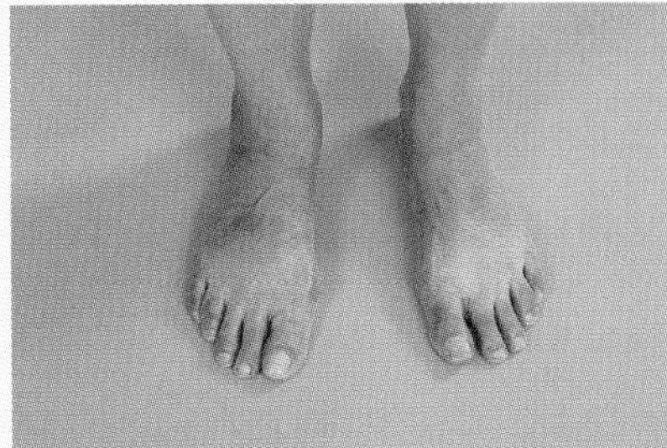

Corns and bunions

Corns are painfully thickened skin over bony prominences and pressure points.

(Continued)

Assessing Joints and Muscles *(Continued)*

ASSESS/NORMAL VARIATIONS	ABNORMAL FINDINGS/RATIONALE
Ankles and Feet (Hinge, Gliding, and Condyloid)	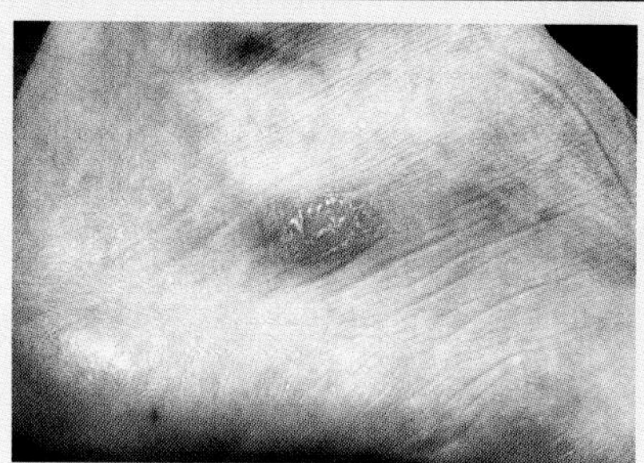 **Callus** A callus is painless, thickened skin that covers pressure points. Plantar warts (verruca vulgaris) are painful warts that occur under a callus. *Tender, painful, reddened, hot, swollen metatarsophalangeal joint of great toe:* Gouty arthritis. *Nodules on posterior ankle:* RA. *Pain and tenderness of metatarsophalangeal joints:* DJD, RA, joint inflammation. **HELPFUL HINT** Many foot problems are caused by poorly fitting shoes.

Additional Tests

You can perform the following additional tests to assess for wrist, spinal, hip, and knee problems.

Tests for Wrist Problems

Phalen's Test: Have the patient flex the hands back to back at a 90-degree angle and hold this position for about 1 minute (Fig. 18–8). If the patient complains of numbness or tingling anywhere from the thumb to the ring finger, the test is positive for carpal tunnel syndrome.

Tinel's Test: Percuss lightly over the median nerve, located on the inner aspect of the wrist (Fig. 18–9). If numbness and tingling occur on the palmar aspect of the wrist and extend from the thumb to the second finger, the test is positive for carpal tunnel syndrome.

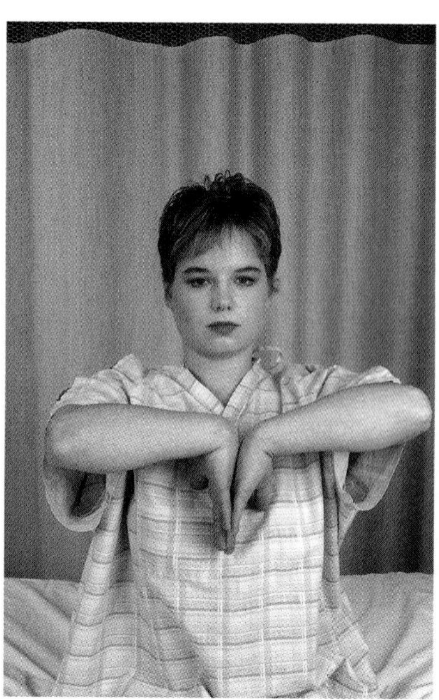

FIGURE 18–8. Phalen's test.

Tests for Arm Problems

Pronator Drift: Perform this test if you detect muscle weakness of the arms. Have the patient stand with arms extended, hands supinated, and eyes open and then

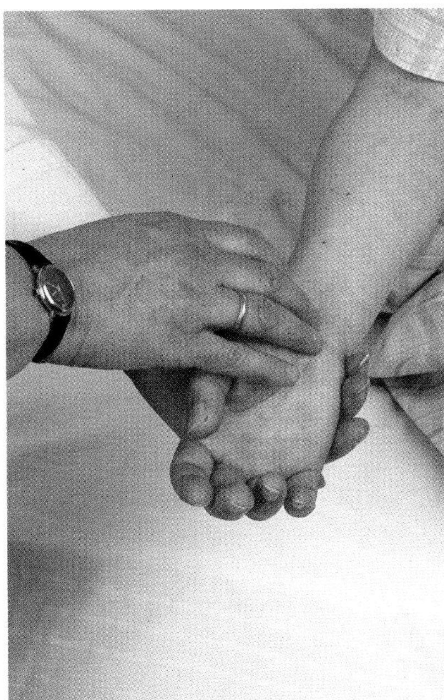

FIGURE 18–9. Tinel's test.

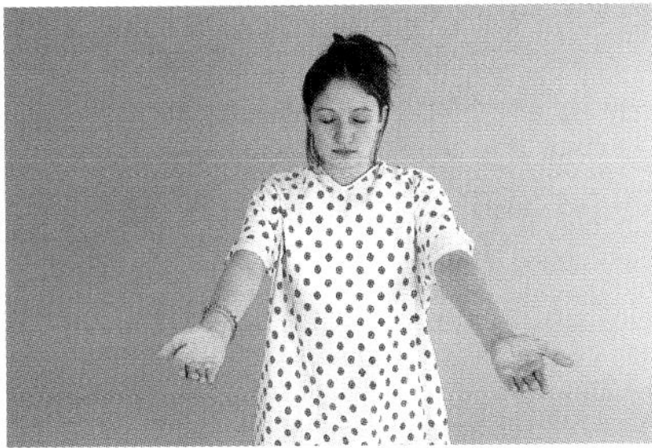

FIGURE 18–10. Assessing for pronator drift.

closed for at least 20 to 30 seconds (Fig. 18–10). Check for downward drift and pronation of the arms and hands. Pronation and drift of one arm is called pronator drift and may indicate a mild hemiparesis. Flexion of the fingers and elbow may accompany pronator drift. A lateral and upward drift may also occur in patients with loss of position sense.If your patient is able to hold his or her arms extended without drift, gently tap downward on the arms. If he or she has normal muscle strength, coordination, and position sense, the arms will return to the horizontal position. A weak arm is easily displaced and does not return to the horizontal position.

You can also assess drifting and weakness by having the patient hold his or her arms over the head for 20 to 30 seconds. Then try to force the arms down to the sides as the patient resists. Drifting or weakness may indicate a hemiparesis.

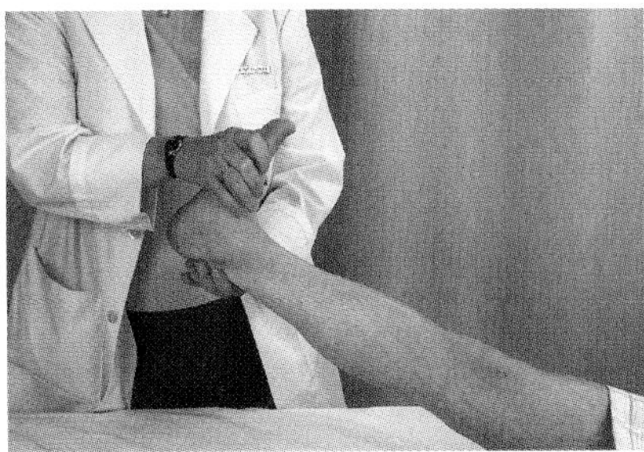

FIGURE 18–11. Straight leg raising.

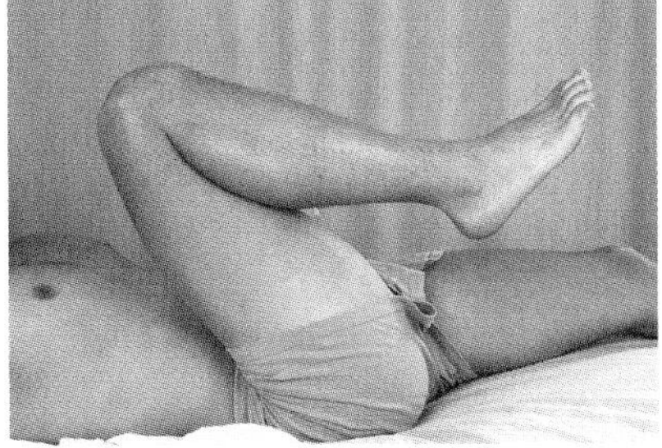

FIGURE 18–12. Thomas test.

Test for Spinal Problems

Straight Leg Raising (Lasègue's Test): Perform this test when the patient complains of low back pain that radiates down the leg (sciatica). This test checks for a herniated nucleus pulposus. Ask the patient to lie flat and raise the affected leg to the point of pain (Fig. 18–11). Pain and sciatica that intensify with dorsiflexion of the foot are a positive sign for a herniated disc.

Tests for Hip Problems

Thomas Test: This test assesses for hip flexure contractures hidden by excessive lumbar lordosis. Have the patient lie supine with both legs extended and then flex one leg to his or her chest (Fig. 18–12). The test is positive if the opposite leg raises off the table. Repeat the same maneuver on the opposite side.

Trendelenburg Test: This test is used to assess for a dislocated hip and gluteus medius muscle strength. Have patient stand erect and check the iliac crest—it should be level. Then have the patient stand on one foot and check again. If the iliac crest remains level or drops on the side opposite the weight-bearing leg, the joint is not stable and there may be a hip dislocation.

Tests for Knee Problems

Perform one of the following two tests if you noted swelling secondary to fluid accumulation or soft tissue damage.

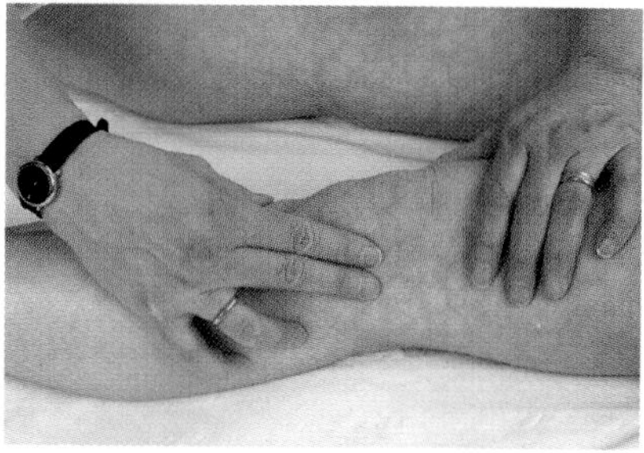

FIGURE 18–13. Bulge test.

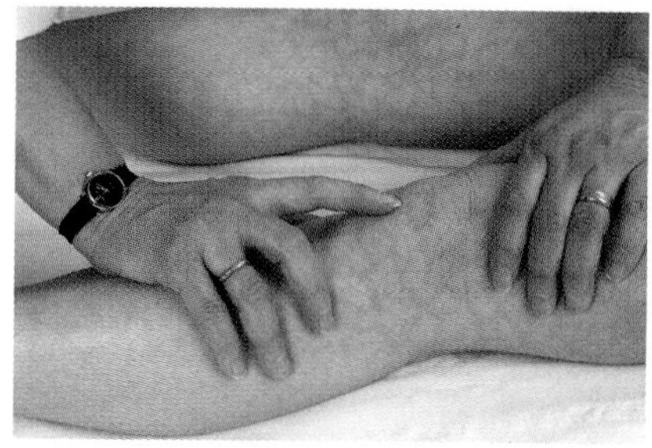

FIGURE 18–14. Patellar ballottement.

Bulge Test: Perform this test if you suspect small amounts of fluid. With the patient supine, stroke the medial side of the knees upward several times to displace the fluid. Then press the lateral side of the knee, and inspect for the appearance of a bulge on the medial side (Fig. 18–13).

Patellar Ballottement: Perform this test if you suspect large amounts of fluid. With the patient supine, press firmly with your left thumb and index finger on each side of the patella (Fig. 18–14). This displaces fluid into the suprapatellar bursa between the femur and patella. Then gently tap on the knee cap. If fluid is present, the patella will bounce back to your finger (floating knee cap).

HELPFUL HINT

Check for hollows on either side of the patella. If hollows are absent, fluid may be present.

Lachman Test: If your patient complains that his or her knee gives way or buckles, test anterior, posterior, medial, and lateral stability. To test medial and lateral stability, have the patient extend the knee and attempt to abduct and adduct it. Normally, no movement should occur if the knee is stable. To assess the anterior and posterior plane, have the patient flex the knee at a 90-degree angle. Stabilize and grasp the leg below the patella, and attempt to move it forward and back. If the joint is stable, no movement should occur (Fig. 18–15).

To test stability of the collateral ligament, have the patient lie supine with the knee slightly flexed. Place your hand at the head of the fibula and apply pressure medially; then reverse and apply pressure laterally. If the joint is unstable, movement will occur and create a palpable medial or lateral gap at the joint.

Perform one of the following tests if your patient complains of clicks or knee-locking and you suspect a torn meniscus.

McMurray's Test: To perform McMurray's test, position the patient supine with his or her knee fully flexed (Fig. 18–16). Place one hand on the heel and the other on the knee and gently internally and externally rotate the foot as you bring the leg to full extension. The test is positive if audible or palpable clicks occur or the knee locks.

Apley's Test: Position the patient supine with his or her knee flexed at 90 degrees (Fig. 18–17). Place one hand on the heel and the other hand on the knee. Apply pressure with both hands and gently rotate the foot. The test is positive if audible or palpable clicks occur.

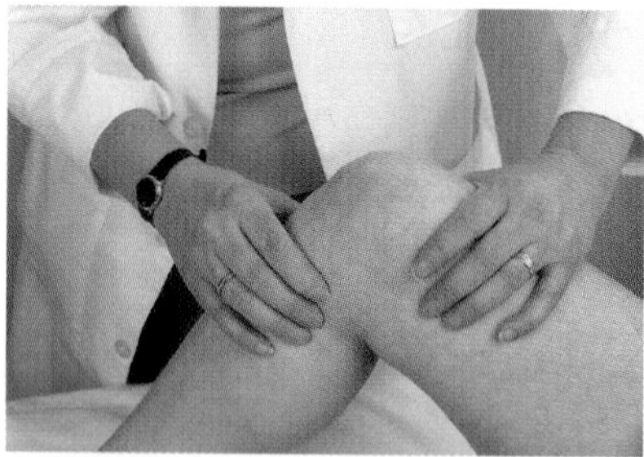

FIGURE 18–15. Lachman test.

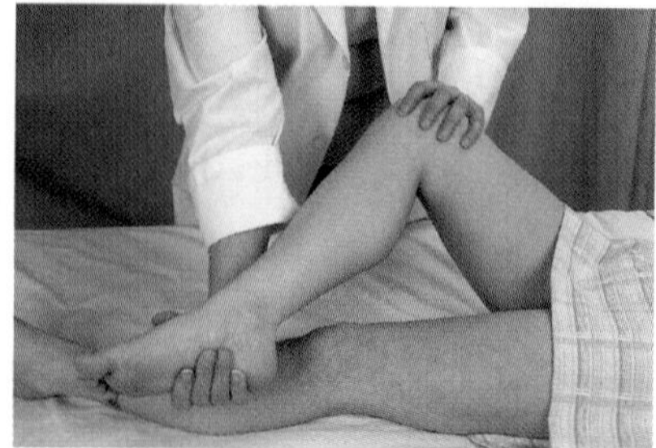

FIGURE 18–16. McMurray's test.

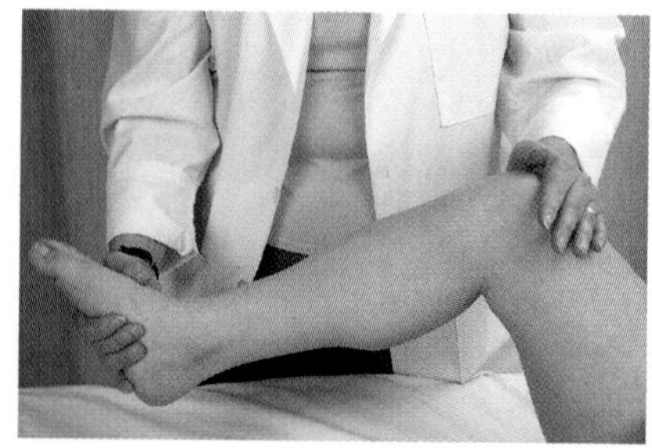

FIGURE 18–17. Apley's test.

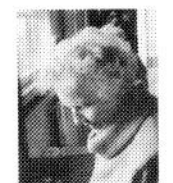

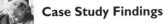

Case Study Findings

Mrs. O'Malley's focused musculoskeletal findings include:

- Gait steady, no support needed for ambulation.
- Mild muscle atrophy noted in quadriceps, all other muscles without atrophy. No involuntary movements.
- Skin intact over joints without rashes, deformities, erythema, ecchymosis, swelling, masses, or nodules.
- Shape and tone of muscles within normal limits.
- Contour smooth over joints; no tenderness, heat, redness, or pain palpated in any joint.
- Full ROM of all joints within normal limits.
- Muscle strength 5/5.
- Leg length 80.5 cm bilaterally, thigh circumference 40 cm bilaterally.
- Mild kyphosis when standing.

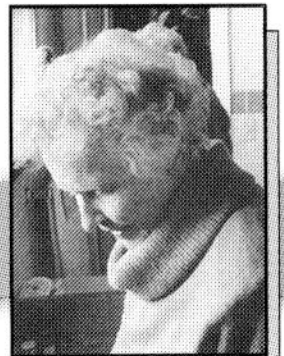

Case Study Analysis and Plan

Now that you have completed a thorough physical assessment of Mrs. O'Malley, list the key history and physical examination findings that will help you formulate your nursing diagnoses.

Nursing Diagnoses

Consider all of the data you have collected during your assessment of Mrs. O'Malley and use this information to identify a list of nursing diagnoses. Some possible ones are provided as follows. Cluster the supporting data.

1. Pain
2. Mobility, impaired physical
3. Injury, risk for
4. Health-Seeking Behaviors

Identify any additional nursing diagnoses.

CRITICAL THINKING ACTIVITY #2

List all of the strengths and areas of concern that have a bearing on Mrs. O'Malley's health status.

CRITICAL THINKING ACTIVITY #3

Now that you have identified some nursing diagnoses for Mrs. O'Malley, select one and develop a nursing care plan and a brief teaching plan for her, including learning objectives and teaching strategies.

Research Tells Us

People who lose inches from their height lose bone mass. Loss of bone mass places people at a high risk for osteoporosis. Nurses should assess height loss as a screening tool for high-risk patients. These data could then serve as the basis for referral and follow-up.

Hip fractures occur most frequently in older adults, particularly women with osteoporosis. In one study, family caregivers of patients discharged from the hospital after repair of a hip fracture had unrealistic expectations about the length of the recovery period. Caregivers reported that the patient's mobility had not improved as quickly as expected. Support and education for family caregivers is essential so that realistic expectations can be discussed. You can play a crucial role in providing this education and support.

Aches and pains are a common musculoskeletal complaint, and they remain the most common symptom pattern for women suffering from fibromyalgia. Symptoms worsen with damp or cool weather, and relaxation and heat are most effective as complementary therapies for pain management. You can assist patients with fibromyalgia to identify disease symptom patterns. Complementary approaches to pain management can be suggested as helpful interventions (Williams et al., 1966).

Health Concerns

More than 25 million people in the United States have osteoporosis to some degree, and the estimated cost of medical care and treatment, direct and indirect, exceeds 10 billion dollars. Identifying those at risk is important for early detection and treatment. Women need to be educated about the importance of calcium in their diets as early as their teens because maximum bone mass is reached during adolescence.

Risk factors for osteoporosis include:

- Female gender (8 times greater in women than men)
- Body build: Thin small frame
- Positive family history of osteoporosis
- Low dietary calcium intake
- Cigarette smoking
- Excessive alcohol intake
- Age: Postmenopausal
- Inactive lifestyle
- Long-term use of steroids and thyroid replacement and anti-seizure medications
- Malabsorption disorders, chronic liver disease, or eating disorders such as bulimia or anorexia nervosa

Common Abnormalities

ABNORMALITY	ASSESSMENT FINDINGS
Anklylosing Spondylitis (Marie-Strümpell Disease) Chronic, progressive disease involving joints. Bilateral sclerosis of the sacroilial joints is a diagnostic sign.	• Males ages 10 to 30 • Familial disorder with genetic predisposition • Low backache • Flattening of lumbar curvature • Decreased joint ROM • Muscle stiffness • Joint swelling and redness • Deformity and immobility • Progressively limited back movement and chest expansion • Decreased spinal ROM with abnormal vertebral alignment, flattened lumbar curve, and dorsal kyphosis • Atrophy of trunk muscles • Fever • Fatigue • Weight loss • Fusion of entire spine in severe cases • Cardiac conduction disturbances in severe and long-standing disease
Carpal Tunnel Syndrome Compression of the medial nerve of the hand	• History of predisposing factors such as wrist trauma or injury, RA, gout, myxedema, diabetes mellitus, leukemia, acromegaly, edema of the hand associated with pregnancy • Pain that worsens after manual activity, especially that involving wrist rotation, or at night • Radiates up the arm • May be intermittent or constant • Causes numbness, burning, or tingling of the thumb and the index and middle fingers • Atrophy of thenar eminence (mass of tissue on the lateral side of the palm) • Positive Tinel's sign (tingling during wrist percussion) • Muscle weakness

Common Abnormalities

ABNORMALITY	ASSESSMENT FINDINGS
Carpal Tunnel Syndrome *(Continued)*	• Dry skin over thumb and first two fingers • Inability to oppose thumb and little finger
Lumbosacral Disc Herniation Prolapse of the nucleus pulposus of a ruptured intervertebral disc into the spinal canal	• Pain on coughing, sneezing, straining, bending, or lifting • Pain increases with sitting • Accompanied by mild to severe low back, buttock, or leg pain • May be associated with spasms • Decreased sensation, paresthesias • Absent or diminished deep tendon reflexes (DTRs) of affected dermatomes • Voiding (particularly urinary retention) or defecating difficulties • History of predisposing factors such as recent spinal trauma, heavy or awkward lifting or occupational stress on back, lack of exercise, obesity, degenerative changes • Decreased spinal ROM • Unequal limb circumference • Abnormal posture, scoliosis, flattening of lumbar curvature • Diminished DTRs of knee and ankle • Positive straight-leg–raising test
Osteoporosis Loss of bone mass density	• Seen mostly in postmenopausal women • History of predisposing factors such as endocrine disorders, inadequate dietary intake of calcium and vitamin D, malabsorption, inadequate exercise, prolonged immobility, decreased estrogen levels, excessive smoking or alcohol and caffeine intake, family history of osteoporosis, small stature • Possible fractures of involved bones, collapse of vertebrae, increasing kyphosis • Evidence of fracture: loss of height, wedging of dorsal or anterior vertebrae, uneven shoulder and iliac crest levels, lateral curvature of spine with rotational deformity, thoracic and flank of deformities (humps)
Swan-Neck Deformity Deformity of a finger	• Flexion of distal interphalangeal joints • Hyperextension of proximal interphalangeal joints • Seen in rheumatoid arthritis

Summary

- This chapter taught you how to make a thorough musculoskeletal assessment, including a health history and physical examination.
- It also covered how to analyze your findings to identify actual and potential health problems and to write nursing diagnoses and a plan of care.

19

Assessing the Sensory-Neurological System

Before You Begin

INTRODUCTION TO THE SENSORY-NEUROLOGICAL SYSTEM

The human nervous system is a unique system that allows the body to interact with the environment as well as maintain the activities of internal organs. It is composed of structures that transmit electrical and chemical signals between the body's systems and the brain. The multiple functions of the nervous system are so automatic that most people are unaware of their magnitude until a problem occurs.

An impaired nervous system can manifest in many ways, from subtle weakness to drastic loss of mobility. The nervous system acts as the main "circuit board" for every body system. Because the nervous system works so closely with every other system, a problem within another system or within the nervous system itself can cause the nervous system to "short-circuit."

A major goal of nursing is early detection to prevent or slow the progression of disease. So it is important for nurses to accurately perform a thorough neurological assessment and to understand the implications of subtle changes in assessment findings. By doing so, you can initiate timely interventions that can save lives.

Because of the complexity of this system, assessment can be challenging, especially for beginning nurses. All body organs and most tissues are innervated; therefore, neurological activity affects functioning within all body systems. For example, the nervous system responds to stress by increasing the heart rate, resulting in increased blood pressure, whereas it responds to the sight or smell of food by increasing the production of digestive juices. Furthermore, a seemingly straightforward neurological symptom such as headache, insomnia, or forgetfulness can have a wide range of causes, contributing factors, and consequences.

Another assessment challenge may be interacting with the patient. Neurological impairment can reduce the ability to communicate, cause confusion, alter personality, and otherwise confound your attempts to obtain an accurate health history. Finally, factors such as drug and alcohol use, medication interactions, diet, amount of sleep, and other self-care factors can influence neurological health. Therefore careful sleuthing is required when taking the health history and gathering and evaluating the physical findings.

The previous chapter discussed neuromuscular function, just one aspect of the highly complex neurological system. This chapter presents the sensory-neurological assessment, including information on assessing cerebral function, cranial nerves (CNs), sensation, and reflexes. Throughout the assessment, you will identify risk factors for neurological impairment and health promotion teaching needs. Remember to document all findings, including normal data, precisely and thoroughly, to provide a baseline against which future neurological function can be measured. This baseline data is critically important for evaluating degeneration in patients with progressive neurological disease, as well as for evaluating patients' progress toward rehabilitation after neurological trauma and other acute problems.

Anatomy and Physiology Review

Before beginning the neurological assessment, you need to understand the anatomy and physiology of the system, including its anatomical and functional divisions and the type and extent of its interaction with other body systems. In addition to the motor aspects discussed in Chapter 18, general functions of the neurological system include:

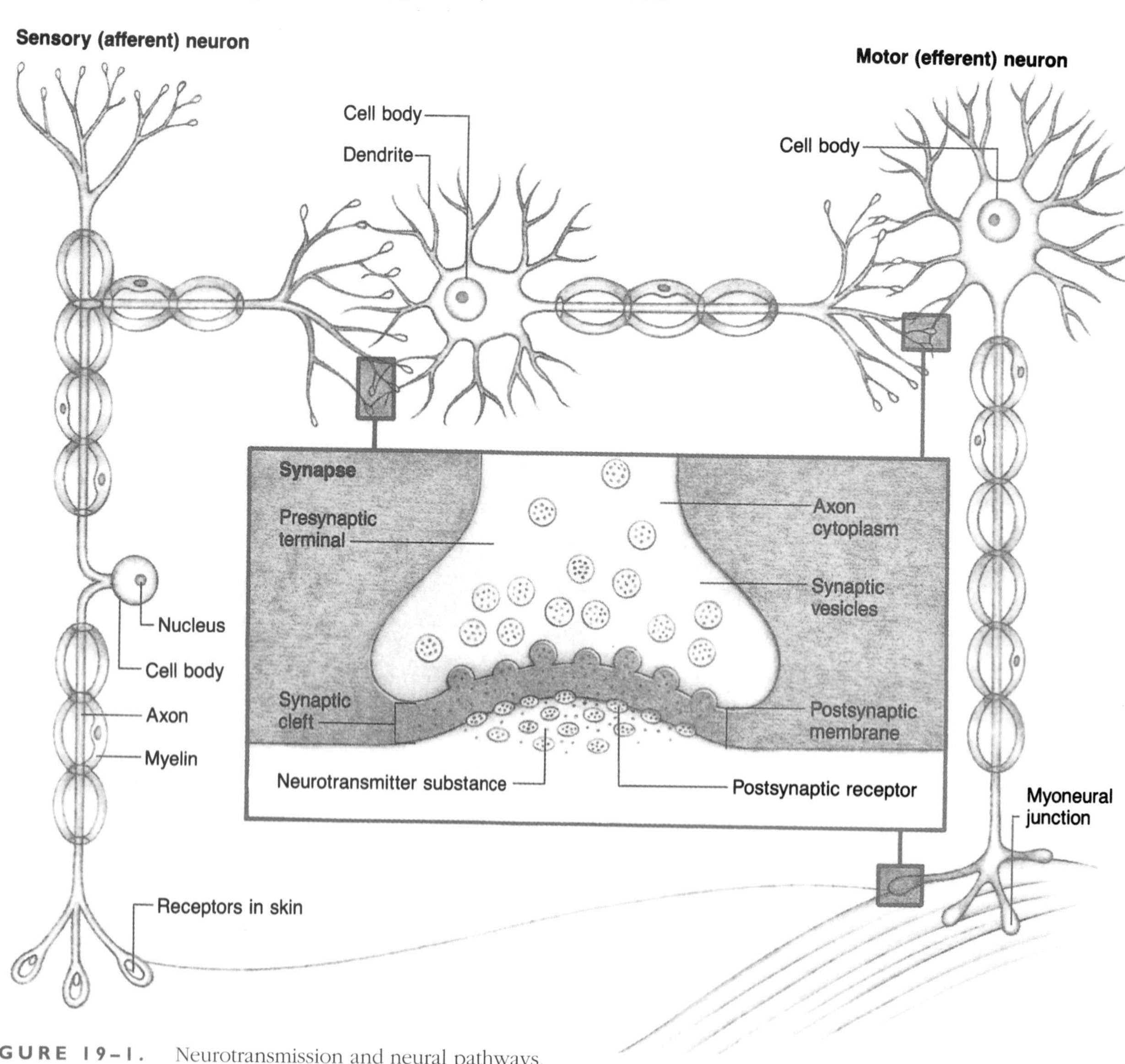

FIGURE 19-1. Neurotransmission and neural pathways.

- Cognition, emotion, and memory
- Sensation, perception, and the integration of sensory-perceptual experience
- Regulation of homeostasis, consciousness, temperature, blood pressure, and other bodily processes

Structures and Functions of the Sensory-Neurological System

There are two types of nerve cells: neuroglia and neurons. Neuroglia act as supportive tissue, nourishing and protecting the neurons. They also maintain homeostasis in the interstitial fluid around the neurons and account for about 50 percent of the CNS volume. Neuroglia have the ability to regenerate and respond to injury by filling spaces left by damaged neurons.

Neurons have the ability to produce action potentials or impulses (excitability or irritability) and to transmit impulses (conductivity). They are composed of a cell body, dendrites, and axons. The cell body contains the nucleus. Dendrites are short, branchlike structures that receive and carry impulses to the cell body. Axons are long fibers that carry the electrical impulses generated by the cell bodies. Some axons are covered with a myelin sheath that allows rapid impulse transmission.

For neurons to communicate with one another, the axon of one neuron has to convey its impulse to the dendrite of the next neuron across a space called a **synapse.** It does this with the help of **neurotransmitters,** chemicals released by the axon that carry the impulse to the receiving dendrite. The impulses conveyed by neurons include sensory data about what the body is seeing, hearing, feeling, and so on, as well as motor data telling the muscles how to respond.

Sensory impulses are transmitted to the brain through **afferent** or ascending pathways. Motor impulses are transmitted from the brain to muscles through the **efferent** or descending pathways (Fig. 19–1).

Neurons band together into peripheral nerves, spinal nerves, the spinal cord, and the tissues of the brain. These structures make up the neurological system, which is divided into the **central nervous system** (CNS) and the peripheral nervous system (PNS).

The Central Nervous System

The CNS consists of the brain and spinal cord.

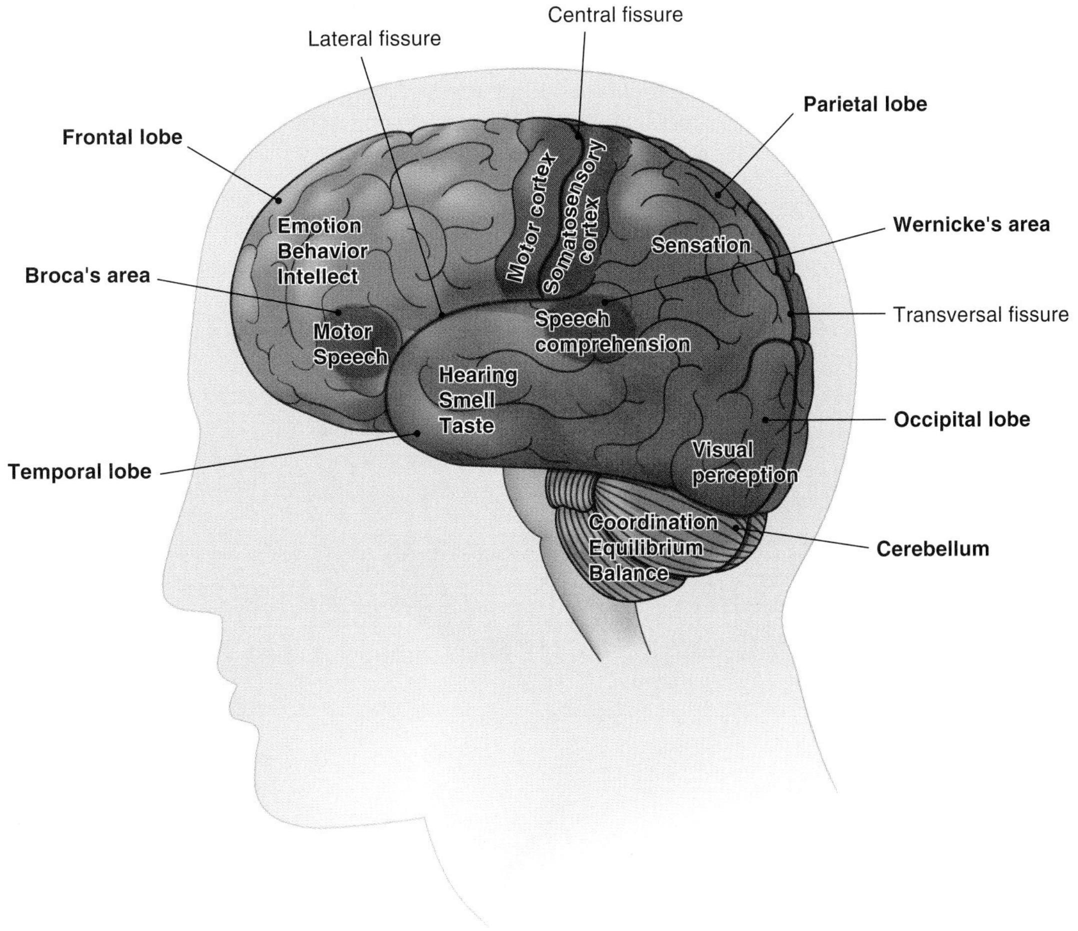

FIGURE 19–2. Lobes of the brain.

The Brain

The **brain** is composed of gray matter made up of neuronal cell bodies and white matter composed of axons and dendrites. The brain consists of four major structures: the cerebrum, diencephalon, cerebellum, and brainstem. These and other components of the brain are shown in Figure 19–2 and described in the accompanying table.

Structures and Functions of the Brain

STRUCTURE	FUNCTION
Cerebrum	Largest part of the brain. Consists of two hemispheres connected by a band of neurons called the corpus callosum, the great commissure of the brain. Each hemisphere has four lobes.
Cerebral Cortex	Outermost layer of cerebrum. Consists of a ridge of gray matter formed from clustered cell bodies of neurons. Folds of the cerebral cortex are called convolutions or gyri, and the grooves between them are called fissures or sulci. Controls most conscious processes.
Frontal Lobes	Regulate emotional expression, behavior, intellect; influence personality; control voluntary movement. Contain Broca's area (left lobe in most people), which controls expressive language function.
Temporal Lobes	Influences hearing, smell, taste, and memory. Left temporal lobe (in most people) contains Wernicke's area, which allows language comprehension. Contains limbic system.
• *Limbic System*	Lies deep in frontal and temporal lobes. Influences emotional and sexual arousal, behavioral expression, recent memory, smell.
Parietal Lobes	Perceive and interpret sensory input, such as pain, temperature, touch, texture, and proprioception.
• *Insula (central lobe)*	Located beneath the parietal, frontal, and temporal lobes. Involved with gastrointestinal (GI) and visceral activity.
Occipital Lobes	Perceive and interpret visual stimuli, including spatial relationships.
Reticular Activating System	Diffuse network of hyperexcitable neurons in brainstem and cerebral cortex that screens and channels incoming sensory input. Helps maintain consciousness or wakefulness.
Diencephalon	Connects cerebrum to brainstem. Contains thalamus and hypothalamus.
Thalamus	Clusters multiple sensory stimuli (e.g., the warmth, smell, and taste of tea) into a coherent whole before sending it to the cerebral cortex for perception. Tunes out continuing unimportant stimuli (e.g., sound of distant radio when you are reading).
Hypothalamus	Controls and integrates autonomic nervous system and pituitary gland activities. Regulates production of several hormones; stimulates visceral responses, such as heart rate, in response to emotions; regulates temperature by prompting shivering and sweating. Helps regulate how much we eat, producing feelings of hunger or satiation in response to changes in cellular levels of nutrients. However, the conscious mind can overrule this feeling. Also helps establish and maintain wake/sleep patterns.
Cerebellum	Located at posterior base of the brain. Regulates involuntary aspects of movement, such as coordination, muscle tone, kinesthetics, posture, equilibrium.
Brainstem	Anterior to cerebellum and superior to spinal cord. Includes midbrain, medulla, and pons. Responsible for involuntary survival behaviors, such as breathing, heart rate, coughing, vomiting. Also transmits impulses from spinal cord to brain. Attachment site for 10 of the 12 cranial nerves.

Structures and Functions of the Brain

STRUCTURE	FUNCTION
Midbrain	Regulates visual, auditory, and other reflexes and controls eye movements, focusing, and pupil dilation.
Medulla	Regulates heart and respiratory rate, blood pressure, and protective reflexes such as swallowing, vomiting, sneezing, and coughing.
Pons	Helps control respiratory function, facial movement and sensation, and eye movement.
Meninges	Three connective tissue membranes that cover and protect brain and spinal cord. Pia mater: Inner layer, contains blood vessels. Arachnoid: Middle layer, provides space for cerebrospinal fluid Dura mater: Outer layer that adds support and protection.
Ventricles	Four cavities within the brain whose capillaries continuously produce and reabsorb **cerebrospinal fluid** (CSF) from blood plasma. CSF cushions the brain, delivers nutrients, and removes wastes. CSF circulates in the subarachnoid space between the arachnoid mater and pia mater.

The Spinal Cord

The **spinal cord** descends through the foramen magnum (large aperture) of the occipital bone of the skull, through the first cervical vertebra (C1), and through the remainder of the vertebral column to the first or second lumbar vertebra. At this point, the cord itself terminates and its roots branch off into the cauda equina ("horse's tail").

A cross-section of the spinal cord reveals gray matter composed of neuronal cell bodies clustered into an "H" shape, with two anterior and two posterior "horns." This gray matter is surrounded by white matter composed of myelinated axons and dendrites. Cord fibers associate into **ascending tracts,** which carry sensory data to the brain, and **descending tracts,** which carry motor impulses from the brain.

Sensory Pathways

Sensory (ascending or afferent) pathways allow sensory data, such as the feeling of a burned hand, to become conscious perceptions. The pathways by which a variety of somatic sensations travel to the cerebral cortex are illustrated in Figure 19–3. The two major sensory pathways are the lateral and anterior spinothalamic tracts and the posterior column. The lateral and anterior spinothalamic tracts transmit nerve impulses for pain, temperature, itching, tickling, pressure, and crude touch, whereas the posterior column transmits nerve impulses for proprioception, discriminitive sensations, and vibrations. Some visceral sensory neurons also enter the spinal cord as shown in the figure; however, other visceral stimuli are carried by the vagus nerve or another of the cranial nerves and enter the brainstem directly, bypassing the spinal cord.

All somatic sensory stimuli—for example, sensations of pain, heat, or pressure—are conveyed from the body periphery into the spinal cord via the posterior root of the appropriate spinal nerve. At that point, sensations of fine touch, **proprioception,** and vibration continue into the posterior column of the spinal cord and into the brainstem. Here they cross to the opposite side of the brainstem before they continue into the thalamus and from there to the sensory areas of the cerebral cortex.

In contrast to this, sensations of pain, temperature, crude touch, and pressure enter the posterior horn and cross the spinal cord into the opposite side of the cord before they begin their ascent. Pain and temperature are carried in the **lateral spinothalamic tract,** whereas crude touch and pressure are carried in the **anterior spinothalamic tract.** These tracts continue to ascend straight upward, entering the thalamus and then the cerebral cortex.

As you might imagine, a patient with a particular type of sensory loss may have a neurological impairment affecting a particular column or tract. For example, someone who loses the ability to perceive vibration and changes in positioning may have a lesion in the posterior column.

Motor Pathways

Motor pathways (descending or efferent) transmit impulses from the brain to the muscles. The three major motor pathways of the CNS are the corticospinal (pyramidal or direct), including the corticobulbar; the extrapyramidal or indirect; and the cerebellum. The descending pathways can be direct or indirect. Direct (pyramidal) pathways carry impulses from the cerebral cortex to lower motor neurons that innervate the skeletal muscles, resulting in voluntary movement. The direct pathways include the anterior and lateral corticospinal and corticobulbar tracts. The corticospinal tracts control voluntary skilled movement of

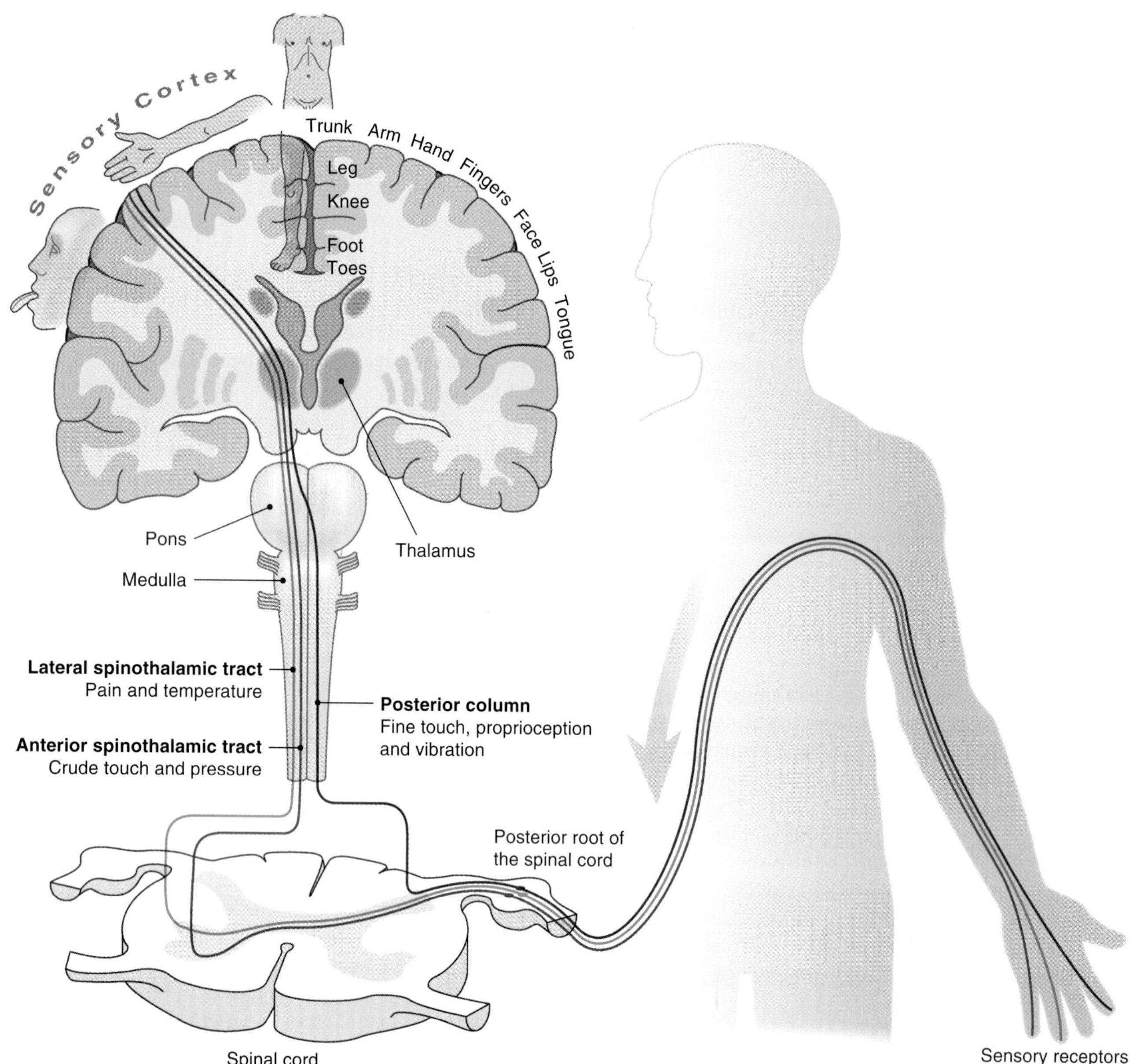

FIGURE 19–3. Sensory pathways.

Major Sensory Tracts

TRACT	SENSATION
Lateral Spinothalamic	Pain and temperature
Anterior Spinothalamic	Light (crude) touch
Posterior Column	Touch-pressure, two-point discrimination, vibratory sensation, position sense (proprioception), and some light (crude) touch

the extremities and fine movement of the fingers. The corticobulbar tract connects the motor cortex to lower motor neurons of the cranial nerves. The indirect (extrapyramidal) pathways carry impulses from the brainstem and other parts of the brain, resulting in automatic movement, coordination of movement, and maintaining skeletal muscle tone and posture. The indirect pathways consist of the reticulospinal, rubrospinal, tectospinal, and vestibulospinal tracts. The possible pathways of the corticospinal system are shown in Figure 19–4. The cerebellar system, which is involved primarily in coordination, equilibrium, and posture, is not shown. Also note that this discussion pertains to somatic, not visceral, motor neurons.

From the motor cortex, all somatic motor impulses descend via one of three tracts through the thalamus and into the brainstem, at which point the configuration of the three tracts resembles a pyramid. The anterior corticospinal and corticobulbar (uncrossed pyramidal tract) and the reticulospinal and vestibulospinal (uncrossed extrapyramidal tract) continues straight down into the spinal cord. There the impulse must cross over to the opposite anterior horn before it can exit the spinal cord via the anterior root of the spinal nerve. The lateral corticospinal (crossed pyramidal tract) and the rubrospinal (crossed extrapyramidal tract) both cross to the opposite side of the brainstem before descending directly into the anterior horn and exiting into the anterior root of the spinal nerve.

Motor impulses from the motor cortex to the periphery are controlled by upper and lower motor neurons. The upper motor neurons are located in the cerebral

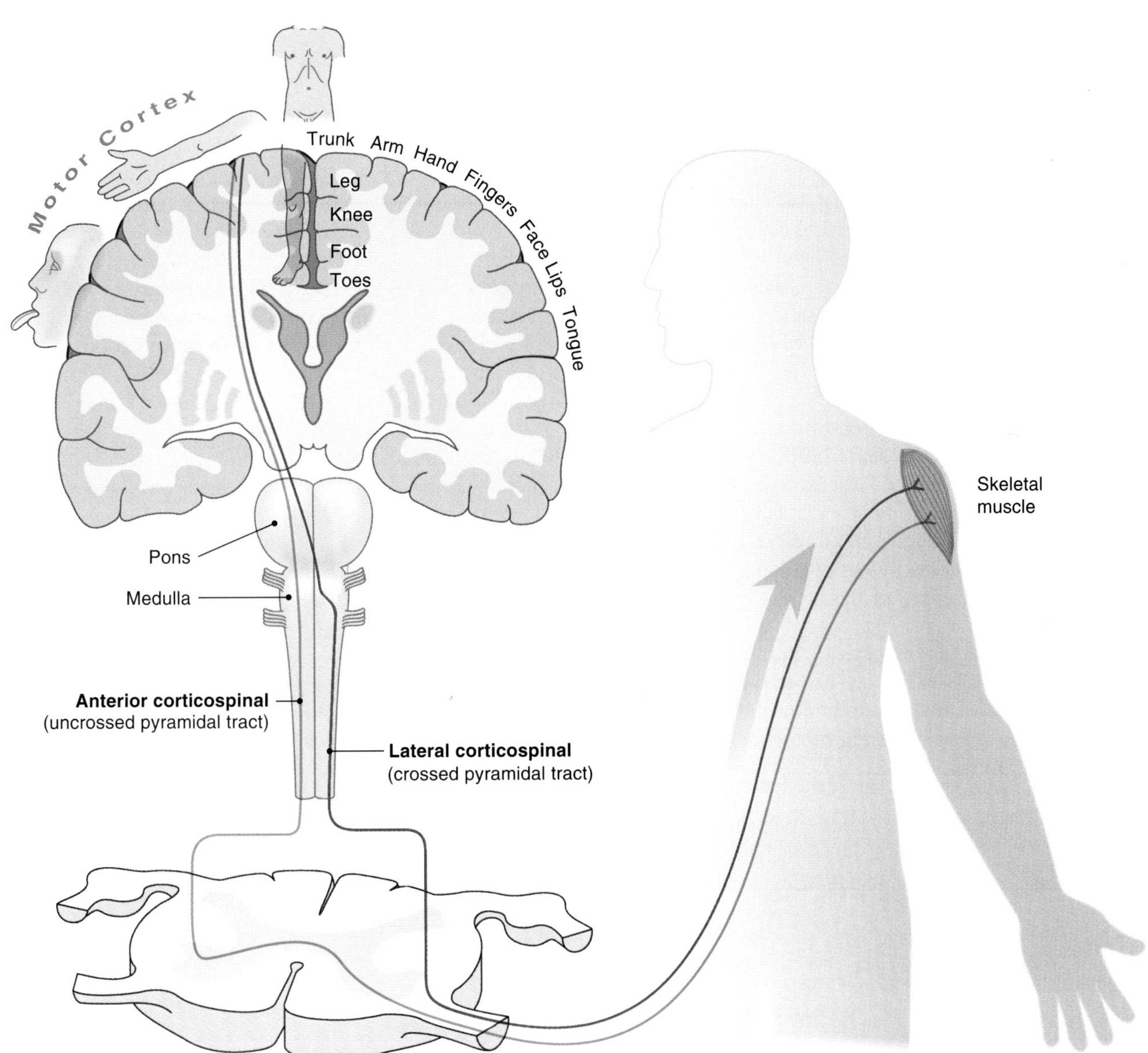

FIGURE 19–4. Motor pathways.

Major Motor Tracts

TRACT	MOTOR EFFECT
Lateral Corticospinal (Crossed Pyramidal)	Major tract controlling movement of extremities, fine movements of fingers
Anterior Corticospinal (Uncrossed Pyramidal)	Voluntary movement of axial muscles
Corticobulbar (Uncrossed Pyramidal)	Cranial nerves
Rubrospinal (Crossed Extrapyramidal)	Control and coordination of skilled muscle movement Minor influence on movement
Reticulospinal (Uncrossed Extrapyramidal)	Integration of axial body movements Maintenance of body posture Integration of body and limb movements Minor influence on movement
Vestibulospinal (Uncrossed Extrapyramidal)	Maintenance of body posture Integration of body and limb movements

cortex and brainstem and regulate the responses of the lower motor neurons. The lower motor neuron cell bodies lie in the anterior horn of the spinal cord, then exit the cord through the nerve roots. The lower motor neurons are the final link between the central nervous system and the skeletal muscles. An upper motor neuron lesion causes increased muscle tone (spasticity) and hyperreflexia. A lower motor neuron lesion causes decreased tone, flaccidity, and absent reflexes or hyporeflexia.

Spinal Reflexes

Spinal reflexes do not depend on conscious perception and interpretation of stimuli, nor on deliberate action; in other words, they do not involve the brain. They occur involuntarily, with lightning speed, and are identical in all healthy children and adults, although they are less developed in infants. When we experience a spinal reflex, we are not aware of the reflexive activity itself, only its result.

The simplest spinal reflexes are known as **deep tendon reflexes** (DTRs). They are **monosynaptic,** involving just one sensory neuron communicating across a single synapse to one responding motor neuron. A reflex arc is shown in Figure 19–5.

The classic example of a deep tendon reflex is the **patellar reflex,** commonly called the "knee-jerk reflex." The patellar reflex is an example of a stretch reflex. The patellar tendon is tapped with a reflex hammer, triggering a stretch response in the sensory fibers of the quadriceps femoris muscle. This stimulus is received by a sensory neuron, which carries it to the anterior horn of the spinal cord, where it is conveyed across a synapse to a motor neuron that then causes the muscle to contract. Because of the simplicity of the reflex arc, this contraction occurs within less than a second after the hammer tap.

Slow or absent deep tendon reflexes could indicate a health problem affecting the peripheral nerves, such as a degeneration of their myelin sheaths. Spinal cord trauma or lesions also commonly affect reflexes; therefore, it is helpful to know the specific spinal cord segment associated with each specific reflex. The box entitled Spinal Reflexes identifies the five deep tendon reflexes, as well as three superficial reflexes involving stimulation of the skin, along with the segmental level at which they occur. Assessment of these reflexes is discussed later in the chapter.

In addition to the monosynaptic reflexes, the body exhibits protective **flexor (or withdrawal) reflexes,** which help minimize trauma from harmful stimuli. For

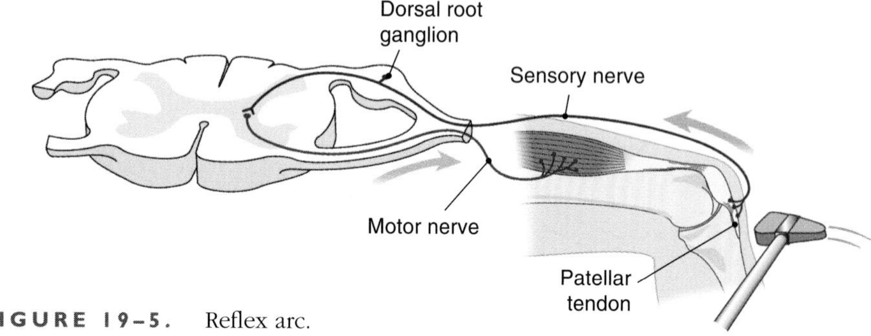

FIGURE 19–5. Reflex arc.

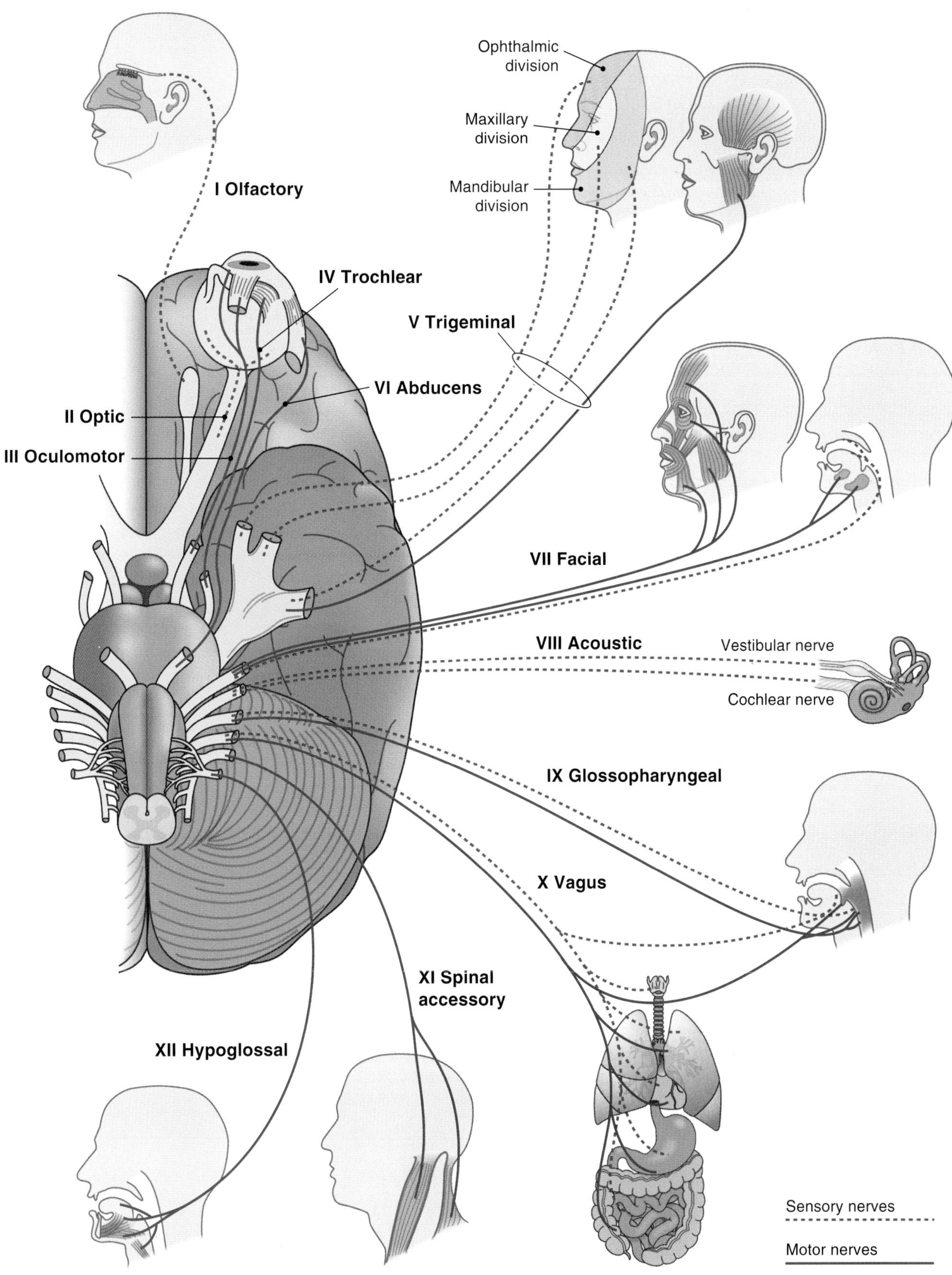

FIGURE 19–6. Origin of cranial nerves.

Spinal Reflexes

Reflex	Spinal Cord Segment Involved
Deep Tendon Reflexes	
Achilles Reflex (plantar flexion at ankle)	S1 and S2
Patellar Reflex (knee extension)	L2, 3, and 4
Biceps Reflex (elbow flexion)	C5 and 6
Triceps Reflex (elbow extension)	C6, 7, and 8
Brachioradialis Reflex (forearm flexion and supination)	C5 and 6
Superficial Reflexes	
Upper Abdominal Reflex	T8, 9, and 10
Lower Abdominal Reflex	T10 and 11
Plantar Reflex	L5, S1 and 2
Cremasteric Reflex	L1, 2
Bulbocavernosus Reflex	S3, 4
Anal Reflex	S3, 4, 5

example, these reflexes allow speedy, involuntary withdrawal from a heat source. Flexor reflexes require a sensory neuron to interact with an intermediate neuron or **interneuron** in the spinal cord. This interneuron, in turn, sends the impulse across a synapse to the receiving motor neuron.

Peripheral Nervous System

The **peripheral nervous system** consists of the cranial and spinal nerves and the peripheral autonomic nervous system. The peripheral nervous system can also be divided into the somatic and the visceral nervous systems. The somatic system has both afferent and efferent divisions. The afferent division receives, processes, and transmits sensory information from the skin and the musculoskeletal system, eyes, tongue, nose, and ears. The efferent division has lower motor neurons and regulates voluntary muscle contraction.

The visceral system also has afferent and efferent divisions. The afferent division is responsible for processing information from the visceral organs. The efferent division is responsible for the motor responses of the smooth muscle, cardiac muscle, skin glands, and viscera.

Function of Cranial Nerves

Number	Name	Type and Function
CN I	Olfactory	*Sensory:* Smell
CN II	Optic	*Sensory:* Sight
CN III	Oculomotor	*Motor:* Opening eyelid; moving eye superiorly, medially, and diagonally; constricting pupils
CN IV	Trochlear	*Motor:* Moving eye down and laterally
CN V	Trigeminal	*Mixed:* *Motor:* Chewing and jaw opening and clenching *Sensory:* Conveying sensory data from eyes (cornea), nose, mouth, teeth, jaw, forehead, scalp, and facial skin
CN VI	Abducens	*Motor:* Moving eye laterally
CN VII	Facial	*Mixed:* *Motor:* Closing eyes, closing mouth, moving lips and other muscles of facial expression, salivation and lacrimation (secreting saliva and tears) *Sensory:* Tasting on anterior tongue
CN VIII	Acoustic	*Sensory:* Hearing, equilibrium
CN IX	Glossopharyngeal	*Mixed:* *Motor:* Swallowing, gag sensation, secretion of saliva *Sensory:* Tasting on posterior tongue
CN X	Vagus	*Mixed:* *Motor:* Palate. Pharynx, larynx (speaking and swallowing) *Sensory:* Sensations in pharynx and larynx *Sensorimotor:* Cardiovascular, respiratory, and digestive systems
CN XI	Accessory	*Motor:* Contracting muscles of neck and shoulders
CN XII	Hypoglossal	*Motor:* Tongue movement, articulating with tongue, swallowing

The efferent system is known as the autonomic nervous system.

Cranial Nerves

The 12 pairs of **cranial nerves** originate from the brain and are called the peripheral nerves of the brain. As shown in Figure 19–6, these nerves originate from the cerebrum, diencephalon, and brainstem. The function of each of the cranial nerves is indicated in the accompanying box.

Spinal and Peripheral Nerves

Branching from the spinal cord are 31 pairs of **spinal nerves:** 8 cervical pairs, 12 thoracic, 5 lumbar, 5 sacral, and 1 coccygeal (Fig. 19–7). The spinal nerves contain both ascending and descending fibers, and although there is some overlap, each is responsible for innervation of a particular area of the body. As shown in Figure 19–8, **dermatomes** are regions of the body innervated by the cutaneous branch of a single spinal nerve. For example, nerve C6 innervates a portion of the lateral (thumb) side of the arm and hand. Although there is some individual variation, it is useful to know which spinal nerves typically innervate which segments of the body so that neurological deficits can be more easily associated with lesions of particular nerves.

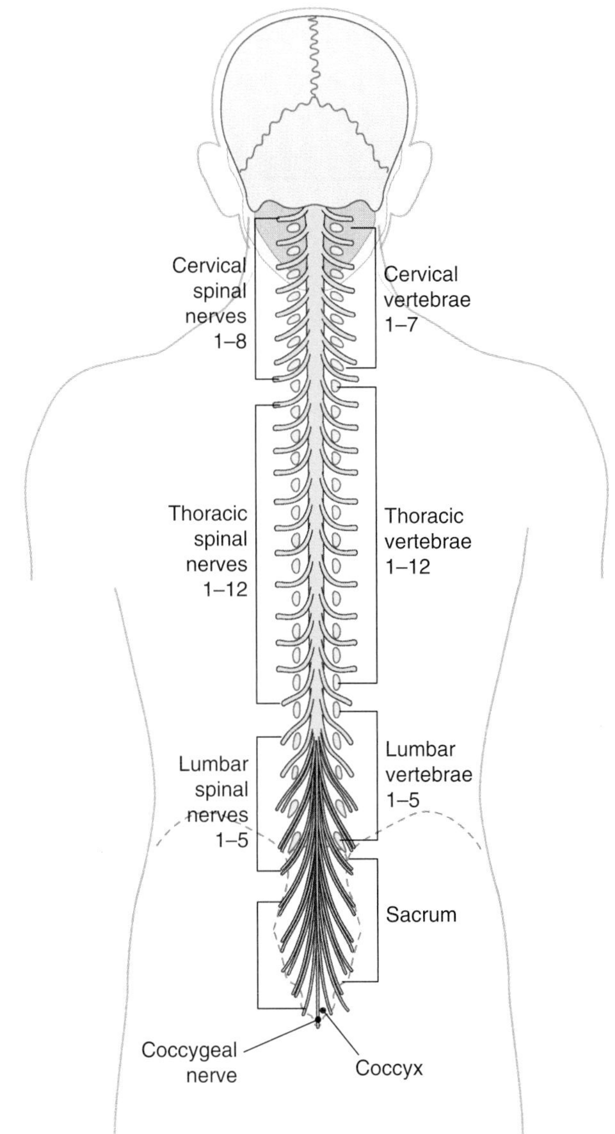

FIGURE 19–7. Spinal nerves.

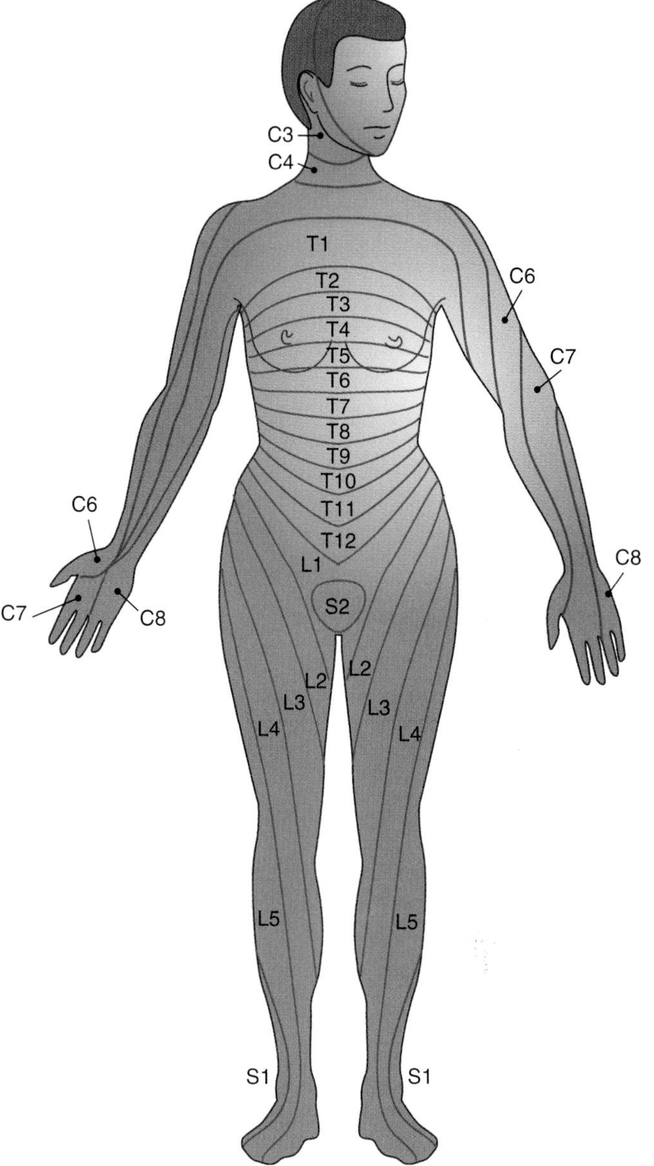

FIGURE 19–8. Dermatomes.

Each spinal nerve emerges from the spinal cord from two distinct roots. The posterior (dorsal) root contains afferent fibers that receive sensory information from the body periphery and convey it to the CNS. The anterior (ventral) root contains efferent fibers that convey motor impulses from the CNS to the muscles of the

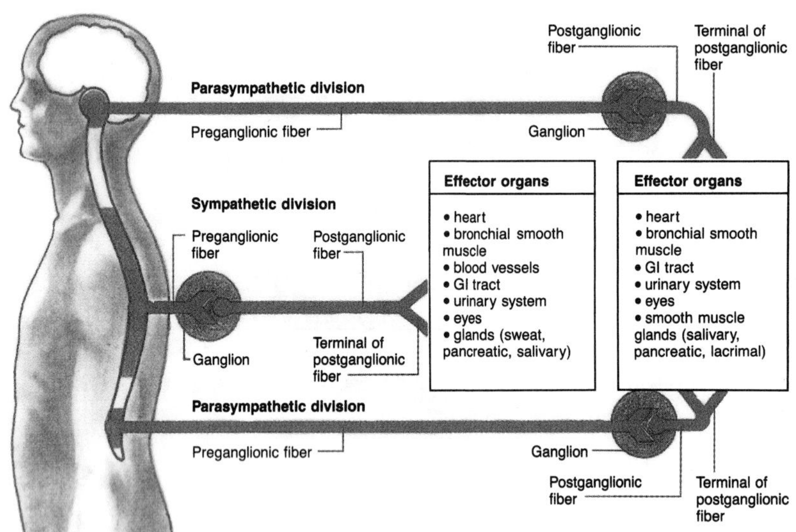

FIGURE 19–9. Autonomic nervous system.

body, directing and refining movement. These anterior and posterior roots then merge just distal to the cord to form one mixed spinal nerve capable of both sensory and motor functioning. Spinal nerves branch further to form the **peripheral nerves** of the body, most of which also carry both sensory and motor fibers.

The autonomic nervous system is divided into the sympathetic and parasympathetic, with efferent fibers to muscle, organs, or glands. Usually, the two systems work opposite each other. The sympathetic allows the body to respond to stressful situations. The parasympathetic functions when all is normal. The sympathetic nerves exit the spinal cord between the level of the first thoracic and second lumbar vertebrae. The preganglionic nerves descend the cord and exit, and then enter a relay station known as the sympathetic chain. The impulse is then transmitted to a postganglionic neuron that goes to the target organ to stimulate a response.

Sympathetic responses include vasoconstriction; increased BP, heart rate, and contractility; increased respiratory rate; smooth muscle relaxation of bronchioles, GI tract, and urinary tract; sphincter contraction; pupillary dilatation; increased sweat, and decreased pancreatic secretion.

The parasympathetic fibers leave the CNS by way of the cranial nerves from the midbrain and medulla, and between the second and fourth sacral vertebrae. A long preganglion fiber exits to an area near the target organ, and then synapses to form a postganglionic nerve, which in turn leads to a response. Parasympathetic responses include decreased heart rate, contractility and velocity; smooth muscle constriction of bronchioles; increased GI tract tone and peristalsis with sphincter relaxation; urinary sphincter relaxation and increased bladder tone; vasodilation of external genitalia causing male erection; pupillary constriction, and increased pancreatic, lacrimal, and salivary secretions. There is little effect on mental and metabolic activity. Figure 19–9 illustrates the autonomic nervous system.

Interaction with Other Body Systems

Because the nervous system is the main circuit board for the body, all body systems interact with it in some way.

The Cardiovascular System

Although the conduction system of the heart is completely independent of extrinsic neural control, cardiac centers in the medulla influence heart rate. Also, the vagus nerve can exert significant influence over both heart rate and vessel constriction, thereby influencing blood pressure.

The Respiratory System

Respiratory centers in the medulla of the brainstem regulate inspiration and expiration. Centers in the pons regulate respiratory drive. The vagus nerve relays data on blood gas levels to the medulla. Voluntary regulation of breathing can be achieved via motor neurons, which can stimulate the respiratory muscles.

The Endocrine System

The secretion of some endocrine glands, such as the adrenal glands, is regulated by nerves. Some neurons in

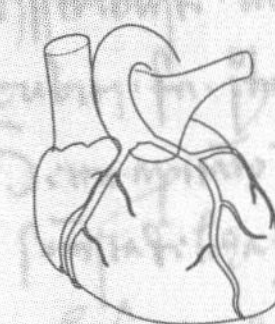

CARDIOVASCULAR

CV system supplies nutrients and removes wastes.

Nervous system can affect heart rate, blood pressure, and contractility.

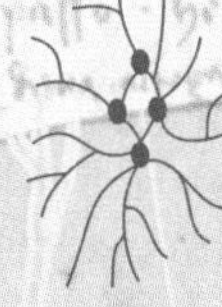

LYMPHATIC

Protects against infections and helps with tissue repair.

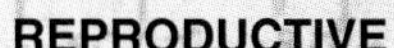

REPRODUCTIVE

Sex hormones can influence behavior.

Nervous system controls sexual function and behavior.

ENDOCRINE

Hormones released by endocrine system affect CNS metabolism.

Endocrine system secretes antidiuretic hormone (ADH) and oxytocin.

Reproductive hormones can affect CNS development and behavior.

Nervous system controls pituitary gland and many other endocrine glands.

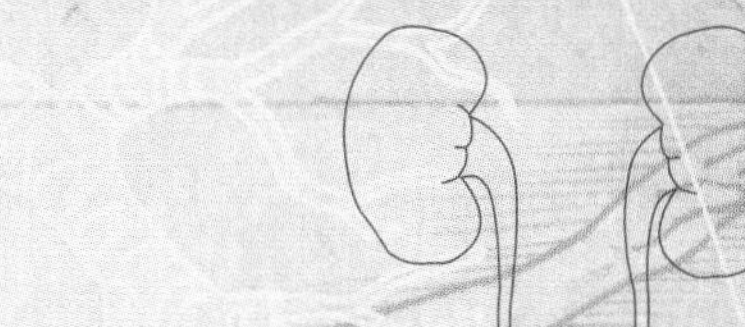

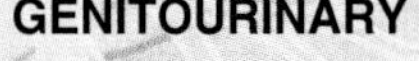

GENITOURINARY

GU system removes wastes and helps regulate pH and electrolytes.

Nervous system also helps regulate pH and can adjust renal blood flow.

Nerves of bladder sense fullness and control emptying.

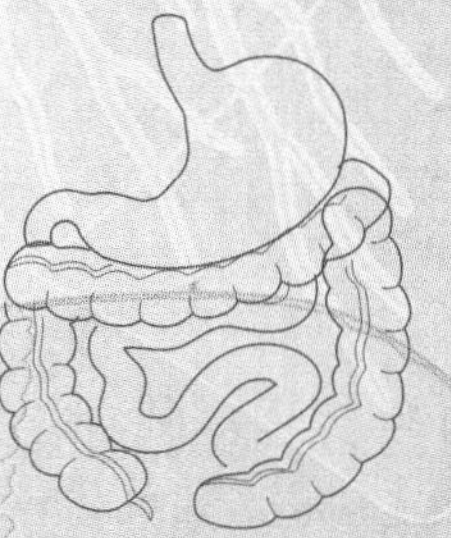

RESPIRATORY

Respiratory system supplies oxygen and removes carbon dioxide.

Nervous system can change the rate and depth of respirations.

GASTROINTESTINAL

GI system provides nutrients to nervous system.

Nervous system controls peristalsis and GI secretions.

Somatic motor nerves allow control of defecation.

MUSCULOSKELETAL

MS system protects brain and spinal cord.

MS system provides calcium if needed for neural impulse transmission.

MS system allows for verbal/nonverbal communication.

Nervous system controls muscle contraction and proprioception.

INTEGUMENTARY

Skin has receptors for sensations of touch, pain, temperature, texture, and pressure.

Skin and hair protect and insulate skull, brain, and peripheral nerves.

Nervous system controls contraction of erector pili muscles and sweat gland secretion.

Neural responses regulate blushing, sweat production, etc.

Relationship of the Sensory-Neurological System to Other Systems

the hypothalamus actually act as endocrine cells, secreting antidiuretic hormone, which stimulates the kidneys to reabsorb water and oxytocin, a reproductive hormone. Some other hormones, notably parathyroid hormone, affect metabolism of electrolytes, which in turn affects neurological function.

The Musculoskeletal System

Somatic and visceral motor neurons receive impulses from the cerebral cortex to carry out both voluntary and reflexive movements.

Developmental, Cultural, and Ethnic Variations

Newborns and Infants

Although neurological development is not complete until toddlerhood, neurological screening to detect the presence or extent of obvious pathologies such as spina bifida and fetal alcohol syndrome is performed on most newborns within the first 24 hours after birth. This screening includes assessment of appearance, alertness, motor and sensory function, and pain. In addition, newborns are assessed for a set of protective reflexes that disappear later in infancy, including the palmar grasp, stepping reflex, and rooting reflex (for more information, see Chapter 22, Assessing the Newborn and Infant).

Injury to the facial nerve during vaginal birth can cause a transient palsy. Down's syndrome is a genetic disorder that causes mild to severe mental retardation. Maternal use of drugs and alcohol during pregnancy, as well as dietary deficiencies, antepartal infections, systemic diseases, and birth trauma can result in neurological disorders such as mental retardation, blindness, deafness, seizures, and neuromuscular impairments.

Children and Adolescents

You can usually examine children past toddlerhood in a manner similar to that used for adults, with obvious adaptations for developmental stage. In most cases, any chronic neurological pathologies will have been discovered during infancy. However, childhood injuries and later-onset disorders, such as obsessive-compulsive disorder and hyperactivity, may only become apparent during the preschool years. Changes in behavior may also signal abuse.

If the parent reports seizure activity, assess for whether it is associated with signs of infection, such as a runny nose, high temperature, or recent immunizations. Fevers in toddlers and preschoolers occasionally cause seizures. Repeated episodes of seizure activity may indicate epilepsy.

If the parent reports that the child complains of headache or eye pain, assess for signs of sinusitis, meningitis, or concussion. If parents express concern over attention deficit disorder, hyperactivity, or other learning disorders, ask whether the child consumes caffeine or sugar daily, because some children are extremely sensitive to these substances. If the family lives in an older home, also assess for signs of lead poisoning, which can cause severe neurological problems.

Finally, observe for behavioral indicators that may signal child abuse. Even in the absence of bruises or other signs of trauma, perform a special assessment for child abuse if a child is inappropriately uncommunicative for his developmental level, extremely apprehensive or clingy, unable to show emotion, makes little or no eye contact, or responds inappropriately or not at all to painful procedures.

Pregnant Women

Ask pregnant patients if they are taking folic acid supplements, and if so, at what point in the pregnancy they began. Folic acid deficiency, especially in the first trimester, is closely linked to neural tube defects such as spina bifida. Other nutrients are also important to support the fetus's neurological development.

During pregnancy, the woman may experience transient episodes of neurological pain, including carpal tunnel syndrome, foot and leg cramps, numbness or tingling in the thighs, and frequent headaches. These usually resolve spontaneously after childbirth. Hyperactive reflexes during the later stages of pregnancy may signal preeclampsia, a hypertensive disorder that can be accompanied by seizures.

Older Adults

Neurons are continually lost during our lives, and with advanced age, neural impulses slow down. However, the common belief that intelligence, memory, and discrimination normally decrease with advanced age is simply not true. Research has shown that creative, critical, and abstract thinking, as well as problem-solving ability, are more typically *increased* in older adults. For this reason, you should carefully evaluate neurological deficits in the older adult for the presence of underlying factors.

Neurological deficits in older adults are commonly caused by:

- Adverse effects of medications or medication interactions
- Nutritional deficiencies
- Dehydration
- Cardiovascular disease affecting cerebral perfusion
- Diabetes and other endocrine disorders

- Neurological trauma
- Brain tumors or metastatic disease
- Stroke (CVA)
- Degenerative neurological diseases, such as Alzheimer's disease and Parkinson's disease
- Alcohol or drug abuse
- Isolation
- Psychiatric disorders
- Abuse or neglect

Also bear in mind that the number and sensitivity of sensory neurons decrease with age, leading to a diminished sense of touch. Reflexes also diminish; for example, the Achilles tendon reflex may be symmetrically diminished or absent in older adults. Abdominal reflexes also may be decreased or absent, and the plantar reflex may be decreased because of musculoskeletal changes in the feet.

People of Different Cultures and Ethnic Groups

Take care not to mistake language barriers or cultural variations in communication styles for evidence of neurological impairment, especially during the mental status examination. Also, make sure your questions are not culturally specific. For example, do not ask a first-generation Mexican-American patient to recite the names of the last four United States presidents.

Some cultures have a tendency for specific neurological diseases; for example, African-Americans have a higher incidence of hypertension and subsequently a higher incidence of stroke. The Irish have a high incidence of neural tube defects. Navajo Native Americans have a unique neuropathy that causes complete absence of myelinated fiber, weakness, hypotonia, areflexia, loss of sensation in extremities, corneal ulcers, and painless fractures. It usually causes death by age 24.

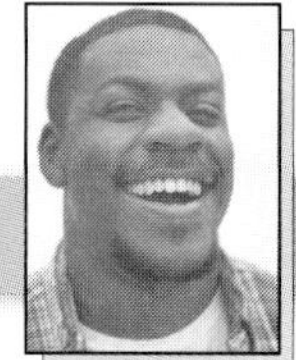

Introducing the Case Study

Leon Webster is a 21-year-old African-American college senior who plays football. Friday night, he and several friends went to a local club to celebrate the team's winning season. While driving home, Leon lost control of his car and hit a tree. He was brought to the emergency room (ER) by ambulance. He was alert and oriented but complaining of a headache and neck pain. He had a 3-inch laceration on his forehead where his head hit the rear-view mirror. He was not wearing a seat belt.

Performing the Sensory-Neurological and Cranial Nerve Assessment

A complete assessment of the patient's neurological system requires you to take a detailed health history, perform a mental status examination, assess the cranial nerves, assess the sensory system, and test deep tendon and superficial reflexes.

Health History

Before you begin the health history, keep in mind that the patient may be experiencing confusion, impaired verbal communication, memory loss, personality changes, or other deficits. This may affect his or her ability to provide reliable information, so verifying subjective data with a family member or friend may be wise. Rather than asking a long series of questions, it may be best to encourage the patient to tell his story without interruption. You can learn a great deal from the content of the story and also by listening to the way it is told.

Biographical Data

As always, review the patient's biographical data for clues that relate to the neurological system. Obviously, the patient's age and educational level will influence the questions you ask and the type and extent of teaching you provide. Keep in mind that certain neurological disorders are age related. For example, the incidence of cerebrovascular accident (CVA) increases with age, and neurological diseases such as myasthenia gravis (MG) and multiple sclerosis (MS) usually attack young women with a peak age between 20 and 30 years. Spinal cord injuries occur more frequently in young people because of the higher rate of accidents. Also, some neurological disorders are gender related. For example, women have a higher incidence of hemorrhagic stroke, whereas men have more thrombic strokes; before age 40, MG occurs in women two to three times more often than in men; and the incidence of MS is higher in women than in men. Even geographic locale influences some types of neurological diseases. For instance, MS occurs most often in colder climates such as the northeastern, Great Lakes, and Pacific Northwestern states. Also, the incidence of CVA is higher in the "stroke belt" states of Alabama, Arkansas, Georgia, Indiana, Kentucky, Louisiana, Mississippi, North Carolina, South Carolina, Tennessee, and Virginia.

Ask adolescents and adults about their job history. Could they have been exposed to neurotoxins? Have they had a head or back injury? Marital status, such as a recent divorce or death of a spouse, can certainly influence neurological findings. A patient's spiritual beliefs may also influence how he perceives illness (e.g., as a punishment) and how he deals with illness (e.g., the Christian Science belief in healing through mental and spiritual means).

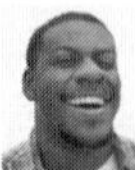

Case Study Findings

Reviewing Mr. Webster's biographical data:

- 21 years old
- African-American
- Baptist religion
- Senior in college; business major
- Insured under family's medical plan while in college
- Lives on campus during school year; home is 1 hour from school
- Contact person: Janet Webster, mother
- Source: Self, seems reliable

Current Health Status

The current health status focuses on the patient's chief complaint. If he or she has a neurological problem, begin with the chief complaint. Major neurological symptoms to watch for are headache, memory loss, confusion, dizziness, loss of consciousness, numbness, sensory loss, and problems with any of the five senses. Explore these complaints using the PQRST format.

ALERT

Establishing time of onset of symptoms is critical if you suspect a CVA. If the patient is a candidate for tissue plasminogen activator (tPA), there is a 3-hour window in which tPA must be administered.

Symptom Analysis

Symptom Analysis tables for all of the symptoms described in the following paragraphs are available on the Web for viewing and printing. In your Web browser, go to http://www.fadavis.com/detail.cfm?id=0882-9 and click on Symptom Analysis Tables under Explore This Product.

Headache

Headache is the most common neurological symptom. The causes are many. The pain may be mild or severe, acute or chronic, localized or generalized. Ninety percent of all headaches are benign in nature, caused by muscle contraction (tension) and/or vascular (migraine and cluster); the other 10 percent have underlying pathology. Because a headache may be a symptom of a serious medical problem, a careful, thorough symptom analysis is needed to determine the cause.

Mental Status Changes

Mental status changes are an early indication of a change in neurological status. The changes may be very subtle and difficult to detect. They may begin slowly as forgetfulness, memory loss, or inability to concentrate, or rapidly proceed to unconsciousness. Causes include neurological problems, fluid and electrolyte imbalance, hypoxia, low perfusion states, nutritional deficiencies, infections, renal and liver disease, hyper- or hypothermia, trauma, medications, and drug and alcohol abuse. If your patient's mental status is severely impaired, ask family members to describe the changes that have occurred.

Dizziness, Vertigo, and Syncope

Dizziness, vertigo, and **syncope** are common neurological signs and symptoms that warrant further investigation. Dizziness is a "fainting" sensation, whereas vertigo is a sensation that the surroundings are spinning around (objective vertigo) or that the person is spinning around (subjective vertigo). Vertigo is often accompanied by nausea and vomiting, nystagmus, and tinnitus. Dizziness can lead to syncope, which is a temporary loss of consciousness. The patient may say that he or she "blacked out" or "had a spell." Although the underlying cause of these signs and symptoms may be benign, they may also indicate a serious problem, such as an impending CVA, and need to be investigated thoroughly.

Numbness or Loss of Sensation

Numbness or tingling is referred to as paresthesia. Possible causes include diabetes and neurological, metabolic, cardiovascular, renal, and inflammatory diseases. Determine the area affected and the onset and progression of symptoms.

Deficits in the Five Senses

Assess changes in any of the five senses. Intact cranial nerves are essential for many of the senses. CN I (olfactory) is responsible for the sense of smell; CN II (optic), III (oculomotor), IV (trochlear), and VI (abducens) are responsible for visual acuity, pupillary constriction, and extraocular movement (EOM); CN VII (facial) and IX (glossopharyngeal) control taste; CN VIII (acoustic) controls hearing; and CN V (trigeminal) and dermatomes control somatic sensations.

Visual problems are a frequent symptom associated with neurological disorders and should be further assessed. Visual changes can result from ocular, neurological, or systemic problems, eye or head trauma, or adverse effects from drugs. The anatomical position of the cranial nerves that control the eye makes the nerves vulnerable to increases in ICP. These visual changes can be total loss of vision, visual field cuts, blurred vision, diplopia (double vision), photosensitivity, and amaurosis fugax (unilateral vision loss, as if a shade were being pulled down, resulting from insufficient blood supply to the retina and lasting up to 10 minutes). The visual deficit may have an acute or gradual onset and be permanent or temporary.

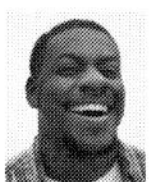

Case Study Findings

Mr. Webster's current health status includes:

- Complains of headache and neck pain from hitting head in motor vehicle accident.
- Had a few beers earlier in night.
- Felt a little confused after accident and is not sure what happened. Does not know whether he lost consciousness.

CRITICAL THINKING ACTIVITY #1

What other questions would you ask Mr. Webster to further assess his chief complaints?

Past Health History

The purpose of the past medical history is to compare it with the patient's present neurological status or uncover risk factors that might predispose the patient to neurological disorders. The following questions will guide you in exploring specific areas related to the sensory-neurological system.

Past Health History

RISK FACTORS/ QUESTIONS TO ASK	RATIONALE/SIGNIFICANCE
Childhood Illnesses	
Do you have a history of head injury or seizures?	Neurological problems in childhood may have permanent effects.
Surgery	
Have you ever had surgery or other treatment involving the nervous system?	Provides baseline information for physical assessment and explains physical findings.
Hospitalizations/Diagnostic Procedures	
Have you ever been treated for a neurological problem?	Helps identify potential or recurring neurological problem.
Serious Injuries	
Have you ever had a serious injury? If so, can you describe it? What treatment was given, and do you have any residual effects from the injury?	Information on past injuries provides baseline data for physical assessment. Postconcussion syndrome can present 1 to 2 weeks postinjury and persist up to a year. Minor head injury in older adults can cause a subdural hematoma that may be asymptomatic for weeks to months. Spine and back injuries may explain peripheral neurological problems.
Serious/Chronic Illnesses	
Do you have any other medical problems?	One-third of people who experience TIAs will have a CVA. CVA increases risk for another CVA 10 times. Determine residual deficits. HTN increases risk for CVA 6 times. Diabetes increases CVA risk 2 to 4 times. Atrial fibrillation increases CVA risk 17 times. Diabetic neuropathies can lead to sensory losses. Tertiary syphilis can cause neurosyphilis.

(Continued)

Past Health History *(Continued)*

RISK FACTORS/ QUESTIONS TO ASK	RATIONALE/SIGNIFICANCE
Serious/Chronic Illnesses *(Continued)* Do you have any other medical problems?	Recent upper respiratory infections may precede meningitis. History of seizures may explain current neurological findings. *New onset of seizures between ages 20 and 30:* Trauma, tumor, vascular disease. *New onset of seizures after age 50:* CVA or metastatic cancer. Three-fourths of all epilepsy is **idiopathic** (exact cause unknown).
Immunizations What immunizations have you had and when?	Diphtheria, pertussis, and tetanus (DPT) vaccine contraindicated in patients who have experienced encephalopathy within 7 days of DPT administration. Administer DPT cautiously in patients who had seizures within 3 days after previous administration. Immunization information can aid in differential diagnoses. *Haemophilus influenzae* type B (HiB) vaccine prevents bacterial meningitis. Meningococcal (menomune) vaccine is also available and is highly recommended for college-bound adolescents.
Allergies Do you have any allergies, and if so, what are they?	Iodine allergy may prohibit use of invasive studies that require contrast dyes.
Medications Are you taking any prescribed or over-the-counter (OTC) medications? Herbal products? Anticoagulants or antiplatelet medications?	Certain medications can affect the neurological system (see box, Drugs That Adversely Affect the Sensory-Neurological System). Anticoagulants or products that affect bleeding may increase risk for intracranial bleeding. They may also prevent treatment of CVA patients with tPA.
Birth control pills (BCP) or hormone replacement therapy (HRT)?	BCP and HRT may increase risk for CVA.
Recent Military Service Were you exposed to toxic chemicals during military service?	Veterans returning from Operation Desert Storm had many neurological complaints.

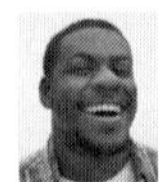

Case Study Findings

Mr. Webster's past health history reveals:

- No hospitalizations or surgeries
- Concussion in high school while playing football, otherwise negative for neurological problems
- Fractured fibula freshman year while playing football; injury casted and healed without problem
- Thinks immunizations are up to date but unsure of last tetanus shot
- No known food, drug, or environmental allergies
- No medications or other medical problems

Drugs That Adversely Affect the Sensory-Neurological System

Drug Class	Drug	Possible Adverse Reactions
Adrenergics	albuterol sulfate, epinephrine, isoproterenol hydrochloride, terbutaline sulfate	Nervousness, tremors, dizziness, restlessness, insomnia
Adrenergic blockers	ergotamine tartrate, methysergide maleate	Lightheadedness, vertigo, insomnia, euphoria, confusion, hallucinations, numbness and tingling of fingers and toes

Drugs That Adversely Affect the Sensory-Neurological System

Drug Class	Drug	Possible Adverse Reactions
Antianginals	diltiazem hydrochloride	Headache, fatigue
	isosorbide dinitrate, nitroglycerin	Throbbing headache, dizziness, weakness, orthostatic hypotension
	nifedipine	Headache, dizziness, lightheadedness, flushing
	verapamil hydrochloride	Headache, dizziness
Antiarrhythmics	lidocaine hydrochloride	Lightheadedness, dizziness, paresthesia, tremors, restlessness, confusion, hallucinations, headache
Antimicrobials	aminoglycosides	Neuromuscular blockade; ototoxicity causing vertigo, hearing impairment, or both
	acyclovir	Myoclonus, seizures
	isoniazid, nitrofurantoin	Peripheral neuropathy
	penicillin G	
	penicillin G	Delirium, headaches, mania, coma
Anticonvulsants	carbamazepine	Dizziness, drowsiness, ataxia, confusion, speech disturbances, involuntary movements
	phenytoin sodium	Dose-related headache, confusion, ataxia, slurred speech, lethargy, drowsiness, nervousness, insomnia, blurred vision, diplopia, nystagmus
Antidepressants	tricyclic antidepressants	Drowsiness, weakness, lethargy, fatigue, agitation, nightmares, restlessness; confusion, disorientation (especially in elderly clients)
	monoamine oxidase inhibitors	Restlessness, insomnia, drowsiness, headache, orthostatic hypotension, hypertension
Antihypertensives	clonidine hydrochloride	Drowsiness, sedation, dizziness, headache, nightmares, depression, hallucinations
	hydralazine hydrochloride	Headache
	methyldopa	Drowsiness, sedation, decreased mental acuity, vertigo, headache, psychic disturbances, nightmares, depression
	propranolol hydrochloride	Fatigue, lethargy, vivid dreams, hallucinations, depression
Antineoplastic agents	fludarabine	Dysarthrias, paresthesias, weakness, seizures, paralysis
	procarbazine hydrochloride	Paresthesis, neuropathy, confusion
	vinblastine sulfate	Paresthesis, numbness
	vincristine sulfate	Peripheral neuropathy, loss of deep tendon reflexes, jaw pain
Antiparkinsonian agents	amantadine hydrochloride	Psychic disturbances, nervousness, irritability, fatigue, depression, insomnia, confusion, hallucinations, difficulty concentrating
	levodopa, pramipaxole, rophirole	Psychic disturbances, decreased attention span, memory loss, nervousness, vivid dreams, involuntary muscle movements
Antipsychotics	haloperidol, phenothiazines	Extrapyramidal reactions, tardive dyskinesia, headache, lethargy, confusion, agitation, hallucinations
Cholinergic blockers	atropine sulfate, benztropine mesylate, glycopyrrolate	Blurred vision, headache, nervousness, drowsiness, weakness, dizziness, insomnia, disorientation
Corticosteroids	dexamethasone, hydrocortisone, methylprednisolone, prednisone	Mood swings, euphoria, insomnia, headache, vertigo, psychotic behavior
Gastrointestinal agents	cimetidine	Confusion (especially in elderly clients), depression
	metoclopramide hydrochloride	Restlessness, anxiety drowsiness, lassitude, extrapyramidal reactions, tardive dyskinesia
Narcotic analgesics	morphine sulfate, hydromorphone hydrochloride, meperidine hydrochloride, methadone hydrochloride, oxycodone hydrochloride	Sedation, dizziness, visual disturbances, clouded sensorium
	butorphanol tartrate, nalbuphine hydrochloride, pentazocine hydrochloride	Sedation, headache, dizziness, vertigo, light-headedness, euphoria

(Continued)

Drugs That Adversely Affect the Sensory-Neurological System *(Continued)*

Drug Class	Drug	Possible Adverse Reactions
Nonsteroidal anti-inflammatory agents	ibuprofen, indomethacin	Headache, drowsiness, dizziness
Sedatives and hypnotics	barbiturates	Drowsiness, lethargy, vertigo, headache, depression, "hangover," paradoxical excitement in elderly clients, hyperactivity in children
	benzodiazepines	Drowsiness, dizziness, ataxia, daytime sedation, headache, confusion
Skeletal muscle relaxants	baclofen	Drowsiness
	chlorzoxazone	Drowsiness, dizziness
	cyclobenzaprine hydrochloride	Drowsiness, dizziness, headache, nervousness, confusion
Miscellaneous agents	lithium carbonate	Lethargy, tremors, headache, mental confusion, dizziness, seizures, difficulty concentrating

Family History

The family history identifies any predisposing or causative factors for neurological problems.

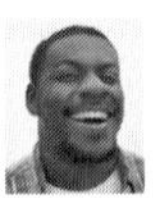

Case Study Findings

Mr. Webster's pertinent family history reveals:

- Father, age 55, has HTN.
- Paternal uncle, age 60, has HTN.
- Paternal grandfather, died at 80 from CVA.
- Maternal aunt, age 50, has HTN.
- Maternal grandfather died at 75 from CVA.

Review of Systems

The review of systems (ROS) allows you to assess how the neurological system affects or is affected by every other system. Often you may uncover an important fact that your patient failed to mention earlier.

Family History

RISK FACTORS/ QUESTIONS TO ASK	RATIONALE/SIGNIFICANCE
Familial/Genetically Linked Neurological Problems	
Do you have a family history of hypertension, stroke, multiple sclerosis, seizures, amyotrophic lateral sclerosis (ALS), Huntington's chorea, Alzheimer's disease, or cancer?	Positive family history for these diseases increases risk to patient.
Do you have a family history of substance abuse or psychiatric problems?	

Review of Systems

SYSTEM/QUESTIONS TO ASK	RATIONALE/SIGNIFICANCE
General Health Survey	
How have you been feeling?	Look for affective changes such as depression. Lethargy, emotional lability seen with CVA.
Have you had a fever?	Associated with meningitis.
Integumentary	
Have you had any changes in or loss of sensation? Rashes?	*Loss of sensation:* TIA, CVA, neuropathies. *Skin rash, petechiae:* Meningococcal meningitis.

Review of Systems

SYSTEM/QUESTIONS TO ASK	RATIONALE/SIGNIFICANCE
HEENT/*Head and Neck*	
Do you have a change in any of your senses?	
Headaches?	*Headaches:* HTN, intracranial bleeding.
Upper respiratory infections (URIs)? Enlarged glands or lumps in your neck?	*URI, enlarged lymph nodes:* Systemic infection that may precede meningitis.
Do you have thyroid disease?	Hypo- or hyperthyroidism can affect patient's mood.
Speech changes or difficulty speaking?	*Dysarthria:* Lack of articulation of speech.

HELPFUL HINT

Patients with dysarthria often have dysphagia (difficulty swallowing) as well.

Aphasia: Total loss of comprehension and use of language. Can be receptive (inability to comprehend what is being said, also called Wernicke's or sensory aphasia) or expressive (inability to conceptualize what words one wants to say, also called Broca's or motor aphasia).
Dysphasia: Impairment of speech. Speech can be nonfluent, slow, deliberate, with few words, or fluent, with intact speech that lacks meaning.

SYSTEM/QUESTIONS TO ASK	RATIONALE/SIGNIFICANCE
HEENT/*Eyes, Ears, Nose, Throat*	
Do you have difficulty swallowing, vision changes, hearing changes, or ringing in your ears (tinnitus)?	Associated with TIA and CVA.
Respiratory	
Do you have any breathing problems?	Mental status changes can occur with COPD as a result of hypoxia or hypercapnea.
Cardiovascular	
Do you have any cardiovascular problems?	Positive history of CV disease increases risk for stroke.
Have you ever been told that you have an irregular heartbeat?	Atrial fibrillation, a common dysrhythmia in older adults, increases risk for CVA.
Do your hands become numb, tingle, or change color in response to cold?	Raynaud's and Buerger's diseases can cause paresthesia.
Gastrointestinal	
Do you have nausea, vomiting, or trouble swallowing?	Nausea is often seen with neurological problems such as head trauma and increased ICP. Dysphagia may occur with CVA, MS, MG, ALS.

ALERT

Patients who have difficulty swallowing are at higher risk for aspiration.

SYSTEM/QUESTIONS TO ASK	RATIONALE/SIGNIFICANCE
Do you have any bowel or bladder problems or loss of sensation?	*Bowel problems, incontinence, loss of bowel function:* Cauda equina syndrome caused by compression of sacral nerve, can occur with herniated disc or spinal stenosis. *Transient loss of bowel and bladder function:* CVA or spinal cord dysfunction. *Incontinence:* Tonic-clonic seizures.

(Continued)

Review of Systems *(Continued)*

SYSTEM/QUESTIONS TO ASK	RATIONALE/SIGNIFICANCE
Reproductive	
Have you had any sexually transmitted diseases (STDs)?	Tertiary syphilis can cause neurosyphilis.
Males: Do you have any problems with sexual performance?	Loss of sensation and inability to achieve erection may be neurological in origin. Problems with erection can occur with neuropathies and CNS disease such as Parkinson's disease.
Females: When was your last menstrual period? Have you had miscarriages? Are you taking birth control pills?	Hypercoagulable states increase the risk for CVA.
Musculoskeletal	
Do you have any loss of sensation, numbness, or weakness?	Associated with many neurological disorders. Neuropathies may be associated with DM.
Have you experienced paralysis?	Paralysis can lead to muscle atrophy from disuse.
Endocrine	
Do you have diabetes mellitus or thyroid disease?	Diabetes can cause neuropathies and muscle wasting. Hypothyroidism can cause weakness, lethargy, flat affect, and labile affect.
Lymphatic/Hematologic	
Do you have any blood disorders? Do you bruise easily?	Bleeding disorders may increase risk for CVA. Patients with platelet count <100,000 and INR >1.7 are not candidates for tPA.

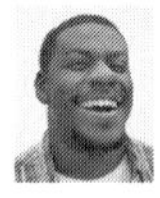

Case Study Findings

Mr. Webster's review of systems reveals:

- **General Health Survey:** Usual state of health good until accident
- **Integumentary:** No changes
- **HEENT:** Headache and neck pain; a little "dizzy"
- **Respiratory:** No problems
- **Cardiovascular:** No problems
- **Gastrointestinal:** Appetite usually good, but felt "a little sick after accident." No vomiting
- **Genitourinary:** No problems
- **Reproductive:** Does not wish to discuss
- **Endocrine:** No problems
- **Lymphatic/Hematologic:** No problems

Psychosocial Profile

The psychosocial profile reveals patterns in the patient's life that may affect the neurological system and put him or her at risk for neurological disorders. It may also identify teaching needs.

Psychosocial Profile

CATEGORY/QUESTIONS TO ASK	RATIONALE/SIGNIFICANCE
Health Practices and Beliefs/ Self-Care Activities	
What activities do you engage in to promote the health of your neurological system?	Helps identify health promotion and preventative activities.
Do you get an annual physical exam?	
Do you wear seat belts? Do you own a gun? Do you wear protective equipment when playing sports?	Motor vehicle accidents, falls, gunshot wounds, and sports injuries are the most common causes of spinal cord trauma.

Psychosocial Profile

CATEGORY/QUESTIONS TO ASK	RATIONALE/SIGNIFICANCE
Health Practices and Beliefs/ Self-Care Activities *(Continued)*	
Do you understand proper body mechanics?	Back injuries can cause herniated discs and subsequent neurological deficits.
Typical Day	
How would you describe your typical day? Are you able to perform self-care activities? Do you have difficulty performing activities of daily living (ADLs)?	Neurological system impairment may hinder patient's ability to perform ADLs. Assess correct use of assistive devices.
Nutritional Patterns	
What did you eat in the last 24 hours?	*Vitamin B deficiency:* Paresthesia in feet and hands, gait disturbances. *Vitamin B_{12}, niacin, folic acid deficiencies:* Peripheral neuropathy.
Are you on any special diets?	Foods that can trigger headaches include those with amines (cheese and chocolate) and nitrites (hot dogs), vinegar, onions, fermented or marinated foods, monosodium glutamate, caffeine, and ice cream. High-cholesterol diet is risk factor for vascular disease.
Activity and Exercise Patterns	
Do you exercise? If so, what type and how much?	Strenuous activity increases risk for injury.
Recreation/Hobbies	
Do you participate in contact sports or activities that require heavy lifting? If so, do you wear protective equipment?	Recreational activities may increase risk for injury. Use of protective equipment decreases risk.
What are your hobbies?	Certain hobbies increase risk for exposure to toxic substances (e.g., lead exposure when working with stained glass).
Sleep and Rest Patterns	
How many hours of sleep do you get per night?	Sleep deprivation can affect cerebral function. Increased somnolence may indicate an increase in ICP. Neurological problems may interfere with sleep. Patients with pain associated with herniated discs may have difficulty finding comfortable sleep position.
Personal Habits	
Do you smoke, drink alcohol or caffeinated beverages, or use drugs?	Cigarette smoking is risk factor for cerebrovascular disease. Alcohol, caffeine, and drug use can alter cerebral function.
Occupational Health Patterns	
What type of work do you do? Does it involve lifting, repetitive movements, or exposure to chemicals or toxins?	Occupations that increase risk for head or back injury may result in neurological problems. Neurological disorders may prevent patient from returning to previous work. Exposure to toxic substances can cause neurological problems. Radiation and carcinogens increase risk for brain tumors. Arsenic and mercury can cause ataxia.
Environmental Health Patterns	
Where do you live?	Helps determine discharge planning needs.
How many floors are there in your house?	

(Continued)

Psychosocial Profile *(Continued)*

CATEGORY/QUESTIONS TO ASK	RATIONALE/SIGNIFICANCE
Roles/Relationships/Self-Concept	
How do you see yourself? How did you see yourself before you had this problem, and how do you see yourself now?	Disabling/crippling problems or deformities associated with some neurological disorders may cause body image disturbances and affect patient's self-image and self-esteem.
What is your role in the family, and has it changed?	Neurological problems such as MS may alter patient's role in family.
Religious/Cultural Influences	
What are your religious practices and beliefs or cultural influences in regard to health care?	May affect patient's healthcare practices.
Sexuality Patterns	
Have physical problems interfered with your usual sexual activity?	Neurological problems may interfere with sexual activity.
Social Supports	
Who are your supports?	Helpful in planning care.
Have physical problems interfered with your ability to interact with others?	Chronic neurological problems can disable a patient, impair socialization, and affect independence.
Stress and Coping	
How do you deal with stress?	Stress can cause headaches and trigger an exacerbation of MS.

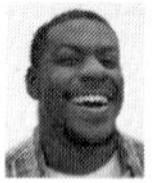

Case Study Findings

Mr. Webster's psychosocial profile includes:

- Gets yearly physical exam for sports.
- Typical day consists of awakening at 9 AM, grabbing some breakfast, and heading to class. Goes to football practice from 3 PM to 6 PM 7 days a week, has dinner, relaxes, and does school work until about midnight. Usually goes to bed by 1 AM.
- Usually eats well; diet high in carbohydrates and protein.
- Practices football with team 3 hours a day, 7 days a week. Wears protective gear.
- Usually gets at least 8 hours of sleep a night.
- Denies use of drugs or nicotine. Admits to drinking alcohol on weekends; amount varies.
- Does well in school (grade point average 3.0).
- Does not wish to discuss sexuality patterns.
- Friends and family are supports.
- Copes with stress by exercising, partying with friends on weekends.
- Attends church occasionally, no religious or cultural influence on health.

Focused Sensory-NeuologicalHistory

Your patient's condition or time restraints may prohibit taking a detailed neurological history. If so, ask questions that focus on a history of neurological problems, the presence of neurological symptoms, identification of risk factors, and health promotion activities. The patient's response to these questions will help direct your assessment. Key questions include the following:

- Do you have any neurological problems?
- Do you have any other medical problems?
- Are you taking any medications?
- Do you have a history of head trauma, loss of consciousness, dizziness, headaches, or seizures?
- Do you have memory problems or changes in your senses?
- Do you have weakness, numbness, or paralysis?
- Do you have problems walking or performing ADLs?
- Do you have mood problems or depression?
- Do you use drugs or alcohol?
- Do you have allergies?
- Have you ever been treated for a neurological or psychiatric problem?
- When did your symptoms start?

Case Study Evaluation

Before you move on to the physical examination, pause a moment and consider what you have learned from your interview with Leon Webster by documenting the sensory-neurological history related to Mr. Webster.

 CRITICAL THINKING ACTIVITY #2

From the subjective information that you have obtained from Leon's history, what neurological problem is he at risk for? What factors contribute to this situation?

Physical Assessment

Once you have obtained the subjective data, focus on collecting the objective data by performing the physical examination. The components of the neurological examination include tests of the patient's:

- Mental status
- Cranial nerve function
- Sensory function
- Reflex function

As a nurse, you will perform an abbreviated screening neurological examination more often than the comprehensive neurological examination described here. Although it is briefer, the screening examination still addresses each area of the neurological assessment and includes:

Evaluation of LOC with brief mental status examination and evaluation of verbal responsiveness

Testing of selected cranial nerves (usually CN II, III, IV and VI)

- Motor screening, including strength, movement, and gait (see Chapter 18, Assessing the Musculoskeletal System).
- Sensory screening, including tactile and pain sensations on upper and lower extremities.
- Reflexes

If the patient's condition warrants it, continue to assess neurological status by performing rapid, repeated checks to evaluate LOC, pupil size and reaction, responsiveness, extremity strength and movement, and vital signs. Remember, one of the earliest indicators of increased ICP is a subtle change in LOC, a loss of detail, forgetfulness, restlessness, or sudden quietness. Be alert for these changes! Early detection with prompt intervention may not only prevent major neurological damage, but may also save your patient's life.

Approach

The neurological physical assessment sequence is different from that for other body systems, but you still use inspection, palpation, and auscultation. The main difference is that this examination consists of a series of tests. Even though the physical assessment establishes the objective database, many of the findings are still somewhat subjective, based on the patient's perception.

Because the exam is lengthy, make sure that the patient is seated comfortably, preferably in a chair with back support rather than on an examination table. Check from time to time to be sure that he or she is not becoming fatigued.

The patient with a neurological disorder may find it difficult to understand instructions and participate fully in the exam. In these cases, limit tests that require a lengthy explanation and active cooperation. If the patient is lethargic or exhibits any other possible alteration in LOC, then it is critical to perform an assessment for LOC.

When assessing older adults, keep in mind that their responses to questions and directions may be slower and that you may need to adjust the pace of the examination. Because of the normal changes of aging and the possibility of paresis, stay close to patients to prevent them from falling, and help with position changes.

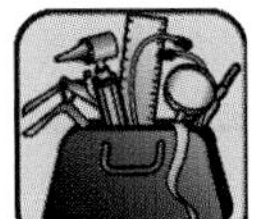

Toolbox

Assemble the following equipment for a routine neurological examination: stethoscope and BP cuff; penlight; nonsterile gloves; wisp of cotton; sharp object such as toothpick or sterile needle; objects to touch, such as a coin, button, key, or paper clip; something fragrant, such as rubbing alcohol or coffee; something to taste, such as lemon juice (sour substance), sugar, salt, and quinine (bitter substance); tongue blade; two test tubes or other vials; a reflex hammer; and an ophthalmoscope.

Performing a General Survey

Before you begin the specific neurological assessment, perform a general survey, including scanning your patient from head to toe and taking vital signs. Look at every system as it relates to the neurological system. If you detect any changes, investigate further as you perform the specific neurological examination.

The general survey can provide immediate and important information about the patient's neurological status. Affect, hygiene, grooming, speech, posture, and body language can provide clues to your patient's general level of functioning, as well as any pain or impairment. Ask yourself: Does the patient appear his or her stated age? Is his or her affect or mood appropriate for the situation? Are his or her responses appropriate? Is he or she following the interview? Is he or she well groomed and neatly dressed? Are his or her clothes stained with food? Is a female patient's make-up appropriately applied? Scan for symmetry, especially in the face. Ask your patient to smile, and look for symmetry of facial features.

Are there any abnormal movements? Shake your patient's hand and note muscle strength. Look at facial expression and eye contact. Is his or her speech clear or slurred? Are responses slow and deliberate or one-word?

Poor grooming, food on clothing, or inappropriate make-up can reflect visual deficits such as visual field cuts; motor deficits, such as weakness or paralysis; impaired cerebral function, such as confusion; and affective problems such as depression. Poor posture or facial asymmetry (ptosis or droopy smile) may be a sign of weakness or hemiparesis. Abnormal movements or balance and coordination problems may indicate a cerebellar dysfunction. Weak hand grip may reflect weakness of a neurological nature. Inappropriate responses, short attention span, or poor eye contact may indicate an underlying cerebral function disorder or a psychiatric problem.

HELPFUL HINT

Two places to assess for symmetry of facial features are the nasolabial fold (smile crease) and the palpebral fissures (distance between the eyelids).

ALERT

Charcot's triad—widening pulse pressure, bradycardia, and irregular breathing patterns—is a late sign of increasing ICP and impending brain herniation.

Vital Signs

Because the neurological system plays a vital role in the regulation of vital signs, a change in vital signs can reflect a change in the neurological system. For example:

- *BP:* HTN is a risk factor for CVA. A widened pulse pressure is a Charcot's sign of increased ICP.
- *Pulse:* Bradycardia is a Charcot's sign indicating increased ICP; atrial fibrillation increases the risk for CVA.
- *Respirations:* Irregular breathing patterns with periods of apnea is a Charcot's sign of increased ICP.
- *Temperature:* A temperature elevation may be associated with infection, meningitis, or brain abscess. A slight temperature elevation may occur after a CVA as a result of the inflammatory response, and a high temperature can occur as a result of a brainstem CVA.

Stroke Assessment Scales

Cincinnati Prehospital Stroke Scale:

- Can be used to quickly assess for signs of stroke.
- Look for facial droop: Have patient smile or show teeth.
- Test for motor weakness: Have patient perform pronator drift (see Chapter 18, Assessing the Motor-Musculoskeletal System).
- Listen for speech problems: Have patient say, "You can't teach an old dog new tricks."

National Institute of Health Stroke Scale:

Quantifies severity of stroke. Has 12 categories with total range of score from 0 (normal) to 42 (most severely impaired). Categories include:

- LOC
- LOC questions
- LOC commands
- Gaze abnormalities
- Visual loss
- Facial weakness
- Motor weakness in arms and legs
- Limb ataxia
- Sensory loss
- Language
- Dysarthria
- Extinction and inattention

Performing a Head-to-Toe Physical Assessment

The neurological system affects the functioning of all other body systems. Therefore it is essential to examine the patient from head to toe to note any unusual findings. Although not every abnormality you note will be related to neurological dysfunction, you should consider a variety of possibilities. For example, a bruise on the forehead may be caused by an injury sustained when a patient with a preexisting neurological impairment experienced a loss of consciousness. On the other hand, the patient may have been healthy before the injury, and the injury may be causing the current symptoms of pain and disorientation.

Performing a Head-to-Toe Physical Assessment

SYSTEM/NORMAL FINDINGS	ABNORMAL FINDINGS/RATIONALE
General Health Survey *INSPECT* No acute distress, AAO × 3, responses clear and appropriate, affect pleasant, well groomed.	*Changes in LOC:* Early sign of developing CNS disorder. *Dysarthria:* Associated with many neurological disorders.

Performing a Head-to-Toe Physical Assessment

SYSTEM/NORMAL FINDINGS	ABNORMAL FINDINGS/RATIONALE
General Health Survey *(Continued)*	
INSPECT	Inability to care for self as reflected by poor grooming may be caused by a neurological problem, such as hemiparesis, or a psychiatric problem, such as depression.
Integumentary	
INSPECT	
Superficial sensations intact.	*Peripheral neuropathies, spinal cord injuries, and CVA:* Can cause sensory deficits.
No rashes or lesions.	*Skin rash and petechiae:* Meningitis.
HEENT/*Head and Neck*	
INSPECT	
Facial expression appropriate and symmetrical, lymph nodes not palpable.	*Asymmetrical facial features:* CVA.
Cranial nerves intact.	*Masklike facial expression:* Parkinson's disease.
Gag reflex intact (CN IX and X intact).	*Enlarged lymph nodes:* Infection. *Abnormal cranial nerves:* Neurological problem.
HEENT/*Eyes*	
INSPECT	
Eyes clear and bright; pupils equal, round, and reactive to light accommodation (PERRLA); pupils direct and consensual; EOM intact; peripheral vision intact; no papilledema (CN II, III, IV, and VI).	*Visual changes:* Increased ICP. *Peripheral field deficits:* Neurological problems. *Papilledema:* Increased ICP.
Respiratory	
AUSCULTATE	
Respiratory rate 18 per minute. Lungs clear.	*Irregular breathing pattern:* Increased ICP. Hypoxia can cause confusion and increased ICP.
Cardiovascular	
AUSCULTATE	
Regular heart rate and rhythm.	Atrial fibrillation increases risk for embolic stroke.
No carotid bruits or thrills.	Bradycardia is a sign of increased ICP. Carotid bruits or thrills reflect carotid stenosis, increasing risk for thrombotic stroke.
Gastrointestinal	
INSPECT/AUSCULTATE/PALPATE	
Swallowing intact.	Dysphagia can occur with neurological disease.
Positive bowel sounds. Abdomen soft, nontender.	Decreased bowel sounds and constipation are most common bowel problem in stroke patients.

(Continued)

Performing a Head-to-Toe Physical Assessment *(Continued)*

SYSTEM/NORMAL FINDINGS	ABNORMAL FINDINGS/RATIONALE
Genitourinary/Reproductive	
INSPECT	
Bladder function intact.	STDs such as syphilis can cause neurosyphilis. Poor bladder control or incontinence frequently occur during acute phase of CVA. Can also occur with spinal cord injuries and other neurological disorders.
Musculoskeletal	
INSPECT/PALPATE	
Muscle strength +5. Movements smooth and coordinated.	*Decreased sensations and numbness:* Neuropathies. Paralysis can result in muscle atrophy.
Gait balanced and fluid, with conformity of phases.	*Balance problems:* Cerebellar dysfunctions.
Negative Romberg test.	Spatial perception problems can result from a stroke.

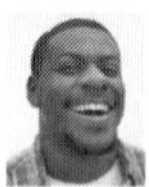

Case Study Findings

Mr. Webster's physical assessment findings include:

- **General Health Survey:** Well groomed, speech clear, posture erect but guarding neck, affect appropriate, appears stated age. 2″ laceration of forehead, alcohol on breath. In no acute distress, but grimacing in pain.
- **Vital Signs:** Temperature 98°F; pulse 88 BPM and regular; respirations 20/min; BP 130/80; pulse oximetry 98% room air.
- **Integumentary:** 2″ sutured laceration on forehead; otherwise negative.
- **HEENT:** Facial features symmetrical, visual acuity intact, pupils 3 mm, PERRLA, EOM intact, fundoscopic negative.
- **Respiratory:** Lungs clear.
- **Cardiovascular:** Heart sounds 80 BPM and regular; no extra sounds.
- **Gastrointestinal:** Abdomen soft, nontender, positive bowel sounds.
- **Musculoskeletal:** +5/5 strength of upper and lower extremities, decreased ROM of neck, gait steady, balance intact.

HELPFUL HINTS

- If your patient has a spatial perception problem, be aware that he may have **neglect,** a spatial perception problem in which he does not see the affected side as part of his body.
- Remember: Problems with the right side of the brain will be clinically manifested on the left side, and vice versa.
- Before allowing a patient with suspected CVA to eat, test gag, swallow, and cough reflexes to avoid aspiration.

ALERTS

- Safety is an issue for patients with right-side brain injury because they tend to be impulsive and not know their own limits.
- When assessing a possible stroke patient, remember that if your patient has dysarthria, he or she may also have dysphagia.

Performing a Focused Neurological Assessment

Once you have completed the head-to-toe scan, zero in of the specifics of the sensory-neurological examination. Begin by assessing cerebral function, and then assess cranial nerve function, sensory function, and reflexes. The motor neurological system was assessed in the previous chapter.

Cerebral Function

Assessment of cerebral function includes LOC, mental status and cognitive functioning, and communication.

Level of Consciousness

Evaluating LOC involves assessing **arousal** (wakefulness) and **orientation** (ability to receive and accurately interpret sensory stimuli).

Assessing Arousal

Determine the arousal state first, using minimal stimuli and increasing intensity as needed. Start with auditory stimuli, move to tactile stimuli, and then use painful stimuli as a last resort.

Auditory and Tactile Stimuli. To assess auditory stimuli, determine whether the patient is sleeping or awake. If the patient is awake, what is he or she doing? If the patient is sleeping, call him or her by name in a normal tone of voice. If he or she does not respond, speak louder. If auditory stimuli fail, try tactile. Gently touch the patient's hand. If he or she does not respond, gently shake his or her shoulder.

Painful Stimuli. If your patient does not respond to tactile stimuli, you will have to resort to painful stimuli. There are acceptable and unacceptable ways to elicit a response to pain. Never perform a nipple twist! Avoid using a pin or needle, because if the skin breaks, you risk infection. Also remember to rotate sites—repeated stimulation at the same site may cause bruising.

Painful stimuli may be central or peripheral. Central painful stimuli include the trapezius squeeze, the sternal rub, supraorbital pressure, and mandibular pressure. Peripheral painful stimuli include nail pressure and the Achilles tendon squeeze. Apply the stimulus for 15 to 30 seconds. A responsive patient will experience pain and move in response to these stimuli:

- *Trapezius squeeze:* Pinch 1 to 2 inches of the trapezius muscle and twist.
- *Sternal rub:* With the knuckles of your dominant hand, apply pressure in a grinding motion to the sternum. Do not use this site repeatedly because it will cause bruising.
- *Supraorbital pressure:* Apply firm pressure with your thumbs at the notch at the center of the orbital rim below the eyebrows. Because a nerve runs in the notch, pressure to this area will cause sinus pain. Use this stimulus carefully to avoid damage to the eyes.
- *Mandibular pressure:* With your index and middle finger, apply inward and upward pressure at the angle of the jaw.
- *Nail pressure:* Apply pressure over the moon of the nail with a pen or pencil.
- *Achilles tendon squeeze:* Squeeze the Achilles tendon between your thumb and index finger.

Documenting Arousal

When documenting your findings, record *how* your patient responds rather than simply giving the response a label. For example, charting that a patient responds slowly to verbal stimuli but drifts back to sleep is much more descriptive than simply writing "lethargic." Because a change in LOC is an early sign of a neurological problem, you need to be able to detect subtle changes in your patient. Describing the response to the stimuli is more objective, and allows better comparisons during follow-up assessments.

TERMS USED TO DESCRIBE LOC

- *Alert:* Follows commands in a timely fashion.
- *Lethargic:* Appears drowsy, may drift off to sleep during examination.
- *Stuporous:* Requires vigorous stimulation (shaking, shouting) for a response.
- *Comatose:* Does not respond appropriately either to verbal or painful stimuli.

The Glasgow Coma Scale provides a more objective way to assess the patient's LOC. It evaluates best eye response, best motor response, and best verbal response on a scale of 3 to 15. Fifteen (highest score) indicates that the patient is awake, alert, oriented, and able to follow simple commands. Three (lowest score) indicates that the patient does not respond to any stimulus and has no motor or eye response, reflecting a very serious neurological state with poor prognosis.

Assessing Orientation

Next, test orientation to time, place, and person. Purpose is also sometimes included as a fourth area of orientation. Avoid asking questions that require only a "yes" or "no" response. Start with specifics; then be more general, if necessary. For example, if your patient does not know the specific date, ask him or her what month it is, and if he or she does not know the month, ask what season it is. If he or she was once oriented to place and is not the next time you ask, this may be an early sign of a deteriorating neurological status.

HELPFUL HINT

When an older patient is disoriented to time, he or she usually thinks it is an earlier date, not a later one.

Glasgow Coma Scale

Observation	Response Elicited	Score
Eye response	■ Opens spontaneously	4
	■ Opens to verbal command	3
	■ Opens to pain	2
	■ No response	1
Motor response	■ Reacts to verbal command	6
	■ Reacts to painful stimuli	
	• Identifies localized pain	5
	• Flexes and withdraws	4
	• Assumes flexor posture	3
	• Assumes extensor posture	2
	■ No response	1
Verbal response	■ Is oriented and converses	5
	■ Is disoriented, but converses	4
	■ Uses inappropriate words	3
	■ Makes incomprehensible sounds	2
	■ No response	1

Eye and verbal responses are self-explanatory. Under motor responses, "Identifies localized pain" denotes that the patient is not fully conscious but is aware enough to respond to an annoying stimulus. "Flexes and withdraws" is a lower-level motor response and indicates that the patient pulls away from painful stimuli. Be sure to apply the stimulus long enough to elicit more than just a reflex response.

Posturing is a still lower level of response and indicates abnormal positions of flexion or extension of the arms with legs extended and internally rotated and feet plantarflexed. It is an ominous sign that usually has a poor prognosis. In **flexion (decorticate) posturing,** the arms are flexed to the chest and the hands are clenched and internally rotated as a result of a lesion at or above the brainstem in the cerebral cortex. In **extension (decerebrate) posturing,** the arms are extended and the hands are clenched and hyperpronated as a result of a midbrain (brainstem) lesion. This is the more serious of the two.

ALERT

If the patient's responses are bizarre—such as thinking it is the year 2050—consider a psychiatric problem.

Time: Ask the patient to state the date, including the year and day of the week. Hospitalized patients—especially older adults—can easily become disoriented to time, but they usually reorient easily. Be sure your documentation reflects this.

Place: Ask your patient to state where he or she is. Can he or she identify environmental cues (e.g., bed, equipment, sound of bells or buzzers) to determine location? A person who is usually oriented but becomes confused when hospitalized often temporarily mistakes the hospital room for home. You will need to address safety concerns with patients who are disoriented both at home and in the hospital; for example, those with Alzheimer's disease, who tend to wander.

Person: Ask the patient to state his or her name. Self-identity usually remains intact the longest, making disorientation to person an ominous sign.

Mental Status and Cognitive Function

Once you have determined that your patient is arousable, assess level of awareness. Level of awareness reflects mental status and cognitive function. It is the functional state of the mind as judged by a person's behavior, appearance, response to stimuli, speech, memory, and judgment. It reflects the person's connection with his or her environment. These areas are at a higher level of functioning than LOC and reflect the cerebral cortex's ability to process and respond. Be sure to explain to your patient that you need to ask questions that have obvious answers to accurately assess his or her neurological status.

Like the general survey, a mental status screening is often integrated into the health history interview. A typical screening consists of 10 questions that address each area of the detailed mental status examination. (See box, Mental Status Screening Questions page 000). However, you will need to perform a rigorous mental status examination in the following situations:

- If data from patient or patient behavior during the health history interview suggests an abnormality
- If family members or caregivers report changes in the patient's personality or behavior
- If the patient has a history of head injury, stroke, dysphasia or aphasia, or mental illness

Mental Status Screening Questions

Question	Function Screened
What is your name?	Orientation to person
What is today's date?	Orientation to time
What year is it?	Orientation to time
Where are you now?	Orientation to place
How old are you?	Memory
Where were you born?	Remote memory
What did you have for breakfast?	Recent memory
Who is the U.S. president?	General knowledge
Can you count backward from 20 to 1?	Attention and calculation skills
Why are you here?	Judgment

A mental status and cognitive function assessment includes: memory, general knowledge and vocabulary, mathematical and calculative skills, and thought process/abstract reasoning/judgment.

Memory

Assess immediate, recent, and remote memory. Test immediate memory by asking your patient to repeat a series of numbers. Test recent memory by asking what the patient had for breakfast or by asking him or her to name three objects—for example, a pen, a tree, and a ball—and then asking him or her to recall them later. To test remote memory, ask birth dates or anniversary dates if someone can validate the information; if not, ask dates of major historical events.

General Knowledge and Vocabulary. Before you assess general knowledge and vocabulary, you need to consider the developmental level, educational level, and cultural background of your patient so that you can phrase and direct your questions accordingly. To test general knowledge, ask about current events, the name of the president of the United States, or common knowledge questions, such as the number of months in a year or days in a week. To test vocabulary, ask the patient to define words. Begin with easy, familiar words, such as "orange," and proceed to more difficult or abstract words, such as "dictatorial."

Mathematical and Calculative Skills. To test mathematical and calculative skills, have your patient solve a simple math problem. Counting backward from 100 by 7s (serial 7s) is frequently used, but this is difficult for many people, especially those dependent on calculators. As an alternative, have the person count backward by 3s or 4s, or ask him or her to solve a simple problem. An example is: "If you purchased a magazine for $1.50, and you have $2.00, how much change would you get back?" Whichever method you use, make sure the problem is appropriate for the patient's educational level.

Thought Process/Abstract Reasoning/Judgment. To assess thought process, examine the appropriateness, organization, and content of your patient's responses throughout the entire assessment. Be alert for any sensory-perceptual experiences, feelings, or false beliefs that are not based on reality and may indicate illusions, hallucinations, or delusions.

Assess abstract reasoning by asking your patient to explain a simple proverb, such as "People in glass houses shouldn't throw stones." If the person's age or cultural background make using proverbs inappropriate, use a phrase such as "It's raining cats and dogs!" Note the degree of concreteness or abstractness of his or her interpretation. You can further assess abstract ability by asking him or her to group similar objects; for example, ask "What do an apple, an orange, and a pear have in common?" Then determine whether the responses are appropriate.

Sound judgment involves considering options and choosing appropriate actions. Assess your patient's judgment by observing his or her response to the current situation or by giving him or her a hypothetical situation. For example, say: "If you were walking down the street and witnessed a car accident, what would you do?" Then decide whether the response is appropriate and reasonable.

Assessing Communication

When assessing speech, evaluate not only the ability to speak, but also the content, appropriateness, speed, and quality of speech. Identify the patient's primary language, and solicit an interpreter if needed. Various speech problems are associated with neurological disorders, and the type of problem depends on which area of the brain is affected. Increasing language difficulties may reflect a turn for the worse in your patient's neurological status that warrants further medical evaluation. The inability to communicate can be frustrating for both of you, so be patient, allow your patient time to respond, and make referrals to speech therapy as needed.

To pinpoint the exact location of the neurological problem, assess further for spontaneous speech, sound recognition, auditory-verbal comprehension, visual recognition, visual-verbal comprehension, motor speech, automatic speech, naming, vocabulary, writing, and copying figures. This assessment can also be used to develop an effective speech therapy plan for your patient.

Cranial Nerve Function

Evaluation of the cranial nerves is an essential part of the neurological examination. However, like other portions of the exam, it depends upon an alert patient who is emotionally, cognitively, and physically able to participate. Assessment techniques are described in the following section. See Chapter 10, Assessing the Eye and Ear, for assessment techniques for CN II, III, IV, VI, and VIII.

Neurological Problems

Agnosia: Inability to recognize object by sight (visual agnosia), touch (tactile agnosia), or hearing (auditory agnosia).
Akinesia: Complete or partial loss of voluntary muscle movement.
Aphasia: Absence or impairment of ability to communicate through speech, writing, or signs.
Expressive (motor) aphasia: Inability to express language even though person knows what he or she wants to say (also called Broca's or motor aphasia). Frontal lobe affected.
Fluent aphasia: Words can be spoken but are used incorrectly.
Nonfluent aphasia: Slow, deliberate speech, few words.
Receptive (sensory) aphasia: Inability to comprehend spoken or written words (also called Wernicke's or sensory aphasia). Temporal lobe affected in auditory-receptive; parieto-occipital nerve affected in visual-receptive.
Apraxia: Inability to carry out learned sequential movements or commands.
Circumlocution: Inability to name object verbally, so patient talks around object or uses gesture to define it.
Dysarthria: Defective speech; inability to articulate words; impairment of tongue and other muscles needed for speech.
Dysphasia: Impaired or difficult speech.
Dysphonia: Difficulty with quality of voice; hoarseness.
Neologisms: Made-up, nonsense, meaningless words.
Paraphrasia: Loss of ability to use words correctly and coherently; words are jumbled or misused.
Tremors: Involuntary movement of part of body.
Intension tremor: Involuntary movement when attempting coordinated movements.
Fasiculation: Involuntary contraction or twitching of muscle fibers.

Assessing Cerebral Function

COMPONENT/TECHNIQUE/NORMAL VARIATIONS	ABNORMAL FINDINGS/RATIONALE
Behavior *Watch patient's facial expression as he or she responds to questions.* *Note his or her posture, grooming, and affect.* Well-groomed, erect posture, pleasant facial expression, appropriate affect.	*Lack of facial expression/ inappropriate expression for speech content:* Possible psychological disorder (e.g., depression or schizophrenia) or neurological impairment affecting cranial nerves.
Normal findings vary depending on situation (e.g., if patient is in pain, then his or her behavior should reflect this).	*Masklike expression:* Parkinson's disease. *Poor grooming/slumped posture:* Depression if psychological in origin; or CVA with hemiparesis if physiological in origin.
LOC *Test orientation to time, place, and person.* Awake, alert, and oriented to time, place, and person (AAO × 3).	Disorientation may be physical in origin, such as exhaustion, anxiety, hypoxia, fluid and electrolyte imbalance, drugs, or a neurological problem. Disorientation can also be psychiatric in origin such as with schizophrenia.

Assessing Cerebral Function

COMPONENT/TECHNIQUE/NORMAL VARIATIONS	ABNORMAL FINDINGS/RATIONALE
Mental Status and Cognitive Function *Memory:* *Test immediate recall:* Ask patient to repeat three numbers, such as "4, 9, 1." If patient can do so, ask him or her to repeat a series of five digits. *Test recent memory:* Ask what patient had for breakfast. *Test long-term memory:* Ask patient to state his or her birthplace, recite his or her Social Security number, or identify a culturally-specific person or event, such as the name of the previous United States president or the location of a recent natural disaster. Immediate, recent, and remote memory intact. HELPFUL HINTS ■ Avoid using number sequences with a meaningful arrangement, such as 2, 4, 6, 8. ■ If you ask your patient for his or her birthday or dates of other events, be sure that you can validate them.	Memory problems can be benign or signal a more serious neurological problem such as Alzheimer's disease. Forgetfulness—especially for immediate and recent events—is often seen in older adults. With benign forgetfulness, person can retrace or use memory aids to help with recall. Pathological memory loss, as in Alzheimer's disease, is subtle and progressive until ability to function is impaired. Temporary memory loss may occur after head trauma. **Retrograde amnesia** is memory loss for events just preceding illness or injury. Postconcussion syndrome can occur 2 weeks to 2 months after injury and may cause short-term memory deficits.
Mathematical and Calculative Ability: Ask patient to perform a simple calculation, such as adding 4 + 4. If successful, proceed to more difficult calculation, such as 11 × 9. Mathematical/calculative ability intact and appropriate for patient's age, educational level, and language facility.	Inability to calculate at level appropriate to age, education, and language ability requires evaluation for neurological impairment.
General Knowledge and Vocabulary: Ask how many days in a week and months in a year.	
Thought Process: Ask patient to define familiar words such as apple, earthquake, chastise. Begin with easy words and proceed to more difficult ones. Remember to consider the patient's age, educational level, and cultural background. Assess throughout assessment. Difficult to assess in children younger than age 7 or 8 without advanced training. Thought process intact.	Incoherent speech, illogical or unrealistic ideas, repetition of words and phrases, repeatedly straying from topic, and suddenly losing train of thought are examples of altered thought processes that indicate need for further evaluation. Inability to define familiar words requires further evaluation.
Thought Process:	Alteration in thought process can be caused by a physical disorder such as dementia, a psychiatric disorder such as psychosis, or drugs and alcohol.

(Continued)

Assessing Cerebral Function *(Continued)*

COMPONENT/TECHNIQUE/NORMAL VARIATIONS	ABNORMAL FINDINGS/RATIONALE
Mental Status and Cognitive Function *(Continued)*	
Abstract Thinking:	
Ask patient to interpret a culturally-appropriate proverb. Able to generalize from specific example and apply statement to human behavior. Children should be able to distinguish like from unlike as appropriate for their age and language facility.	*Impaired ability to think abstractly:* Dementia, delirium, mental retardation, psychoses.
Judgment:	
Observe patient's response to current situation. Ask patient to respond to a situation or hypothetical situation. Judgment appropriate and intact.	Impaired judgment can be associated with dementia, psychosis, or drug and alcohol abuse.
Communication	
Speech and Language:	
Listen to patient's rate and ease of speech, including enunciation. Speech flows easily; patient enunciates clearly. Sophistication of speech matches age, education, and fluency.	*Hesitancy, stuttering, stammering, unclear speech:* Lack of familiarity with language, deference or shyness, anxiety, neurological disorder. *Dysphasia/aphasia:* Neurological problems such as CVA. Drugs and alcohol can also cause slurred speech.
Spontaneous Speech:	
Show patient a picture and have him or her describe what he or she sees. Spontaneous speech intact.	*Impaired spontaneous speech:* Cognitive impairment.
Motor Speech:	
Have patient repeat, "do, ray, me, fa, so, la, te, do." Motor speech intact.	*Impaired motor speech (dysarthria):* Problem with CN XII.
Automatic Speech:	
Have patient say something that is committed to memory, such as days of week or months of year. Automatic speech intact.	*Impaired automatic speech:* Cognitive impairment or memory problem.
Sound Recognition:	
Have patient close eyes and identify familiar sound such as clapping hands. Sound recognition intact.	*Impaired sound recognition (auditory agnosia):* Temporal lobe affected.
Auditory-Verbal Comprehension:	
Ask patient to follow simple directions or explain meaning of a series of words. Auditory-verbal comprehension intact.	*Impaired auditory-verbal comprehension:* Temporal lobe affected. *Expressive aphasia:* Frontal lobe affected. *Auditory-receptive aphasia:* Temporal lobe affected.

Assessing Cerebral Function

COMPONENT/TECHNIQUE/NORMAL VARIATIONS	ABNORMAL FINDINGS/RATIONALE
Visual Recognition: Have patient identify familiar object by sight (e.g., cup, pencil, pen). Visual recognition intact.	*Impaired visual recognition (visual agnosia):* Parieto-occipital lobe affected.
Visual-Verbal Comprehension: Have patient read sentence from newspaper and explain meaning. Visual-verbal comprehension intact.	*Impaired visual-verbal comprehension (visual-receptive aphasia)*: Cognitive impairment.
Writing: Have patient write name, address, simple sentence, one word with eyes open and then closed, name of an object. Writing ability intact.	*Impaired writing ability.*
Copying Figures: Show patient several figures and ask him or her to copy them, increasing in complexity. (e.g., circle, X, square, triangle, star). Able to copy figures.	*Impaired figure copying ability.*

Assessing the Cranial Nerves

NERVE/TECHNIQUE/NORMAL VARIATIONS	ABNORMAL FINDINGS/RATIONALE
CN I—Olfactory Nerve	

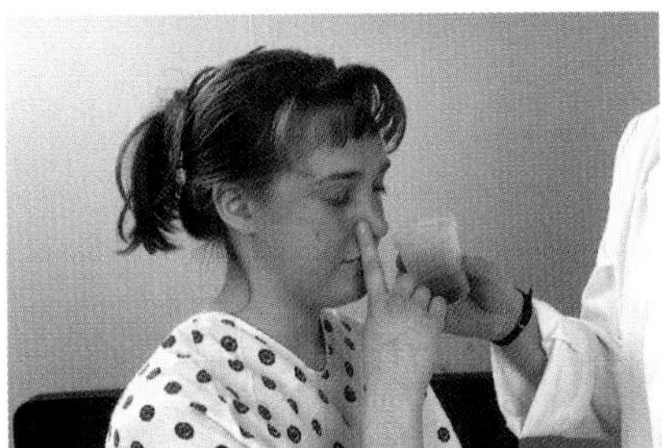

Testing olfactory nerve

NERVE/TECHNIQUE/NORMAL VARIATIONS	ABNORMAL FINDINGS/RATIONALE
Before testing nerve function, ensure patency of each nostril by occluding in turn and asking patient to sniff. Once patency is established, ask patient to close eyes. Occlude one nostril and hold aromatic substance such as coffee beneath nose. Ask patient to identify substance. Repeat with other nostril. Patient is able to identify substance. Bear in mind that some substances may be unfamiliar, especially to children.	**Anosmia** is loss of sense of smell. It may be inherited and nonpathologic, or may result from chronic rhinitis, sinusitis, heavy smoking, zinc deficiency, or cocaine use. It may also indicate cranial nerve damage from facial fractures or head injuries, disorders of base of frontal lobe such as a tumor, or

(Continued)

Assessing the Cranial Nerves *(Continued)*

NERVE/TECHNIQUE/NORMAL VARIATIONS

CN I—Olfactory Nerve (Continued)

CN II, III, IV, and VI—Optic, Oculomotor, Trochlear, and Abducens Nerves

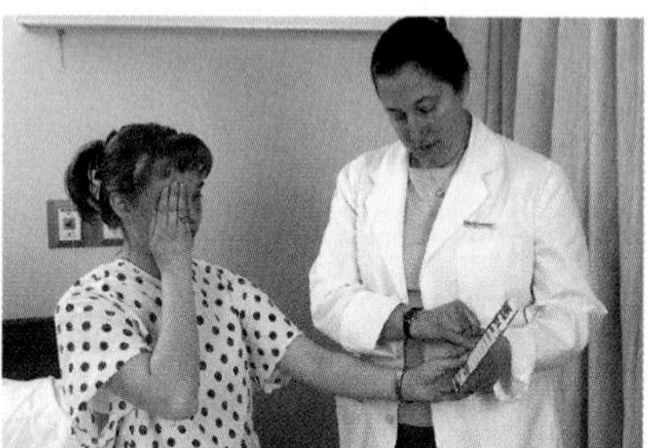

Testing visual acuity

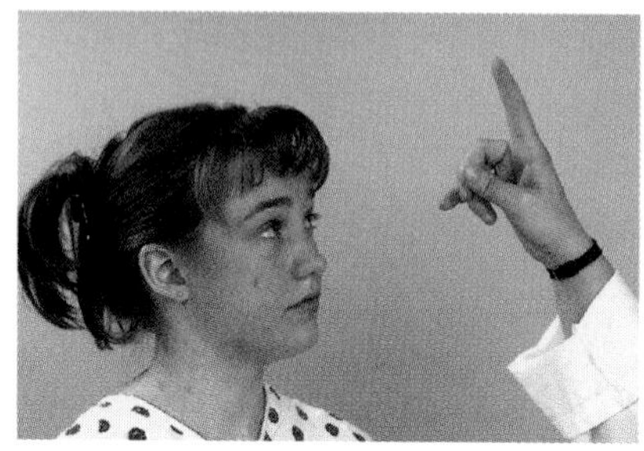

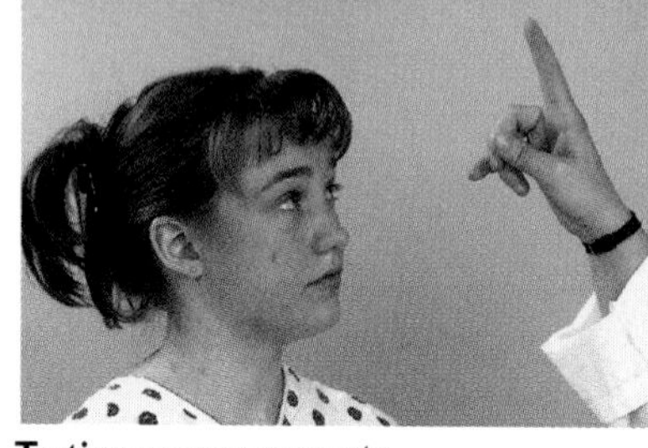

Testing eye movements

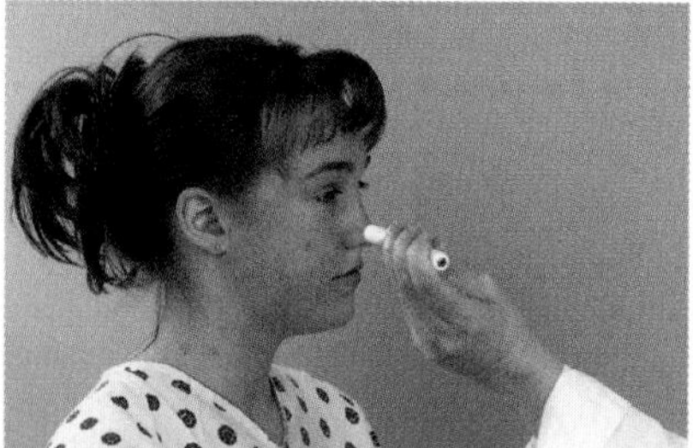

Testing pupil accommodation

Test visual acuity, peripheral vision, eye movements, and pupil accommodation as discussed in Chapter 10.

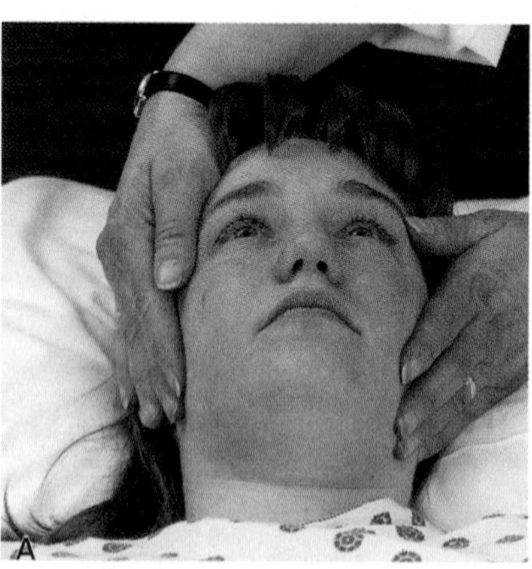

A and B. Testing oculocephalic reflex

Test oculocephalic reflex ("doll's eyes") in unresponsive patient. Rotate head quickly from side to side.

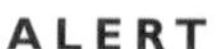

ALERT

Never perform this test on a patient with suspected neck injury!

Visual acuity intact 20/20, both eyes; PERRLA direct and consensual; EOM intact.

Hippus phenomenon—brisk constriction of pupils in reaction to light,

ABNORMAL FINDINGS/RATIONALE

artherosclerotic changes. Persons with anosmia usually also have taste problems.

CN II deficits can occur with CVA or brain tumor.

Changes in pupillary reactions can signal CN III deficits. Increased ICP causes changes in pupillary reaction. As pressure increases, response becomes more sluggish until pupils finally become fixed and dilated.

Abnormal doll's eyes (eyes fixed): Damage to oculomotor nerves (CN III, IV, VI) or brainstem.

Assessing the Cranial Nerves

NERVE/TECHNIQUE/NORMAL VARIATIONS	ABNORMAL FINDINGS/RATIONALE

CN II, III, IV, and VI—Optic, Oculomotor, Trochlear, and Abducens Nerves (Continued)

followed by dilation and constriction—may be normal or sign of early CN III compression.

Normal doll's eyes: Eyes deviate to side opposite from way head is turned.

CN V—Trigeminal Nerve

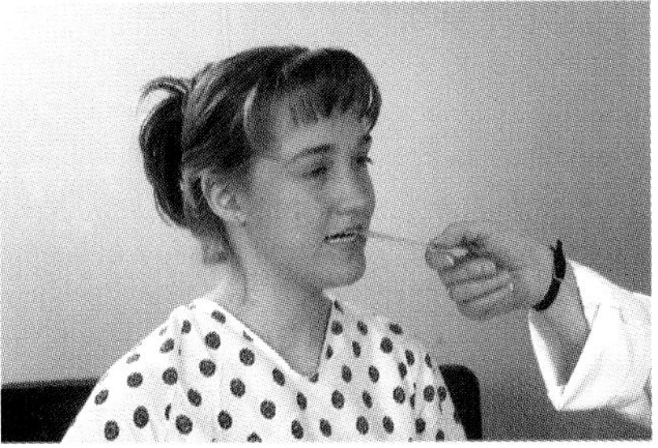

Testing CN V motor function

Testing motor function: Ask patient to move jaw from side to side against resistance and then clench jaw as you palpate contraction of temporal and masseter muscles, or to bite down on a tongue blade.

Weak or absent contraction unilaterally: Lesion of nerve, cervical spine, or brainstem.

ALERT

Food may collect in cheek on patient's affected side, increasing risk for aspiration.

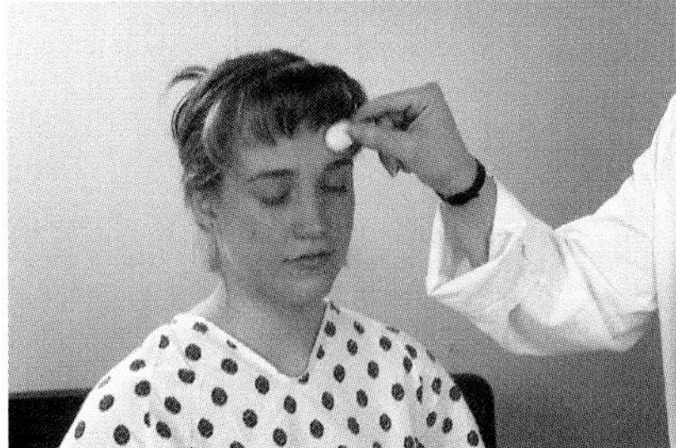

Testing CN V sensory function

Testing sensory function: Ask patient to close eyes and tell you when he or she feels sensation on the face. Touch jaw, cheeks, and forehead with cotton wisp. Touch same areas with toothpick. Compare both bilaterally.

Full range of motion (ROM) in jaw and +5 strength.

Patient perceives light touch and superficial pain bilaterally.

Inability to perceive light touch and superficial pain may indicate peripheral nerve damage.

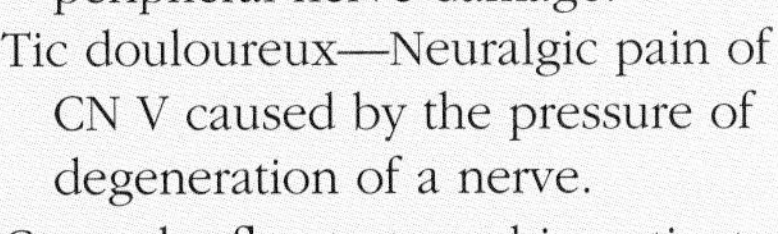

Tic douloureux—Neuralgic pain of CN V caused by the pressure of degeneration of a nerve.

Corneal reflex test used in patients with decreased LOC to evaluate integrity of brainstem.

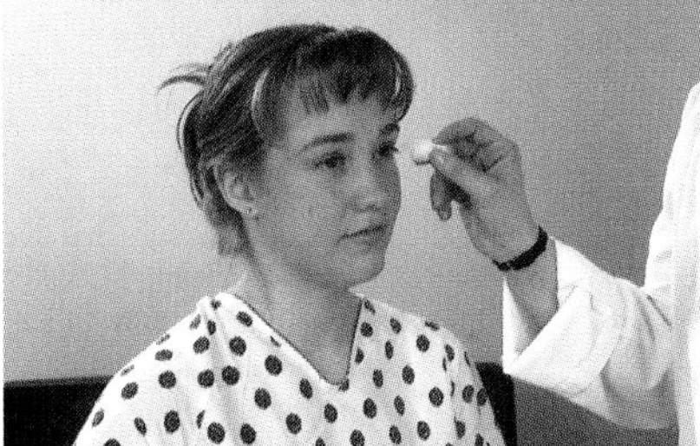

Testing corneal reflex

Testing corneal reflex: Gently touch cornea with cotton wisp.

HELPFUL HINT

Touching cornea can cause abrasions. Alternative approach is to puff air across cornea with a needle and sterile syringe, or gently touch eyelash and look for blink reflex.

(Continued)

Assessing the Cranial Nerves *(Continued)*

NERVE/TECHNIQUE/NORMAL VARIATIONS

CN VII—Facial Nerve

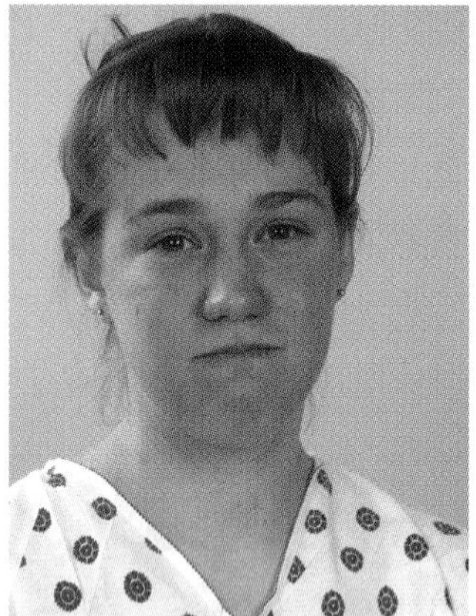

Testing CN VII motor function

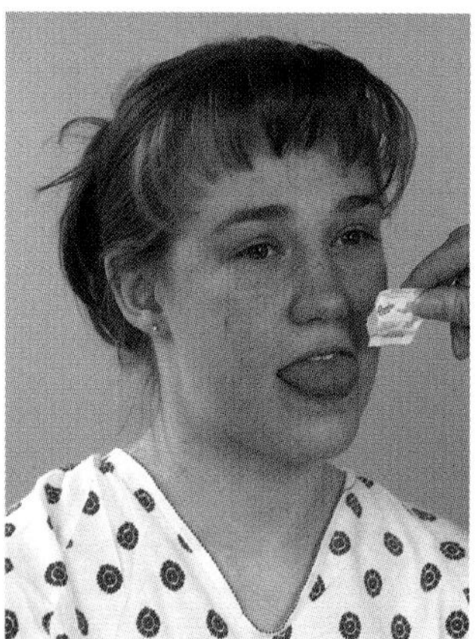

Testing taste sensation

Testing motor function: Ask patient to perform these movements: smile, frown, raise eyebrows, show upper teeth, show lower teeth, puff out cheeks, purse lips, close eyes tightly while nurse tries to open them.

Testing sensory function: Test taste on anterior 2/3 of tongue for sweet, sour, salty.

HELPFUL HINT

Sweet: Tip of the tongue
Sour: Sides of back half of tongue
Salty: Anterior sides and tip of tongue
Bitter: Back of tongue

Facial nerve intact; able to make faces. Taste sensation on anterior tongue intact.
Taste decreased in older adults.

CN VIII—Acoustic Nerve

Perform Weber and Rinne tests for hearing (see Chapter 10, Assessing the Eye and Ear).

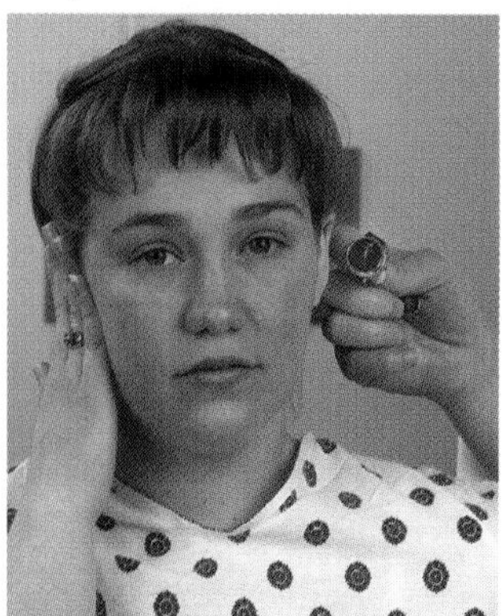

Watch-tick test

Perform watch-tick test by holding watch close to patient's ear.
Perform Romberg test for balance (see Chapter 13, Assessing the Musculoskeletal System).

ABNORMAL FINDINGS/RATIONALE

Asymmetrical or impaired movement: Nerve damage, such as that caused by Bell's palsy or CVA.

Impaired taste/loss of taste: Damage to facial nerve, chemotherapy or radiation therapy to head and neck.

Hearing loss, nystagmus, balance disturbance, dizziness/vertigo: Acoustic nerve damage.
Nystagmus: CN VIII, brainstem, or cerebellum problem or phenytoin (Dilantin) toxicity.

Assessing the Cranial Nerves

NERVE/TECHNIQUE/NORMAL VARIATIONS	ABNORMAL FINDINGS/RATIONALE
CN VIII—Acoustic Nerve	
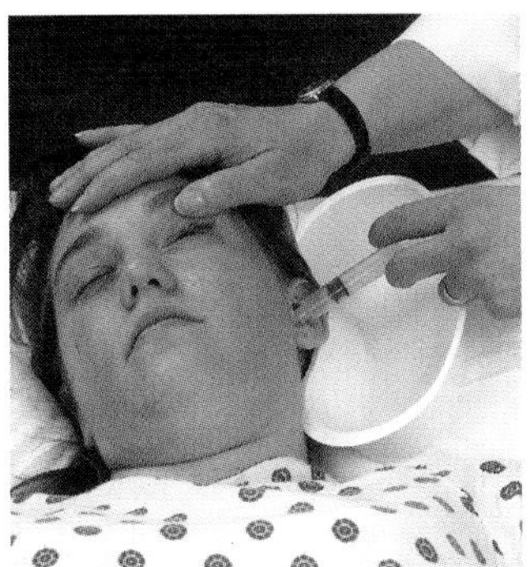 **Cold caloric test** If patient is unresponsive, perform cold caloric test for oculovestibular reflex (tests CN III, VI, and vestibular portion of VIII): Irrigate external ear canal with ice-cold water. Normal response is **nystagmus** (involuntary, rhythmic eye movement) toward irrigated ear.	*Abnormal cold caloric test (no eye movement)*: Damage to CN III, VI, and VIII.
ALERT Do not irrigate an ear unless you are sure the tympanic membrane is intact.	
Hearing intact. Negative Romberg test. Normal cold caloric test.	
CN IX and X—Glossopharyngeal and Vagus Nerves	
Observe ability to cough, swallow, and talk.	*Unilateral movement:* Contralateral nerve damage.
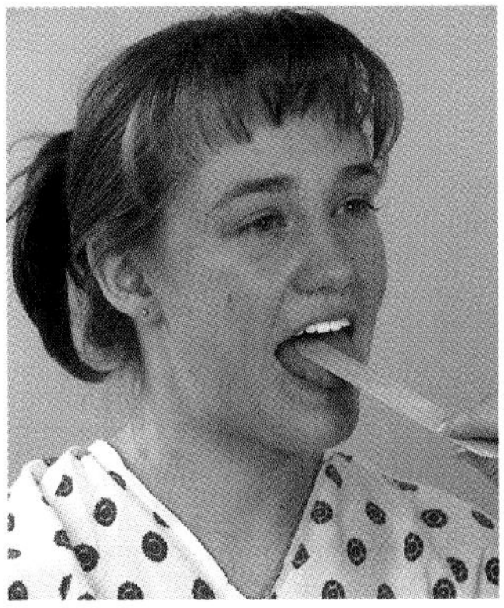 **Testing CN IX and X motor function**	
Testing motor function: Ask patient to open mouth and say "ah" while you depress the tongue with a tongue blade. Observe soft palate and uvula. Soft palate and uvula should rise medially. Test sensory function of CN IX and motor function of CN X by stimulating gag reflex. Tell patient that you are going to touch interior throat, then lightly touch tip of tongue blade to posterior pharyngeal wall. Observe movement. Test taste on posterior portion of tongue.	Damage to CN IX and X also impairs swallowing. *Changes in voice quality (e.g., hoarseness):* CN X damage. CN X damage may also affect vital functions, causing arrhythmias because vagus nerve innervates most of viscera through parasympathetic system.

(Continued)

Assessing the Cranial Nerves *(Continued)*

NERVE/TECHNIQUE/NORMAL VARIATIONS	ABNORMAL FINDINGS/RATIONALE
***CN IX and X—Glossopharyngeal and Vagus Nerves** (Continued)*	
Swallow and cough reflex intact. Speech clear. Elevation and constriction of pharyngeal musculature and tongue retraction indicate positive gag reflex. Taste on posterior tongue intact.	*Diminished/absent gag reflex:* Nerve damage. Evaluate further because patient is at increased risk for aspiration. *Impaired taste on posterior portion of tongue:* Problem with CN IX.
CN XI—Accessory Nerve 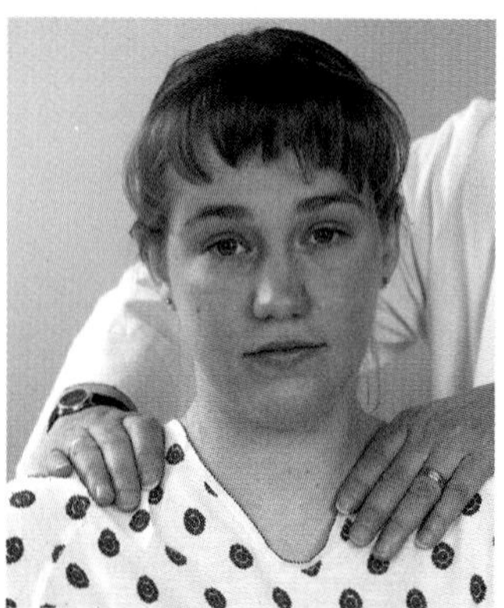 **Testing CN XI motor function** Test motor function of shoulder and neck muscles: Ask patient to shrug shoulders upward against your resistance. Then ask him or her to turn head from side to side against your resistance. Observe for symmetry of contraction and muscle strength. Movement symmetrical, with patient moving against resistance without pain. Full ROM of neck with +5/5 strength.	*Asymmetrical/diminished/absent movement/pain/ unilateral or bilateral weakness:* Peripheral nerve CN XI damage.
CN XII—Hypoglossal Nerve Precise articulation indicates proper functioning, so further assessment is indicated only when speech is impaired. Have patient say "d, l, n, t" or a phrase containing these letters, such as the phrase in the Cincinnati Prehospital Stroke Scale. The ability to say these letters requires use of the tongue.	
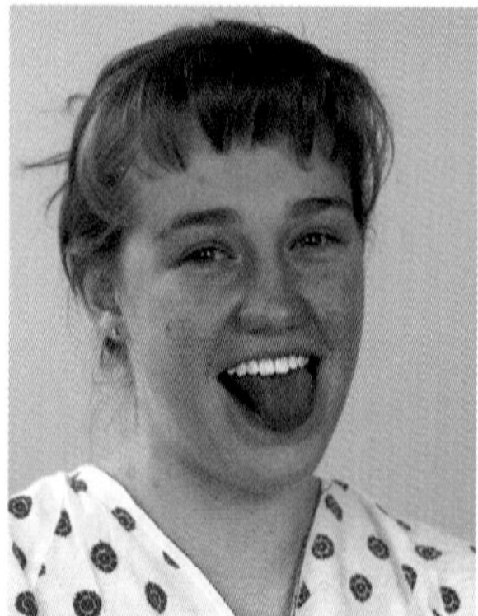 **Testing CN XII motor function** Ask the patient to protrude the tongue. Observe any deviation from midline, tumors, lesions, or atrophy. Now ask the patient to move the tongue from side to side	*Asymmetrical/diminished/ absent movement/deviation from midline/protruded tongue:* Peripheral nerve CN XII damage.
Can protrude tongue medially. No atrophy, tumors, or lesions.	Tongue paralysis results in dysarthria.

Sensory System Function

Assess the patient's sensory function using tests of light (superficial) touch, pain, temperature, vibration, position sense, **stereognosis** (ability to recognize the form of solid objects by touch), **graphesthesia** (ability to recognize outlines, numbers, words, or symbols written on skin), two-point discrimination, point localization, and extinction. Light touch, pain, and temperature are superficial sensations and travel the spinothalamic tracts of the anterolateral system. Vibration, position sense, stereognosis, graphesthesia, two-point discrimination, point localization, and extinction are highly localized and travel the dorsal column-medial lemniscal pathway of the posterior column-medial lemniscal pathway.

Before beginning this portion of the examination, inform the patient that you will apply various stimuli, and that he or she should close the eyes during the entire exam. Instruct him or her to say "now" whenever he or she perceives a sensation. Avoid asking leading questions, such as, "Can you feel anything here?" Also avoid using any recognizable pattern, but do test symmetrical regions. If you notice an area of altered sensation, stimulate areas close to it until you have delineated its borders. Record your findings with a diagram of the area.

The extent of the sensory assessment depends on your findings. For screening purposes, include the upper and lower extremities and the trunk. If you detect a deficit, perform a more thorough assessment.

Assessing Sensory Function

COMPONENT/TECHNIQUE/NORMAL VARIATIONS	ABNORMAL FINDINGS/RATIONALE
Light Touch	
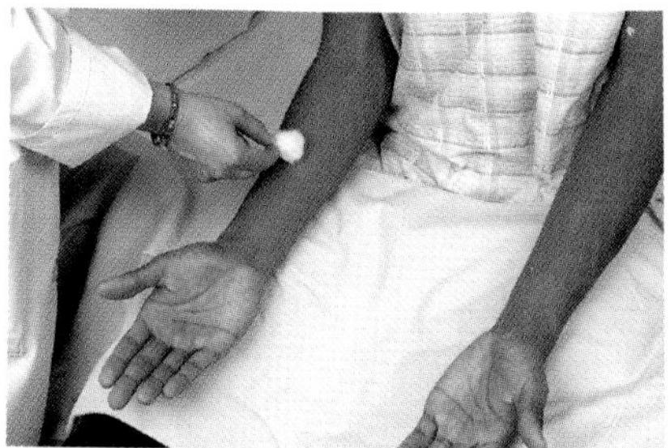 **Testing superficial touch** Brush a light stimulus such as a cotton wisp over patient's skin in several locations, including torso and extremities.	*Diminished/absent cutaneous perception:* Peripheral nerve damage or damage to posterior column of spinal cord. Peripheral neuropathies can also cause sensory deficits.
HELPFUL HINT: If light touch sensation is intact distally, do not assume that it is intact proximally.	
Identifies areas stimulated by light touch.	*Hypesthesia:* Increased sensitivity. *Paresthesia:* Numbness and tingling. *Anesthesia:* Loss of sensation.
Pain 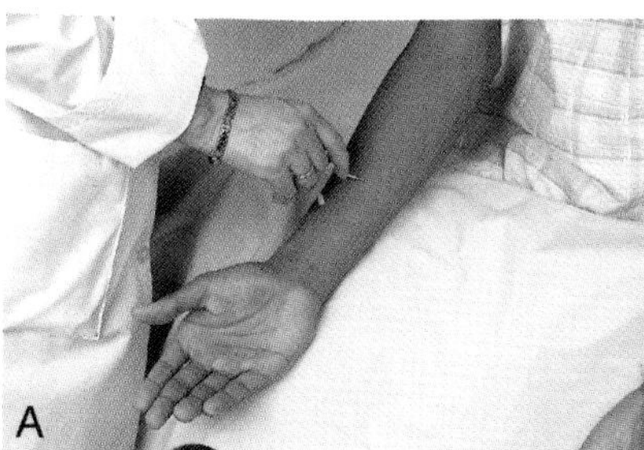 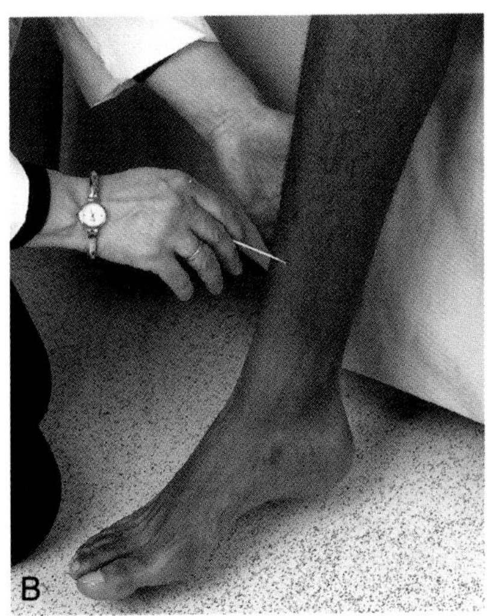 **A. Assessing pain in upper extremity, B. Assessing pain in lower extremity**	*Diminished or absent pain perception:* Peripheral nerve damage or damage to lateral spinothalamic tract.

(Continued)

Assessing Sensory Function *(Continued)*

COMPONENT/TECHNIQUE/NORMAL VARIATIONS	ABNORMAL FINDINGS/RATIONALE
Pain (Continued) Stimulate skin lightly with sharp and dull ends of toothpick. Apply stimuli randomly and ask patient to identify whether sensation is sharp or dull. Identifies areas stimulated and type of stimulation.	**Hyperalgia:** Increased pain sensation. **Hypoalgesia:** Decreased pain sensation. **Analgesia:** No pain sensation.
Temperature	*Diminished/absent temperature perception:* Peripheral nerve damage or damage to lateral spinothalamic tract.

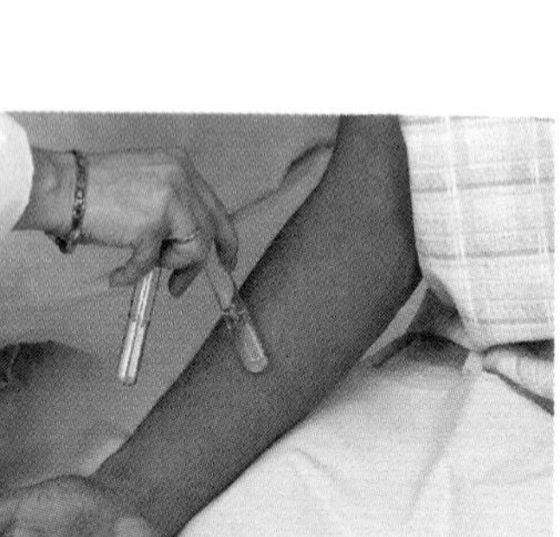

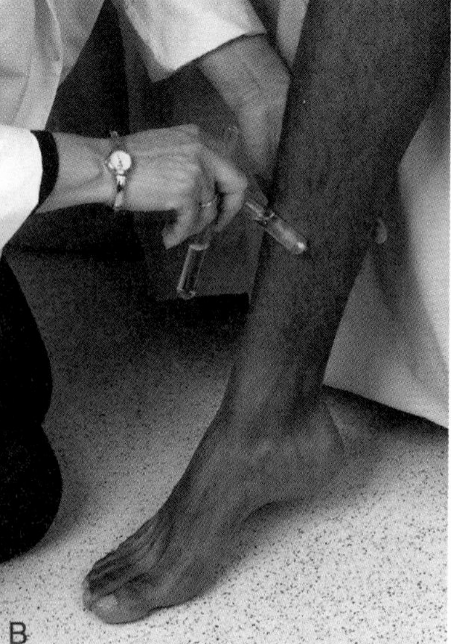

A. Testing temperature in upper extremity, B. Testing temperature in lower extremity

Test temperature only if patient's perception of pain is abnormal. Touch patient's skin with test tubes filled with hot or cold water. Apply stimuli randomly, and ask patient to identify whether sensation is hot or cold.

HELPFUL HINT

If pain sensation is intact, there is no need to test temperature, because temperature and pain run along the same tract.

Identifies areas stimulated and type of stimulation.

COMPONENT/TECHNIQUE/NORMAL VARIATIONS	ABNORMAL FINDINGS/RATIONALE
Vibration	*Diminished/absent vibration sense:* Peripheral nerve damage caused by alcoholism, diabetes, or damage to posterior column of spinal cord.

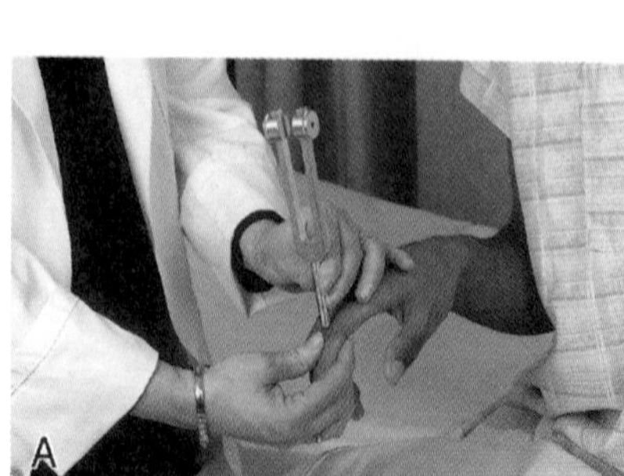

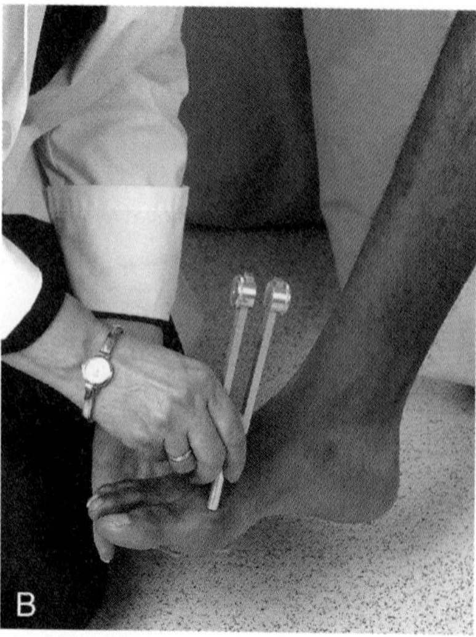

A. Vibrating upper extremity, **B. Vibrating lower extremity**

Assessing Sensory Function

COMPONENT/TECHNIQUE/NORMAL VARIATIONS	ABNORMAL FINDINGS/RATIONALE

Vibration (Continued)

Place a vibrating tuning fork over a finger joint, and then over a toe joint. Ask patient to tell you when vibration is felt and when it stops. If patient is unable to detect vibration, test proximal areas as well.

HELPFUL HINT

If vibratory sensation is intact distally, it is intact proximally.

Vibratory sensation intact bilaterally in upper and lower extremities.

Kinesthetics (position sense)

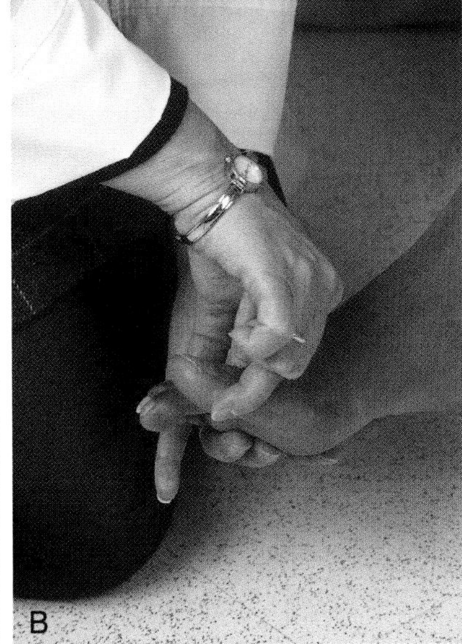

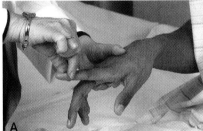

A. Testing position sense in finger, B. Testing position sense in toe

Determine patient's ability to perceive passive movement of extremities. Hold fingers on sides and move up and down. Have patient identify direction of movement. Flex and extend patient's big toe. Ask patient to describe movement as up or down.

Diminished or absent position sense: Peripheral nerve damage or damage to posterior column of spinal cord.

HELPFUL HINTS

- Avoid moving the patient's finger by placing your finger on top of the patient's because the patient may sense the pressure of your finger rather than a true position change.
- If position sensation is intact distally, it is intact proximally.

Position sensation intact bilaterally in upper and lower extremities.

Stereognosis

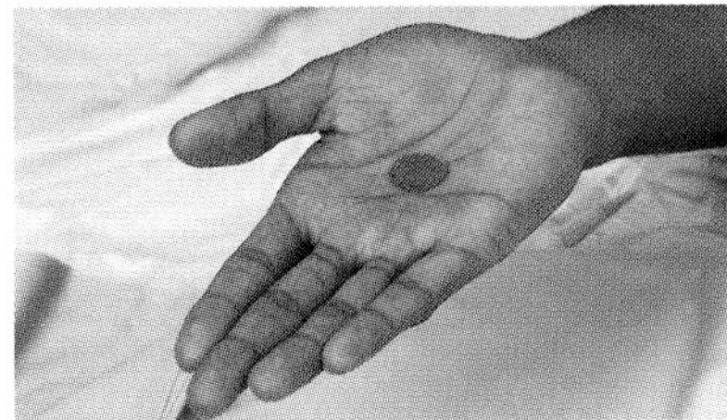

Testing stereognosis

With patient's eyes closed, place a familiar object, such as a coin or a button, in patient's hand. Ask patient to identify it. Test both hands using different objects.

Abnormal findings suggest a lesion or other disorder involving sensory cortex or a disorder affecting posterior column.

(Continued)

Assessing Sensory Function *(Continued)*

COMPONENT/TECHNIQUE/NORMAL VARIATIONS	ABNORMAL FINDINGS/RATIONALE
Stereognosis *(Continued)* Stereognosis intact bilaterally.	
Graphesthesia	Abnormal findings suggest lesion or other disorder involving sensory cortex or disorder affecting posterior column.

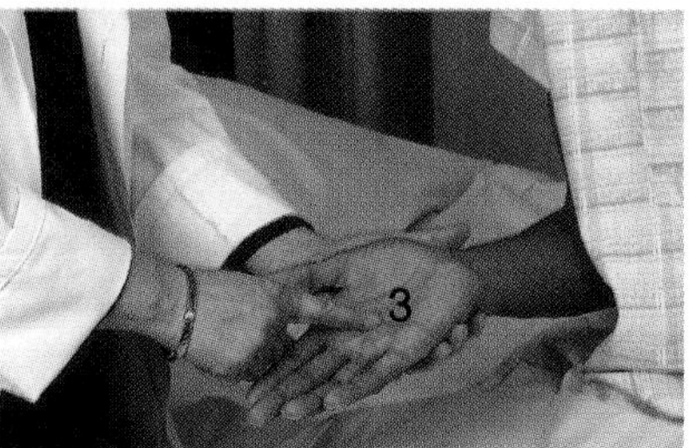

Testing graphesthesia

With patient's eyes closed, use point of a closed pen to trace a number on patient's hand. Ask patient to identify the number.

Graphesthesia intact bilaterally.

COMPONENT/TECHNIQUE/NORMAL VARIATIONS	ABNORMAL FINDINGS/RATIONALE
Two-Point Discrimination (ability to differentiate between two points of simultaneous stimulation)	Abnormal findings suggest lesion or other disorder involving sensory cortex or disorder affecting posterior column.

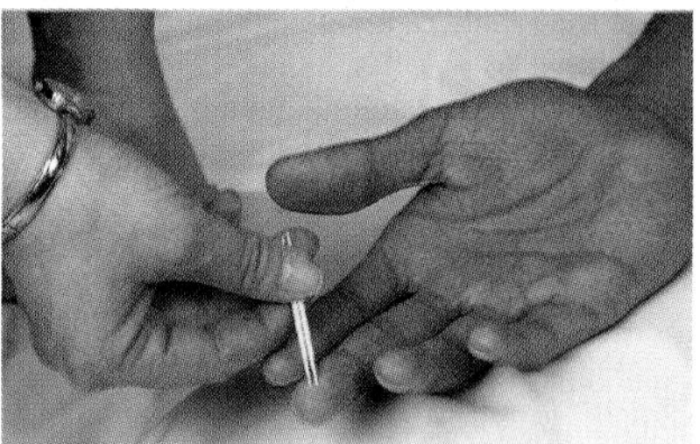

Testing 2-point discrimination

Using ends of two toothpicks, stimulate two points on fingertips simultaneously. Gradually move toothpicks together, and assess smallest distance at which patient can still discriminate two points (minimal perceptible distance). Document distance and location.

HELPFUL HINT

The normal discriminatory distance depends on the area tested, with the fingertips being the most discriminating.

Discriminates between two points on fingertips no more than 0.5 cm apart and on hands no more than 2 cm apart.

COMPONENT/TECHNIQUE/NORMAL VARIATIONS	ABNORMAL FINDINGS/RATIONALE
Point Localization (ability to sense and locate area being stimulated)	Abnormal findings suggest lesion or other disorder involving sensory cortex or disorder affecting posterior column.

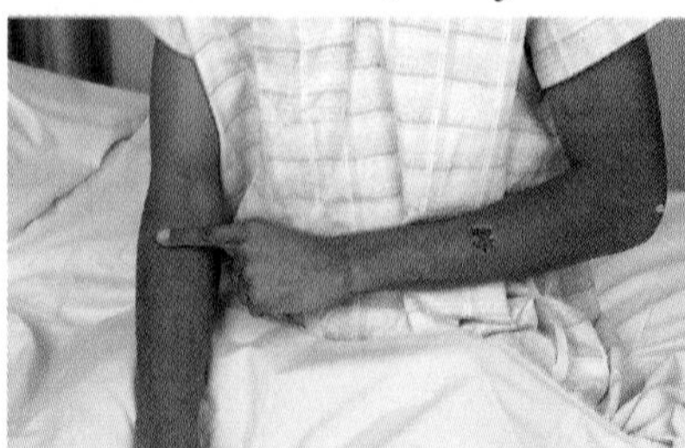

Testing point localization

With patient's eyes closed, touch an area; then have patient point to where he or she was touched. Test both sides and upper and lower extremities.

Point localization intact.

Assessing Sensory Function

COMPONENT/TECHNIQUE/NORMAL VARIATIONS	ABNORMAL FINDINGS/RATIONALE
Sensory Extinction	
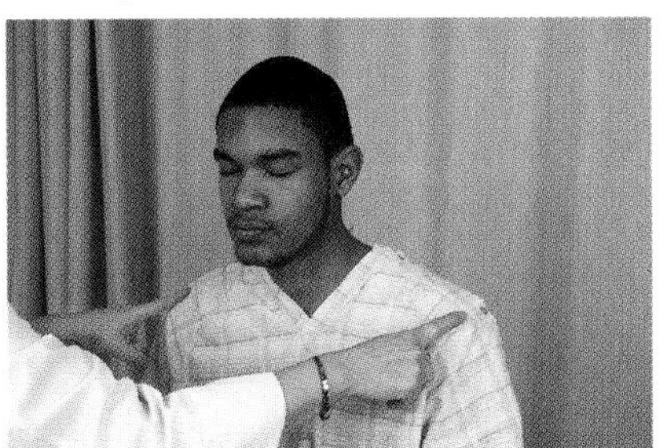 **Testing extinction** Test by simultaneously touching both sides of patient's body at same point. Ask patient to point to where he or she was touched. Extinction intact.	Identification of stimulus on only one side suggests lesion or other disorder involving sensory cortical region in opposite hemisphere.

Reflexes

Reflex assessment evaluates the intactness of the spinal cord. Intact sensory and motor systems are required for a normal reflex response. Normal reflexes include deep tendon reflexes (DTRs) and superficial reflexes. Reflexes that normally occur in newborns are termed pathological or primitive reflexes when they occur in adults.

Deep Tendon and Superficial Reflexes

Deep tendon reflexes include the biceps (C5, C6), triceps (C7, C8), brachioradialis (C5, C6), patellar (L2, L3, L4) and Achilles (S1, S2). Superficial reflexes include the plantar (L4 to S2), abdominal (T8, T9, T10), anal (S3, S4, S5), cremasteric (L1, L2), and bulbocavernous (S3, S4).

To test deep tendon reflexes, use a rubber percussion hammer to swiftly tap a slightly stretched tendon to elicit contraction of an associated skeletal muscle. Keep your wrist loose so that immediately upon impact, it swings back spontaneously. As with other neurological assessments, test reflexes bilaterally. Then grade DTRs on a scale from 0 to 4. Stick figures are often used to chart DTR findings (Fig. 19–10).

Because the normal response for a DTR is muscle contraction, eliciting a response may be difficult if your patient is tense and the muscles are contracted. Through **cognitive inhibition,** the patient can override and suppress the peripheral reflex response. Tell your patient to relax and let you support the limb being tested. If you are still having difficulty eliciting a DTR response, use a reinforcement technique to enhance the response. One technique, distraction maneuvers, allows the patient to concentrate on something other than the reflex being tested, thereby relaxing the area and eliminating unintentional cognitive inhibition. The other technique, isometric maneuvers, overrides the inhibitory message from the brain and increases reflex response. Two isometric maneuvers are having your patient clench his or her teeth (enhances upper extremity reflexes) and having the patient interlock his or her hands and push (enhances lower extremity reflexes). These techniques are shown in Figure 19–11. If you use a reinforcement technique, be sure to document it.

When assessing superficial reflexes, use a tongue blade, the base of the reflex hammer, or the back of your thumbnail and stroke the body briskly, without pressing into the underlying organs. Superficial reflexes are graded as positive or negative. Deep tendon reflexes are graded as follows:

- 0: No response detected
- 1: Response present but diminished (hypoactive)
- 2: Response normal
- 3: Response somewhat stronger than normal
- 4: Response hyperactive with clonus.

Grades 1 and 3 are usually considered normal. Even grade 0 may occur symmetrically in some patients in the absence of any underlying neurological disorder. For example, a patellar reflex may be difficult to elicit on a patient who has had knee surgery. Grade 4 usually indicates pathology. **Clonus** is the presence of rhythmic involuntary contractions, most often at the foot and ankle. Sustained clonus confirms CNS involvement.

Pathological or Primitive Reflexes

Pathological or primitive reflexes usually indicate a severe underlying neurological problem. They reflect cerebral degeneration or late-stage dementia and are referred to as primitive reflexes because they are normally

Documenting reflex findings

Use these grading scales to rate the strength of each reflex in a deep tendon and superficial reflex assessment.

Deep tendon reflex grades
0 absent
\+ present but diminished
\+ + normal
\+ + + increased but not necessarily pathologic
\+ + + + hyperactive or clonic (involuntary contraction and relaxation of skeletal muscle)

Superficial reflex grades
0 absent
\+ present

Record the client's reflex ratings on a drawing of a stick figure. The figures here show documentation of normal and abnormal reflex responses.

Normal

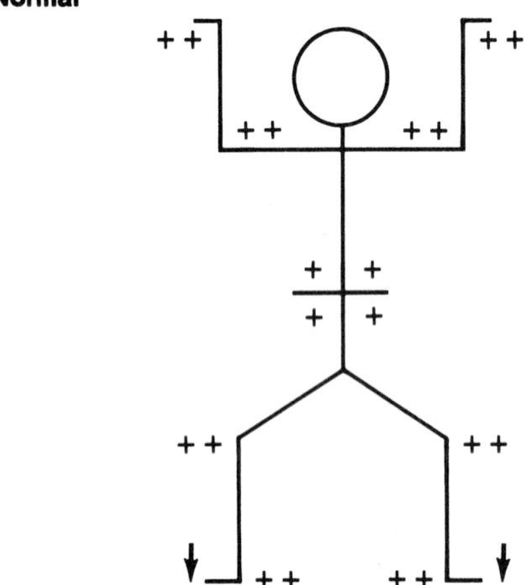

Abnormal

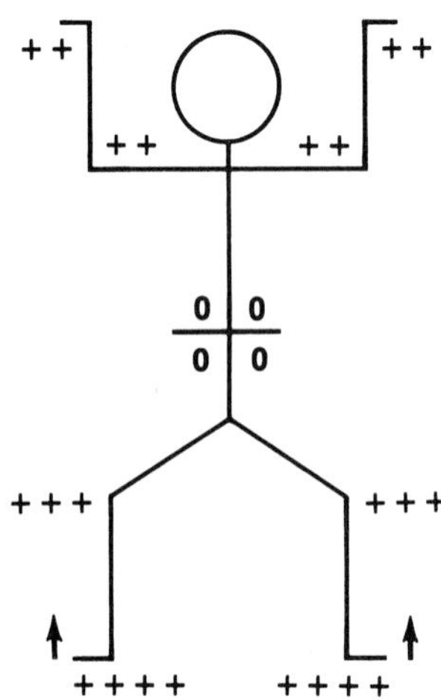

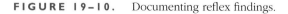

FIGURE 19–10. Documenting reflex findings.

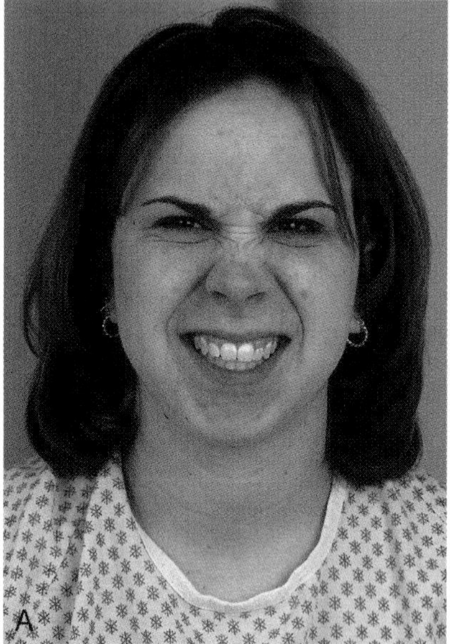

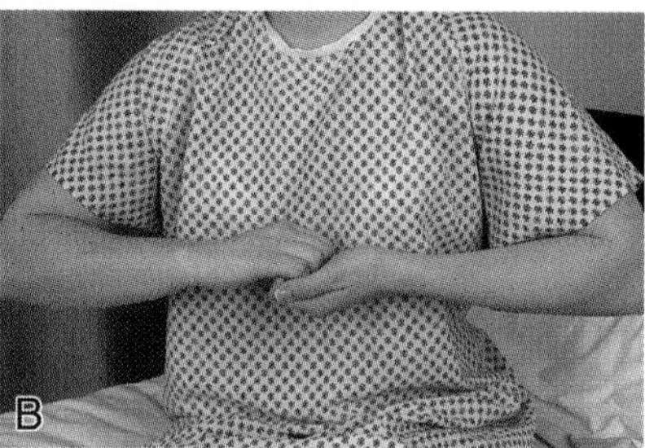

FIGURE 19–11. Isometric maneuvers. (*A*) Clenching teeth. (*B*) Interlocking hands.

seen in a newborn with an immature neurological system. Family members may be misled by these reflexes, which may seem like a sign of improvement. Therefore be sure to explain that these are reflexive responses and provide support for the family.

Primitive reflexes include the following:

- **Grasp:** Place your fingers in palm of patient's hand. Patient will close his fingers and grasp yours.
- **Sucking:** Gently stimulate patient's lips with a mouth swab. Patient will start sucking.
- **Snout:** Gently tap oral area with finger. Patient's lips will pucker.
- **Rooting:** Gently stroke side of patient's face. Patient will turn toward stimulated side.
- **Glabellar:** Gently tap on patient's forehead. Patient will blink.
- **Babinski:** Stroke lateral aspect of sole of foot. Dorsiflexion of great toe and fanning of toes will occur.

Meningeal Signs

Classic signs of meningitis include nuchal rigidity (extension of neck with resistance to flexion), fever, photosensitivity, headache, nausea, and vomiting. If you suspect

(Text continues on p. 689).

REFLEX/LOCATION/TECHNIQUE/NORMAL VARIATIONS	ABNORMAL FINDINGS/RATIONALE
Deep Tendon Reflexes *Biceps Reflex*	*Absent/diminished DTRs:* Degenerative disease; damage to peripheral nerve such as peripheral neuropathy; lower motor neuron disorder, such as ALS and Guillain-Barré syndrome. *Hyperactive reflexes with clonus:* Spinal cord injuries, upper motor neuron disease such as MS.

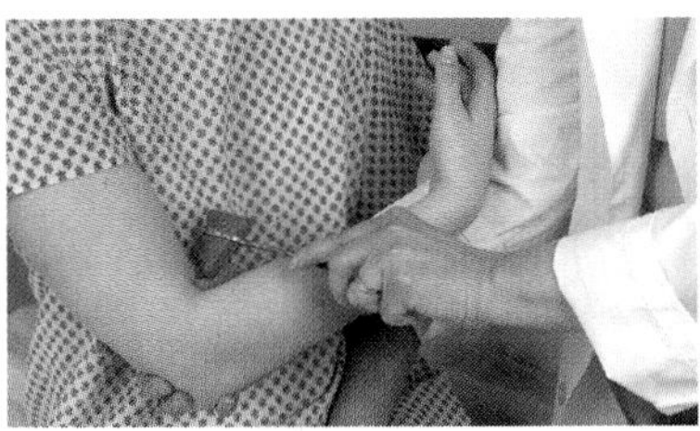

Testing biceps reflex

Rest patient's elbow in your nondominant hand, with your thumb over biceps tendon. Strike your thumbnail.

Contraction of biceps with flexion of forearm.

+2

Triceps Reflex

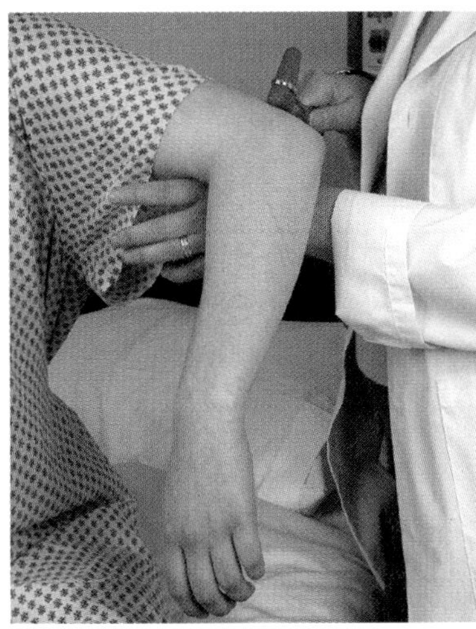

Testing triceps reflex

Abduct patient's arm and flex it at the elbow. Support the arm with your nondominant hand. Strike triceps tendon about 1–2 inches above olecranon process, approaching it from directly behind.

Contraction of triceps with extension at elbow.

+2

Brachioradialis Reflex

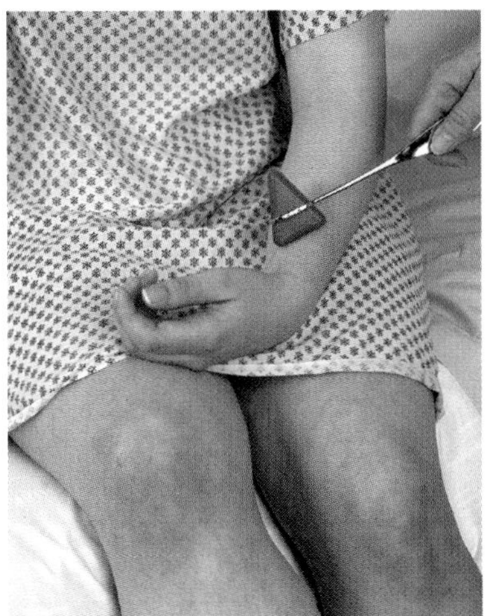

Testing brachioradialis reflex

(Continued)

Assessing Reflexes *(Continued)*

REFLEX/LOCATION/TECHNIQUE/NORMAL VARIATIONS	ABNORMAL FINDINGS/RATIONALE

Brachioradialis Reflex (Continued)

With your nondominant hand, support patient's hand and palpate brachioradialis tendon 3 to 5 cm above wrist. Simultaneously strike styloid process of radius.

Flexion at elbow and supination of forearm. You may also notice flexion of fingers.

+2

Patellar Reflex

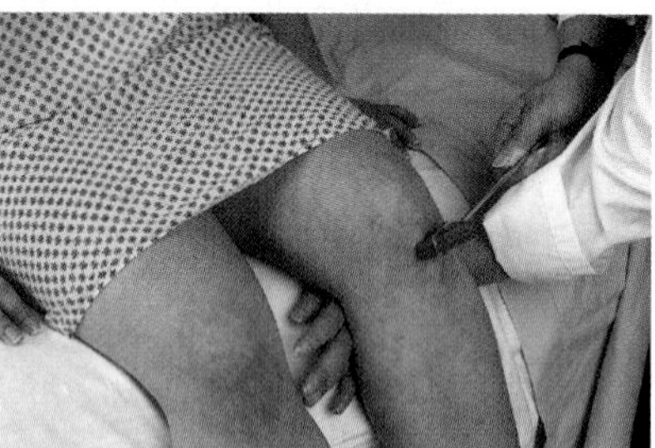

Testing patellar reflex

Have patient sit with legs dangling. Strike tendon directly below patella.

Contraction of quadriceps with extension of knee.

+2.

Achilles Reflex

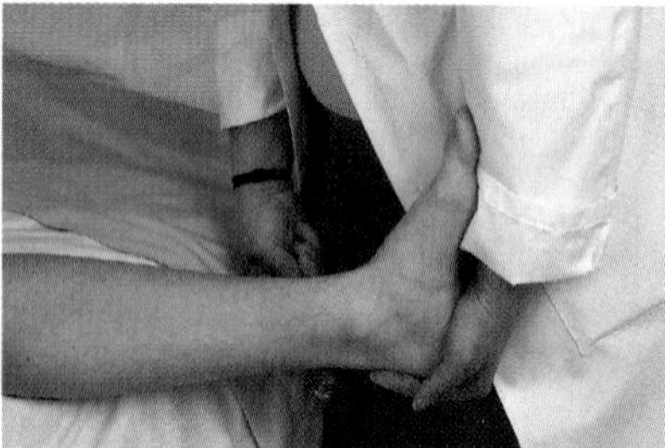

Testing Achilles reflex

Have patient lie supine or sit with one knee flexed. Holding patient's foot slightly dorsiflexed, strike Achilles tendon.

Plantarflexion of foot.

+2

Ankle Clonus

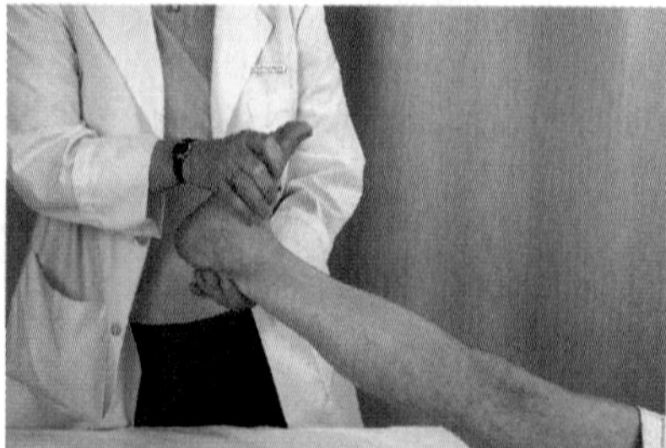

Testing for clonus

If you get +4 reflexes while supporting leg and foot, quickly dorsiflex foot.

No contraction

Abnormal findings/rationale (Ankle Clonus): Rhythmic contraction of leg muscles and foot is positive sign of clonus and indicates upper motor neuron disorder.

Assessing Reflexes

REFLEX/LOCATION/TECHNIQUE/NORMAL VARIATIONS	ABNORMAL FINDINGS/RATIONALE
Superficial Reflexes *Abdominal Reflex* 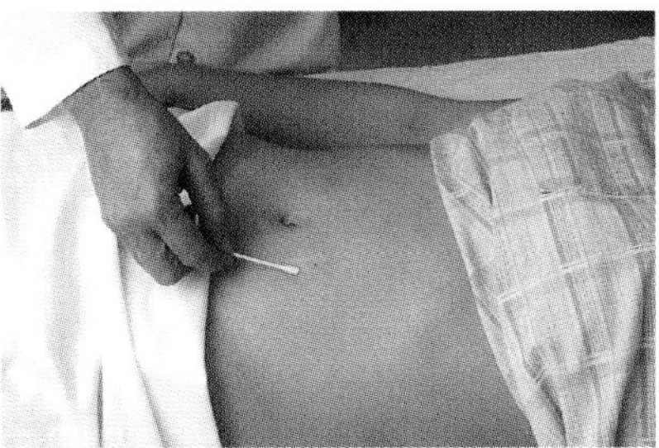 **Testing abdominal reflex** Stroke patient's abdomen diagonally from upper and lower quadrants toward umbilicus. Contraction of rectus abdominis. Umbilicus moves toward stimulus. Obesity and pregnancy can mask this reflex.	Absence of superficial reflexes may indicate pyramidal tract lesions.
Anal Reflex Gently stroke skin around anus with gloved finger. Anus puckers.	
Cremasteric reflex Gently stroke inner aspect of a male's thigh. Testes rise.	
Bulbocavernosus Reflex Gently apply pressure over bulbocavernous muscle on dorsal side of penis. Bulbocavernosus muscle contracts.	
Plantar Reflex (Babinski's response) 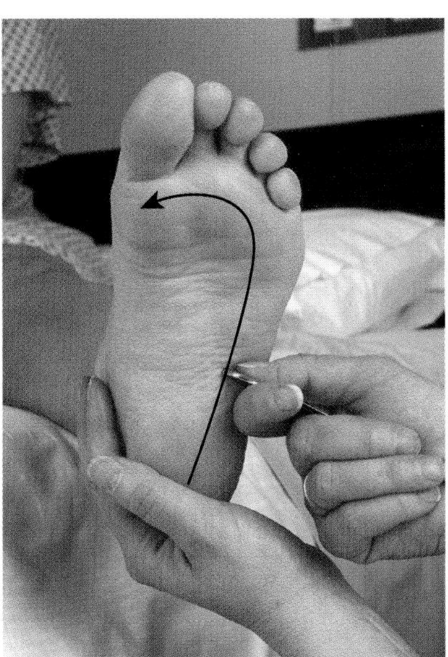 **Testing plantar reflex** Stroke sole of patient's foot in an arc from lateral heel to medial ball. Flexion of all toes.	*Babinski's response:* Dorsiflexion of big toe, with or without fanning of other toes. In absence of drug or alcohol intoxication, it suggests pathology involving upper motor neurons.

AREA/SYSTEM	SUBJECTIVE DATA
General	*Ask about:* General health Fever
Integumentary	*Ask about:* Rashes Changes in sensations
HEENT	*Ask about:* Changes in sense of smell, taste, sight, hearing, touch Headaches Changes in speech or swallowing
Respiratory	*Ask about:* Breathing difficulty
Cardiovascular	*Ask about:* History of CV problems
Gastrointestinal	*Ask about:* Nausea, vomiting Changes in bowel function Difficulty swallowing
Genitourinary/ Reproductive	*Ask about:* History of STDs Changes in sexual activity, desire, ability Changes in bladder function
Musculoskeletal	*Ask about:* Muscle weakness Paralysis Problems walking Balance problems
Endocrine	*Ask about:* History of diabetes mellitus and thyroid disease
Lymphatic/ Hematologic	*Ask about:* Fever Bruising

AREA/SYSTEM	OBJECTIVE DATA
General	*Measure:* Vital signs *Observe:* Mental status, grooming, affect, behavior, symmetry
Integumentary	*Inspect:* Rashes or petechiae *Test:* Superficial sensations
HEENT	*Inspect:* Symmetry of facial features *Palpate:* Lymph nodes, thyroid *Examine:* Optic disk *Test:* Cranial nerves
Respiratory	*Auscultate:* Lungs
Cardiovascular	*Auscultate:* Heart sounds, noting rhythm Carotids for bruits and thrills
Gastrointestinal	*Auscultate:* Bowel sounds
Genitourinary/ Reproductive	*Inspect:* Lesions *Palpate:* Bladder distention
Musculoskeletal	*Inspect:* Gait *Test:* Muscle strength ROM Cerebellar function

Assessment of the Sensory-Neurological System,s Relationship to Other Systems

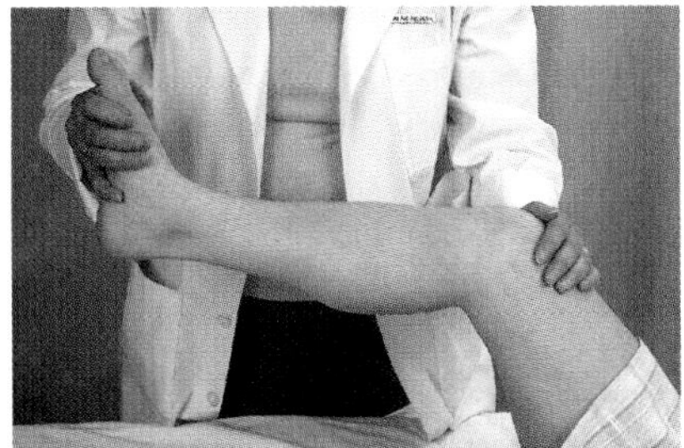

FIGURE 19–12. Kernig's sign.

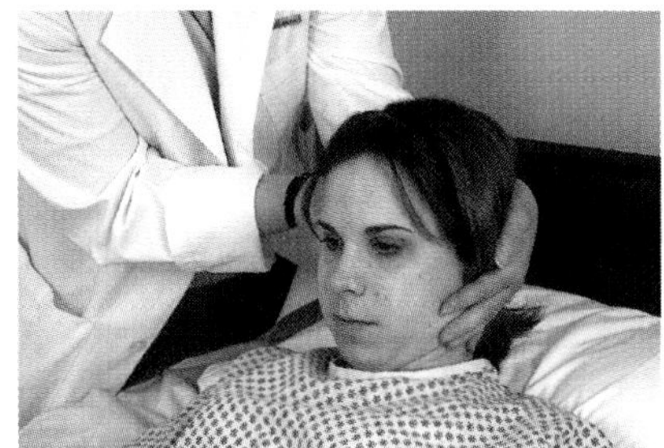

FIGURE 19–13. Brudzinski's sign.

that your patient has meningitis, assess for Kernig's and Brudzinski's signs.

To assess for Kernig's sign (Fig. 19–12) have the patient lie supine with one leg flexed. Tell him or her to try to extend the leg while you apply pressure to the knee. Contraction and pain of the hamstring muscles and resistance to extension are positive signs of meningitis.

To assess for Brudzinski's sign (Fig. 19–13), have the patient lie supine with his head flexed to his chest. Flexion of the hips is a positive sign of meningitis.

Case Study Findings

Mr. Webster's focused sensory-neurological system findings include:

- LOC: AAO × 3; Glasgow Coma Scale 15.
- Communication: Intact
- Memory: Immediate and remote intact, but doesn't remember events of accident.
- Cognitive functions: Intact
- Cranial nerves I XII:\: Intact
- DTR +2; positive plantar

Case Study Analysis and Plan

Now that you have completed a thorough assessment of Leon Webster, document your health history and physical examination findings:

List key history and physical examination findings that will help you formulate your nursing diagnoses.

Nursing Diagnoses

After you complete the assessment, formulate nursing diagnoses. The following are possible diagnoses. Cluster the supporting data for each.

1. Pain, related to injuries
2. Risk for altered cerebral tissue perfusion related to head injury
3. High risk for injury related to risky behavior

Identify any additional nursing diagnoses.

CRITICAL THINKING ACTIVITY

Now that you have identified some nursing diagnoses for Mr. Webster, select one and develop a nursing care plan and a brief teaching plan for him, including learning objectives and teaching strategies.

Research Tells Us

Stroke (CVA) is the third leading cause of death in the United States. New treatment modalities have been successful in reversing and preventing some of the long-term disabling effects associated with stroke. Although tPA has long been used for the treatment of acute myocardial infarction, it has only recently been used for the treatment of stroke. The key to successful treatment of stroke with tPA is to identify patients who are candidates for treatment within a 3-hour window from the onset of symptoms. The 3-hour window is based on the increased risk for intracranial hemorrhage beyond 3 hours.

Ringleb et al. (2002) performed a meta-analysis on major trials using tPA beyond the 3-hour window. Within 3 to 6 hours, one study reported that, although there was a slight increase in intracranial hemorrhage, the results were not significant, and the results of tPA administrations were positive. Another study with a 3- to 5-hour window failed to show the benefits of treatment, but also failed to readjust the treatment criteria. The researchers concluded that to limit stroke treatment to 3 hours is unjustified. These researchers recommend development of better patient selection methods to identify and individualize the time window for each patient.

The implications for nursing are twofold: First, accurate stroke assessment is crucial to ensure prompt treatment. Second, nurses are ideally positioned to educate patient, family, and the community to recognize and respond at the first signs and symptoms of stroke. Time is brain!

Health Concerns

Although the mortality rate for stroke is alarming, the physical, emotional, and financial cost for those who survive is just as alarming. You cannot put a price on the physical and emotional toll, but the direct and indirect financial costs exceed $41 billion annually. According to the National Institutes of Health Neurological Institute, stroke risk reduction and prompt treatment could decrease stroke by 80 percent by the end of the decade. Identifying risk factors is the first step!

Risk Factors for Stroke:

- ***Nonmodifiable:*** Age, gender, race, previous stroke or TIA, asymptomatic carotid stenosis, heredity.
- ***Modifiable:*** HTN; diabetes mellitus; cardiovascular disease; abnormal serum lipid, triglyceride, cholesterol, LDL, and HDL levels; cigarette smoking; excessive alcohol; drug abuse.
- ***Other factors:*** Obesity, migraines, oral contraceptive use, hypercoagulable states.

Common Abnormalities

ABNORMALITY	ASSESSMENT FINDINGS
Alzheimer's Disease A chronic, progressive disorder that accounts for 50% of all dementias	• Most common in people over 65 • Pathological changes in the brain including plaques and neuronal tangles • Begins with mild memory loss • Progresses to deterioration of intellectual function, personality changes, and speech and language problems • Repeated head trauma • Exposure to aluminum • Previous CNS infection • Family history • Emotional lability • Weight loss, anorexia, malnutrition • Incontinence • Poor hygiene • Gait instability, weakness • Inability to perform ADLs • Awakening frequently during night with daytime naps • Forgetfulness • Inability to solve problems • Depression, suicidal ideation • Disheveled appearance • Agitation • Memory loss (early sign) that is progressive • Disorientation to time

Common Abnormalities

ABNORMALITY	ASSESSMENT FINDINGS
Alzheimer's Disease *(Continued)*	• Flat affect • Impaired cognitive functioning • Nocturnal wandering • Repetitive behaviors • Stubbornness, paranoia *More advanced disease:* • Aphasia, agnosia, apraxia • Seizures • Limb rigidity, flexor posturing
Brain Tumor An intracranial mass that can be neoplastic, cystic, inflammatory (abscess), or syphilitic	• Early morning headache • Subtle personality changes or dysphasia • Papilledema, possibly leading to visual loss • Changes in pupil size and response • Disorders of extraocular movement • Focal deficits • New onset of seizures
Cerebrovascular Accident Stroke, caused by either ischemia or hemorrhagic lesions	• Hemiparesis or hemiparalysis (loss of tactile sensation on affected side of body) • Hypertension; atherosclerosis; family history of cardiovascular or cerebrovascular disease • Sudden onset of symptoms with or without warning signs • Intact or altered mental activity; emotional lability • Hemiparesis or hemiparalysis, usually affecting the arm more than the leg • Facial sagging on affected side • Impaired swallowing • Homonymous hemianopia (vision defect in the right halves or left halves of the visual fields in both eyes) • Language disturbance and aphasia with right-sided weakness • Perceptual disturbance and altered visual-spacial perceptions with left-sided weakness • Loss of sensation on affected side • Disturbed stereognosis, body scheme, and visual-spacial skills
Chronic Subdural Hematoma A swelling or mass of blood beneath the dura, usually caused by head injury	• Personality changes • Gradual progressive decrease in level of consciousness; headache • History of trivial head injury weeks or months earlier • Progressive deterioration in mental activity and level of arousal • Disorientation • Focal deficit
Guillain-Barré Syndrome Acute autoimmune inflammatory destruction of the myelin sheath leading to rapid, progressive symmetrical loss of motor function with no sensory loss, usually triggered by a viral infection	• Muscle weakness that affects the lower extremities • First flaccid paralysis, little or no sensory loss • History of recent surgery, cancer, pregnancy, childbirth, infection, or vaccination • Respiratory insufficiency • Labile blood pressure • Tachycardia • Vasomotor flushes • Hyperpyrexia and increased sweating • Tracheobronchial secretions • Paralytic ileus • Blurred vision or diplopia

(Continued)

Common Abnormalities *(Continued)*

ABNORMALITY	ASSESSMENT FINDINGS
Guillain-Barré Syndrome *(Continued)*	• Facial weakness; impaired swallowing • Symmetrical flaccid paralysis, usually beginning in legs and progressing upward • Absent deep tendon reflexes
Herniated Intervertebral Disc Prolapse of the nucleus pulposus of a ruptured intravertebral disc into the spinal canal	• Sharp, severe pain in the back, which may radiate down extremity (in a pattern that reflects the nerve involved) and may be intensified by such actions as coughing, sneezing, straining, and moving • History of recurring symptoms • Decreased muscle tone in affected area • Mild motor weakness • Paresthesia in affected area • Intact, absent, or diminished brachioradialis, biceps, and triceps reflexes, depending on the level of lesion • Diminished or absent patellar and Achilles reflexes
Meningitis Inflammation of the membranes of the brain or spinal cord	• Headache, nuchal rigidity • Elevated temperature (up to 105°F) • Irritability, restlessness, photophobia, confusion • History of adjacent infection, neurosurgery, head trauma, systemic sepsis, or immunosuppression • Restlessness, disorientation, lethargy, stupor, coma • Decreased visual acuity or loss • Brudzinski's sign, Kernig's sign • Generalized seizures • Opisthotonos (abnormal posture characterized by back arching and wrist flexion) as a late sign • Hyperalgesia, photophobia, increased reflexes • Elevated temperature • Altered respiratory pattern; weak, rapid pulse • Vomiting
Migraine, Classic An often familial symptom complex of periodic attacks of vascular headache, usually temporal and unilateral in onset	• Throbbing headache lasting 2 to 12 hours, often preceded by a visual disturbance or scotomata lasting 15 to 20 minutes • Anorexia; nausea; vomiting • Diarrhea • Photophobia • Dizziness • Syncope • Scalp tenderness • History of stress, fatigue, hormonal changes, menstruation, change in amount of sleep, or other predisposing factors • Ingestion of certain foods (such as aged cheese, red wine, or chocolate) or oral contraceptives that seem to trigger symptoms • Perfectionist, compulsive, intelligent, rigid personality type; family emphasis on achievement • Transient mood and personality changes • Prodromal transient neurologic deficits such as hermiparesis, aphasia, ophthalmoplegia, and photophobia
Parkinson's Disease Chronic nervous system disease characterized by a fine, slowly spreading tremor, muscular weakness and rigidity, and a peculiar gait	• Akinesia • Cogwheel rigidity • Resting tremor • Gait disturbance • Impaired swallowing • Flat affect

Common Abnormalities

ABNORMALITY	ASSESSMENT FINDINGS
Parkinson's Disease *(Continued)*	• Monotonous speech • Decreased blinking • Increased sweating and salivation • History of cerebral arteriosclerosis, cerebral hypoxia, trauma, toxin ingestion (carbon monoxide, manganese, or mercury), or use of illegal drugs • Slow onset and gradual progression of signs and symptoms • Emotional lability, depression, or paranoia • Diminished facial movements, decreased blinking, impaired swallowing, and abnormal muscle tone • Bradykinesia with difficulty initiating movement, intermittent "freezing," and pill-rolling tremor of hands • Small, jerky, cramped handwriting (micrographia) • Abnormal gait that is slow to start, includes short and shuffling steps, gradually accelerates, and is difficult to stop • Low, monotonous speech; involuntary repetition of words (echolalia) or sentences (palilalia) spoken by others
Spinal Cord Tumor Swelling or mass of the spinal cord that can be neoplastic, cystic, or inflammatory	• Pain and local tenderness throughout the sensory nerve root • Motor weakness below level or lesion • Slow progression of sensory and motor dysfunction: initially unilateral, eventually bilateral • Dysfunction of cranial nerves VIII through XII (with lesion at C4 or above) • Spastic weakness or paralysis below the lesion • Flaccid paralysis or weakness at level of lesion • Respiratory failure or difficulty, occipital headache, nystagmus, and stiff neck with lesion at C4 or above • Sensory loss below the level of the lesion • Loss of pain and temperature sensation below and contralateral to lesion when only one side of cord is affected • Loss of tactile, position, and vibration sensations ipisilateral to lesion • Band of hyperesthesia just above level of lesion • Increased deep tendon reflexes below level of lesion • Absent reflexes at level of lesion; intact reflexes above lesion; positive Babinski reflex

Summary

- This chapter taught you how to take a thorough sensory-neurological assessment, including a health history and physical examination.
- It also covered how to analyze your findings to identify actual and potential health problems, as well as write nursing diagnoses and plan of care.

20

Putting It All Together

Before You Begin

INTRODUCTION TO DOING A COMPLETE HEALTH ASSESSMENT

Now that you have learned what questions to ask and how to examine each body system, how do you combine the steps into a format for performing a complete assessment of your client? A complete assessment is a very individualized process that depends on many factors, including your client's age, developmental level, presenting symptoms, cultural background, and health needs. Your aim is to identify abnormalities, symptoms, health maintenance issues, teaching and learning needs, and your client's strengths, so you can use them in planning client care. Once health needs are identified, you can help your client find appropriate resources to meet them. As a professional nurse, you will also be looking for health problems to address in a care plan, using the nursing process and nursing diagnoses.

In previous chapters, you learned about the many developmental, cultural, and ethnic variations to consider when assessing a client. To illustrate how to "put it all together," this chapter focuses on assessing a female client in the developmental stage of menopause.

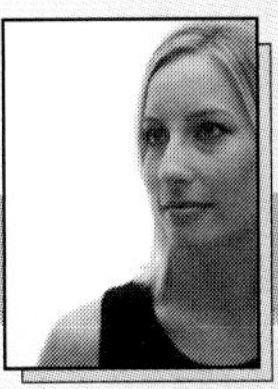

Introducing the Case Study

Marcia Malone is a 40-year-old woman who comes to you for a health screening. She is seeking information about routine health screenings recommended for her age group. She is concerned about her risk for osteoporosis and has several questions about **menopause.**

Developmental Considerations

The focus of this assessment is an adult female client who is approaching menopause.

Developmental Stage Issues

At age 40, Marcia Malone is at the generativity vs. stagnation stage of development, with a focus on being a productive member of both her family and society. Tasks for this developmental stage include raising a family and contributing to the community, usually through work or volunteer efforts. Because this stage marks the halfway point in life, people often reflect back on what they have done and look forward to what they hope to accomplish in relationships, self-development and career. Toward the end of this stage, a person who has successfully raised a family may be confronted with the "empty nest syndrome." Some people have a difficult time and search for meaning in life, whereas others see an opportunity to further fulfill personal and career goals. Midlife is also a time when role reversals occur with parents. With life expectancy increasing, caring for aging parents may become a major concern.

Perimenopause and Menopause

Menopause is a developmental change that occurs in adult women. It is defined as the permanent cessation of menstruation as a result of loss of ovarian follicular activity. It usually occurs at about age 51. Although most women have minimal discomfort at this time, many still have concerns about the increased risk of cancer, cardiovascular disease, stroke, and osteoporosis, as well as the physical and neurological effects of menopause. They may also feel anxious because so many myths surround menopause. You can help your clients by debunking these myths, discussing the real concerns of menopause, and helping them to be active participants in maintaining their health into old age.

Perimenopause is a period of up to 10 years before and after menopause, during which signs and symptoms of ovarian involution are present. Symptoms in perimenopausal women are variable but include:

- Vasomotor
  - Hot flashes
  - Night sweats
  - Dizziness
  - Nausea
  - Lightheadedness
  - Palpitations
  - Nervousness
- Genitourinary
  - Vaginal dryness and itching
  - Urinary frequency
  - Urinary urgency and stress incontinence
  - Decreased libido and sexual response
  - Irregular or missed periods
  - Decreased menstrual flow
- Emotional and cognitive
  - Decreased concentration
  - Forgetfulness
  - Depression
  - Irritability
  - Emotional lability
  - Tension
  - Heightened stress response
- Physical
  - Headache
  - Insomnia
  - Sleep disturbances
  - Fatigue (related to sleep disorders)
  - Breast tenderness
  - Musculoskeletal aching
  - Appetite changes
  - Constipation

During perimenopause, women need preventive health screenings and education. Components of a comprehensive midlife healthcare program include the following:

- Complete history and physical examination
- Blood work that includes a lipid panel, blood chemistries, and CBC
- Thyroid function test
- Pap smear
- Hemoccult test
- Mammography
- Psychosocial screening
- Flexibility and exercise screening
- Bone density screening
- Dietary profile

All women in midlife benefit from educational programs focused on menopause, osteoporosis, mammography, and breast self-examination. Selected clients also benefit from individualized health education for incontinence, heart disease, smoking cessation, skin cancer, and fibrocystic breast disease.

Performing the Assessment

A complete assessment begins with a comprehensive health history. Findings from the health history provide clues to actual or potential health problems to watch for as you perform the physical examination. During the physical examination, keep the key history findings in mind. If a problem area is revealed, perform a more thorough assessment of that area. The health history and physical examination are based on the client's concerns and needs. Together, they provide you with a complete picture of her health status.

Health History

A complete health history includes obtaining biographical data, current health status, past health history, family history, a review of systems, and a psychosocial profile. By the end of the history, you should have a good idea of appropriate nursing diagnoses for the client. You may also uncover concerns by asking age-appropriate or systems-review questions.

Biographical Data

Your client's age, occupation, family or living situation, religion, ethnic background, and hobbies provide clues about his or her current health. For example, some diseases are age related, and some changes occur normally with aging. Religion, ethnic background, and family or living situation affect how a client deals with illness and health care. Certain occupations and hobbies put a client at risk for health problems.

As you establish rapport with your client, also remember to take note of his or her clothing, hygiene, and mental status.

As you talk with Mrs. Malone, you note that she is dressed appropriately and that her hygiene is good. She is oriented to person, place, and time; has appropriate affect; has well-developed language; and presents her ideas and concerns in a relaxed, coherent, and logical manner. She appears well nourished and healthy. Her biographical data, although unremarkable, give a few important clues to her current health status.

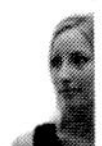

Case Study Findings

Reviewing Mrs. Malone's biographical data:

- 40-year-old woman
- Northern European extraction
- Protestant religion
- Married, with three children, ages 12, 15, and 18
- Has a full-time, sedentary job as an accountant
- Source: Self; seems reliable

Current Health Status

Your client's current health status focuses on her chief complaint. She may seek health care because of a diagnosed illness or a set of worrisome symptoms. Or she may feel well and need information about maintaining her current good health. If she identifies an illness, obtain a chronological account of its appearance and development. Be sure to include a symptom analysis (PQRST) of any problems identified.

Mrs. Malone denies any current health problems. Rather, her main concern is staying healthy. She states, "I'm concerned about 'the change' because my mother had so many problems at that time. I want to know what I can do at my age to stay healthy and avoid osteoporosis."

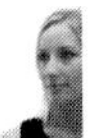

Case Study Findings

Mrs. Malone's current health status includes:

- No current health problems.
- Concerned about physiological changes of approaching menopause and health care recommended for her age.
- Occasionally takes acetaminophen for tension headaches. No other medications.

Past Health History

A past health history tells you about any diseases, injuries, or medications in the client's past that might affect her current health. Mrs. Malone has been healthy all her life, so her past health history is uncomplicated.

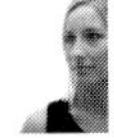

Case Study Findings

Mrs. Malone's past health history reveals:

- Had chickenpox, measles, mumps, and rubella as a child. Also had frequent bouts of strep throat as a child.
- Had an appendectomy at age 15. Was hospitalized for birth of her three children. Had a tubal ligation at age 35 for fertility control. Has never had a serious injury requiring hospitalization.
- No history of medical problems.
- No drug, environmental, or food allergies. Has taken penicillin without a reaction.
- Had all childhood immunizations. Last diphtheria-tetanus shot 10 years ago. Negative skin test 5 years ago.
- Has not traveled in a foreign country within last year. Has never served in the armed services.

Family History

Familial health problems are an important indicator of your client's current and future health. Mrs. Malone is well versed in her family's health history and provides you with detailed information.

Case Study Findings

Mrs. Malone's family history reveals:

- Client, age 40, alive and well
- Husband, age 45, alive and well
- Son, age 18, alive and well
- Daughter, age 15, alive and well
- Daughter, age 12, alive and well
- Mother, age 76, had breast cancer at age 54, osteoporosis and fractured hip at age 63.
- Father, age 78, has history of hypertension and had a myocardial infarction (MI) at age 68.
- Younger brother died in car accident at age 35.
- Two sisters, ages 42 and 50, alive and well.
- Maternal grandmother died of breast cancer at age 78.
- Maternal grandfather died of MI at age 81.
- Maternal aunt, age 78, has history of breast cancer and osteoporosis.
- Maternal uncle, age 80, has history of hypertension (HTN).
- Paternal grandmother died of cerebrovascular accident at age 82.
- Paternal grandfather died of MI at age 86.
- Paternal aunt, age 65, alive and well.
- Paternal aunt, age 69, history of breast cancer.
- Paternal uncle, age 71, history of HTN.

Mrs. Malone's genogram is shown in Figure 20–1.

Review of Systems

The review of systems takes the client's chief complaint and relates it to every other body system to determine its impact on the client's total health. Asking your client questions about every body system may also trigger her memory so that she asks more questions and voices more concerns.

Mrs. Malone reports no serious problems during your review of systems. By all indications, she is healthy and is experiencing normal changes for a woman in midlife.

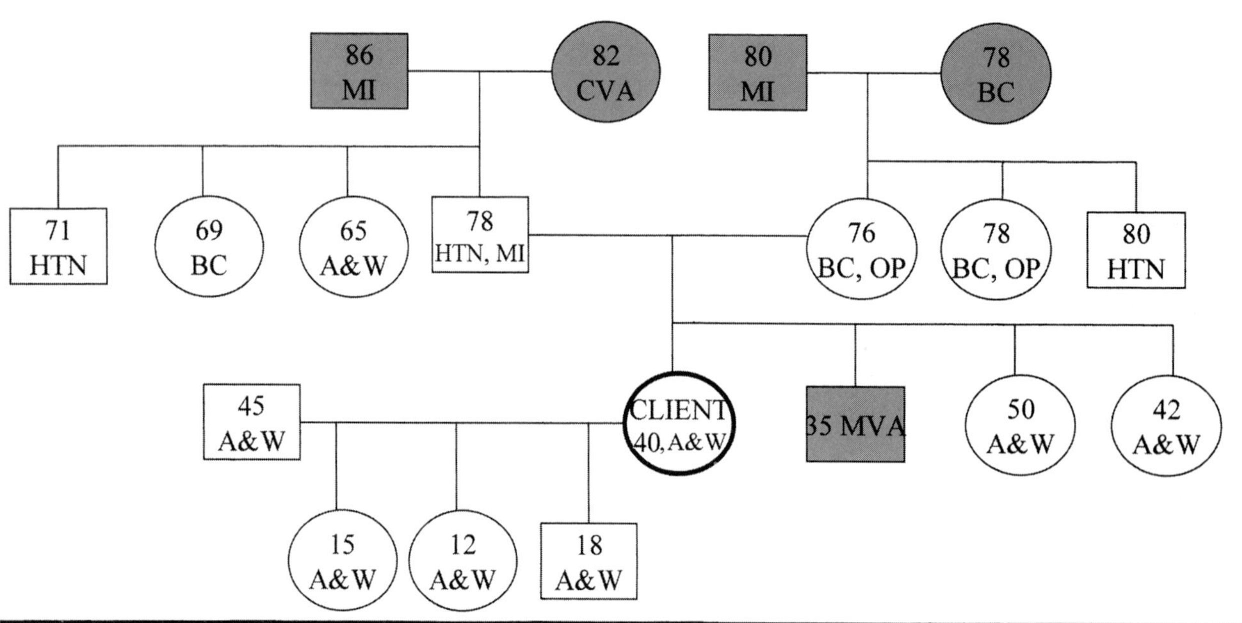

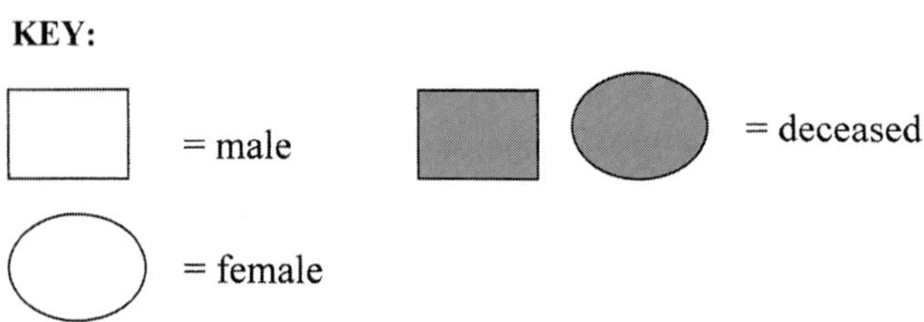

A&W = alive and well
MI = myocardial infarction
CVA = cerebral vascular accident
HTN = hypertension
BC = breast cancer
OP = osteoporosis
MVA = motor vehicle accident

FIGURE 20–1. Genogram for Mrs. Malone.

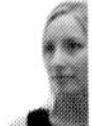

Case Study Findings

Mrs. Malone's review of systems reveals:

- **General Health Status:** Client feels that her overall health is good. No fever, chills, fatigue, depression, or anxiety. She has occasional colds and has gained 10 lb in the last year without a change in diet.
- **Integumentary:** No rashes, lesions, mole changes, or bruising. Skin is dry and hair is graying slightly.
- **HEENT:** No headaches; frequent sore throats; hoarseness; or problems with vision, hearing, or sinuses.
- **Respiratory:** No shortness of breath, wheezing, or productive or nonproductive cough.
- **Cardiovascular:** No history of HTN, heart problems or murmurs, blood clots or phlebitis, chest pain, palpitations, edema, orthopnea, or claudication.
- **Breasts:** Performs breast self-examination (BSE) occasionally, when she remembers. No breast pain, tenderness, masses, nipple discharge, or change in nipples. Has breast pain 7 days before menstrual cycle. Breastfed all 3 children.
- **Gastrointestinal:** No nausea/vomiting, abdominal pain, dysphasia, heartburn, jaundice, hemorrhoids, or blood in stool. Has daily bowel movement, brown in color.
- **Genitourinary:** No dysuria, frequency, or urgency, although she reports occasional stress incontinence.
- **Reproductive:** Last menstrual period 21 days ago. Menarche at age 14. Gravida 3, para 3. Menses are irregular, ranging from 23 to 45 days (cycle used to be 28 to 30 days). Menses last 5 days with moderate-to-heavy flow. Contraception method is tubal ligation. Satisfied with sex life except for increasing vaginal dryness.
- **Musculoskeletal:** No joint pains, swelling, or muscle weakness.
- **Neurological:** No dizziness, vertigo, syncope, head injuries, seizures, numbness, or tingling of extremities. Reports forgetfulness and difficulty concentrating. Has never been treated for mental disorders, depression, or anxiety, although she did visit a counselor about a family problem 3 years ago.
- **Endocrine:** No diabetes, thyroid disease, polyuria/polydipsia, or heat or cold intolerance. Weight gain of 10 lb last year.
- **Immune/Hematologic:** No current infections, allergies, cancer, bleeding, anemia, or blood transfusions. Blood type A+.

Psychosocial Profile

The psychosocial profile reveals patterns in the client's lifestyle that affect her health, increase her risk for health problems or influence her adaptation to them. Mrs. Malone's psychosocial profile pinpoints some behaviors that increase her risk for illness.

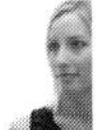

Case Study Findings

Mrs. Malone's psychosocial profile includes:

- Does not usually seek routine health care or screenings. Feels that she is healthy and does not need health care unless she is sick. Does not know her cholesterol level, has never had a mammogram, has not had a Pap smear or physical examination in 3 years.
- Typical day consists of arising at 6:00 AM, getting her children off to school and then going to work. She works from 8:00 AM to 5:00 PM 5 days a week. After work, she makes dinner for her family and reads or watches television. She goes to bed at 11:00 PM each night.
- Reports that she eats a balanced diet with foods from each of the major food groups each day, including 3 vegetables and 2 fruit servings. Admits to eating sweets every day. Evaluation of daily calcium intake reveals that she usually ingests 500 mg/day. Has had an unexplained 10-lb weight gain in last year.
- 24-hour recall shows the following: Breakfast was two fried eggs, two slices of bacon, two slices of white toast with butter, one 4-oz glass of orange juice, and a cinnamon bun with butter. Lunch was a chicken salad sandwich with mayonnaise on two slices of white toast, potato chips, two chocolate chip cookies, an 8-oz cola, and a chocolate candy bar. Snack was one apple. Dinner was steak, baked potato with butter, string beans, tossed salad with Russian dressing, apple pie with ice cream, and 8 oz of 2 percent lowfat milk.
- Admits that her only exercise is walking from her car to her office twice a day and walking up and down two flights of stairs several times a day. She walked on a daily basis in the past but stopped this year because of lack of time and inability to fit it into her schedule. For recreation she reads, does housework, and gardens on weekends.
- Hobbies include reading and gardening. Has a house cat.
- States that she usually sleeps well for 7 to 8 hours a night. Has occasional night sweats that awaken her.
- Has never smoked and is not exposed to smoke at home. Has smoke and carbon monoxide detectors at home. Drinks a glass of wine with dinner two to three times a week. Denies ever using illicit drugs.
- Identifies no occupational risks. Is not exposed to smoke at work. Drives 40 miles round trip to work each day. Wears seatbelt when driving.

- Attends church weekly with family. No religious or cultural influences that affect health practices.
- States that her marriage is supportive and comfortable. Describes good relationships with children, siblings, and parents.
- Uses prayer, friendships, and family support to deal with stress.

 CRITICAL THINKING ACTIVITY #1

What problems can you identify for Mrs. Malone after completing her health history?

 CRITICAL THINKING ACTIVITY #2

Based on information provided in Mrs. Malone's health history, what will you include in your physical assessment?

Case Study Evaluation

Before you move on to the physical examination, review and summarize the key information from Mrs. Malone's health history.

Physical Assessment

Once you have completed the subjective data collection, begin to collect objective data by means of the physical examination. Keep the key history findings in mind. These findings, along with those from the physical examination to come, will complete the assessment picture. Then you can analyze the data, formulate nursing diagnoses, and develop a plan of care for Mrs. Malone.

The purpose of the physical assessment is to find signs of disease or abnormalities that the client may or may not have reported in the history or review of systems.

Approach

Two methods are used for completing a total physical assessment. These methods are a systems approach and a head-to-toe approach. Each approach is systematic and complete, and obtains the same data. The advantages of each assessment method relate to the preferences of the individual nurse, the client population, and the setting for the assessment. Some nurses find it easier to conceptualize and perform the assessment according to systems, and others are comfortable with a head-to-toe (or regional) approach.

A systems approach allows a thorough assessment of each system, doing all assessments related to one system before moving on to the next. This approach works well when you are performing a focused assessment. A head-to-toe assessment includes the same examinations as a systems assessment, but you assess each region of the body before moving on to the next. With this method, the client does not need to change positions as often, and you can also compare regions of the body for symmetry. This approach is best suited for a complete physical examination. No matter which approach you use, be systematic and consistent.

For the purposes of this text, a convenient head-to-toe approach is demonstrated. All four assessment techniques—inspection, percussion, palpation, and auscultation—are used to perform a complete examination.

- Inspect for abnormalities and normal variations of visible body parts.
- Palpate to identify surface characteristics, areas of pain or tenderness, organs, and abnormalities, including masses and fremitus.
- Percuss to determine the density of underlying tissues and to detect abnormalities in underlying organs.
- Auscultate for sounds made by body organs, including the heart, lungs, intestines, and vascular structures.

Assessment data are usually charted by systems (e. g., respiratory or neurological) and by regions to a limited extent (e.g., head/neck). Your documentation can focus only on positive findings or on both positive and negative findings. No matter which format you use, always be brief and to the point and avoid generalizations.

Performing a Focused Physical Assessment

When your client's condition or time restraints do not permit a comprehensive assessment, perform a focused assessment. This assessment focuses only on systems that relate to your client's problem. Because it is only a partial assessment, less data are collected during the examination.

A focused physical assessment should include the following:

- A general survey with vital signs and weight
- Assessment of level of consciousness
- Assessment of skin color, temperature, and texture
- Testing of gross motor balance and coordination
- Testing of extraocular movements
- Testing of pupillary reaction
- Testing of gross vision and hearing
- Inspection of oral mucosa as client says "ah"
- Auscultation of anterior and posterior breath sounds
- Palpation of apical impulse, point of maximal impact (PMI)
- Auscultation of heart sounds
- Percussion of abdomen
- Palpation of abdomen
- Palpation of peripheral pulses
- Testing sensation to touch on extremities

- Palpation of muscle strength of upper and lower extremities

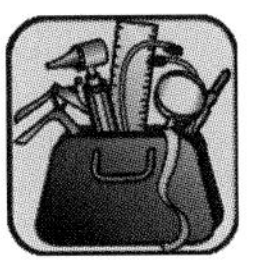

Toolbox

Because you are performing a complete head-to-toe examination, you will use all four techniques and most of the assessment tools previously described in this text. The tools you use depend on the client's problems and age and the extent of the examination. You will definitely need a stethoscope, sphygmomanometer, tongue blades, tuning fork, reflex hammer, gloves, supplies for a rectal examination, supplies for a vaginal examination if your client is a woman, an otoophthalmoscope, Snellen charts or visual acuity tests as available, and an audiometer for a hearing acuity test. Be sure to wear gloves when assessing the mucous membranes, genitalia, rectal area, and any area that might expose you to body fluids (such as lesions), infections, or infestation.

Performing a General Survey

The first part of the physical assessment is the general survey. At this time, you will take the client's vital signs, height, and weight and note his or her overall appearance. Observe nutritional status, emotional status, body habitus, and general appearance, including hygiene and clothing.

Performing a Head-to-Toe Physical Assessment

Now, keeping the client's chief complaint in mind, examine him or her for specific signs of diseases affecting other organ systems. Have the client change into a gown and ensure privacy by closing the door or pulling the curtain. Drape the client, exposing only the area being assessed. As you perform the assessment, tell him or her what you are planning to do and why.

Here are some other helpful hints to keep in mind:

- Wash your hands before you begin!
- Listen to your client!
- Provide a warm environment.
- If your client has a problem, start at that point.
- Work from head to toe.
- Compare side to side.
- Let your client know your findings.
- Use your time not only to assess but also to teach your client.
- Leave sensitive or painful areas until the end of the examination.

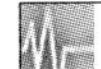

CRITICAL THINKING ACTIVITY #3

What are Mrs. Malone's strengths? Are there any areas of concern?

Below is a head-to-toe physical assessment by region for Mrs. Malone.

Performing a Head-to-Toe Physical Assessment

AREA/REGION EXAMINED AND TECHNIQUE USED	FINDINGS FOR MRS. MALONE
General Health Survey *INSPECT*	
• Age: Appearance vs. stated.	• Appears younger than stated age (40 years).
• General health appearance, including nutritional status, hygiene, odors, clothing.	• Well-developed, well-nourished woman, neatly dressed and well groomed.
• Level of consciousness, speech, affect	• Oriented to person, place, and time; appropriate affect. Speech clear and responds appropriately.
• Signs of distress.	• No acute distress at this time.
• Motor activity, gait, posture, gross deformities.	• Moves all extremities well, gait balanced and coordinated.
MEASURE	
• Anthropometric data and vital signs.	• Height 5′5″; weight 145 lb • Vital signs: Temperature, 98.8°F; pulse, 74; respirations,18; BP 128/80.

(Continued)

Performing a Head-to-Toe Physical Assessment *(Continued)*

AREA/REGION EXAMINED AND TECHNIQUE USED	FINDINGS FOR MRS. MALONE
Integumentary *INSPECT/PALPATE*	
• Inspect visible skin for color and lesions throughout examination. • Palpate skin temperature, texture, moisture, turgor	• Skin even in color, warm, dry, positive turgor, no suspicious lesions. 3-cm white scar from appendectomy on right lower quadrant (RLQ).
• Inspect/palpate hair for texture, color, distribution.	• Hair clean, coarse, slightly graying, evenly distributed.
• Inspect/palpate nails for texture, color, refill, and angle of attachment.	• Nails pink, brisk capillary refill, no clubbing.
HEENT/*Head/Face* *INSPECT/PALPATE*	
• Inspect size, shape, position.	• Normocephalic, erect, midline.
• Palpate scalp mobility, tenderness, lesions, masses.	• Scalp mobile, no lesions, tenderness, or masses.
• Inspect nasolabial folds and palpebral fissures for facial symmetry. • Note facial expression and ability to frown, smile (cranial nerve [CN] VII).	• Facial features symmetrical
• Palpate temporomandibular joint (TMJ); test range of motion.	• No TMJ tenderness, locking, or clicking.
• Palpate temporal arteries.	• + 2 temporal arteries.
• Test facial sensation (CN V)	• CN V intact
HEENT/*Eyes* *INSPECT/PALPATE/ FUNDOSCOPIC*	
• Test visual acuity with Snellen or pocket vision screener (CN II).	• Snellen: R: 20/20; L: 20/20; both: 20/20.
• Test color vision with color bars on Snellen chart.	• Color vision intact.
• Test near vision.	• Difficulty noted with near vision.
• Test peripheral vision by confrontation.	• Visual fields normal by confrontation.
• Test extraocular movements (EOMs) by 6 cardinal fields of gaze (CN III, IV, VI).	• EOMs intact; no nystagmus.
• Test corneal light reflex, corneal blink reflex.	• Corneal light reflex symmetrical bilaterally.
• Perform cover-uncover test.	• No drifting.
• Note general appearance of eyes, eyelids, sclera, conjunctiva.	• Eyes clear and bright; positive blink reflex; no lid lag, ectropion or entropion, lesions on lids; sclera white; conjunctivae clear and glossy.
• Inspect cornea, anterior chamber, iris, lens with oblique lighting.	• Cornea, iris intact; anterior chamber.
• Palpate lacrimal glands and ducts.	• Lacrimal glands and ducts nontender.
• Test pupillary reaction: direct, consensual, convergence.	• Pupils 3 mm, PERRLA (see chapter 10) direct and consensual; positive constriction and convergence.

Performing a Head-to-Toe Physical Assessment

AREA/REGION EXAMINED AND TECHNIQUE USED	FINDINGS FOR MRS. MALONE
• Perform fundoscopic examination and check for red reflex (darken room).	• Red reflex present bilaterally, discs flat with sharp margins, vessels present without crossing defects, retina even in color without hemorrhages or exudates, macula even in color.
HEENT/*Ears* *INSPECT/PALPATE/OTOSCOPIC*	
• Inspect/palpate external ear.	• Skin of external ear intact with no masses, lesions, or discharge.
• Check angle of attachment.	• Angle of attachment <10 degrees. Tragus, mastoid, helix nontender.
• Perform Weber, Rinne, whisper tests (CN VIII).	• Positive whisper test. Weber test: no lateralization. Rinne test: ac>bc bilaterally.
• Perform otoscopic examination of canals and tympanic membrane.	• External ear canals clear without redness, swelling, lesions, or discharge. Tympanic membranes intact, pearly gray, with light reflex and landmarks visible.
HEENT/*Nose/Sinuses* *INSPECT/PALPATE*	
• Palpate sinuses for tenderness.	• Frontal, maxillary sinuses nontender.
• Palpate nasal patency.	• Nares patent.
• Test sense of smell (CN I).	• Client recognizes familiar odor.
• Inspect nasal mucus membranes, septum, turbinates with speculum.	• Nasal mucosa pink, septum intact with no deviation.
HEENT/*Mouth* *INSPECT/PALPATE*	
• Inspect/palpate lips, oral mucosa.	• Lips, oral mucosa, gingivae pink and without lesions.
• Inspect teeth, gingiva.	• Teeth all present and clean; dental work present; no obvious caries.
• Inspect pharynx, tonsils, palate.	• Pharynx pink, tonsils +1, palate intact.
• Inspect tongue, test taste on anterior/posterior tongue (CN VII, IX).	• Tongue smooth, pink, symmetrical with no lesions; taste intact.
• Check mobility of tongue (CN XII).	• Full range of motion (ROM).
• Test gag, swallow reflexes (CN IX, X).	• Symmetrical rise of the uvula, positive gag and swallow reflex.
• Palpate parotid and submandibular glands.	• Glands nonpalpable.

(Continued)

Performing a Head-to-Toe Physical Assessment *(Continued)*

AREA/REGION EXAMINED AND TECHNIQUE USED	FINDINGS FOR MRS. MALONE
HEENT/*Neck*	
INSPECT/PALPATE/AUSCULTATE	
• Inspect/palpate thyroid gland.	• Thyroid nonpalpable.
• Palpate/auscultate carotid pulses. Inspect/measure jugular venous pressure (JVP).	• Carotid pulses equal, + 2. No bruits, thrills, or jugular venous distention (JVD). JVP 2 cm at 45-degree angle.
• Palpate nodes in head, neck.	• No lymphadenopathy of head, neck.
• Note deviation of trachea, abnormal masses, pulsations.	• Trachea midline, no abnormal masses or pulsations.
• Note ROM of neck.	• Full ROM of neck.
• Test neck muscle strength. (CN XI)	• +5 muscle strength.
Posterior Thorax/*Lungs*	
INSPECT/PALPATE/PERCUSS/AUSCULTATE	
• Palpate excursion and fremitus.	• Equal excursion, no lag; equal fremitus.
• Percuss diaphragmatic excursion. • Auscultate breath sounds	• Resonance percussed bilaterally. Posteriorly, diaphragmatic excursion 2 inches (5 cm) separate. Lungs clear, no adventitious sounds.
Posterior Thorax/*Spine*	
INSPECT/PALPATE/PERCUSS	
• Inspect normal curves of spine (cervical, thoracic, lumbar, sacral)	• Normal curves of spine.
• Inspect and test for scoliosis, kyphosis, lordosis.	• No scoliosis, kyphosis, lordosis.
• Check ROM of spine.	• Full ROM.
• Palpate paravertebral muscles and posterior thorax for tenderness, masses.	• Paravertebral muscles nontender.
• Fist/blunt percuss costovertebral angle (CVA) tenderness.	• No CVA tenderness.
Anterior Thorax	
INSPECT/PALPATE	
• Breasts and lymph nodes (axillary and epitrochlear) with client in various positions.	• Breasts symmetrical, no masses or retraction, no nipple discharge, no lymphadenopathy.
INSPECT/PALPATE/PERCUSS/AUSCULTATE	
• Precordium	• Anteroposterior transverse diameter; respirations 16/minute unlabored.
• Lungs	• Chest expansion symmetric, no tenderness, scars, masses, lesions.
AUSCULTATE	
• Lungs, heart	• Equal excursion; equal tactile fremitus. • Resonant percussion sound over lung fields. • Lungs clear; no adventitious breath sounds.

Performing a Head-to-Toe Physical Assessment

AREA/REGION EXAMINED AND TECHNIQUE USED	FINDINGS FOR MRS. MALONE
	• PMI 1 cm at 5th intercostal space at midclavicular line.
	• Heart rate 85 BPM and regular, S_1, S_2; no S_3, no S_4, murmurs, gallops, or thrills present.
Upper Extremities *INSPECT/PALPATE*	
• Palpate brachial, radial, ulnar pulses.	• + 2 pulses.
• Perform Allen's test, if indicated.	
• Perform Tinel or Phalen test for carpal tunnel syndrome, if indicated.	• Negative Phalen test.
• Check nails for color, temperature, capillary refill, deformities, clubbing.	• Nails pink, brisk capillary refill, no clubbing.
• Inspect hands for joint deformities.	• No deformities, full ROM
• Palpate skin temperature and test hand grip.	• Hands warm, equal + 5 hand grip.
• Measure arm lengths and circumferences, note dominant side.	• Client right-handed, arm lengths and circumferences equal
• Check ROM and strength of upper extremities and hands.	• Full ROM of upper extremities, +5 muscle strength OK.
• Test for pronator drift.	• Negative pronator drift.
• Test for coordination with rapid alternating movement (RAM) and finger-thumb opposition.	• Positive RAM of hands and finger-thumb opposition.
• Test for accuracy of movements with point-to-point localization.	• Accuracy of movements intact.
• Test superficial and deep sensations of arms and hands.	• Superficial and deep sensations intact.
• Test biceps, triceps brachioradialis deep tendon reflex (DTR).	• +2 DTR of upper extremities.
Abdomen *INSPECT/AUSCULTATE/PERCUSS/PALPATE*	
• Inspect for shape, scars, movements, respirations, pulsations, peristalsis, abnormalities. Test for hernias.	• Abdomen flat, no masses or pulsations, surgical scar on right lower quadrant. Tympany in all four quadrants.
• Auscultate for bowel sounds, vascular sounds.	• Bowel sounds present, no vascular sounds heard.
• Percuss abdomen and organs. If ascites is suspected, percuss for shifting dullness.	• Abdomen soft, no hepatomegaly, splenomegaly, masses, tenderness.
• Palpate liver, kidneys, spleen, aorta.	• Liver 8 cm at right midclavicular line (RMCL) kidneys not palpable, aorta 2 cm.
• Test superficial abdominal reflexes	• Negative abdominal reflexes.
• Palpate inguinal nodes.	• No palpable lymph nodes in inguinal area.
• Palpate/auscultate femoral arteries.	• No femoral bruits; pulses 2 + and equal.

(Continued)

Performing a Head-to-Toe Physical Assessment *(Continued)*

AREA/REGION EXAMINED AND TECHNIQUE USED	FINDINGS FOR MRS. MALONE
Lower Extremities *INSPECT/PALPATE*	
• Inspect skin color, hair distribution, varicose veins.	• Skin warm, hair on both lower legs, no varicose veins.
• Perform Trendelenburg test or manual compression test to check venous circulation, if indicated.	
• Palpate pedal pulses, temperature	• + 2 pedal pulses.
• Inspect feet for deformities, toenail condition, lesions.	
• Test ROM in lower extremities.	• Full ROM in lower extremities, no crepitus.
• Measure leg lengths and circumferences.	• Leg lengths and circumferences equal.
• Perform straight leg test for herniated disc, if indicated. • Perform patellar tap or bulge sign if fluid is suspected. • Check for draw sign if torn anterior cruciate ligament suspected. • Perform Apley's or McMurray's test if torn meniscus suspected.	
• Test muscle strength and superficial and deep sensations.	• Muscles well developed, +5 muscle strength, superficial and deep sensations intact.
• Inspect gait, toe walk, heel walk, deep knee bend.	• Gait steady and coordinated, heel and toe walk, deep knee bend without difficulty.
• Perform Romberg test. • Have client toe tap and run heel down shin. • Test patellar and Achilles DTR and plantar reflex.	• +2 DTR, positive plantar flexion. • Joints and muscles symmetrical.
	ALERT Put on gloves for this part of the examination.
Female Genitalia/Rectum *INSPECT/PALPATE*	
• Inspect and palpate external and internal genitalia.	• External genitalia without lesions or abnormalities. • Vaginal mucosa pale pink/dry with few rugae. • Cervix pale pink, no lesions or discharge. • Nontender, uterus midline, normal size. • Adnexa without masses or tenderness • Perianal area intact without hemorrhoids.
• Inspect/palpate rectum for masses.	• Rectal wall smooth without masses or tenderness.
• Test stool for occult blood.	• Stool brown, occult blood negative.

Once you have completed your assessment, document your findings. You performed the physical assessment by region; now document your findings by system.

Documenting the Physical Assessment Findings

Area/System	Findings
General Health Survey	• Appears younger than stated age (40 years) • Well-developed, well-nourished woman, neatly dressed and well groomed • Oriented to person, place and time; appropriate affect • Speech clear and responds appropriately • No acute distress at this time • Moves all extremities well, gait balanced and coordinated • Height 5′5″; weight 145 lb • Vital signs: Temperature 98.8°; Pulse 74; Respirations 18; Blood pressure 128/80
Integumentary	• Skin even in color, warm, dry, positive turgor, no suspicious lesions • White scar from appendectomy on RLQ • Hair clean, coarse, slightly graying, evenly distributed • Nails pink, brisk capillary refill, no clubbing
Head/Face/Neck	• Normocephalic, erect, midline • Scalp mobile, no lesions, tenderness, or masses • Facial features symmetrical • Thyroid not palpable • No palpable lymph nodes
Eyes	• Snellen: R: 20/20; L: 20/20; Both: 20/20 • Color vision intact • Difficulty noted with near vision • Visual fields normal by confrontation • EOMs intact, no nystagmus • Corneal light reflex symmetrical bilaterally • No drifting • Eyes clear and bright; positive blink reflex; no lid lag, ectropion/entropion, or lesions noted on lids; cornea, iris intact; anterior chamber clear • Sclera white, conjunctivae clear and glossy • Lacrimal glands and ducts nontender • Pupils 3 mm, PERRLA direct and consensual • Positive constriction and convergence • Red reflex present bilaterally, discs flat with sharp margins, vessels present without crossing defects, retina even in color without hemorrhages or exudates, macula even in color
Ears/Nose/Throat	• Skin of external ear intact with no masses, lesions, or discharge • Angle of attachment <10 degrees • Tragus, mastoid, helix nontender • Positive whisper test • Weber test: No lateralization • Rinne test: ac>bc bilaterally • External ear canals clear without redness, swelling, lesions, or discharge • Tympanic membranes intact, pearly gray with light reflex and landmarks visible • Frontal and maxillary sinuses nontender • Nares patent; client recognizes familiar odor • Nasal mucosa pink, septum intact with no deviation
Mouth	• Lips, oral mucosa, gingivae pink and without lesions • Teeth all present and clean; dental work present, no obvious caries • Pharynx pink, tonsils +1, palate intact • Symmetrical rise of uvula, positive gag and swallow reflex • Tongue smooth, pink, symmetrical, no lesions, taste intact, full ROM • Glands nonpalpable.
Respiratory	• Respirations 16/minute unlabored, trachea midline • AP< transverse diameter • Chest expansion symmetrical; no tenderness, scars, masses, lesions

(Continued)

Documenting the Physical Assessment Findings *(Continued)*

Area/System	Findings
	• Equal excursion, no lag, equal tactile fremitus • Resonant percussion sound over lung fields, diaphragmatic excursion 2 inches (5 cm) • Lungs clear; no adventitious breath sounds
Cardiovascular	• PMI 1 cm at 5th ICS at midclavicular line • Heart rate 85 BPM and regular; S_1, S_2; no S_3, S_4, murmurs, gallops, or thrills present • Pulses +2, no bruits or thrills, no varicose veins • JVP 2 cm at 45-degree angle
Breasts	• Symmetrical, no masses, nipple retraction, nipple discharge, lymphadenopathy
Abdomen	• Abdomen flat, no masses or pulsations • Surgical scar on R lower abdomen • Bowel sounds present, no vascular sounds heard • Tympany in all four quadrants • Liver 8 cm at RMCL • Abdomen soft, no hepatomegaly, splenomegaly, masses or tenderness • Negative abdominal reflexes • Kidneys nonpalpable; no palpable lymph nodes in inguinal area • Aorta 2 cm • No CVA tenderness
Reproductive	• External genitalia without lesions or abnormalities • Vaginal mucosa pale pink, dry with few rugae • Cervix pale pink, no lesions or discharge • No cervical motion tenderness; uterus midline, normal size • Adnexa without masses or tenderness • Perianal area intact, without hemorrhoids • Rectal wall smooth without masses or tenderness • Stool brown, occult blood negative
Musculoskeletal	• Normal curves of spine; no scoliosis, kyphosis, lordosis • Joints and muscles symmetrical, nontender; no deformities • Right side dominant, arm and leg lengths and circumferences equal, equal hand grasp • Muscles well developed, +5 muscle strength • Full ROM in upper and lower extremities, no crepitus
Neurological	• Awake, alert, oriented to time, place, person; cooperative; responds appropriately • CN I through XII intact • Gait steady and coordinated; no pronator drift; negative Romberg; able to heel and toe walk and do deep knee bends without difficulty • Point-to-point localization intact • Superficial and deep sensations intact • + 2 DTR, + plantar flexion, negative abdominal reflexes

Case Study Analysis and Plan

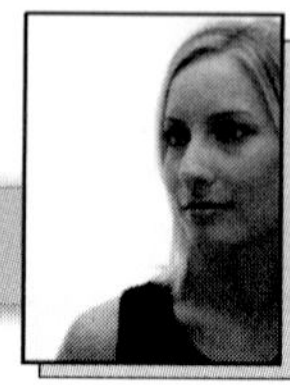

Now that you have completed Mrs. Malone's assessment, document your key history and physical examination findings.

List key history findings and key physical examination findings that will help you formulate your nursing diagnoses.

Nursing Diagnoses

Consider all of the data you have collected during your assessment of Mrs. Malone. Now use this information to identify a list of nursing diagnoses. Some possible ones are provided below; cluster the supporting data.

1. Nutrition: imbalanced, more than body requirements
2. Knowledge, deficient, related to need for age-appropriate health activities

Collaborative Nursing Diagnoses

Identify any collaborative nursing diagnoses, and be specific as to what the desired outcome of each would be.

CRITICAL THINKING ACTIVITY #4

Now that you have identified some nursing diagnoses for Mrs. Malone, select one from the list above and develop a nursing care plan and a brief teaching plan for her.

Referrals

Mrs. Malone's health history and physical examination findings warrant several referrals to either a physician or practitioner. Identify what needs to be done at each referral and the reasons behind it.

Research Tells Us

Osteoporosis is a major health problem for the older population in this country, especially women. It places people at risk for fractures as a result of low bone mass and deterioration of bone tissue. The first manifestation of the disease is usually a fracture, most often in the hip, spine, or wrist. Loss of height over 1 inch and spinal deformity are also indicators of osteoporosis. Fractures cause morbidity in the elder population and have psychological effects such as depression, anxiety, fear, and anger.

Osteoporosis has both modifiable and nonmodifiable risk factors. Modifiable risk factors include a sedentary lifestyle, low calcium intake, low body weight, high alcohol consumption, smoking, and estrogen deficiency. Nonmodifiable risk factors include being a white or Asian female over age 65 and having a slight build, a family history of osteoporosis, premature or surgical menopause, and endocrine or chronic disease.

Treatments and techniques for diagnosing osteoporosis have improved in recent years. Techniques include dual x-ray absorptiometry, quantitative computed tomography, and quantitative ultrasound. Treatments include antiresorptive therapies, such as hormone replacement therapy, bisphosphonates, and selective estrogen receptor modulators. Encourage your clients to discuss evaluation and treatments with their healthcare providers.

Prevention continues to focus on health education. Nurses can encourage women to modify risk factors through adequate diet and weight control, adequate calcium intake, exercise, and avoidance of smoking and alcohol.

Summary

- A comprehensive health history and a physical examination are important components of a health maintenance program.
- Time intervals for a health assessment vary depending on age and the presence of chronic health problems. Standard recommendations are made by various organizations and the U.S. Preventive Services Task Force (1996).
- The content of periodic health examinations varies with age because of the risks of health problems in different age categories.
- In addition, certain age-specific health screenings, client counseling, and preventive health activities occur during the health assessment. Much like nursing diagnoses and care plans, these screenings are highly individualized, based on client need and presentation in the clinical setting.
- Begin your assessment by obtaining a health history. The health history guides your physical assessment.
- After you have completed the health history, perform the physical examination. For a complete assessment, work head to toe by regions.
- Once you have completed your assessment, document your findings. When possible, organize and document the physical assessment findings by systems.
- Remember to share the information with your client so that you can develop an effective plan of care.

UNIT IV

Adapting Assessment to Special Populations

CHAPTER 21

Assessing the Mother-to-Be

Before You Begin

INTRODUCTION TO ASSESSING THE MOTHER-TO-BE

Pregnancy is usually an exciting and special time in a woman's life. The duration of human pregnancy is 9 calendar months, 10 lunar months, 40 weeks, or 280 days. The length of pregnancy is divided into 3 trimesters, or 3-month periods. Each trimester is characterized by its own unique and predictable developments for the mother and her baby. To accommodate the changes taking place throughout the gestational period, the pregnant woman's body undergoes changes in size and shape, and all of her organ systems modify their various functions to create an environment that is protective and nurturing for the growing fetus.

Anatomy and Physiology Review

The female body undergoes many physiologic and anatomical changes during pregnancy. Several factors are responsible for the woman's adaptation to pregnancy. Hormonal influences, mechanical pressure arising from growth of the fetus inside the uterus, and the mother's physical adaptation to her changing body all account for the changes that take place during pregnancy. The majority of these changes are brought about by the hormones of pregnancy, primarily **estrogen** and **progesterone**. Although the most dramatic changes occur in the reproductive system, every other body system is also affected by pregnancy.

Although pregnancy is a normal event, problems can occur. Therefore you need an understanding of normal maternal physiology so that you can recognize potential or actual problems that warrant attention. Also, your understanding of the normal physiologic and psychological events that take place during pregnancy will assist you in teaching your client and her family about changes that are normal and expected, and how to identify signs and symptoms that should be reported to her healthcare provider.

Normal Changes Associated with Pregnancy

SYSTEM/STRUCTURE/CHANGES	CLINICAL SIGNS AND SYMPTOMS
Integumentary/*Skin*	
• Changes result from hormones and mechanical stretching. Increased skin thickness and hyperpigmentation are caused by increased secretion of melanotropin, an anterior pituitary hormone.	• **Chloasma**, the "mask of pregnancy," is a brownish hyperpigmentation of the skin over the cheeks, nose, and forehead. It appears in 50% to 70% of pregnant women and occurs most often in those with dark complexions, usually after the 16th week. Sunlight enhances the heightened pigmentation, which generally fades after delivery. • Darkening of the nipples, areolae, axillae, and vulva also occur, and scars and moles may darken. • The **linea alba** may become pigmented (**linea nigra**) and extends from the symphysis pubis to the umbilicus.
• Increased action of adrenocorticosteroids, occurs in 50% to 90% of pregnant women, causing cutaneous elastic tissue to become more fragile.	• Stretch marks (**striae gravidarum**)—pinkish-red streaks with slight depressions in the skin—may appear over the abdomen, thighs, breasts, and buttocks, fading to silvery or white after pregnancy.
• Increased estrogen results in color and vascular changes.	• **Angiomas**, or "vascular spiders," are tiny, branched, pulsating end-arterioles on the neck, chest, face, and arms. These skin lesions are bluish, do not blanch with pressure, and usually disappear after the baby's birth. • **Palmar erythema** is characterized by a pinkish red, diffuse mottling over the palms of the hands.
• Increased sebaceous gland secretions	• The skin develops increased oiliness and acne, or takes on a "healthy glow."
• Increased blood supply to skin, increased basal metabolic rate, and progesterone-induced increased body temperature	• Increased perspiration and feeling "hotter."
Integumentary/*Hair*	
• Increased hair growth during pregnancy as a result of hormonal influences	• Some women may have excessive hair growth in unusual places (**hirsutism**). Increase in fine body hair growth also occurs, but disappears after delivery. Increase in brittle hair growth usually does not. Excessive scalp oiliness or dryness may also occur.
Integumentary/*Nails*	
• Changes in nail growth and texture as a result of hormonal influences	• Nails may grow longer or soften or thin.

Normal Changes Associated with Pregnancy

SYSTEM/STRUCTURE/CHANGES	CLINICAL SIGNS AND SYMPTOMS
HEENT/*Ear*	
• Increased vascularity of upper respiratory tract may cause swelling of the tympanic membrane and eustachian tube.	• Decreased hearing, a sense of fullness in the ears, or earaches.
HEENT/*Nose*	
• Estrogen-induced edema and vascular congestion of the nasal mucosa and sinuses	• Nasal stuffiness and **epistaxis** (nosebleed).
HEENT/*Mouth/Throat*	
• Edema of the larynx	• Some women may experience vocal changes.
• Higher estrogen levels increase vascularity and connective tissue proliferation.	• Gum hypertrophy and bleeding of gums while brushing teeth is common. **Epulis**—raised, red nodules on gums that bleed easily—may develop, but generally regress after delivery.
Respiratory	
• Estrogen promotes relaxation of the ligaments and joints of ribs.	• Increase in transverse diameter by 2 cm with a total circumference increase of 6 cm. Increase in the costal angle >90 degrees. • Thoracic breathing as pregnancy progresses. • The diaphragm becomes displaced as pregnancy progresses.
• Increase in oxygen consumption by 15%–20%	• Slight increase in respiratory rate. • 30%–40% increase in tidal volume. • Increase in inspiratory capacity. • Decrease in expiratory volume. • Total lung capacity slightly decreased.
• Higher levels of progesterone increase sensitivity of respiratory receptors, increasing tidal volume, which results in respiratory alkalosis with compensated mild metabolic acidosis.	• Decrease in PCO_2 (27–32 mm Hg) leads to increase in pH (more alkaline) and decrease in bicarbonate (18–21 mEq/L).
Cardiovascular	
• Increase in cardiac output and maternal blood volume by approximately 40%–50%. Because the heart must pump harder, it actually increases in size. The body adapts to increase in blood volume with peripheral dilatation to maintain blood pressure (BP). Hormones cause peripheral dilatation.	• Heart rate may increase by 10 to 15 beats per minute, and systolic murmurs may be heard. Increase in blood volume may cause physiologic or "pseudo" anemia because the plasma increase exceeds red blood cell production. Sinus arrhythmias and premature atrial or ventricular contractions may occur. BP is normal in first and third trimester; systolic and diastolic BP drops 5–10 mm Hg during second trimester.
• Compression of vena cava impairs venous return and results in decreased cardiac output when woman is supine during second half of pregnancy.	• Orthostatic hypotension can occur as a result of decreased venous return and decreased cardiac output. **ALERT** *Watch for signs of* ***supine hypotension (vena caval syndrome),*** *which may occur when pregnant client lies in a supine position. Weight of abdominal contents may compress vena cava and aorta, causing a 30 mm Hg drop in BP with reflex tachycardia. Signs and symptoms include pallor, dizziness, faintness, breathlessness, tachycardia, nausea, and clammy skin. Reposition client on left side until signs and symptoms subside and vital signs return to within normal limits.*

(Continued)

Normal Changes Associated with Pregnancy *(Continued)*

SYSTEM/STRUCTURE/CHANGES	CLINICAL SIGNS AND SYMPTOMS
Cardiovascular *(Continued)*	
• Compression of iliac veins and inferior vena cava increases venous pressure and decreases blood flow to extremities.	• Dependent edema, varicose veins in legs and vulva, hemorrhoids.
Breasts	
• Increase in estrogen and progesterone soon after conception causes many changes in mammary glands.	• Breasts may feel full, with increased sensitivity, tingling, and heaviness. Increased nipple erectility and hypertrophy of **Montgomery's tubercles** (glands).
• Increased blood supply to breasts.	• Blood vessels become more visible.
• Increased growth of mammary glands.	• Increase in breast size. • **Striae gravidarum** (stretch marks) on breasts.
• Increase in luteal and placental hormones leads to increase in lactiferous ducts and lobule-alveolar tissue.	• Breasts become softer, looser, and nodular. **Colostrum** produced by 16th week.
Gastrointestinal	
• Increased levels of hCG and altered carbohydrate metabolism.	• Morning sickness during first trimester.
• Change in senses of taste and smell.	• May result in decreased appetite or unusual food cravings (**pica**).
• Decreased swallowing and increased stimulation of salivary glands by starch ingestion.	• Nausea. • Some women develop **ptyalism**, or excessive salivation.
• After the 7th month of pregnancy, the upper portion of the stomach may herniate.	• **Hiatal hernia** is more likely to occur in older, obese, or **multiparous** women.
• Increased progesterone decreases tone and motility of smooth muscles.	• Esophageal regurgitation, reverse peristalsis, and delayed stomach emptying result in heartburn (**pyrosis**).
• Increased estrogen leads to decrease in hydrochloric acid.	• Peptic ulcers rarely occur.
• Increased progesterone decreases muscle tone and peristalsis.	• Constipation can be caused by hypoperistalsis, increased water absorption from large intestines, decreased physical activity, displacement of intestines, abdominal distention, and iron supplements.
• Gallbladder becomes increasingly distended because of decreased muscle tone. Emptying time is prolonged and bile thickens.	• Increased risk for gallstones.
• Displacement of intestines by uterus.	• Abdominal changes include round ligament tension, flatulence, distention, cramping, pelvic heaviness, and contractions.
Genitourinary	
• Changes caused by increased estrogen and progesterone. By 10th week of pregnancy, renal pelvis and ureters have already begun to dilate. As pregnancy progresses, smooth muscle walls of ureters undergo hypertrophy	• Increased risk for urinary tract infections.

Normal Changes Associated with Pregnancy

SYSTEM/STRUCTURE/CHANGES	CLINICAL SIGNS AND SYMPTOMS
Genitourinary *(Continued)*	
and hyperplasia and muscle tone relaxes. Ureters become elongated and tortuous, resulting in larger volume of urine held in pelvis and ureters, slower urine flow rate, and urinary stasis.	
• Increased vascularity in pelvic area.	• Hyperemia of bladder and urethra.
• Decreased bladder tone.	• Increased bladder capacity to 1500 mL.
• Increased pressure on bladder by uterus.	• Increased urge to void.
• Increase in renal blood flow.	• Increased glomerular filtration rate.
• Decrease in renal blood flow in latter part of pregnancy	• Physiologic/dependent edema.
Reproductive	
• Increased pelvic congestion	• Softening of cervix (**Goodell's sign**). Bluish coloration of cervix and vaginal mucosa (**Chadwick's sign**). • Hypertrophy of glands in cervical canal. Softening and compressibility of lower end of uterus (**Hegar's sign**). • Vaginal smooth muscle and connective tissue loosen up and expand to accommodate passage of fetus through birth canal.
• Increased levels of estrogen and progesterone	• Uterus undergoes cell hypertrophy and hyperplasia and grows to a capacity of approximately 1000 grams. Once conception occurs, ovulation ceases, uterine endometrium thickens, and number and size of uterine blood vessels increases. As fetus grows, uterus continues to enlarge throughout pregnancy.
Musculoskeletal	
• Increase in abdominal size with decreased muscle tone and increased weight-bearing capacity	• Causes forward tilting of pelvis and changes in posture and walking style. To maintain balance, the lumbosacral curve becomes more exaggerated, and woman develops exaggerated anterior flexion of head.
• Increased mobility of pelvic joints	• Facilitates labor and birth process.
• Abdominal musculature stretches as uterus enlarges.	• Rectus abdominis muscles may stretch to the extent that a permanent separation occurs **(diastasis recti abdominis)**.
Neurological	
• Hypoglycemia, postural hypotension, or vasomotor instability	• **Syncope** and lightheadedness, often seen in early pregnancy.
• Anxiety	• Tension headaches may be related to anxiety.
• Hormonal changes	• Emotional lability.
• Edema compresses median nerve beneath carpal ligament of wrist, producing paresthesia and pain radiating to **thumb, index, middle and part of ring fingers**, especially in dominant hand.	• Carpal tunnel syndrome.
• Inadequate calcium intake	• Leg cramps or **tetany**.
• Enlarged uterus may compress pelvic nerves.	• Sensory changes in lower extremities.

(Continued)

Normal Changes Associated with Pregnancy *(Continued)*

SYSTEM/STRUCTURE/CHANGES	CLINICAL SIGNS AND SYMPTOMS
Neurological *(Continued)*	
• Accentuated lumbar curve **(lordosis)** compresses or pulls lumbar nerve roots.	• Low back pain.
• Stoop-shouldered posture puts pressure on brachial plexus	• Numbness and tingling in hands **(acroesthesia)**.
• Change in body's center of gravity during pregnancy	• Body's base of support widens.
Endocrine/*Pituitary and Placental Hormones*	
• Decreased follicle-stimulating hormone	• Amenorrhea. • Fat deposits in subcutaneous tissue over abdomen, back, and thighs.
• Increased progesterone relaxes smooth muscles, which results in decreased uterine contractions and prevents spontaneous abortion.	• Maintains pregnancy.
• Increased estrogen	• Enlarges uterus, breasts, and genitals; increases vascularity.
• Increased prolactin	• Causes lactation.
• Increased oxytocin	• Causes uterine contractions at time of delivery and let-down milk reflex.
• Human placental lactogen or human chorionic somatotropin acts as a growth hormone and decreases glucose metabolism and increases fatty acids.	• Contributes to breast development.
Endocrine/*Thyroid*	
• Basal metabolic rate (BMR) gradually increases throughout pregnancy.	• May cause heat intolerance, fatigue, and lassitude.
• Hyperplasia and increased vascularity of thyroid gland.	• Enlargement of thyroid gland.
Endocrine/*Parathyroid*	
• Increased parathyroid hormone peaks between 15 and 35 weeks gestation to meet increased requirements for calcium and vitamin D for fetal skeletal growth.	• Slight hyperparathyroidism develops.
Endocrine/*Pancreas*	
• As fetus grows, it requires increasing amounts of glucose.	• As mother's glucose stores are depleted, she experiences decreasing blood glucose levels.
Endocrine/*Adrenals*	
• Increase in cortisol	• Increases production of insulin and mother's resistance to insulin.
Immune/Hematologic	
• Increased coagulability results from increases in clotting factors VII, VIII, IX, X, and fibrinogen. Fibrinolytic activity is depressed to minimize risk of bleeding.	• Increased risk for thrombus formation.

Normal Changes Associated with Pregnancy

SYSTEM/STRUCTURE/CHANGES	CLINICAL SIGNS AND SYMPTOMS
Immune/Hematologic *(Continued)*	
• Increase in blood volume 40%–50% > nonpregnant state, about 1500 mL; 1000 mL is plasma, 500 RBCs.	• Hemodilution causes physiologic anemia.
• Increase in WBCs during second and third trimester.	• Increase is seen in granulocytes.

Developmental, Cultural, and Ethnic Variations

Adolescents

Physical assessment of the teenage mother-to-be is essentially the same as for the adult pregnant woman. However, careful attention to the baseline blood pressure is necessary because teenagers have lower systolic and diastolic pressures than older women. Also, when conducting the physical examination, look for signs of physical and sexual abuse in the young adolescent, who may be ashamed or afraid to share this important information. Remember that adolescent girls are very modest and usually anxious during pelvic examinations. Conducting the examination in a calm, unhurried manner, along with instructions for relaxation techniques should be helpful.

Also, the diets of adolescents are often lacking in essential nutrients, such as calcium and iron, needed during pregnancy. Additional problems associated with teen pregnancy are related to growth changes occurring in the teenager during the pregnancy. Because the mother and the fetus are both growing, they compete for nutrients. Cephalopelvic disproportion is a common problem for teen pregnancy because the growth of the pelvis lags behind growth in stature. For these reasons, pregnant teens are at increased risk for complications.

Older Women

In general, the risk for maternal or fetal complications increases with the client's age. Pregnant women over age 35 have an increased risk of developing gestational diabetes, pregnancy-induced hypertension (PIH), gestational bleeding, abruptio placentae, and intrapartal fetal distress. They also have an increased risk for conceiving a child with chromosomal abnormalities. In addition, older women are more likely to have pre-existing medical conditions, such as diabetes and hypertension. In fact, pre-existing conditions appear to pose a greater risk for maternal well-being and pregnancy outcome than the mother's age.

People of Different Cultures or Ethnic Groups

When obtaining the biographical information, it is important to establish your client's ethnicity because certain ethnic populations are more likely to experience race-related genetic disorders. Blacks and Southeast Asians are at risk for sickle cell disease; Jewish women are at risk for Tay-Sachs disease; Mediterranean, Italian, and Greek women are at risk for beta-thalassemia, and Asians are at risk for alpha-thalassemia. Women from these ethnic groups may need to be referred for prenatal screening. Aside from screening for genetic disorders related to specific ethnic groups, assessment of your client's cultural background may identify pregnancy and childbearing practices specific to a particular cultural/ethnic group. You will need to explore and identify your client's cultural views and practices on fertility and pregnancy. Specific prescriptive, restrictive, and taboo practices related to pregnancy, birthing, and postpartal care need to be identified and considered when caring for your client.

Pregnancy and Childbearing Practices of Various Ethnic Groups

CULTURAL GROUP	PRACTICES/BELIEFS
African-American	Oral contraceptives most popular type of birth control. High rate of teen pregnancy. Primary advisors are grandmother and maternal relatives. Geophagia (eating of earth or clay) common practice.

(Continued)

Pregnancy and Childbearing Practices of Various Ethnic Groups *(Continued)*

CULTURAL GROUP	PRACTICES/BELIEFS
African-American *(Continued)*	Taboos/beliefs: If food cravings not met, baby is marked. Labor is induced by a bumpy ride, a big meal, castor oil, or sniffing pepper. Photographing pregnant woman causes stillbirth or captures baby's soul. Lifting hands over head causes cord to wrap around baby's neck. Amniotic sac over baby's face denotes that baby has special powers. Child born after set of twins, the seventh child, or a child born with a physical condition has special powers from God.
Amish	Children are a gift from God. Average number of children per family is 7. Women have high status because of their role as child producer. Birth control seen as interfering with God's will. Prenatal care by Amish lay-midwives. Fathers expected to be involved and present during delivery and to participate in prenatal classes. No major taboos, but showing emotions is considered inappropriate, so woman labors quietly without expressing discomfort. Childbirth is not viewed as medical condition, so few have health insurance, keeping hospitalizations very short. Family and community are expected to care for mother and baby.
Appalachian	Contraceptive practices similar to those of general public, but a common belief is that laxatives facilitate abortion. Believe that healthy living during pregnancy leads to a healthy baby. Taboos/beliefs: Boys are carried high, girls low; photo taking causes stillbirth; reaching over head causes cord strangulation; wearing an opal ring may harm baby; birth marks are caused by eating strawberries or citrus fruit; experiencing a tragedy during pregnancy leads to congenital anomalies. Birthing is considered a natural process to be endured. Family members are expected to care for mother and child during postpartum period. A band may be placed around the baby's abdomen to prevent umbilical hernias and an asafetida bag around the neck to prevent contagious diseases.
Arab-American	Believe that God decides family size and God provides. Procreation is the purpose of marriage, resulting in high fertility rates. Irreversible means of contraception and abortions are considered unlawful. Sterility may lead to rejection or divorce. With emphasis on fertility and bearing a son, pregnancy occurs early in marriages. Pregnant women are pampered. Unmet cravings are thought to result in birthmarks. Pregnant women are excused from fasting during sacred days. Men are excluded from labor and delivery. Deliveries are often performed at home by midwives because of limited access to hospitals. Breathing and relaxation techniques are not practiced, and labor pain is openly expressed. Baby's stomach is wrapped after birth to prevent exposure to cold. Male circumcision is a Muslim requirement. Postpartum bathing is avoided for fear of mother being exposed to cold. Breastfeeding is delayed until second or third day to allow mother to rest. Postpartum foods include lentil soup to increase milk production and teas to cleanse the body.
Chinese-American	To control population, Chinese government has one-child law. Contraception is free; abortion common. Pregnancy is seen as positive experience. Men not very involved in process. Female midwives often preferred because of modesty of Chinese women.

Pregnancy and Childbearing Practices of Various Ethnic Groups

CULTURAL GROUP	PRACTICES/BELIEFS
Chinese-American *(Continued)*	Dietary beliefs: Adding meat to diet makes blood "strong" for fetus. Shellfish cause allergies. Iron makes delivery more difficult. Fruits and vegetables should be avoided during postpartum period because they are "cold" foods. Mother drinks rice wine to increase strength and has 5 to 6 meals a day with rice, soups, and 7–8 eggs. 5–7 day hospital stay after delivery, 1 month for recovery. Chinese government allows 6 months maternity leave with full pay. If mother is breastfeeding, work time is allowed for feedings. Many mothers avoid "cold"—do not go outside or bathe, and wear many layers of clothes even in warm weather. **ALERT** *Wine may increase bleeding time.*
Cuban-American	Cuba has lowest birth rate in Latin America because of high labor-force participation for women and high divorce rate. Childbirth is a celebration. Beliefs: Must eat for two during pregnancy (leads to excessive weight gain); eating coffee grounds cures morning sickness; eating fruit ensures that baby will have smooth complexion; wearing necklaces causes umbilical cord to wrap around neck. During postpartum period, family members care for mother for 4 weeks. Mother should avoid ambulation and exposure to cold because this is seen as risk for infection. Prefer breastfeeding but wean at 3 months and start solid foods. Believe that a fat child is a healthy child.
Egyptian-American	Must have children to make family complete. Three children ideal number. Woman expected to conceive within first year of marriage, and there is much stress until pregnancy occurs. Inability to conceive is grounds for divorce. Pregnancy brings security and respect. Birthing, especially of a son, has status and power. Beliefs: Curtail activities during pregnancy to prevent miscarriage; eat for two; cravings must be met or baby will be marked with the shape of the craved food. Maternal mother is expectant mother's source of support during labor and delivery. Men excluded from birthing process. In postpartum period, mother should avoid cold, such as bathing. Postpartum period is 40 days, and family tend to mother and baby.
Filipino-American	Fertility practices influenced by Catholic faith; rhythm is only acceptable method of contraception; abortion is a sin. Child-centered culture. Pregnancy is normal; expectant mothers are pampered. Maternal mother is great source of support and often serves as labor coach. Beliefs: Uses healthcare providers but also a message therapist. Cravings should be met to avoid harm to baby. Baby takes on characteristics of craved foods, (e.g., dark-colored foods, dark skin). If mother has a sudden scare or stress, it can harm fetus. Postpartum beliefs: Chicken soup stimulates milk production. Showers may cause arthritis, but sponge baths are allowed. Family cares for new mother and baby during postpartum period.
French-Canadian	Fertility practices influenced by Catholic faith. Abortion considered morally wrong by many. Fear of labor and delivery. Fathers encouraged to be present during delivery. Use of analgesia high. Breastfeeding has regained popularity. Both maternity and paternity leaves are available.

(Continued)

Pregnancy and Childbearing Practices of Various Ethnic Groups *(Continued)*

CULTURAL GROUP	PRACTICES/BELIEFS
French-Canadian *(Continued)*	Beliefs: Washing floors can trigger labor; so can full moon. Hyperglycemia during pregnancy means that mother is likely to give birth to a boy. Hyponatremia during pregnancy means that mother is likely to give birth to a girl.
Greek-American	Family size is limited because of desire to provide for family and ensure education for children. Greek Orthodox faith condemns birth control and abortion. Infertility causes great stress. Pregnant woman is greatly respected and protected. Birthing usually by midwife or female relatives; fathers remain uninvolved. Mother considered impure and susceptible to illness for 40 days postpartum. Remains at home. Breastfeeding common. Beliefs: Encouraged to eat foods high in iron and protein. Child will be marked if food cravings are unmet. Breastfeeding mothers who shower may cause diarrhea or milk allergy in baby. Silver objects or coins placed in crib bring good luck.
Iranian-American	Hot and cold influence pregnancy practices. Women are expected to have children early in marriage. Infertility blamed on woman. Breastfeeding used as method of contraception. Bearing a child, especially a boy, is prestigious. Beliefs: Cravings must be met with balance for hot and cold foods. Heavy work causes miscarriages. Much support from female relatives. Father usually not present during delivery. Postpartum period 30–40 days. Postpartum beliefs: Baby boys are "hotter" than girls. Baby may be kept at home for first 40 days until strong enough to defend against environmental pathogens. Ritual baby bath given between 10th and 40th day.
Irish-American	Fertility practices influenced by Catholicism. Sexual relationships often seen as a duty. Abstinence and rhythm only acceptable methods of birth control, and abortion considered morally wrong. Beliefs: Eating well-balanced diet during pregnancy important; not eating right leads to deformities. Lifting hands above head wraps cord around baby's neck. Experiencing a tragedy during pregnancy results in congenital anomalies. Going to bed with wet hair or wet feet causes illness in pregnant woman.
Jewish-American	Children are a gift and duty; males are more important. Sterility is a curse. Birth control pill is acceptable form of contraception. Orthodox Jews condone abortion if mother's health is at risk. Reform Jews believe that women have control over their own bodies, therefore it is their decision. Hasidic husband not allowed to touch mother during delivery or view her genitals, therefore may only give verbal support or choose not to be present during delivery. Male circumcision performed on the 8th day by a mohl, a person trained in circumcision, asepsis, and the religious ritual.
Mexican-American	Fertility practices influenced by Catholicism. Abstinence and rhythm acceptable methods of birth control. Breastfeeding also seen as method of birth control. Abortion morally wrong. Multiple births common; childbearing age between 19 and 24 is seen as best time; may be considered too old if over 24. Large family equates with man's virility. Pregnancy is natural and desirable condition, so many do not seek prenatal care; extended family provides advice and support. Beliefs: Hot food provides fetus with warmth; cold foods should be eaten during postpartum period. Pregnant women sleep on back to prevent harm to baby.

Pregnancy and Childbearing Practices of Various Ethnic Groups

CULTURAL GROUP	PRACTICES/BELIEFS
Mexican-American *(Continued)*	Frequent intercourse during pregnancy keeps vaginal canal lubricated and eases delivery. Walking in moonlight and viewing lunar eclipses leads to deformities. Avoid becoming cold. Lifting hands over head causes cord to wrap around baby's neck. Pregnant mother may wear safety pin or metal object to prevent deformities. Father not included in delivery. Mothers are very verbal during labor and do not practice breathing techniques. Mother puts legs together after delivery and wears cotton binder or girdle to prevent air from entering womb. Postpartum period 40 days, warmth preferred, showers avoided. Lactating mothers exposed to pesticides have decreased milk production and increased risk of breast cancer. Postpartum beliefs: Cutting baby's nails causes blindness and deafness.
Navajo Native American	Large families are favorable; many do not practice birth control. Having twins is not favorable and traditionally one must die; now however, one may be placed for adoption. Beliefs: Reluctant to deliver in hospital because hospitals are associated with sickness and death. Birthing necklaces worn during labor to ensure a safe birth. Mother holds onto woven sash when ready to push. Chanting may occur during delivery. Mother does not buy baby clothes before the baby's birth. Postpartum beliefs: Placenta is buried after birth to protect baby from evil spirits. Baby is given special mixtures after birth to rid mouth of mucus.
Vietnamese-American	High fertility rate because of long period of childbearing (up to age 44). Taboos/beliefs: Dietary practices influenced by hot/cold, wind/tonic. Wind foods are cold, tonic foods are hot and sweet. Maintaining balance between hot and cold restores bodily balance. In first trimester, woman is considered weak and cold, so she eats hot foods. Second trimester is neutral state. In third trimester, woman is considered hot, so she eats cold foods. Woman remains physically active but avoids heavy lifting and raising hands above head (thought to pull on placenta). Sexual intercourse late in pregnancy thought to cause respiratory distress. Taboo to attend weddings and funerals while pregnant. Early prenatal care is not the norm. Labor usually short, woman may prefer squatting or walking while in labor. Prenatal beliefs: Head of mother and baby considered sacred, so should not be touched. Placenta is buried to protect baby's health. Ritual cleansing of mother without water. Mother avoids showers because of cold influence for a month after delivery. Family helps care for mother and child. Breastfeeding common practice, but colostrum may be discarded. May alternate breast with bottle because of hot/cold influence (hot foods benefit mother's health; cold foods promote healthy breast milk).

Source: Adapted from Purnell and Paulanka, 1998.

CRITICAL THINKING ACTIVITY #1

Consider each of the cultural perspectives just described. How might they influence your approach in planning your client's care during the antepartal, intrapartal, and postpartal periods?

CRITICAL THINKING ACTIVITY #2

For each of the cultures described above, identify an intervention that incorporates your client's cultural beliefs into her care.

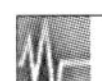

CRITICAL THINKING ACTIVITY #3

What questions should you ask your client to identify the cultural impact on her health?

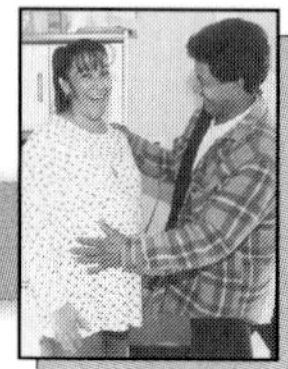

Introducing the Case Study

Mrs. Rosa Ramirez arrives at the Women's Clinic for confirmation of pregnancy. She is a 24-year-old Hispanic-American who has missed two menstrual periods. During the interview, Mrs. Ramirez states that she has experienced fatigue, nausea, and occasional vomiting over the past 3 weeks and has noticed an increase in breast size as well as breast tenderness and tingling. She also mentions that she has urinary frequency. Mrs. Ramirez is 65 inches tall and weighs 125 pounds. She states that she usually weighs between 126 and 128 pounds.

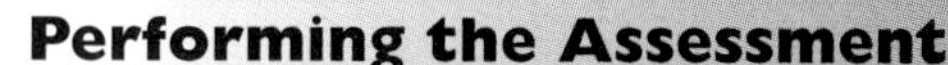

Performing the Assessment

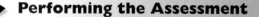

Your client's prenatal workup includes a health history and physical assessment. A complete health history is essential in providing optimal care for the pregnant woman. If there is no recent complete health history available, you should perform one before proceeding with the specific pregnancy-related questions.

After the health history comes the physical examination. Keep the key history findings in mind as you perform it. Taken together, the history and physical examination form a complete picture of your client's prenatal health.

Health History

This section focuses specifically on the current pregnancy. The first prenatal visit involves collection of baseline information about your client and her partner and identification of risk factors.

Key points to remember when obtaining a prenatal history:

- Focus on the current pregnancy and the presenting presumptive symptoms. Take a detailed obstetric/gynecologic history.
- Use the past medical history to identify anything that would affect or be affected by pregnancy.
- Pay special attention to the nutritional history.
- Pay special attention to the use of prescribed, over-the-counter, and illegal drugs; it may have a major impact on the developing fetus.
- Determine the client's reaction to pregnancy—was it planned?
- Identify major supports—family, spouse, significant other.
- Assess for history or risk of physical abuse.
- After you have completed your questions, ask the client if she has any problems or concerns that have not been covered, and give her an opportunity to discuss them.

Biographical Data

A careful review of the biographical data will be helpful in identifying actual or potential problems. Collecting this data also allows your client to answer uncomplicated questions comfortably and sets the tone for the remainder of the interview.

First, clarify your client's name, address, and date of birth. Geographic location may have a bearing on pregnancy outcome because women residing in the southern and western regions of the United States have a higher incidence of **preeclampsia**. Women who will be age 35 or older at the time of delivery should be offered genetic counseling and testing. Determine what effect the client's occupation may have on her pregnancy. Also identify the client's religious preference and cultural/ethnic group and incorporate them into her care, if appropriate. Biographical data will also be helpful in identifying your client's supports.

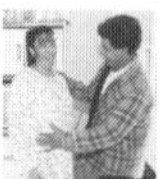

Case Study Findings

Reviewing Mrs. Ramirez's biographical data:

- 24 years old, married, first pregnancy
- College graduate, full-time social worker
- Born and reared in the United States, Hispanic descent, Catholic religion
- Health insurance through own and husband's work plan.
- Referral: Routine prenatal care
- Source: Self, seems reliable

Current Health Status

The current health status includes verifying the client's pregnancy, performing a symptom assessment, and calculating the estimated date of birth (EDB) or "due date."

Documenting Pregnancy

It is useful to document the client's pregnancy before proceeding with the initial comprehensive prenatal evaluation. Both urine and serum pregnancy tests are based on levels of **human chorionic gonadotropin (hCG),** which are secreted into the mother's bloodstream and then excreted into the urine.

Urine pregnancy tests are 95 percent to 98 percent accurate and are sensitive within 7 days after implantation. The test is inexpensive and widely available without a prescription, so many women test themselves at home. The first voided specimen of the morning is best to use for testing because concentrated urine improves the pregnancy detection rate. Serum pregnancy tests do not indicate pregnancy until levels rise above baseline values—usually around 25 to 30 metric International Units (mIU)/mL. The hCG is detectable in serum as early as 7 to 9 days after ovulation, or just after implantation. During the first 3 to 4 weeks after implantation, the hCG level doubles every 2 days, then peaks at 60 to 70 days.

The diagnosis of pregnancy is based on the following indicators:

- Presumptive signs (experienced by the client)
- Probable signs (observed by the examiner)
- Positive signs (attributed only to the presence of the fetus)

Symptom Assessment

The presenting symptoms usually relate to the presumptive signs of pregnancy. Your client may present with multiple symptoms and vague complaints, all related to the pregnancy. Because pregnancy affects every system of the body, the review of systems will address every presenting sign and symptom. Remember to perform a symptom analysis (PQRST) for all presenting symptoms.

Calculating the Estimated Date of Birth

Once the pregnancy has been confirmed, the EDB, also termed the estimated date of confinement (EDC), is calculated. Establishing the baby's due date involves obtaining accurate information regarding the mother's menstrual history, including the last menstrual period (LMP).

To calculate the EDB, apply **Naegele's rule:** Add 7 days to the first day of the LMP, and then subtract 3 months from that date. Considerations in calculating the EDB include the following:

- Find out the first day of the LMP. Make sure that the client is sure of the date because the EDC is based on the LMP. Conception usually occurs around 2 weeks after the LMP in a 28-day cycle.
- Review the client's menstrual history, including frequency of menses, length of flow, normalcy of the LMP, and contraceptive use.
- Ultrasound studies may also be used to estimate the gestational age.

Signs and Symptoms of Pregnancy

Signs And Symptoms	Description/Time Frame
Presumptive Signs	
Cessation of menses **(amenorrhea)**	Uterine lining does not slough off; women may experience spotting during implantation.
Nausea, vomiting	From weeks 2–12; usually subsides after 12 weeks.
Frequent urination	Bladder irritability caused by enlarging uterus.
Breast tenderness	Starts at 2–3 weeks; soreness; tingling.
Perception of fetal movement **(quickening)**	Occurs at 16–18 weeks; sensation of "fluttering" in abdomen perceived by mother-to-be.
Skin changes	Increased pigmentation; **striae gravidarum.**
Fatigue	Starts at 12 weeks.
Probable Signs	
Abdominal enlargement	Palpated at 12 weeks.
Piskacek's sign	Palpated at 4–6 weeks; uterus asymmetric with soft prominence on implantation side.
Hegar's sign	6 weeks; palpable softening of the lower uterine segment.
Goodell's sign	Palpated at 8 weeks; softening of the cervix.
Chadwick's sign	Seen at 6–8 weeks; bluish hue on vulva, vagina, cervix from increased venous congestion.
Braxton Hicks contractions	Painless, irregular, intermittent uterine contractions that typically start after the fourth month and last through remainder of pregnancy.
Pregnancy test	Positive 7–10 days after conception.
Ballottement	Occurs at 16–18 weeks, passive movement of the unengaged fetus.
Positive Signs	
Fetal heartbeat	By ultrasound, fetal heart motion is noted by 4–8 weeks after conception; by Doppler, auscultated by 10–12 weeks; by fetal stethoscope, auscultated by 17–19 weeks.
Visualization of the fetus	By ultrasound, at 5–6 weeks; by radiograph, by 16 weeks (but rarely used to diagnose pregnancy because of teratogenic effects).

Case Study Findings

Mrs. Ramirez's current health status and presenting symptoms include:

- Fatigue
- Nausea and vomiting for 3 weeks
- Breast enlargement, tingling, and tenderness
- Urinary frequency
- Amenorrhea

CRITICAL THINKING ACTIVITY #4

From what you have learned about Mrs. Ramirez, calculate her EDB using Naegele's rule.

CRITICAL THINKING ACTIVITY #5

Identify the presumptive signs of pregnancy Mrs. Ramirez has experienced.

Past Health History

The purpose of the past health history is to uncover diseases or other risk factors that could affect the woman's health or the fetus's well-being during pregnancy. Allergies to food, drugs, or environmental factors need to be noted because they can be exacerbated during pregnancy. Ask about exposure to toxins (e.g., radiation or chemicals) in the environment or at work, because this can affect fetal health. Is your client on any medications? Identify all prescribed and over-the-counter drugs (including alcohol and tobacco) your client took before and during her pregnancy for their potential effects on the developing fetus.

Also take an obstetric history. Has your client had previous pregnancies? If so, ask how many and if complications occurred during pregnancy or labor. Also ask about neonatal complications, such as birth defects, jaundice, infection, or death. Be sure to follow up on unclear or vague answers, and remember that sometimes rewording the question may help the client find a relevant response.

Ask your client if she has any of the diseases listed in the following paragraphs, which pose a particular risk to the expectant mother and/or fetus:

Diabetes

If your client has diabetes, ask about the age of onset. If she is insulin dependent, ask what type and amount of insulin she takes. If her diabetes is diet controlled, ask about use of oral hypoglycemics. If she has had other pregnancies, did she have gestational diabetes? Uncontrolled diabetes in pregnancy can cause congenital anomalies, fetal overgrowth (**macrosomia**), intrauterine fetal death, delayed fetal lung maturation, and neonatal death. Oral hypoglycemics may cause fetal damage and are contraindicated. Women with a history of gestational diabetes are more likely to develop it again with subsequent pregnancies.

Hypertension

If your client has chronic hypertension, ask how she controls it. Does she take antihypertensive medication? If so, explain that these drugs may be contraindicated in pregnancy. Hypertension may result in decreased placental perfusion and intrauterine fetal growth restriction. PIH may recur.

Cardiac Disease

Clients with mitral valve prolapse may need prophylactic antibiotics during labor to prevent streptococcal infections and subsequent bacterial endocarditis and valve disease.

Liver Disease

If your client has hepatitis B, the infant may require treatment (hepatitis B immunoglobulin and hepatitis vaccine) after birth.

Cancer

Clients with cervical cancer who were treated with cone biopsy (cone-shaped section of the cervix is removed for examination) are at risk for preterm labor.

Infectious Diseases

Rubella, mononucleosis, and other viral infections in the first trimester can cause fetal abnormalities.

Pulmonary Disease

Medications and inhalers used for asthma may be harmful to the fetus or may affect anesthesia used during labor. Inhalants and general anesthesia may be contraindicated for clients with asthma.

Gastrointestinal Disease

Ask about previous abdominal surgery and note the type of scarring; this may influence the type of delivery. Colitis and other bowel problems may be exacerbated in pregnancy.

Other Medical Problems

Varicosities and renal, gallbladder, genitourinary, autoimmune, neurologic, and psychiatric conditions may be exacerbated in pregnancy.

Gynecologic Diseases and STDs

Vaginitis should be identified and treated early to prevent intrauterine complications. Untreated STDs, such as genital herpes and gonorrhea, can be transmitted to the fetus during passage through the birth canal. The transmission rate for babies born to HIV-infected mothers is 20 to 35 percent.

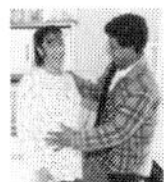

Case Study Findings

Mrs. Ramirez's past health history reveals:

- Usual childhood illnesses
- No surgeries, hospitalizations, or allergies
- Immunizations current
- Takes one multivitamin with iron daily; no other medications
- Physical examinations yearly since 18 years; normal Pap smears
- Used oral contraceptives for 5 years without problems; discontinued them 8 months ago to attempt pregnancy
- No previous pregnancies

Family History

The purpose of the family history is to identify potential physical and emotional complications of pregnancy and familial patterns of health or illness. Ask specific questions to pinpoint inherited diseases. For example, "Was anyone in your family diagnosed with heart disease before age 50?" (Cardiovascular disease or heart defects may be inherited.) "Does anyone in your family have lung disease, tuberculosis, or asthma?" (Pulmonary disorders may be familial; tuberculosis is contagious.) "Do any family members have diabetes?" (Endocrine problems are genetically linked.) "Cancer?" (There is a genetic component with certain types of cancer.) "Birth defects, inherited genetic disorders, blood disorders, or mental retardation?" (There is a genetic risk for Down syndrome, spina bifida, brain defects, anencephaly, heart defects, muscular dystrophy, cystic fibrosis, hemophilia, thalassemia, and other disorders.) "Did your mother or sisters have complications during pregnancy or labor?" (Daughters and sisters of preeclamptic women have a higher tendency toward preeclampsia.)

Be sure to consider your client's race/ethnic background when taking a family history. For example, children of African-American women are at risk for sickle cell disease. Identification of sickle cell disease will prevent a crisis; testing the mother-to-be is appropriate if status is uncertain.

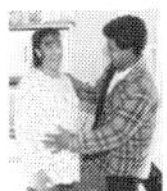

Case Study Findings

Mrs. Ramirez's family history reveals:

- Grandmother, age 64, takes medication to control high blood pressure.
- All other relatives alive and well; two older sisters married with children and experienced no complications during pregnancies; one younger sister is single.

Review of Systems

Normal changes that occur during pregnancy have an impact on every body system. The Review of Systems (ROS) will help you to identify normal physiologic changes as well as alert you to abnormal findings.

Review of Systems

AREA/QUESTIONS TO ASK	RATIONALE/SIGNIFICANCE
General Health Survey	
How have you been feeling?	Feelings of fatigue and ambivalence are normal during the first trimester. During the second trimester, mothers-to-be are introspective and energetic. The third trimester is characterized by restlessness, mood swings, and interest in preparing for the baby.
	ALERT *Denial of the pregnancy, withdrawal, depression, or psychosis signal psychological problems that warrant referral.*
General Health Survey/*Body Weight*	
What is your normal weight (before pregnancy)? Have you lost or gained weight since a year ago? How much?	Optimal weight gain during pregnancy depends on client's height and normal weight. Recommended weight gain in pregnancy is: Underweight client: 28–40 lb Normal weight client: 25–35 lb Overweight client: 15–25 lb Twin gestation: 35–45 lb

(Continued)

Review of Systems *(Continued)*

AREA/QUESTIONS TO ASK	RATIONALE/SIGNIFICANCE
General Health Survey/*Body Weight* *(Continued)*	**ALERT** *Low pregnancy weight and inadequate weight gain during pregnancy contribute to fetal growth restriction and low birth weight.*
Integumentary	
Have you noticed any changes in your skin, hair, or nails?	Hormonal changes cause hyperpigmentation of skin (chloasma, linea nigra), thin nails, oily hair.
HEENT/*Eyes*	
Do you have any vision problems?	Excessive tearing may be associated with allergies; blurred vision or spots before the eyes may indicate preeclampsia.
HEENT/*Ears*	
Do you have any hearing problems?	Decreased hearing, earaches, or sense of fullness in ears occurs because tympanic membranes swell as a result of increased vascularity.
HEENT/*Nose*	
Do you have nasal stuffiness? Nosebleeds?	Increased vascularity from increased estrogen causes nasal edema.
HEENT/*Neck*	
Have you noticed any masses in your neck?	Slight thyroid enlargement is normal; marked enlargement may indicate hyperthyroidism.
HEENT/*Mouth/Throat*	
Do you have any trouble with your throat? Since your last menstrual period, have you had a fever or chills without a cold? Do you have a cough that doesn't go away or frequent chest infections?	Prolonged nasal congestion with sore throat, fever, and chills may be an upper respiratory infection. Fetal exposure to viral illnesses is associated with fetal growth restriction, developmental delays, hearing impairment and mental retardation. Persistent cough and frequent chest infections may indicate pneumonia or tuberculosis.
Do your gums bleed? When was your last dental exam?	Gum hypertrophy is common; bleeding during tooth brushing may be associated with gum disease and warrants further dental evaluation.
Increased saliva?	**Ptyalism** (excessive saliva) often occurs within 2–3 weeks after the first missed period and is not associated with pathology.
Respiratory	
Do you have shortness of breath? Dyspnea? Other breathing problems?	Thoracic breathing, slight hyperventilation, and shortness of breath occur in late pregnancy. Dyspnea may be associated with respiratory distress; dyspnea with markedly decreased activity tolerance may indicate cardiovascular disease.
Cardiovascular	
Do you have a history of cardiovascular disease? Palpitations? Dizziness?	Pregnant women with pre-existing cardiovascular disease, such as mitral valve prolapse, can decompensate as a result of increased workload of the heart. Be alert for cardiovascular changes associated with PIH and eclampsia. Supine hypotension can occur from vena caval compression. **ALERT** *Lying supine compresses vena cava and aorta, decreasing cardiac output. Advise client to lie on left side to increase renal perfusion and output and reduce edema.*
Do your ankles swell?	Dependent edema and varicose veins in legs frequently occur in pregnancy, but may also be associated with PIH and eclampsia.

Review of Systems

AREA/QUESTIONS TO ASK	RATIONALE/SIGNIFICANCE
Breasts	
Have you noticed pain, lumps, or fluid leaking from your breasts?	Fullness, increased sensitivity, tingling, and heaviness are common early in pregnancy; however, lumps and pain may also indicate breast disease. Colostrum secretion from breasts is normal during pregnancy and varies in color.
Gastrointestinal	
Do you have nausea and vomiting that do not go away? Are you more thirsty than usual?	Excessive nausea and vomiting may be associated with **hyperemesis gravidarum**; sudden, excessive weight gain could indicate a multifetal gestation or fluid retention associated with PIH. Abdominal pain or cramping may be related to **round ligament pain** or may signal impending miscarriage. Hydration must be maintained because the client may be at risk for **hypovolemia**, **cholecystitis**, or **cholelithiasis**. **ALERT** *Appendicitis during pregnancy may be difficult to diagnose because the appendix is displaced upward and laterally.*
Do you ever notice black or bloody stools? Do you have diarrhea or trouble passing stools?	Blood in the stools or a change in bowel habits may indicate constipation or hemorrhoids.
Genitourinary	
Do you ever have burning or pain when you urinate? Do you have to urinate more often than normal?	Urinary urgency and frequency are common during pregnancy and are not cause for concern unless accompanied by pain or burning, which may signal a urinary tract infection (UTI). During pregnancy, women may have **asymptomatic bacteriuria.** UTIs must be promptly diagnosed and treated because untreated UTIs predispose client to complications such as preterm labor, pyelonephritis, and sepsis.
Reproductive	
When was your last menstrual period?	Needed to determine EDC.
Do you have increased vaginal discharge?	Increased white vaginal discharge (**leukorrhea**) is normal during pregnancy. Discharge accompanied by a foul odor, itching, or burning may indicate infection.
Have you experienced any vaginal bleeding, leakage of fluid, or unusual vaginal discharge?	Vaginal bleeding, fluid leakage, or vaginal discharge may indicate **placenta previa**, rupture of membranes, or vaginal infection. Untreated vaginal infections predispose client to preterm labor or fetal infections.
Musculoskeletal	
Do you have leg cramps?	Leg cramps may indicate calcium deficiency.
Do you have back pain?	Curvature of the lumbar spine may be accentuated during pregnancy, resulting in backache. Severe back pain may be associated with disc disease.
Neurological	
Do you have a history of depression, difficulty sleeping, loss of appetite?	Emotional lability can occur during pregnancy; however, these symptoms also may indicate psychological disorders. **ALERT** *Clients with a history of psychological disorders must be continually monitored for signs and symptoms and referred when appropriate.*

(Continued)

Review of Systems *(Continued)*

AREA/QUESTIONS TO ASK	RATIONALE/SIGNIFICANCE
Neurological *(Continued)*	
Have you experienced light-headedness, dizziness, or fainting?	Fainting may indicate anemia.
Do you have wrist pain, numbness, or tingling?	Wrist pain, especially in the dominant hand, may indicate carpal tunnel syndrome.
Endocrine	
Do you have increased fatigue or heat intolerance?	Common symptoms associated with increase in BMR and hormonal changes.
Do you have a history of diabetes or gestational diabetes?	Positive history of diabetes calls for close monitoring.
Immune/Hematologic	
Do you have a history of anemia?	Physiologic anemia may occur during pregnancy. As a result, pre-existing anemia may worsen.
History of thrombophlebitis?	Increase of clotting factors increases risk of thrombus formation.

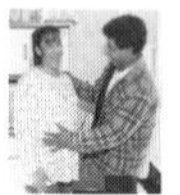

Case Study Findings

Mrs. Ramirez's review of systems reveals:

- **General Health Survey:** Very tired for past couple of months, needs to take a nap every day when she gets home from work. Body weight 125 lb, on the low end of her reported range of 126 to 128 lb. Has lost 2 lb since becoming pregnant.
- **Integumentary:** Noticed nipples getting darker and line on abdomen. Hair very oily.
- **HEENT:** No changes in head/neck. Has nasal stuffiness but no colds, allergies, or flu. Gums bleed with brushing; last dental exam 6 months ago. No eye changes.
- **Respiratory:** No changes.
- **Cardiovascular:** No history of mitral valve prolapse (MVP), palpitations, or edema.
- **Breasts:** Enlargement, tenderness, and tingling sensation.
- **Gastrointestinal:** Nausea and vomiting in the morning, usually subsides by noon; says certain foods "just turn my stomach;" reports constipation.
- **Genitourinary:** Reports frequency of urination, no burning.
- **Reproductive:** LMP 4/10/01.
- **Musculoskeletal:** No changes.
- **Neurological:** Occasional "lightheadedness;" no history of depression; excited at possibility of being pregnant.
- **Endocrine:** No history of gestational diabetes; reports heat intolerance.
- **Immune/Hematologic:** No history of anemia.

CRITICAL THINKING ACTIVITY #6

List strategies that may help combat Mrs. Ramirez's morning sickness.

Psychosocial Profile

The psychosocial profile is an important component of the assessment because it lays the groundwork for a trusting nurse-client relationship. The profile provides an opportunity to explore the client's reactions to the pregnancy and to identify lifestyle patterns that may pose a threat to her or her baby's well-being.

Start by asking your client about her health practices and beliefs. Is she proactive (getting regular preventive health care) or reactive (seeking health care only when ill)? Also inquire about self-care, such as breast self-examinations (BSEs). Determine the client's acceptance of the prenatal care plan and understanding of recommended actions, including the need for regular prenatal visits.

Next, ask about your client's typical day. What constitutes a usual day's activities? How has pregnancy affected her daily lifestyle pattern?

Inquire about nutrition and weight loss or gain. Weight loss often occurs in the first trimester as a result of morning sickness. Failure to gain enough weight in the second and third trimesters may be associated with fetal growth restriction. Rapid, sudden weight gain may indicate PIH.

Ask if the client takes vitamins and supplements. Supplementation may be necessary to ensure adequate intake and should be started before conception. The

Centers for Disease Control (CDC) recommend 0.4 mg of folic acid per day for the prevention of neural tube defects; it is best to begin 1 month before conception and continue through the first 3 months of pregnancy. Pregnant women should also receive prenatal vitamins with 30 mg of ferrous iron daily.

Question the client about the amount and type of exercise she does. Daily exercise is highly recommended as long as it is well tolerated by the client. Women in good physical condition tend to have easier labors than those who are not physically fit.

Ask about pets. If the client has a cat, warn her to wear gloves when changing litter boxes because of the risk of **toxoplasmosis** infection. Suggest that other family members change the cat litter, and encourage the client to wash her hands well after petting the cat.

Ask about sleep and rest. How much uninterrupted sleep does the client get every night? Does she take naps? Does she suffer from insomnia? Adequate rest is important in assuring optimal health for the mother and fetus. Difficulty sleeping during the third trimester is common and may be treated with massage, tub baths, or warm milk.

Inquire about personal habits. Does the client currently smoke? Does she take recreational drugs, such as cocaine, speed, or marijuana? Does she drink alcohol? Cigarette smoking during pregnancy is associated with increased perinatal mortality, preterm delivery, premature rupture of membranes, **placental abruption,** stillbirth, and bleeding during pregnancy. Cocaine use is associated with a higher rate of spontaneous abortions and placental abruption. Alcohol use during pregnancy is associated with low birth weight, stillbirth,and **fetal alcohol syndrome,** the leading cause of mental retardation. There is no known safety level for alcohol use during pregnancy.

Find out where the client works and what she does for a living. Does it involve heavy lifting, toxic exposure, or anything else that might harm the fetus? Can she take rest periods? Physiologic changes during pregnancy place a tremendous amount of stress on the body, and frequent rest periods are encouraged.

Ask about environmental hazards such as secondhand smoke and paternal exposure to toxins and industrial pollutants. There is an increased incidence of preeclampsia in women residing in southern and western states. Smoke and industrial chemicals are hazardous to the fetus. Paternal exposure to workplace toxins has been associated with an increased risk of spontaneous abortion. Also ask about living conditions. Ascertain whether the client's home is adequate for the expanding family, and work with her to improve the situation, if needed. Refer to community agencies, if appropriate.

Ask about cultural and religious influences in the client's life. How do they affect her healthcare practices, especially during pregnancy and delivery?

Ask about the client's family relationships. Does she have a spouse or partner? Does she have any other children? How old are they? Education and preparation for the baby can offset potential problems with sibling rivalry. Encourage sibling classes. Also ask about support systems outside the immediate family. Does she have relatives or friends to rely on during pregnancy and the postpartum period?

Ask the client about stress and coping. How has the pregnancy affected her emotional well-being? Many women experience mood swings during pregnancy, but signs of clinical depression must be evaluated and referred.

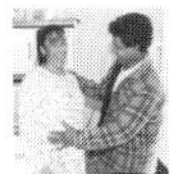

Case Study Findings

Mrs. Ramirez's psychosocial profile includes:

- Client is proactive regarding health care. Has yearly physical examination and Pap smear. Performs monthly BSE. Believes people are responsible for maintaining their own health.
- Typical day consists of arising at 6:30 AM and eating breakfast with husband. (Lately unable to enjoy usual breakfast of cold cereal and juice because of nausea.) Drives 4 miles to office 5 days a week and works from 8 AM to 5 PM at desk part of time and interviews clients in a clinic located on the ground floor of her office building for rest of time. Loves her work. Evenings she and husband prepare and eat supper, clean up dishes, take a walk in the neighborhood, then relax by watching television, playing cards, or reading. Client showers and goes to bed around 10 PM.
- Usually eats a healthy diet, but lately has been skipping breakfast because of nausea. As day progresses, is gradually able to eat bland food, such as baked chicken, potatoes, and steamed vegetables.
- Walks daily for 45 minutes with husband.
- Has no pets. Recreation includes daily walk with husband, dinner at restaurant or movie once a week, family get-togethers. Hobbies include reading and needlework.
- Sleeps around 8 1/2 hours normally, but lately gets very sleepy at work, especially in mid-afternoon. Combats sleepiness with a walk outside her office and an afternoon snack of fruit and yogurt or crackers. Takes a short nap after work. No problems falling asleep.
- Does not smoke, use drugs, or drink alcoholic beverages.
- No chemical exposure at work.
- Lives in a 1-story, 2-bedroom single-family home in suburbs; has hot water, heating, and air

conditioning; negative for radon gas. Will convert guest room into baby's room. No recent travel outside local community.

- Catholic religion, Hispanic nationality (third generation). No religious or cultural influences that affect health care, pregnancy, or delivery.
- Supportive, caring husband (nonsmoker) who is computer analyst for national company; married 5 years; attempted pregnancy for 6 months.
- Mother, mother-in-law, and three sisters live in same community and will assist with infant care. Client plans to breastfeed and stay at home for 6 weeks after birth and then return to job.
- Copes with stress by walking, talking with husband and family members, doing needlework.

 CRITICAL THINKING ACTIVITY #7

Based on the subjective information you have obtained, identify positive lifestyle factors that will enhance Mrs. Ramirez's pregnancy and birthing experience.

Focused Obstetrical History

If your client's condition or time prohibits a detailed obstetrical history, and the current pregnancy has been confirmed, just ask these key questions. They focus on significant past pregnancy events, current pregnancy status, identification of risk factors, and health promotion activities. The client's response will help to direct your assessment.

- How many times have you been pregnant? What were the outcomes of these pregnancies? Did you experience any problems during these pregnancies?
- When was your last menstrual period? Was this a normal period?
- When is this baby due? How was your due date determined?
- Since you became pregnant this time, have you:
  - Had any x rays? If yes, when and why?
  - Been exposed to any viral illnesses, such as German measles (rubella)? If yes, when?
  - Experienced any other childhood illnesses? If yes, describe.
  - Had a fever? If yes, when, and how high was your temperature?
- Have you used any medications: prescribed, over-the-counter, home remedies/herbal preparations, vitamin or mineral supplements?
- Have you had any bleeding or leakage of fluid from your vagina? When?
- Have you had any prenatal care? If yes, where and when?
- Do you have any medical conditions (hypertension, diabetes, etc.)?
- How much weight have you gained so far during this pregnancy?

Case Study Evaluation

Before performing the physical examination, document what you have learned about Mrs. Ramirez so far.

Physical Assessment

Now that you have completed the subjective data collection, begin to collect objective data by means of the physical examination. Keep the history findings in mind. These findings, along with those from the physical examination, will complete the assessment picture. Then you can analyze the data, formulate nursing diagnoses, and develop a plan of care.

Approach

You will begin the physical examination with inspection, then proceed to palpation, percussion, and finally, auscultation. Remember that normal findings may vary somewhat from one pregnant client to another; thus a systematic approach is essential. Explain to your client that after the examination is complete, she will go to the laboratory for initial prenatal blood tests.

PRENATAL LABORATORY TESTS

Urine Tests

One of the first laboratory tests to obtain (preferably before beginning the physical examination) is the clean-catch midstream urine specimen, which will be tested for glucose (to assess for diabetes), protein (to assess for PIH), and nitrites and leukocytes (to assess for infection).

Blood Tests

Initial prenatal blood tests include complete blood count, blood type and screen, Rh status, rubella titer, serologic test for syphilis, and hepatitis B surface antigen. Clients of African ancestry are also referred for a sickle cell anemia screen. Additionally, clients who are at high risk for infection with human immunodeficiency virus (HIV) should be screened for this disease.

Between 16 and 18 weeks gestation, a multiple marker or "triple screen" is usually obtained. This blood test measures the maternal serum level of alpha-fetoprotein (MSAFP), human chorionic gonadotropin (hCG), and unconjugated estriol (uE3). High levels of alpha-fetoprotein are associated with neural tube defects, low triple screen values with Down syndrome, and other chromosomal abnormalities. MSAFP screening can detect approximately 80% to 85% of all open neural tube defects (NTDs) and open abdominal wall defects early in pregnancy. AFP is produced by the fetal liver, GI tract, and embryonic yolk sac and readily crosses the placenta and fetal membranes into the mother's bloodstream, resulting in a rise in the maternal serum. The AFP level can be measured by taking a sample of the mother's blood between 15 and 21 weeks gestation; measurement at 17 weeks is ideal.

Toolbox

The tools for the obstetric assessment include a stethoscope, light for the pelvic examination, tape measure, fetoscope or fetal Doppler, and equipment for the pelvic exam: speculum, gloves, lubricant, glass slides, KOH, normal saline, and cytology fixative. Also, sharpen your senses because you will use all of them during the obstetric examination.

Performing a General Survey

The first part of the physical assessment focuses on the general survey, including a measurement of height and weight (Fig. 21–1). At the initial visit, it is important to establish a baseline height, weight, pulse, respirations, and blood pressure; on subsequent prenatal visits, the weight, pulse, respirations, and blood pressure (taken in a sitting position) are also recorded.

Throughout each prenatal examination, observe your client's behavior. During the first trimester, she is likely to appear tired and even ambivalent about her pregnancy. The second trimester is usually characterized by excitement, enthusiasm, and energy. The third trimester is marked by periods of restlessness, self-doubts, and concerns about the upcoming birth experience.

HELPFUL HINT

Consider your client's position and anxiety level when assessing BP. BP is highest when sitting and lowest when supine. So always take BP in the same arm and in the same position.

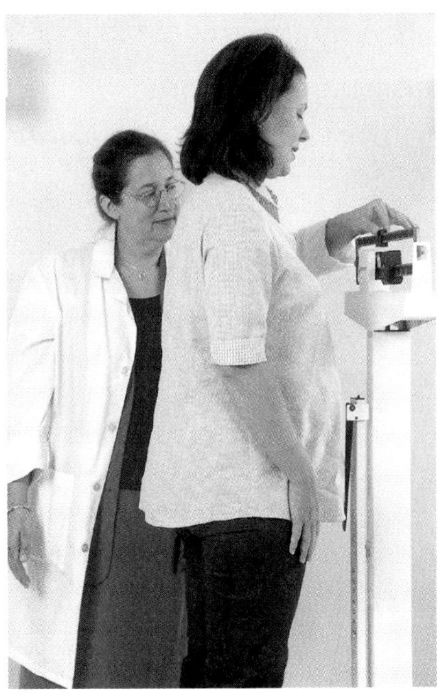

FIGURE 21–1. Establishing baseline weight.

Performing a Head-to-Toe Physical Assessment

Because physiologic changes occurring during pregnancy affect every other body system, physical signs may be seen in any system. You will need to perform a full head-to-toe examination, including a pelvic examination. Pelvic cultures obtained with this examination include a Pap smear and gonorrhea and chlamydial cultures.

For the next component of the assessment, the client should be comfortably seated on the examining table. She should be wearing a gown and adequately draped to ensure privacy. Explain to her what you will be doing and why, and what she may expect to feel just before and during each part of the examination. As you progress through your initial physical assessment, remember that pregnancy affects every other body system and that you will need to be able to differentiate normal changes from abnormal changes.

Performing a Head-to-Toe Physical Assessment

SYSTEM/NORMAL VARIATIONS	ABNORMAL FINDINGS/RATIONALE
Integumentary/*Skin, hair, nails* *INSPECT* • Linea nigra, striae gravidarum, chloasma, spider nevi, palmar erythema • Increased growth, softening, thinning of hair and nails	• *Pale skin:* Anemia.

(Continued)

Performing a Head-to-Toe Physical Assessment *(Continued)*

SYSTEM/NORMAL VARIATIONS	ABNORMAL FINDINGS/RATIONALE

Integumentary/*Skin, hair, nails (Continued)*

ALERT
Your client is anemic if hemoglobin drops below 10 g/dL.

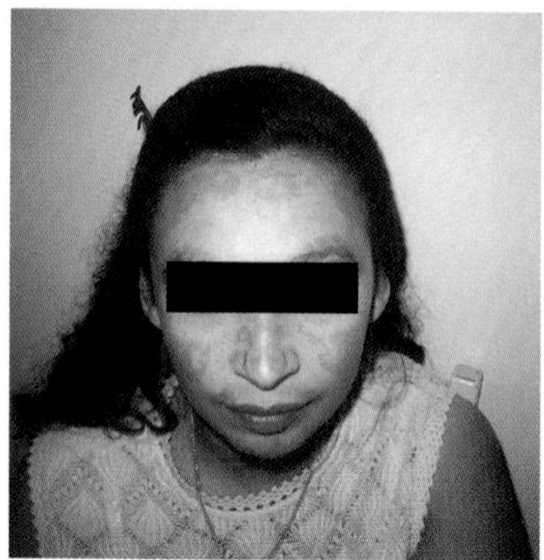

Chloasma

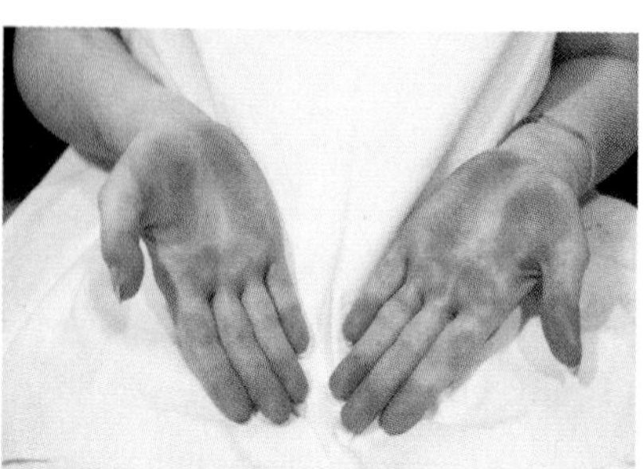

Palmar erythema

HEENT/*Head and Neck*
PALPATE

- Palpable smooth, nontender small cervical chain lymph nodes. Slight thyroid gland enlargement.
  - *Hard, tender, fixed or prominent cervical nodes:* Cancer.
  - *Marked thyroid enlargement:* Hyperthyroidism.

HEENT/*Ear*
INSPECT

- Tympanic membranes clear, landmarks visible
  - *Tympanic membranes red and bulging with pus:* Infection.

HEENT/*Nose*
INSPECT

- Mucosal swelling and redness, epistaxis (nosebleeds) common because of increased estrogen
  - *Purulent discharge:* Upper respiratory infection.

HEENT/*Mouth/Throat*
INSPECT

- Gums: Gingival hypertrophy and **epulis** usually regress spontaneously after delivery.
  - *Bleeding gums:* Gingivitis.
  - *Redness:* Exudate present.
  - *Enlarged tonsils:* Infection.

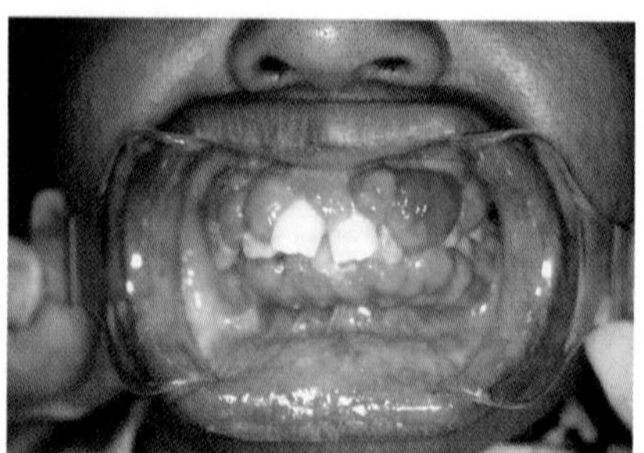

Gingival hypertrophy

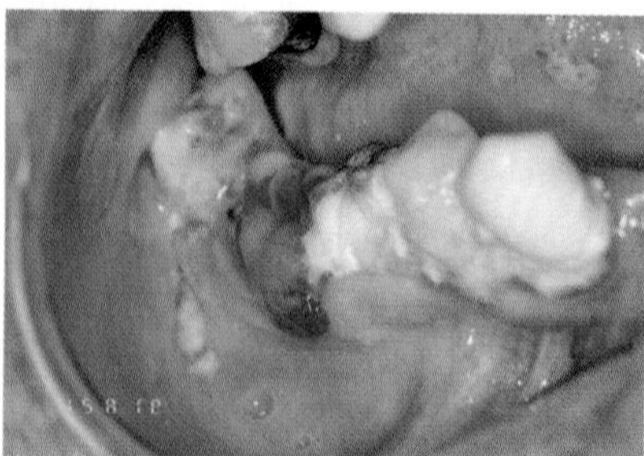

Epulis

- Throat: Pink, no redness or exudates

Performing a Head-to-Toe Physical Assessment

SYSTEM/NORMAL VARIATIONS	ABNORMAL FINDINGS/RATIONALE
Respiratory *INSPECT/PALPATE/PERCUSS/AUSCULTATE* • Increased anteroposterior chest diameter, thoracic breathing, slight hyperventilation, shortness of breath in late pregnancy, lung sounds clear bilaterally	• *Dyspnea, crackles, rhonchi, wheezes, rubs, absence of breath sounds, unequal breath sounds, respiratory distress:* May indicate pulmonary complications, such as pulmonary edema or acute respiratory distress syndrome.
Cardiovascular/*Heart* *PALPATE/AUSCULTATE* • Point of maximal impulse (PMI) may be displaced upward and laterally in the latter stages of pregnancy. • Normal sinus rhythm	• *Enlarged PMI:* May be associated with hypertension. • *Irregular rhythm:* Cardiac disease. • *Dyspnea, palpitations, markedly decreased activity tolerance:* Cardiovascular disease.
• Soft systolic murmur caused by increased blood volume	• *Midsystolic click and late systolic murmur:* MVP.
Breasts *INSPECT/PALPATE* • Venous congestion with prominence of Montgomery's tubercles. Increased size and nodularity; increased sensitivity; colostrum secretion in the third trimester. • Hyperpigmentation of nipples and areolar tissue.	• Nipple inversion may be problematic for breastfeeding women. • *Localized redness, pain, and warmth:* Mastitis. • *Bloody nipple discharge and skin retraction:* Cancer.
Gastrointestinal ***Abdomen*** *INSPECT/AUSCULTATE/PALPATE* • Note cesarean scars and location; obtain previous pregnancy records to confirm type and location of uterine incision. • Note linea nigra, striae.	
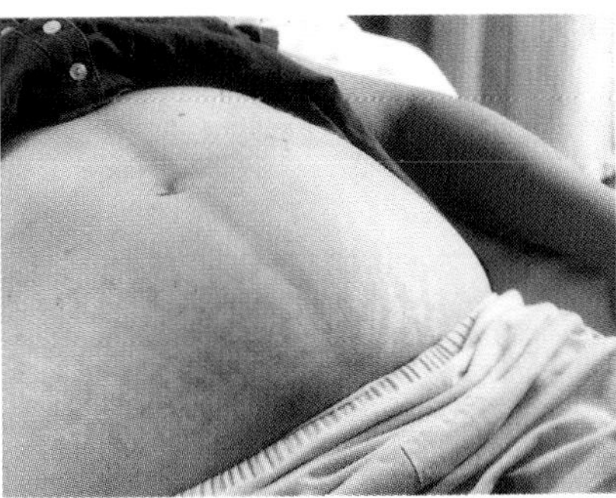 **Linea nigra** 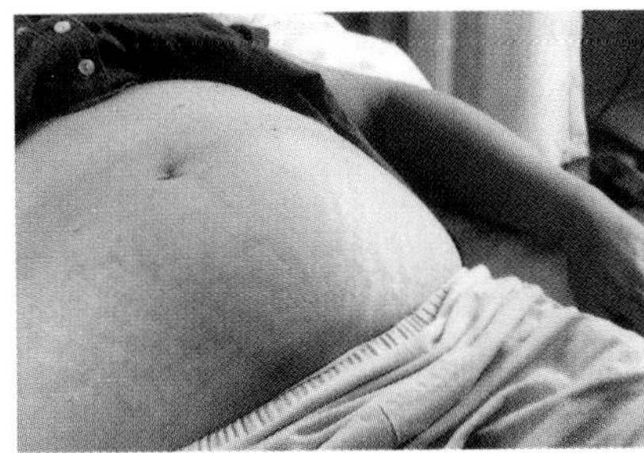 **Striae**	• Note any scars that may indicate previous abdominal surgery and influence type of delivery.

(Continued)

Performing a Head-to-Toe Physical Assessment *(Continued)*

SYSTEM/NORMAL VARIATIONS	ABNORMAL FINDINGS/RATIONALE

Gastrointestinal *(Continued)*

- Abdominal enlargement caused by fetus; in later pregnancy, uterine shape may suggest fetal presentation and position. Palpable uterus at 10–12 weeks.
- Fetal movement noticed by mother at 18–20 weeks (earlier for multipara).
- *Uterine contractions* may be present; intensity is described as mild, moderate, or firm to palpation.

- *Abnormal palpable masses:* Uterine fibroids or hepatosplenomegaly.
- *No fetal movement felt:* Wrong EDC or fetal demise.
- *Regular contractions before 37 completed weeks of gestation:* Preterm labor.

HELPFUL HINT

How long are the client's contractions? Time them from beginning to end of same contraction. How frequent are they? Time them from beginning of one contraction to beginning of next.

- *Fundal height measurement:* Place zero point of tape measure on symphysis pubis and measure to top of fundus. Fundal measurement should approximately equal number of weeks gestation; measurements may vary by 2 cm; measurements by different examiners should be approximately the same.

- Measurements greater than 4 cm from the estimated gestational age warrant further evaluation.

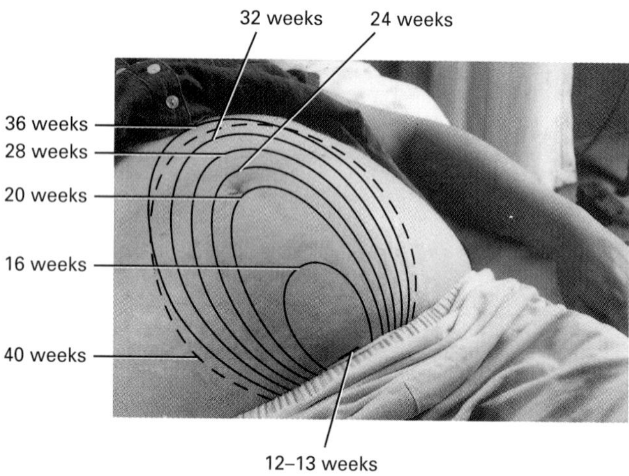

Fundal height assessment

- Measurements greater than 4 cm from the estimated gestational age warrant further evaluation.
- *Greater than expected:* Multiple gestation; **polyhydramnios**; fetal anomalies; macrosomia.
- *Smaller than expected:* Fetal growth restriction.

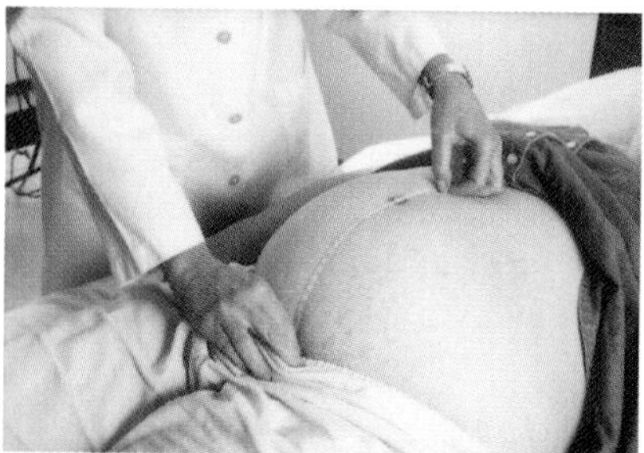

Fundal height measurement

- *Fetal heart tones* (FHTs) are best auscultated through the back of the fetus. A fetal Doppler can be used after 10–12 weeks gestation; a fetoscope may be used after 18 weeks gestation.

Performing a Head-to-Toe Physical Assessment

SYSTEM/NORMAL VARIATIONS	ABNORMAL FINDINGS/RATIONALE

Gastrointestinal *(Continued)*

- Fetal heart rate (FHR) range: 120–160 beats per minute. In third trimester, FHR accelerates with fetal movement.

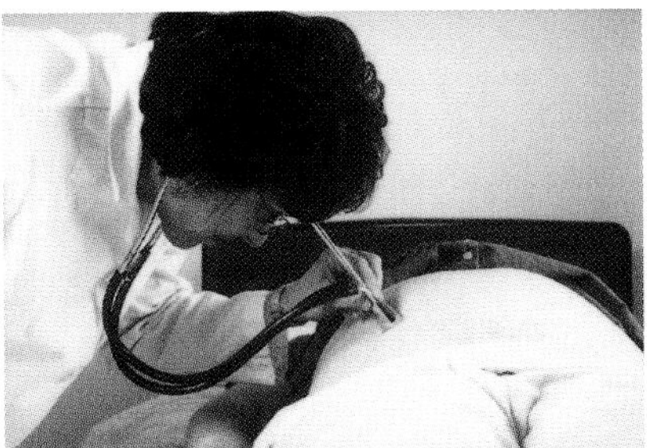

Auscultating FHT with fetoscope

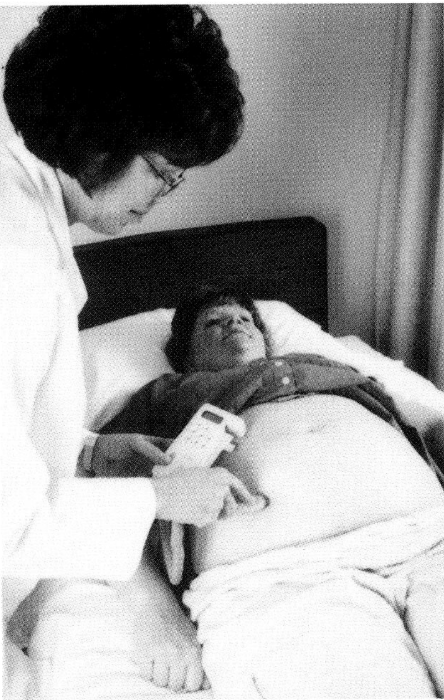

Auscultating FHT with Doppler

- *Inability to auscultate FHT with a fetal Doppler at 12 weeks:* Retroverted uterus; uncertain dates; fetal demise; false pregnancy.
- *Fetal heart rate decelerations:* Poor placental perfusion.

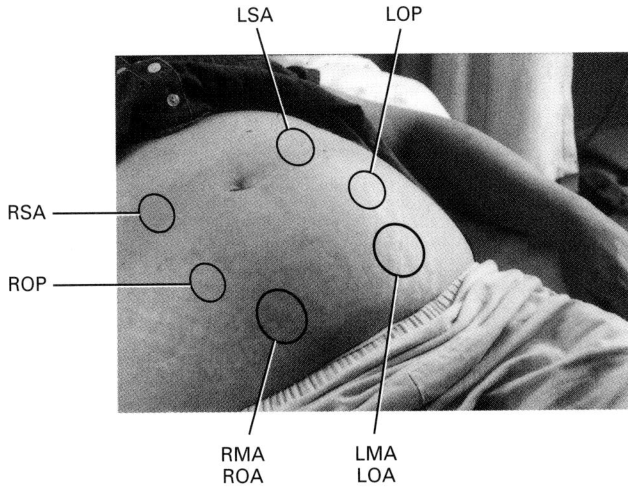

Fetal heart tones
Intensity varies according to fetal position. RSA = right sacrum anterior, LSA = left sacrum anterior, ROP = right occipitoposterior, LOP = left occipitoposterior, RMA = right mentum anterior, LMA = left mentum anterior, ROA = right occipitoanterior, LOA = left occipitoanterior

- *Fetal position:* Use Leopold's maneuvers to palpate the fundus, lateral aspects of the abdomen and lower pelvic area. Leopold's maneuvers assist in determining: **fetal lie** (body of fetus in relation to mother's back), **presentation** (fetal presenting part into the maternal pelvis), size, and position. A longitudinal lie (fetal spine axis is parallel to mother's spine axis) is expected. Fetal presentation may be cephalic, breech, or

- *Oblique or transverse lie:* Breech presentation.

(Continued)

Performing a Head-to-Toe Physical Assessment *(Continued)*

SYSTEM/NORMAL VARIATIONS | **ABNORMAL FINDINGS/RATIONALE**

Gastrointestinal *(Continued)*

shoulder. Fetal size is estimated by measuring fundal height and by palpation.

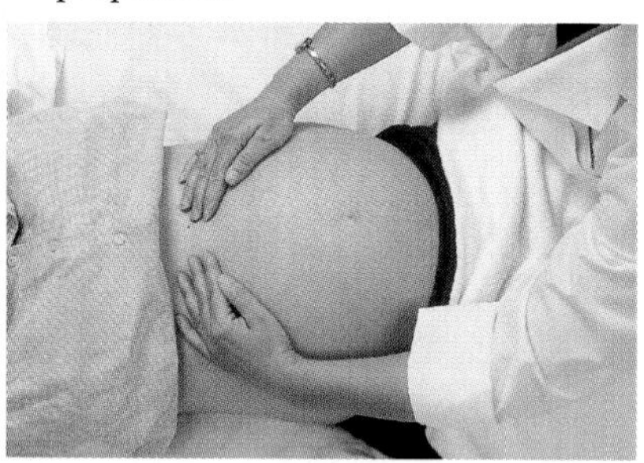

First Leopold's maneuver

- *First maneuver:* Face the client's head and place your hands on the fundal area. You should palpate a soft, irregular mass in the upper quadrant of the mother's abdomen. The soft mass is the fetal buttocks; the round, hard part is the fetal head.

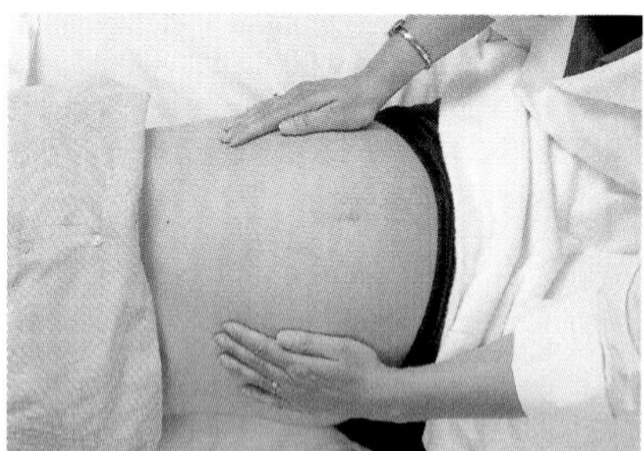

Second Leopold's maneuver

- *Second maneuver:* Next, move your hands down to the lateral sides of the mother's abdomen. On one side of the abdomen you will palpate round, irregular nodules—the fists and feet of the fetus. Expect to feel kicking and movement. The other side of the mother's abdomen feels smooth—this is the fetus's back.

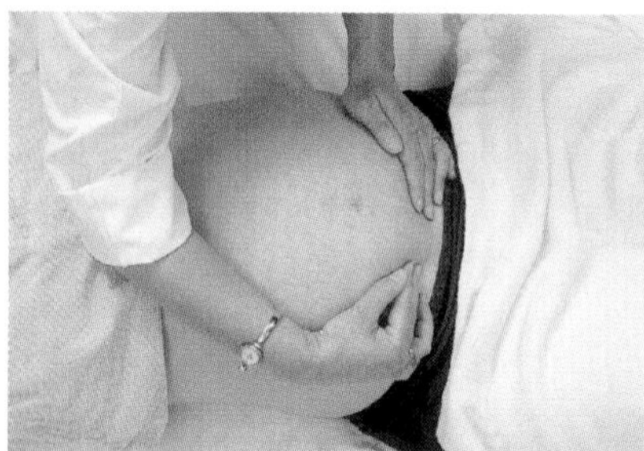

Third Leopold's maneuver

- *Third maneuver:* Now move your hands down to the mother's lower pelvic area and palpate the area just above the symphysis pubis to determine the presenting part of the fetus. Grasp the presenting part with your thumb and third finger. If the presenting part is the head, it will be round, firm, and ballottable; if it is the buttocks, it will be soft and irregular.

HELPFUL HINT

If you hear fetal heart sounds above the umbilicus, it is a breech presentation; below the umbilicus, a vertex presentation.

Performing a Head-to-Toe Physical Assessment

SYSTEM/NORMAL VARIATIONS | **ABNORMAL FINDINGS/RATIONALE**

Gastrointestinal *(Continued)*

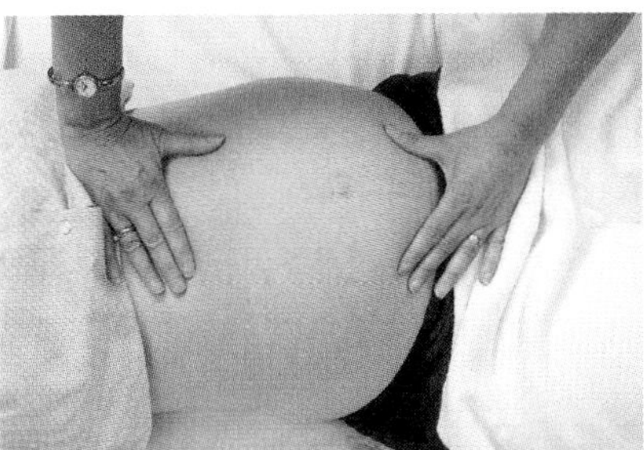

Fourth Leopold's maneuver

- *Fourth maneuver:* Last, place your hands on her upper and lower abdomen and try to move your hands toward each other while applying downward pressure. If your hands move together easily, the fetal head is not descended into the mother's pelvic inlet. If your hands do not move together and stop because of resistance, the fetal head is engaged into the mother's pelvic inlet.

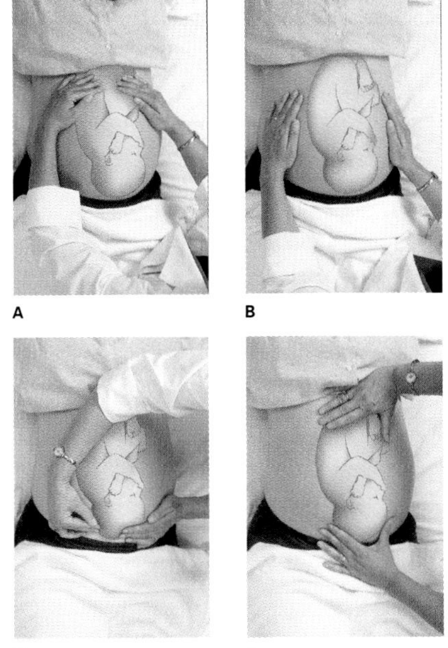

Fetal presentation/position

(Continued)

Performing a Head-to-Toe Physical Assessment *(Continued)*

SYSTEM/NORMAL VARIATIONS	ABNORMAL FINDINGS/RATIONALE
Extremities *INSPECT/PALPATE* • In third trimester, dependent edema is normal; varicose veins may also appear.	• *Calf pain, positive Homans' sign, generalized edema, diminished pedal pulses:* deep vein thrombophlebitis (DVT).
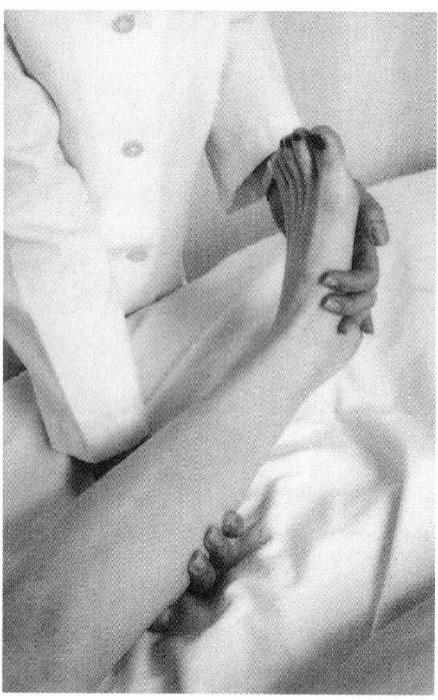 **Homans' assessment**	
Genitourinary INSPECT/PALPATE *External genitalia* • Labial and clitoral enlargement; parous relaxation of introitus; scars from episiotomy or perineal lacerations (multiparous women)	• *Labial varicosities:* Venous congestion.
Genitourinary/*Bartholin's and Skene's Glands* • No discomfort or discharge	• *Discharge and tenderness:* infection.
Genitourinary/*Vaginal orifice* • Small amount of whitish discharge (leukorrhea)	• *Thick, purulent vaginal discharge:* Gonorrheal infection. • *Thick white, cheesy discharge:* Yeast infection. • *Gray-white discharge, sweet smell, positive clue cells:* Bacterial vaginosis infection.
Genitourinary/*Cervix* • Smooth, pink, or bluish, long, thick, closed; 2.3–3 cm long. Softening of lower uterine segment (Hegar's sign) should be present. Bluish color (Chadwick's sign) indicates increased blood flow to pelvic area and is probable sign of pregnancy.	

Performing a Head-to-Toe Physical Assessment

SYSTEM/NORMAL VARIATIONS	ABNORMAL FINDINGS/RATIONALE
Genitourinary/*Cervix (Continued)*	• *Effaced, opened cervix:* Preterm labor or incompetent cervix if not a term gestation.

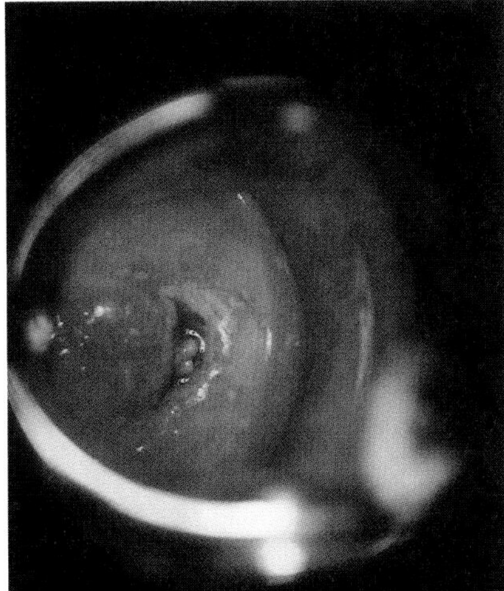

Chadwick's sign

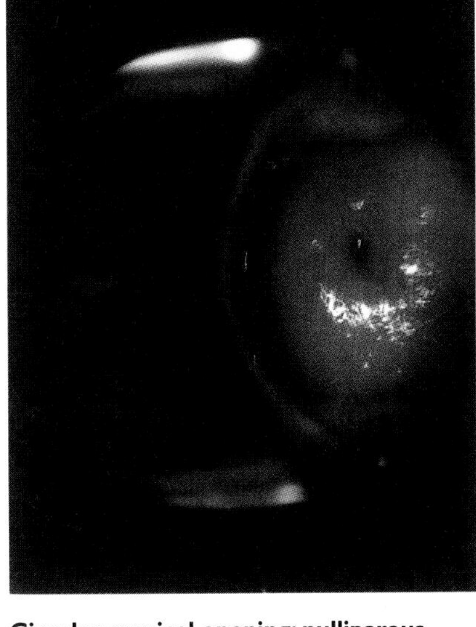

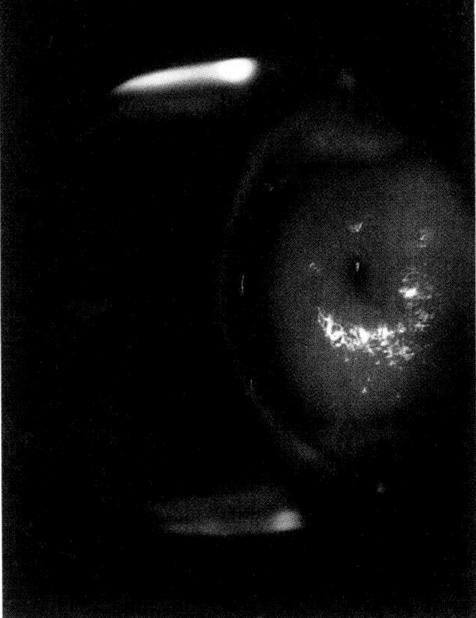

Circular cervical opening: nulliparous

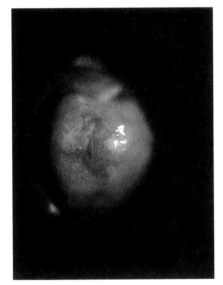

Slitlike cervical opening: multiparous

SYSTEM/NORMAL VARIATIONS	ABNORMAL FINDINGS/RATIONALE
Genitourinary/*Uterus*	
• Uterus is size of orange at 10 weeks; grapefruit at 12 weeks.	• *Uterine size not consistent with dates:* Wrong dates, fibroids, multiple gestation.
• No masses in left and right adnexa; some discomfort caused by stretching of round ligaments.	• *Palpable masses:* Ectopic pregnancy.
Musculoskeletal	
• Accentuated lumbar curve (lordosis) • Wider base of support	• *Diastasis recti abdominis:* Separation of abdominal muscles from pregnancy.

(Continued)

Performing a Head-to-Toe Physical Assessment *(Continued)*

SYSTEM/NORMAL VARIATIONS	ABNORMAL FINDINGS/RATIONALE
Musculoskeletal *(Continued)*	
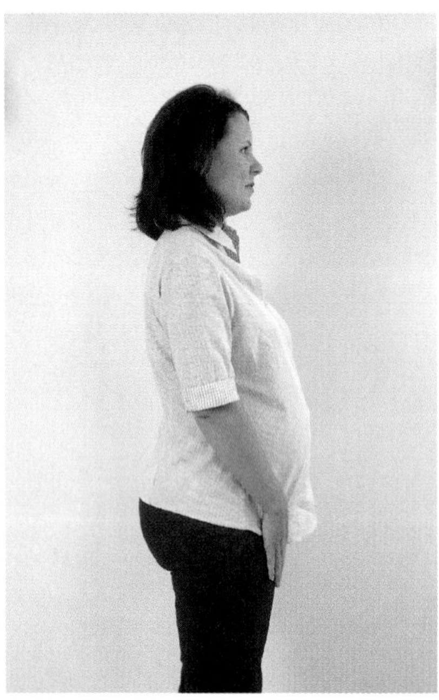 **Accentuated lumbar curve**	
Neurological	
• + 1–2 deep tendon reflex (DTR)	• *Hyperreflexia, clonus:* Preeclampsia, eclampsia.
• Negative Phalen's or Tinel's sign	• *Positive Phalen's or Tinel's sign:* Carpal tunnel syndrome.
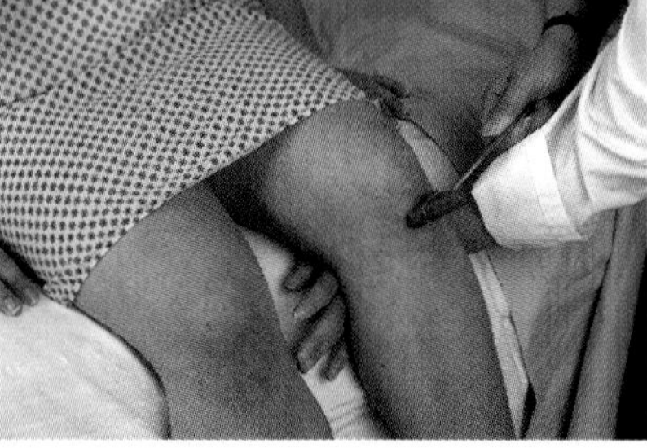 **DTR assessment**	

Case Study Analysis and Plan

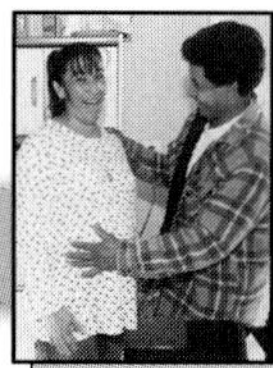

Now that you have completed a thorough assessment of Mrs. Ramirez, document your key history and physical examination findings. List key history findings and key physical examination findings that will help you formulate your nursing diagnoses.

 CRITICAL THINKING ACTIVITY #8

What are Mrs. Ramirez's strengths? Are there any areas of concern?

 CRITICAL THINKING ACTIVITY #9

As with most pregnant women, Mrs. Ramirez's readiness to learn is high. What information about her pregnancy would be important to share with her at this time?

 CRITICAL THINKING ACTIVITY #10

How often do you expect Mrs. Ramirez to be seen in the prenatal clinic? Which components of the examination will be repeated at each prenatal visit?

CRITICAL THINKING ACTIVITY #11

What questions will you ask Mrs. Ramirez on each visit?

Nursing Diagnoses

Your next step is to analyze the data from Mrs. Ramirez's history and physical assessment and develop nursing diagnoses. The following are possible nursing diagnoses for this client. Cluster the supporting data for each diagnosis.

1. Knowledge, deficient, related to plan for prenatal visits during the remainder of pregnancy
2. Nutrition: imbalanced, less than body requirements, related to nausea
3. Fluid Volume Imbalance, risk for, related to vomiting and weight loss associated with early pregnancy
4. Fatigue, related to early pregnancy
5. Health-Seeking Behaviors

Identify any possible additional nursing diagnoses.

 CRITICAL THINKING EXERCISE #12

Now that you have identified some nursing diagnoses for Mrs. Ramirez, develop a brief teaching plan for her, selecting a diagnosis from the previous section. Include learning outcomes and teaching strategies.

Case Study Follow-Up

Subsequent Prenatal Visits

Mrs. Ramirez is seen at regular intervals throughout her pregnancy. As described previously, her routine prenatal assessments include an interview to determine her general physiologic and emotional well-being, to answer questions, and to revise the birth plan, if needed. At each visit, Mrs. Ramirez is reminded of danger signs and symptoms and encouraged to continue her physical activity. Her physical examination consists of measurement of weight, pulse, respirations, blood pressure (sitting), and fundal height; and abdominal inspection and palpation. A clean-catch urine to test for glucose, protein, nitrites, and leukocytes is obtained. A hematocrit is obtained frequently. At 25 weeks, a routine glucose challenge screening for gestational diabetes is conducted and is within normal limits. Fundal height measurements show normal fetal growth and an ultrasound examination at 26 weeks reveals a healthy fetus.

Childbirth

In her 39th week, Mrs. Ramirez begins to experience regular uterine contractions that intensify with activity. Two hours after she arrives at the hospital, her membranes rupture; the following morning, she gives birth to a healthy baby girl, Carmen Lucretia, who weighs 7 pounds, 6 ounces. After the birth, Mrs. Ramirez and Carmen experienced no problems, and were discharged from the hospital 2 days later.

The Postpartal Assessment

Mrs. Ramirez, her mother, and Carmen arrive at the Women's Clinic 6 weeks later for the postpartal examination. Mrs. Ramirez is breastfeeding without difficulty, and reports that Carmen is gaining weight appropriately. She has had no problems and is smiling and cooing over the baby. Measurement of her weight reveals a 15-pound loss (her total weight gain during pregnancy was 26 pounds); her pulse, respirations, and blood pressure are all within normal limits. A clean-catch urine specimen is obtained and is negative. Her hemoglobin/hematocrit levels are consistent with her prenatal values. During the interview, she has no complaints, and states that she plans to return to work in 4 more weeks. Her mother and older sister will share child care, and she will continue to breastfeed Carmen. She is still taking prenatal vitamins. She is interested in the diaphragm as a method of contraception. She has not had a menstrual period since her delivery, and reports that her lochia progressed through the normal stages of lochia rubra, lochia serosa, and lochia alba, and now has ceased.

When conducting her physical assessment, you proceed from head to toe, beginning with her general appearance and vital signs.

Mrs. Ramirez is fitted with a diaphragm, instructed in its use and insertion and removal technique, which she is able to complete without difficulty. Because her prenatal Pap smear was normal, she is given a return appointment for 6 months for a routine follow-up visit.

Postpartal Physical Assessment

AREA/NORMAL VARIATIONS	ABNORMAL/RATIONALE
HEENT/*Neck*	
• Thyroid nonpalpable	• Thyromegaly. • *Palpable nodules:* Thyroiditis, hypothyroidism.
Respiratory	
• Equal bilateral breath sounds	• *Unequal bilateral breath sounds:* Infection.
Cardiovascular/*Heart*	
• Normal sinus rhythm	• Murmurs.
Extremities	
• Nontender, no swelling, no increased warmth to any area	• Phlebitis; varicosities.
Breasts	
• Lactating: Full, milk expressible	• Erythema, masses. • *Lymphadenopathy:* Mastitis.
• Nonlactating: Soft, without lymphadenopathy; bilateral galactorrhea (up to 3 months)	• *Hard, masses, lymphadenopathy:* Mastitis.
Gastrointestinal/Musculoskeletal	
• No tenderness, masses, hernias, enlarged lymph nodes; diastasis recti; uterus nonpalpable	• *Costovertebral angle tenderness (CVAT):* Kidney infection, subinvolution.

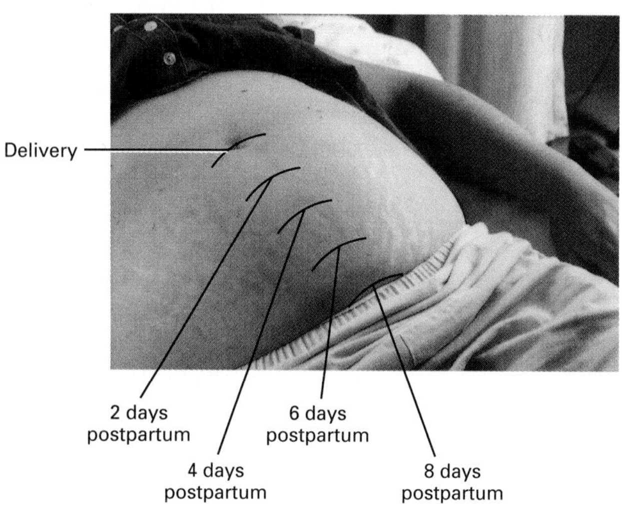

Fundal heights postpartum

AREA/NORMAL VARIATIONS	ABNORMAL/RATIONALE
Genitourinary/*External/Internal Genitalia*	
• No edema, lesions, tenderness; episiotomy site intact; internal cervical os closed; uterine corpus nonpregnant size	• Infection.

Research Tells Us

Saunas and hot tubs should be avoided during pregnancy and preconception because of embryo/fetal risks associated with hyperthermia. Because facilities that offer hot tubs and saunas often do not post pregnancy warnings, nurses have an important role in informing expectant women about the possible teratogenic effects of hyperthermia (Rogers & Davis, 1995).

Health Concerns

Complications can occur during each trimester of pregnancy.

Complications of Pregnancy

Signs/Symptoms	Possible Causes
First Trimester:	
Severe vomiting	Hyperemesis gravidarum
Chills, fever	Infection
Burning on urination	Infection
Abdominal cramping, bloating, vaginal bleeding	Spontaneous abortion, miscarriage
Second and Third Trimesters:	
Severe vomiting	Hyperemesis gravidarum
Leakage of amniotic fluid from vagina before labor begins	Premature rupture of membranes (PROM)
Vaginal bleeding, severe abdominal pain	Miscarriage, placental separation
Chills, fever, diarrhea, burning on urination	Infection
Change in fetal activity	Fetal distress, intrauterine fetal demise
Uterine contractions before due date (EDD)	Preterm labor
Visual disturbances: blurring, double vision, spots	Hypertensive disorders: PIH
Swelling of face, fingers, eye orbits, sacral area	PIH
Severe, frequent, or continuous headaches	PIH
Muscular irritability or convulsions (seizures)	PIH
Severe stomachache (epigastric pain)	PIH
Glucosuria, positive glucose tolerance test result	Gestational diabetes mellitus

Summary

- A thorough prenatal assessment provides invaluable data regarding the client's overall health status.
- Remember that the initial evaluation includes a thorough review of the client's health history as well as a careful physical examination. This first visit provides an excellent opportunity to screen for possible complications of pregnancy, as well as to lay the groundwork for a trusting relationship with the pregnant woman.
- Also keep in mind that pregnancy affects every body system. Before you begin the assessment, review normal anatomy and physiology, as well as changes that routinely occur during pregnancy so that you will be able to recognize abnormal findings.
- Always work in a systematic manner from apex to base and side to side. Establish a baseline, using the client as her own control (i.e., as a comparison throughout the pregnancy).
- After completing the assessment, document your findings; the plan for prenatal care should flow from your assessment and your findings with your client. This provides an excellent opportunity for teaching, and is an important beginning of the development of an individualized birth plan that meets the mother's needs and promotes a healthy pregnancy.
- Once the initial prenatal comprehensive assessment has been completed, routine follow-up prenatal visits usually include assessment of maternal weight, pulse, respirations, blood pressure (same arm, with the client sitting), urinalysis (glucose, protein, nitrites, and leukocytes), edema, fundal height, fetal heart tones. and fetal movement.

CHAPTER 22

Assessing the Newborn and Infant

Before You Begin

INTRODUCTION TO ASSESSING THE NEWBORN AND INFANT

Each newborn (birth to 30 days) arrives as a unique person with the energetic desire to grow and learn. For approximately 40 weeks, the fetus has enjoyed a warm, comfortable uterine environment with all needs met. At birth, he or she is totally dependent on the caretaker. Because the newborn is unable to directly communicate his or her needs, the nurse must learn assessment skills to identify abnormal findings and promote a healthy environment.

Infants (1 month to 11 months) have few communication skills. As they grow, they can smile, frown, point, and even say "no," but it will be several years before they can communicate well enough to provide information during a patient history. Until then, parents, siblings, and extended family are fine sources of information. Healthy families usually raise healthy babies, so take every opportunity to offer education and support during your assessment.

Anatomy and Physiology Review

Before you begin to examine a newborn or infant, you must have an understanding of the basic characteristics of this age group. These findings may vary slightly from child to child and change according to age and development. Use of standard measurement guidelines and physiologic assessments will assist you in your task.

Many physiologic changes occur at birth. Newborns begin their own oxygenation and circulatory efforts, and they must thermoregulate their bodies, ingest food, process nutrients, and expel wastes. They begin to interact mentally and physically with the surroundings.

Normal Newborn Physiologic Changes

AREA/SYSTEM CHANGE	CAUSES/RATIONALE
Integumentary	
• *Acrocyanosis (peripheral cyanosis):* Normal for 12 hours after birth	• Caused by thermoregulation adjustments.
• *Vernix caseosa:* White, cheesy substance of sebum and desquamated epithelium, seen in small amounts in skin folds of full-term babies	• Protects skin in utero.
• Desquamation (peeling of skin)	• As skin dries after delivery, peeling is normally seen within 2 days.
• *Cutis marmorata (mottled skin):* Seen in early infancy. If it persists, it may indicate congenital problems.	• Dilation of superficial vessels, not chilling.
• *Harlequin sign:* Dependent side red and nondependent side pale	• Positional color changes seen in low–birth-weight newborns.
• *Lanugo:* Fine, downy hair on face, shoulders, and back	• More common in premature infants.
Head	
• Bruises, lacerations, and temporary scalp and skull swelling may occur.	• Caused by physical stress of birth process. Increase in swelling may be caused by a hematoma or hydrocephalus.
Respiratory	
• Rapid, periodic breathing required for extrauterine life. Newborns begin nose breathing immediately at birth. Breathing helps remove birth fluids from respiratory tract. Respiration permits oxygenation.	• Respiration initiated by chemical and mechanical events of birth.
Circulatory	
• Onset of breathing stimulates transportation of oxygen. Shortly after first cry, heart rate accelerates.	• Blood pressure is highest immediately after birth.
Hepatic	
• At birth, liver takes a major role in iron storage, red cell production, carbohydrate metabolism, bilirubin conjugation, and coagulation.	• Immature liver often does not function well, resulting in high levels of bilirubin.

Normal Newborn Physiological Changes

AREA/SYSTEM CHANGE	CAUSES/RATIONALE
Gastrointestinal	
• Newborn has necessary enzyme activity and peristalsis to digest simple carbohydrates, fat, and protein. Stomach capacity is 50–60 mL. Stools are passed, often after a feeding.	• Feeding promotes peristalsis. Cardiac sphincter of stomach is immature and may be cause of regurgitation after feedings.
Urinary	
• Urination often occurs at birth or shortly after.	• Newborns are less able than adults to concentrate urine. Fluid intake enhances urination.
Musculoskeletal	
• Increased body movements are noted during reactive, awake phases.	• Behavioral and sensory abilities trigger movement and exploration.
Thermoregulation	
• Newborn strives to maintain body temperature. The large body mass enhances heat loss, which consumes oxygen and may cause respiratory distress.	• Body heat loss is caused by: • Convection: From body to cooler air. • Radiation: From body to cooler surfaces not in direct contact. • Evaporation: From body moisture to vapor. • Conduction: From direct skin to cooler surface.
Neurological	
• During first period of reactivity, newborns are alert and active.	• This phase lasts 30 minutes and is the natural inclination to search for a feeding.
• A sleep phase occurs after 30 minutes.	• This restorative phase lasts 2 to 4 hours.
• During second period of reactivity, newborn is awake and alert.	• Readiness for feeding is observed.

Circulatory Adaptation

Major changes occur at birth to transition blood flow from fetal to newborn circulation. Aortic pressure increases and venous pressure decreases. Systems pressure increases and pulmonary pressure decreases. Closure of the foramen ovale, ductus arteriosus, and ductus venosus occurs. Any variations in these changes may cause hypoxia and cyanosis. Figure 22–1 shows fetal circulation.

Hepatic Adaptation

Newborns have immature livers that cannot break down products of hemolysis easily. Bilirubin, a byproduct of this process, consequently builds up in the blood and cannot be excreted well though urine and feces. This results in jaundice—yellow-tinged skin, sclera, or mucous membranes. Prolonged high levels of bilirubin can cause mental and developmental delays. Physiologic jaundice does not become apparent until after the newborn is 24 hours old.

Developmental, Cultural, and Ethnic Variations

As you perform your assessment, keep in mind the rapid developmental changes that occur during the first year of life and note any variations from the norm. Also remember that infants of different races and ethnic groups have different physical characteristics. Last, be aware of cultural variations that may affect parenting.

Developmental Considerations

During the first year of life, the infant experiences rapid growth and developmental changes. Many physical, gross motor, fine motor, primitive reflex, sensory, communication, and socialization changes are seen. During the first year of life, psychosocial development focuses on establishing trust. Trust is established trust when the infant senses that his or her needs are being met.

Cognitive development during the first year of life is also called the sensorimotor phase of development. The

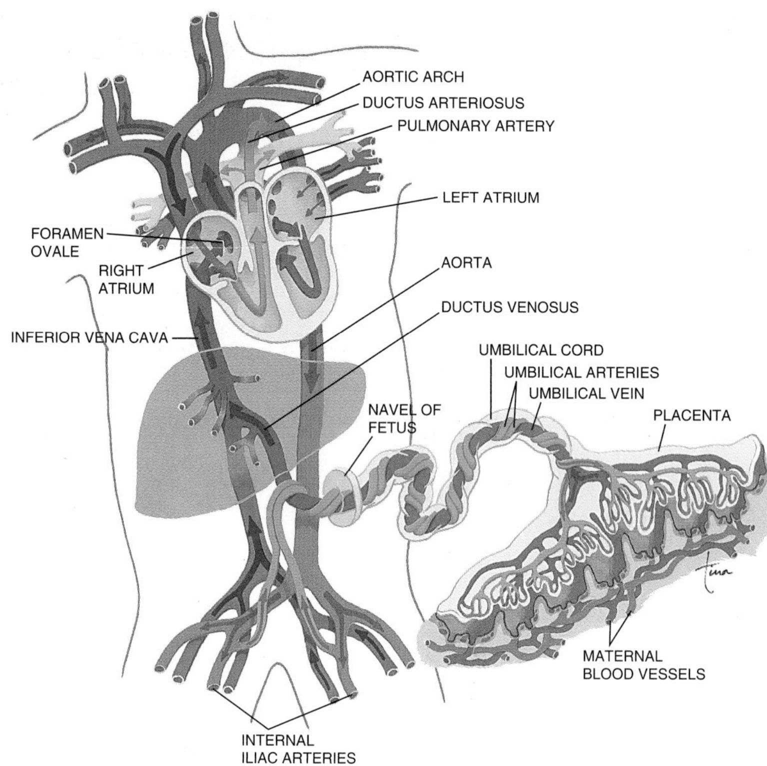

FIGURE 22–1. Fetal circulation.

three major tasks during this phase are separation, realizing that self is separate from other objects; object permanence, realizing that objects are permanent even when not in sight; and mental representation, recognizing symbols of objects without actually experiencing the object. The infant also is developing a body image by exploring and playing with different parts of his or her body.

Social development at this age includes developing attachment to parents or caregivers and experiencing separation anxiety and fear of strangers.

Communication and language development also occurs during the first year. The Denver Developmental Screening Test–II (DDST-II) and growth charts are frequently used to assess and track the growth and development of the infant during well-baby checkups.

As you assess the infant, be sure to note if his or her physical development is appropriate for his or her age and whether he or she is performing appropriate developmental tasks for that age. Because growth and development are so rapid during the first year of life, even the slightest developmental delay may signal an underlying problem and warrant further investigation.

Key physical changes include:

- Birth weight doubles by 6 months, triples by 12 months.
- Height increases by 1 inch per month for first 6 months.
- Fontanels are closing.
- Lumbar curve develops with a lordosis once the infant begins to walk.
- Drooling and teething occur.
- Primitive reflexes disappear as neurological system matures.

Gross motor changes include:

- Rolls, crawls
- Pulls self up to sit
- Begins to walk
- Achieves head control

Fine motor changes include:

- Grasps objects
- Puts objects in mouth
- Holds bottle
- Plays with toes
- Develops pincer grasp

Sensory changes include:

- Develops better vision
- Follows objects with eyes
- Responds to sounds

Communication changes include:

- Initially cries to convey needs
- Babbles

- Laughs
- Says 3 to 5 words by 12 months
- Begins to comprehend simple directions
- Imitates sounds

Socializaton changes include:

- Identifies parents
- Develops social smile
- Is aware of strange situations
- Has increasing difficulty separating from parents
- Becomes more fearful of strangers
- Begins to develop memory
- Shows emotions

Cultural and Ethnic Considerations

Cultural or ethnic influences may affect your assessment findings. You need to be aware of these normal variations so that you do not mistake them for abnormal findings. Cultural or ethnic influences may also affect the relationship between child and parent and define the roles of both parent and child within the family.

Cultural and Ethnic Variations in Infants

CULTURAL GROUP	INFLUENCE
African-American	Mongolian spots and other birthmarks more prevalent than in other ethnic groups.
Amish	Babies seen as gifts from God. Have high birth rates, large families.
Appalachian	Newborns wear bands around abdomen to prevent umbilical hernias and asafetida bags around neck to prevent contagious diseases.
Arab-American	Children "dearly loved." Male circumcision is a religious requirement.
Chinese-American	Children highly valued because of one-child rule in China. Mongolian spots occur in about 80% of infants. Bilirubin levels higher in Chinese newborns than others, with highest levels seen day 5 or 6.
Cuban-American	Childbirth is a celebration. Family takes care of both mother and infant for the first 4 weeks. Tend to bottle-feed rather than breastfeed. If breastfeeding, weaning is early, around 3 months. If bottle feeding, weaning is late, around 4 years.
Egyptian-American	Children very important. Mother and infant cared for by family for the first 50 days.
Filipino-American	Eyes almond shaped, low to flat nose bridge with mildly flared nostrils. Mongolian spots common.
French-Canadian	Five mutations account for 90% of phenylketonuria (PKU) in French Canadians. High incidence of cystic fibrosis and muscular dystrophy.
Greek-American	High incidence of two genetic conditions: thalassemia and glucose-6-phosphate dehydrogenase (G-6PD).
Iranian-American	Believe in hot/cold influences, with baby boys "hotter" than baby girls. Infant may be confined to home for first 40 days. Ritual bath between 10th and 40th day.
Jewish-American	Children seen as valued treasure. High incidence of Tay-Sachs disease. Male circumcision is a religious ritual.
Mexican-American	Wears stomach belt *(ombliguero)* to prevent umbilicus from popping out when infant cries. Believe that cutting nails in the first 3 months after birth causes blindness and deafness.
Navajo Native American	Infants kept in cradle boards until they can walk. Mongolian spots common.
Vietnamese-American	Mongolian spots common.

Source: Purnell and Paulanka, 1998)

Introducing the Case Study

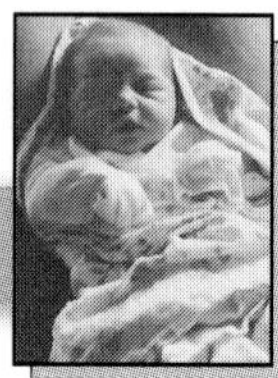

As you recall from the previous chapter, Mrs. Ramirez gave birth to a baby girl, Carmen. Carmen is now 2 hours old. Her mother had a normal vaginal delivery, and you are admitting them both to the postpartum unit. You assessed Mrs. Ramirez and noted normal vital signs, firm uterus, intact perineum, and moderate lochia rubra. She breastfed Carmen in the delivery room. You also obtained Apgar scores for Carmen of 8 at 1 minute and 10 at 5 minutes. Now you will assess Carmen more thoroughly. When you change her diaper, you note that she has voided and passed a meconium stool.

Performing the Initial Newborn Assessment

The initial newborn assessment consists of obtaining an Apgar score immediately after birth, taking a health history, and then performing a physical assessment that includes a general survey, head-to-toe assessment, and tests for reflexes. Depending on the newborn's condition, certain diagnostic and screening tests may also be performed.

Apgar Score

Assess the newborn's physiologic and cardiopulmonary status immediately after birth. The Apgar score assesses five vital areas: heart rate, respiration, color, muscle tone, and reflex irritability. A score from 0 to 2 is assigned to each category for a score range of 0 to 10. This score is obtained at 1 and 5 minutes after birth. A score of 8 to 10 is excellent, 4 to 7 is guarded, and 0 to 3 is critical.

Newborn Health History

The newborn's health history addresses two main areas: prenatal health and labor and delivery. The focus of prenatal health is on the mother's prenatal care, obstetrical history; use of medications; and use of tobacco, alcohol, and drugs. Labor and delivery addresses gestational week at time of delivery, duration of labor, type of delivery, and type of anesthesia.

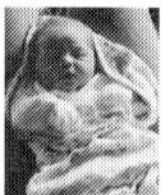

Case Study Findings

Newborn Carmen's health history reveals:

- 39 weeks gestation, gravida 1/para 1

Apgar Score

Heart Rate	0 = absent	1 = <100 beats/ minute	2 = >100 beats/ minute
Respirations	0 = absent	1 = <30, irregular	2 = strong cry, regular
Muscle Tone	0 = flaccid	1 = some flexion in arms and legs	2 = full flexion, active movement
Reflex Irritability	0 = no response	1 = grimace, weak cry	Vigorous cry
Color	0 = pale, blue	1 = body pink, extremities blue	2 = totally pink

Newborn Health History

HEALTH HISTORY	SIGNIFICANCE
• General health, prenatal diseases or conditions, prenatal care, number of pregnancies	• Maternal health problems (e.g., gestational diabetes, cardiac or kidney disease) may cause potential risk factors in newborn.
• Use of prescribed or OTC medications, tobacco, alcohol, illegal drugs	• Medications and other agents may affect physiologic systems (e.g., smoking during pregnancy related to low birth weights, alcohol use related to fetal alcohol syndrome [FAS]).
• Duration of pregnancy and labor, type of anesthesia, type of delivery, complications	• Details of labor and delivery alert nurse to observe for potential newborn problems.

- Positive prenatal care
- Mother generally healthy, no history of medical problems
- No prenatal diseases
- No history of smoking, drug or alcohol abuse in mother
- Prenatal vitamins once a day
- 16-hour labor, uncomplicated vaginal delivery
- Epidural anesthesia
- First-degree laceration and midline episiotomy
- Parents Cuban-American, bilingual.

Newborn Physical Assessment

Now, proceed to the newborn physical assessment. Keep your history findings in mind and combine them with the physical examination findings to form a total picture of the newborn.

Approach

Use your senses of sight, smell, hearing, and touch along with all four techniques of physical assessment. Remember that your equipment and techniques will have to be adjusted for the size of your client. In addition, instead of proceeding from head to toe, adapt your assessment sequence to fit the newborn's needs. For example, move techniques that may evoke crying—such as the otoscopic examination—to the end of the assessment. Also be sure to keep the room and the baby warm.

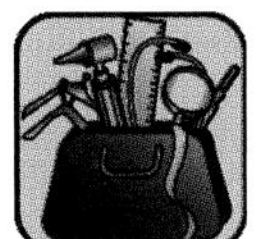

Toolbox

Gather the following equipment: Tape measure, stethoscope, thermometer, blood pressure cuff, penlight, otoscope, and ophthalmoscope. You will also need a baby scale.

Performing a General Survey

Before you perform your head-to-toe assessment of the newborn, ask yourself the following questions and record your observations as baseline data.

- **Integumentary:** Are there any abrasions, lacerations, or birthmarks? If so, describe them, and monitor for infection, bleeding, and trauma.
- **Head/Neck:** Are there masses on the head or neck? These may indicate cephalohematoma or a fractured clavicle.
- **Eyes/Ears/Nose/Mouth/Throat:** Is there exudate in the eyes? If so, monitor for infection. Is the baby blinking? Do his or her eyes follow an object within 8 inches? Is there discharge from the ears, nose, and throat or nose congestion? Fluid may be from delivery or could indicate infection. Does the newborn respond to sound? A reaction to sound should occur.

ALERT

Babies are obligatory nose breathers, so clear secretions from nose to ease breathing.

- **Respiratory Characteristics, Lungs, and Breathing:** Is the newborn congested or gasping for breath? Fetal fluid that remains in the lungs can cause airway obstruction.
- **Cardiovascular Characteristics:** Is there cyanosis? It may denote poor vascular profusion. Is the newborn alert? A newborn in difficulty will demonstrate irritability or be unarousable.
- **Temperature Regulation:** Is body temperature maintained? Newborns are poor regulators of body temperature and are dependent on their environment for warmth. Cold stress can cause respiratory distress.
- **Hepatic Regulation:** Does the newborn have jaundice? Increasing jaundice denotes increased blood bilirubin, which can cause mental deterioration if untreated.

ALERT

Jaundice within 24 hours of birth is pathological jaundice; jaundice after 24 hours is probably physiologic jaundice.

- **Gastrointestinal Adaptation:** Has the newborn passed stool? This proves that an anus is present. Has he or she vomited? Persistent vomiting suggests intestinal obstruction.
- **Genitourinary Adaptation:** Has the baby voided? Voiding denotes kidney function.
- **Neurological Characteristics:** How are extremities moving? Muscle tone should be symmetrical and not flaccid, extremities should be partially flexed; hand-mouth behavior should be evident; and when awake, newborn should demonstrate random, purposeless, bilateral movements. How does cry sound? It should be loud, not high pitched or weak.
- **Endocrine Characteristics:** Is there evidence of fetal or maternal endocrine disease? Is newborn jittery? Maternal diabetes can cause severe hypoglycemia in the newborn. Low glucose levels often manifest as jittery extremities.
- **Immunological Adaptation:** Are defenses maintained? Because the newborn's immune response is not well established, protect portals of entry (umbilical stump and breaks in skin) from infection.

- **Sleep and Rest Patterns:** What is the sleep pattern? Newborns sleep up to 18 hours a day. The long sleep period promotes growth and development. They should awaken for feedings every 3 to 4 hours.
- **Relationships/Psychosocial Profile/Cultural/Ethnic Variations:** How are family members relating to the newborn? The newborn is dependent on the family for its well-being. Parents should demonstrate touching and holding of infant. Assist in the bonding process. Responses may vary depending on cultural/ethnic variations.

Performing a Head-to-Toe Physical Assessment

Next, perform a head-to-toe physical assessment of the newborn.

Performing a Newborn Head-to-Toe Physical Assessment

AREA/SYSTEM/NORMAL VARIATIONS	ABNORMAL FINDINGS/RATIONALE
Posture • Head and extremities flexed.	• *Limp posture with extension of extremities:* Associated with birth injuries, anesthesia, acidosis, hypoglycemia, hypothermia, or congenital problems.
Head Circumference 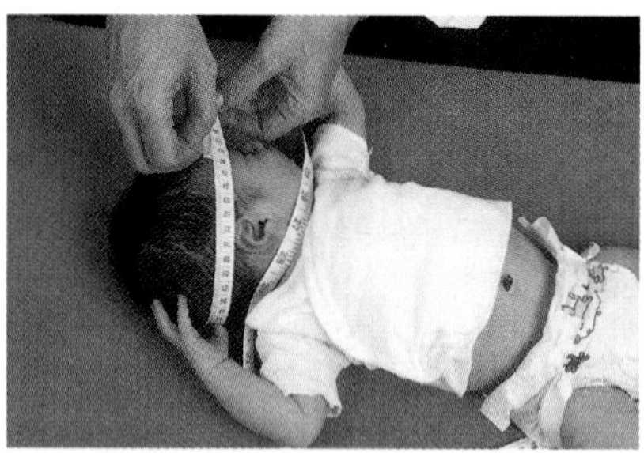 **Measuring head circumference** • 33–35 cm	• *Head circumference < 10% of normal:* Microcephaly related to congenital malformation or infection. • Head *circumference > 90% of normal: Macrocephaly* related to hydrocephalus.

HELPFUL HINT
Measure head circumference from occiput to forehead.

AREA/SYSTEM/NORMAL VARIATIONS	ABNORMAL FINDINGS/RATIONALE
Chest Circumference 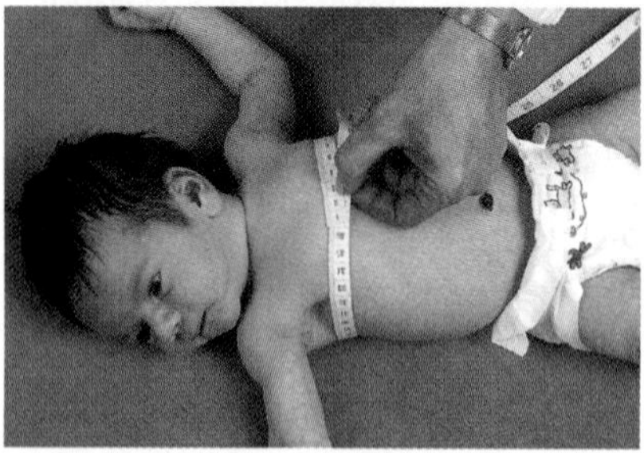 **Measuring chest circumference** • 30.5–33 cm (2–3 cm less than head) • Breast engorgement can affect measurement.	

HELPFUL HINT
Measure chest at nipple line.

Performing a Newborn Head-to-Toe Physical Assessment

AREA/SYSTEM/NORMAL VARIATIONS	ABNORMAL FINDINGS/RATIONALE

Abdominal Circumference

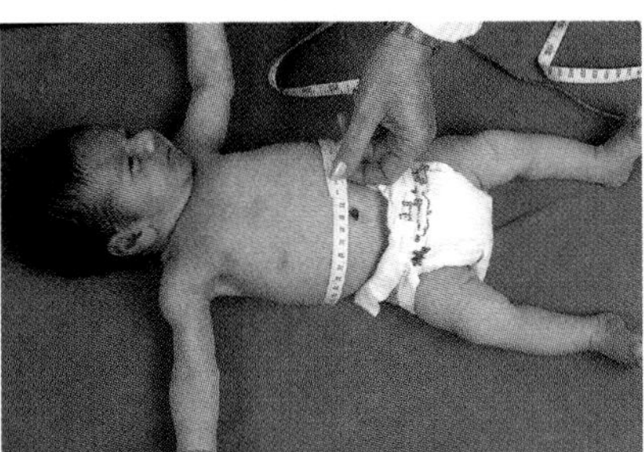

Measuring abdominal circumference

- Similar to chest measurement. Should not be distended.

HELPFUL HINT

Measure abdomen above the umbilicus.

Length

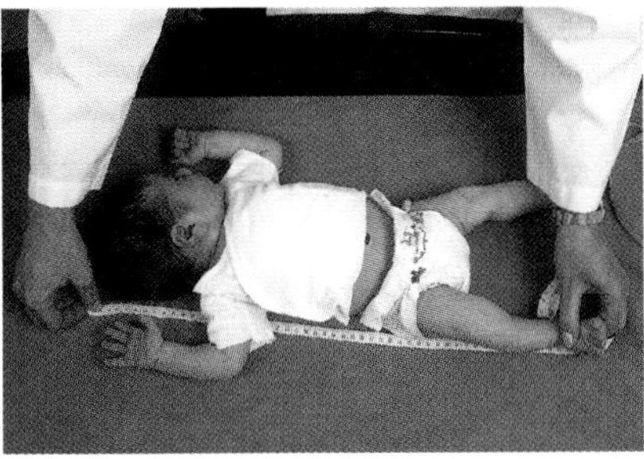

Measuring length

- Crown to rump: 31–35 cm (about equal to head circumference).
- Head to heel: 45–55 cm (18–22 inches) at birth.
- Molding can affect measurement.

Weight

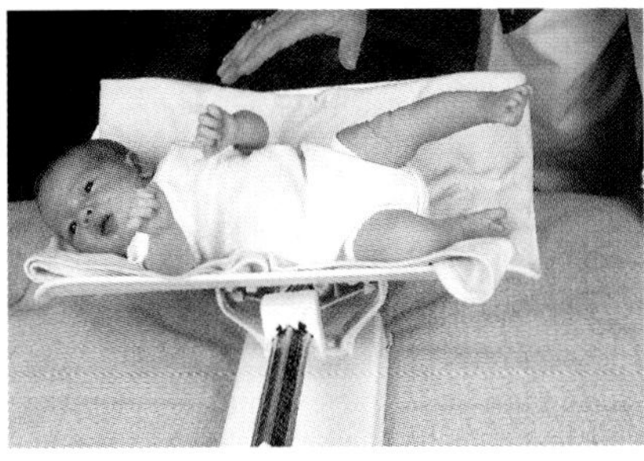

Weighing infant

- Newborn weight is usually between 2500 and 4000 g (5 lb, 8 oz and 8 lb, 13 oz).

Abnormal findings/rationale (Weight):

- Birth weights <10% or >90% are abnormal.
- *Low birth weight (small for gestational age):* Associated with prematurity.

(Continued)

Performing a Newborn Head-to-Toe Physical Assessment *(Continued)*

AREA/SYSTEM/NORMAL VARIATIONS	ABNORMAL FINDINGS/RATIONALE
Weight *(Continued)*	• *Macrosomic infant (large for gestational age):* Associated with gestational diabetes in mother.
Temperature • Axillary: 36.5–37.2°C	• Hypothermia leads to cold stress. Sepsis, environmental extremes, and neurological problems can cause hypothermia or hyperthermia.
Pulse • Apical rate 120–160 BPM • Rate increases with crying and decreases with sleep.	• Irregular rhythms such as bradycardia (<100 BPM) and tachycardia (>160 BPM). • Most murmurs are not pathological and disappear by age 6 months.
Respirations • 30–60 breaths a minute; irregular. • Anesthesia during labor and delivery can affect respirations.	• Respirations <30 or >60 breaths a minute. • Periods of apnea >15 seconds.
Blood Pressure (BP) • Systolic: 50–75 mm Hg • Diastolic: 30–45 mm Hg • Crying and moving increase systolic pressure.	• *Low BP:* May be caused by hypovolemia. • Late clamping of umbilical cord can increase BP because of expanded blood volume from the "placental transfusion."
Integumentary/*Skin* *INSPECT* • Skin may be red, smooth, edematous, mottled (cutis marmorata). • Hands and feet may be cyanotic (acrocyanosis). • Physiologic jaundice occurs after 24 hours. • Color may change with position (Harlequin sign). • Cheesy substance (vernix caseosa) decreases as baby's gestational age increases to term. • Desquamation (peeling), ecchymosis, and petechiae may occur from trauma during delivery. • Milia (white papules) may occur on face. • Miliaria or audamina (papules or vesicles on face) are caused by blocked sweat ducts. • Mongolian spots (bluish discoloration in sacral area) are commonly seen in African, Asian, Latin, and Native American babies. • Telangiectatic nevi • Flat hemangiomas ("stork bites") may be present at nape of neck.	• *Persistent acrocyanosis:* May indicate thermoregulation problem or hypoglycemia. • *Extensive desquamation:* Seen in post-term baby. • Pathological jaundice occurs within first 24 hours. • *Plethora:* May indicate polycythemia. • *Pallor:* May indicate anemia, hypothermia, shock, or sepsis. • *Persistent ecchymosis or petechiae:* May be caused by thrombocytopenia, sepsis, or congenital infection.

Performing a Newborn Head-to-Toe Physical Assessment

AREA/SYSTEM/NORMAL VARIATIONS

Integumentary/*Skin (Continued)*

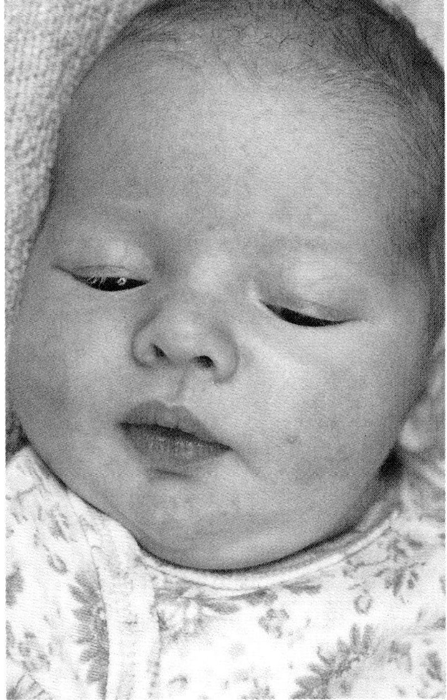

Milia

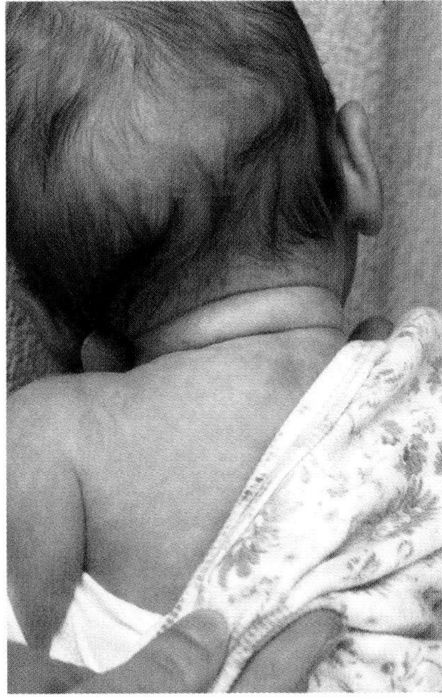

Stork bite

Integumentary/*Hair*

- Some lanugo is normal.

ABNORMAL FINDINGS/RATIONALE

- *Poor turgor:* Intrauterine growth retardation or hypoglycemia.
- *Café-au-lait spots (light brown spots:* If more than 6 or larger than 4 × 6 cm, may indicate neurofibromatosis and can become precancerous with age.
- *Nevus flammeus (port-wine stain):* Disfigures face and may be associated with cerebral vascular malformation.
- Giant hemangiomas and nevus vasculosus ("strawberry marks") tend to trap platelets and lower circulating platelet counts. They usually disappear by age 5.
- Reddish-blue round mass of blood vessels (cavernous hemangioma) must be monitored, and if size increases, surgery may be necessary.
- Erythema toxicum, a common newborn rash of red macules and papules, usually disappears in 1 week.

(Continued)

Performing a Newborn Head-to-Toe Physical Assessment *(Continued)*

AREA/SYSTEM/NORMAL VARIATIONS	ABNORMAL FINDINGS/RATIONALE
Integumentary/*Hair (Continued)*	• *Bullae or pustules:* May indicate infections such as syphilis or staphylococcus. • Thin, translucent skin and vernix caseosa are signs of prematurity. • Genetic disorders may cause extra skin folds. • Abundant lanugo is a sign of prematurity. • Genetic disorders may cause abnormal hair distribution unrelated to gestational age.
Integumentary/*Nails*	• Long nails are seen in post-term babies.
HEENT *Head/Face* *INSPECT/PALPATE*	• Fused sutures. • *Large fontanels:* Associated with hydrocephaly, osteogenesis imperfecta, congenital hypothyroidism. • *Small fontanels:* Associated with microcephaly.

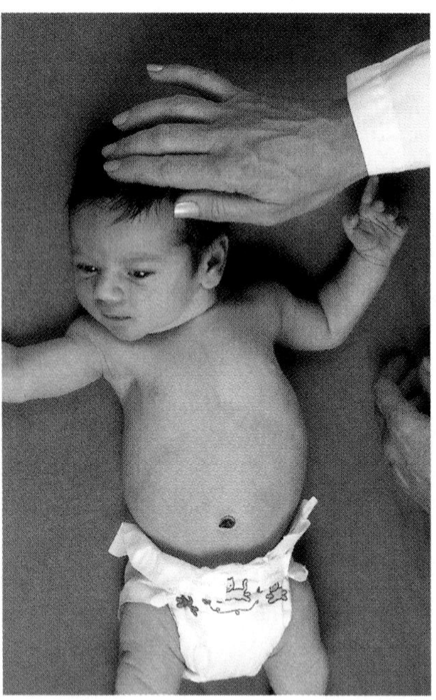

Palpating fontanel

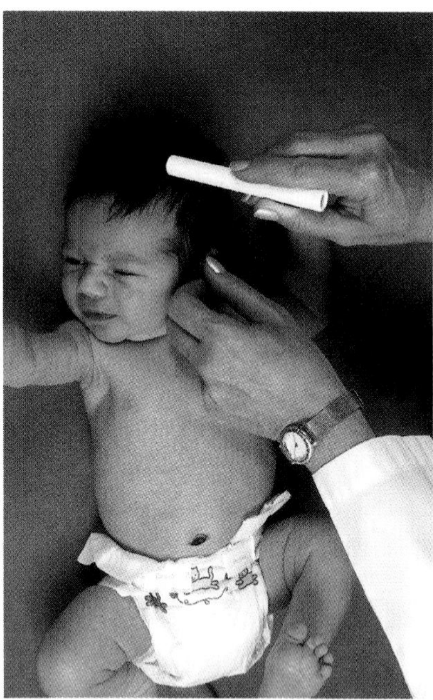

Transilluminating fontanel

- Molding in birth canal may cause asymmetry of face and skull and should resolve within 1 week.
- Anterior fontanel: Diamond shaped, 2.5–4 cm
- Posterior fontanel: Triangle shaped, 0.5–1 cm
- Soft and flat

Performing a Newborn Head-to-Toe Physical Assessment

AREA/SYSTEM/NORMAL VARIATIONS	ABNORMAL FINDINGS/RATIONALE
	• *Bulging fontanels:* May indicate increased intracranial pressure.
• Symmetrical facial movements	• *Depressed fontanels:* Associated with dehydration. • Craniosynostosis (premature closure of the sutures). • Cephalohematoma (hematoma between periosteum and skull with unilateral swelling). • Most uncomplicated cephalohematomas totally resolve within 2 weeks to 3 months. • Caput succedaneum (edema of soft scalp tissue from birth trauma) decreases gradually in several days. • *Asymmetrical facial movements:* May result from damage to facial nerve during forceps delivery.
HEENT/*Neck* *INSPECT/PALPATE* • Positive tonic reflex • Short neck • Able to hold head up with "pull-to-sit" test.	• *Absent tonic reflex:* Erb's palsy if unilateral or dislocation of cervical spine or fractured clavicle. • *Head lag with "pull-to-sit" test:* Muscle weakness. • Torticollis (wry neck).
HEENT/*Eyes* *INSPECT* 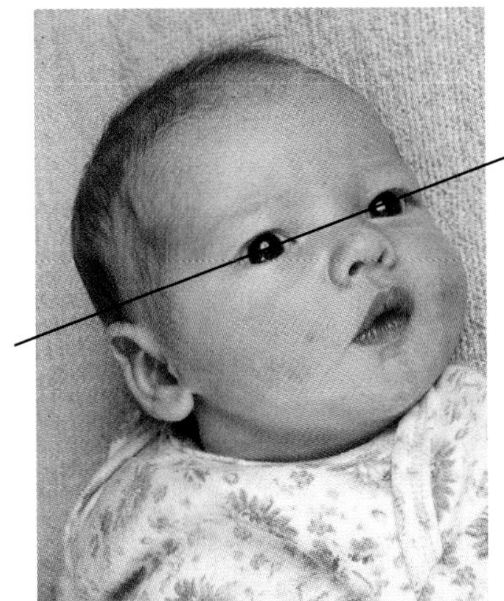 **Normal eye line**	• *Subconjunctival hemorrhage:* Trauma during delivery. • *Brushfield spots (speckling of iris), epicanthal fold, and Mongolian slant:* Down syndrome. • *Absent red light reflex:* May indicate congenital cataract. • *Ptosis:* Neuromuscular weakness. • *Sun-setting (crescent of sclera over iris caused by retraction of upper lid):* Hydrocephalus. • *Yellow sclera:* Jaundice. • *Blue sclera:* Osteogenesis imperfecta.

(Continued)

Performing a Newborn Head-to-Toe Physical Assessment *(Continued)*

AREA/SYSTEM/NORMAL VARIATIONS

HEENT/*Eyes (Continued)*

HELPFUL HINT

Avoid bright light because it will cause the newborn to avoid opening his or her eyes and make assessment difficult.

- Eyes may be edematous after vaginal delivery.
- Eyes equal and symmetrical.
- Blue/gray or brown iris; white or bluish-white sclera.
- Antimongolian slant; Mongolian slant seen in Asian infants.
- Positive red light reflex
- Positive blink reflex
- Positive corneal reflex
- No tears (tear production begins by 2 months).
- Positive fixation on close objects.
- Positive pupillary reaction to light.
- Strabismus and searching nystagmus caused by immature muscular control.

ABNORMAL FINDINGS/RATIONALE

- *Persistent nystagmus, absent blink reflex, inability to follow objects:* May indicate vision problem, such as blindness.
- *Dilated or fixed pupil:* May indicate anoxia or neurological damage.
- Chemical conjunctivitis from eye prophylaxis may occur during first 24 hours.

HEENT/*Ears*

INSPECT/PALPATE/TEST HEARING

- Pinna flexible, without deformity, aligns with external canthus of eyes.
- Positive startle reflex.

American Academy of Pediatrics recommends hearing screening by auditory brainstem response or evoked otoacoustic emissions on newborns before discharge.

- *Low-set ears:* Down syndrome.

ALERT

The ears and kidneys develop at the same time in utero, so malformed ears may be accompanied by renal problems.

- *Absent startle reflex:* Possible hearing problem.

HEENT/*Nose*

INSPECT

- Nares patent
- Small amount of thin white mucus
- Nose may be flattened and bruised from birth

- Because infants are obligatory nose breathers, large amounts of mucus drainage may obstruct nostrils and cause respiratory difficulty.
- *Nasal flaring:* Sign of distress.

Performing a Newborn Head-to-Toe Physical Assessment

AREA/SYSTEM/NORMAL VARIATIONS

HEENT/*Mouth/Throat*

INSPECT

- Mucous membranes pink and moist.
- Frenulum of tongue and lip intact.
- Palate intact, uvula midline
- Strong sucking reflex, positive rooting, gag, extrusion, and swallowing reflexes.
- Minimal saliva
- Strong cry
- Natal teeth may be benign or associated with congenital defects.

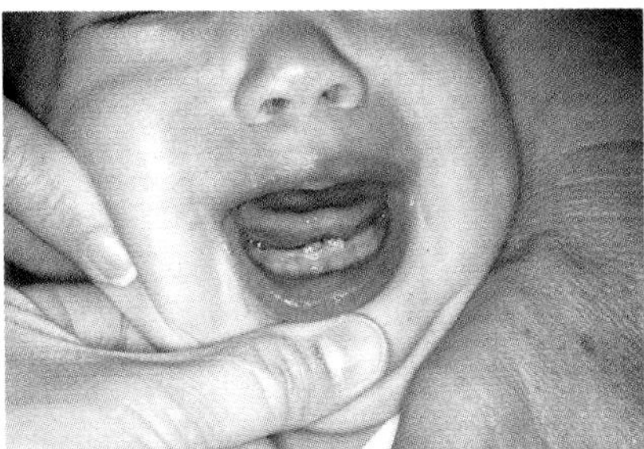

Natal teeth

ALERT

Natal teeth must be removed by a specialist because they usually fall out and can cause choking.

Small white, pearl-like epithelial cysts on the palate (Epstein's pearls) disappear within a few weeks.

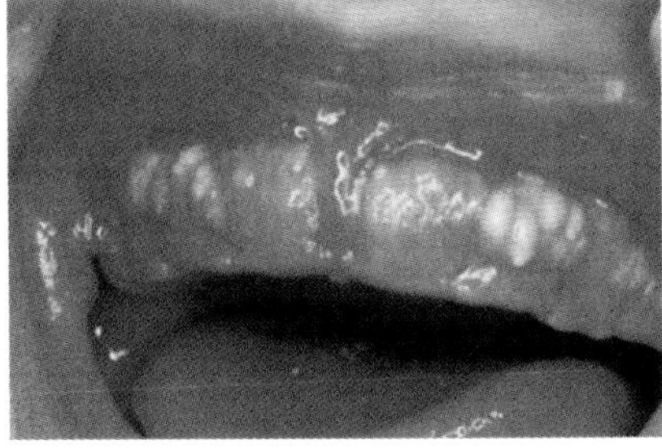

Epstein's pearls

ABNORMAL FINDINGS/RATIONALE

- *Cyanotic mucous membranes:* Hypoxia
- *Candida albicans (thrush):* Contracted during vaginal delivery.

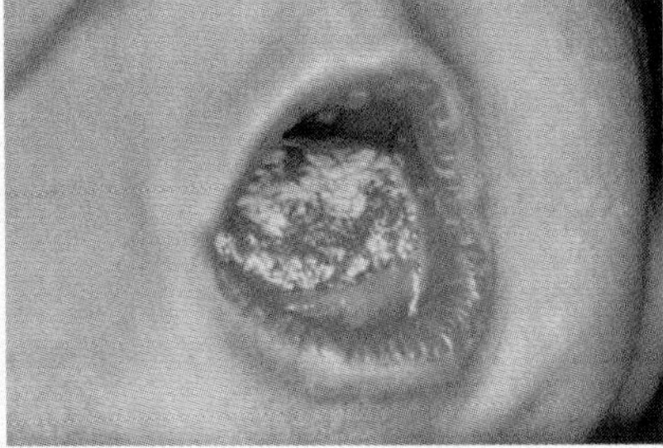

Thrush

Weak sucking, swallowing reflex: May be caused by maternal anesthesia or perinatal asphyxia.

- *Opening in palate or lips:* Cleft palate or lip. Any opening is abnormal. A series of surgical interventions will be necessary.

ALERT

Cleft lip or palate will cause newborn to have difficulty with feeding.

Weak cry: May indicate neuromuscular problem, hypotonia, and prematurity.

(Continued)

Performing a Newborn Head-to-Toe Physical Assessment *(Continued)*

AREA/SYSTEM/NORMAL VARIATIONS | **ABNORMAL FINDINGS/RATIONALE**

Chest

INSPECT/AUSCULTATE

- Anteroposterior: lateral (1:1).
- Equal chest excursion.
- Breast engorgement.
- Clear or milky liquid from nipples ("witch's milk") develops from maternal hormones in utero.
- Supernumerary nipples are a benign finding.

Abnormal findings/rationale:

- Funnel chest *(pectus excavatum):* Congenital anomaly.
- *Pigeon chest (pectus carinatum):* Obstructed respiration in infancy.
- *Asymmetrical excursion, retraction:* Respiratory distress.
- Red, firm nipples.

Respiratory

AUSCULTATE

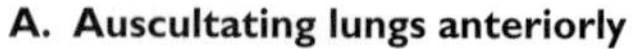

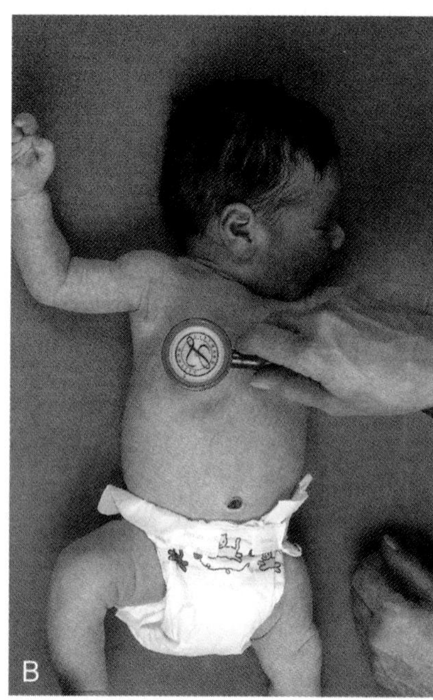

A. Auscultating lungs anteriorly **B. Auscultating lungs posteriorly**

- Lungs clear, bronchial breath sounds audible
- Cough reflex absent at birth, but present 1–2 days later
- Scattered crackles a few hours after birth.

Abnormal findings/rationale:

- Persistent crackles, wheezes, stridor, grunting, paradoxical breathing, decreased breath sounds, prolonged periods of apnea (>15–20 seconds) are signs of respiratory problems.

Cardiac

AUSCULTATE

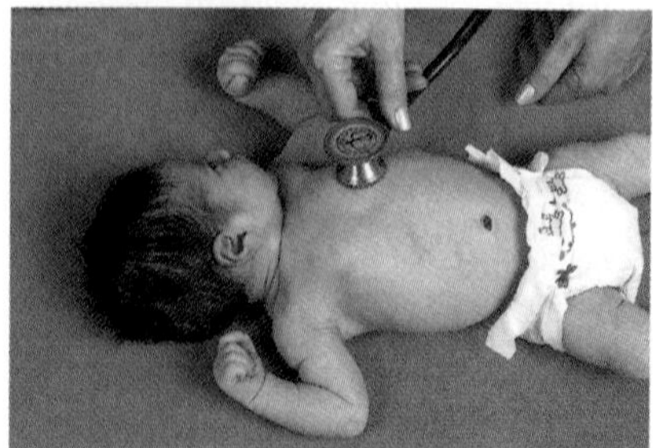

Auscultating heart

Abnormal findings/rationale:

- Dextrocardia (heart on right side).
- *Cardiomegaly:* Displaced PMI.
- Murmurs are often heard at base or along left sternal border, and are usually benign, but need to be evaluated to rule out cardiac disorder.
- Thrills.

Performing a Newborn Head-to-Toe Physical Assessment

AREA/SYSTEM/NORMAL VARIATIONS	ABNORMAL FINDINGS/RATIONALE

Cardiac *(Continued)*

- S_1, S_2, normal rhythm with respiratory variations.
- Point of maximal impulse (PMI) 4th left intercostal space midcostal line (MCL).
- Quiet but clearly audible murmurs occur in 30% of newborns but should disappear in 2 days.

Abdomen

INSPECT/PALPATE

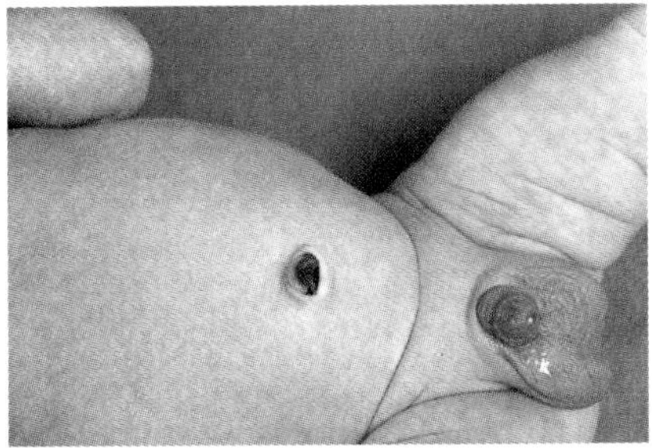

Inspecting cord

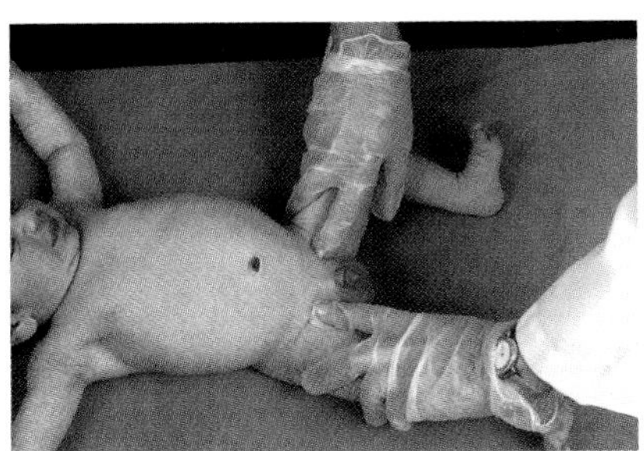

Palpating femoral pulse

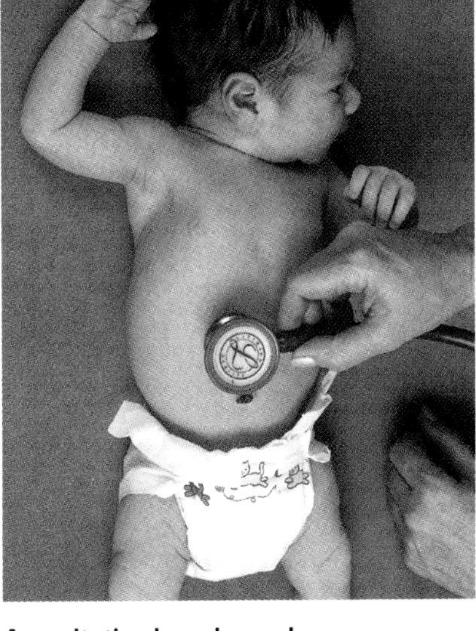

Auscultating bowel sounds

- Abdomen round
- Positive bowel sounds
- Liver edge palpable 2–3 cm
- Tip of spleen, kidneys palpable
- Cord bluish white with two arteries and one vein
- Positive femoral pulses.
- Umbilical hernias and diastasis recti (separation of rectus muscles) more common in African-American infants and often resolves within a year.

Abnormal findings:

- *Abdominal distention, ascites, distended veins:* May indicate portal hypertension.
- *Green umbilical cord:* May indicate infection.
- *Absence of umbilical vessels:* Associated with heart and kidney malformations.

Rectum

INSPECT

- Anus patent
- Passage of meconium stool within 48 hours
- Positive anal reflex ("anal wink")

Abnormal findings:

- Anal fissures or fistulas.
- *No stools:* May indicate malformation in GI tract.

ALERT

Imperforate anus (absent anus) requires immediate surgical repair.

(Continued)

Performing a Newborn Head-to-Toe Physical Assessment *(Continued)*

AREA/SYSTEM/NORMAL VARIATIONS	ABNORMAL FINDINGS/RATIONALE
Female Genitalia *INSPECT/PALPATE* • Urination within 24 hours. • Urinary meatus is midline and an uninterrupted stream is noted on voiding. • Labia majora and minora may be edematous. Place thumbs on either side of labia and gently separate tissues to visualize perineum • Blood-tinged vaginal fluid may be noted (pseudomenstruation). • Note presence of clitoris, vagina, and hymen.	• Fused labia or absent vaginal opening • Ambiguous genitalia • Meconium from vaginal opening • Inability to urinate within 24 hours **ALERT** *A newborn clitoris larger than 0.5 cm is abnormal.*
Male Genitalia *INSPECT/PALPATE* 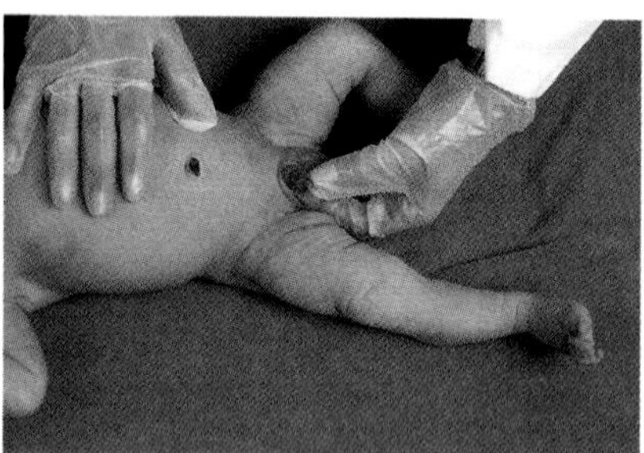 **Palpating scrotum** • Urination within 24 hours • Foreskin retracts • Urethral opening at tip of penis • Scrotum edematous • Smegma • Palpable testes	• Hypospadias (urethral opening on ventral surface of penis) • Epispadias (urethral opening on dorsal side of penis) • Chordee (ventrally curved penis) • Hydrocele (fluid in scrotum) • Inability to urinate within 24 hours • Inability to retract foreskin • Undescended testicles • Inguinal hernia • Ambiguous genitalia • Meconium from scrotum
Musculoskeletal *INSPECT/PALPATE* 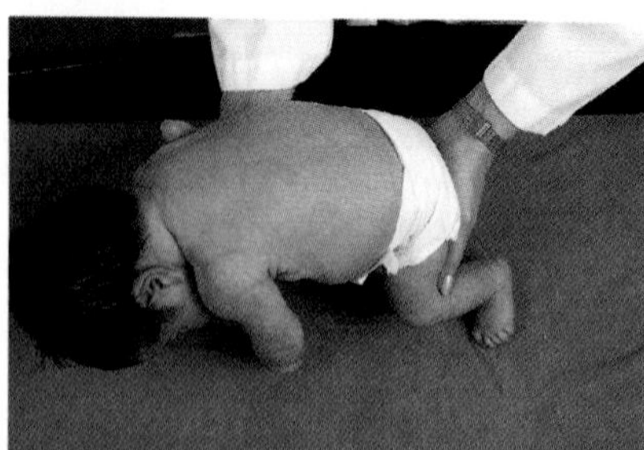 **Checking for C curve** 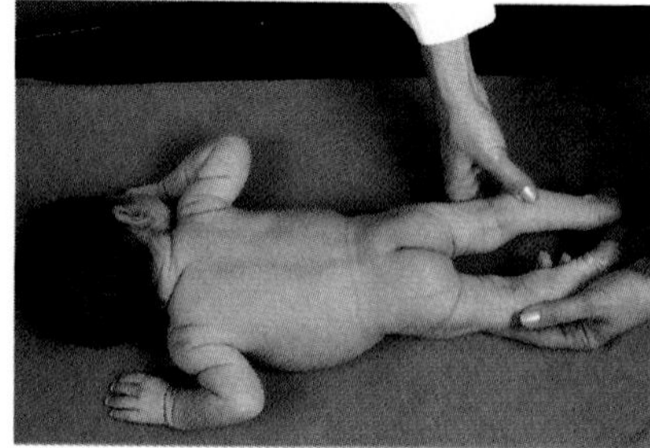 **Checking gluteal folds**	• *Polydactyly:* Extra digits. • *Syndactyly:* Webbed digits. • *Phocomelia:* Hands and feet attached close to chest. • *Hemimelia:* Absence of distal part of extremity. • *Talipes (clubfoot):* Foot permanently twisted out of shape. • Severe bowing of legs is abnormal. • *Unequal gluteal folds and positive Barlow-Ortolani maneuver:* Associated with congenital hip dislocation. Requires immediate referral.

Performing a Newborn Head-to-Toe Physical Assessment

AREA/SYSTEM/NORMAL VARIATIONS

Musculoskeletal *(Continued)*

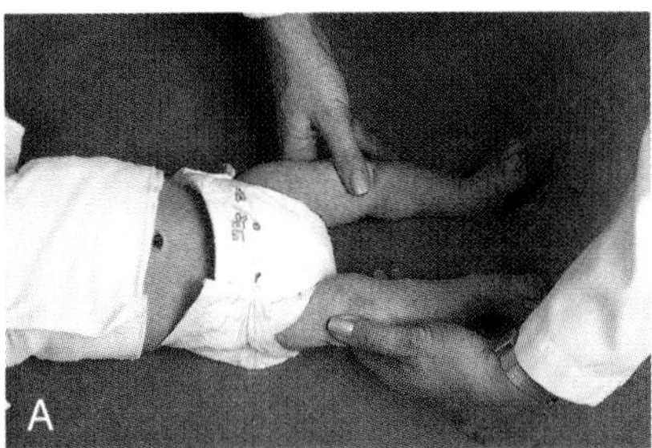

A. Barlow-Ortolani maneuver #1

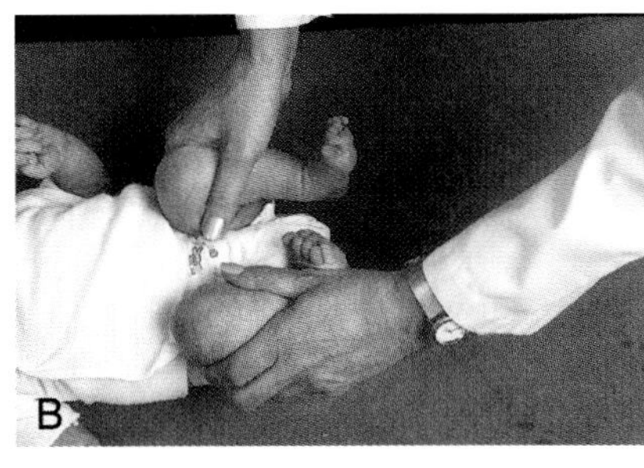

B. Barlow-Ortolani maneuver #2

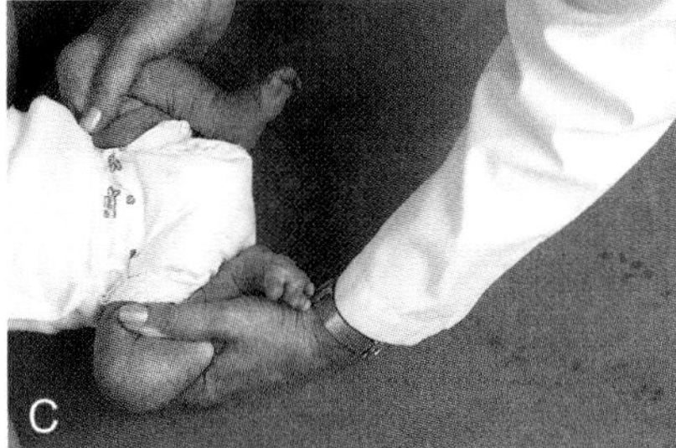

C. Barlow-Ortolani maneuver #3

- 10 fingers and 10 toes
- Full range of movement
- No clicks in joints
- See box on page 766 for Barlow-Ortolani maneuvers
- Equal gluteal folds
- C curve of spine, no dimpling
  - When arms and legs are extended:
  - Muscles symmetrical and with equal muscle tone.
  - Arms and legs symmetrical in size and movement.
  - Hands held as fists until after 1 month, when grasp becomes strong and equal.
  - Position in utero may affect appearance.

ABNORMAL FINDINGS/RATIONALE

- Decreased ROM and muscle tone.
- *Swelling, crepitus, neck tenderness:* Possible broken clavicle.
- *Simian (transverse palmar) creases:* Down syndrome.

Neurological

INSPECT/PALPATE/PERCUSS

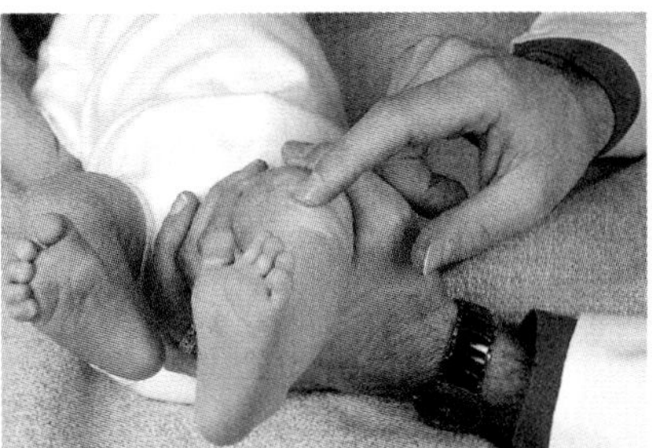

Checking knee reflex

- Positive newborn reflexes
- Positive knee reflex

ABNORMAL FINDINGS/RATIONALE

- *Hypotonia:* Floppy, limp extremities.
- Paralysis.
- Marked head lag.
- Tremors.
- Asymmetrical posture.
- *Hypertonia:* Tightly flexed arms and stiffly extended legs with quivering.
- Opisthotonic posture: Arched back.
- *Dimpling of spine, tuft of hair:* May indicate spina bifida or pilonidal cyst.

Barlow-Ortolani Maneuver

Place the infant supine on a flat surface. Flex his or her knees, holding your thumbs in the inner thighs and your fingers on the outside of the greater trochanters of the hips. Move the legs inward until your thumbs touch. Gently but firmly rotate the hips outward so that the knees touch the flat surface. There should be no clicking or crepitus noted during this procedure. If there is, the joint is unstable.

Testing Reflexes

Infant reflexes are often present at birth and occur because the neurological system is immature. Many of these reflexes disappear as the neurological system develops. Some reflexes are critical for survival, such as rooting, sucking, and swallowing. Other reflexes are protective reflexes and last throughout life. These include the blink or corneal, papillary reaction, sneezing, gag, cough, and yawn reflexes.

HELPFUL HINT

In premature babies, newborn reflexes may persist longer.

Newborn/Infant Reflexes

REFLEX/TECHNIQUE/NORMAL RESPONSE	ABNORMAL RESPONSE
Moro • Present at birth and lasts 1–4 months • *Technique:* Startle infant by suddenly jarring bassinet, or with infant in semisitting position, let head drop back slightly. 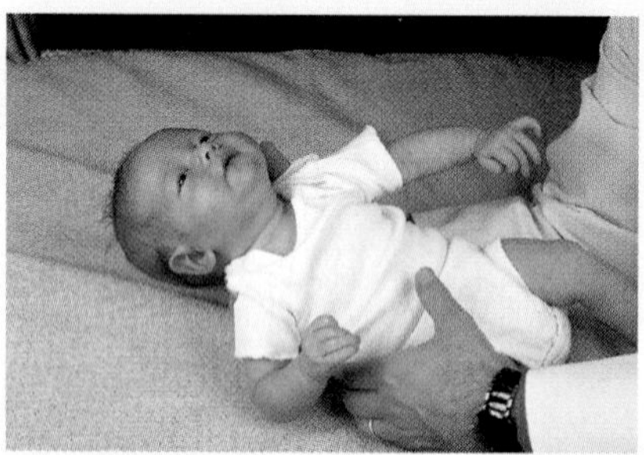 **Moro reflex** • Quickly abducts and extends arms and legs symmetrically. • Makes "C" with index finger and thumb. Legs flex up against trunk.	• Premature or ill infants may have sluggish response. • Positive response beyond 6 months indicates neurological problem. • Asymmetrical response may be caused by injury to clavicle, humerus, or brachial plexus during delivery.
Startle • Present at birth and lasts 4 months • *Technique:* Startle infant by making loud noise. 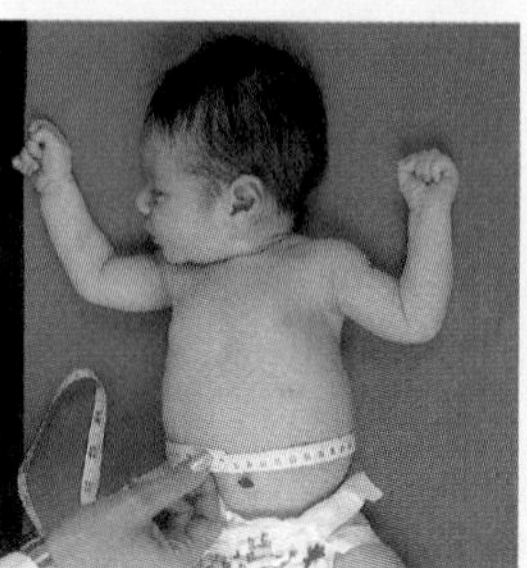 **Startle reflex** • Hands clenched, arms abducted, flexion at elbow.	• Same as Moro.

Newborn/Infant Reflexes

REFLEX/TECHNIQUE/NORMAL RESPONSE	ABNORMAL RESPONSE
Tonic Neck • Present between birth and 6 weeks; disappears at 4–6 months. • *Technique:* With infant supine, rotate head to one side so that chin is over shoulder. 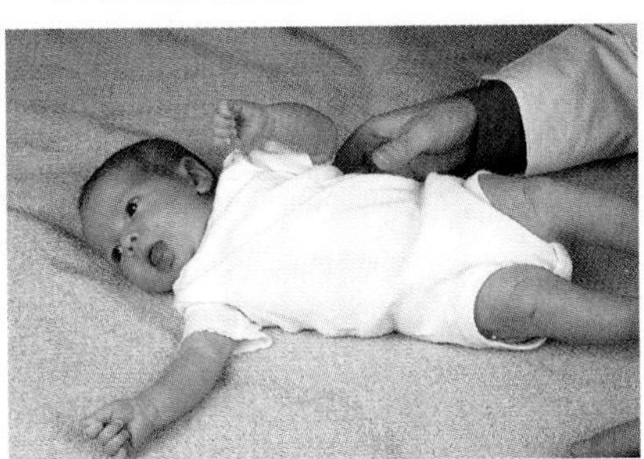 **Tonic neck reflex** • Infant assumes "fencing position," with arm and leg extended in direction to which head was turned.	• Response after 6 months may indicate cerebral palsy.
Palmar Grasp • Present at birth; disappears at 3–4 months. • *Technique:* Place object or finger in palm of infant's hand. 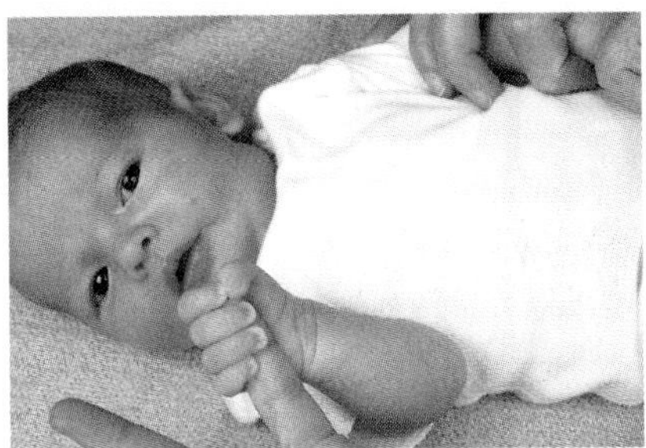 **Palmar grasp reflex** • Infant grasps object tightly. If he or she grasps your fingers with both hands, infant can be pulled to a sitting position.	• Negative grasp seen with hypotonia or prenatal asphyxia.
Plantar Grasp • Present at birth; disappears at 3–4 months. • *Technique:* Place thumb firmly against ball of infant's foot. 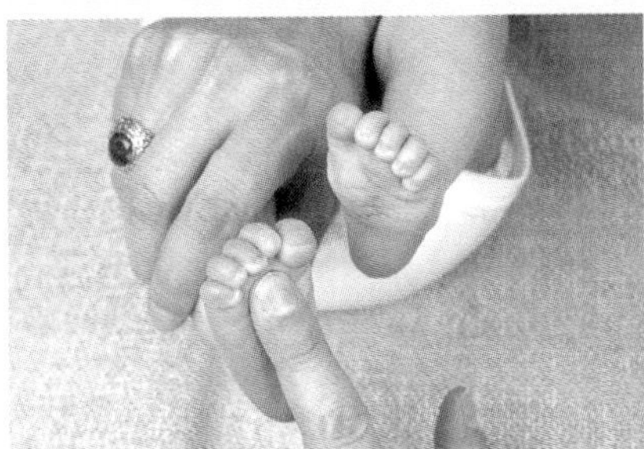 **Plantar grasp reflex** • Toes flex tightly downward in a grasping motion.	• Negative grasp seen with hypotonia or spinal cord injury.

(Continued)

Newborn/Infant Reflexes *(Continued)*

REFLEX/TECHNIQUE/NORMAL RESPONSE	ABNORMAL RESPONSE
Babinski • Present at birth; disappears at 1 year. • *Technique:* Stroke lateral surface of sole of infant's foot. 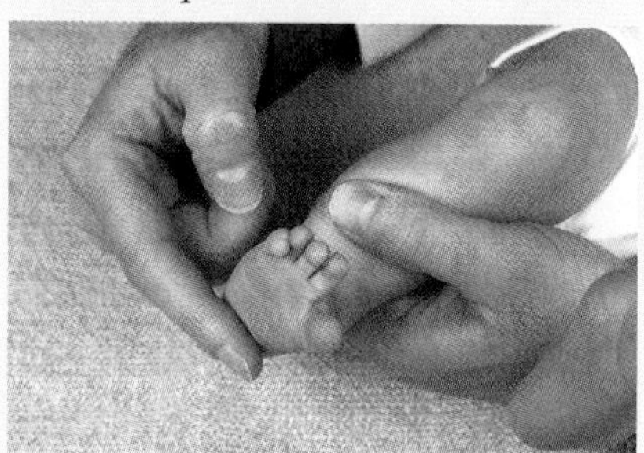 **Babinski reflex** • Toes should fan.	• Diminished response associated with neurological problem.
Stepping or Dancing • Present at birth; disappears at 3–4 weeks. • *Technique:* Hold infant upright with his or her feet touching a flat surface. 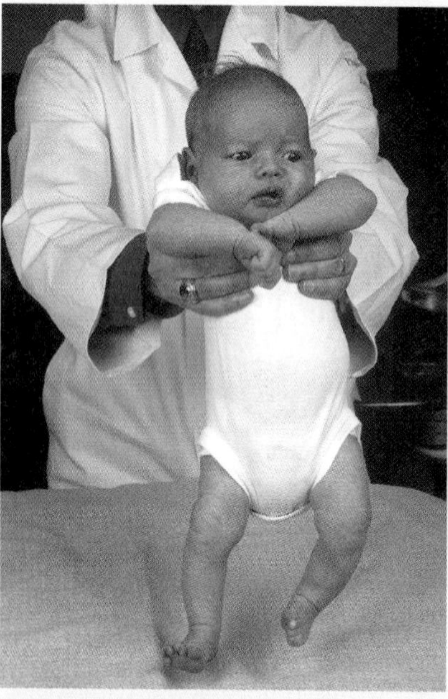 **Stepping or dancing reflex** • Infant steps up and down in place.	• Poor response caused by hypotonia.
Rooting • Present at birth; disappears at 3–6 months. • *Technique:* Brush cheek near corner of mouth. 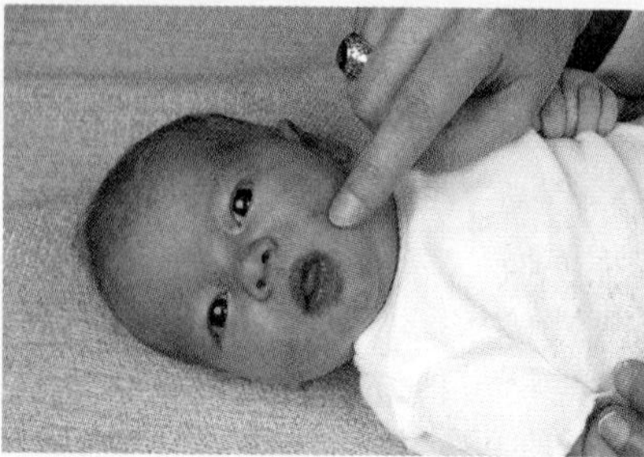 **Rooting reflex**	• Prematurity or neurological problem may cause weak or absent response.

Newborn/Infant Reflexes

REFLEX/TECHNIQUE/NORMAL RESPONSE	ABNORMAL RESPONSE
Rooting *(Continued)* • Infant turns head in direction of stimulus and opens mouth.	
Sucking • Present at birth; disappears at 10–12 months. • *Technique:* Touch lips.	

HELPFUL HINT

Don't check for rooting or sucking responses immediately after a feeding—they will be difficult to elicit.

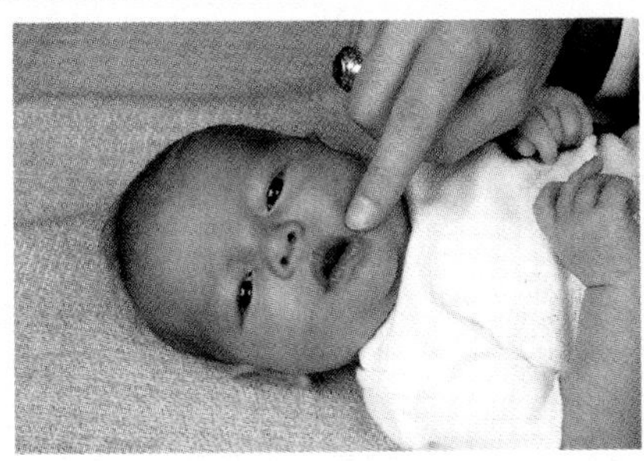

Sucking reflex

REFLEX/TECHNIQUE/NORMAL RESPONSE	ABNORMAL RESPONSE
• Sucking motion occurs.	• Weak or absent response associated with prematurity or neurological defect.
Swallowing • Present at birth and lasts throughout life. • *Technique:* Automatically follows sucking response during feeding. • Sucking and swallowing should occur without coughing, gagging, or vomiting.	• Weak or absent response associated with prematurity or neurological problem.
Extrusion • Present at birth and lasts throughout life. • *Technique:* Touch tip of tongue.	

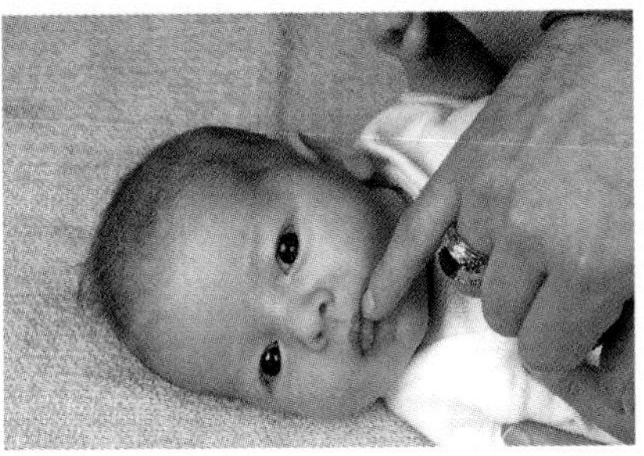

Extrusion reflex

REFLEX/TECHNIQUE/NORMAL RESPONSE	ABNORMAL RESPONSE
• Tongue protrudes outward.	• Absence may indicate neurological problem. • Continued extrusion of large tongue associated with Down syndrome.
Glabellar • Present at birth • *Technique:* Tap on forehead.	• Persistent blinking with repeated taps indicates extrapyramidal problem.

(Continued)

Newborn/Infant Reflexes *(Continued)*

REFLEX/TECHNIQUE/NORMAL RESPONSE	ABNORMAL RESPONSE
Glabellar *(Continued)* 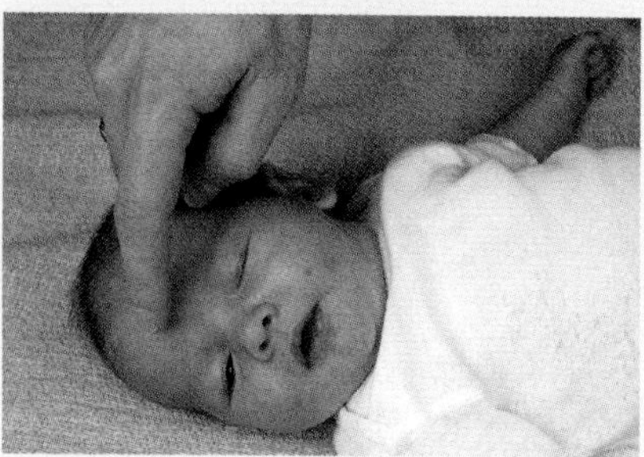 **Glabellar reflex** • Newborn blinks for first few taps.	
Crawling • Present at birth; disappears at 6 weeks. • *Technique:* Place infant on abdomen. 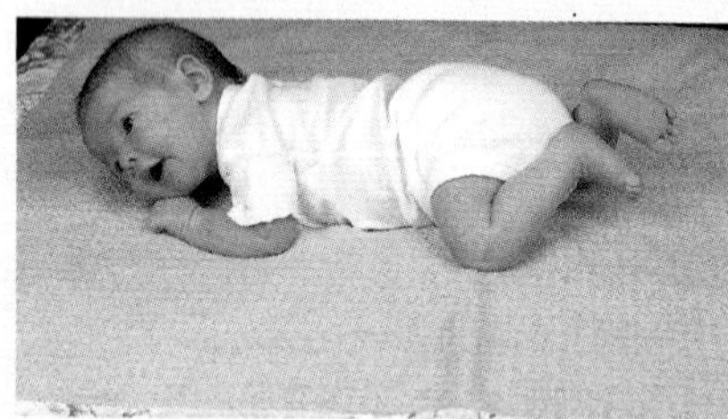 **Crawling reflex** • Newborn attempts to crawl.	
Crossed Extension • Present at birth; disappears at 2 months. *Technique:* Infant supine with leg extended. Stimulate foot. 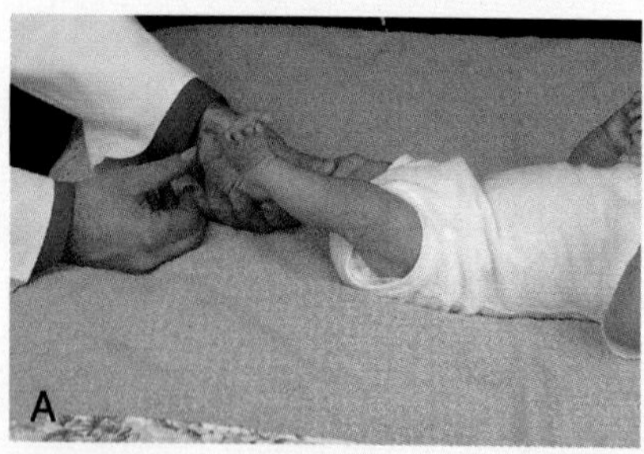 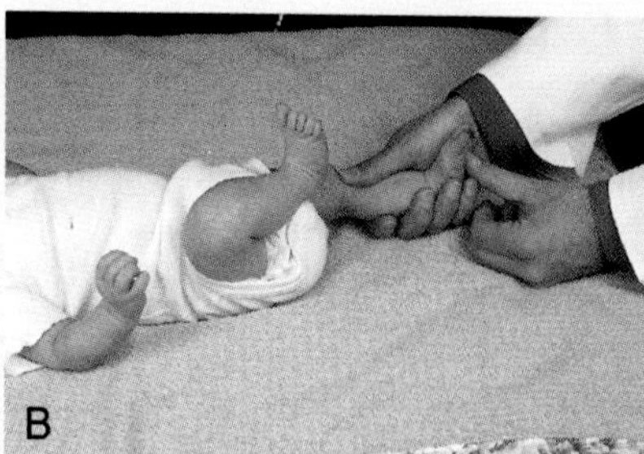 **A. Crossed extension** **B. Stimulate foot** • Flexion, adduction, then extension of opposite leg.	• Peripheral nerve damage causes weak response. • Spinal cord lesion causes absent response.
Pull-to-Sit • Present at birth • *Technique:* Pull infant to sitting position.	

Newborn/Infant Reflexes

REFLEX/TECHNIQUE/NORMAL RESPONSE	ABNORMAL RESPONSE
Pull-to-Sit *(Continued)* 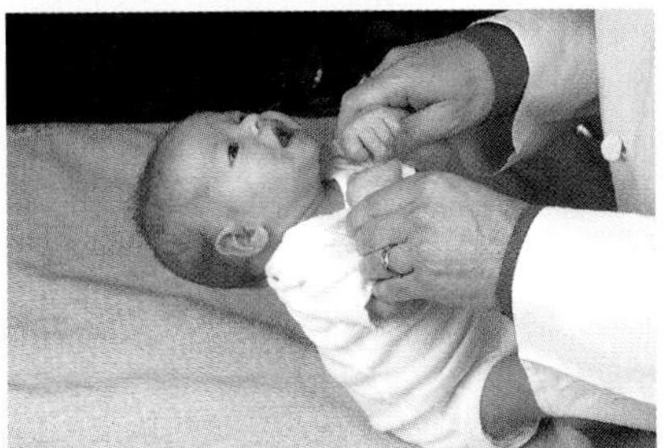 **Pull-to-sit reflex** • Head lags as infant is pulled to sitting position, but then infant is able to hold up head temporarily.	• Inability to hold up head suggests prematurity or hypotonia.
Trunk incurvation • Present at birth; disappears in a few days to 4 weeks. • *Technique:* With infant prone, run finger down either side of spine. 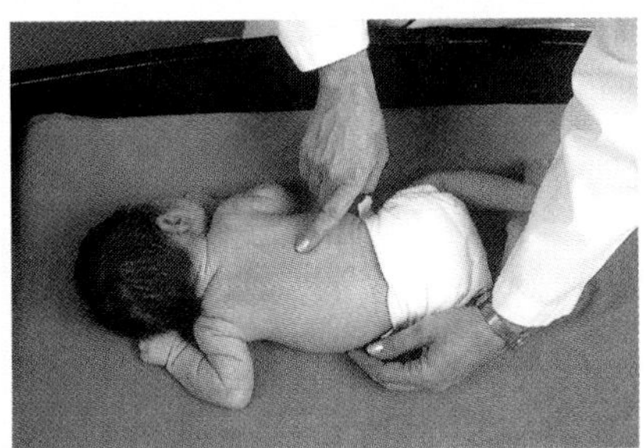 **Trunk incurvation reflex** • Flexion of trunk with hip moving toward stimulated side.	• Absent response indicates neurological or spinal cord problem.
Magnet • Present at birth. • *Technique:* With infant supine, flex leg and apply pressure to soles of feet. 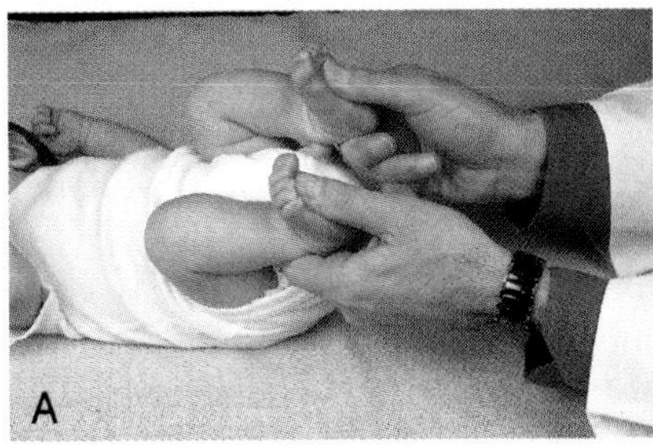 **A. Flex legs** **B. Apply pressure to soles of feet** • Extends legs against pressure.	• Breech birth may diminish reflex. • Absent response caused by spinal cord problem.

Performing Diagnostic/Screening Tests

Depending on the newborn's condition, various diagnostic and screening tests are performed shortly after birth. Mandatory testing varies from state to state.

Diagnostic/Screening Tests for Newborns

Test	Significance
Phenylketonuria: Measures amount of phenylalanine amino acids in blood.	Test is collected after several days of feedings. High phenylalanine levels can cause brain damage.
Galactosemia: Transferase deficiency.	Elevated galactose and low fluorescence may result in mental retardation, blindness, or death from dehydration and sepsis.
Maple Syrup Urine Disease	Elevated leucine can result in acidosis, seizures, mental retardation, and death.
Homocystinuria	Elevated methionine can lead to mental retardation, seizures, and behavioral disorders.
Congenital Adrenal Hyperplasia	Elevated 17-hydroxyprogesterone can lead to hyponatremia, hypokalemia, hypoglycemia, and ambiguous female genitalia.
Biotinidase Deficiency	Decreased activity of biotinidase on colorimetric assay causes mental retardation, skin changes, hearing and vision problems, even death.
Thyroxine	Thyroxine is a thyroid hormone necessary for growth, development, and metabolism. Low values are associated with brain defects.
Blood Type	RH and ABO incompatibility can cause hemolysis and subsequent jaundice. If mother is RH− and newborn is RH+, mother must be treated promptly to avoid sensitization to future RH+ fetuses.
Sickle Cell Anemia	Detects presence of hemoglobin S. Electrophoresis identifies whether infant has the trait or disease.
Audiometric Testing	Identifies hearing disorders early.
HIV: Newborns of mothers with HIV are tested for virus.	Early virus detection can initiate early treatment that may enhance survival.
Gestational Age: Normal gestational age is 38–42 weeks. A newborn less than 38 weeks is premature. A screening test, such as the Ballard test, estimates fetal gestation.	Accurate estimate of gestational age influences care management and special monitoring needs. Full-term infant should have creases over entire sole of foot, full breast areolas, firm ear cartilage. Males should have pendulous testes and deep scrotal rugae. In females, the labia majora should cover the clitoris and labia minora.

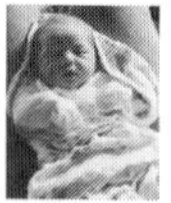

Case Study Findings

Newborn Carmen's physical assessment findings include:

- **General Health Survey/Anthropometric Measurements:** Flexed head and extremities, head 33 cm, chest 31 cm, abdomen 32 cm, length head to heel 50 cm, weight 7 lb, 6 oz.
- **Vital signs:** Axillary temperature 98°F; pulse 144 BPM, respirations 44 and irregular, BP 64/38.
- **Apgars:** 8 and 10.
- **Integumentary:** Skin pink and warm with no jaundice, lanugo on face and shoulders, vernix caseosa in groin skin folds, one 4-cm Mongolian spot on each buttock.
- **Head/Face:** Positive molding, but skull appears symmetrical, fontanels soft and flat.
- **Eyes, Ears, Nose, Mouth, Throat, Neck:** Eyes: Intact, positive red light reflex OU; Ears: React to noise, ears align with external canthus of eyes; Nose/mouth: Small amount of clear mucus in nose and mouth, palate intact, strong sucking reflex.
- **Respiratory:** Irregular, unlabored breathing. Occasional periods of apnea lasting no more than 5 seconds. Lungs clear.
- **Cardiovascular:** No cyanosis. Apical pulse 144 regular. No murmurs. Positive femoral pulses.
- **Gastrointestinal:** Positive bowel sounds, anus patent, meconium stool, positive anal reflex, umbilical cord white with two arteries and one vein, intact with no drainage.
- **Genitourinary:** Voided.
- **Genitalia:** Pink and edematous.
- **Musculoskeletal:** 10 fingers and 10 toes, C curve of spine, no dimpling, equal gluteal folds, full range of motion of extremities, no fractures or dislocations.
- **Neurological:** Good muscle tone, strong cry, positive newborn reflexes.

CRITICAL THINKING ACTIVITY #1

How would you adjust your assessment of Carmen to include the educational needs of her parents? What resources on the hospital unit would you use?

CRITICAL THINKING ACTIVITY #2

Mrs. Ramirez brings 3-day-old Carmen to the pediatric clinic. She states that Carmen nurses for 30 to 40 minutes every 3 to 4 hours but sleeps after each feeding. She is concerned that the baby sleeps 15 to 16 hours a day. Mrs. Ramirez states that she had an uncomplicated pregnancy and delivery and that she feels so good, she cannot understand why Carmen sleeps so much. What information about sleeping and feeding patterns would you offer Mrs. Ramirez?

COMMON HEALTH PROBLEMS

As you gather information, consider some common health problems that affect newborns and infants.

- **Newborns**
  - Heart murmurs
  - Respiratory distress syndrome
  - Mother-to-child disease transmission (e.g., STDs such as HIV and syphilis)
- **Infants**
  - Otitis media
  - Upper respiratory infections
  - Diaper rash
  - Allergies
  - Colic

Case Study Follow-Up

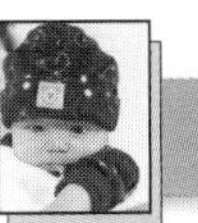

Carmen is now 6 months old. Mrs. Ramirez brings her to the pediatric clinic for her routine checkup. She states that last month Carmen was diagnosed with otitis media and was on an antibiotic for 1 week. Mrs. Ramirez is concerned that Carmen does not appear to be well fed and wonders if formula would help her gain weight. She states that she continues to enjoy her job as a social worker and appreciates her mother's and sister's help with child care while she works.

Performing the Infant Assessment

The initial assessment is performed immediately after birth, while the newborn is still in the hospital. It serves as a baseline. The subsequent history and physical examination are performed when the infant visits the clinic or pediatrician's office for well-baby checkups.

Infant Health History

A complete health history can be obtained from the newborn's chart and from a parent or guardian. Review the chart, paying special attention to prenatal care, gestational or family health problems and supports. Then ask the parent or guardian about developmental milestones, and discuss safety issues and immunizations. The parent or guardian is critical in obtaining a full health history. Encourage discussion of concerns and questions. The interview is also an ideal teaching opportunity.

Developmental Milestones

Ask the parent or guardian about milestones, such as when the infant first rolled over. This information will identify delays that must be addressed.

Home Safety

Ask about safety in the home, including fall prevention, fire and burn prevention, gun and poison control, and car seat restraints. Take every opportunity to educate parents on safety issues.

ALERT

Accidents are a leading cause of death in children.

Immunizations

Immunizations are critical for primary prevention of childhood diseases. Discuss the immunization schedule with the parent or guardian. The following immunizations are recommended:

Hepatitis B: First dose within 2 months of age, second dose 1 month after first dose, and third dose 6 months after second dose.

Diphtheria, Pertussis, Tetanus Toxoid (DPT): Doses at 2 months, 4 months, and between 6 and 18 months.

Haemophilus Influenzae Type B (Hib): Doses at 2 months, 4 months, and 6 months (check with manufacturer if third dose at 6 months is required).

Inactivated Polio Vaccine (IPV): Doses at 2 months, 4 months, and between 6 and 18 months.

Pneumococcal Conjugate (PCV): Doses at 2 months, 4 months, and between 6 and 18 months.

For the most recent information about vaccines, visit the National Immunization Program Home Page at *http://www.cdc.gov/nip/*, or call the National Immunization

Hotline at 800-232-2522 (English) or 800-232-0233 (Spanish).

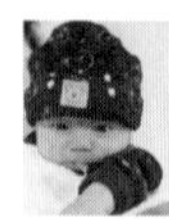

Case Study Findings

Infant Carmen's developmental, safety, and immunization findings include:

- Developmental
  - Sits
  - Bears weight on hands, stands with assistance
  - Rolls over
  - Controls head
  - Grasps objects
  - Is teething
  - Imitates sounds
  - Is attached to parents
  - Has separation anxiety
- Safety
  - Smoke and carbon monoxide detectors
  - Safety gates
  - Cabinet locks
  - Electrical outlet caps
  - Car seats
  - Medications and cleaning solutions out of reach
- Immunizaions
  - Hepatitis B 1 and 2
  - DPT 1 and 2
  - Polio 1 and 2
  - HIB 1 and 2
  - PCV 1 and 2

Review of Systems

The last part of your history is a review of systems. This review will help you identify normal physiologic changes as well as alert you to abnormal findings.

Review of Systems

AREA/QUESTIONS TO ASK	RATIONALE/SIGNIFICANCE
General Health Survey	
How is your infant doing now?	Determining the parents' view of their infant's general well-being provides a baseline for you to begin your assessment.
Body Weight	
Has he or she been gaining weight?	Weight gain within normal parameters is an indicator of nutritional status.
Integumentary	
Does the infant have good skin turgor? Does the skin appear healthy?	Skin tenting denotes dehydration. Scaly skin may be caused by an underlying medical condition or by dryness from soaps or lotions.
Do hair and nails appear healthy or brittle?	Brittle hair and nails may be caused by poor protein intake.
Head and Neck	
Is head shape symmetrical?	Symmetry is normal.
Can infant hold head upright while sitting and move head from side to side?	Head control is a necessary motor development milestone.
Eyes, Ears, Nose, and Throat	
Can infant recognize toys you give him or her? Do eyes focus symmetrically? Is there eye exudate?	Refer infants with signs of visual difficulties to specialist. Infants are highly susceptible to eye infections and may require medications.
Does infant turn head when his or her name is called? Can he or she vocalize?	Ability to hear and speak is critical for development. If you notice signs of hearing/speaking problems, refer infant to specialist.
Is there exudate from the nose?	Nose exudate may signal infection or allergies or may be normal mucus production.
Respiratory	
Is breathing labored?	Monitor abnormal breathing patterns carefully.

Review of Systems

AREA/QUESTIONS TO ASK	RATIONALE/SIGNIFICANCE
Cardiovascular	
Is infant active? Is skin ever blue tinged?	Infants should be active and lively when awake. Lethargy may be related to cardiac difficulties, of which cyanosis is a warning sign.
Gastrointestinal	
How is the infant's appetite? What does he or she usually eat and drink each day?	Good appetite denotes good health. Adequate daily nutrient intake is necessary for growth.
How many bowel movements a day does he or she have?	Regular bowel movements suggest normal gastrointestinal activity.
Genitourinary	
Is urination pattern consistent with fluid intake?	Adequate urination pattern denotes normal kidney function.
How many diaper changes a day?	Usually about 8 diapers a day is normal, depending on fluid intake.
Musculoskeletal	
Does infant roll over, sit unsupported, transfer toy from one hand to the other? Can he or she creep forward or backward on tummy?	Body movements should be within developmental norms.
Neurological	
Have you noticed any unusual movements such as tremors? Problems with sucking, swallowing?	Tremors or other unusual movements may indicate seizures. Diminished sucking or swallowing reflexes may indicate an underlying neurological problem.
Infections	
Has infant had any colds, fevers, infections?	Usual infant infections may not be preventable. However, teach parents infection-control methods.
Development	
Does infant prefer to play with people rather than toys? Does he or she search for an object that is out of sight? Is he or she afraid of strangers?	Deviations from these developmental milestones may impair social activities.
Relationships	
How do you feel about the new baby and about being a mother or father?	Mother may cry, feel irritable, and have loss of appetite and sleeplessness for first 10 days or so after delivery. If these problems persist for more than 2 weeks, they may signal postpartum depression and warrant referral.

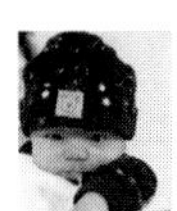

Case Study Findings

Infant Carmen's review of systems reveals:

- **General Health Survey:** Very robust and active infant, healthy appearance.
- **Body weight:** 16 lb, gained 2 lb since last month's visit for otitis media.
- **Integumentary:** No scaly skin.
- **Head and Neck:** Easily holds head upright and in alignment.
- **Eyes, Nose, and Throat:** Eyes: Normal response to visual stimuli, no drainage.
- **Ears:** Normal sound recognition and making sounds. No apparent abnormalities. Otoscope

examination indicated because of recent otitis media.

- **Respiratory:** No breathing problems
- **Cardiovascular:** No apparent distress. Active when awake.
- **Gastrointestinal:** Exclusively breastfed and nurses every 3 to 4 hours during the day, with daily bowel movements, yellow in color.
- **Genitourinary:** Normal urination pattern noted; 8 diapers a day.
- **Musculoskeletal:** Attempts to crawl; rolled over and sat up on her own (normal findings).
- **Neurological:** No abnormal movements, nurses well, no problems.
- **Immunological:** No infection aside from otitis media.
- **Developmental:** Laughs easily with mother but is fearful of examiner. Normal age-related behavior observed.
- **Relationships:** Warm, caring responses noted toward baby from parents. Both parents say they enjoy parenthood very much.

Case Study Evaluation

Before you proceed to the physical assessment, record what you have learned about infant Carmen's health history so far.

Infant Physical Assessment

After the history, perform the physical examination on the infant, considering the important role that the parent or guardian plays in this process. Physical examinations should be conducted in a warm environment. The alert, well-fed newborn is usually a most cooperative client. Involve the family whenever possible because this is a fine opportunity for education and support. Infants after the age of 6 months will most likely fear the practitioner. Therefore conduct as much of the examination as possible with the child in the mother's lap.

Performing a Head-to-Toe Physical Assessment

Next, perform a head-to-toe physical assessment of the infant.

Performing an Infant Head-to-Toe Physical Assessment

AREA/SYSTEM/NORMAL VARIATIONS	ABNORMAL FINDINGS/RATIONALE
Anthropometric Measurements	
• *Head and Chest:* Apply tape measure around widest part of head, just above eyebrows. Measure chest at nipple line.	• Greater-than-normal head circumference may indicate hydrocephalus. Smaller than normal head circumference is microcephaly.
• ***Height and Weight:*** Measure length from head to heels. Weigh without clothing or diaper. Increases by 1.5 cm each month for first 6 months and by 0.5 cm per month until age 12 months. Chest circumference equals head circumference by 12 months. Height should increase 50% by age 12 months. Birth weight should double by 6 months and triple by 12 months.	• Anthropometic measurements deviating from normal may be caused by underlying disease or inadequate eating or nutritional pattern.
Integumentary/***Skin***	
INSPECT • Skin appearance and skin folds • Skin turgor • Axillary temperature	
• Inspect skin appearance throughout your physical exam. Skin pigmentation varies. Newborns of dark-skinned parents may appear light-skinned at birth. True skin color develops by 3 months of age. • Good skin turgor in newborns and infants is a sign of adequate hydration.	• Persistent cyanosis in a warm infant is never normal and requires immediate referral. Other deviations include the following: • *Diaper rash (diaper dermatitis):* Red, excoriated skin. Secondary yeast infection (*Candida*) causes

Performing an Infant Head-to-Toe Physical Assessment

AREA/SYSTEM/NORMAL VARIATIONS	ABNORMAL FINDINGS/RATIONALE
Integumentary/*Skin (Continued)*	bright, round scaling patches. • *Eczema (atopic dermatitis):* Dry, itchy patches on face and skin folds in infants with allergies. • *"Cradle cap"* (seborrheic dermatitis): Flat, greasy scales on scalp that may be caused by infrequent shampooing. Some cultures fear touching fontanel area. • *Depressed fontanels and skin tenting:* Signs of severe dehydration.
• Axillary temperature range for newborns and infants is 35.9°C to 36.7°C (96.6°F to 98.0°F). **ALERT** *Never use a mercury thermometer on a newborn or infant. Mercury is highly toxic.*	• Low temperature suggests hypothermia. • High temperatures can cause seizures in newborns and infants.
Head/Face/Neck *INSPECT/PALPATE* • Face and skull symmetrical. Fontanels flat and soft. At birth, anterior fontanel is 2.5–4 cm across; it closes between 12 and 18 months of age. Posterior fontanel is initially 2 cm and closes by 3 months. • Neck is short and should rotate left to right.	• Sunken fontanel associated with dehydration. Bulging fontanel associated with intracranial pressure.
HEENT/*Eyes* *INSPECT, PALPATE, CHECK VISUAL ACUITY:* *External eye, eyelids, lacrimal ducts, conjunctiva, sclera* • Bilateral blinking. • Corneal reflex positive. • Transient strabismus common.	• Continued strabismus after 6 months is abnormal.
• No tearing in first month. • Sclera may be blue tinged.	• Lack of tears after 2 months may be caused by clogged lacrimal ducts and requires medical attention.
• Pupils constrict with light and are round and equal in size. • Test visual acuity using the DDST II. Infants have full binocular vision.	• Fixed or dilated pupils indicate neurological problem.
HEENT/*Ears* *INSPECT, PALPATE, CHECK HEARING* *External ear, internal ear* • Infant should respond to noise. • Pinna flexible.	• Lack of response to noise may indicate hearing problem.

HELPFUL HINT

To perform otoscopic exam, place infant flat and restrain arms above head. Pull auricle down and back to observe tympanic membrane.

(Continued)

Performing an Infant Head-to-Toe Physical Assessment *(Continued)*

AREA/SYSTEM/NORMAL VARIATIONS	ABNORMAL FINDINGS/RATIONALE
HEENT/*Nose* *INSPECT* • Infants are nose breathers. Check patency by closing one nostril, then the other. • Thin white mucus discharge and sneezing are normal.	• Flaring of nares is sign of respiratory distress. • Bloody discharge or large amount of nasal secretions may obstruct nares.
HEENT/*Mouth/Throat* *INSPECT* *Oral cavity: palate, tongue, gums, tonsils (use light and tongue blade)* • White nodules (Epstein's pearls) may be found on hard palate and usually disappear by 3 months. • Tongue should not protrude from mouth.	• Protruding tongue associated with congenital disorders, such as Down syndrome or hypothyroidism.
• No coating in mouth. • Suck should be strong. • First primary teeth usually appear at 6 to 8 months.	
Chest/Back/Shoulders *INSPECT* • Convex spinal curvature (C curve). • No blemishes or skin openings. • By 12–18 months, lumbar curve develops and lordosis is present as walking begins.	• Limited ROM may result from injury. • Dimpling in spine may be associated with neural tube defects.
Respiratory/*Chest* *INSPECT/PERCUSS/PALPATE/AUSCULTATE* • Percuss lightly. • Palpate back with two fingers while baby is crying. • Auscultate lungs. **HELPFUL HINT** Use direct percussion.	**ALERTS** *Apnea >than 15 seconds accompanied by decreased heart rate is abnormal.* • Stressful breathing with flaring nares and sighing with each breath are signs of respiratory distress and require immediate attention.
• Normal respiratory rate 25–50 breaths per minute. Apnea is less common in infants than in newborns. Normal breath sounds are more bronchial in infants. Infants are abdominal breathers. Anteroposterior: lateral diameter is equal.	• Inspiratory stridor, expiratory grunts, retractions, paradoxical (seesaw) breathing, asymmetrical or decreased breath sounds, wheezing, and crackles are abnormal. • Depressed sternum may affect normal respiration.

Performing an Infant Head-to-Toe Physical Assessment

AREA/SYSTEM/NORMAL VARIATIONS	ABNORMAL FINDINGS/RATIONALE
Cardiovascular/*Heart/Peripheral Pulses* *AUSCULTATE*	
HELPFUL HINT Use a stethoscope with a small diaphragm and perform exam when infant is quiet.	
• Apical pulse felt in fourth or fifth intercostal space just medial to midclavicular line.	
• Heart rate range 80–160 bpm.	• Abnormal heart rate range requires attention. • Murmurs accompanied by cyanosis may indicate congenital heart defects.
• Capillary refill <1 second.	• Capillary refill times longer than 2 seconds may indicate dehydration or hypovolemic shock.
• Peripheral pulses present.	• Evaluate newly discovered murmurs. • Infant eating poorly may have cardiovascular problem.
Gastrointestinal/*Abdomen* *INSPECT/PALPATE/PERCUSS/AUSCULTATE* • Bowel sounds present.	
• Bowel soft. • Tympany may be heard because of air swallowing. • Umbilicus flat.	• Umbilical hernias >2 cm wide may require further evaluation. • Abdominal pain may indicate childhood illnesses.
• Liver edge 1–2 cm below right rib cage (costal margin).	• Enlarged liver or palpable spleen may indicate disease.
Extremities *INSPECT* *Hands, arms, feet, legs, hips* *TEST ROM*	
• Feet flat. • Legs equal in length. • Transfers objects from one hand to other by 7 months.	• Inadequate ROM may indicate congenital malformation or birth injury or may result from pulling or lifting infant.
• Crawls and sits unsupported by 7 months. • Pulls to standing position and holds on to furniture by 11 months.	• Inability to meet developmental milestones may indicate neurological or environmental deficits.
Genitourinary/*Male* *INSPECT/PALPATE* *Penis, urethra* Genitourinary/*Female* *INSPECT* *Exernal genitalia*	
• Note infant's sex.	• Ambiguous genitalia abnormal.

(Continued)

Performing an Infant Head-to-Toe Physical Assessment *(Continued)*

AREA/SYSTEM/NORMAL VARIATIONS	ABNORMAL FINDINGS/RATIONALE
Genitourinary/*Female (Continued)*	
• In uncircumcised male infant, foreskin may not be fully retractable until 1 year. • Urethra midline.	• ***Male Infants:*** Phimosis (tight foreskin) can constrict penis. Instruct parents on gentle retraction of foreskin to prevent phimosis.
• Urine flow straight and strong.	• Weak urine stream or dribbling suggests stricture at urinary meatus.
• No palpable masses in testes.	• Solid scrotal masses are abnormal. Hernias present as scrotal masses.
• Two testes should be palpated in scrotum or brought down from inguinal ring.	• Testes not palpable indicates undescended testicles. • If scrotum is swollen, transilluminate to determine if fluid (hydrocele) present.
• External genitalia of female infant should be pink and moist.	• ***Female Infants:*** Blood-tinged fluid from vagina abnormal after 1 week. • Vaginal discharge or labial redness or itching may be caused by diaper or soap irritation or sexual abuse.
Anus and Rectum *INSPECT*	
• In infants, bowel movements may occur with each feeding. By 1 year, they occur once or twice a day. • Breastfed babies have stools that are mustard colored and soft. • Formula-fed babies have stools that are yellowish-green and more formed.	• Watery stools and explosive diarrhea indicate infection. Constipation or hard stools indicate inadequate hydration or nutrition.
Neurological *INSPECT/TEST* *Muscle strength, function, sensory function, reflex movements*	
• Infant's body stays erect when you support him or her with both hands under axilla. Motor control develops from head to toe. Infant opens eyes to noise and responds to touch.	• Delays in motor or sensory activity may indicate brain damage, mental retardation, illness, malnutrition, or neglect. • Asymmetrical posture or spastic movements need further evaluation.
• Presence of infantile reflexes denotes healthy neurological system.	• Maintenance of infant reflexes past usual age is abnormal.

Performing Diagnostic/Screening Tests

Depending on the infant's condition, certain diagnostic and screening tests are performed. Mandatory screening varies from state to state.

Diagnostic/Screening Tests for Infants

Test	Significance
Developmental testing: Should occur regularly throughout childhood. Denver Developmental Screening Tool 2 assesses skills in areas of personal/social, fine motor, language, and gross motor.	If delays are noted, refer child to specialist for further testing. Medications, malnutrition, neurological and emotional conditions affect test results.
Urine screening: Dipstick screening test is usually sufficient.	Any abnormalities require full urinalysis.
Hemoglobin or hematocrit.	Hemoglobin below 10 g/dL is low and infant is considered anemic. Hematocrit below 29% is low.
Lead screening: Only if environmental exposure is suspected.	Elevated blood lead levels can cause neurological damage.

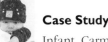

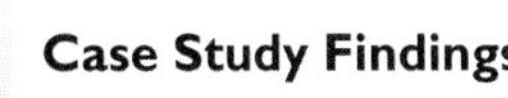

Case Study Findings

Infant Carmen's physical assessment finding's include:

- **General Health Survey:** Well-developed, robust, alert 6-month-old girl sitting upright in mother's lap.
- **Anthropometric Measurements:** Length 66 cm (26 in), Weight 7.25 kg (16 lb), Head circumference 40.5 cm (16 in).
- **Vital Signs:** Temperature 36.7°C (98.0°F), BP 113, Respirations 30, lungs clear.
- **Integumentary:** Skin pink and warm to touch; hair shiny and clean.
- **Head/Face:** Head and skull symmetrical, posterior fontanel closed, anterior fontanel flat and soft.
- **Eyes, Ears, Nose, Mouth, Throat:** Eyes clear, follows objects. External ears intact, piercing for earrings noted. Internal ear intact; no redness or exudate. Responds to noise and when name is called. Mouth and palate intact, two teeth noted.
- **Chest, Neck, Shoulders, and Back:** Intact.
- **Cardiovascular:** Positive peripheral pulses.
- **Gastrointestinal:** Abdomen soft, positive BS+, several soft, yellow stools daily.
- **Extremities:** Legs, feet, arms, and hands intact with symmetrical movement.
- **Genitourinary:** Voids with every feeding. Labia and buttocks excoriated (diaper rash).
- **Musculoskeletal:** Barlow-Ortolani maneuver negative. Equal gluteal skin folds. Sits unassisted. Attempting to crawl. Transfers object from one hand to other.
- **Reflexes:** Tonic neck, plantar grasp, Babinski and suck present.
- **Relationships:** Smiling baby, comfortable with mother.
- **Additional Data:** Immunization and assessment visits on schedule. Nutrition status is good and within normal for age. Mother is breastfeeding but wonders if Carmen's weight is normal.

CRITICAL THINKING ACTIVITY #3

Unfortunately, Mrs. Ramirez's mother and sister are moving to another state. They have both helped with child care and are a major source of support. List community resources that would be of assistance to the family.

Case Study Analysis and Plan

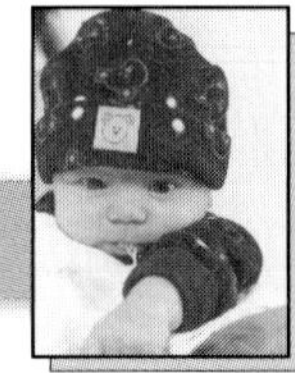

Now that you have completed a thorough assessment of infant Carmen, document the key history and physical examination findings that will help you formulate your nursing diagnoses.

Nursing Diagnoses

Analyze the data on infant Carmen and develop nursing diagnoses. Then cluster the supporting data for each diagnosis. Because the caregiver affects the infant, be sure to include the family in the plan.

1. Tissue Integrity, impaired
2. Infection, risk for
3. Nutrition: imbalanced, risk for more than body requirements
4. Social Isolation, potential for
5. Health-Seeking Behaviors

CRITICAL THINKING ACTIVITY #4

Now that you have identified some nursing diagnoses for infant Carmen, select one and develop a nursing care plan and a brief teaching plan for her mother, including learning outcomes and teaching strategies.

Research Tells Us

According to the U.S. Department of Transportation, 50 percent of all children killed in auto accidents in 1999 were unrestrained. Although all states require restraints for children, research points out the need for further education of families and healthcare providers. When performing health assessments on newborns and infants, take every opportunity to inform parents of car safety issues. An infant car seat testing program is a critical component to infant public health.

Sources: U.S. Department of Transportation; American Academy of Pediatrics; Creehan, P, 2002.

Health Concerns

Health concerns for infants focus on health promotion, such as maintenance of regular well-baby assessments and immunization schedules, supporting and educating parents in their critical role as infant caregivers, and using community resources to enhance the family unit.

Summary

- A thorough newborn and infant assessment is a fundamental component in health promotion and disease prevention for the entire family.
- The baby clinic visit may be the only access point to the healthcare system for the family.
- Because infant health depends on family health, incorporating the total family is critical in your approach to health assessment.
- Encourage parents to keep all scheduled child assessment visits, and take every opportunity to make the necessary referrals for family members.

CHAPTER 23

Assessing the Toddler and Preschooler

Before You Begin

INTRODUCTION TO ASSESSING THE TODDLER AND PRESCHOOLER

The terms "toddler" and "preschooler" refer to children between the ages of 1 and 5. This is a time of challenge, discovery, and learning control. Specifically, the toddler period extends from 12 to 36 months, and the preschool period from 3 to 5 years. The toddler years are often referred to as the "terrible twos" as the child struggles to gain control. During the preschool years, the child matures cognitively and emotionally in preparation for entering school. This chapter will help you effectively assess this age group by familiarizing you with the physical, psychosocial, and cognitive developmental changes that occur.

Before you begin the health assessment, ask yourself:

- How does assessment of the toddler and preschooler differ from assessment of other patients?
- What approach is best for assessing the toddler and preschooler?
- What health concerns should I keep in mind as I proceed with the assessment?

Developmental Changes

Physical Changes

During the toddler and preschool years, physical growth continues at a steadier pace than in infancy. Body systems also develop more mature functioning. The specific physical changes that occur are presented during the physical examination section of this chapter.

Psychosocial and Emotional Changes

During the toddler years, the child struggles to develop a sense of autonomy. He or she works to gain control over bodily functions, tolerate separation from parents, differentiate self from others, develop socially acceptably behavior and verbal communication skills, become less egocentric, and tolerate delay in gratifying needs. Unsuccessful attempts at developing autonomy result in doubt and shame. The negativism associated with this period explains the term the **terrible twos,** when "no" seems to be the only word in the child's vocabulary. But even though the child is trying to achieve control, he or she also looks for consistency within the environment. This gives the child a sense of safety and comfort. During the toddler and preschool years, the child also recognizes sexual differences and roles. Sex role imitation, such as "dressing up," is common during these years, Once the toddler has developed autonomy, he or she moves to the next stage, which Eric Erikson calls initiative versus guilt. This is a time of playing and learning. If the child goes beyond set limits, guilt results. The **superego** or conscience is in its early developmental stages, and the ability to tolerate a delay in satisfying needs reflects ego development. During the preschool years, the superego continues to develop. Behavior is seen as good or bad based on the outcome—reward or punishment.

Rapid cognitive development also occurs during this time. The child develops new skills, constantly building on what he or she has learned. The toddler begins to see causal and spatial relationships, develops object permanence, and imitates household activities and sex-role behavior. Preoperational thought processes develop. During the preschool years, language skills continue to develop, and play becomes an important means of expression and learning.

As the child approaches the preschool years, he or she begins to have some concept of a Supreme Being, having been introduced to the idea at an early age through bedtime or mealtime prayers. Preschoolers' perceptions of the Supreme Being are concrete and based on parental influence.

Health Issues and Risk Factors

As a professional nurse, you are in an ideal position to screen for risk factors and teach parents health prevention. As you proceed with the assessment, stay alert for the following problems that are common in toddlers and preschoolers.

Toilet Training

The child needs to be physiologically and psychologically ready for toilet training, and this usually occurs between 18 and 24 months. Usually the child gains bowel control before bladder control, and full bladder control may not be achieved until age 5.

Sibling Rivalry

Jealousy is a normal reaction in a toddler or preschooler, who may have trouble understanding and accepting a new baby. Talking to children and letting them help prepare for the new baby helps minimize conflict. Because the toddler or preschooler may act out, close supervision is needed once the baby comes home.

Temper Tantrums and Negativism

As the child tries to assert his or her independence, he or she may act out by having temper tantrums and holding breath. Although ignoring this behavior is usually the best approach, emphasize to parents that the child needs to be protected from injury. Negativism (saying "no") can be minimized by avoiding yes-or-no choices.

Fears, Stress, and Regression

A child's fears may be real or imagined. Helping the child deal with fears may help resolve them. Usually, imaginary fears disappear by the time the child reaches school age. Even young children can experience stress. A variety of situations, such as a new baby, being hospitalized, or fighting among family members, can cause stress. But because young children have not yet developed effective skills to deal with stress, they may regress (return to an earlier reaction) when confronted with stressful situations. **Regression** is often seen when the child is hospitalized.

Communicable Diseases

Many communicable diseases can be prevented by proper immunizations. Provide parents with written information on immunization schedules. The hand-mouth activity common with toddlers increases their risk for various intestinal parasitic diseases and stomatitis. Emphasize the importance of washing the hands!

Poisonings and Injuries

The inquisitiveness of toddlers and preschoolers increases the risk for accidents and ingestion of toxic substances. Safety is of the utmost importance. Make sure that parents have the number for the Poison Control Center. Also advise them to have syrup of ipecac in their medicine cabinets in case Poison Control advises them to induce vomiting. Discuss how to childproof the home to decrease risks. Also discuss the use of car seats and bicycle helmets. Emphasize that supervison is the best prevention!

Child Abuse and Neglect

Abuse or neglect can occur at any age, but younger children are dependent on parents for all their needs, both physical and psychological, and are therefore more vulnerable. See Guidelines for Assessing Abuse in Appendix C.

RECOGNIZING ABUSE

Abuse can occur at any age and comes in many different forms. It can take the form of neglect, physical injury, sexual abuse, or psychological abuse. Be alert for the following signs and symptoms of abuse or neglect in children:

- Obvious physical signs of abuse or neglect
- Repeated emergency room visits
- Siblings blamed for injury
- Inconsistent account of how injury occurred
- Report of abuse by child
- Inappropriate response by child or parent to injury
- Inconsistency between physical findings and cause of injury
- Inconsistency between injury and child's developmental level
- Previous history of abuse

ALERT

A sudden change in a child's behavior may reflect an underlying problem that warrants further investigation.

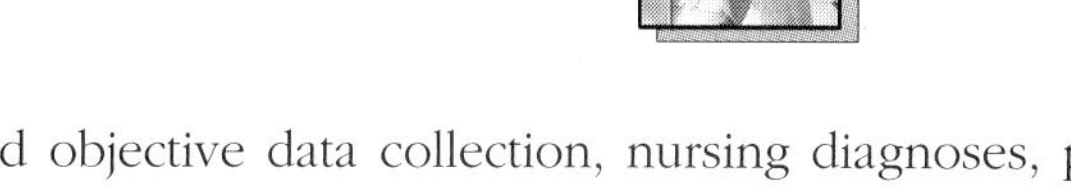

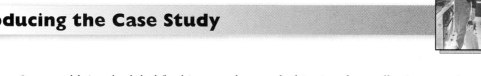

Introducing the Case Study

Travis Harrison, 3 years old, is scheduled for his annual checkup. He sits quietly on his mother's lap but looks wide eyed and anxious as you approach to bring him into the examination room.

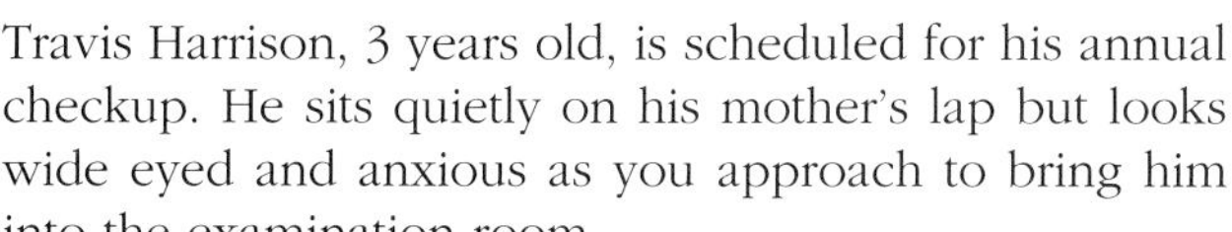

Performing the Toddler and Preschooler Assessment

At this age, the assessment is performed with the parent or guardian present. Even so, you need to explain what you are doing and why. Because the toddler thinks in a very concrete way, keep your explanations very simple. Toys, such as hand puppets, or games can be helpful when examining the toddler or preschooler. If some procedures might cause discomfort—such as the otoscopic examination if the child has an earache—leave them until the end.

As you perform the examination, keep in mind the normal developmental changes affecting this age group. As with all assessments, the process involves subjective and objective data collection, nursing diagnoses, planning, interventions, and evaluation.

Health History

Although the parent will provide most of the history, you may want the child's response to a few questions. For instance, if there is an acute problem, ask the child to describe it in his or her own words. As you perform the assessment, also look for changes in the child's behavior that might reflect his or her health status.

Biographical Data

Begin with the biographical data. Take note of where and with whom the child resides. Also note who is listed as contact person—it may not be the parent. Do not assume anything!

Current Health Status

Ask about the health status of the child. Has he or she been healthy, or is there an acute problem? Be sure to ask about all current prescription and over-the-counter medications the child may be taking.

Past Health History

Besides asking specific health history questions, ask the mother about her pregnancy and the delivery of the child. Problems at this time may affect the child's growth and development. Also, be sure to ask whether the child's immunizations are current. (See Health Concerns, p. 794, for required immunizations.)

Family History

Ask about heart disease, strokes, cancer, and other serious health conditions within the family.

Review of Systems

Go through every system, asking the parent about changes or problems specific to the toddler or preschool child.

Review of Systems

SYSTEM/QUESTIONS TO ASK	RATIONALE/SIGNIFICANCE
General Health Survey	
How has the child been feeling?	Screens for any obvious problems.
Has his or her behavior changed? If so, how?	Good indicator of how child is feeling.
How much does the child weigh?	Monitor weight closely to evaluate normal growth and development.
Integumentary	
Does the child have any skin problems, such as rashes or excessive itching?	**Tinea capitis**, ringworm, and contagious disorders often occur in toddlers and preschoolers, especially if the child is in day care or preschool. **Atopic dermatitis** (eczema) is often associated with allergies and has a familial tendency. **Diaper dermatitis** (diaper rash) occurs from prolonged exposure to an irritant, such as urine or feces. **Pediculosis capitis** (head lice) often occurs in preschoolers in day care or preschool. Playing dress-up or sharing hats increases transmission.
Is the child exposed to the sun? Does he or she wear sunblock?	Excessive sun exposure (ultraviolet rays) without sunblock increases risk for skin cancer later in life.
HEENT/*Eyes*	
Does the child have vision problems? Crossed eyes?	Normal visual acuity is 20/40 for toddlers. Depth perception is still developing.
When was the child's last eye examination?	Test vision routinely during physical exams.
***HEENT/*Ears**	
Does the child have hearing problems?	Test hearing routinely during physical exam.
Does he or she respond to sounds?	
Is he or she talking or making sounds?	
When was the child's last hearing exam?	
Does the child have frequent ear infections?	Toddlers and preschoolers have a high incidence of **otitis media**, with the highest incidence between 6 months and 2 years.
Is the child irritable? Does he or she have a poor appetite or sleep poorly?	
HEENT/*Teeth*	
How many teeth does the child have?	All 20 primary teeth should be in by age 2½.

Review of Systems

SYSTEM/QUESTIONS TO ASK	RATIONALE/SIGNIFICANCE
Has the child had his or her first dental exam?	The first dental exam should occur shortly after primary teeth start erupting. At least one dental exam per year recommended.
Does the child brush his or her own teeth? How often?	Review toothbrushing technique with child and parent.
Is your water fluorinated?	Fluoride decreases tooth decay.
Does the child go to bed with a bottle?	Bedtime bottles, nocturnal breast feeding, or coating pacifiers with a sweet substance can cause **baby bottle caries**, which occurs most frequently between 18 months and 3 years.
	ALERT Fluoride is toxic if ingested. Advise parents to supervise toothbrushing and not allow the child to eat or swallow toothpaste.
Respiratory	
Does the child have a cough, sneezing, runny nose, or fever?	Upper respiratory infections (URIs) are common in toddlers and preschoolers. **Respiratory syncytial virus** (RSV) causes one-half of all bronchiolitis and usually occurs in children under age 2.
Does he or she wheeze or have trouble breathing?	Asthma is the most common disease among children. Onset is usually between ages 3 and 8.
Is the child exposed to air pollutants, such as smoke or second-hand smoke?	Exposure to second-hand smoke increases risk for respiratory and ear infections and asthma attacks.
Cardiovascular	
Were you ever told that the child had a heart murmur?	Although cardiovascular disease is uncommon in children, murmurs are a common finding. Most are innocent, functional murmurs, but follow-up is indicated to rule out pathology.
Has the child ever turned blue?	Change in skin color may indicate cardiopulmonary problem.
Gastrointestinal	
Is the child potty trained?	Bowel control is usually achieved before age 3.
What is his or her bowel pattern?	
Genitourinary	
Does the child have bladder control?	Full bladder control may not occur until age 5.
Musculoskeletal	
Is the child walking?	The child should be able to walk without difficulty by 12 or 13 months.
	ALERT Even though the child can walk, he or she is still at risk for falls because he or she does not have refined coordination or full depth perception.
Neurological	
Is the child speaking? Does he or she use complete sentences?	Cognitive skills continue to develop and speech normally develops between ages 2 and 4.
Does he or she have any fears?	Fear of real and imaginary things is common (e.g., fear of dogs or of the dark).
Does the child have temper tantrums or aggressive behavior?	May need to educate parents about effective ways to deal with child's behavior.
Lymphatic/Hematologic	
Does child have any lumps in the neck, groin, or underarms?	May indicate infection.

Psychosocial Profile

The psychosocial profile should focus on the child's health practices and behaviors that affect health and well-being.

Health Practices

When was the child's last checkup? (Checkups are recommended every year.) Keep in mind that the child may have no control over frequency of health screenings. The parent or guardian usually assumes this responsibility, and health insurance or lack of it may be an influencing factor. You may need to make appropriate referrals or provide information on available health resources.

Typical Day

What is the child's typical day like? Does he or she have a babysitter or go to day care or preschool? If so, does he or she enjoy it? What kind of day-care situation is it (e.g., day-care center, child care in private home, babysitter in your own home)?

Nutritional Patterns

If necessary, provide nutritional education to children and families.

Ask: Is child still nursing or bottle feeding? If yes, how often? Because breast milk contains immunoglobulin A (IgA), and breastfeeding minimizes reflux of milk into the eustachian tube, breastfeeding decreases the risk of otitis media and respiratory viruses and allergies. Ask for a 24-hour diet recall, inquiring about how often child eats breakfast and what he or she usually eats at each meal. Ask the child to name his or her favorite foods and snacks. Also ask about junk food and fast food, which amount to empty calories and contribute to the high incidence of obesity among children.

Toddlers between 12 and 18 months still have high protein and calorie requirements for growth and high calcium, iron, and phosphorous requirements for bone growth. After 18 months, the toddler's appetite decreases (**physiologic anorexia**) in response to decreased nutritional needs. Preschoolers need an average of 1800 calories a day, as well as calcium and minerals for bone growth. They should eat limited fats. During the toddler and preschool years, the child develops taste preferences and may become a picky eater.

Activity and Exercise Patterns

Is the child very active? What does he or she enjoy doing? Is he or she supervised during activities? Toddlers and preschoolers are normally very active and need close supervision.

Recreation and Hobbies

Safety is a major concern for the toddler and preschooler. If recreational activities or hobbies increase the risk for injury, ask if protective measures are used such as bike helmets. Also ask about the parents' hobbies. For example, are there guns in the home? Play for toddlers is parallel (playing next to each other but not together); play for preschoolers is associative, group play, with more social interaction. In both age groups, safety is paramount, supervision is needed, and toys must be appropriate for the child's age.

Sleep and Rest Patterns

Ask about sleep patterns and naps, bedtime rituals, and sleep problems (nightmares, night terrors, somambulance, enuresis). How many hours does the child sleep? Twelve hours a day is normal. Toddlers usually need a nap, but preschoolers do not.

Personal Habits

Ask parents about their and other caregiver's personal habits. Do they smoke, drink alcohol, or use drugs? Exposure to these substances places the child at risk for health problems. If drug and alcohol abuse is an issue, the caregiver's ability and the home environment need to be assessed to ensure the child's safety. Referrals may be warranted.

Roles and Relationships

If there are siblings, ask the parent about the relationship. Sibling rivalry is not uncommon.

Religion and Spirituality

The toddler and preschooler's perception of a Supreme Being is concrete and based on the beliefs and practices of parents and caregivers. Prayers are often part of bedtime rituals and can be a source of comfort for a child.

Sexuality

Toddlers and preschoolers are curious by nature and exhibit sex-role imitation. They are also curious about their own bodies, and it is not uncommon for them to masturbate. How parents address this behavior is important and can have lasting effects.

Stress and Coping

Does the child behave aggressively or have temper tantrums? If the child hurts himself or herself or others, he or she needs to learn effective coping strategies, and a referral may be necessary.

Physical Assessment

After you complete the health history, perform the physical examination. You will use all four assessment techniques (for more information, see Chapter 3, Approach

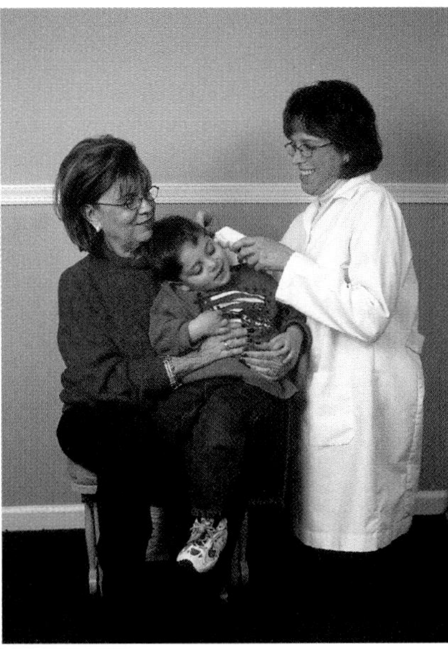

FIGURE 23–1. Taking temperature.

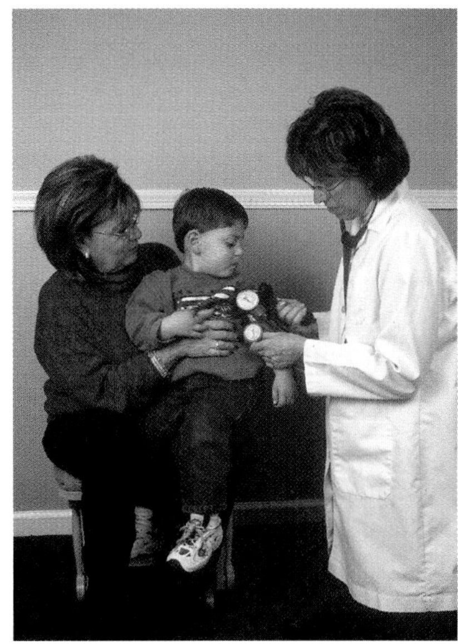

FIGURE 23–2. Taking blood pressure.

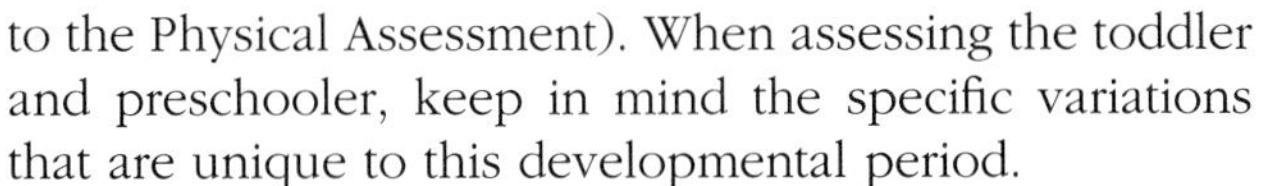

to the Physical Assessment). When assessing the toddler and preschooler, keep in mind the specific variations that are unique to this developmental period.

Begin with a general survey, obtaining height, weight, and vital signs such as temperature and blood pressure (Figs. 23–1 and 23–2). Keep track of the child's growth and development by plotting height and weight on growth charts (see Appendix B) The toddler usually gains 4 to 6 pounds and grows 3 inches a year. Head and chest circumferences are usually equal by age 2. The preschooler gains 5 pounds and grows 2½ to 3 inches a year. Changes in vital signs include a slight, gradual increase in blood pressure (BP) and a slight decrease in temperature, pulse, and respirations.

Performing a Head-to-Toe Physical Assessment

SYSTEM/ASSESSMENT	NORMAL VARIATIONS/ ABNORMAL FINDINGS/RATIONALE
General Health Survey	
INSPECT	
Inspect overall appearance, noting appropriate growth and development for child's age.	Toddler's general appearance: Pot belly and wide base of support. Preschooler loses pot belly and becomes taller and leaner. Note delays or premature maturation. Note obvious weight problems.
Integumentary	
INSPECT	
Inspect skin for lesions.	Lesions, such as tinea capitas or ringworm, need treatment.
Inspect hair and scalp for lice.	Pediculosis is common among preschoolers.

ALERT
Suspect abuse if you find unexplained bruising or injury (see box, Recognizing Abuse, page 785).

(Continued)

Performing a Head-to-Toe Physical Assessment *(Continued)*

SYSTEM/ASSESSMENT	NORMAL VARIATIONS/ ABNORMAL FINDINGS/RATIONALE
HEENT/*Head and Face*	
INSPECT/PALPATE	
Inspect head and face.	Head size growth slows to 1 inch a year by end of age 2; then ½ inch a year until age 5.
Palpate anterior fontanel.	Anterior fontanel closes by 18 months.
HEENT/*Eyes*	
INSPECT	
Test visual acuity.	Visual acuity is normally 20/40 during the toddler years. Begin vision screening between ages 3 and 4. Visual deficits warrant follow-up.
Test for "lazy eye" **(strabismus)** with corneal light reflex or cover-uncover test.	Referral needed for strabismus to prevent **amblyopia.**
HEENT/*Ears*	
INSPECT	
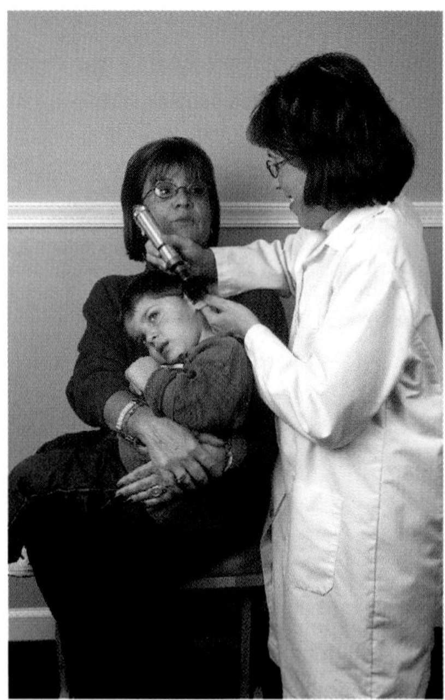 **Inspecting ear with otoscope** Test hearing with pure tone audiometer. Inspect external ear canal and tympanic membrane.	Test hearing by age 3 or 4. Hearing deficits warrant follow-up. Toddlers and preschoolers have a high incidence of otitis media.
HEENT/*Nose*	
INSPECT	
Inspect nasal septum and mucosa.	*Boggy, bluish-purple, or gray turbinates:* Chronic rhinorrhea, which can result from allergic rhinitis.

Performing a Head-to-Toe Physical Assessment

SYSTEM/ASSESSMENT	NORMAL VARIATIONS/ ABNORMAL FINDINGS/RATIONALE
	ALERT When inspecting nares or external ear canal, be alert for foreign objects.
HEENT/*Mouth* Inspect oral mucosa and pharynx. Inspect number and condition of teeth.	Generally, tonsils are large. Eruption of primary teeth is usually complete by age 2½ years. Note baby bottle caries. 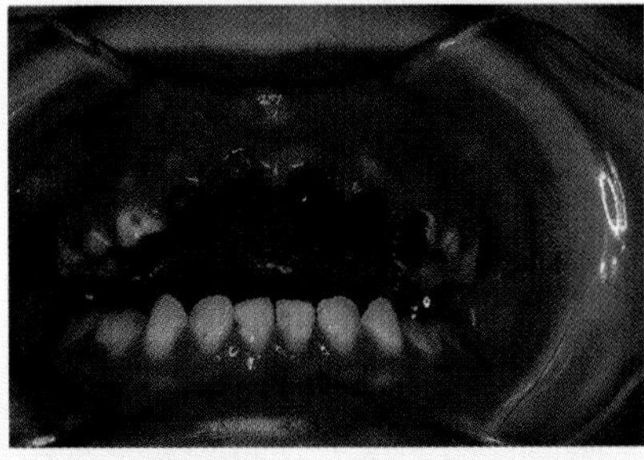 **Baby bottle caries** Review dental hygiene with parent and child.
HEENT/*Neck* *PALPATE* Palpate for lymph nodes.	*Enlarged lymph nodes:* Infection or lymphoma.
Respiratory *INSPECT/AUSCULTATE* Inspect and measure size and shape of chest. 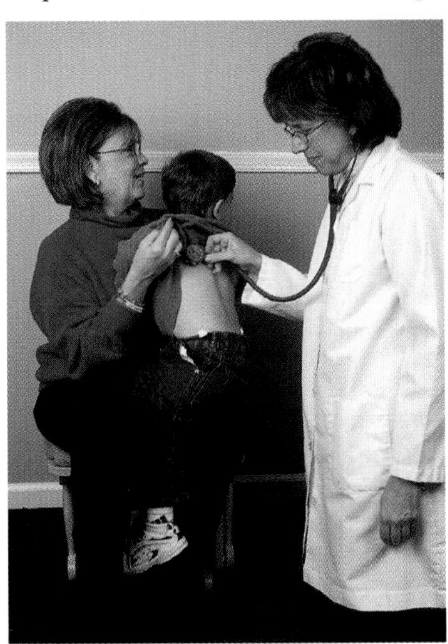 **Auscultating lungs**	Anteroposterior to lateral diameter should be 1:2 by end of second year.

(Continued)

Performing a Head-to-Toe Physical Assessment *(Continued)*

SYSTEM/ASSESSMENT	NORMAL VARIATIONS/ ABNORMAL FINDINGS/RATIONALE
Respiratory (*continued*) Auscultate lungs.	Toddlers and preschoolers have a high incidence of respiratory infections.
Cardiovascular *AUSCULTATE*	
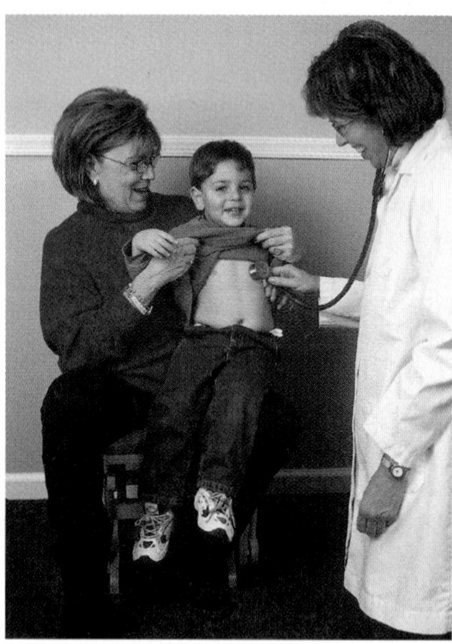 **Auscultating heart** Auscultate heart, noting rate and rhythm.	Children often have a sinus arrhythmia and a split second heart sound that both change with respiration. This is a normal variation. Systolic innocent murmurs and venous hum are common findings. **ALERT** If you detect a murmur, refer the patient for follow-up to rule out pathology.
Gastrointestinal *INSPECT/PALPATE/AUSCULTATE* Inspect, palpate, and auscultate the abdomen.	
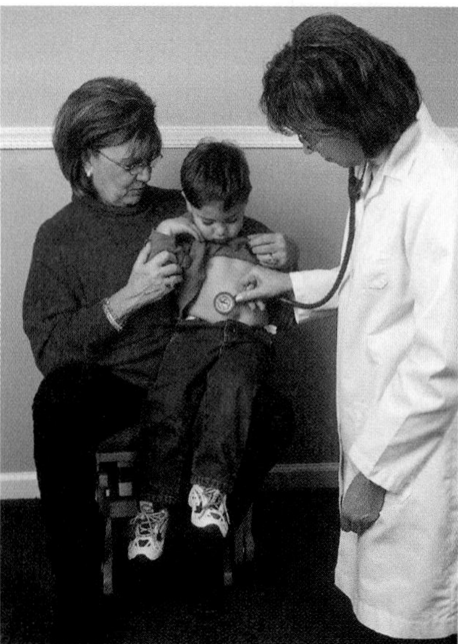 **Auscultating abdomen**	Pot belly normal for toddler; disappears as abdominal muscles strengthen.

Performing a Head-to-Toe Physical Assessment

SYSTEM/ASSESSMENT	NORMAL VARIATIONS/ ABNORMAL FINDINGS/RATIONALE
Genitourinary *INSPECT/PALPATE* Inspect external genitalia.	If child is still in diapers, inspect for diaper dermatitis.
Musculoskeletal *INSPECT* Inspect gait.	Toddlers usually can walk alone by 12 to 13 months. Balance is unsteady with wide base of support. **Valgus** (knock knees) or **varus** (bowlegs) may be present. The preschooler's gait is more balanced, smaller base of support; child walks, jumps, climbs by age 3.
Test muscle strength.	Strength increases during preschool years.
Neurological *INSPECT* Test balance, coordination, and accuracy of movements.	Balance and coordination improve with refinement of fine motor skills.

Once you have completed your assessment, document your findings, identify any nursing diagnoses, and formulate a plan of care.

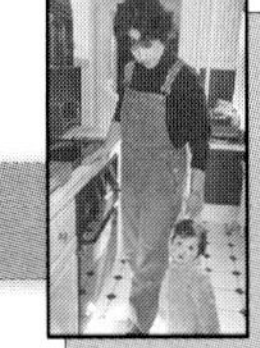

Back to the Case Study

Now that you understand the physical and psychosocial issues surrounding toddlers and preschoolers, apply your knowledge to our case study subject, 3-year-old Travis Harrison, by answering the following questions.

CRITICAL THINKING ACTIVITY #1

How does assessment of the toddler and preschooler differ from assessment of other patients?

CRITICAL THINKING ACTIVITY #2

What approach is best for assessing the toddler and preschooler?

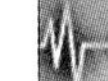

CRITICAL THINKING ACTIVITY #3

What health concerns should I keep in mind as I proceed with the assessment?

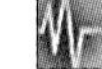

CRITICAL THINKING ACTIVITY #4

List some nursing diagnoses that are appropriate for the toddler and preschooler.

Research Tells Us

Accidents are the leading cause of death in children. Teaching preventive behaviors may reduce the risk of accidents, but what age is appropriate to begin teaching children? The Pre-school Health and Safety Knowledge Assessment (PHASKA) is an instrument used to evaluate the health and safety knowledge of young children in the areas of safety, hygiene, and health and nutrition knowledge.

In this study, 308 preschool children between ages 28 months and 80 months (M = 53.7 months) were tested. Aside from establishing the reliability and validity of this instrument, the PHASKA scores increased with age. These findings suggest that preschoolers are ready and willing learners.

As a nurse, you are in an ideal position to teach children health and safety behaviors. Children who are taught at an early age may well continue healthy behaviors into adulthood.

Mobley, C., & Evanshevski, J. (2000). Evaluating health and safety knowledge of preschoolers: Assessing their early start to begin health smart. *Journal of Pediatric Health Care, 14*(4), 160–165.

Health Concerns

Immunizations needed between ages 1 and 5 include:

- **Polio:** Dose 3 between 12 and 18 months; dose 4 between ages 4 and 6.
- **Diphtheria, Tetanus, Pertussis (DTaP)**: Dose 4 between 12 and 18 months and dose 5 between ages 4 and 6.
- **Measles, Mumps, Rubella (MMR):** Dose 1 between 12 and 15 months and dose 2 between ages 2 and 6.
- **Varicella Zoster (Chickenpox) (VZV):** Between 12 and 18 months or at any age after that if the child has never had chickenpox.
- **Hepatitis B (HepB):** Dose 3 between 6 and 18 months.
- ***Haemophilus influenzae* (Hib):** Dose 4 between 12 and 15 months.

Common Problems

Problems occurring frequently in toddlers and preschoolers include toilet training issues, sleep problems, temper tantrums, sibling rivalry, fears, stress, regression, child abuse and neglect, poisoning, injuries, otitis media, baby bottle caries, nutritional problems, and asthma.

Summary

- Toddlers and preschoolers have their own unique developmental and psychosocial issues.
- Understanding these issues and knowing how to communicate honestly and effectively with children and parents will help you conduct a thorough assessment and develop an effective plan of care.

CHAPTER 24

Assessing the School-Age Child and Adolescent

Before You Begin

INTRODUCTION TO ASSESSING THE SCHOOL-AGE CHILD AND ADOLESCENT

During the period from school age through adolescence, the patient grows and matures from a child to a young adult. Dealing with this age group is a challenging, yet potentially very rewarding aspect of nursing care. To effectively assess and intervene, you must be familiar with the significant physical, psychosocial, and cognitive developmental changes that occur before, during, and after puberty. Although each stage has its own set of milestones, the assessment techniques you use are essentially the same. This chapter covers the complete health history and physical assessment for the school-age patient first, and then moves on to the adolescent.

Assessing the School-Age Child

The school-age child is between the ages of 6 and 12 years. This age span (called the "latency period" by Freud) is like the calm before the storm and both follows and precedes a time of great growth and development. Although this is a slower, more stable period, some major changes do occur. For example, when the child begins school, a whole new world opens up to him or her, and the child begins to develop relationships other than those within the family.

Before beginning your health assessment, ask yourself:

- How does assessment of the school-age child differ from assessment of other patients?
- What approach is best for the school-age child?
- What health concerns should I keep in mind as I proceed?

Developmental Changes

The changes that take place during the school-age years are subtle. Growth and development are both physical and psychosocial. Before you can detect any abnormalities, you need to understand the normal changes that occur in this age period.

Physical Changes

As the school-age child grows, his or her measurements become more proportional as baby fat disappears. The neuromuscular system continues to develop, and the child becomes more agile and coordinated. For specific physical changes that occur, see the Physical Assessment section.

Psychosocial and Emotional Changes

Psychosocial changes also occur at an even pace. Erikson describes this stage as industry versus inferiority. The child becomes more independent, developing skills and competencies. Social skills also develop as the child becomes more involved in school and community activities. With each success at school, at home, or in the community, confidence and independence grow. The child learns to cooperate, work, and compete with others. It is important that both adults and peers recognize the child's accomplishments.

Health Concerns and Risk Factors for School-Age Children

Injuries and Accidents: These are the most frequent cause of morbidity and mortality in children. The school-age child is very active and involved in many activities. Participation in sports especially increases the risk for injury. Injury can result from overuse or from engaging in activities not yet suitable for the child's age. Common injuries include tendonitis, osteochondritis, Osgood-Schlatter disease (osteochondritis of the epiphysis of the tibial tuberosity), and stress fractures.

Drug, Alcohol, and Nicotine Use: Although the use of drugs, alcohol, and nicotine occurs more frequently among adolescents, experimentation often begins during the school-age years and may continue into adolescence. Remember, peer pressure exerts great influence on a child's behavior. Prevention works best, so education needs to begin at an early age.

Eating Disorders: Obesity is an increasing problem among American children. Eating habits are established at an early age, and psychosocial and cultural factors can influence them. Eating may be associated with nurturing. The effects of obesity are not only physical; they also can affect the child's self-image. If obesity continues through adolescence into adulthood, the effects can be long lasting, increasing the person's risk for cardiovascular disease, hypertension, hyperlipidemia, diabetes, degenerative joint disease, sleep apnea, and colon cancer.

Learning Problems: During the school-age years, learning problems become apparent. Attention deficit hyperactivity disorder (ADHD) and learning disability (LD) are common. ADHD is characterized by developmentally inappropriate inattention, impulsiveness, and hyperactivity; LD is difficulty with reading, writing, listening, reasoning, speaking, mathematical skills, and social skills. Care must be taken not to prematurely label a child as having ADHD or LD because many children exhibit one or more of these behaviors. The symptoms of ADHD begin before age 7, and children exhibit 6 or more symptoms for at least 6 months. As a nurse, you will need to make appropriate referrals as indicated, and help with the education and therapeutic management of children with ADHD and LD.

Lying, Cheating, and Stealing: Children may lie to avoid punishment or cheat to win a game. These common behaviors usually occur in this age group and diminish as the child becomes older and more responsible for his or her behavior.

Emotional Problems: Children commonly experience stress. The source can be the home, school, or community. Children also experience various types of emotional problems, such as school phobia, recurrent abdominal pain, conversion reactions, depression, and even schizophrenia. Often, the emotional problem is triggered by a traumatic event, such as an illness, the loss of a parent, or a major family crisis such as divorce. Be alert for signs of stress that warrant further assessment such as headaches; stomachaches; sleep problems; enuresis; changes in eating habits; changes in behavior, such as aggressiveness; poor performance in school; isolation or withdrawal from participation; and regression. The key is to identify the problem and respond promptly to avoid further ill effects.

Peer acceptance becomes especially important. The child needs a sense of belonging and of "fitting in." Peers often have a greater influence on a child than his or her parents. Sex roles are established through peer relationships, and same-sex friendships develop. School provides the child with the opportunity to see different perspectives and to argue, negotiate, resolve conflicts, work together, and develop friendships. Belonging to clubs, teams, and peer groups is important.

Even though peer influence seems greater than parental influence, parents still play a major role in the child's development. Children test parents, so it is important that parents set limits to give the child a sense of security.

Team play becomes important, either on sport teams or in quiet games. Both involve rules and rituals that children strongly adhere to. Watching sports, creating artwork, reading, collecting things, cooking, sewing, and similar activities are also important activities that often carry through adolescence into adulthood. As the child progresses through this stage, his or her self-concept further develops. For a positive self-concept to develop, the child needs to feel special.

The child also moves from preconceptual thinking to conceptual thinking. Piaget calls this stage of cognitive development "concrete operations," when the child begins using thought processes to perceive the world. The child masters the tasks of conservation and classifications. Reading is the most important skill that develops during this stage.

During the school-age years, the child becomes less egocentric and begins to develop a conscience. Initially, his or her views were black and white, right or wrong based on the parents' moral values. But as the child grows and matures, he or she incorporates different points of views before making judgments. The Supreme Being is seen in concrete terms. Illness or injury may be seen as a punishment.

As you proceed with the assessment, stay alert for the following health problems and risk factors common in school-age children.

Cultural and Ethnic Variations

Various cultures have different perspectives on children and their role in the family. You need to understand any cultural influences that might have an impact on your patient's plan of care.

Cultural and Ethnic Variations in School-Age Children

CULTURAL GROUP	INFLUENCE
Amish	Children are seen as gift from God. Parents very directive of child throughout school.
Appalachian	Parents believe in physical punishment. Having children is associated with sense of importance.
Arab-American	Child's character and success depend on parental influence. Children are taught conformity and cooperation. A "good" child is obedient; behavior that would bring dishonor is avoided. Parents believe in physical punishment.
Chinese-American	Boys and girls play together when young but are separated when older. Children are pressured to succeed. Males are more valued than females. Children are expected to help out at home.
Cuban-American	Children are expected to study and respect their parents.
Egyptian-American	Children are expected to be studious and goal oriented as well as respectful and loyal to family.
Filipino-American	Children are expected to honor and respect their parents.
French-American	Children are well educated and a source of pride for the family.
Greek-American	Children are the center of the family. Parents use teasing as a form of discipline to toughen children and make them aware of public opinion.
Iranian-American	This is a child-oriented society. Children are expected to be respectful.
Irish-American	Boys are expected to be more aggressive than girls. Children are expected to show self-restraint, discipline, respect, and obedience.

(Continued)

Cultural and Ethnic Variations in School-Age Children *(Continued)*

CULTURAL GROUP	INFLUENCE
Jewish	Children are seen as a valued treasure. Children are expected to respect and honor parents.
Mexican-American	Children are highly valued but must respect parents.
Navajo Native American	Children are allowed to make own decisions, such as taking medicine, which might seem irresponsible on part of parents.
Vietnamese-American	Children are prized and valued. Children are expected to be obedient and devoted.

Introducing the Case Study

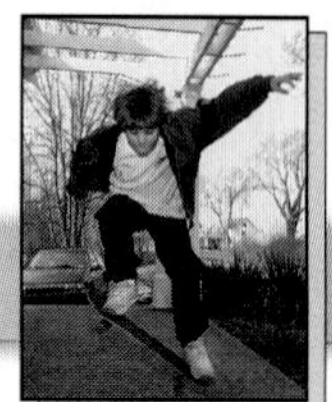

Joshua Goldfarb, age 6, is starting first grade this fall. He is in the pediatrician's office for his required physical examination. Joshua is sitting close to his mother and seems a little anxious. He asks you, "Do I have to get any shots?"

Performing the School-Age Child Assessment

Now that you understand the major issues affecting this age group, you can begin the actual assessment. The process is similar to that for an adult. To communicate with this age group, be honest, open, and nonjudgmental. School-age children often need an adult to look up to, and you are in an ideal position to serve as a role model. You are also in an ideal position to screen for risk factors and teach healthy lifestyle behaviors.

As with all assessments, the process involves data collection (both subjective and objective), diagnosis, planning, interventions, and evaluation.

Health History

Follow the history format used for an adult, but keep in mind the normal developmental changes and the issues confronting the school-age child. Although the parent or guardian usually provides most of the history, you may want the child's response to a few questions. For example, if there is an acute problem, you should ask the child to describe it in his or her own words. Because most of the health history is identical to an adult's, the sections that follow contain only information that is especially important to ask the school-age child or that is specific to this age group.

Biographical Data

Begin with the biographical data, noting where and with whom your client resides. Also note who is listed as contact person—it may not be a parent. Do not assume anything!

Current Health Status

Ask the parent or guardian about all prescription and over-the-counter medications.

Past Health History

Ask the parent or guardian specific past health history questions. An immunization history is especially important (see Health Concerns, p. 807, for required immunizations).

Family History

Ask the parent or guardian about heart disease, strokes, cancer, and other serious health conditions within the family. Be sure to ask if anyone died at an early age (under 35) from a sudden heart attack. This may be a risk factor for sports participation and may require additional investigation.

Review of Systems

Go through every system, asking about changes or problems specific to the school-age child. Although the questions that follow are addressed to the child, you will need to question the parent or guardian in the case of younger children.

Review of Systems

SYSTEM/QUESTIONS TO ASK	RATIONALE/SIGNIFICANCE
General Health Survey	
How have you been feeling?	Screens for obvious problems.
Have you lost or gained weight recently?	Changes in weight, especially gains, may indicate poor eating habits.
Integumentary	
Do you have any skin rashes or lesions? Excessive itching?	Tinea capitis; ringworm; verruca (warts); contact dermatitis; and poison ivy, oak, and sumac frequently seen in school-age children. Pediculosis capitis (head lice) common in school-age children.
Are you exposed to the sun? Does you use sunblock?	Excessive sun exposure (UV rays) without sunblock increases risk for skin cancer later in life.
HEENT/*Eyes*	
Do you have any visual problems?	Visual acuity reaches 20/20 by school age.
Do you wear glasses? If yes, do you wear them consistently, especially while at school?	Children may not consistently wear glasses for fear of being teased by other children.
Do you wear contact lenses?	May identify teaching needs regarding care of contact lenses.
When was your last eye exam?	Eyes should be tested routinely during physical examinations.
HEENT/*Ears*	
Do you have any hearing problems? Do you listen to loud music?	Cochlear damage can result from excessive exposure to loud noise, such as CD players and rock concerts. May identify health teaching need regarding noise pollution's effect on hearing.
When was your last hearing exam?	Hearing should be tested routinely during physical exams.
HEENT/*Teeth*	
How many second teeth do you have?	Primary teeth are lost during school-age years and replaced by secondary teeth. These years are called the "age of the loose tooth" or "ugly duckling stage," because secondary teeth are initially too big for the face.
When was your last visit to the dentist? Do you see an orthodontist?	Should have at least an annual dental exam. Common dental problems include dental caries, periodontal disease, malocclusion, and dental injury.

(Continued)

Review of Systems *(Continued)*

SYSTEM/QUESTIONS TO ASK	RATIONALE/SIGNIFICANCE
	ALERT In secondary tooth evulsion, the tooth should be replanted as soon as possible. If it is replanted within 30 minutes, replantation is 70% successful.
Respiratory Do you have asthma?	Asthma is the most common respiratory disease in children. Allergies and asthma often become apparent during school-age years.
Do you ever have trouble breathing or wheeze when exercising or running? Are you exposed to air pollutants, smoke, or second-hand smoke?	*Exercise-induced bronchospasm:* Acute, reversible, self-terminating airway obstruction that occurs after vigorous exercise, peaks 5–10 minutes once activity stops, and then ceases within 30 minutes.
Cardiovascular Do you have any chest pain? Does your heart ever skip a beat?	Although cardiovascular disease is not common in children and adolescents, it can occur. Prolonged QT syndrome can cause sudden cardiac death in a seemingly healthy child.
Gastrointestinal Do you have any stomach problems? How often do you have a bowel movement?	**Encopresis** (fecal incontinence and voluntary or involuntary loss of bowel control) is more common in boys, usually secondary to constipation. Recurrent abdominal pain is common during childhood and is often psychosomatic. Child usually has poor self-image. School can precipitate attacks. **ALERT** If child presents with recurrent abdominal pain, rule out physiologic causes first.
Genitourinary Do you have bladder control? Do you wet the bed?	Noctural bedwetting is more common in boys and often ends by ages 6 to 8.

Review of Systems

SYSTEM/QUESTIONS TO ASK	RATIONALE/SIGNIFICANCE
Musculoskeletal Do you have any back problems? Have you ever been told you had a spinal problem?	Heavy backpacks are associated with low back problems in children. **Scoliosis** (lateral curvature of spine) occurs more often in girls than boys. Screening usually occurs in middle school and high school. If present, determine whether scoliosis is structural or postural (see Chapter 18, Assessing the Musculoskeletal System). Physical maturity varies and does not always correlate with emotional or social maturity.
Neurological How would you describe your mood?	Stress, anxiety, and fear are seen in children. Depression, conversion reactions, and even schizophrenia can occur during childhood and can be difficult to detect.
Lymphatic/Hematological Have you been tired? Do you have any lumps in your neck, underarms, or groin?	Non-Hodgkin's lymphomas occur most frequently in children before age 15.

Psychosocial Profile

The psychosocial profile focuses on the child's health practices and on behaviors that affect health and well-being. Although the questions below are addressed to the child, you will need to question the parent/guardian with younger patients.

Health Practices

When did the child have his or her last checkup? Check-ups are recommended every 2 years, more frequently if child has an existing health problem or is involved in sports. Keep in mind that the child may have no control over frequency of health screenings. The parent or guardian usually assumes this responsibility, and health insurance or lack of it may be an influencing factor. You may need to make appropriate referrals or provide information on available health resources.

Typical Day

What is a typical day like? How is the child doing in school? This allows you to see the patient through his or her own eyes and possibly identify stresses confronting him or her in everyday life. A change in academic performance or a sudden disinterest in school may reflect a more serious problem. What subjects does the child like and dislike? If he or she is having problems with a particular subject, has he or she sought help? How many days of school does he or she usually miss every term? ADHD and LD may become more apparent once the child starts school, and you should make appropriate referrals. School phobias are common at age 10, with somatic complaints such as nausea, headache, or abdominal pain. These complaints quickly subside once the child is assured that he or she doesn't have to go to school. If the patient is a "latchkey child," ask what he or she does with the time until the parent or guardian returns home. Children who are left home alone are at a higher risk for injury or delinquent behavior.

Nutritional Patterns

Ask for a 24-hour diet recall. Inquire about eating patterns, asking, "How often do you eat breakfast?" "What so you usually have for lunch?" "What are your favorite snacks?" Junk food and fast food amount to empty calories and contribute to the high incidence of obesity among children. Take this opportunity to provide nutritional education to children and families.

Activity and exercise patterns

Ask what the child enjoys doing outside the home. Does he or she play any sports? If so, what? Contact sports increase the risk for injury. Does he or she wear protective equipment? What does the child like to do with his or her friends? How often does he or she watch TV during the week? How much time does he or she spend on the computer? You may identify a need for health education about the importance of routine exercise.

ALERT

If a child is active in sports, he or she should engage in those that are appropriate for his or her age.

Recreation/Hobbies

What does the child do for fun? What hobbies does he or she have? If recreational activities or hobbies increase the risk for injury, ask if he or she uses protective measures such as a bike helmet. Ask whether there are weapons in the home. If there are guns, ask if child has taken gun or hunting safety courses.

Sleep/Rest Patterns

Ask when the child usually goes to bed and when he or she awakens. Children from ages 8 to 11 may resist going to bed. Does the child have a bedtime routine? Does he or she wet the bed? Enuresis can continue into adolescence.

Personal Habits

Substance abuse is occurring at younger and younger ages; so many school-age children have already tried smoking or alcohol. Experimentation is common in this age group, and peer pressure can be great. So inquire about drug, alcohol, and nicotine use. Ask: "If you smoke cigarettes, how many do you smoke in an average day?" "If you use alcohol, how much do you usually drink during the week?" "If you use drugs, what type and what method (e.g., smoking, snorting, huffing, ingesting, or injecting)? Asking questions in this way is less threatening to the child; so he or she will be more likely to give an honest response.

Roles/Relationships/Self-Concept

Ask the child, "Who lives at home with you?" If he or she has siblings, ask about their relationship. Also ask, "Is there an adult in your life whom you feel comfortable talking with?" Teachers can have a major influence on a child's development, either positively or negatively. Ask about peer relationships. Does the child have a special friend, and what do they enjoy doing together? During the school-age years a child develops close same-sex friendships.

Ask the child to describe himself or herself by saying, "Tell me about yourself." Self-image and body image are often influenced by a child's perception of how he or she is seen by others. Anything out of the norm may become an easy target for teasing, and such teasing can have lasting effects.

Religious and Spiritual Influences

The school-age child's values and beliefs are often guided by those of the parents. The Supreme Being is thought of in concrete terms. Illness may be perceived as a punishment. Prayer can be a source of comfort for a child; for example, prayers are often part of bedtime rituals.

Sexuality Patterns

The school-age child is curious by nature, and it is not unusual for school-age children to incorporate some form of sexuality into play. This is the best time to begin sex education, and you are in an ideal position to educate both children and parents.

Stress and Coping

Ask questions such as: "What makes you angry?" What do you do when you get angry?" "What do you do to have fun or relax?" This identifies if the child has healthy coping strategies to deal with life's stresses. Violence is ever present in our society, at home, at school, and within the community. If the child uses violence as a coping mechanism, you need to help him or her to develop more effective coping strategies or make appropriate referrals.

Physical Assessment

After you complete the history, perform the physical examination. Physical assessment of the school-age child does not differ greatly from that of the adult—you use all four assessment techniques and the same tools (for more information, see Chapter 3, Approach to the Physical Assessment.) However, there are specific variations that are unique to this developmental period.

Begin with a general survey, obtaining height and weight. Plot the patient's height and weight on growth charts to note growth and development (see Appendix B for growth charts). School-age children grow about 5 cm a year and gain about 4½ to 6½ lb a year. Boys and girls are relatively equal in size until they reach preadolescence; then girls usually surpass boys in both height and weight. Until the boys catch up during adolescence, this growth discrepancy can be distressing for both boys and girls.

Also take vital signs (Figs. 24–1 and 24–2). Be aware that as children age, their pulse and respiration rates decrease and their blood pressure (BP) increases compared to what they were during infancy.

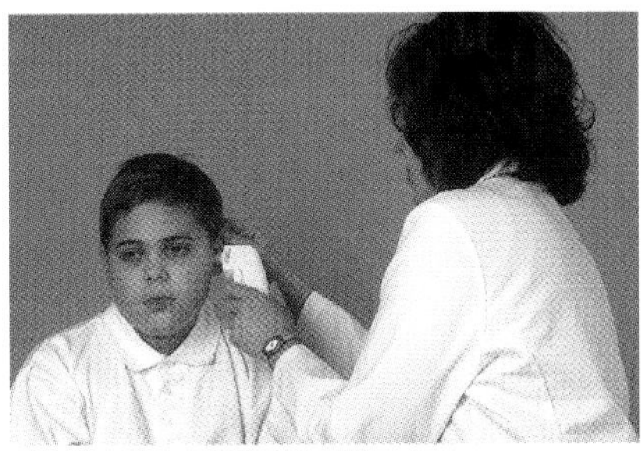

FIGURE 24–1. Taking temperature.

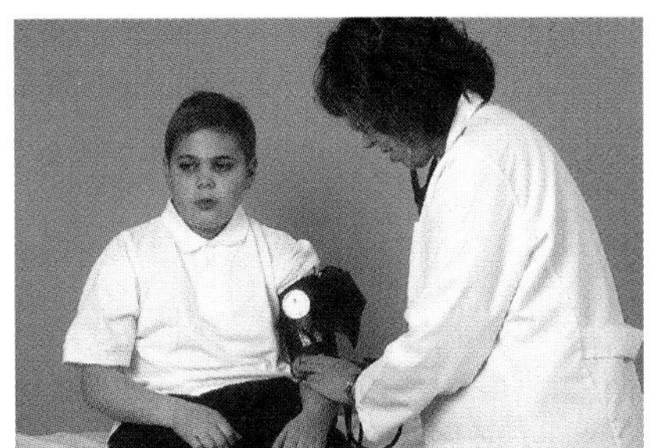

FIGURE 24–2. Taking blood pressure.

Performing a Head-to-Toe Physical Assessment

SYSTEM/ASSESSMENT	NORMAL VARIATIONS/ABNORMAL FINDINGS/RATIONALE
General Health Survey *INSPECT* Inspect overall appearance, noting appropriate growth and development for child's age.	General appearance becomes more slender; baby fat disappears. Note delays or premature maturation. Note obvious weight problems.
Integumentary *INSPECT* 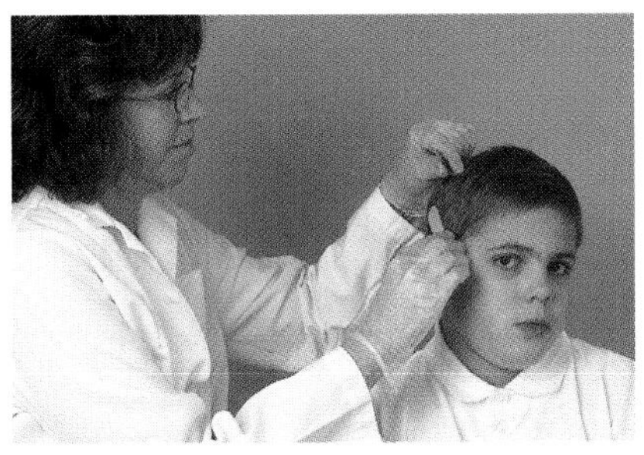 **Inspecting hair and scalp** Inspect skin for lesions. Inspect hair and scalp for lice.	Lesions, such as tinea capitis or ringworm, need treatment. Pediculosis is common among school-age children.
HEENT/*Head and Face* *INSPECT/PALPATE* Inspect head and face.	Head size becomes more proportionate to body.
HEENT/*Eyes* *INSPECT* 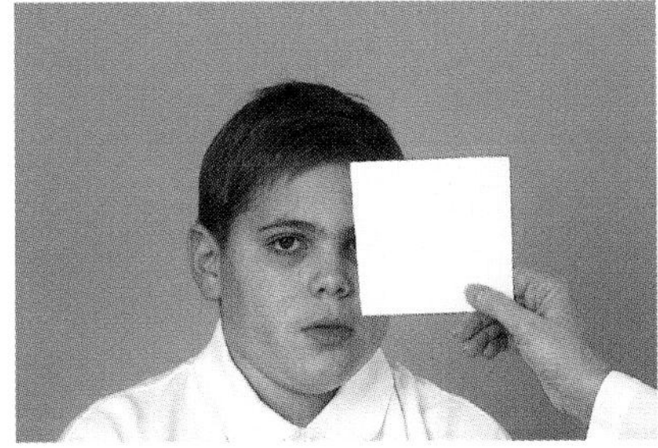 **Testing visual acuity** Test visual acuity.	Visual acuity should be 20/20 by age 6. Visual deficits warrant follow-up.

(Continued)

Performing a Head-to-Toe Physical Assessment *(Continued)*

SYSTEM/ASSESSMENT	NORMAL VARIATIONS/ABNORMAL FINDINGS/RATIONALE
HEENT/*Ears* *INSPECT*	
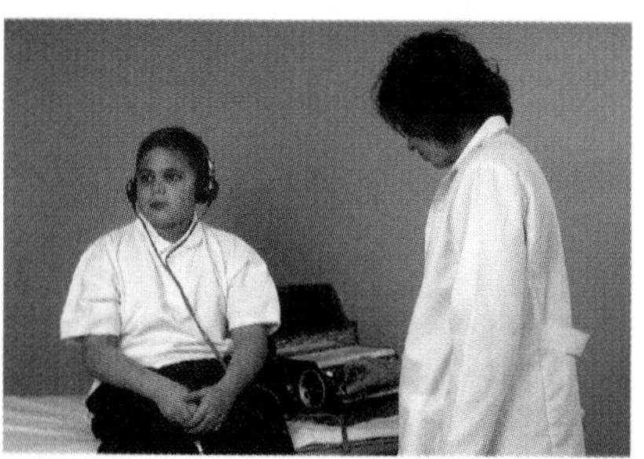 **Testing hearing** Test hearing with pure tone audiometer.	Hearing deficits warrant follow-up. Take this opportunity to teach hazards of listening to loud music.
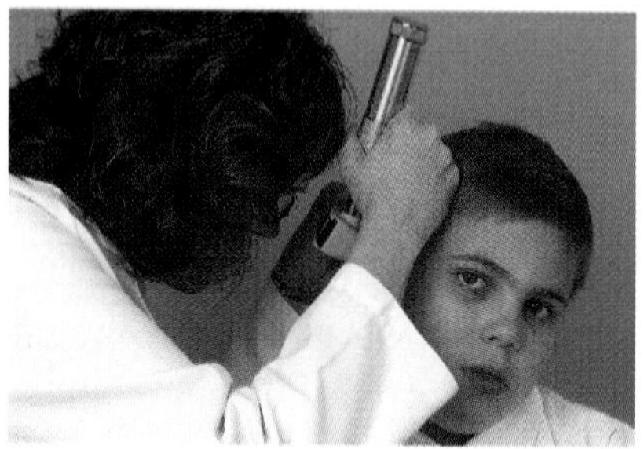 **Examining ear with otoscope** Examine ear with otoscope.	*Discharge, red tympanic membrane:* **Otitis media** (inflammation of middle ear). Common in children. Foreign bodies in ear are common.
HEENT/*Nose* *INSPECT* Inspect nasal septum and mucosa.	*Boggy, bluish-purple, or gray turbinates:* Allergic rhinitis. Can result in chronic rhinorrhea.
HEENT/*Mouth and Throat* *INSPECT*	
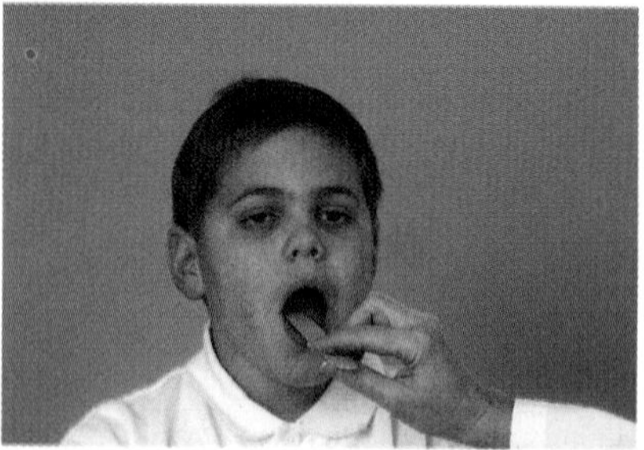 **Examining mouth and throat** Inspect oral mucosa and pharynx. Inspect occlusion, number of teeth.	Tonsils are usually large. If malocclusion present, may need to make referral to orthodontist. Child loses first teeth during this time. Secondary teeth begin to erupt around age 6 (6-year molars), and most secondary teeth are in by the time 12-year molars erupt. Also assess for orthodontic devices and brushing technique around them.

Performing a Head-to-Toe Physical Assessment

SYSTEM/ASSESSMENT	NORMAL VARIATIONS/ABNORMAL FINDINGS/RATIONALE
HEENT/*Neck* *PALPATE* 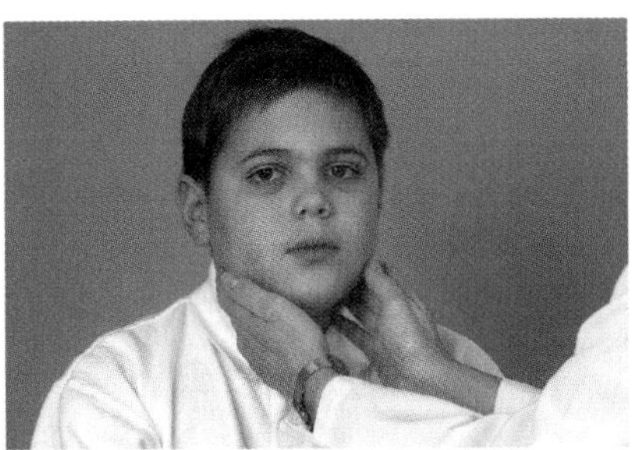 **Palpating lymph nodes** Palpate lymph nodes.	*Enlarged lymph nodes:* Infection or lymphoma.
Respiratory *AUSCULTATE* Auscultate lungs.	Children with exercise-induced asthma (EIA) require bronchodilators before activity. Usually, albuterol via a metered dose inhaler is given 20 to 30 minutes before exercise.
Cardiovascular *AUSCULTATE* Auscultate heart, noting rate and rhythm. 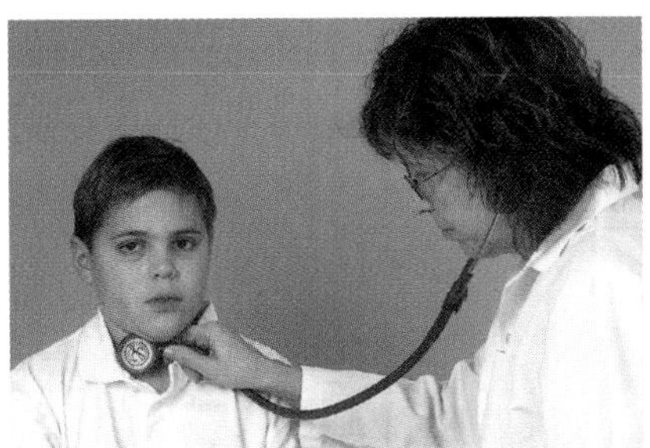 **Auscultating for venous hum** Auscultate for venous hum and murmurs.	Children often have sinus arrhythmia and split second heart sound, which change with respiration. This is a normal variation. Jugular venous hum is a normal, common finding in children. Murmurs are also common in children. They are often innocent and functional, but should be followed up to rule out pathology.

HELPFUL HINT

Be careful not to confuse a venous hum with a murmur. Remember: Jugular venous pulsations are easily obliterated!

SYSTEM/ASSESSMENT	NORMAL VARIATIONS/ABNORMAL FINDINGS/RATIONALE
Gastrointestinal *INSPECT/PALPATE/AUSCULATE* Inspect, auscultate, and palpate the abdomen.	Appendicitis is the most common illness during childhood that requires surgery.

(Continued)

Performing a Head-to-Toe Physical Assessment *(Continued)*

SYSTEM/ASSESSMENT	NORMAL VARIATIONS/ABNORMAL FINDINGS/RATIONALE
Genitourinary/Reproductive	
INSPECT	
Inspect external genitalia.	*Precocious puberty:* Sexual development before age 8 in girls and age 9 in boys warrants follow-up evaluation
Musculoskeletal	
INSPECT/PALPATE	
Inspect and palpate spinal curves.	Scoliosis is a major variation within musculoskeletal system.
Test for spinal deformities (see Chapter 18, Assessing the Musculoskeletal System).	Screening should be done in the preadolescent period, generally when the child is in the fifth to sixth grade. Significant curvature should be referred for evaluation and follow-up.
Test muscle strength.	Strength doubles during school-age years.
Neurological	
INSPECT	
Test balance, coordination, and accuracy of movements.	Balance and coordination greatly improve, with refinement of fine motor skills.

Once you have completed your assessment, document your findings, identify any nursing diagnoses, and formulate a plan of care. If you identify problem areas, actively involve both the child and his or her parents in the plan of care.

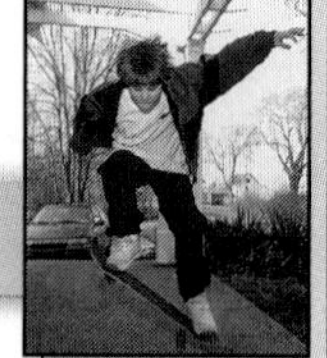

Back to the Case Study

Now that you understand the physical and psychosocial issues surrounding school-age children, apply your knowledge to our case study subject, 6-year-old Joshua Goldfarb, by answering the following questions.

 CRITICAL THINKING ACTIVITY #1

How does assessment of the school-age child differ from assessment of other patients?

 CRITICAL THINKING ACTIVITY #2

What approach is best for assessing the school-age child?

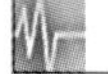 CRITICAL THINKING ACTIVITY #3

What health concerns should I keep in mind as I proceed with the assessment?

 CRITICAL THINKING ACTIVITY #4

List some nursing diagnoses that are appropriate for the school-age child.

Research Tells Us

More and more families in the United States are becoming homeless. An estimated 40 percent of children live below the poverty level and account for 25 percent of all homeless people. One recent study compared the health status of children using a school-based health center (SBHC) for comprehensive care. Of the 308 children seen at the SBHC, 76 lived in shelters and 232 lived in homes. The 308 charts were reviewed to identify health problems and medical coverage. The findings revealed that homeless children had significantly more health problems than children who lived at home. The authors concluded that homeless children were at higher risk for health problems and lack of medical coverage, and that SBHC is an effective means for providing health services to an increasingly underserved population. These findings are not surprising and have great implications for nursing. Support of SBHC would allow nurses to provide health care to this group.

Source: Berti, Zylbert and Rolnitzky, 2001.

Health Concerns

Immunizations needed between ages 6 and 12 include:

- **Polio:** Dose 4 by age 6.
- **Diptheria, Tetanus, Pertussis (DTaP):** Between ages 4 and 6.
- **Tetanus-Diphtheria "Booster" (Td):** After age 7 for children who have not gotten at least three doses of any tetanus and diphtheria vaccine; whenever child suffers a wound, if booster has not been received in last 5 years.
- **Measles, Mumps, Rubella (MMR):** Between ages 11 and 12 if second MMR shot was not received between ages 4 and 6.
- **Varicella Zoster (Chickenpox) (VZV):** Any time between ages 6 and 12 if child has never had chickenpox.
- **Hepatitis B (HepB):** Any time if child was not immunized during infancy or school-age years. Children between ages 11 and 15 may need only two doses, 4 to 6 months apart.
- ***Hemophilus influenzae* (Hib):** Not necessary unless child has special health concerns, such as sickle cell disease, HIV/AIDS, removal of spleen, bone marrow transplant, or cancer treatment with drugs.

Common Problems

Problems occurring frequently in school-age children include behavioral problems (e.g., school phobias, learning problems, and lying, cheating, or stealing); injuries and accidents; skin problems, such as ringworm, pediculosis, and contact dermatitis; asthma, nocturnal bedwetting (mainly boys); malocclusion; and eating disorders (including poor nutrition).

Summary

- School-age children have their own unique developmental and psychosocial issues.
- Understanding these issues and knowing how to communicate honestly and effectively with children and parents will help you conduct a thorough assessment and develop an effective plan of care.

Assessing the Adolescent

The term *adolescence* literally means "growing to maturity." In the past, the terms "adolescent" and "teenager" were considered synonymous. Today, however, the span of adolescence is considered not so much a specific range of years (13 to 19), but rather a time period marked by specific developmental tasks, both physical and psychosocial. With this definition, adolescence can extend from age 8 or 9 to age 21 or 22. Before assessing an adolescent, ask yourself these questions:

- How does assessment of the adolescent differ from assessment of other patients?
- What approach is best for assessing the adolescent?
- What health concerns should I keep in mind as I proceed with the assessment?

Developmental Changes

Many physical changes take place during adolescence. Height, weight, and muscle mass increase rapidly. Sexual maturation also occurs. You need to understand the normal changes that occur in order to detect abnormalities.

Stages of Adolescence

Many authorities divide adolescence into early, middle, and late (based on specific developmental tasks), or **prepubescence, puberty,** and **postpubescence** (based on physical changes). Early adolescence begins at puberty (as early as age 8 or 9 but more typically age 11 to 14 for girls and age 12 to 16 for boys). This period of rapid physical growth corresponds with the onset of menstruation in girls and sperm production in boys. Middle adolescence typically ranges from age 14 to 16 in girls and age 16 to 18 in boys. Females have generally achieved their adult height by this stage, but males may continue their linear growth. Late adolescence typically starts around age 17 and can continue into the early 20s. This rapid period of both physical growth and psychosocial development is what makes the adolescent period so complex and challenging for health care providers.

Prepubescence is defined as the 2-year period before puberty in which preliminary physical changes occur. Puberty is the point when sexual maturity occurs, reproductive organs begin to function, and secondary sexual characteristics develop. Postpubescence occurs 1 to 2 years after puberty, when skeletal growth is complete and reproductive function is regular.

Physical Changes

For girls, the first sign of sexual maturation is breast development. Menstruation generally begins within 2 years after the onset of breast development. For boys, sperm production (**spermatogenesis**) corresponds with increased testicular size and penile enlargement. Nocturnal emissions ("wet dreams") typically start about 1 year after the penis begins to enlarge in size. Sexual maturity can be tracked using the Tanner scale. The achievement of Tanner Stage 5 for both girls and boys corresponds with adult sexual maturity. (See Chapter 14, Assessing the Breasts, and Chapter 17, Assessing the Male Genitourinary System, for Tanner scales.)

Rapid physical growth is responsible for much of the clumsiness and awkwardness associated with this age period. Adolescents are faced with adjusting to rapidly changing physical bodies that may not always have the agility and grace associated with younger years. They often feel uncoordinated and ill at ease with their rapidly changing physiques. A number of other physical changes occur that will be addressed later in this chapter.

Psychosocial and Emotional Changes

From a psychosocial perspective, Eric Erikson describes this period as one of "identity versus identity diffusion." Adolescents become preoccupied with others' opinions of them in an attempt to be accepted. The focus of influence shifts from family to peer group, and the adolescent begins to forge a sense of identity with the peer group. This is a normal developmental progression but one with potential conflicts, depending on the chosen peer group. If the peer group supports a sense of self-identity and self-worth, the outcome tends to be a positive one. But if the peer group discourages such internalization of values (such as with gangs), the adolescent does not progress in the direction of independent thought and decision making. Ideally, the adolescent moves through this stage developing a set of personal values and a sense of self-competency while beginning to plan for a future career.

Jean Piaget describes cognitive development during adolescence as the "formal operational stage." This means that the adolescent begins a process of more logical thinking. He or she begins to hypothesize, wondering "what if?" and starts to reflect on outcomes to specific hypotheses. Previously, thought was based on very concrete concepts—what could be readily visualized or experienced. Concepts such as right versus wrong and good versus bad now become more abstract and situational. Other people's concepts and views become more important, which only adds to the decision-making dilemma. This is a time when conflicts with parents begin to occur. Traditional family values may be challenged by the exposure to new ideas and values from peers.

During this time the adolescent also struggles to develop his or her own set of moral principles by questioning established moral codes. Peers often have more

Health Concerns and Risk Factors for Adolescents

Be alert for the following health problems as you perform the assessment:

Injuries and Accidents: Accidents, especially motor vehicle accidents, are the leading cause of death among adolescents,. Alcohol is often a contributing factor. Sports injuries are also common.

Eating Disorders: Body-image issues contribute to eating disorders. **Anorexia** and **bulimia** are more common in girls, but they are also seen in boys. Anorexia usually involves almost totally abstaining from food, resulting in extreme weight loss, electrolyte imbalance, and loss of lean muscle tissue (including organ tissue such as heart muscle). It can also include obsessive exercise and is the client's way of taking control over her life. Bulimia involves bingeing on large quantities of food and then purging, through either vomiting or laxative use. This also results in electrolyte imbalance as well as dental erosion. Boys with eating disorders are usually involved in sports that strictly limit weight categories, such as wrestling or boxing. Girls are more affected by the media, where the emaciated model is the desired female ideal. Family or self-pressure to be successful (e.g., to be a straight-A student) can also be a factor. Early identification and referral is critical to prevent serious sequelae.

Obesity: Now seen in over 30 percent of United States adolescents, obesity is largely caused by decreased physical activity, increased TV and computer time, and too many high-fat foods.

Pregnancy: The United States has the highest rate of adolescent pregnancy of any developed country in the world, although rates have decreased slightly. One cause includes the "it can't happen to me" mind-set common in this age group. Pregnancy may also be intentional or an outcome of sexual abuse. All states provide confidential referral of adolescents to family planning centers for counseling and education on abstinence and contraception. Services are generally free and completely confidential, regardless of the patient's age.

Sexually Transmitted Diseases (STDs): Thousands of sexually active adolescents have STDs, which may cause long-term negative effects. Chlamydia, the most common and least recognized STD, is the major cause of pelvic inflammatory disease (PID) and can result in fertility problems. Human papillomavirus (HPV) is the most common cause of abnormal Pap tests in adolescent females and is a major cause of cervical cancer. Confidential services are available nationwide for the diagnosis and treatment of STDs and can be located through country or city health departments. Generally free of charge, these services also provide counseling related to safe sex and supplies such as condoms.

Emotional Disorders: Depression, bipolar disorders, conduct disorders, and obsessive-compulsive disorders can have serious outcomes, including suicide if undiagnosed and untreated. Early detection and prompt referral for treatment is crucial. In many states, adolescents can "self-refer" for diagnosis and treatment of mental illness.

Substance Abuse: Alcohol is the most commonly reported substance of abuse, but marijuana, cocaine, methamphetamine, and some "designer drugs" such as "ecstasy" are also widely used. More than 30 percent of teens also report using cigarettes or smokeless tobacco. Education is a valuable tool, but to be effective, information must be presented factually and scare tactics avoided. In most states, adolescents can self-refer for treatment.

Violence: Violent acts involving adolescents continue to increase. School shootings and random gang violence give some young people a fatalistic view. They think, "I'm going to die anyway, so what's the big deal?" Those without a strong sense of self-worth and purpose are most likely to be involved in violence, either as recipients or perpetrators. Although recent studies fail to reveal any one identifiable personality trait of violent adolescents, those who are withdrawn, noncommunicative, angry, and "loners" may be at greater risk. Talking to the client about behaviors of this type may open the door for therapeutic interventions.

influence than parents, but often pre-established values and morals persist. This is also a time for questioning spiritual beliefs, and many adolescents turn away from formal religion, eventually resolving the questions and identifying their sense of spirituality.

Adolescence is also a time of increased risk taking. This is a result of several factors: the desire to separate from parental influence, peer pressure and the need to belong, and a feeling of invulnerability or "it can't happen to me." Unprotected sexual activity, substance use, and unsafe driving are examples of risky behavior. Understanding this phenomenon is essential to effective counseling and education in the area of risk reduction.

Cultural and Ethnic Variations

Cultural influences may affect adolescent behaviors by establishing expectations.

Cultural and Ethnic Variations in Adolescents

CULTURAL GROUP	INFLUENCE
Amish	Adolescent may want to break away from cultural norms (e.g., dress), but this is considered experimental. Teen expected to eventually assume adult role and adhere to prescribed norms.

(Continued)

Cultural and Ethnic Variations in Adolescents *(Continued)*

CULTURAL GROUP	INFLUENCE
Appalachian	Formal education not stressed, but teen expected to work and support family. Marriage at ages as young as 13 to 15 common. Having children associated with sense of importance. Underage alcohol abuse common.
Arab-American	Chastity and decency expected.
Chinese-American	Expected to score well in national tests by age 18. Must make career choice during adolescent years. Teenage pregnancy not common. Teens expected to respect elders.
Cuban-American	Boys expected to learn a trade; girls expected to keep themselves honorable and prepare for marriage. "Rite of passage" (ready for courting) celebration at age 15 for girls. Unmarried couples may have chaperones.
Egyptian-American	Loss of virginity affects marriageability, so parents are very strict.
Filipino-American	Short courtships.
Greek-American	Girls have less dating freedom than boys. Dating often prohibited until late adolescence.
Iranian-American	Girls expected to maintain virginity.
Irish-American	Expected to remain loyal to family.
Jewish-American	Rite of passage at age 13 for boys, age 12 for girls.
Native American	Menarche for teenage girl seen as passage to adulthood. Older children taught to be stoic and not complain.
Vietnamese	Teens expected to respect elders.

Introducing the Case Study

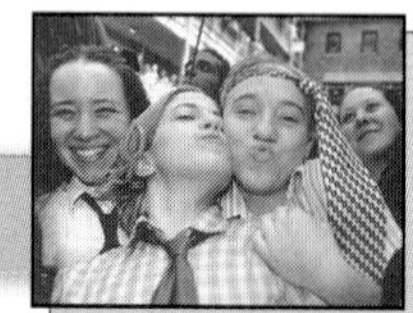

Margaret Chung, a pretty 14-year-old, has been in your school health office 4 times in the last 2 weeks, each time with a different vague complaint. So far, you have been unable to assess any specific malady. Today when you ask what brings her there, she says that she just wants to talk. Several other students are waiting, so you escort Margaret to one of the private examination rooms and explain that you will return shortly, after seeing the students who were there first. After attending to them, you place an "Exam In Progress—Do Not Disturb" sign on the door, and then you begin your assessment.

Performing the Adolescent Assessment

Assessing an adolescent is similar to assessing an adult. As you begin the process, keep in mind the normal developmental changes and issues affecting adolescents. Communicating during the assessment can be a challenge, but many adolescents are looking for an adult who will listen and not preach or talk down. For tips on talking to adolescents, see the box, Communicating with Adolescents, on page 811.

As with all assessments, the process involves subjective and objective data collection, diagnosis, planning, interventions, and evaluation.

Health History

Interview the adolescent alone, at least for some part of the examination. If a parent is present, explain that it is appropriate for young people to begin having independent relationships with their healthcare providers in preparation for managing their health care as adults. Because the history is essentially the same as for an adult, in this section differences will be presented as they relate specifically to the adolescent.

COMMUNICATING WITH ADOLESCENTS

As a professional nurse, you may be the only receptive adult in an adolescent's life. Many young people feel that they have no adult to communicate with. Or they may be separating themselves from parental authority and moving toward self-autonomy, but still want and need adult guidance. The guidelines below will help you communicate with adolescents:

1. **Listen Actively:** This may be the most effective strategy of all. Adolescents understand that adults will not always agree with them, but they desperately want a solid "sounding board." Listening can help you understand the issues at hand, even if you do not condone them. Here are some tips for active listening:
   - Start with less sensitive subjects and work your way up to more sensitive ones.
   - Make sure you and your patient understand each other, clarify as needed, and never assume.
   - Use gender-neutral terms and open-ended questions, and restate if necessary.
   - Show true concern and respect for the adolescent's perspective and opinion.
   - Be nonjudgmental.
2. **Help with Decision Making:** Listening actively puts you in a position to summarize the issues or questions and then help the adolescent verbalize the pros and cons of each side. This way, he or she can more objectively deal with the issue at hand and is more likely to make a logical, informed decision.
3. **Avoid Scare Tactics:** Adults often use these in an attempt to control behavior. Most young people know that one puff on a cigarette will not addict them for life, but adults often make statements like this. Such comments can destroy your credibility and make the patient less likely to follow your advice on other health issues.
4. **Maintain Confidentiality.** This is a major issue. Make sure the female patient knows she is guaranteed confidentiality in pregnancy testing, contraceptive services, and diagnosis and treatment of STDs. Then keep your promises. If the patient has expressed the desire to harm himself or herself or others, be sure that he or she knows this is one problem you *cannot* keep confidential.

Biographical Data

Begin with standard biographical data, but also take note where the client lives and with whom. Note who is listed the contact person—it may not be the parent. Do not assume anything!

Current Health Status

Be sure to ask about all prescription and over-the-counter (OTC) medications. Many adolescents (especially those involved in athletics) take vitamin or protein supplements, so assessing for these is important. Ask girls if they are on birth control pills (oral contraceptives), take monthly "shots" (Depoprovera), or have a contraceptive implant (Norplant). Also ask girls if they take the acne medication Acutane. If they do, tell them that taking Accutane while pregnant can cause serious birth defects, and counsel them about pregnancy prevention.

Past Health History

Because the adolescent may not be aware of all his or her past health history, you may need to check with a parent or guardian for specifics such as immunizations (see Health Concerns, p. 820 for required immunizations).

Family History

If the adolescent is being interviewed alone, he or she may have limited knowledge in this area. Many, however, will be aware of heart disease, stroke, cancer, and other serious health conditions within the family. It is also important to ask if anyone in the family died before age 35 from a sudden heart attack. This may be a risk factor for sports participation and may require additional investigation.

Review of Systems

Review every system, keeping in mind changes or problems specific to the adolescent.

Review of Systems

SYSTEM/QUESTIONS TO ASK	RATIONALE/SIGNIFICANCE
General Health Survey	
How have you been feeling?	Screens for any obvious problems.
Have you had any weight changes?	*Weight loss or gain:* May indicate eating disorder.
Integumentary	
Do you have any skin problems, such as acne?	Adolescents are very self-conscious about appearance, and acne may affect self-image.

(Continued)

Review of Systems *(Continued)*

SYSTEM/QUESTIONS TO ASK	RATIONALE/SIGNIFICANCE
Integumentary (*continued*)	
Have you had changes in body hair growth?	Secondary sexual changes include increase in body hair—pubic hair, axilla and leg hair, and facial hair for boys.
Do you have piercings or tattoos?	*Body piercing and tattooing:* Increased risk for HIV or hepatitis B.
Do you use sunscreen? Do you lie in the sun or go to tanning salons?	*Excessive exposure to sun (UV rays) without sunscreen:* Increased risk for skin cancer later in life.
HEENT/*Eyes*	
Do you have any vision problems?	Visual refractive problems peak during adolescence.
Do you wear glasses or contact lenses?	Identifies teaching need regarding care of contact lenses.
When was your last eye exam?	Test visual acuity routinely during physical exams.
HEENT/*Ears*	
Do you have any hearing problems?	Identifies teaching need regarding noise pollution's affect on hearing.
Do you listen to loud music?	Cochlear damage can result from excessive exposure to loud noise such as CD players and rock concerts.
When was your last hearing exam?	Test hearing routinely during physical exams.
HEENT/*Mouth*	
When was your last visit to the dentist?	Should have at least annual dental exam.
Do you go to an orthodontist?	Need for orthodontia usually becomes apparent during adolescence and can make patient even more self-conscious about appearance.
Respiratory	
Do you have asthma?	Asthma is the most common disease among children.
Do you ever have trouble breathing or wheeze when you exercise or run?	Exercise-induced bronchospasm is an acute, reversible, self-terminating airway obstruction that occurs after vigorous exercise. It peaks 5 to 10 minutes after activity stops, and then stops within 30 minutes.
Are you exposed to air pollutants, such as smoke and second-hand smoke?	
Cardiovascular	
Do you have chest pain?	Although cardiovascular disease is not common in adolescents, it can occur.
Does your heart ever skip a beat?	Prolonged QT syndrome can cause sudden cardiac death in a seemingly healthy adolescent.
Breasts	
Girls:	
Are your breasts tender? Have they increased in size? Are they growing equally?	Determines whether normal breast development is occurring. May identify areas for health teaching. Initially, breasts may develop asymmetrically, but they should even out eventually.
Boys:	
Have your breasts enlarged?	During early puberty, boys may experience temporary **gynecomastia** (breast enlargement), which usually disappears within 2 years. Because their appearance is of great concern, gynecomastia can be very alarming for boys and make them very self-conscious.
Gastrointestinal	
Do you have any stomach problems?	Identifies underlying eating disorder.

Review of Systems

SYSTEM/QUESTIONS TO ASK	RATIONALE/SIGNIFICANCE
Gastrointestinal (*continued*)	
How often do you have a bowel movement? Do you use laxatives?	Excessive use of laxatives associated with eating disorders.
Genitourinary/Reproductive	
Girls:	
Did your periods start? When? How often do you have them? How heavy is the flow?	Identifies start of menarche and determines if cycle is normal.
Do you use pads or tampons?	Tampon use has been associated with risk for toxic shock syndrome (TSS).
Do you have burning when you go to the bathroom?	May identify health teaching needs.
Have you had urinary tract infections (UTIs)?	Frequent UTIs in girls can be caused by sexual activity and require follow-up.
Girls and boys:	
Are you sexually active? Have you ever had sex? Are you practicing safe sex?	Identifies health teaching need.
Musculoskeletal	
Do you have any back problems?	Heavy backpacks are associated with low back problems in children and adolescents.
Have you ever been told you had a spinal problem?	Scoliosis (lateral curvature of spine) occurs more frequently in girls than boys. Screening usually occurs in middle school and high school. If it is present, determine if problem is structural or postural (see Chapter 18, Assessing the Musculoskeletal System).
Neurological	
How would you describe your usual mood? Do you feel sad a lot?	Adolescence is a time of change, and emotional response to these changes varies. Depression or suicidal ideations must be identified and treated.
Endocrine	
Do you have any swelling in your neck? Difficulty swallowing? Hoarseness?	The thyroid is more active during puberty. *Enlarged thyroid:* Hypo- or hyperthyroid disease. Lymphocytic thyroiditis (Hashimoto's disease or juvenile autoimmune thyroiditis) is most common in children after age 6 and reaches peak occurrence in young people during adolescence. Graves' disease occurs in young people between ages 12 and 14. If sexual maturation is not progressing, consider endocrine problems.
Lymphatic/Hematologic	
Have you been tired?	Rapid growth and poor dietary habits increase risk of iron deficiency anemia.
Do you have any lumps in your neck, underarms, or groin?	Hodgkin's lymphoma is prevalent between ages 15 and 19. Non-Hodgkin's lymphomas occur more frequently before age 15.

Psychosocial Profile

The psychosocial profile focuses on how the adolescent's health practices and behaviors affect his or her health and well-being.

Health Practices and Beliefs and Self-Care Activities

When did the patient have his or her last health examination (every 2 years is recommended). More frequent examinations may be needed if he or she has an existing health problem or is involved in sports. Keep in mind that adolescents may have no control over the frequency of their health screenings. The parent or guardian often assumes this responsibility, and health insurance or the lack of it may be an influencing factor. You may need to make appropriate referrals or provide information on available health resources.

Typical Day

What constitutes a usual day's activities? How is the adolescent doing in school? What subjects does he or she like and dislike? Has the adolescent sought help for subjects that he or she is having problems with? This allows you to identify stresses confronting the patient in everyday life. A change in academic performance or a sudden disinterest in school may reflect a more serious problem. How many days of school has he or she missed this term? High absenteeism (except for serious illness) correlates with other risky behaviors.

Nutritional Patterns, Weight Loss and Weight Gain

Ask for a 24-hour diet recall. Then ask questions about body image, such as "How much do you think you should weigh?" Further explore this issue if the response is unrealistic. Ask about eating patterns, such as "How often do you eat breakfast?" "What is a usual lunch for you?" and "What are your favorite snacks?" These open-ended questions will provide a much clearer picture of the adolescent's nutritional status and potential risks.

Vitamin and Mineral Supplements

At this age, dietary needs for calcium, iron, and zinc are greater. Calcium is needed for bone growth and bone mass development during adolescence; it also influences the development of osteoporosis later in life. Assess both overeating and undereating problems. Girls are usually more concerned about losing weight, whereas boys may want to "bulk-up" and improve strength.

Activity and Exercise Patterns

Ask what the patient enjoys doing outside of the home. What sports does he or she play? What does he or she like to do with his or her friends? How much TV does he or she watch? How much time does he or she spend on the computer? You may identify a need for health education about the importance of routine exercise. If the teen does participate in sports, ask if he or she uses protective equipment and if it is a contact sport. Contact sports may increase the risk for injury.

Recreation and Hobbies

What does the client do for fun? If activities increase the risk for injury, ask if protective measures are used, such as bike helmets. Also ask about weapons in the home and hunting safety courses, if appropriate.

Sleep and Rest Patterns

What time does the client usually go to bed and wake up? Does he or she feel refreshed in the morning or still tired? How does this pattern change on weekends? Even though sleep needs increase during growth spurts, teens often get less-than-ideal amounts of sleep during the week and sleep late on weekends. This can disrupt healthy sleep patterns. Also ask about bedwetting, which is not entirely uncommon at this age, specially in boys. Phrase your question in a nonthreatening way to decrease embarrassment. For example, say: "Many young people find they sometimes wet themselves during their sleep. Does this ever happen to you?"

Personal Habits

Ask if the client uses drugs, alcohol, or nicotine, and phrase your questions in a nonthreatening way to increase the likelihood of an honest response. For example, say: "If you smoke cigarettes, how many do you smoke in an average day?" "If you use alcohol, how much do you usually drink during the week?" "If you use drugs, what type and what method (e.g., smoking, snorting, huffing, ingesting, or injecting)?

Risky Behavior

Accidents are the leading cause of death among teenagers, especially motor vehicle accidents. If the patient drives, ask if he or she attended a driver's education program. Does he or she wear a seat belt? Is he or she aware of the hazards of driving under the influence of drugs or alcohol? Take this opportunity to reinforce the importance of not driving under the influence or riding with someone under the influence. If drug or alcohol use is identified, make appropriate referrals.

Roles, Relationships, and Self-Concept

Ask the young person to tell you what he or she likes best about himself or herself and what he or she would like to change. Remember that adolescence is a time of great change. These questions will help you identify how satisfied the patient is with the changes that have occurred. Also ask about family relationships. For example, ask: "Who lives at home with you?" "How do you get along with your family?" "Is there an adult in your life whom you feel comfortable talking with?" Ask about peer relationships. Does the patient have a special friend, and what things does he or she enjoy doing with that friend? Does he or she date?

Religious and Spiritual Influences

Ask the adolescent what is important to him or her and whether he or she believes in God or a higher power. Established spiritual beliefs may be a source of support and influence behavior.

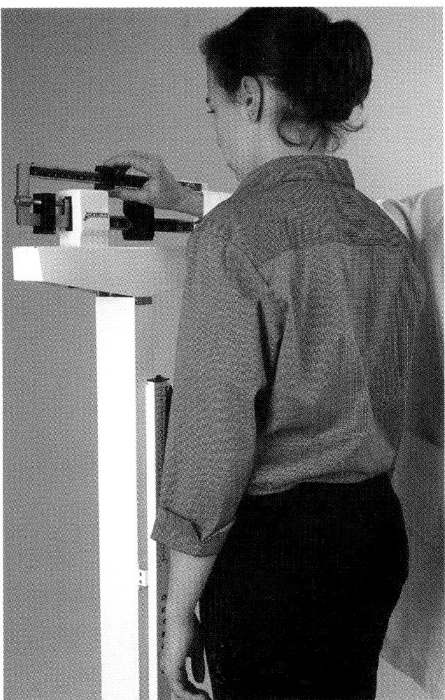

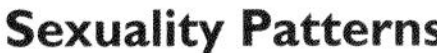

FIGURE 24–3. Weighing patient.

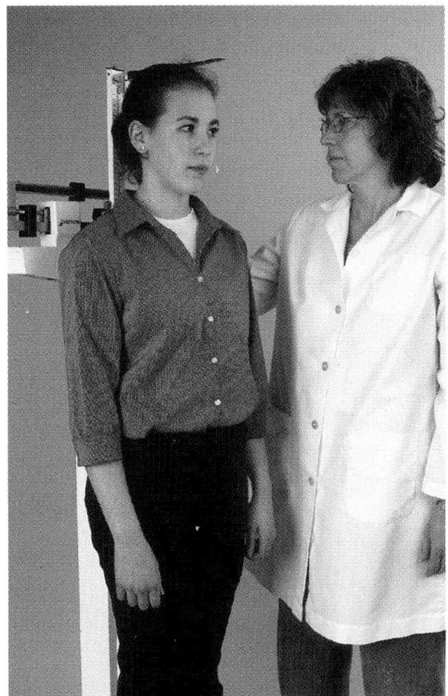

FIGURE 24–4. Measuring patient.

Sexuality Patterns

Ask girls if they have any questions or concerns about menstrual issues. Ask boys if they have any questions about physical changes. Inquire about sexual activity. You might ask: "If you are sexually active, how do you protect yourself against sexually transmitted diseases and unwanted pregnancy?" Keep in mind that sexual preferences become apparent during adolescence, and gay or bisexual teens may be confronted with homophobic attitudes.

Stress and Coping

Ask: "What do you do when you get angry?" "What makes you angry?" "What do you do to relax?" Identify whether the adolescent has healthy coping strategies to deal with life's stressors. Violence is on the rise among teenagers. If your patient uses violence as a coping mechanism, you may need to make referrals to help him or her develop more effective coping strategies.

Physical Assessment

After you complete the history, perform the physical examination. Physical assessment of the adolescent does not differ greatly from that of the adult—you use all four assessment techniques and the same tools (for more information, see Chapter 3, Approach to the Physical Assessment).

Begin with a general survey, obtaining height and weight (Figs. 24–3 and 24–4.. Also take vital signs, which are essentially the same as for adults. Then perform a head-to-toe physical examination.

HELPFUL HINT

Always weigh adolescents in private. When weighing is done in front of other people—for example, in school settings—it is a source of anxiety for teens, especially those who are overweight or think they are.

Performing a Head-to-Toe Physical Assessment

SYSTEM/ASSESSMENT	NORMAL VARIATIONS/ABNORMAL FINDINGS/RATIONALE
General Health Survey	
INSPECT	
Inspect overall appearance, noting appropriate growth and development for age of client.	Detects delays or premature sexual maturation. Detects obvious weight problems.

(Continued)

Performing a Head-to-Toe Physical Assessment *(Continued)*

SYSTEM/ASSESSMENT	NORMAL VARIATIONS/ABNORMAL FINDINGS/RATIONALE
Integumentary	
INSPECT	
Inspect skin for lesions.	Acne is common problem and major concern. This condition should be treated and not dismissed as insignificant. Severe acne can result in permanent scarring. Many effective treatments are now available.
Note piercings and tattoos.	Increase risk for HIV and hepatitis B.
Note body hair distribution.	Absent or excessive body hair may relate sexual maturation problem.
HEENT/*Eyes*	
INSPECT/PALPATE	
Test visual acuity.	Many teenagers have some degree of myopia (nearsightedness) but are reluctant to wear prescribed eyeglasses.
HEENT/*Ears*	
INSPECT	
Test hearing with pure tone audiometer.	Listening to loud music, especially with earphones, can cause early hearing loss. Use opportunity to teach hazards of listening to loud music.
HEENT/*Nose*	
INSPECT	
Inspect nasal septum and mucosa.	*Boggy, bluish-purple turbinates:* Chronic rhinorrhea caused by allergic rhinitis. *Mucosal damage:* Possible cocaine use, which also causes rhinorrhea.
HEENT/*Mouth*	
INSPECT	
Inspect oral mucosa and pharynx.	Hypertrophied tonsils of early childhood have usually shrunk to more normal proportions.
Inspect occlusion.	If malocclusion is present, refer to orthodontist.
Inspect number of teeth and check for wisdom teeth.	Should have 28 permanent teeth. Third molars ("wisdom teeth") may erupt during this period. May need referral if wisdom teeth are impacted.
Assess for orthodontic devices and brushing technique around them.	*Improper brushing:* Increased risk for gum problems and cavities.

Performing a Head-to-Toe Physical Assessment

SYSTEM/ASSESSMENT	NORMAL VARIATIONS/ABNORMAL FINDINGS/RATIONALE
HEENT/*Neck* *PALPATE* Palpate thyroid.	*Tender, enlarged thyroid gland:* Acute throiditis.
Respiratory *AUSCULTATE* Auscultate lungs.	Adolescents with exercise-induced asthma (EIA) require bronchodilators before activity (usually albuterol via a metered dose inhaler 20 to 30 minutes before exercise).
Cardiovascular *AUSCULTATE* 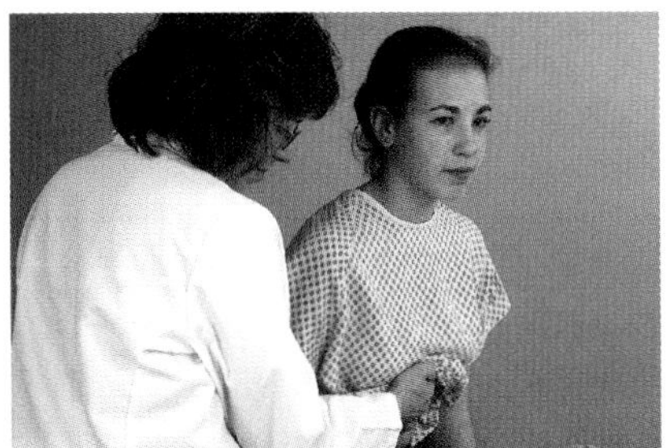 **Auscultating heart** Auscultate heart and note rate and rhythm.	Sinus arrhythmia and split second heart sound that change with respiration are normal variations.
Breasts *INSPECT/PALPATE* Inspect and palpate breasts.	Breast examinations should begin during adolescence, along with instruction in breast self-examination. Gynecomastia occurs in about ⅓ of boys.
Gastrointestinal *INSPECT/PALPATE/ AUSCULTATE* Inspect, auscultate, and palpate the abdomen.	Except for pregnancy, no specific variations occur with the abdomen. It is not unusual to detect pregnancy during a routine exam in an adolescent who is denying it. By 20 weeks' gestation, the fundus is at level of the umbilicus.
Genitourinary/Reproductive *INSPECT/PALPATE* Inspect external genitalia.	Examine sexually active adolescents for STDs.

(Continued)

Performing a Head-to-Toe Physical Assessment *(Continued)*

SYSTEM/ASSESSMENT	NORMAL VARIATIONS/ABNORMAL FINDINGS/RATIONALE
Boys: Perform testicular exam. *Girls:* Perform pelvic exam at age 18 or earlier if sexually active.	Instruct boys in testicular self-exam. Note Tanner stage for boys and girls. *Pubertal delay for girls:* No breast development by age 13 or no menarche within 4 years of initial breast changes. *Pubertal delay for boys:* No changes in testes or scrotum by age 13½ to 14 or incomplete genital growth within 4 years of initial change.
Musculoskeletal *INSPECT/PALPATE*	
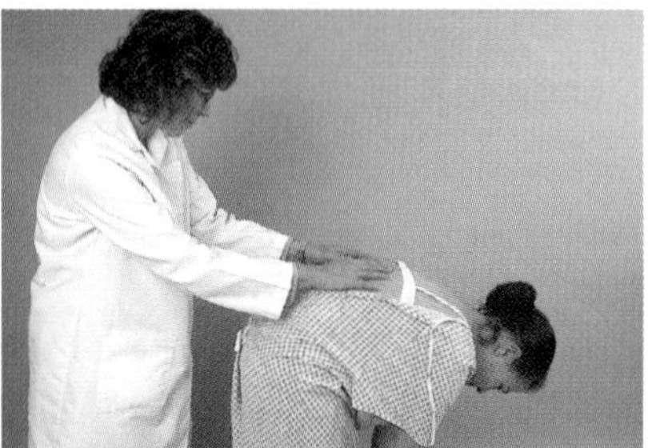 **Inspecting for scoliosis** Inspect and palpate spinal curves. Test for spinal deformities.	Scoliosis is a major variation within the musculoskeletal system. Screening should be done in the preadolescent period, generally during fifth and sixth grade. Refer children with significant curvature for evaluation and follow-up.
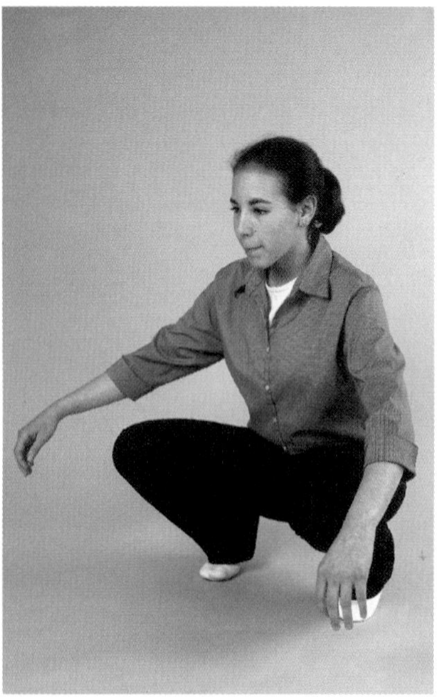 **Testing knee strength and stability** If patient is active in sports, test knee strength and stability.	

Performing a Head-to-Toe Physical Assessment

SYSTEM/ASSESSMENT	NORMAL VARIATIONS/ABNORMAL FINDINGS/RATIONALE
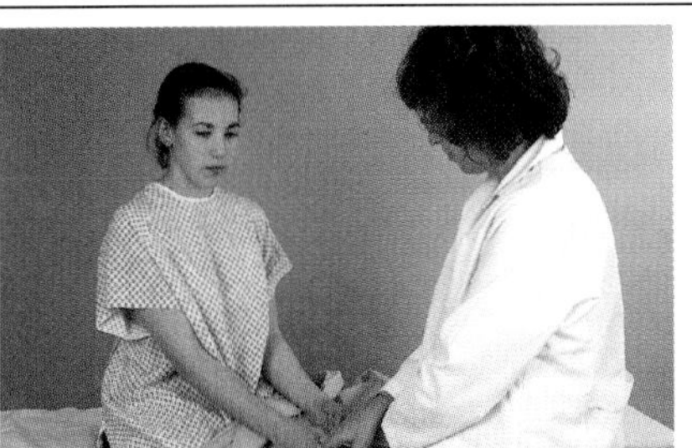 **Testing muscle strength**	
Test muscle strength grip.	For more information on testing for scoliosis and muscle strength, see Chapter 18, Assessing the Musculoskeletal System.
Neurological *INSPECT* Focus on affect and cognitive functioning.	Depression and suicidal ideations warrant immediate intervention.

Now that your assessment is over, analyze your data and formulate nursing diagnoses. If you identify problem areas, actively involve both the adolescent and his or her parents in the plan of care.

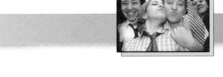

Back to the Case Study

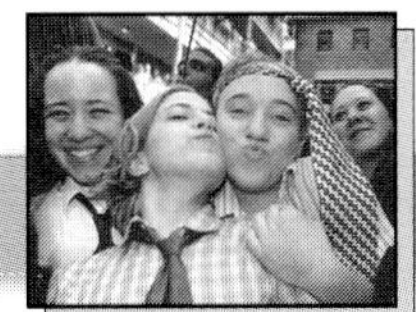

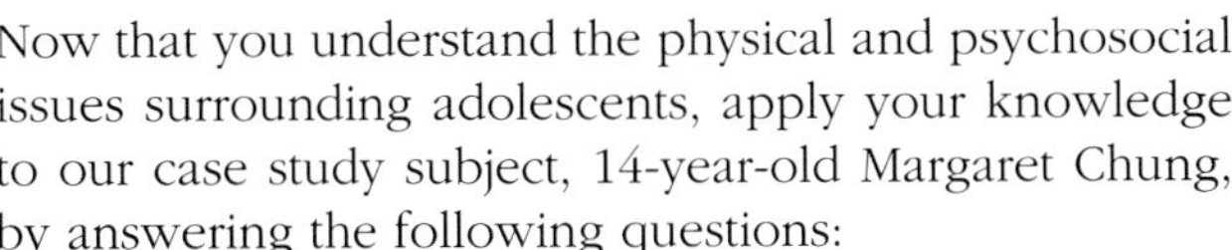

Now that you understand the physical and psychosocial issues surrounding adolescents, apply your knowledge to our case study subject, 14-year-old Margaret Chung, by answering the following questions:

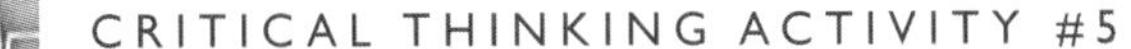

CRITICAL THINKING ACTIVITY #5

How does assessment of the adolescent differ from assessment of other patients?

CRITICAL THINKING ACTIVITY #6

What approach is best for assessing the adolescent?

CRITICAL THINKING ACTIVITY #7

What health concerns should I keep in mind as I proceed with the assessment?

CRITICAL THINKING ACTIVITY #8

Some nursing diagnoses are appropriate for all adolescents. What are they?

Research Tells Us

One study examined the relationship of substance abuse to sexual risk-taking behaviors in late adolescence into adulthood. Subjects completed substance abuse and sexual behavior questionnaires. The authors reported that adolescent substance abusers were more likely to engage in risky sexual behavior and then continue this behavior into adulthood as long as the substance abuse persisted.

These findings stress the importance of including sex education with substance abuse education and treatment. Nurses need to be proactive by beginning such education at an earlier age with adolescents.

Source: Tapert, S., Aarons, G., Sedlar, G, & Brown, S. (2001). Adolescent substance use and sexual risk-taking behavior. *Journal of Adolescent-Health, 28*(3): 181–189.

Health Concerns

Immunizations recommended during adolescence include:

- **Tetanus-Diphtheria "Booster" (Td):** Between ages 11 and 12 and every 10 years thereafter; whenever person suffers a wound, if booster not received within past 5 years.
- **Measles, Mumps, Rubella (MMR):** Between ages 11 and 12 if second MMR not given between ages 4 and 6.
- **Varicella Zoster (Chickenpox) (VZV):** At any age if person has never had chickenpox; if vaccine not given until age 13 or older, should get 2 doses, 4 to 8 weeks apart.
- **Hepatitis B (HepB):** Any time between ages 6 and 12, if not immunized during infancy. Children between ages 11 and 15 may need only two doses, 4 to 6 months apart.
- ***Hemophilus influenzae* (HiB):** Not recommended for healthy adolescents. Children over age 5 usually do not need this vaccine unless they have special health concerns, such as sickle cell disease, HIV/AIDS, removal of spleen, bone marrow transplant, or cancer treatment with drugs.
- **Meningitis (Menomune):** Before starting college.

Common Problems

Common problems in this age group include acne, eating disorders, scoliosis, pregnancy, STDs, injuries and accidents, substance abuse, malocclusion, EIA, and pubertal delay.

Summary

- Managing adolescent health care presents challenging issues for the nurse.
- The key to success lies in effective communication and understanding the developmental and psychosocial issues related to adolescence.
- Having a foundational understanding of these concepts will help you develop an effective plan of care.

25

Assessing the Older Adult

Before You Begin

INTRODUCTION TO ASSESSING THE OLDER ADULT

Obtaining an accurate and useful history and physical assessment is a vital skill in working with all adults, but it is particularly challenging in working with older adults. This challenge is a result of the normal changes that occur with aging, the tendency of older people to present with disease in an atypical fashion, their long medical histories, and common communication problems caused of hearing loss, **aphasia,** or cognitive impairment. The actual assessment process does not differ from that used with any other adult. You just need to focus your attention on the changes that occur with aging. Understanding the normal changes that occur with age and how they interrelate with disease and its presentation will improve your assessment skills and facilitate the diagnosis and management of common problems in older clients.

Anatomy and Physiology Review

In evaluating the older adult, it is often difficult to differentiate between normal changes and those caused by environmental factors, lifestyle, or disease. For example, skin changes such as wrinkling, which were once believed to be related exclusively to aging, are now believed to be influenced by sun exposure. Understanding the normal changes associated with aging in each body system and being familiar with them are essential in assessing older adults.

Normal Changes Associated with Aging

SYSTEM OR STRUCTURE/CAUSES	CHANGES
Integumentary/*Skin*	
• Decreased collagen and subcutaneous fat	• Increased wrinkling • Decreased elasticity
• Atrophy of sweat glands and decreased function	• Increased dryness • Pruritus
• Decline in fibroblast proliferation, cell production, and epidermal turnover	• Thinning • Increased healing time
• Capillary fragility and decreased vascularity	• Bruising
• Decreased sensory receptors and increased thresholds	• Decreased sensory perception • Decreased vitamin D production • Increased skin lesions
Integumentary/*Hair*	
• Decreased **melanocytes**	• Graying of body hair • Uneven skin color
• Decreased hair follicle density	• Loss and thinning of hair
Integumentary/*Nails*	
• Hypo/hyperplasia of nail matrix	• Increased longitudinal ridges • Nails thick and brittle
• Decreased blood supply to nails	• Growth slow
Head, Eyes, Ears, Nose, and Throat (HEENT)/*Eyes*	
• Decreased orbital fat	• Sunken eyes
• Decreased elasticity of lids	• Ectropion or entropion
• Decreased tears	• Dry eyes
• Decreased corneal sensitivity	• Decreased corneal reflex
• Increased lipid deposits around cornea	• Arcus senilis
• Decreased aqueous humor	• Decreased lens accommodation
• Atrophy of ciliary muscles	• Decreased peripheral vision
• Decreased elasticity of lens	• Decreased ability to adapt to light and dark
• Increased density of lens	• Glare intolerance
• Decreased color of iris	• Impaired night vision
• Decreased pupil size	• Decreased visual acuity
• Increased vitreous debris	• Floaters

Normal Changes Associated with Aging

SYSTEM OR STRUCTURE/CAUSES	CHANGES
HEENT/*Ears*	
• Increased external canal hair in men • Decreased cerumen • Degeneration of middle ear bones • Thickened tympanic membrane	• Conductive hearing loss
• Decreased hair in inner ear • Atrophy of cochlea and organ of Corti	• Decreased speech discrimination • Difficulty hearing higher-frequency sound
HEENT/*Nose*	
• Atrophic changes	• Vasomotor rhinitis • Decrease in sense of smell and ability to distinguish odors
Respiratory	
• Rigid ribs and thoracic wall	• Increased anterior-posterior diameter • Senile kyphosis
• Decreased muscle strength	• Decreased vital capacity • Increased residual lung capacity
• Atrophy of cilia	• Reduced cough and clearing
• Decreased elastic recoil	• Decreased lung compliance
• Decreased pulmonary bed	• Decreased ventilation and perfusion
• Thickening and decrease in number of alveoli	• Decreased $Pa0_2$ and 0_2 saturation
• Decreased response to hypoxia/hypercarbia	• More difficulty in maintaining acid-base balance
Cardiovascular/*Heart*	
• Decreased cardiac output and cardiac index • Decreased response to beta-adrenergic stimulation	• Decreased stroke volume and output
• Decreased heart muscle with increase in fat and collagen	• Increased myocardial oxygen demands
• Thickening of ventricular walls • Decreased compliance • Increased dependence on atrial contraction	• Ventricular hypertrophy • S_4 (see Chapter 12)
• Calcification of valves • Decreased sinoatrial node pacer cells and bundle of His fibers	• Murmurs • Arrhythmias • Slower rates in response to stress
Cardiovascular/*Arteries*	
• Decreased elastin and smooth muscle • Decreased compliance and stiffness of vessels • Increased peripheral vascular resistance • Aortic dilatation	• Increased blood pressure
• Decreased baroreceptor response • Rigidity of arteries leading to decreased peripheral circulation	• Orthostatic hypotension • Decreased pulses • Cool temperature
Cardiovascular/*Veins*	
• Increased tortuosity	• Varicosities

(Continued)

Normal Changes Associated with Aging *(Continued)*

SYSTEM OR STRUCTURE/CAUSES	CHANGES
Gastrointestinal/*Mouth and Teeth*	
• Decreased dentine • Gingival recession	• Potential loss of teeth
• Decreased papillae on tongue • Increased threshold for tasting salt and sugar	• Decreased sense of taste
• Decreased saliva	• Dry oral mucous membranes
Gastrointestinal/*Esophagus*	
• Decreased sphincter pressure • Decreased motility	• Heartburn • Dysphagia • Increased risk for hiatal hernia, gastroesophageal reflux disease (GERD), and aspiration
Gastrointestinal/*Stomach*	
• Decreased gastric acid and hydrochloric acid	• Decreased absorption of iron, B_{12}, and calcium
• Atrophy of mucosa • Decreased blood flow	• Food intolerance
• Delayed emptying	• Decreased hunger • Weight changes
Gastrointestinal/*Small Intestine*	
• Decreased villae, enzymes, and motility	• Decreased absorption of nutrients and fat-soluble vitamins
Gastrointestinal/*Large Intestine*	
• Decreased blood flow and motility • Decreased sensation of need to defecate	• Constipation • Increased risk for diverticular disease
Gastrointestinal/*Liver*	
• Decrease in number and size of cells • Decreased protein synthesis • Decreased regeneration	• Decreased drug metabolism and ability to detoxify
Gastrointestinal/*Pancreas*	
• Decreased lipase and reserve	• Impaired fat absorption • Possible glucose intolerance
Genitourinary/*Kidneys*	
• Decreased renal mass, nephrons, glomerular filtration rate, blood flow	• Decreased ability to concentrate urine, resulting in loss of free water and increased sensitivity to salt • Decreased creatinine clearance • Increased blood urea nitrogen • Decreased toxins and drug clearance
Genitourinary/*Bladder*	
• Decreased smooth muscle and elastic tissue	• Decreased control and possible incontinence • Decreased capacity
• Decreased sphincter control	• Increased frequency, urgency, and **nocturia**

Normal Changes Associated with Aging

SYSTEM OR STRUCTURE/CAUSES	CHANGES
Genitourinary/*Female Reproductive*	
• Decreased hormones • Decreased size of ovaries and uterus • Decreased pelvic elasticity • Atrophy and fibrosis of cervical and uterine walls • Decreased elasticity of vagina • Vaginal secretions pH alkaline • Involution of mammary gland tissue • Decreased elasticity and subcutaneous tissue • Increased adipose tissue	• Thin, pale vaginal mucosa • Decreased vaginal secretions • Decreased intensity of sexual response • Potential for prolapses and infections • Sagging of breasts • Possible stringy feeling of mammary ducts
Genitourinary/*Male Reproductive*	
• Enlarged prostate • Decreased sperm count and seminal fluid volume	• Prostatic hypertrophy • Decreased intensity of sexual response
• Seminal vesicles atrophy • Increased estrogen levels • Decreased testosterone • Reduced elevation and decreased size of testes	• Increased time to achieve erection • Decreased force of ejaculation • Tendency of testes to hang lower • Gynecomastia
Musculoskeletal/*Bones*	
• Narrow intervertebral discs	• Loss of height (1 to 4 inches) • Kyphosis • Wider pelvis
• Increased cartilage in nose and ears	• Increased length of nose and ears
• Decreased bone mass, bone growth, and osteoblastic activity	• Increased risk for osteoporotic fractures
Musculoskeletal/*Muscles*	
• Decreased number of muscle fibers • Muscle **atrophy** • Increased fat in muscles • Slow muscle regeneration	• Decreased strength
• Stiffening of ligaments and tendons • Increased contraction and latency time	• Decreased agility
Musculoskeletal/*Joints*	
• Decreased cartilage • Increased erosion and calcium deposits	• Decreased ROM and mobility • Osteoarthritis
Neurological/*Brain*	
• Decreased brain size, weight, and volume • Decreased neurons, glial cells, and conduction of nerve fibers • Neurofibrillary tangles • Hypoperfusion • Atrophy • Decreased neurotransmitters, dopamine, norepinephrine, serotonin, and acetylcholine • Elevated cortisol, sodium, and monoamine oxidase levels • Decreased deep sleep and REM sleep	• Decreased processing and reflexes • Delayed reaction time • Decreased psychomotor performance • Depression • Altered pain response • Decreased **proprioception** • Increased balance problems • Decreased sensory input • Increased periods of being awake and difficulty falling asleep • Decreased dreaming

(Continued)

Normal Changes Associated with Aging *(Continued)*

SYSTEM OR STRUCTURE/CAUSES	CHANGES
Endocrine	
• Decreased basal metabolic rate	• Increased weight
• Decreased sensitivity to hormones	• Decreased insulin response, glucose response, glucose tolerance and sensitivity of the renal tubules to ADH
• Decreased febrile response	• Decreased shivering and sweating
• Decrease in hormones (e. g., growth, thyroid)	• Effects of hormonal change
Immune/Hematologic	
• Decreased immunoglobulin IgA	• Decreased ability to reject foreign substances
• Involuted thymus	• Increased autoimmune disorders
• Decreased thymopoietin,	• Delayed hypersensitivity reactions
• lymphoid, antibodies, T lymphocytes	• Decreased response to acute infection
• Increased autoantibodies	
• Decreased memory of previous antigenic stimuli	• Increased incidence of malignancy
• Decreased responsiveness to immunizations	
• Increased anergy	• Recurrent latent herpes zoster or tuberculosis

Source: Adapted from Lewis et al., pp 225–260.

Developmental, Cultural, and Ethnic Variations

Assessing your client's developmental status is part of the assessment process. All humans continue to grow and develop throughout their lifetime. Erikson's psychosocial development theory identifies the final stage of development as ego integrity versus despair. Ideally, adults over age 65 will be able to do a life review with a sense of satisfaction and accomplishment and be able to accept their own mortality. This stage of life correlates well with Maslow's Hierarchy of Human Needs self-actualization need, in which self-fulfillment of one's potential is actualized. Many factors over a lifetime influence whether the older adult will attain self-actualization, a sense of accomplishment and satisfaction or despair. You need to be sensitive to your client's response to aging and assist him or her in achieving successful resolution of this final stage of development.

The definition and value of aging are dependent on culture. Aging can be defined in years, functional abilities, or social mores. Understanding this cultural influence may be helpful in planning care of the older client.

CRITICAL THINKING ACTIVITY #1

Consider the different cultural perspectives that follow. What impact do you think each of these perspectives has on the way families provide health care for their elderly members?

Cultural Perspectives on Aging

CULTURAL GROUP	VIEW OF AGING
African-American	Elderly people are valued and treated with respect. The grandmother has a central role and often offers economic support and child care. Grandchildren are often raised by the grandmother.
Appalachian	Elderly people are respected and honored, live close to their children, and participate in care of grandchildren.
Brazilian-American	Elderly parents live with children and are included in all activities.
Chinese-American	Elderly people are highly valued and respected and are considered very wise. Children are expected to care for parents.

Cultural Perspectives on Aging

CULTURAL GROUP	VIEW OF AGING
Cuban-American	Elderly parents live with children. Multigenerational households are common.
Egyptian-American	Elderly people are respected and thought to become wiser with age. Family is expected to take care of elders. Women gain status with age and childbearing; however, elderly women are expected to care for elderly men.
European-American	Value is on youth and beauty; elderly people are seen as less important than young people, and little attention is paid to their problems.
Filipino-American	Multigenerational households are common. Grandparents act as surrogate parents while parents work.
Greek-American	Elders are well respected. Children are expected to care for parents, who actively participate in family activities.
Iranian-American	Believe that with age comes experience, worldliness and knowledge; therefore elderly persons are seen with respect. Caring for elderly parents is children's obligation.
Irish-American	Elderly people are well respected and opinions are valued. Elderly parents are cared for in home.
Jewish-American	Elderly people are respected and seen as having wisdom. Honoring and caring for parents is important. Old age is a state of mind.
Korean-American	60 is considered old and persons over that age are expected to retire.
Mexican-American	Elderly parents live with children. Large extended family.
Navajo Native American	Elderly people with many children are seen with respect. Elderly people have important role in teaching and keeping rituals to children and grandchildren.
Vietnamese-American	Elders are honored, have key role in family activities. Elders are consulted on major family decisions.

Source: Data from Purnell, L., and Paulanka, B: Transcultural health care: A culturally competent approach. F. A. Davis, Philadelphia, 1998.

Introducing the Case Study

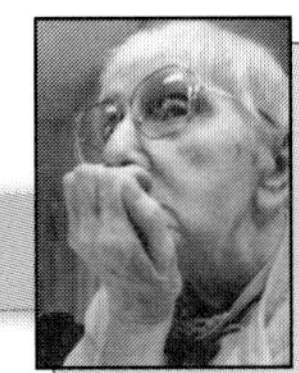

Mrs. Nurick, an 80-year-old widow, comes into the health office of the continuing care retirement community where she has lived for the past 8 years. She complains of vague fatigue, not being able to participate in her walking group over the past few weeks, decreased appetite, and general malaise. She says that she just doesn't feel like herself. She has been forcing herself to eat small amounts, take care of her cat, and do other necessary things. She still goes down to the dining room for dinner, and most weekends one of her four daughters takes her to mass and to lunch at a restaurant or dinner at her home. She has no specific complaints of bowel or bladder changes or problems, cough or shortness of breath, indigestion, or pain.

Performing the Assessment

A complete history and physical examination are essential in providing comprehensive, holistic care for the older adult. If the client has a long and complicated medical history, you may need to do the history and physical examination on separate visits and schedule an hour for each visit. You may also need to allow more time to help your client into the examination room and with dressing and undressing. When obtaining a history, ask one question at a time and allow enough time for your client to respond. You may also need to repeat questions and confirm answers.

Remember that older adults may not present in the same way as younger people when they are ill. When performing your assessment, keep these three factors in mind:

- Older adults may minimize or ignore symptoms.
- They often have several concurrent medical problems.
- They often present with atypical signs and symptoms of disease.

Symptom Reporting

Although some older adults are "health pessimists" who exaggerate their symptoms, the opposite is more often true. Many older adults are "health optimists" who downplay symptoms and give a more positive evaluation of their overall health status in the face of disease and disability. Unfortunately, failing to report symptoms or explaining them away can lead to late recognition of serious medical problems.

Older adults are also the least likely of all clients to take action in response to symptoms of serious illness. Instead they may attribute symptoms to normal aging and then simply wait and watch what happens, accept the changes they are experiencing, deny any danger associated with the symptoms, and delay seeking help. Many older adults worry that if they report symptoms to their healthcare provider, they may end up in a nursing home or in a more restrictive level of care. The cost of health care is also a major concern for many older adults. Also, when older adults do complain of a particular problem, they are more likely to identify a specific disease than younger clients.

Multiple Pathologies

Another major challenge in doing a history and physical examination in an older adult is the likelihood of multiple pathologies. Active medical problems frequently interact with one another and can confuse the clinical picture. For example, uncontrolled diabetes in an older woman can result in a urinary tract infection, which causes subsequent urinary incontinence. The urinary incontinence may then result in the client slipping on the wet bathroom floor and fracturing her hip. When moved to an acute-care setting, this same client may develop atrial fibrillation.

Alternately, older adults may have unidentified multiple pathologies that interact with the current treatment of a newly diagnosed problem. These are referred to as disease-treatment interactions. An older man who presents with insomnia and is given an antihistamine to help him sleep at night may return to the office with acute urinary retention because of an underlying enlargement of his prostate that was previously undetected.

Disease Presentation

You should also recognize when doing a history and physical on an older adult that these clients do not always present with the typical signs and symptoms of disease found in younger clients. Illness in older persons is not likely to be signaled by a single specific symptom or sign that points to the organ with the pathology. Older persons are much more likely to present with nonspecific problems such as a change in cognition or functional performance, a fall, decreased appetite and intake, new-onset incontinence, dizziness, or vague weakness and lethargy.

Vulnerable systems, such as the brain, are likely to **decompensate** as a result of systemic impact of disease anywhere in the body. Older clients often present with blunted or atypical signs and symptoms of specific disease states. For example, an older client may have a myocardial infarction without pain or pneumonia without cough, shortness of breath, or fever. He or she may complain only of "not feeling well."

Health History

The format for history taking with older clients is similar to that used with younger clients. However, the history should also include a functional assessment and investigation into advanced directives. Even though the formats are similar, some liberalization of the traditional interpretation of these components of the history is necessary to be relevant to the needs of the older adult.

Traditionally, the client is the primary source of information for the history. However, many older adults are unable to provide comprehensive medical information because of cognitive changes or a lack of interest or knowledge about their medical problems. When working with these clients, it may be necessary to get information from medical records (from an acute-care hospital stay or an outclient or nursing home chart) or from family, friends, and hospital or nursing home staff. The choice to have a family member present during the history and examination should be based on the client's wishes. If a family member is present, it should be made clear that the client is to answer the questions when possible and not the relative. The relative can clarify points and augment findings at the end of the history.

Even clients with known cognitive impairment or known to be unreliable in terms of their ability to provide information should be given an opportunity to answer questions and describe their symptoms. It is, however, essential to evaluate the client's cognitive status to determine his or her ability to provide reliable health information. Even in severe dementia, the client's response to questions regarding current symptoms may yield useful information, and it is important to establish a caring relationship by listening to what the client has to say.

To quickly establish an overall sense of the client's cognitive status, begin the history taking with questions that focus on orientation and past information. For example, ask questions that test time and place orientation and ask about the reasons for the visit, previous healthcare contacts, biographical data, and medication use.

Key points to remember when obtaining a history:

- Realize that age differences between you and your client may influence his or her response.
- Be aware of your own views and values associated with aging.
- Explain what you are doing and why.
- Allow more time than you do with younger clients.
- Realize that you may need to obtain the history over several visits.
- Ask the client if he or she can hear you clearly.
- Sit in front of and at the same level as the client without invading his or her personal space.
- Maintain eye contact.
- Speak slowly and clearly; the lower the pitch the better.
- Set time limits for your interview.
- Redirect the interview as needed, but respect the client's need to reminisce.
- Allow the client to respond to each question before asking another.
- Listen to what your client is saying and be alert for any signs of fatigue or discomfort.
- Use lay terminology that is culturally relevant to elicit more comprehensive information (e.g., "sugar" rather than "glucose" in diabetes).

Biographical Data

Begin by scanning the biographical data. The client's age and gender will identify any risk factors. His or her address, contacts, cultural or religious factors, and financial status may signal an underlying problem, explanation of a problem, or need for referral.

Case Study Findings

A review of Mrs. Nurick's biographical data reveals the following information:

- 80-year-old widow with four daughters
- Widowed since 1988
- Resident of continuing care retirement community for 8 years
- Catholic religion, Polish ancestry
- Not referred by doctor—came to outclient office of her own accord
- Source: Self, seems reliable

Current Health Status

Begin by determining the reason for seeking treatment. Remember that the older client often has more than one presenting symptom and is more likely to have multiple medical problems with associated multiple symptoms and complaints. The complaints may also be overlapping and nonspecific. It is useful to develop a list of chief complaints rather than focusing on one complaint. Help your client prioritize the problems according to which ones are the most distressing.

Symptom Assessment

As with chief complaints, there may be a history relevant to numerous lesser complaints, and each of these needs to be explored. In exploring them, it may be possible to find some connections among complaints and help identify the problem and relieve symptoms. For example, the client may describe a sudden onset of right knee pain and also report increased urinary urgency. On further questioning, you may learn that the knee pain resulted in decreased functional ability, causing the client to limit fluid intake so that he or she would not have to go to the bathroom very often. Limiting fluids resulted in strong, concentrated urine that caused the sensation of urgency in this client.

The chronology of events is particularly challenging when assessing older adults who have some cognitive impairment or are retired and less focused on the days, dates, and timing of events. It is sometimes necessary to use a calendar to review the sequence of events or to relate the onset of symptoms to timing of the client's activities. For example, you might ask if the pain started before the client went to church this week, or after her friend's birthday party.

When expanding on the present illnesses of older adults, it is important to use open-ended questions. Older clients look to the healthcare provider to have the answers and will probably follow your lead. Rather than asking if the pain was throbbing or stabbing, ask the client to describe the pain. If the client is unable to describe the pain in his or her own words, provide a choice of adjectives to describe it rather than asking the client to respond to yes or no questions. It is also important to repeat questions and confirm findings frequently.

Medications

Older adults often take many prescribed and over-the-counter medications, so **polypharmacy** may account for many of your client's symptoms. Determine your client's understanding of the medications and whether additional teaching may be needed. Also determine if the medications are being taken as prescribed, or if use of over-the-counter medications is affecting the desired action of prescription medications. Visual impairment may also cause mistakes in medication use. Ensuring safe administration of medication is a primary concern.

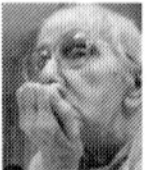

Case Study Findings

Mrs. Nurick's current health status includes:

- Complaints of vague fatigue all day, decreased appetite, and inability to engage in usual activities such as walking group. Fatigue has been present for several weeks and has grown worse in the past week even though the client has been going to bed around 9 PM and getting up at 8 AM. Is forcing herself to participate in social activities such as going to the dining room with friends for dinner. However, has no desire to eat.
- Is taking Lasix 20 mg po qd for hypertension and Tamoxifen 20 bid to prevent recurrence of breast cancer.

CRITICAL THINKING ACTIVITY #2

How might Mrs. Nurick's reactions to medications be affected by the changes associated with aging?

Past Health History

It is not uncommon for older adults to have an extensive medical history. Taking the time to obtain a comprehensive medical history is essential to prevent recurrence of past problems. Begin by asking your client about known medical problems, providing prompts such as, "Do you remember being told you had a problem with your heart?" Next, ask about specific diseases, asking questions such as, "Have you ever been told you have diabetes?" Another way to prompt your client's memory is to ask about past hospitalizations and the reasons for them. Do not focus on childhood illnesses, with the exception of asking about any childhood illness that kept the client in bed or out of school for an extended period of time. This question will help identify, for example, a history of rheumatic fever, which may cause rheumatic heart disease later in life.

Surgery

With regard to surgical history, it may also be necessary to prompt older clients' memory with questions about common surgeries that occur with age, such as cataract surgery, joint replacements, or removal of skin lesions. It is also necessary to ask specifically about the removal of organs such as the gallbladder, appendix, uterus, or prostate. During the physical examination, confirm any obvious scars with the surgical history given, and question the client about any unexplained scars you identify.

Medications

Reviewing medications is a good way to stimulate the older adult to recall previous diagnoses and medical problems. For example, if a client is on amiodarone (Cordarone) but does not report any cardiac history, it is helpful to ask specifically if the client knows why he or she is taking that medication and if he or she ever had an irregular heart rate.

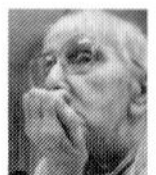

Case Study Findings

Mrs. Nurick's past health history reveals:

- Medical History
  - Breast cancer 20 years ago
  - Hypertension controlled by diuretics
  - Degenerative joint disease (DJD), mostly in hips
- Surgical History
  - Cataract surgery, 1990 (right eye) and 1991 (left eye)
  - Lumpectomy, right breast, 1979
  - Elective left total hip replacement, 1985

Family History

Asking older adults about causes of mortality among parents and other relatives is usually irrelevant. Aside from a known history of Alzheimer's disease or nonspecified dementia, most other familial diseases are present before the person reaches old age. Therefore, don't spend a long time reviewing family health histories.

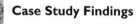

Case Study Findings

Mrs. N's family history reveals no known history of cognitive problems. She believes that both of her parents died of heart disease in their 70s and 80s, and does not know of any family history of cancer.

Review of Systems

In addition to the usual review done with all adult clients, the review of systems (ROS) with older adults should focus on problems that are particularly prevalent in this population. Specifically, these problems include a change in cognition, urinary or bowel incontinence, falls (see box on page 837), immobility, insomnia, dysphagia, and sensory changes. Positive responses to questions about any of these problems can be a useful starting point for a more comprehensive evaluation of the problem and the identification of more serious underlying problems

Review of Systems

SYSTEM/QUESTIONS TO ASK	RATIONALE/SIGNIFICANCE
General Health Survey	
How would you describe your usual state of health? Are you able to do what you usually do?	Helps to identify current heath status and activity tolerance
Have you noticed any changes in your height or weight? Do you notice any difference in how your clothes fit?	Loss of height (normally 6–10 cm) occurs with aging. Changes in weight distribution occur with age; a decrease of subcutaneous fat is seen on the face and extremities with an increase on the abdomen and hips. Differences in the way clothes fit may signal subtle changes in weight that warrant further investigation.
Integumentary/*Skin*	
Have you noticed any changes in your skin; e.g., dryness, itching, rashes, blisters?	There are many age-related changes in the skin, some of which are also caused by the environment. They result in uncomfortable symptoms such as pruritus and **xerosis** (dry skin), which occurs frequently in elderly people during the winter.
How often do you bathe? What type of soap do you use? Do you use lotions, sunscreens?	Skin care practices, sun exposure, and occupational history may influence current skin condition.
Have you been in the sun a great deal? What type of work did you do?	
Have you noticed any skin changes such as changes in size of growths, or open, sore, cracked, itchy, bleeding areas that won't heal?	The incidence of skin cancer increases with age.
Have you noticed any new rough areas of your skin that do not seem to go away?	Remember that visual changes that occur with aging may make early recognition of skin changes more difficult.
Integumentary/*Hair*	
Any hair loss, increased hair growth, graying, dry scalp, or other hair changes? What are your usual patterns of hair care? Have you undergone hair replacement treatments?	Changes in hair growth and distribution are commonly associated with aging. Dry scalp is a normal and common complaint. Hair loss may be distressing for both men and women. Women may also be concerned about increased facial hair. You need to differentiate normal changes from possible disease.
Integumentary/*Nails*	
How do you care for your nails? Do you cut them yourself? Do you see a podiatrist?	Nails thicken with age and may be more difficult to trim. Fungal nail infections are common. A podiatry consult may be indicated, especially if the client has a history of diabetes or vascular disease.
HEENT	
Do you have facial pain?	Increased incidence of **temporal arteritis** in elderly people may exhibit pain over temporal artery.
HEENT/*Head and Neck*	
Can you move your head easily?	Range of motion (ROM) in the head and neck may be limited by musculoskeletal changes or osteoarthritis.

(Continued)

Review of Systems *(Continued)*

SYSTEM/QUESTIONS TO ASK	RATIONALE/SIGNIFICANCE
HEENT/*Eyes*	
Have you noticed any changes in your vision? Can you read normal-sized print or large-print materials? Do you have problems going from light to dark areas? Do you drive at night?	Common problems (e.g., cataracts, macular degeneration, and glaucoma) can affect vision. Normal age changes include increased sensitivity to glare and decreases in visual acuity, lens elasticity, peripheral vision, color intensity (specifically blue, green, and purple), night vision, accommodation to changes in lighting, tear production and viscosity, depth perception, and near vision (presbyopia).
Do your eyes feel dry?	Dry eyes are very common. They may be caused by decreased tear production or blocked tear ducts, so further investigation is warranted.
Do you have floaters? Do you see flashes of light? Does it look like a shade is being pulled over your eye?	There are several eye complaints that require immediate attention, such as a sudden onset of floaters or flashes of light seen peripherally, with decreased visual acuity. The client may describe this as being like a curtain coming down over the field of vision (amaurosis fugax). These symptoms indicate retinal detachment, transient ischemic attack (TIA), or cerebrovascular accident (CVA). A complaint of a sudden onset of painless unilateral loss of vision also requires immediate attention because this may be a result of retinal vein occlusion.
HEENT/*Nose*	
Have you noticed any changes in your sense of smell?	**Anosomia**—a decreased ability to identify and discriminate odors—occurs with aging.
Do you have a runny nose (rhinorrhea)? Do you sneeze frequently? Do you have postnasal drip?	Atrophic changes associated with aging may cause vasomotor rhinitis.
HEENT/*Mouth and Throat*	
Do you have difficulty chewing, swallowing, tasting, smelling, or enjoying food?	Age-related changes on the surface of the tongue and atrophy of taste buds affect the ability to eat and enjoy food. In particular, there is a decrease in the ability to taste sweets and salt. Gums become thinner and recede, resulting in loose teeth and exposure of the roots.
Do you wear dentures? Do they fit properly? Do you have any sores in your mouth? When was the last time you saw your dentist?	Poorly fitted dentures may lead to poor nutrition and mouth sores. May identify need for referral.
When you are eating, do you ever cough or choke? Does this occur with liquids and/or solids? Do you have problems swallowing?	**Dysphagia**, defined as the mechanical interruption of eating, may be related to a variety of underlying problems and is not a normal part of aging. It warrants further investigation.
Does your mouth always feel dry with a bad taste? Do you have difficulty swallowing dry food or difficulty speaking for long periods?	Dry mouth (**xerostomia**) is a very common problem in older adults and can be caused by medication, decreased production of saliva, inadequate fluid intake, atrophy of the oral mucosa, vitamin deficiencies, poor nutrition, and poor oral hygiene. Burning mouth syndrome is also common in the older adult. It causes dry mouth, altered taste, thirst, difficulty swallowing, swelling in the face and cheeks, and altered sense of smell.
Respiratory	
Do you have any difficulty breathing? If yes, when does it occur and with how much exertion? Has it affected your ability to perform usual activities?	Respiratory disorders are common in the older adults. Clients may describe themselves as having breathing difficulties, trouble getting a deep breath or sufficient air. With chronic obstructive pulmonary disease (COPD), dyspnea is usually insidious in onset and progressive.

Review of Systems

SYSTEM/QUESTIONS TO ASK	RATIONALE/SIGNIFICANCE
Respiratory *(Continued)*	
Do you have a cough?	Lung cancer most frequently occurs between ages 55 and 74. There is a recent increase in tuberculosis among elderly people. If there is a new-onset cough, determine if the client has been exposed to a change in environment or has taken any new medications, such as angiotension converting enzyme (ACE) inhibitors.
Cardiovascular	
Do you get short of breath when walking or making the bed? Do you have swelling in the feet, hands, face, or abdomen; weight gain; or shoes or clothing that no longer fit? Does the swelling get worse as the day goes on and disappear in the morning?	Cardiovascular disease is not a normal change associated with aging, but it is the most common problem. Unfortunately it often does not exhibit the typical signs and symptoms found in younger people. For example, an older adult may present with atrial fibrillation but have no symptoms at all or complain vaguely of just not feeling right. If the client reports swelling, explore if this is related to his or her activity level or a change in medication or diet.
Do you get dizzy? When? Does the dizziness get worse when going from lying to standing, or is it worse with exertion? Are there any changes in your energy level?	Dizziness is a very common complaint and may be described as lightheadedness or a woozy feeling. Vague symptoms of dizziness may indicate postural (orthostatic) hypotension or a more serious underlying medical problems such as atrial fibrillation or congestive heart failure.
Do you have a cough? Is it worse at night? Do you get more short of breath when lying flat? Do you need to sleep with several pillows?	Cough may be related to congestive heart failure or a cardiac medication. Vascular disease increases with age.
Do you have headaches?	Headaches may be associated with hypertension, stroke, or temporal artery disease.
Do you have leg pain when walking? Skin changes, swelling, ulcers, or varicose veins in your legs?	**Intermittent claudication** (pain in legs when walking) and skin changes (thin, shiny and hairless) suggest arterial vascular disease. There is a high incidence of venous disease in elderly people.
Gastrointestinal	
What is your typical diet for a day? Any change? Any food intolerance?	Food intolerance is a common complaint and may be associated with hiatal hernia and esophageal reflux.
What are your usual bowel patterns? What is your diet and fluid intake? What medications, prescribed and over-the-counter, do you take?	Constipation is one of the most common digestive complaints in older adults, and accounts for 2.5 million physican visits annually. The prevalence of constipation increases with age, is more common in women than in men, in nonwhites than in whites, and in people with lower family income and less education. Constipation may have dangerous complications in older adults, including acute changes in cognition, urinary retention, urinary incontinence, and fecal impaction. Fecal impaction can result in intestinal obstruction, ulceration, and urinary problems. Chronic straining to defecate can have adverse effects on cerebral, coronary, and peripheral vascular circulation. Constipation can be categorized as functional (slow transit of stool) or rectosigmoid outlet delay (anorectal dysfunction, 10 minutes or more needed to defecate). Bowel changes associated with bleeding and weight loss suggest a malignancy.

(Continued)

Review of Systems *(Continued)*

SYSTEM/QUESTIONS TO ASK	RATIONALE/SIGNIFICANCE
Genitourinary/*Urinary*	
Do you have trouble getting to the bathroom on time? Do you need to wear a pad? If so, how many times a day do you have to change it? Does the incontinence occur with coughing or sneezing, on the way to the bathroom, or at night? Does it interfere with your ability (or desire) to do daily activities or engage in social activities?	Urinary incontinence is not a normal aspect of aging, but it is a common problem. Approximately 10 million Americans suffer from urinary incontinence. Report of new-onset incontinence, loss of appetite, vomiting, falls, nocturia, difficulty urinating, or behavioral and cognitive changes should alert you to a possible urinary tract infection. Prostate enlargement can cause incontinence. See box for types of incontinence.
Ask men about frequent urination, hesitancy, weak or intermittent stream, a sensation of incomplete emptying of the bladder, dribbling after voiding, and nocturia.	
Genitourinary/*Female Reproductive*	
Do you have any vaginal discharge? If so, what is the type, color, odor, and consistency of the discharge?	Changes in vaginal secretions, amount, and pH increase the risk for vaginal infections.

Types of Incontinence

Type of Incontinence	Definition	Pathophysiology	Signs and Symptoms
Stress	Involuntary loss of urine caused by urethral sphincter failure with increases in intra-abdominal pressure.	Usually caused by weakness and laxity of pelvic floor musculature or bladder outlet weakness. Also may be caused by urethral hypermobility.	Urine is lost during coughing, sneezing, laughing.
Urge	Leakage of urine because of inability to delay voiding after sensation of bladder fullness is perceived.	Associated with detrusor hyperactivity, central nervous system disorders, or local genitourinary conditions.	Urine is lost on the way to the bathroom or as soon as the urge to void is felt.
Overflow	Leakage of urine resulting from mechanical forces on an overdistended bladder.	Results from mechanical obstruction or an acontractile bladder.	Variety of symptoms, including frequent or constant dribbling, increased incontinence at night, frequency, and urgency.
Functional	Urine leakage caused by inability to get to toilet because of cognitive or physical impairment.	Cognitive and physical functional impairment.	Client is aware of the need to void but urine is lost on the way to the bathroom.

Review of Systems

SYSTEM/QUESTIONS TO ASK	RATIONALE/SIGNIFICANCE
Genitourinary/*Female Reproductive (Continued)*	
Do you have vaginal pressure, or an uncomfortable, bearing-down sensation, in addition to symptoms of urinary incontinence?	
Do you have any vaginal bleeding? Are you taking hormone replacement therapy? When did you go through menopause? When was your last Pap test?	Bleeding may be related to hormone replacement therapy. If client is not on hormones, bleeding that occurs after 1 year postmenopause is abnormal and needs follow-up. Symptoms may be related to the presence of a uterine prolapse, cystocele, or rectocele.
Do you do breast-self-examinations?	
When was your last mammogram? Do you get them yearly?	Incidence of breast cancer increases with age. Yearly mammograms are recommended for women over age 50. May identify teaching needs.
Are you satisfied with your sexual activity? Do you have pain during intercourse (**dyspareunia**) or vaginal dryness?	Older adults continue to be sexually active, unless they no longer have a sexual partner, have a disease, or are exposed to a treatment that decreases libido or makes intercourse uncomfortable. None of the age-related changes in either men or women preclude the continuation of a satisfying sex life. Decreased vaginal secretions may may result in dyspareunia. If this is present, an appropriate plan of care should be developed.
Have you ever had a sexually transmitted disease? Do you practice safe sex?	Because older women do not fear pregnancy, they are less likely to ask their partners to use condoms as a form of protection.
Genitourinary/*Male Reproductive*	
When was the last time you had your prostate checked?	Increased incidence of prostate cancer in older men. Yearly prostate exams should begin at age 40. May identify need for health teaching.
Have you ever had a Prostate Specific Antigen (PSA) test? Do you have any urinary changes or problems?	
Are you satisfied with your sexual activity? Have you been feeling more tired than usual?	Sexuality does not normally decrease with age. However, the physical act and response may require more time and be less intense. Be alert for vague complaints. Give men the opportunity to talk about impotence and associated feelings so that individualized plans can be developed.
Musculoskeletal	
Do you have pain, stiffness, joint enlargement, decreased range of motion and functional changes?	**Osteoarthritis** is the most common joint disease in the older adult and affects over 80% of people age 65 and over (Nesher & Moore, 1994). **Rheumatoid arthritis** also increases with age. **Gout** is also common, exacerbated by use of diuretics or alcohol.
Do you have pain, stiffness, and decreased range of motion in the neck, shoulders, or hips persisting for at least one month? Do you have severe headache, visual loss, scalp tenderness, and mouth pain?	Common problems in older adults include **polymyalgia rheumatica**, a syndrome that involves the musculoskeletal system; **giant cell arteritis**, a vasculitic disorder of the cranial arteries associated with polymyalgia rheumatica; and osteoporosis.

(Continued)

Review of Systems *(Continued)*

SYSTEM/QUESTIONS TO ASK	RATIONALE/SIGNIFICANCE
Musculoskeletal ***(Continued)***	
Have you had any fractures, bone pain, and loss of height? Do you take calcium and vitamin D? Do you exercise? If so, what type of activity do you do? Are you taking any additional bone building medication?	Identifies participation in measures to prevent further bone loss and possible teaching needs.
Do you have balance problems or a history of falls?	Refer to the checklist *Evaluating the Risk Factors for Falls*. This can help determine whether the fall is caused by gait or balance disorder or another underlying problem for which the client needs to be evaluated and treated.
Do you have any foot problems? How do your shoes fit? Do you see a podiatrist? How do you care for your feet?	Foot problems are common in elderly people and may result from poorly fitted shoes or poor foot care. Referrals may be warranted.
Neurological	
Do you have problems with balance, mobility, coordination, sensory interpretations, level of consciousness, intellectual performance, personality, communication, comprehension, emotional responses, and thoughts?	Changes in the neurological system may be normal or caused by disease. CVA (stroke) is the most common neurological problem in elderly people. Parkinson's disease is the most common extrapyramidal problem.
Do you have dizziness? Do you feel that the room is spinning or you're spinning?	**Vertigo** is a common problem, and diagnosis is based mainly on clinical symptoms.
Do you have a known history of seizures? Do you have repetitive shaking or muscle contractions, brief lapses of consciousness, or any abnormal sensations?	Incidence of seizures significantly increases in people over age 65 because of an increase in strokes, tumors, subdural hematomas, metabolic disorders, **dementia**, and medications.
Endocrine	
Have you been feeling depressed? Experiencing weight loss or gain?	Thyroid disease presents differently in older adults than in younger adults. Signs of hyperthyroidism include apathy, depression, and emaciation rather than hyperactivity. Atrial fibrillation also often occurs. Hypothyroidism is the most frequent thyroid disorder in elderly persons, but it is easy to miss because signs (dry skin and hair, hypotension, slow pulse, sluggishness, depressed muscular activity, goiter, weight gain) are often attributed to aging.
Does your heart ever flutter, race or skip beats?	
Do you have increased thirst, urination and appetite?	The incidence of diabetes mellitus increases with age.
Immune/Hematologic	
Have you been feeling more tired than usual?	When an elderly person becomes sick, symptoms may be vague because of changes in the immune system. Fatigue may be associated with anemia, a common problem in elderly people, usually caused by iron deficiency.

Drug-Nutrient Interactions

MEDICATION	POTENTIAL EFFECT ON NUTRIENTS
Mineral oil	Decreased absorption of fat-soluble vitamins A, D, E, and K
Anticonvulsants	Reduced storage of vitamin K and absorption of calcium and vitamin D
Antacids with aluminum	Reduced absorption of phosphorous and fluoride and increased calcium excretion
Antacids with aluminum or magnesium	Reduces absorption and increases intestinal elimination of phosphate
Antacids with sodium bicarbonate	Sodium overload and water retention
Gentamicin	Increased potassium and magnesium excretion
Penicillin	Increased potassium excretion
Tetracycline	Decreased absorption of iron, calcium, zinc, and magnesium
Aspirin	Decreased folate and ascorbic acid, causing iron deficiency as a result of blood loss
Corticosteroids	Decreased calcium and phosphorous absorption Increased need for pyridoxine, folate, ascorbic acid and vitamin D
Potassium supplements	Decreased vitamin B_{12} absorption as a result of decreased acidity in the ileum
Laxatives	Hypokalemia, hypoalbuminemia, decreased calcium absorption, malabsorption with steatorrhea
Cholestyramine	Decreased absorption of fat-soluble vitamins and calcium
Cimetidine	Decreased absorption of vitamin B_{12} as a result of hypochlorhydria
Neomycin	Decreased absorption of fat, lactose, nitrogen, calcium, iron, potassium, and vitamin B_{12}
Isoniazid	B_6 and niacin deficiency
Hydralazine	B_6 deficiency

Source: Miller, pp 301–302, with permission.

ration and severity, and how the change in sleep impacts his or her life. Ask about difficulty falling and staying asleep, feeling rested in the morning, snoring, and movement, pain or jerking in the leg that either prevents the client from falling asleep or wakes him or her during the night.

HOW AGE AFFECTS SLEEP

- Longer time to fall asleep
- Increased time in stages 1 and 2 sleep
- Decreased time in deeper stages of sleep (stages 3 and 4)
- Decreased rapid eye movement (REM) sleep
- Increased and shorter repetition of sleep cycle
- Increased nighttime awakenings
- Altered circadian rhythm with a need to fall asleep earlier and awaken earlier

Also ask if the client is having any associated symptoms that are influencing sleep, such as chest pain, indigestion, back pain, or urinary frequency. Review bedtime routines, caffeine use, and exercise/activity as they relate to sleep behavior. Be sure to ask the client if he or she naps during the day, the approximate length of the naps, and the amount of time he or she spends in bed not sleeping. Roommates, caregivers, and spouses or significant others should also be asked about the client's snoring or changes in breathing patterns (which might provide a clue to an underlying problem such as sleep apnea), and excessive leg movement or jerking during the night (which might interrupt normal restful sleep patterns).

Self-Care Responsibilities

The health history should also include questions about health promotion and prevention practices. There is evidence to suggest that older people benefit just as much from primary and secondary health promotion activities as middle-aged people. Exercise and reducing cholesterol levels improve overall health status and physical fitness, including aerobic power, strength, balance, and flexibility and help prevent acute medical problems such as fractures, myocardial infarctions, and cerebrovascular accidents. Mammograms, Pap tests, digital examinations for monitoring prostate size, and yearly evaluations of stool specimens for occult blood can help reduce mortality and morbidity among older adults.

Unfortunately, with age there is a general decline in primary and secondary preventive behaviors, particularly in regard to mammography, Pap tests, having stools checked for occult blood, and monitoring cholesterol. Reasons include advanced age, unwillingness to undergo treatment if given a positive finding, and not being referred for testing by a primary healthcare provider. During history taking, healthcare providers should take an individualized approach, discussing the pros and cons of primary and secondary prevention activities and helping older adults make decisions about participation in these activities. Once clients have been educated, it is important that healthcare providers listen to the clients' wishes and respect their decisions. For example, if an older woman says that she will not undergo surgery for a breast mass, it may not be appropriate to send her for mammography.

Personal Habits

Ask about the use of nicotine, alcohol, and street drugs. Rather than asking the older adult if he or she drinks alcohol, ask how much alcohol he or she drinks. Assuming that an older adult drinks alcohol regularly reduces the feeling that judgment is being passed. It is also helpful to use screening instruments to explore alcohol use in the older client. The CAGE is a short four-item questionnaire that helps identify people at risk for alcohol abuse. A positive response to any of the questions indicates further assessment of an alcohol abuse or dependency problem.

CAGE

- Have you ever felt you should cut down on your drinking?
- Have people annoyed you by criticizing your drinking?
- Have you ever felt bad or guilty about your drinking?
- Have you ever had a drink first thing in the morning to steady your nerves or get rid of a hangover?

Source: Mayfield et al., pp 1121–1123, with permission.

Support Systems

Information on support systems is a relevant part of the client history because it is necessary to understand what personal and community support the older client has to help with ADLs. Determining if the client lives alone or with others and what type of setting he or she lives in is important, as is information about the client's community at large. Explore all potential social supports with the client and determine what type of interaction is available (phone calls or visits).

Environmental Structure and Hazards

Ask the client to describe his or her home, the presence and condition of any stairs, the accessibility of the bathroom and kitchen, and household activities with which he or she currently needs assistance (e.g., grocery shopping, cooking, cleaning, laundry). Assessment of your client's home environment may identify needs for assistive devices or referrals.

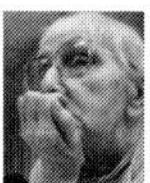

Case Study Findings

Mrs. Nurick's psychosocial history reveals:

- Typical day starts around 8 AM. She fixes herself breakfast in her efficiency apartment, feeds her cat, then has coffee and watches television. Does laundry, light housecleaning, and "putters around" apartment. At midmorning usually goes to the activity room to socialize or play cards with other residents. Fixes own lunch. Until recently, walked 20 minutes 3 times a week with walking group in afternoon. Goes on planned outings with other residents. Sees daughters every weekend for lunch or dinner, shopping, and mass on Sunday. Previously went to bed at 11 PM but has been retiring at 9 PM for past few weeks because of fatigue.
- Doesn't smoke and rarely has a glass of wine socially.

Functional Assessment

A very important component of the history in older adults is exploring functional performance. Functional evaluations should include ADLs such as eating, bathing, dressing, transferring, toileting, and ambulation. Instrumental activities of daily living (IADLs) include activities such as taking medications, paying bills, using the telephone, and using public transportation. Use of a functional status instrument will help you obtain baseline information that you can follow from year to year on your client. Many such instruments are available, and the decision to use one over the other may depend on the client. For example, the Katz Index is a basic measure that describes the client as dependent, semi-dependent, or independent in ADLs but does not identify small changes over time.

Conversely, the Barthel Index gives weighted scores for each ADL and allows the nurse to recognize small changes over time. A score of less than 60 on this index indicates that the client needs assistance with ADLs. Duke University provides an example of a common measure used to review IADLs. Reviewing these items with the client allows you to determine his or her level of functioning and make appropriate referrals for care.

The Katz Index of ADL

Abbreviations: I=independent; A=assistance; D=dependent

1. Bathing (sponge, shower, or tub)
   I: Receives no assistance (gets in and out of the tub)
   A: Receives assistance in bathing only one part of the body
   D: Receives assistance in bathing more than one part of the body
2. Dressing
   I: Gets clothes and gets completely dressed without assistance
   A: Gets clothes and gets dressed without assistance except in tying shoes
   D: Receives assistance in getting clothes or in getting dressed or stays partly or completely undressed
3. Toileting
   I: Goes to bathroom, cleans self, and manages clothes without assistance (may use an assistive device)
   A: Receives assistance in going to bathroom or in cleaning self, managing clothes, or emptying a bedpan
   D: Doesn't go to bathroom for elimination
4. Transfer
   I: Moves in and out of bed or chair without assistance (may use assistive device)
   A: Moves in and out of bed or chair with assistance
   D: Doesn't get out of bed
5. Continence
   I: Controls urination and bowel movements independently
   A: Has occasional accidents
   D: Urine or bowel control maintained with supervision; client is incontinent or has catheter
6. Feeding
   I: Feeds self without assistance
   A: Feeds self except for cutting meat or buttering bread
   D: Receives assistance in feeding or is fed partly or completely by tubes or intravenous fluids

Source: Adapted from Katz et al, 1963.

The Barthel Index

LEVEL OF CARE	INTACT	LIMITED	HELPER	NULL
Self-Care				
1. Feed	10	5	3	3
2. Dress (upper extremities)	5	5	3	0
3. Dress (lower extremities)	5	5	2	0
4. Don brace	0	0	−2	0
5. Grooming	4	4	0	0
Cleanse Perineum	4	4	2	0
Sphincters	Completely Voluntary	Urgency/Appliance	Some help needed	Frequent accidents
6. Bladder	10	10	5	0
7. Bowel	10	10	5	0
Mobility/Transfer	Easy/No device	With difficulty or uses device	Some help needed	Dependent
1. Chair	15	15	7	0
2. Toilet	6	5	3	0
3. Tub	1	1	0	0
4. Walk 50 yds	15	15	10	0
5. Stairs	10	10	5	0
6. Wheelchair 50 yds	15	5	0	0

Source: Adapted from Barthel et al., pp 61–65.

Instrumental Activities of Daily Living (IADL)

Abbreviations:
I=independent; A=assistance, and D=dependent

1. Telephone:

   I: Able to look up numbers, dial, receive, and make calls without help

   A: Able to answer phone or dial operator in an emergency, but needs special phone or help in getting number or dialing

   D: Unable to use the telephone

2. Traveling:

   I: Able to drive own car or travel alone on bus or taxi

   A: Able to travel but not alone

   D: Unable to travel

3. Shopping:

   I: Able to take care of all shopping with transportation provided

   A: Able to shop but not alone

   D: Unable to shop

4. Preparing meals:

   I: Able to plan and cook full meals

   A: Able to prepare light foods, but unable to cook full meals alone

   D: Unable to prepare any meals

5. Housework:

   I: Able to do heavy housework (e.g., scrubbing floors)

   A: Able to do light housework, but needs help with heavy tasks

   D: Unable to do any housework

6. Medication:

   I: Able to take medications in the right dose at the right time

   A: Able to take medications, but needs reminding or someone to prepare it

   D: Unable to take medications

7. Money:

   I: Able to manage buying needs, write checks, pay bills

   A: Able to manage daily buying needs, but needs help managing checkbook and paying bills

   D: Unable to manage money

Source: Duke University Center for the Study of Aging and Human Development, pp 169–170, with permission.

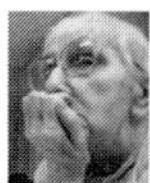

Case Study Findings

Mrs. Nurick's functional assessment reveals:

- Performs all of her personal care independently. Does her own laundry, shopping, finances, and cleaning aside from the vacuuming, which is done by the facility every 2 weeks.
- Walks independently with a rolling walker. Has been participating in a walking group and until recently was walking for 20 minutes 3 times per week.

Advance Directives and Preferences for Care

Directives for acute and end-of-life care are not traditionally part of the client history. But in the current healthcare arena it is essential to address these issues with older adults. The 1990 Client Self-Determination Act (PSDA), which requires that clients be asked about the existence of advance directives at the time of enrollment or admission to a healthcare facility, increased awareness of the right to determine acute and end-of-life care options. Unfortunately, discussions and decisions about these care options with older adults have only increased moderately since the PSDA. A large number of older adults still do not have advance directives. Moreover, many written advance directives have care options that are poorly delineated, so the proxy is not aware of the client's specific wishes.

With regard to directives for care, old-old people (90 years of age and older) usually express a decreased interest in receiving aggressive medical interventions for acute and end-of-life care. It is not uncommon when working with old-old clients to have them report a feeling of satisfaction with a long life lived, yet a desire for this life to end quietly. Certainly these wishes need to be acknowledged. Older adults are also more likely to want to be hospitalized for treatment of an acute illness, but are less likely to want treatment for a potentially life-threatening injury. They do not want life prolonged if their function and quality of life will be impaired.

Unfortunately, 6 to 20 percent of older adults defer decisions regarding acute and end-of-life care to their primary healthcare providers or the people who have power of attorney. It has been shown repeatedly that proxy decisions are different from the client's wishes. Older adults should be encouraged to exercise their moral and ethical right to determine their care. Healthcare providers have a responsibility to educate them about these rights, to provide accurate, up-to-date information, and to correct misinformation about acute and end-of-life care options. Discussions about care decisions, executing a living will, and designating a proxy decision maker and durable power of attorney for health care will help older adults make sure that their wishes are carried out if they can no longer dictate their own care.

Case Study Evaluation

Before performing the physical examination, document what you've learned about Mrs. Nurick so far.

 CRITICAL THINKING ACTIVITY #4

What are Mrs. Nurick's strengths? Are there any areas of concern?

Physical Assessment

Once you have completed the health history, collect objective data through your physical examination.

Approach

When examining the older client, make sure the environment is as safe and appropriate as possible. To ensure a senior-friendly environment, do the following:

- Keep examination rooms warm (between 70° and 80°).
- Use bright but nonglaring lights.
- Keep background noise to a minimum.
- Provide higher than standard seating (because clients might have trouble getting up, and if they have DJD or have had joint replacement, they shouldn't flex the joint more than 90 degrees) with arm rests on all chairs.
- Use examination tables that mechanically elevate the client from lying to sitting and vice versa and a broad-based step stool to help clients get onto the table.
- Use a private examination room, if possible, or at least pull the privacy curtain if there is a roommate.
- Minimize position changes to keep the client from getting tired.
- Uncover only the area being assessed, making sure that client is warm and covered with blankets or drapes.
- Provide reading materials with large print.
- Allow more time than usual for the examination. The complete examination may need to be scheduled over several meetings.
- Make safety a priority. If your client can't tolerate or perform what is expected for the examination, then adapt the examination to meet his or her needs.
- Take the time to explain everything you are doing to your client.

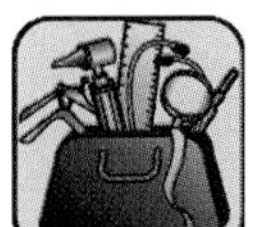

Toolbox

To perform the physical examination, you will need all the tools of assessment.

Performing a General Survey

The physical examination of the older client begins as soon as you meet. During the client history, you observed the functional mobility of your client, his or her overall appearance (particularly hygiene), emotional status, body habitus, and so on. As you begin the physical examination, note the client's ability to transfer from a chair to the examination table and to dress and undress. Look at your client's posture. A common problem is senile kyphosis (dowager's hump or widow's hump), an accentuated thoracic curve in which the head tilts back and the neck shortens, giving a rounded "e" profile. A wide base of support may signal balance problems. Note if there are any other obvious problems or signs of distress, such as suspicious skin lesions or shortness or breath. Also obtain vital signs and height and weight in a standardized fashion. If the scale requires a step up, be sure to help the client. In light of the increased risk and incidence of hypothermia in older adults, it is important to have a reliable low-reading thermometer. To check for orthostatic hypotension, take blood pressures in the supine position after a least 10 minutes of rest, then immediately upon standing, and then 3 minutes after standing. Evaluating the heart rate response to postural changes at the same time provides important information about the cause of orthostatic hypotension. A rise of less than 10 beats per minute with a drop in blood pressure suggests baroreceptor reflex impairment.

Performing a Head-to-Toe Physical Assessment

You will use all four techniques of physical assessment and all of your senses when you perform the examination. As you examine your client, keep in mind the changes that normally occur with aging so that you can differentiate them from abnormal changes.

Performing a Head-to-Toe Physical Assessment

SYSTEM/NORMAL VARIATIONS

Integumentary/*Skin*

INSPECT

- Skin color uneven in areas, increased creases, wrinkle lines and skin lesions. Some common wrinkle lines and skin lesions. Some common lesions include **seborrheic keratosis**, **lentigines** (liver spots), and **acrochordons. Senile purpura**, commonly found on hands and forearms, is caused by frail capillaries.

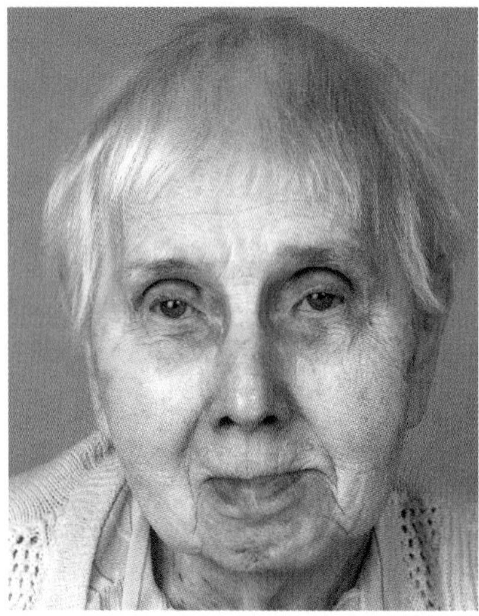

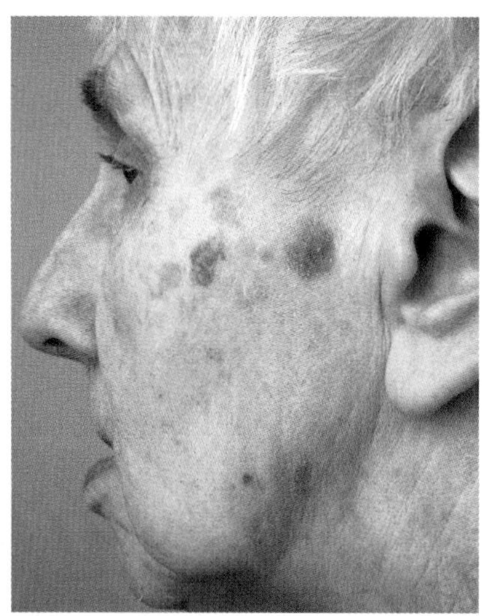

Seborrheic keratosis

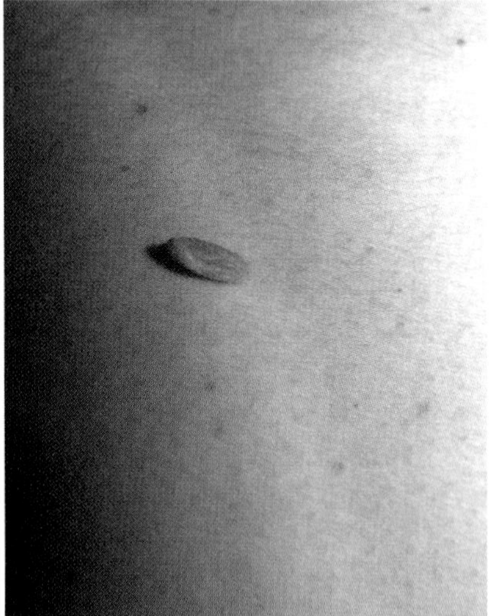

Acrochordon

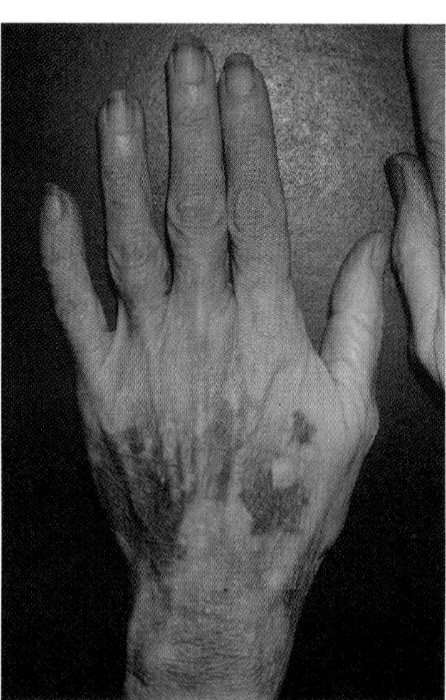

Senile purpura

HELPFUL HINT

An easy way to measure skin lesions is to apply a piece of Scotch tape over them and trace the outline of the lesion onto the tape. Place the tape in the client's chart and re-evaluate over time.

ABNORMAL FINDINGS/RATIONALE

- Areas of pressure or pressure sores from immobility or splints/appliances.
- Elderly clients are more apt to have body folds and develop intertrigo (inflammatory, moist erythema and scaling lesions) or fungal infections. The box on page 845 describes common skin lesions associated with aging.

ALERT

If you detect excessive bruising, consider the possibility of elder abuse.

Performing a Head-to-Toe Physical Assessment

SYSTEM/NORMAL VARIATIONS	ABNORMAL FINDINGS/RATIONALE

Common Skin Lesions Associated with Aging

Skin Lesion	Description
Lentigines	Hyperpigmented macular lesions (liver spots)
Ichthyosis	Dry, scaly, fishlike skin
Acrochordons	Small, benign polyp-growths (skin tags)
Actinic keratosis	Rough precancerous skin macule or papule from sun exposure
Seborrheic keratosis	Benign pigmented lesions with a waxy surface on face and trunk
Senile purpura	Vascular lesion of ecchymoses and petechiae on arms and legs caused by the frail nature of capillaries and decreased collagen support
Venous lakes	Bluish-black papular vascular lesion
Senile ectasias	Red-purple macule or papule lesions (senile or cherry angiomas)
Basal cell carcinoma	Pearly, papular, or plaquelike cancerous lesions that may be ulcerated in the center; associated with sun exposure
Squamous cell carcinoma	Erythematous, indurated areas that may be scaly or hyperkeratotic, associated with sun exposure, and tend to grow more rapidly than basal cell carcinomas

Integumentary/*Skin (Continued)*

PALPATE

- Temperature: Warm, but hands and feet may be cool.
  - Cool extremities may signal vascular disease. Unilateral cool temperature may indicate an occlusion and warrants medical attention.
- Turgor: Normally decreased. Not a marker of hydration status.
  - Decreased turgor increases risk for injury and skin breakdown.
- Hydration/texture: Dry, flaky, and thin.
  - Excessive dryness may indicate dehydration.

Integumentary/*Hair and Scalp*

INSPECT/PALPATE

- Hair color/distribution: Graying in both sexes; thinning/balding especially in men.
  - Changes in hair may also relate to endocrine problems or may occur as a side effect from medications.
- Increased facial hair (hirsutism) in women.
- Coarse, dry hair and dry flaky scalp (senile xerosis).

Integumentary/*Nails*

INSPECT/PALPATE:

- Yellow, dry, brittle nails with longitudinal ridges.
  - Yellow, thick nails may also be caused by disease or a fungal infection.

(Continued)

Performing a Head-to-Toe Physical Assessment *(Continued)*

SYSTEM/NORMAL VARIATIONS	ABNORMAL FINDINGS/RATIONALE
HEENT *INSPECT/PALPATE* ***Head/Neck*** • May have decreased ROM caused by musculoskeletal changes.	• Decreased ROM of the neck may also be associated with DJD.
HEENT/*Lymph Nodes* • Lymph tissue decreases in size with aging and should be nonpalpable.	• Palpable nodes warrant referral.
HEENT/*Thyroid* • Nonpalpable.	• Palpable thyroid may signal thyroid disease (common in elderly people) and warrants referral.
HEENT/*Temporal Artery* • Palpable and nontender.	• Pain, nodularity, and presence of a pulse may indicate temporal arteritis.
HEENT/*Eyes* *INSPECT* • Decreased near vision (presbyopia) may cause difficulty reading.	• Loss of central vision, halos, and eye pain may indicate glaucoma and warrant referral. Visual changes may also occur with cerebrovascular disease.
• Far vision may be intact. • Decreased peripheral vision. • Dry eyes.	• Basal cell carcinoma frequently found on inner third of lower lid.
• Enophthalmus (recession of eyeball into orbit). • Arcus senilis: white to yellow deposit at outer edge of the cornea, along with xanthelasma (yellowish, raised tumor on upper or lower lids).	• Yellow or opaque lens associated with increased incidence of cataracts.

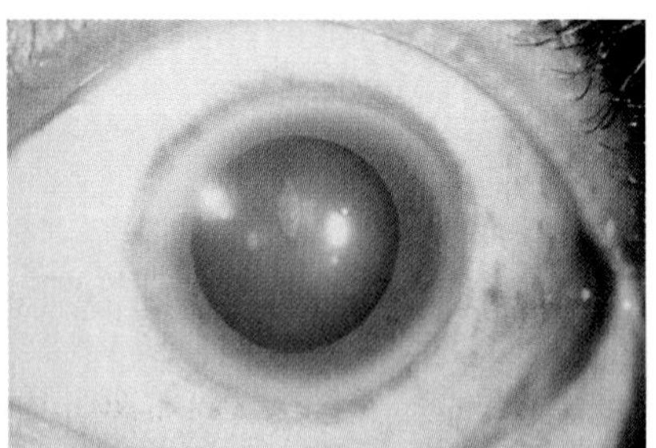

Arcus senilis

SYSTEM/NORMAL VARIATIONS	ABNORMAL FINDINGS/RATIONALE
• **Senile entropion** (inversion of the lashes).	• Entropion increases the risk of corneal abrasions.
• **Senile ectropion** (eversion of the lashes).	• Ectropion increases risk of dryness and conjunctivitis.
• Xanthelasma (lipid deposits) on lids. • Pale or yellow-tinted conjunctiva; pale iris; pingueculae (clear to yellow fleshy lesion on conjunctiva).	

Performing a Head-to-Toe Physical Assessment

SYSTEM/NORMAL VARIATIONS	ABNORMAL FINDINGS/RATIONALE
HEENT/*Eyes (Continued)* *INSPECT* • Pterygium: similar to pingueclae, but extends over cornea • Increased stimulation needed to elicit corneal reflex • Small pupils; reaction equal but may be less brisk	
• Fundoscopic—Retina and optic disc become paler with age.	• Macular degeneration. • Check for diabetic and hypertensive retinal changes because the incidence of these diseases increases with age.
HEENT/*Ears* *INSPECT* Internal • Gross hearing intact but diminished with decreased pitch discrimination. • Potential conductive hearing loss (presbycusis). • Increased difficulty hearing high-pitched sounds, especially s, t, f, and g. • Difficulty understanding speech.	
• Equilibrium-balance problems.	• Balance problems and tinnitus may indicate a neurological problem. • Balance problems increase risk for falls and injury.
External • Lobes elongate.	• Dry ears with scratch marks related to senile pruritus.
• Increased external ear canal hair in men. Otoscopic	
• Dry **cerumen**. • Diminished cone of light.	• Cerumen impaction can decrease hearing acuity by 40 to 45 dB; removal of cerumen corrects the impairment. • Hearing aids can cause contact dermatitis.
HEENT/*Nose* • Elongated nose. *INSPECT* • Increased nasal hair. • Decreased sense of smell (CN I).	• Vasomotor rhinitis causes pale nasal mucosa and boggy turbinates.
HEENT/*Mouth and Throat* • "Purse-string" appearance of mouth.	• Gum recession and bleeding (atrophic gingivitis).
INSPECT • Teeth may show staining, chipping, or erosion. Some teeth may be loose or missing.	• Chewing and swallowing difficulty may be caused by poor dentition or poorly fitted dentures, or more serious problem such as CVA.
• Buccal mucosa and gums thin and pale. • Oral mucosa dry, causing halitosis. • Decreased sense of taste (CN VII and CN IX).	• Leukoplakia (white precancerous lesion) in mouth, particularly under tongue.

(Continued)

Performing a Head-to-Toe Physical Assessment *(Continued)*

SYSTEM/NORMAL VARIATIONS	ABNORMAL FINDINGS/RATIONALE
HEENT/*Mouth and Throat (Continued)* • Decreased gag reflex (CN IX and CN X). • Decreased papillae on tongue. • Varicose veins under tongue (caviar spots).	
Respiratory *INSPECT/PALPATE/AUSCULTATE* • **Senile kyphosis** (increased anterior to posterior diameter) caused by MS changes, barrel chest appearance. • Decreased respiratory excursion. • Cheyne-Stokes breathing may occur during sleep. • Breath sounds may be decreased with few crackles at bases.	• Respiratory changes increase risk for pulmonary problems, such as pneumonia.
Cardiovascular *INSPECT/PALPATE/AUSCULTATE* • Increase in premature beats and irregular pulse. • Decreased pedal pulses. • Stiffer arteries. • Slight increases in blood pressure and wider pulse pressure. • Orthostatic drops in BP more common in elderly people.	• Increased incidence of vascular disease. If present, carotid bruit present and carotid thrills may be palpable. • Increased varicosities. • Abnormal heart sounds: Rate irregular with ectopic beats., S_4 common, systolic murmurs associated with aortic stenosis. • Differentiate arterial insufficiency from venous insufficiency.
Gastrointestinal *INSPECT/PALPATE/PERCUSS/AUSCULTATE* • Abdomen very soft because of decreased musculature, so organs may be easier to palpate. • Bowel sounds may be slightly decreased.	• Palpable bladder with retention. • Palpable intestines if filled with stool. • A pulsatile mass in the abdomen may be an aneurysm. Incidence of abdominal aortic aneurysms increases with age.

HELPFUL HINT

When assessing the mouth, be sure to remove dentures and partial plates and evaluate for bacterial plaque, food debris, and pressure areas.

HELPFUL HINT

Here's how to differentiate a radiating murmur from a carotid bruit: A murmur is usually heard bilaterally and diminishes as you move away from the heart; a carotid bruit is unilateral and increases in intensity as you move away from the heart.

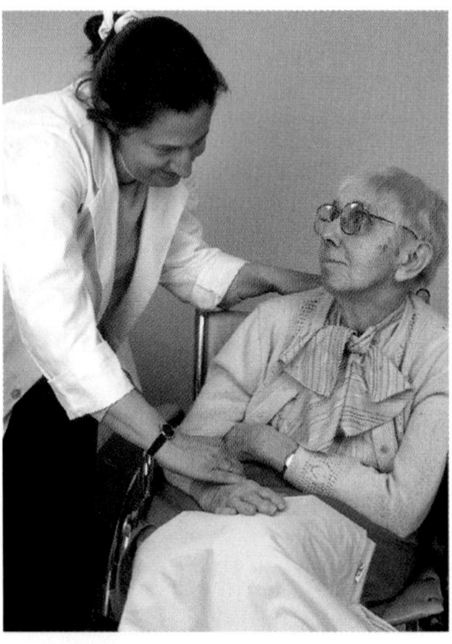

HELPFUL HINT

Check for old scars—they may provide information about surgeries the client forgot to mention in the history.

Performing a Head-to-Toe Physical Assessment

SYSTEM/NORMAL VARIATIONS	ABNORMAL FINDINGS/RATIONALE
Gastrointestinal *(Continued)* *INSPECT/PALPATE/PERCUSS/AUSCULTATE*	An aneurysm may have lateral as well as anteroposterior pulsation. Aneurysms are usually wider than 3 cm and often have an associated bruit. Surgical evaluation may be appropriate, particularly if aneurysm is greater than 5 cm. • Dullness over bladder may signal urinary retention; dullness over bowel may signal stool retention. Do a follow-up physical examination to determine that dullness is not caused by a tumor. • Bruits may be heard over stenotic arteries or aneurysms.
• Rectal examination: Stool negative for occult blood; no fecal impaction; prostate soft and smooth and not enlarged.	• Incidence of colorectal cancer peaks between ages 85 and 92 and accounts for 20% of all cancers found in persons age 90 and above. • Risk of benign prostatic hypertrophy (BPH) and prostatic cancer increases with age. If prostate feels abnormal, refer client for urological evaluation.
Female Reproductive *INSPECT/PALPATE* • Decreased elasticity, breast sag, cordlike feel to breasts.	• Palpable ovaries, masses, rectocele, cystocele, or prolapsed uterus require referral.
• Decrease and graying of pubic hair. • External genitalia decrease in size and skin becomes thin, inelastic, and shiny. • Pelvic exam reveals pale vaginal walls and narrow, thick, glistening cervix as a result of decreased estrogen. • Uterus and ovaries decrease in size. Ovaries should not be palpable.	

HELPFUL HINT

Elderly women may not be able to assume the full lithotomy position because of arthritic or cardiovascular changes. Adjust the position to ensure comfort, and use a smaller speculum for the pelvic exam.

(Continued)

Performing a Head-to-Toe Physical Assessment *(Continued)*

SYSTEM/NORMAL VARIATIONS	ABNORMAL FINDINGS/RATIONALE
Male Reproductive *INSPECT/PALPATE*	
• **Gynecomastia** may be seen • Decrease and graying of pubic hair. • Scrotum and penis decrease in size. • Testes hang lower and have fewer rugae.	• Any mass requires referral.
Musculoskeletal *INSPECT/PALPATE*	
• About half of people over 65 have decreased arm swing during gait; a wider base of support; a decline in step length, stride length, and ankle range of motion; decreased vertical and increased horizontal head excursions; decrease in spinal rotation and arm swing; increased length of double support phase of walking, and a reduction in propulsive force generalized at the push-off phase. Decrease in sensory input, slowing of motor responses, and musculoskeletal limitations result in an increase in unsteadiness or postural sway under both static and dynamic conditions. • Thoracic curvature (senile kyphosis).	• Musculoskeletal changes associated with aging increase the risk for falls and injury.
• ROM decreased.	• **Heberden's nodes**, involving the distal interphalangeal joints, are commonly seen with osteoarthritis or DJD but are rarely inflamed.

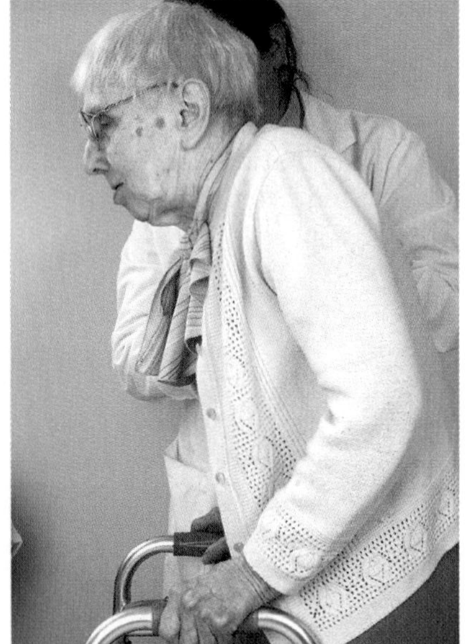

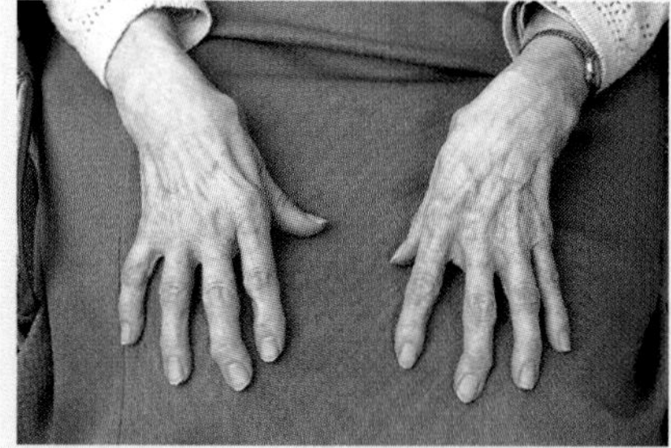

Heberden's nodes

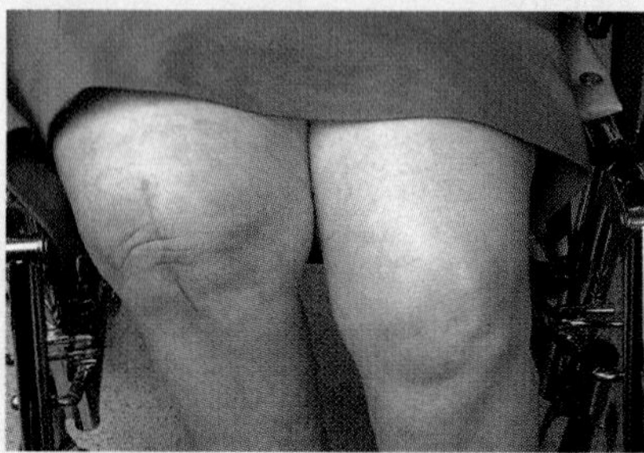

Degenerative joint disease (osteoarthritis)

Performing a Head-to-Toe Physical Assessment

SYSTEM / NORMAL VARIATIONS — **ABNORMAL FINDINGS/RATIONALE**

Musculoskeletal *(Continued)*

INSPECT/PALPATE

- Crepitation, stiffness with ROM.
- Decreased muscle strength and tone. Muscle strength depends on muscle mass. Strong equal hand grip usually remains intact.
  - Asymmetrical decrease in strength and tone may be associated with TIA or CVA.

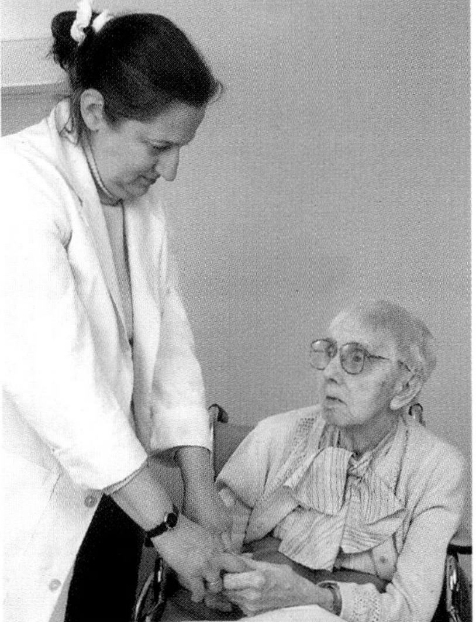

HELPFUL HINT

An easy way to test upper extremity function is having the client touch the back of his or her head with the hands, pick up a penny, and shake hands.

- Shoes fit well, wear evenly. No lesions, calluses or deviations noted. Toenails well groomed.
  - Diabetes-related ulcerations, fungal infections of the feet or toenails, calluses, bunions, **hallus valgus** (a lateral deviation of the large toe), and other deformities are very common and can affect function.

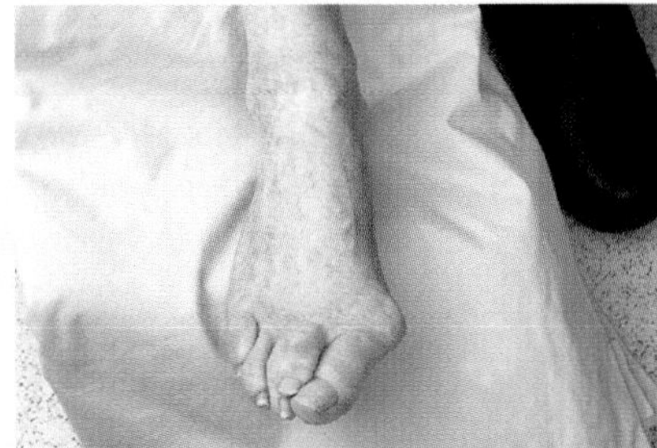

Hallus valgus and bunions

Neurological/*Mental Status*

INSPECT

- Cognitive ability intact; benign forgetfulness; short-term memory and long-term memory for new information may decrease with age.
  - Confusion may be caused by delirium, an underlying dementia, or depression. These conditions may be difficult to differentiate and may occur independently or together.
  - Clients with dementia work hard to answer questions and **confabulate** answers. Delirium causes difficulty concentrating

HELPFUL HINT

To assess depression quickly, use the single-item Yale Depression Screening Tool, which simply asks, "Do you often feel sad or depressed?" This tool has been shown to correlate very closely with the 15-item GDS.

(Continued)

Performing a Head-to-Toe Physical Assessment *(Continued)*

SYSTEM/NORMAL VARIATIONS	ABNORMAL FINDINGS/RATIONALE
Neurological/*Mental Status* INSPECT *(Continued)*	on the questions and attending to the task. Clients with depression often are unwilling to try to complete the task or answer the question. Detection of dementia, delirium, or depression warrants referral. Several bedside screening tools are available to differentiate between dementia, delirium, and depression and to evaluate cognitive function. See boxes below and on pages 853 and 855.

Neurological/*Cranial Nerves*
• Slower response time bilaterally
  • CN I Olfactory—decreased
  • CN II Optic—decreased visual acuity
  • Presbyopia
  • Fundoscopic changes
  • CN III Oculomotor—Pupils smaller and reaction to light not as brisk
  • CN III Oculomotor, CN IV Trochlear, CN VI Abducen } Extraocular movements intact
  • CN V Trigeminal—Increased stimulation needed to elicit corneal reflex
  • CN VII Facial—decreased taste
  • CN VIII Acoustic—Presbycusis, increased loss of hearing of high-pitched sounds progresses to loss of all frequencies
  • CN IX Glossopharyngeal—decreased taste
  • CN X Vagus—decreased gag reflex
  • CN XI Spinoaccessory—No change, but ROM and strength depend on MS changes
  • CN XII Hypoglossal—no change
	• Diminished response time on only one side warrants further investigation.

ALERT

Know the symptoms of depression! They can be easily misread as normal changes associated with aging.

Characteristics of Dementia, Delirium, and Depression

Feature	Dementia	Delirium	Depression
Onset	Gradual (months to years)	Abrupt (hours to a few weeks)	Either
Prognosis	Irreversible	Reversible	Variable
Course	Progressive	Worse in PM	Worse in AM
Attention	Normal	Impaired	Variable
Memory	Impaired recent and remote	Impaired recent and immediate	Selective impairment
Perception	Normal	Impaired	Normal
Psychomotor Behavior	Normal/Apraxia	Hypo/Hyperkinetic	Retardation/Agitation
Cause	Caused by many diseases, including alcoholism, AIDS, cerebral anoxia, and brain infarcts	Caused by acute illness, fever, infection, dehydration, electrolyte imbalance, medications, and alcoholism	Usually coincides with life event, such as death in the family, loss of a friend or a pet, or a move.

Performing a Head-to-Toe Physical Assessment

SYSTEM/NORMAL VARIATIONS	ABNORMAL FINDINGS/RATIONALE
Neurological/*Muscle Function Movements* • Positive drifting with minimal weakness. • No abnormal movements.	• Tremors are common in older clients. Types include: • Postural or physiologic—benign fine tremors • Intention, essential, familial and senile—visible tremor associated with intentional movements, diminishes with rest • Rest—visible tremor at rest but absent or diminished with movement; "pill-rolling;" associated with Parkinson's disease • Action—large, irregular tremors of limbs, associated with cerebellar dysfunction (e.g., in multiple sclerosis)
Neurological/*Cerebellar Function* *INSPECT* ***Reflexes*** • Romberg sign—slight swaying normal • Loss of balance (positive Romberg sign) may be associated with Parkinson's disease	

Geriatric Depression Scale

*Are you basically satisfied with your life?
*Have you dropped many of your activities and interests?
*Do you feel that your life is empty?
*†Do you often get bored?
Are you hopeful about the future?
Are you bothered by thoughts that you just cannot get out of your head?
*Are you in good spirits most of the time?
*Are you afraid that something bad is going to happen to you?
*Do you feel happy most of the time?
*†Do you often feel helpless?
Do you often get restless and fidgety?
*†Do you prefer to stay at home rather than going out and doing new things?
Do you frequently worry about the future?
*Do you feel you have more problems with memory than most?
*Do you think it is wonderful to be alive now?
Do you often feel downhearted and blue?
*†Do you feel pretty worthless the way you are now?
Do you worry a lot about the past?
Do you find life very exciting?
Is it hard for you to get started on new projects?
*Do you feel full of energy?
*Do you feel that your situation is hopeless?
*Do you think that most people are better off than you are?
Do you frequently get upset over little things?
Do you frequently feel like crying?
Do you have trouble concentrating?
Do you enjoy getting up in the morning?
Do you prefer to avoid social gatherings?
Is it easy for you to make decisions?
Is your mind as clear as it used to be?

Source: Yesavage, et al., pp 37–47.
*Items included in the 15-item Geriatric Depression Scale
†Items included in the 5-item Geriatric Depression Scale

(Continued)

Performing a Head-to-Toe Physical Assessment *(Continued)*

SYSTEM/NORMAL VARIATIONS	ABNORMAL FINDINGS/RATIONALE
Neurological/*Cerebellar Function (Continued)*	
• Deep tendon reflex (DTR) may be increased or decreased (+1 or +3) • Achilles reflex more difficult to elicit. May need to use reinforcement techniques to elicit response.	• Asymmetrical reflexes may indicate an underlying problem.
• Superficial abdominal reflexes disappear with age. • Older adults may demonstrate the release of some primitive reflexes including the snout, glabella, and palmomental.	• Positive primitive reflexes may also indicate a severe neurological assault.

HELPFUL HINTS

- Vibratory testing is more reliable on the malleolus (protuberance on both sides of the ankle joint) than on the great toe.
- Aging may cause decreased vibratory sense in the lower extremities and fingers. To test functioning of the posterior column, check position sense rather than vibratory sense. Keep in mind that position sense of the great toe may also be decreased.

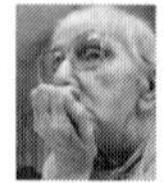

Case Study Findings

Mrs. Nurick's physical assessment findings include:

- **General Health Survey:** 80-year-old woman who is well groomed and dressed, pleasant, and appropriate in behavior during the interview.
- **Vital Signs:** Temperature 97°F; B/P 130/70; Height: 5ft. 2 inches and weight 140 lbs. Body mass index of 22.
- **Integumentary:** Skin intact throughout without evidence of growths or lesions. Skin is dry, especially on extremities. Toenails are thick and yellow on all nails bilaterally.
- **HEENT:** Hair is gray and thin. Pupils equal and react to light and accommodation. Conjunctiva white and no drainage or tearing noted. Fundoscopic exam revealed intact retina with no signs of hemorrhage. Vision 20/30 in the right eye and 20/20 in the left eye with corrective lenses. Able to read normal-size print. Able to hear normal tone of voice but unable to repeat three whispered words. Ear canals bilaterally without evidence of impacted cerumen and tympanic membrane normal. Neck has full range of motion without evidence of dizziness during range.
- **Respiratory:** Respirations 16 and unlabored
- **Cardiovascular:** Rate 72 regular without S_3, S_4 or murmur. Carotid upstroke normal. No bruits bilaterally. See below for pulses.
- **Gastrointestinal:** Normal bowel sounds in all four quadrants. Abdomen soft with slight tenderness in right upper quadrant. Liver edge palpable and tender. No bruits noted.
- **Genitourinary/Reproductive:** Vaginal mucosa dry and pale but skin intact. No evidence of discharge. Speculum exam/Pap test refused because of age, and she would not do anything even if the test were abnormal. No evidence of **prolapse.** Has urinary leakage with bearing down when lying and also when standing and coughing or bearing down. Incisional scar on left breast. Breasts symmetrical and no masses or tenderness noted. No nipple retraction or discharge.

PULSES	RADIAL	BRACHIAL	DORSALIS PEDIS	POSTERIOR TIBIALIS	POPLITEAL	FEMORAL
Right	2+	2+	2+	2+	2+	2+
Left	2+	2+	2+	2+	2+	2+

- **Musculoskeletal:** Slight enlargement of distal interphalanges (Heberden's nodules), but no evidence of warmth or tenderness. Full range of motion in upper extremities with strength 5/5 in upper proximal and distal extremities and 4/5 in lower proximal and distal extremities. Increased curvature of thoracic spine. Gait steady with walker with 6-inch base of support. Positive accentuated thoracic curve (kyphosis).
- **Neurological:** Sensation intact to light touch, localization, and pin prick. Position sense intact. Cerebellar intact finger to nose, heel to shin, and rapid hand movement. Romberg negative. Reflexes symmetrical and 2+ throughout with Babinski downgoing. Scored a 29/30 on the Mini-Mental Status Exam. Scored a 1/15 on the Geriatric Depression Scale.

Signs and Symptoms of Depression

Typical

- Changes in appetite
- Changes in sleep patterns
- Social withdrawal
- Loss of motivation
- Constipation
- Pessimism
- Guilt
- Decreased self-esteem
- Feelings of helplessness
- Hostility
- Agitation
- Aggression

Atypical

- Vague somatic complaints—such as constipation, joint pain, fatigue, and memory changes—that seem to be out of proportion to the actual problem.
- Client may become obsessed with the problems and feel that if the problems are relieved, he or she will be fine.

Mini-Mental Status Examination

Have the client answer the following questions or follow these instructions:

What is the season, month, day, and year? .... 5 points
(subtract 1 point for each item left out)

Where are you (state, county town, hospital floor)? .... 5 points
(subtract 1 for each item left out)

I will say the names of three objects. Repeat the names. .... 3 points
(subtract 1 point for each word client forgets)

Counting backwards from 100, subtract 7 five times (serial 7s).
Or spell "world" backwards .... 5 points

Recall the same three objects from a few minutes ago (question 3) .... 3 points
(subtract 1 point for each word client forgets)

I will show you two common objects. Tell me what they are. .... 2 points

Repeat the phrase "no ifs, ands, or buts." .... 1 point

I am going to give you a blank piece of paper. Take this paper,
put it in your right hand, fold it in half, and put it on the floor .... 3 points

I am going to print on a piece of paper. (Print "Close your eyes.")
Read it and do it. .... 1 point

Write a sentence of your own .... 1 point

Copy a pair of intersecting pentagons on a piece of paper .... 1 point

Scoring:
24–30: no cognitive impairment
23–18: mild cognitive impairment
0–7: severe impairment

Source: Adapted from Folstein et al., pp 196–198.

Clock Scoring

Give the client a piece of paper and ask him or her to draw a circle. Instruct the client to draw the face of a clock inside the circle, putting the numbers in the correct positions. Then ask him or her to draw the hands to indicate 10 minutes after 11 or 20 minutes after 8.

Scoring:

Assign 1 point for each of the following:

- Draws closed circle
- Places numbers in correct positions
- Includes all 12 numbers in correct positions
- Places clock hands in correct positions.

There are no specific cutoff scores. If performance on clock drawing is impaired, consider a complete diagnostic evaluation for dementia.

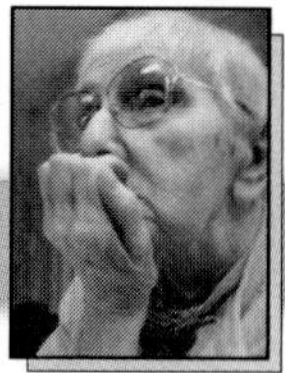

Case Study Analysis and Plan

Now that your examination of Mrs. Nurick is complete, document your key history and physical examination findings.

List key history findings and key physical examination findings that will help you formulate your nursing diagnoses, and physical examination findings.

Nursing Diagnoses

Consider all of the data you have collected during your assessment of Mrs. Nurick, and then use this information to identify a list of nursing diagnoses. Some possible ones are provided below; cluster the supporting data.

1. Nutrition: imbalanced, less than body requirements, related to loss of appetite
2. Injury, risk for, related to altered mobility and fatigue
3. Activity intolerance, risk for, related to fatigue
4. Fatigue

Identify any additional nursing diagnoses.

CRITICAL THINKING ACTIVITY #5

Now that you have identified some nursing diagnoses for Mrs. Nurick, select a nursing diagnosis from above and develop a nursing care plan and a brief teaching plan for her, including learning outcomes and teaching strategies.

Research Tells Us

Aging has been defined as the process of change that occurs in people over the course of time.

Declines in vision, hearing, immune function, maximum oxygen consumption, and renal blood flow are all examples of changes that occur. Potentially, these changes occur in everyone; however, they seem to vary greatly from person to person. Some people note changes at relatively young ages, others when they are much older, and still others note no changes at all. The Baltimore Longitudinal Study on Aging (BLSA) has provided very useful information to help differentiate between what is normal and what is disease in older adults.

Cross-sectional studies have generally suggested that systolic blood pressure increases with age, the heart remodels with a thickening of the ventricular wall, the contractile process slows, and cardiac output decreases. The BLSA, however, demonstrated that when people with disease were excluded from the study, cardiac output was maintained into the seventh and eighth decades (Rodcheffer et al, 1994). Likewise, muscle quality, when evaluated longitudinally, did not normally decline with age (Metter et al., 1997). Sensory changes do seem to change with chronological age, although these changes can be modified by environmental interventions, such as decreasing glare. (Morrell et al., 1996; Pearson et al., 1995; Ship et al., 1996). Research is currently ongoing to better establish what is normal aging and what is disease. This information will help us to suggest interventions to retard any potentially avoidable declines in function for each body system.

Health Concerns

The screening tests recommended for adults are especially important for older adults because of their increased risk of disease. The following box describes the pros and cons of several of these tests.

Pros and Cons of Health Screening Tests and Preventive Treatments

ACTIVITY SUGGESTED	FREQUENCY	PROS	CONS
Immunization: *Pneumonia* *Flu* *Tetanus*	 Every 6 years Every year Every 10 years	• Disease prevention, particularly to prevent an epidemic. • Decreased morbidity and mortality associated with pneumonia or flu.	• Side effects such as local irritation or flulike symptoms.
Pap test	Every year for high-risk women; otherwise, every 3 years	• Risk for cervical cancer increases with age. • Older women may not have had the opportunity to get regular Pap tests and may want this early screening. • Pursue only if woman is willing to undergo treatment if disease is identified. • Noninvasive treatment may improve quality of life by detecting and managing problems such as atrophic and dry vaginal mucosa.	• Cervical cancer develops slowly and is unlikely to be cause of death in women over age 90. Less risk of cervical cancer if client is not sexually active. • Testing can be difficult and uncomfortable in older women, particularly those no longer (or never) sexually active.
Mammogram	Every year	• Breast cancer risk increases with age. These tumors are generally estrogen receptor positive and treatable. • Pursue only if woman is willing to undergo treatment if disease is identified.	• New-onset breast cancer is not likely to be cause of death in women age 90 and older. Tumors in older women tend to grow slowly. • Discomfort associated with mammogram.
Prostate exam	Digital rectal exam and PSA every year	• Risk for prostate cancer increases with age. • Pursue only if man is willing to undergo treatment if disease is identified. Survival rates increase dramatically with early detection.	• Controversy persists with regard to effectiveness of treatment options and usefulness of treatment, especially for men with < 10 years' life expectancy.
Fecal Occult Blood Testing (FOBT)	Every year	• Early detection of a cancer that could cause discomfort and impact quality of life if left untreated. • Easily performed with no discomfort to client. • FOBT has better predictive value in older adults than in young adults.	• False positives, which may result in additional testing and anxiety for client.
Cholesterol Monitoring/ Interventions	Initial and then as appropriate	• Although not tested in clients age 90 and above, decreasing cholesterol reduces mortality and cardiac events in clients over 65.	• Diet restrictions may affect quality of life. May be no advantage to restricting dietary fat in those age 90 and over. Focus should be to eat a healthy diet low in fat and high in fruits, vegetables, and grains.

(Continued)

Pros and Cons of Health Screening Tests and Preventive Treatments *(Continued)*

ACTIVITY SUGGESTED	FREQUENCY	PROS	CONS
Cholesterol Monitoring/ Interventions *(Continued)*			• Lipid-lowering medications may have unpleasant side effects and/or interfere with other medications.

Source: Adapted from Resnick, 2001.

Summary

- The history and physical examination of the older adult should take into consideration the normal changes associated with aging and focus strongly on function.
- Every system clearly plays a role in the older adult's ability to perform ADLs. As you evaluate the systems, your goal is to identify problems that can treated to improve function.
- Pay special attention to gait disorders, incontinence, sensory problems, cognitive status, and mood changes because these problems often reflect the presentation of a much more serious condition.

APPENDIX A

Chapter Feedback

CHAPTER 1

Page 11: Critical Thinking Activity #1

- **Headache:** Subjective
- **BP 170/110:** Objective
- **Nausea:** Subjective
- **Diaphoresis:** Objective
- **Equal pupillary reaction:** Objective
- **Tingling sensation:** Subjective
- **Dizziness:** Subjective
- **Decreased muscle strength:** Objective
- **Slurred speech:** Objective
- **Numbness of left arm:** Subjective

Page 12: Critical Thinking Activity #2

- **Primary data source:** Patient, Eileen Ploransky
- **Secondary data source:** Husband, prenatal records
- **Subjective data:** Contractions like "severe cramps." Husband says, "I think her water broke on the way to the hospital."
- **Objective data:** 29-year-old woman, contractions 5 minutes apart, 6 cm dilated, fetal hear rate (FHR) 120 BPM, VS 140/80, 90, 22. H & H 12.0, 45, blood type AB+.

Page 20: Critical Thinking Activity #3

- **Physiological:** Tissue Perfusion, ineffective; Nutrition: imbalanced; Elimination, alterations in
- **Safety:** Mobility, Impaired Physical; Injury, Risk for
- **Love and belonging:** Social Interaction, impaired; Role Performance, Ineffective
- **Self-esteem:** Self-esteem, Risk for Situational Low; Body Image, Disturbed
- **Self-actualization:** Spiritual Well-Being, Readiness for Enhanced; Spiritual Distress; Health-Seeking Behaviors

Page 20: Critical Thinking Activity #4

- **Bleeding:** Primary
- **Fatigue, pallor, hemoglobin 7.0:** Secondary
- **Nausea and vomiting:** Secondary
- **Grieving:** Tertiary
- **Sleep disturbance, fever, night sweats:** Secondary
- **Knowledge, deficient, on self-administration of insulin:** Tertiary
- **Impaired mobility, fractured hip:** Secondary
- **Irregular heart rate >140 BPM:** Primary
- **BP 70/40:** Primary
- **New parent role:** Tertiary

CHAPTER 2

Page 25: Critical Thinking Activity #1

- Where is the chest pain? Point to where it hurts.
- What does it feel like?
- Did you ever have this before?
- What were you doing before the pain started?
- Does it go anywhere else?
- Does anything make it better?
- When did it start? How long did it last?

Page 25: Critical Thinking Activity #2

- **Past Health History:** Did you ever have this before? Do you have a history of heart disease or high blood pressure?
- **Family History:** Do you have a family history of heart disease, heart attack, or high blood pressure?
- **Review of Systems:** Do you have any breathing problems? Nausea or other gastrointestinal complaints?
- **Psychosocial Profile:** How has this problem affected your activities of daily living, ability to work, or ability to have fun?

Page 32: Critical Thinking Activity #3

- Cardiovascular disease
- HTN
- MVP
- Breast cancer

CHAPTER 3

Page 67: Critical Thinking Activity #1

With a blind client, explaining exactly what you plan to do is even more important. Letting the client feel the equipment before you use it may also help put him or her at ease.

Page 70: Critical Thinking Activity #2

- Color changes such as cyanosis or pallor
- Diaphoresis
- Grimacing
- Guarding because of pain

CHAPTER 4

Page 87: Critical Thinking Activity

At the end of the lesson, Lucas will be able to put on and remove a condom according to the effective condom use checklist.

CHAPTER 5

Page 95: Case Study Analysis and Plan

Jan (age 16) is a junior in high school. She had screenings for vision, dental, hearing, height, weight, hemoglobin and hematocrit, vital signs, and stress. She was assessed for current vaccinations and received educational materials on exercise, nutrition, weight management, safe sex, accident prevention (such as driving and seat belt use), and drug and alcohol abuse.

Mrs. Chen had her height, weight, body mass index (BMI), vision, cholesterol, pulse, respiration, and blood pressure checked. She was also assessed for history of immunizations such as tetanus and hepatitis B. She received educational materials on menopause, nutrition, prevention of osteoporosis, self-assessment of risk for cancer, and heart disease.

Mrs. Wong had her height, weight, BMI, vision, and vital signs checked. In addition, she had a screening bone mineral density (BMD) test of her heel to detect signs of osteoporosis, which would indicate whether more extensive testing (for example, hip and spine) was needed. Her immunization history (e.g., tetanus, hepatitis B, influenza, and pneumonia) was also taken. She received educational materials on nutrition, especially the need for calcium and vitamin D, osteoporosis, use and abuse of medications and alternative therapies, safe exercise, fall prevention, and screening for heart disease, cancer, and depression.

CHAPTER 6

Page 100: Critical Thinking Activity #1

- **Illnesses that interfere with food intake:** These include dental disease, anorexia nervosa, and diseases or treatments that cause anorexia.
- **Lack of suitable foods:** Grocery stores in urban areas may not stock perishable items such as fresh fruits and vegetables.
- **Intake habits that favor deficiencies:** Busy schedules have engendered a preference for fast foods that are quick and tasty but high in calories, salt, and fat; and lacking in nutrients.
- **Inability to afford necessary food for an adequate diet:** This is a principal reason for primary malnutrition among poor and older adults.
- **Knowledge deficiency:** Lack of knowledge about good nutrition.

Page 100: Critical Thinking Activity #2

Chronic and hereditary conditions may impair digestion and absorption of nutrients from the GI tract or cause competition for nutrients at the cellular level. Acute medical conditions (e.g., GI infection or inflammatory bowel disorders), multiple trauma, serious burns, and major abdominal surgery are causes of secondary malnutrition.

Page 111: Case Study Evaluation

Biographical Data

- 78-year-old African-American male
- Widowed, lives alone in urban area
- Retired postal worker
- Baptist religion
- Medicare/Medicaid insurance
- Daughter is primary contact

Current Health Status

- Vague complaints of not feeling well, being very tired, and having no energy. Weight loss of 10 lb since wife's death.
- Current medications are Lasix 40 mg od and Vasotec 5 mg bid. No over-the-counter (OTC) medications except occasional milk of magnesia (MOM) for constipation. No illegal drug use.

Past Health History

- Positive history of HTN for 10 years
- Hospitalized last year for uncontrolled HTN
- Appendectomy at age 12
- No allergies to food, drugs, or environmental factors
- Medications listed previously

Family History

- Daughter, age 50, alive and well
- Wife deceased age 74, breast cancer
- Mother deceased age 75, HTN,CVA
- Father deceased age 80, HTN, MI
- Sister, age 70, HTN
- Sister age 73, alive and well
- Brother, age 75, DM, HTN, CAD
- Maternal aunt deceased age 80, CAD, MI
- Maternal uncle deceased age 78, CVA
- Paternal aunt deceased age 82, colon cancer
- Paternal uncle deceased age 81, CVA

Review of Systems

- **General Health Survey:** 10-lb weight loss, fatigue.
- **Integumentary:** Dry, flaky skin.
- **HEENT:** Wears dentures.
- **Respiratory:** No changes.
- **Cardiovascular:** No chest pain; positive history of HTN.
- **Gastrointestinal:** Bowel movement every 2 to 3 days, brown and formed. Takes MOM as needed.
- **Genitourinary/Reproductive:** On Lasix; no problems with urination; voids about 8 timesa day. Not sexually active since wife died.

- **Musculoskeletal:** Weakness and occasional cramping in legs.
- **Neurological:** No sensory changes. Very lonely since wife's death.
- **Lymphatic:** No allergies or recent infections

Psychosocial Profile

- Wife used to prepare meals, finds it hard to cook for one person.
- Says dentures are a little loose since he lost weight.
- Visits doctor every 6 months for BP check.
- Typical day: Awakens at 7 am, has breakfast, walks to corner for newspaper, takes midmorning nap, usually skips lunch, watches TV, has dinner around 5 pm, watches TV after dinner, usually falls asleep while watching TV, goes to bed after the 10 pm news.
- Has three 8 oz. glasses of water a day, not trying to lose weight. Eats out about once a week, likes fried foods. Not much appetite since wife died. Usually eats alone.
- Daily walk to corner for paper, no other scheduled exercise.
- Sleeps 7 to 8 hours a night. Awakens at least once to go to bathroom. Takes two 20- to 30-minute naps during day.
- Never smoked or used drugs. Occasional alcoholic drink about 2 times a month.
- Retired postal worker on fixed income with government pension; able to meet financial needs.
- Most close friends have passed away.
- No cultural or religious influence on dietary habits.
- Says life is "pretty routine without much stress."
- Daughter is main source of support; lives 1 hour away, visits once a week, takes patient shopping.

24-Hour Recall

- Breakfast: 8 ounces black coffee, 8 ounces water, bowl of Cheerios with whole milk
- No lunch
- Afternoon snack: 4 pretzels
- Dinner: Frozen dinner of Salisbury steak, potatoes, and corn, piece of apple pie, 8 ounces water, 8 ounces black coffee.

Page 111: Critical Thinking Activity #3

- Recent loss of wife
- Fact that he lives alone
- Weight loss
- Reports that it is hard to prepare meals for himself and that he skips
- Diuretic use and urination patterns
- Fatigue
- Dry, flaky skin.

Page 116: Key history findings

- Wife died 6 months ago
- Lives and eats alone
- 10-lb weight loss in past 6 months
- Says it is hard to cook for 1 person; skips lunch, eats frozen dinners; not much appetite
- Dry, flaky skin
- Wears dentures

Page 116: Key physical examination findings

- 10-lb weight loss since last examination
- Increased heart rate
- Sad affect, poor eye contact
- Dry, flaky skin
- Dry mucous membranes
- Dentures poorly fitted
- Decreased muscle strength

Page 116: Nursing diagnoses clustered supporting data

- 24-hour recall, weight loss, dry mucous membranes, patient's admission that he does not eat regularly and that it is hard to cook for one.
- Limited intake, urination patterns, dry mucous membranes, increased heart rate.
- 24-hour recall, weight loss, skipped meals, fluid intake, diuretic use.

CHAPTER 7

Page 125: Critical Thinking Activity #1

Recognizing the range of different traditions, the best approach would be to ask the client and/or family how you might best assist in providing comfort to the client. For example, you may discover that the client wishes to wash before praying or that he or she would like to have religious symbols pinned to his or her hospital gown or visible in the room.

Page 125: Critical Thinking Activity #2

- Who are your support people?
- What provides you with strength and hope?
- What gives your life meaning and purpose?
- How is your faith important to you?

The answers to these questions will demonstrate the importance of spiritual issues in your client's care. For example, the client may mention a clergyperson or fellow church (temple, mosque) member as important in his or her spiritual life. If the client mentions only family members, then connectedness to others rather than organized religion is more important (but still spiritual in nature). The presence of religious symbols, such as the Bible, Qur'an (Koran), or prayer books; wearing of jewelry with religious symbols; presence of other objects such as crystals; or listening to inspirational or religious music will also signify the impact of spirituality on your client's life. These behaviors will give the client strength for enduring or recovering from illness.

Page 125: Critical Thinking Activity #3

- **African-Americans:** Allow privacy when clergy visits, offer to read Bible passages for client or pray with client.
- **Amish:** Allow time for prayer before meals, rather than rushing client to start eating. Allow for consultation with religious leader and family.
- **Appalachians:** Realize that client may refuse some types of therapies, including preventive measures because of fatalistic viewpoint. Allow privacy for prayer. May need to reassure client that it is all right to pray in hospital.
- **Arab-Americans:** Provide for washing and hygiene before prayers (5 times a day). Help client to face East. Also realize that client may prefer to endure pain rather than expect relief from it.
- **Chinese-Americans:** Allow privacy for prayer.
- **Cuban-Americans:** Realize that fatalism may interfere with planned medical and nursing therapies. Although many are Catholic, may rely on folk medicine as well. Allow use of folk remedies as long as they have been cleared as safe.
- **Egyptian-Americans:** Allow practice of Christian or Muslim rituals as appropriate.
- **Filipino-Americans:** Prayer is important; provide privacy. Usually Catholic. Use of religious symbols (rosary, crucifix) is source of comfort. Realize that client may be fatalistic, making treatment difficult. Respect client's decisions.
- **French-Canadians:** Although prayer is important, there is little acceptance of spirituality as important to health. Because family is important source of strength, provide for adequate visiting.
- **Greek-Americans:** Encourage display of icons of family saint or Virgin Mary. Allow for daily prayer.
- **IranianAmericans:** Allow for Muslim prayers (5 times a day). Help client to face East and provide for washing before prayers. Fatalistic, so respect client's decisions not to pursue therapies.
- **Irish-Americans:** Most are Catholic. Encourage symbols of faith (rosary, crucifix). Offer to call priest as needed. Provide privacy for prayer.
- **Jewish-Americans:** Provide for observance of dietary laws if this is important to client. Allow time for prayer. Orthodox men may wear yarmulke at all times or only when praying.
- **Mexican-Americans:** Usually Catholic. Similar to Cuban-Americans and Filipino-Americans. Folk medicine is important and should be allowed if not contraindicated. Encourage use of cultural symbols of the spirit and discussion of the soul.
- **Navajo Native Americans:** Provide for healing ceremonies by tribal shaman as complementary to traditional medicine. Provide privacy. Arrange room assignments to permit visibility of outdoors.
- **Vietnamese-Americans:** Allow modified altar (without candles lighted) in room, if possible. Arrange for family visits; family and prayer are major sources of strength.

Page 127: Critical Thinking Activity #4

Strengths:

- Close relationship with sister
- Church affiliation (active in church before hospitalization).

Areas of concern:

- Not geographically close to daughter
- Does not drive
- Feels isolated from church community

Page 127: Case Study Evaluation

Biographical Data

- 68 years old
- Husband died 1 year ago
- One grown daughter who lives in California with her husband and two sons, ages 4 and 6
- Lives in 2-story home; sister lives across the street in her own home
- Born in Grady Falls, Pennsylvania
- African-American
- Episcopal religion
- MS in education, retired from teaching elementary school
- Has Medicare with supplemental HMO from teacher's union
- Hospital admission for congestive heart failure
- Good historian; alert and seems reliable

Current Health Status

- Difficulty breathing at rest, lower extremity edema, change in sleep patterns, uses two pillows.
- Currently hospitalized for exacerbation of congestive heart failure.
- Also has hypertension.
- Current medications are lisinopril (Prinivil), 10 mg a day, for hypertension.

Past Health History

- Congestive heart failure for 3 to 5 years
- Hypertension, treated for 15 years

Family History

- Father died of heart failure at age 89.
- Mother died at age 70 from complications of a stroke.

Psychosocial Profile

- Typical day starts at 7:00 AM, when Mrs. Mays arises, makes her bed, eats breakfast, and reads the paper. Usually does light housework, such as dusting and washing breakfast dishes. She then rests because the activity leaves her short of breath. Generally calls her sister to come over for lunch and watch soap operas. Sister leaves by 4 PM to get dinner for her husband. Mrs. Mays usually eats a light supper and then does needlework until 10 PM, when she watches the news. Goes to bed at 10:30 PM.
- Eats three meals a day. Lunch is her main meal, and she enjoys it most because she usually has her sister for company. Doesn't like to cook just for herself, so eats a light supper.
- Until last week, walked to the corner store for her daily paper. Now has it delivered because the walk is too difficult. Also unable to walk to services at her church, which is three blocks away. Does not drive.
- Goes to bed at 10:30 PM and arises at 7 AM. Not sleeping well because of breathing problems caused by CHF.
- Sees her doctor regularly for hypertension and CHF.
- Sister lives across the street, and they spend most weekday afternoons together. Only child and two grandchildren live in California. They talk on the phone weekly, but she sees them rarely. Attended church and taught Sunday school and vacation Bible school until recently.
- Retired teacher.
- Hobbies are needlepoint, reading, watching television.
- Lives in two-story house with bedroom on second floor.
- Has never smoked; doesn't drink alcohol.
- Says she doesn't like to make a "big fuss" over her health problems or "burden anyone" with them.

Page 134: List key history findings

- 68-year-old widow (1 year).
- Lives alone.
- Episcopal religion.
- Only child lives in distant state.
- Retired from teaching.
- CHF for 3–5 years; recent hospitalization for exacerbation.
- Hypertension for 15 years.
- Mother died of CVA-related causes at age 70.
- Shortness of breath makes walking difficult, so can't attend church.

Page 134: List key spiritual assessment findings

- BP elevated despite medication.
- Lies in bed with face turned away from door, hands folded, and lips moving silently.
- Says, "I'm no use now."
- No visitors in 2 days; wonders why sister hasn't come.
- Wears cross, has Bible on nightstand.

Page 134: Nursing diagnoses clustered supporting data

- Questions meaning of suffering and meaning of own existence; verbalizes concern about God's plan; unable to practice usual religious rituals; has alteration in behavior or mood as evidenced by withdrawal and anxiety.
- Hospitalizations necessary about every 6 weeks; statement about how her life has changed.
- Unable to get to church; lack of visitors; lack of relationship with pastor.

Page 134: Additional Nursing Diagnoses

- Grieving, Anticipatory
- Coping, Ineffective

Page 136: Nursing Interventions/Rationales

- Demonstrate respect for and acceptance of Mrs. Mays' values and beliefs. To foster a therapeutic nurse/client relationship, the nurse must be accepting of the client and her beliefs and values.
- Adapt nursing activities to accommodate values and religious beliefs (e. g., Mrs. Mays' desire for visit from clergyperson and privacy to receive communion).
- Maintain and respect client's preferences during hospitalization.
- Allowance for rituals provides spiritual comfort. Encourage family (sister) to bring significant symbols to Mrs. Mays (Bible, religious jewelry).
- Promote comfort.

CHAPTER 8

Page 153: Critical Thinking Activity #1

- Fair skin
- Family history of basal cell carcinoma and malignant melanoma
- Only occasional use of sunscreen

Page 153: Critical Thinking Activity #2

- Usual state of health good
- Nutritious diet
- Motivation and health-seeking behaviors

Page 153: Case Study Evaluation

Biographical Data

- 48-year-old Caucasian female, married, with two adult children (22 and 27 years old)
- Works part time in retail sales
- Born in the United States, of English-Scottish descent
- Protestant religion
- Husband is accountant, health insurance provided by his employer

Current Health Status

- Feels that she is in very good health. No current problems.
- Has recently started taking estrogen and progesterone (Prempro) for menopause symptoms. Is tolerating therapy well.
- Occasionally takes aspirin or acetominophen for headache or back/shoulder discomfort, but not monthly.

Past Health History

- Usual childhood diseases, without sequelae.
- One miscarriage at 10 weeks of pregnancy, age 22.
- Hospitalized for two childbirths, with uncomplicated vaginal deliveries; cholecystectomy 2 years ago.
- No history of allergies or skin disorders.
- No recent exposures to people with infections.
- Unsure about immunization status. Received all childhood immunizations but cannot recall tetanus or other shots.

Family History

- Mother died of breast cancer at age 65, had previously had two basal cell lesions remved.
- Brother (age 45) has HTN and a history of childhood asthma.
- Father (age 73) has "bordeline" blood pressure and adult-onset diabetes, but is in generally good health. He has also had two basal cell cancers on his face and has several "sun spots."
- Two older siblings (ages 49 and 50) are in good health, although one had a small malignant melanoma between two toes, which was surgically removed 3 weeks ago, with no lesions or spread detected.
- Children are both in good health.

Review of Systems

- **General Health Survey:** Feels well generally.
- **Integumentary:** Skin is somewhat dry, itches occasionally. No sores or rashes. No changes in hair or nails.
- **HEENT:** No runny nose or itchy eyes.
- **Respiratory:** No shortness of breath, congestion, or cough.
- **Cardiovascular:** No chest pain.
- **Gastrointestinal:** No abdominal discomfort, nausea, or change in bowel habits.
- **Genitourinary:** No change in bladder habits. Last menstrual period was about 1.5 years ago. Before that, periods were regular until the final year, when they fluctuated a little.
- **Musculoskeletal:** No joint pain except mild discomfort after extensive gardening.
- **Neurological:** No dizziness or headache.
- **Endocrine:** No problems.
- **Lymphatic/Hematologic:** No problems.

Psychosocial Profile

- Bathes or showers daily, usually with very warm water. Shampoos her hair every other day and rarely uses any hair spray, mousse, or other hair cosmetics. Nails closely filed with clear polish. Wears cosmetics daily and has never had problems tolerating them. Colored her hair in the past but does not do so now.
- Is often out in the Florida sun as she walks and gardens, but only occasionally wears sunscreen. Does not reapply sunscreen when she has been out in the sun for extended time. Worries about damage to skin now that her sister has had skin cancer.
- Typical day starts at 7:00 AM, when her alarm wakens her. On days when she works (2 to 3 days a week), she showers, dresses, eats breakfast, and works from 9 AM to 5 PM. On her nonworking days, she cleans her house, works in the yard/garden when weather permits, and just "keeps busy" until about 5 PM. She then fixes dinner and watches TV or does needlework in the evening. She generally goes to bed at 10:30 to 11:00 PM.
- Eats three meals a day with foods from all categories. Feels that she should lose 10 to 15 lb, which she has gradually gained over the past 10 years. Tries to remember to drink several glasses of wter daily, but sometimes drinks only 1 or 2 8-oz glasses.
- Gardening is one of her main forms of exercise. Also walks 2 or 3 miles a day 3 or 4 times a week.

- Sleeps very well, with rare interruptions to void (2 or 3 times a week).
- Only medications are those mentioned previously. Drinks 1 cup of coffee and 4 to 5 glasses of iced tea daily. Rarely drinks colas. Has never smoked but was exposed to second-hand cigarette smoke until her husband quit smoking 5 years ago. Does not drink alcohol or use recreational drugs.
- Is not exposed to chemicals or unusual environmental situations at work, but uses various chemicals in gardening (fertilizers, pesticides, and weed killers). Does not always wear gloves, masks, or other protective equipment.
- Has no pets. Has lived in current ranch-type home for 12 years. House is adequate for needs and has central air and heat.
- Enjoys meeting customers at work and has several close friends with whom she often has lunch or shops. Has close and caring relationship with husband and good relationship with their children, who live nearby. Father and siblings live 600 miles away, but she sees them 2 or 3 times a year for an enjoyable visit. Is not currently involved in any specific community group and rarely attends church.

Page 185: List key history findings

- Takes estrogen and progesterone.
- Has no allergies or skin disorders.
- Mother and father both had 2 basal cell lesions removed.
- Brother had childhood asthma.
- Gardens and walks for exercise.
- Rarely wears sunscreen.
- Sometimes uses fertilizers, pesticides, and weed killers without protection.
- Exposed to husband's second-hand smoke until 5 years ago.

Page 185: List key physical examination findings

- Well-developed, 48-year-old, fair-skinned female, appearance consistent with stated age
- No signs of distress, appears comfortable and provides history with no difficulty
- Temperature 97.4°F, pulse 82 and regular, respirations 14 and unlabored, BP 134/82, left arm
- Height 5′4″, weight 138 lb
- Hair
  - Generally brown with scant amount of gray interspersed and distributed evenly over scalp
  - Cut short and well groomed
  - Shiny, with no signs of damage
  - No areas of excess hair growth on body
- Nails
  - Short, with smooth edges
  - Coat of clear, glossy polish present
  - Nailbed pink, firm to palpation
  - No hemorrhages or discoloration of nails or surrounding tissues
  - No clubbing
- Skin
  - Warm, with good turgor indicated by brisk recoil
  - Generally intact, with smooth texture
  - Coloring symmetrical: pale pink on unexposed areas, moderately tanned on exposed areas, with diffusely scattered freckles, consistently light brown and all 0.2 to 0.4 cm in diameter
  - Approximately 30 moles, 0.2 to 0.4 com in diameter, with well-circumscribed, regular borders, all dark brown and consistent in color
  - Three patches if slightly pink, scaly, flat skin, approximately 0.8 cm each (two on right forearm, one on left forearm); no telangiectasia, ulcerations of the sites, or changes in surrounding skin

Page 185: Nursing diagnosis clustered supporting data

- Expresses concern about skin cancer history among relatives and past exposures to environmental skin irritants
- Frequent sun exposure with failure to use sunscreen consistently
- Frequent use of gardening-related chemicals without protective equipment
- Expresses fear regarding potential for skin cancer related to family history and sun exposure

Page 185: Additional nursing diagnoses

- Infection, risk for, related to impaired skin integrity
- Injury, risk for, related to environmental conditions, exposures, trauma
- Skin Integrity, impaired, related to various external environmental or internal factors
- Tissue Perfusion, ineffective, related to interrupted arterial or venous circulation
- Pain (itching), related to chemical or inflammatory stimulation of superficial nerves
- Body Image, disturbed, related to real or perceived disfigurement of skin, hair, or nails
- Social Isolation, related to alterations in physical appearance

CHAPTER 9

Page 212: Case Study Evaluation

Biographical Data

- 17-year-old unmarried male.
- Works part-time in fast food restaurant.

- Born in the United States, was adopted immediately after birth.
- Protestant religion.
- Adoptive father is computer salesman and adoptive mother is radiology technician.
- Source: Self, reliable.

Past Health History

- Usual childhood illnesses, without complications.
- Tonsils and adenoids removed at age 4 after frequent throat infections.
- Tympanoplasty at age 3 after frequent bouts of ear infections.
- Immunizations are up to date. Tetanus updated last year when client stepped on a piece of glass while wading on a shoreline.
- Seasonal hay fever since childhood.
- Takes over-the-counter antihistamines when he has no prescribed antihistamines on hand, but usually takes Claritin (fexophenidine) during seasonal allergy attacks. Has always taken one multivitamin daily. Takes no other medications.
- No recent exposures to known infections, but notes that he works in a busy restaurant and attends public school, so could be exposed to "whatever's going around."

Family History

- Biological family history is unknown; would like to know his family health history, but has been told this is not available.
- Adoptive parents are both in good health.

Review of Systems

- **General Health Survey:** States that health is usually good. No changes in weight or energy level.
- **Integumentary:** No changes in skin, hair, and nails. No skin rashes.
- **HEENT:** No swollen nodes or masses in head or neck. "Allergy attack" causes ear fullness; nasal congestion and clear drainage; postnasal drip; sneezing; and scratchy/itchy throat, eyes, and nose. Vision 20/20, no problems reported.
- **Respiratory:** No cough, SOB, or wheezing.
- **Cardiovascular:** No chest pain or history of cardiovascular disease.
- **Gastrointestinal:** Appetite good, no dietary restrictions, no nausea or vomiting, has daily bowel movement.
- **Genitourinary:** No history of renal disease.
- **Reproductive:** Heterosexual, not currently sexually active, is aware of safe sex practices.
- **Musculoskeletal:** No weakness reported.
- **Neurological:** No headaches, dizziness, tremors or paresthesia.
- **Endocrine:** No changes in weight or shoe size (shoe size 11)
- **Lymphatic/Hematologic:** Positive seasonal allergies, no bleeding disorders.

Psychosocial Profile

- Bathes daily; uses no cosmetics on face other than occasional over-the-counter acne medication; sees doctor and dentist for checkup once a year.
- Typical day starts at 6:45 AM, when his mother awakens him to get ready for school. Attends school from 8 AM until 3:15 PM on weekdays, and works 5 PM until 11 PM Monday and Friday nights and noon until 6 PM on Saturday. Goes to bed at 11:30 PM on school nights and 1 AM on weekends.
- Eats three meals plus 1 or 2 snacks daily. Breakfast consists of cereal, milk, and juice. Lunch is fast food, obtained between classes. Dinner is usually a cooked meal, shared with his parents. No specific dietary restrictions or food intolerances.
- Plays baseball and competes on swim team; practices 1 to 2 hours a day, depending on time of year. Wears protective gear while playing baseball. Tolerates swimming well, wearing goggles. Does some amount of physical activity daily, and this is well tolerated.
- Normally sleeps well and awakens rested. During "allergy season" sometimes has sleep difficulty. When he takes OTC antihistamines, they make it difficult to sleep and he awakens frequently during the night. If he takes no antihistamines or decongestants, he often awakens with congestion and/or sinus pressure.
- No medications other than seasonal use of antihistamines and daily vitamin. Uses no recreational drugs. Admits to rare use of alcohol (beer).
- Works 5 PM until 11 PM Monday and Friday nights and noon until 6 PM on Saturday. Exposed to second-hand smoke in the restaurant where he works; otherwise not generally around smokers or exposed to any known chemicals. Tries to avoid exposure to smoke because he is concerned about the potential health hazards.
- Lives in a single family, two-story home described as "more than adequate" for his family.
- Has many friends and enjoys spending time with groups. Dates, but has no steady girlfriend.
- Does well in school and has been accepted to the state university. No major yet chosen.
- Not currently sexually active.

Page 212: Critical Thinking Activity #1

John's history identifies several conditions or behaviors that might place him at risk for injury to this system:

- Sports activity, even with protective gear, can result in major injury to the head, neck, and specific structures of the face.
- Work in a public setting and school attendance provide exposure to various infectious agents.
- Use of OTC and prescribed antihistamines and occasional alcohol use puts client at risk for traumatic injury while driving.
- Recurrent allergic episodes increase the risk of injury to the upper airway structures and infection.
- Although his history indicates he is not current sexually active, the potential for sexual activity in adolescent males places John at risk for exposures to STDs, which affect the head and neck.
- Plans to participate in diving activities, which increase risk for injury of decompression illness, as well as barotrauma to the sinus or middle ear.
- The absence of a family history makes a comprehensive risk assessment incomplete.

Page 212: Critical Thinking Activity #2

John's history includes several areas of potential strength. These include:

- Wearing protective equipment during athletic activities
- Awareness of sexual activity-related risks
- Healthy dietary practices
- Daily physical activity
- Adequate rest habits
- Obtaining necessary health care and immunizations in the past
- Desire to maximize his health
- Adequacy of family financial resources

Page 239: Key history findings

- Current "good health" in "health-directed" young man
- Frequent exposure to potential injury, with protection, during sports participation
- History of seasonal "hay fever," treated with antihistamines
- Rare allergy symptoms, including congestion, sneezing, sleep disturbance
- Up-to-date immunization status
- Unknown family history
- Exposure to second-hand smoke
- Occasional alcohol intake
- Desires clearance for deep-sea diving class

Page 239: Key physical assessment findings

- Mildly pale nasal mucosa, with slightly enlarged turbinates

Page 239: Critical Thinking Activity #3

Strengths:

- Healthful outlook
- Positive behaviors (e.g., healthy diet, rest, activity, protection)
- Health-seeking activities
- Strong adoptive family
- Ability to learn and understand instructions and guidance

Areas of concern:

- Potential for sexual and casual exposures to infectious diseases
- Chronic, recurrent allergic symptoms that cause intermittent distress
- Risks associated with the various athletic and recreational activities
- Absence of biological family history
- Chronic changes to nasal mucosa and turbinates
- Occasional use of medications and alcohol that may alter mental status and safety

Page 239: Nursing diagnoses clustered supporting data

- Verbalizes interest to maximize health; reports good health; practices health-directed behaviors with diet and participation in regular physical activity; responsibly maintains up-to-date immunizations; avoids exposures to tobacco smoke as able; takes daily vitamin; made appointment for proper clearance before new activity.
- Participates in team sports and recreation associated with some risks (baseball, future diving).
- 17-year-old driver; uses substances that can affect mental status (occasional alcohol, although no indications of drinking while driving, and antihistamines).
- Describes difficulty sleeping after OTC antihistamines and frequent awakening during episodes of congestion/sinus pressure.

Page 239: Additional nursing diagnoses

- Activity Intolerance, related to discomfort, respiratory impairment
- Nutrition: imbalanced, less than body requirements, related to poor dentition, oral pain, or difficulty swallowing
- Fluid Volume, deficient, related to difficulty swallowing, oral pain
- Swallowing, impaired, related to inflammatory throat pain
- Body Image, disturbed, related to real or perceived disfigurement of the head, face, or neck
- Social Isolation, related to altered physical appearance
- Oral Mucous Membrane, impaired, related to

infection, ulcerations, dehydration, effects of medications, or inflammation

- Pain, acute, related to inflammation of the mucous membranes
- Airway Clearance, ineffective, related to swelling of the mucous membranes and nasal congestion
- Sensory Perception, disturbed (olfactory), related to swelling of nasal mucosa

CHAPTER 10

Eye

Page 255: Critical Thinking Activity #1

Considering Mrs. Scammel's age of 55, you might expect to observe greater laxity of the eyelids and periorbital tissues, and pupils that are smaller at rest than a younger adult's and are slower to react to light and accommodation. Also, she may be less likely to focus clearly on near objects, and the general background of her eyes may be paler.

Page 256: Critical Thinking Activity #2

In chronic hypertension, the ophthalmic examination of the fundus may reveal papilledema or blurred, nondistinct margins of the optic disk, alteration in A/V ratio, and cotton-wool spots on the general background. In diabetes, eye changes may include diminished visual acuity, diminished peripheral vision, and microhemorrhages on the fundus.

Page 261: Case Study Evaluation (Mrs. Scammel)

Biographical Data

- 55-year-old Caucasian widow and mother of one child, age 30.
- Works full-time as a secretary at a large law firm.
- Has major medical insurance coverage through her employer. Does not have coverage for dental or vision examinations.
- Catholic, of Irish-Italian descent.

Current Health Status

- Complains of blurred vision that has increased over the past month. Blurred vision is constant and worsened by fatigue. States that nothing seems to cause the problem or has helped relieve it. Wonders if she needs new glasses.
- Typically works at a computer for at least 4 hours each day.
- Blurred vision has not prevented her from caring for herself at home; however, it is difficult to read the material she is typing on the computer screen, even with reading glasses.
- Denies tearing, ear pain, drainage, double vision, sensitivity to light, or changes in the appearance of the eyes. Currently takes Lasix 20 mg bid, Captopril 25 mg bid, Glucatrol 5 mg bid, and 400 to 600 mg of ibuprofen as needed for joint pain nearly every day.

Past Health History

- History of hypertension for past 10 years and poorly controlled adult-onset diabetes diagnosed 3 years ago.
- Denies trauma or surgery affecting the eyes or hospitalizations except for childbirth. One child, no abortions.
- Denies allergies to foods, drugs, or environment.
- Last physical examination 10 months ago; last eye examination 5 years ago. Mammogram and Pap smear negative.

Family History

- Has one child, age 30, alive and well.
- Only sibling, a brother, died 2 years ago at age 50 of a myocardial infarction.
- Father had history of colon cancer and died of heart failure at age 56.
- Mother, age 68, lives in nursing home and has history of non–insulin-dependent Type II diabetes, multiple sclerosis, and stroke 4 years ago.
- No family history of glaucoma or vision loss.

Review of Systems

- **General Health Survey:** States that she is usually in good health.
- **Integumentary:** No skin lesions or allergies.
- **HEENT:** No eye tearing or drainage. No history of headache or head injury. No symptoms of upper respiratory infection.
- **Respiratory:** No history of respiratory disease.
- **Cardiovascular:** No history of cardiac symptoms; positive history of hypertension.
- **Gastrointestinal:** No history of liver or kidney disease.
- **Musculoskeletal:** No joint pain or deformity or rheumatoid arthritis.
- **Neurological:** No muscle weakness, parasthesia, MS, or myasthenia gravis.
- **Endocrine:** Positive history Type II diabetes; no history of thyroid disease.
- **Lymphatic:** No history of HIV, chemotherapy, or immunotherapy.

Psychosocial Profile

- Last physical exam 10 months ago; last eye exam 5 years ago. Gets yearly mammograms and Pap tests.
- Typical day includes: Rises at 6:30 AM, showers and dresses, has breakfast (bagel and coffee), leaves for work at 8 AM. Works 8:30 AM to 5 PM Monday through Friday. Eats lunch (sandwich) at diner most days. Usually returns home by 6 PM unless she runs errands or shops for groceries. Rarely cooks a full dinner unless her son visits. Watches TV or reads after dinner. Goes to bed at 11 PM. Spends weekends gardening in warm weather, visiting mother in nursing home, visiting son, running errands, doing housework. Goes to movies with friends occasionally.
- Admits difficulty following prescribed diabetic and low sodium diets. Tries to eat regularly but has a limited appetite and finds it difficult to cook balanced meals for one person.
- Main source of exercise is gardening and yard work.
- Since loss of her husband, has tried to become more involved in her favorite hobbies: reading, watching TV, and gardening.
- Generally sleeps 8 hours a day without napping.
- Drinks socially 3 to 4 times a year. Smoked 1 pack of cigarettes a day since age 18 until 10 years ago when diagnosed with high blood pressure.
- Was a full-time homemaker during her 22-year-marriage, but returned to workforce after husband died of a heart attack 2 years ago. Now works full time as a secretary, with occasional overtime. Reports using computers for an average of 4 hours a day.
- Lives in a rural community just outside of town, in her own home. Commutes 30 minutes to and from work.
- Sees son once a week (lives in a neighboring town). Visits mother in nursing home once a week.
- Is Catholic, but is not currently active in church. Denies any specific ethnic or cultural practices.
- Main social supports are friends from neighborhood and son and daughter-in-law.
- Stress and coping mechanisms include gardening and talking over problems with son and longtime friends from neighborhood.

Page 261: Critical Thinking Activity #3

Mrs. Scammel's visual problems may affect her ability to function safely and independently at home and at work. Diminished visual acuity and peripheral vision may affect her ability to drive safely to and from work, so she might limit her driving only to essential trips, which decreases her sense of independence. Diminished visual acuity may also affect her ability to engage in her favorite pastimes, such as reading and watching TV, and may make performing her secretarial duties more difficult.

Page 261: Critical Thinking Activity #4

Mrs. Scammel may need to make modifications at work that will enable her to function optimally. For example, she might use magnifying devices, print items to be proofed in large or bold print, and take frequent breaks from close-range computer work to reduce eye strain. She will also need more frequent eye examinations and close monitoring of blood sugar levels and blood pressure.

Page 261: Critical Thinking Activity #5

Mrs. Scammel's strengths include her desire to be active and independent, as evident in her returning to work after her husband's death. She has a variety of interests outside of work and generally engages in healthy habits of getting enough sleep, not smoking, and drinking in moderation only. When confronted with health problems that can benefit from a change in lifestyle, she is usually successful in changing. She was successful in quitting smoking and tries to avoid foods that would worsen her hypertension and diabetes.

Page 261: Critical Thinking Activity #6

Both of Mrs. Scammel's medical diagnoses of hypertension and diabetes have effects on the eyes. Her last eye exam was 5 years ago. During the interim, she may have experienced some irreversible damage to the eyes. Also, her past smoking history may have narrowed or damaged the vasculature of the eyes.

Page 278: Critical Thinking Activity #7

The bulbar conjunctiva is clear and covers the sclera, which is white. When the conjunctiva becomes inflamed during an infection such as conjunctivitis, the blood vessels that normally are not visible become irritated, more prominent, and more visible against the white sclera.

Page 284: Key history findings

- Age 55.
- Overweight.
- Complains of blurred vision.
- History of HTN and NIDD.
- Insurance does not cover eye exams.
- Wears corrective lenses.
- Works at computer 4 hours a day.
- Positive family history of DM, MS, cardiovascular disease, and cerebrovascular disease.

Page 284: Key physical examination findings

- Overweight
- BP 170/108

- Near vision blurred
- Decreased peripheral vision in temporal fields
- Hazy cornea OD
- Arcus senilis
- Abnormal fundoscopic findings (nicking, blurred disc margins, and scattered dot hemorrhages)

Page 284: Nursing diagnoses supporting data

- Sensory Perception, disturbed (visual): Complaint of blurred vision; near vision blurred; decreased peripheral vision in temporal fields; hazy cornea; fundoscopic changes.
- Injury, risk for: Complaint of blurred vision; near vision blurred; decreased peripheral vision in temporal fields; fundoscopic changes; drives to work 30 minutes each way.
- Social Interaction, impaired: Visual changes; widowed; lives alone.

Page 284: Additional nursing diagnoses

- Knowledge, deficient (management of diabetes, hypertension)
- Health Maintenance, ineffective

Ear

Pages 298–299: Case Study Evaluation (Mr. Arnez)

Biographical Data

- Married, 42-year-old father of two (ages 14 and 16).
- Full-time construction supervisor with bachelor's degree.
- Family's main source of financial support; wife is disabled.
- Carries HMO insurance through his employer that covers entire family.
- Native American and Spanish descent.
- Catholic religion
- Source of Biographical Data is client, who appears reliable.

Current Health Status

- Chief complaint is intermittent fullness and pressure in both ears for past 2 weeks.
- Denies precipitating factors, such as recent upper respiratory infection or recent altitude changes.
- Related symptoms include intermittent, bilateral hearing loss described as "like hearing in a tunnel" and intermittent dizziness.
- Rates severity of his ear fullness and pressure as 7 on a 10-point scale.
- Denies ear pain, drainage, or recent trauma to the ears.

Past Health History

- History of frequent ear infections as an infant and young child. Treated with antibiotics.
- Hospitalized once at age 3 with pneumonia and concurrent bilateral otitis media.
- Denies asthma, diabetes, or hypertension.
- Received polio, measles/mumps/rubella, tetanus, and diphtheria vaccinations.
- Allergic to sulfa, penicillin, dust, and pollen.
- Current medications include an over-the-counter allergy medication.

Family History

- Father, age 68, has controlled hypertension.
- Mother, age 60, diagnosed with MS at age 45, currently in remission.
- One sister, age 40, diagnosed with neurofibromatosis with acoustic neuroma.
- One brother, age 36, recently diagnosed with hypertension.
- Client has two teen-aged girls, ages 14 and 16, both alive and well.

Review of Systems

- **General Health Survey:** Denies fatigue or recent weight loss. Health is usually good.
- **Integumentary:** Denies rashes, lesions, or slow wound healing.
- **HEENT:** Denies ear pain, drainage, tinnitus, or ear trauma. Reports recent upper respiratory infection 4 weeks ago, with earache, resolved with antibiotics. History of frequent childhood ear infections and occasional ear infections as an adult, occurring yearly or less often. Environmental allergy to dust and pollen.
- **Gastrointestinal:** Denies nausea, vomiting, diarrhea, or recent changes in bowel habits.
- **Genitourinary:** Denies changes in bladder habits.
- **Neurological/Musculoskeletal:** Intermittent problem with balance since onset of ear pressure. Denies vertigo, muscle weakness, or paresthesia.

Psychosocial Profile

- Last physical examination was 6 months ago. Last ear exam was 4 weeks ago during recent ear infection. Denies ever having a hearing test.
- Typical day: Rises at 5:30 AM on workdays (works 7–3 shift). Showers, has breakfast (cereal and coffee), leaves for work by 6:15 AM. Eats quick lunch in hospital cafeteria. Returns home by 4 PM most days unless he has errands to run. Cooks

dinner for wife and two daughters, then often drives daughters to various school or social activities. Spends evenings watching TV. Goes to bed by 10 PM. Spends weekends attending sporting events, running errands, chauffeuring daughters. (Wife cannot drive because of disability.)

- Ear pressure and fullness have caused intermittent problems in work environment and socializing. States that he can usually compensate for the hearing loss at home.
- States that hearing loss causes difficulties at work.
- Denies chronic or recent exposure to loud noise at home or at work.

Page 299: Critical Thinking Activity #9

Factors in Mr. Anez's history that may explain his hearing problem include a history of recurrent ear infections in childhood and as an adult and a family history of acoustic neuroma and multiple sclerosis.

Page 299: Critical Thinking Activity #10

Hearing loss may make Mr. Arnez less confident in work and in social situations in which verbal communication is emphasized. Intermittent dizziness may make him fearful of being injured and more reluctant to be active or drive a car.

Page 299: Critical Thinking Activity #11

Strengths that Mr. Arnez possesses include independence and being the sole financial support for his family. His level of education will facilitate understanding of his medical condition and its treatment. He also has insurance coverage and family members nearby for emotional support.

Page 310: Key history findings

- 42-year-old construction supervisor, sole support of family.
- Complains of intermittent fullness and pressure in ears for past 2 weeks, severity 7/10, dizziness; describes hearing as "hearing in a tunnel" and reports hearing loss.
- Recent upper respiratory infection.
- Frequent ear infections as a child.
- Positive family history of HTN, MS, and acoustic neuroma.
- Positive environmental allergies.
- Hearing problems have affected work and socialization.

Page 310: Key physical examination findings

- Scarring of TM
- Rinne test AC < 2 × BC
- Dizziness with head rotation
- Positive Romberg's test

Page 310: Nursing diagnoses supporting data

- Reports changes in hearing like "hearing in a tunnel." Difficulty hearing when auscultating.
- Rinne test AC < 2 xs BC. Scarring on TM.
- Complains of pressure and fullness in ears, severity 7/10.
- Recent upper respiratory infection; fullness and pressure in ears.

Page 310: Additional nursing diagnoses

- Diversional Activity, deficient
- Communication, impaired verbal
- Social Interaction, impaired
- Injury, risk for

CHAPTER 11

Page 327: Case Study Evaluation

Biographical Data

- 38-year-old Caucasian female
- Married, mother of three children, ages 10, 8, and 4
- Part-time accountant; BA degree in accounting.
- Born and raised in United States, Baptist religion.
- Healthcare insurance (HMO) through husband's work.
- Referral: Preadmission workup for surgery
- Source: Self, seems reliable

Current Health Status

- Brief morning cough for past 5 years, productive of small amount of thin, whitish-gray mucus, no odor or bad taste. Cough does not occur with activity or exercise. Positive history of smoking.
- No dyspnea or chest pain.
- No edema, loss of usual energy, change in sleeping patterns (except when gallbladder discomfort awakens her).

Past Medical History

- Frequent upper respiratory infections (URIs) as a child.
- No history of asthma, pneumonia, or TB.
- Never had surgery. Hospitalized only for childbirth: uncomplicated vaginal delivery of three children.
- No known exposure to people with respiratory infections.
- Denies allergies to food, drugs, or environmental factors.
- No medical problems except for gallbladder disease.

- Immunizations up to date. Last PPD a year ago was negative.
- Denies taking prescribed drugs. Takes acetaminophen about twice a month for headache relief.

Family History

- Grandfather smoked and died of lung cancer at age 63.
- Father, age 65, recently quit after smoking a pack a day for 40 years (40 pack-years). Diagnosed with lung cancer a year ago.
- All other known relatives alive and well.

Review of Systems

- **General Health Survey:** States that usual health is good. Has gained 15 lb in past 2 years.
- **Integumentary:** No changes in skin, hair, or nails.
- **HEENT:** Head/Neck: No swelling or masses. Eyes/Ears: Vision 20/20; hearing good. Nose/Throat: Productive morning cough with whitish-gray mucous. Has occasional cold.
- **Cardiovascular:** No chest pain.
- **Gastrointestinal:** Appetite good, no nausea or vomiting. Daily bowel movement.
- **Urinary:** No changes reported.
- **Reproductive:** Is in a monogamous relationship; satisfied with sexual performance.
- **Musculoskeletal:** No weakness or muscle wasting reported.
- **Neurological:** Memory good. No changes noted. No tremors.
- **Immune/Hematologic:** No allergies or anemia.

Psychosocial Profile

- Has a physical exam and Pap smear every 2 years. Made a special appointment when she noticed RUQ colicky abdominal pain after eating high-fat meals. Scheduled surgery as soon as recommended by physician.
- Typical day consists of arising at 6 am, having breakfast with family, and getting children off to school. Walks 5 blocks to and from work at CPA office 4 days a week. Works 8 AM to 4 PM at desk with computer. Spends evenings playing with children, helping them with homework, shopping, fixing dinner, doing housework, visiting with husband, watching TV, or reading. Showers, then goes to bed at 11 PM.
- Usually eats a healthy diet, but has gained about 15 lb over the past 2 years. Attributes this to sedentary job, "sweet tooth," and lack of exercise.
- Walks to and from work and likes to ride a bike, but does not have much time because of family, home, and work responsibilities.
- No pets; hobbies include reading and biking.
- Sleeps about 6 to 7 hours a night, uninterrupted, with one pillow. Denies problems falling asleep, but awakens with morning cough.
- Has smoked one pack a day of filtered cigarettes for past 10 years (10 pack-years). Lived with smokers all her life. Has tried to quit by cutting back without success. Drinks alcohol about 3 times a month at social events. Denies recreational drug use.
- Denies respiratory irritants at work.
- Lives in 2-story, single-family home in suburbs with ample living space for five people; has hot water heating and air conditioning; home negative for radon gas; denies recent travel outside local community. Will stay in downstairs bedroom for the first week after surgery.
- Supportive, caring husband; good relationship with children. Concerned about father's prognosis and mother's ability to care for him. Aware of health risks of second-hand smoke for children, so tries not to smoke at home. Husband also smokes, both would like to "kick the habit." No community involvement at this time, but has several friends who will help out after surgery.
- Copes with stress by talking with husband or friends or by ignoring it; also by smoking.

Page 327: Critical Thinking Activity #1

History of smoking and type of surgery place her at risk for altered respiratory function, hypoventilation and a potential complication, atelectasis.

Page 327: Critical Thinking Activity #2

Strengths are understanding risks associated with smoking, willingness to stop smoking, supportive family, health-seeking behaviors.

Page 327: Critical Thinking Activity #3

Encourage coughing and deep breathing, control pain, early ambulation, and adequate hydration.

Page 327: Critical Thinking Activity #4

Because the gallbladder is located in the RUQ. So postoperatively, Mrs. Kane may tend to hypoventilate because taking deep breaths may increase pain.

Page 348: Key history findings

- Brief morning cough for past 5 years, productive of small amount of thin, whitish-gray mucus.
- Frequent URIs as a child.
- Family history of lung cancer (grandfather and father).
- Has smoked one pack a day of filtered cigarettes for past 10 years (10 pack-years).

- Family history of cigarette smoking and long-term exposure to second-hand smoke.
- Wants to stop smoking. Has tried to quit by cutting back without success. Accepts difficulty of quitting smoking.
- Understands potential health effects of smoking on self and family.
- Sedentary occupation, walks to and from work.
- 15-lb weight gain over 2 years.
- RUQ pain from gallbladder disease. Understands potential for postsurgical discomfort.

Page 348: Key physical examination findings

- Skin pink, warm and dry, good turgor; mucous membranes pink and moist.
- Nails pink, firm, capillary refill < 3 seconds, nicotine stains on fingers and nails, no clubbing.
- Trachea midline.
- Chest: AP:lateral 1:2, costal angle < 90 , equal chest excursion, normal spinal curvatures, skin intact, no use of accessory muscles, no retraction.
- Chest nontender, symmetrical chest excursion, no masses, crepitus.
- Tactile fremitus equal anterior and posterior to mid thorax.
- Resonance noted throughout lung fields. Diaphragmatic excursion 4 cm bilaterally.
- Lungs CTA except for expiratory wheezing that clears with coughing; no crackles or rubs.

Page 348: Nursing diagnoses clustered supporting data

- Scheduled for cholecystectomy. States that she is frightened. Asking questions about pre- and postoperative course.
- RUQ pain from gallbladder disease. Expiratory wheeze that clears with coughing. 10–pack-year smoking history.
- Brief morning cough for past 5 years productive of small amount of thin, whitish-gray mucus. Unsuccessful at attempting to stop smoking.
- Desires to stop smoking; previously unsuccessful attempts. Walks to and from work. Aware of effects of second-hand smoke on children.
- Frequent URIs as a child. Family history positive for lung cancer. Grandfather smoked and died of lung cancer at age 63. Father, age 65, recently quit after smoking one pack a day for 40 years (40 pack-years); diagnosed with lung cancer a year ago.
- Weight gain of 15 lb over past 2 years. Sedentary occupation.

Page 349: Additional nursing diagnoses

- Infection, risk for
- Activity Intolerance
- Fatigue
- Breathing Pattern, ineffective
- Pain, self-management
- Anxiety

Page 349: Collaborative nursing diagnoses

- Potential complication: atelectasis.
- Scheduled for cholecystectomy with general anesthesia. Smoking history.

CHAPTER 12

Page 381: Critical Thinking Activity #1

Risk factors

- Age
- Male gender
- Family history
- Newly diagnosed HTN
- Diet; 60 lb overweight
- Sedentary lifestyle
- Work schedule
- Lack of exercise
- Alcohol intake
- Stress

Modifiable

- HTN controllable
- Diet
- Weight
- Lack of exercise
- Sedentary lifestyle
- Alcohol intake
- Work schedule
- Stress

Unmodifiable

- Age
- Male gender
- Family history

Page 382: Case Study Evaluation

Biographical Data

- 68-year-old Caucasian male, married, father of seven grown children, self-employed entrepreneur. Born and raised in the United States, Italian descent
- Catholic religion
- BS in engineering
- Blue Cross/Blue Shield Medical Insurance Plan
- Referral: Follow-up by PCP
- Source: self, reliable

Current Health Status

- Denies chest pain, dyspnea, palpitations, or edema
- Reports fatigue, loss of energy, and occasional dizzy spells

Past Health History

- No history of rheumatic fever in childhood
- No history of murmurs
- No history of injuries
- Inguinal hernia repair
- EKG revealed left ventricular hypertrophy
- Hospitalized 3 weeks ago for HTN
- No known food, drug, or environmental allergies
- Immunizations up to date
- No prescribed medications except Vasotec (enalapril) 5 mg bid and weekly use of antacid for indigestion.

Family History

- Positive for HTN and CVA. Mother had HTN and died at age 78 from CVA. Paternal uncle died at age 79 from MI.

Review of Systems

- **General Health Survey:** reports fatigue, weight gain of 60 lb over past 3 years.
- **Integumentary:** Reports feet cold, thick nails, tight shoes.
- **HEENT:** Reports 2 dizzy spells over past 6 months. Eyes: wears glasses, no visual complaints, yearly eye exam.
- **Respiratory:** Reports being "short winded" with activity.
- **Gastrointestinal:** Indigestion on weekly basis.
- **Genitourinary:** Awakes at least once a night to go to bathroom.
- **Male Reproductive:** Little sexual activity because he is "too tired;" also states that it is becoming difficult to have an erection.
- **Musculoskeletal/Neurological:** General weakness, cramps in legs on walking.

Psychosocial Profile

- Typical day starts at 7 AM, when patient showers, has breakfast, then goes to work. Returns home by 6 PM, eats dinner, watches TV until 11:30 PM, but usually fall asleep before news is over. Usually in bed by 12:00 midnight. Usually works 7 days a week.
- 24-hour recall reveals a diet high in carbohydrates and fats and lacking in fruits and vegetables. Heavy-handed with saltshaker. Admits he has gained weight over the years and is 60 lb overweight.
- No exercise program; states that he is "too busy running my business."
- Sleeps about 7 hours a night but usually feels he is not getting enough sleep, lately is more and more tired. Wife states that he snores.
- Does not have routine checkups. States, "I only go to the doctor's when I'm sick."
- Has never smoked. Drinks a bottle of wine every night with dinner.
- Hobbies include reading, crossword puzzles, and antique collecting.
- Has a large, close, caring family. Feels that running his own business can be very stressful, but feels he can handle it alone and doesn't need anyone to help him.
- Lives with wife of 45 years in a two-story, single home in suburbs with ample living space.

Page 404: Critical Thinking Activity #2

HTN increases the work of the heart so that it has to pump against greater resistance. This could lead to left ventricular hypertrophy.

Page 404: Critical Thinking Activity #3

Left-sided CHF can result from left ventricular hypertrophy that developed secondary to hypertension. Clinical signs of left CHF include breathing difficulties, such as SOB, DOE, or PND.

Page 404: Critical Thinking Activity #4

The carotid pulsation is normally palpable because the arterial system is a high-pressure system. The venous system is a low-pressure system, so although the jugular venous pulsation may be visible, it is not palpable. The jugular venous pulse is obliterated with palpation.

Page 405: List key history findings

- 68-year-old Caucasian male
- Positive fatigue and dizzy spells
- Newly diagnosed with hypertension
- Vasotec (enalapril) 5 mg bid
- Use of antacids weekly
- Positive family history of HTN, CVA, MI
- Diet high in fats, carbohydrates, and salt
- Weight gain, 60 lb overweight
- Sedentary lifestyle
- Lack of routine activity or exercise program
- SOB with activity
- Changes in skin
- Intermittent claudication
- Indigestion weekly
- Change in sexual activity

- Lack of restful sleep, snoring, nocturia
- Lack of health promotion and prevention activities
- Alcohol intake
- Large, close, caring family

Page 405: List key physical examination findings

- BP 150/90
- Arcus senilis, AV nicking, and cotton-wool spots
- +1 pedal pulses; skin cool, pale, dry, thin, and hairless with trace of edema
- +3 carotids
- Sustained pulsation displaced lateral to apex, PMI 3 cm
- Accentuated S_2, $+S_4$

Page 405: Critical Thinking Activity #5

Strengths:

- Usual state of health good.
- Blood pressure is more stable.
- Supportive family.

Areas of concern:

- Newly diagnosed HTN
- Family history of cardiovascular disease
- Overweight
- Unsatisfactory diet
- Sedentary lifestyle
- Stress
- Inactivity, lack of routine exercise
- Arcus senilis and fundoscopic changes
- +1 pedal pulses with skin changes
- 3-cm PMI with displacement
- S_4 and accentuated S_2

Page 405: Nursing diagnoses clustered supporting data

- Positive pedal pulses; skin and nail changes in extremities; blood pressure
- 60 lb overweight; diet high in fats and carbohydrates; high salt intake
- HTN, EKG with LVH; S_4; enlarged and displaced PMI
- Newly diagnosed with HTN

Page 406: Additional Nursing Diagnoses

- Health Maintenance, ineffective, related to lack of knowledge regarding risk factors for heart disease
- Activity Intolerance, related to fatigue secondary to cardiovascular disease
- Coping, ineffective, related to stress of work
- Sleep pattern, disturbed, related to snoring (sleep apnea)
- Sexuality patterns, ineffective, related to activity intolerance

CHAPTER 13

Page 422: Case Study Evaluation

Biographical Data

- 38-year-old African-American female, married, one child
- Works full-time as a secretary.
- Born and raised in United States, Baptist religion.
- High school graduate, interested in attending community college when her baby gets older.
- Healthcare insurance, PPO, through husband's work plan.
- Husband is firefighter.
- Referral: private practice, internal medicine office.
- Source: self, seems nervous but reliable.

Current Health Status

- 6-day history of dull, aching pain and tenderness in left leg that is progressively getting worse.
- Pain is worse when standing and walking and is minimally relieved by rest and elevation.
- Aspirin has not helped.
- Denies chest pain or SOB.

Past Medical History

- Delivered premature baby 1 week ago.
- Prolonged bed rest 2 months before delivery.
- No history of surgery. Hospitalized only for childbirth. Uncomplicated vaginal delivery; baby's gestational age is 31 weeks.
- No history of chronic illness.
- Denies prescribed drugs.
- Has smoked 1 pack of cigarettes a day for 22 years (22 pack-years).

Family History

- Mother, age 65, has HTN and is obese.
- Father, age 67, had MI at age 50; quit smoking 17 years ago.
- All other known relatives alive and well.

Review of Systems

- **General Health Survey:** General health good, feeling tired since delivery of baby.
- **Integumentary:** Inflammation and swelling of left calf.
- **HEENT:** Head/neck: No swelling or masses, no sore throat.

- **Respiratory:** No breathing problems.
- **Cardiovascular:** No chest pain.
- **Gastrointestinal:** No complaints, daily bowel movement.
- **Genitourinary:** No nocturia since delivery of baby.
- **Reproductive:** Has not been sexually active for about the past 3 months because of complications of pregnancy. No problems before this. Plans to bottle-feed baby.
- **Musculoskeletal:** Tenderness in left calf.
- **Neurological:** No numbness, tingling, or loss of sensation.
- **Endocrine:** No history of thyroid disease or diabetes

Psychosocial Profile

- Has PAP smear by gynecologist every year. Last complete physical exam 5 years ago.
- Typical day consists of arising at 7 AM, showering and dressing, and having breakfast with husband. Takes train to work. Works 8 AM to 5 PM 5 days a week as secretary, which involves mostly sitting at desk with computer. Spends evenings watching TV, reading, going out socially with husband. This routine was dramatically altered 2 months ago because of premature labor and bed rest.
- Usually eats lots of fast foods but has worked hard to maintain a healthy diet during her pregnancy. Gained 50 lb during pregnancy, which she attributes primarily to 2 months of bed rest.
- Likes to walk and continued this activity throughout pregnancy until she was put on bed rest. Before pregnancy, played tennis once a week with husband.
- Normally sleeps about 8 hours nightly without difficulty. During pregnancy, sleep was interrupted because of need to void.
- No pets. Hobbies include walking, tennis, sewing, and reading.
- Has smoked one pack a day of filtered cigarettes for past 22 years (22 pack-years). Has tried behavior modification, cold turkey, and nicotine patches without success.
- Drinks wine with dinner on weekends, but none since pregnancy. Denies recreational drug use.
- Sits for long hours in front of computer at work. Denies other occupational hazards.
- Lives in ranch home in suburbs with ample living space, air conditioning, and hot water heating. Denies travel outside of state.
- Has supportive, caring husband who worries about premature baby who will be coming home from hospital shortly. Visits baby daily. Concerned about client's ability to care for baby with her leg problem. Would like her to quit smoking before baby comes home from hospital.
- Denies religious or cultural influences on health.
- Denies any sexual problems. Had sexual relations with husband until bed rest was ordered.
- Copes with stress by smoking and talking with husband and friends.

Page 422: Critical Thinking Activity #1

- Circulatory problem: Thrombophlebitis
- Contributing factors: Prolonged bed rest, pregnancy, smoking

Page 422: Critical Thinking Activity #2

Child care for newborn, parent-newborn relationship.

Page 436: Key history findings

- Six-day history of dull, aching pain and tenderness in left leg that is progressively getting worse.
- Delivered premature baby 1 week ago. Uncomplicated vaginal delivery; baby's gestational age is 31 weeks.
- Prolonged bed rest 2 months before delivery.
- 50-lb weight gain with pregnancy.
- Sedentary occupation. Understands need to resume previous exercise regime.
- Concerned over new role as mother of premature child.
- 22–pack-year smoking history. Attempts to stop smoking unsuccessful in past. Understands potential health effects of smoking on self and family.

Page 436: Key physical examination findings

- Positive Homans' sign.
- Left leg edematous and warm to touch, slightly cyanotic.
- Femoral and popliteal pulses strong; left posterior and pedal pulses difficult to locate.
- Left leg circumference 41 cm; right leg circumference 38 cm.
- Temperature 99.8°F.

Page 436: Nursing diagnoses clustered supporting data

- Describes pain as dull and achy with progressive worsening over 1 week. Pain gets worse with standing or walking and is only minimally relieved by rest and leg elevation. Positive Homan's sign.
- Appears anxious. States she is worried about having DVT and about how it will affect her ability to care for her baby. Also worried about her new role as mother, especially with a premature baby. This is her first child.
- States that she is having difficulty walking and standing because of leg pain. Is aware that

management of DVT requires bed rest and limb elevation.
- States that she wants to stop smoking despite previous unsuccessful attempts. Desire to stop smoking is enhanced by wanting a good environment for her child. Also wants to lose weight gained during pregnancy. Past behaviors included both exercise and balanced diet.
- Gained 50 lb with pregnancy. States that she wants to lose weight. Has sedentary occupation but exercised before complications of pregnancy. Is aware that medical management of DVT requires additional bed rest.

Page 438: Additional nursing diagnoses

- Coping, ineffective, related to necessary lifestyle changes
- Family Processes, interrupted, related to loss of income and inability to work secondary to DVT and recent childbirth
- Mobility, impaired physical, related to intermittent claudication and fatigue
- SleepPattern, disturbed, related to rest pain
- Diversional Activity, deficient, related to prolonged immobility
- Injury, risk for, related to diminished arterial flow
- Skin Integrity, risk for impaired, related to decreased oxygenation of tissues secondary to vasospasm and arterial occlusion.
- Therapeutic regimen: ineffective management
- Noncompliance, related to failure to stop smoking cigarettes.
- Tissue Integrity, impaired, caused by ineffective flow of fluid in the lymphatic vessels
- Body Image, disturbed, related to accumulation of fluid in the extremities
- Self care deficit, related to limb enlargement secondary to lymphedema.

Page 438: Collaborative nursing diagnoses

- Potential complication: pulmonary embolus
- Risk for bleeding

CHAPTER 14

Page 450: Critical Thinking Activity #1

After ovulation, the breasts become engorged with blood and fluid because of the influence of progesterone. This causes them to become painful and/or tender.

Page 450: Critical Thinking Activity #2

- When did your husband first notice the lump?
- Do you have breast pain?
- Have you noticed and changes in your breasts?

Page 455: Case Study Evaluation

Biographical Data

- 46-year-old married woman
- No pregnancies, no children
- Caucasian, Catholic religion, Polish descent
- College graduate; employed as high school teacher
- Contact person: Husband, Edward Kobrynski, a steelworker.
- Insurance from full-time work
- Source of information: Self, seems reliable

Current Health Status

- Chief complaint is that her husband thinks she has a lump.
- Does not perform monthly BSE.

Past Health History

- Menarche at age 12; menstrual cycles have always been regular—every 28 days and lasting for 3 days.
- Had lumpectomy for benign breast lesion; otherwise negative.
- No pregnancies; no history of infertility.
- No known food, drug, perfume, or deodorant allergies.
- Does not take any medications other than occasional Tylenol for headache. No history of BCP.
- No other medical problems. Does not examine breasts and has never had a CBE or mammogram.

Past Health History

- Positive for ductal breast cancer.
- Maternal grandmother deceased age 87; diagnosed with ductal breast cancer at age 85.
- Mother had benign breast lesion at age 57.
- Client has two younger sisters, both alive and well.
- One maternal aunt, alive and well.
- No other cancer history in family.

Review of Systems

- **General Health Survey:** Usual state of health good
- **Integumentary:** No dimpling, redness, or rashes on breasts or axillae
- **Cardiovascular:** Reports no problems or medications
- **Reproductive:** Menarche at age 12; menstrual cycle regular every 28 days, lasting 3 days; no history of BCP or HRT.

Psychosocial Profile

- Has not had physical exam in 5 years; has never had a mammogram; does not perform BSE; has not had CBE in 5 years.
- Typical day consists of awakening at 6 AM, showering and dressing, eating breakfast with husband, and driving 30 minutes to school. Works 8 AM to 3:30 PM Monday through Friday. Returns home by 4 PM, takes a walk or relaxes, fixes dinner. After dinner corrects papers, watches TV, or reads. Spends weekends catching up on housework, shopping and running errands, socializing with friends.
- Usually eats well, although diet premenstrually tends to be high in fats and salt. Temporarily gains 5 lb before she gets her period; otherwise, weight stable for past 10 years.
- Walks 3 miles, 3 to 4 times a week.
- Usually gets 8 hours sleep; no difficulty sleeping.
- Denies use of alcohol and caffeine.
- Employed full time, likes job, which does not require lifting.
- Satisfied with sex life.
- Married 15 years, husband and friends are supports.
- Goes to church weekly; religion is an important aspect of her life.

Page 455: Critical Thinking Activity #3

- Problem: Breast cancer
- Risk factors: Family history of breast cancer; fact that she has never been pregnant; high-fat diet.

Page 465: List key history findings

- Age 46
- No pregnancies
- Husband thinks she has lump in breast
- Does not perform BSE
- Had lumpectomy for benign breast lesion
- Has never had a CBE or mammogram
- High-fat diet
- Maternal grandmother died of ductal breast cancer at age 87

Page 465: List key physical examination findings

- Healthy-appearing 46-year-old Caucasian female, appears stated age.
- Temperature 98.4°F; pulse 72 BPM; respirations 18/min; BP 110/68; height 5′4″; weight 116 lb
- Day 7 of menstrual cycle.
- *Breasts:* Right breast slightly larger than left; uniform and symmetrical; ovoid in shape; no skin lesions noted; no redness or dimpling. Small, pea-sized (0.5 cm), easily movable, rubbery, smooth-edged lesion palpated in right breast at 2 o'clock; 4 cm from aerola in the right upper outer quadrant; no lesions palpated in left breast.
- *Nipple:* No lesions observed or palpated; nipples erect and point in same direction; no inversion or eversion; patient denies discharge from nipple; unable to elicit discharge from either nipple; no specimens sent
- *Axillae:* No lesions or thickening noted.

Page 465: Nursing diagnoses clustered supporting data

- Does not perform BSE.
- Has not had physical for 5 years; never had a mammogram.
- Lump in left breast, slightly anxious
- Possible need for breast surgery

CHAPTER 15

Page 479: Critical Thinking Activity #1

Appendicitis causes both visceral and parietal pain. The visceral pain results from distention of the appendix and results in umbilical pain; the parietal pain results from inflammation of the appendix and consequent inflammation of the peritoneum, which produces severe, localized pain that increases with movement.

Page 488: Case Study Evaluation

Biographical Data

- 56-year-old divorced woman, mother of 2 grown children
- French-Canadian descent, speaks English and French
- Roman Catholic religion
- High school graduate and mill worker
- Source of information: self, reliable

Current Health Status

- No bowel movement in 4 days.
- Dull, intermittent lower abdominal pain rated 2 on a 0-to-10 point scale. Walking around makes it better and nothing makes it worse.
- Denies visible red blood in stool, black stool, or symptoms in other body systems.
- Says she has had problems with constipation for the past few years.

Past Health History

- Positive for varicella and measles
- No history of GI problems as a child

- Cholecystectomy 5 years ago; appendectomy 50 years ago
- Denies having any GI assessment procedures or blood transfusions
- Denies lactose intolerance or any allergies to substances, foods, or medications
- Denies having any other health problems
- Up to date on all immunizations; had hepatitis B series, pneumovax, and tetanus 5 years ago, yearly flu shot last fall
- Takes no prescribed medications
- Takes no OTC medications now. Has used laxatives to relieve constipation over past few years.
- Uses no herbal preparations.

Family History

- Mother and brother died of colon cancer.
- Father died of congestive heart failure.
- No family history of obesity or diabetes.

Review of Systems

- **General Health Survey:** No changes in energy level, just feels "bloated"
- **Integumentary:** No changes
- **HEENT:** No problems with head, neck, eyes, ears, nose, mouth, throat; no difficulty swallowing, last dental exam 6 months ago
- **Respiratory:** No breathing difficulties
- **Cardiovascular:** No problems
- **Genitourinary:** No burning, frequency, or incontinence, no history of renal disease
- **Neurological:** No loss of sensation, bowel and bladder control intact
- **Musculoskeletal:** No changes, no history of arthritis
- **Immune/Hematologic:** No allergies
- **Endocrine:** No history of thyroid disease or diabetes
- **Reproductive:** Postmenopausal

Psychosocial Profile

- Typical day begins at 5:30 AM, when she bathes, eats breakfast, and gets ready for work at the textile mill. Works 7 AM to 3 PM. Goes grocery shopping after work, prepares supper, does housework, calls her sister, and then relaxes by watching TV. Goes to bed at 10 PM every night.
- 24-hour recall reveals that Mrs. Robichaud likes "junk food," especially high-fat dishes traditional to the French culture. Breakfast usually consists of pancakes with butter and syrup; for lunch she has chips and a sandwich; and for dinner, baked beans and brown bread. Says desserts are her weakness. She eats 1 serving of fruit; 1 serving of vegetables; 3 servings of meat; 1/2 serving of milk; 2 servings of white breads/pasta/rice/grains, and at least 5 fats a day. She reports that her usual weight is 175 lb and she is 5′3″.
- No exercise program; uses car to get to work.
- Sleeps 7.5 hours a night, longer on weekends.
- Goes for yearly physical examination.
- Does not drink alcohol or smoke cigarettes.
- Likes to make stained-glass objects in her spare time.
- Mother of two adult children, lives by herself and calls her sister every day. Has no pets.
- Lives alone in an apartment in a part of town where she doesn't feel safe walking alone.
- Mill where she works has been laying off employees, and she is worried that she will be next. Has been talking with her sister and other mill workers about this concern.
- Works in a textile mill, but does not know what chemicals she may be exposed to. Her apartment was built in 1985.

Page 488: Critical Thinking Activity #2

- Age and weight
- History of abdominal surgery
- Family history of colon cancer
- History of constipation
- Use of laxatives
- High-fat diet
- Lack of routine exercise
- Lead exposure from stained-glass hobby
- Possible occupational exposure risk

Page 488: Critical Thinking Activity #3

- Abdominal discomfort as a result of no BM for past 4 days
- Bloated feeling
- Lack of exercise
- History of constipation
- Use of laxatives
- History of abdominal surgery
- Unsatisfactory diet

Page 514: List key history findings:

- Age 56, weight 175 lb
- Lower abdominal discomfort, dull intermittent 2/10
- No BM for 4 days
- History of cholecystectomy, appendectomy
- Use of laxatives
- Positive family history of colon cancer
- Junk food eater, high-fat diet
- No routine exercise
- Lead exposure from stained-glass hobby
- Possible occupational exposure risk

Page 514: List key physical examination findings:

- Temperature 98.8°F; pulse, 86 and regular; respirations 22; B/P 168/98; height 5′2″, weight 175 lb
- Well-nourished, obese, 56-year-old woman who appears older than her years.
- In no acute distress, but mildly anxious; posture erect; pleasant and cooperative; provides history with ease.
- Abdomen uniformly light pink in color, protruberant and slightly distended in lower half, soft with complaints of slight tenderness in the lower quadrants.
- No striae, bruises, or hernias noted, umbilicus centered. Scar noted from previous cholecystectomy.
- No aortic pulsations, peristalsis noted.
- Hypoactive bowel sounds in the four quadrants.
- No bruits, friction rubs, or venous hums auscultated.
- Liver span 6.5 at MCL.
- Unable to percuss the bladder or spleen.
- Negative CVA tenderness.
- Liver, spleen, kidneys, bladder, and inguinal nodes not palpable.
- Abdominal aorta approximately 2 cm, palpable just left of the midline.
- Superficial abdominal reflexes intact.
- Negative fluid.

Page 514: Nursing diagnoses clustered supporting data

- Abdominal discomfort rated 2/10; abdomen slightly distended and tender in lower quadrants
- Dietary history of junk foods, fatty foods
- High-fat, low-fiber diet
- Family history of colon cancer; personal risk for colon cancer related to diet and lack of exercise

Page 514: Additional nursing diagnoses

- Activity Intolerance
- Nutrition: imbalanced, more than body requirements
- Pain
- Constipation
- Fatigue
- Knowledge, deficient, regarding diet and exercise

Page 514: Collaborative diagnoses

Prevention of colon cancer through screening tests.

Page 514: Critical Thinking Activity #5

- What is your daily fluid intake?
- Do you have trouble walking?
- How do you usually treat your constipation?
- Do you use laxatives?
- What medications are you on (may have a side effect of constipation)?

Page 514: Critical Thinking Activity #6

- Increase fluid and fiber intake.
- Increase exercise.
- Respond promptly to defecation urge.

CHAPTER 16

Page 537: Case Study Evaluation

Biographical Data

- 29-year-old African-American female
- Married, mother of a 4-year-old girl
- American by birth; Protestant religion.
- Attended 1 year of college after high school; homemaker at present. Husband is stockbroker for investment banking company.
- Healthcare insurance with husband's company.
- Source of referral: Self, seems reliable

Current Health Status

- Scant midcycle vaginal bleeding for the past 2 months with no other complaints at present.
- Seeking care for annual Pap smear, gynecological examination and renewed prescription for oral contraceptives.

Past Health History

- Rheumatic fever at age 7.
- Usual childhood illnesses except for measles, mumps and rubella.
- Denies any previous surgeries or serious injuries.
- Has taken oral contraceptives since birth of child 4 years ago. No other medications except occasional aspirin.
- No history of STDs.
- Gravida 1, para 1, no complications with pregnancy or vaginal delivery.
- Menarche at age 12, LMP 21 days ago. Menses last 5 days with moderate to light flow and occurs every 21 to 23 days. Denies dysmenorrhea.
- Denies exposure to DES.

Family History

- No gynecological carcinomas or maternal exposure to DES.
- Parents are alive and well.
- Has two healthy female siblings, ages 33 and 35.

Review of Systems

- **General Health Survey:** Usual state of health good, no changes in weight or energy level
- **Integumentary:** No changes in skin, hair, or nails
- **HEENT:** No sore throat, headaches, lumps or masses in neck
- **Respiratory:** No history of respiratory disease
- **Cardiovascular:** No history of CV disease
- **Gastrointestinal:** Appetite good, no GI problems
- **Musculoskeletal:** No weakness, joint pain, or fractures
- **Neurological:** No history of neurological problems.
- **Endocrine:** No history of diabetes or thyroid disease
- **Lymphatic/Hematologic:** No lymphatic or hematologic disorders

Psychosocial Profile

- Last gynecological examination and Pap smear 1 year ago with no abnormalities found. Had one cold in past year without seeking medical attention. Bathes daily and does not douche.
- Typical day includes waking at 6:00 AM, preparing family breakfast, and performing household chores. Daughter goes to daycare 2 days a week while client volunteers at indigent healthcare facility.
- Eats three meals a day, drinks two cups of coffee. Does not eat at restaurants often and attempts to make healthy meals.
- Exercise and leisure activities include gardening, reading and outside activities with family.
- Family pet is a 1-year-old beagle.
- Asleep by 10:30 PM (7-1/2 hours a night).
- Does not smoke, drinks one glass of wine occasionally with evening meals, denies recreational drug use.
- Lives in a suburban house of adequate size for a large family.
- No cultural or religious influences on health care. Family attends church most Sundays.
- Describes loving relationship with spouse and states that they intend to have three more children. Enjoys being a homemaker.
- Copes with stress by communicating with spouse.

Sexual history:

- Sexually active in a monogamous, heterosexual relationship with husband.
- Satisfied with sexual performance.
- Uses oral contraceptives.

Page 537: Critical Thinking Activity #1

Pelvic examination and Pap test.

Page 552: Key history findings

- Scant midcycle bleeding
- Uses oral contraceptives

Page 552: Key physical examination findings

Normal gynecological examination without significant findings.

Page 552: Critical Thinking Activity #2

- Knowledge of oral contraceptives, side effects, and so forth.
- Compliance with taking oral contraceptives.

Page 552: Nursing diagnoses clustered supporting data

- Waited until annual Pap smear was due to mention midcycle bleeding. Lack of concern over midcycle bleeding.
- Midcycle vaginal bleeding could indicate a uterine or vaginal infection, hormonal disturbance, or malignancy.

Page 552: Additional nursing diagnoses

- Infection, risk for
- Sexuality Patterns, ineffective
- Growth and Development, delayed
- Sexual Dysfunction
- Role Performance, ineffective
- Self-Esteem, risk for situational low
- Pain, management
- Tissue Integrity, impaired, related to lesions

Page 552: Collaborative nursing diagnoses

Alteration in menstrual cycle patterns related to oral contraceptive use.

CHAPTER 17

Page 572: Case Study Evaluation

Biographical Data

- 35-year-old Caucasian male
- American by birth; Protestant religion
- Recently divorced, has a 10-year-old daughter.
- Employed as telephone lineman for 10 years; healthcare insurance through work.
- High school education.
- Source of referral: self, seems reliable.

Current Health Status

- Onset of dysuria 3 days ago. Clear urethral discharge occasionally at end of urine stream.

- Denies low back pain, blood in urine, or recent trauma.
- Denies suprapubic discomfort.
- Has had two different sex partners within the past 6 months.
- Uses condoms "sometimes."

Past Health History

- Usual childhood illnesses except for measles, mumps, and rubella
- Tonsillectomy in 1967, no other surgeries or hospitalizations
- Had chlamydia approximately a year ago and received antibiotics
- No history of renal calculi
- Immunizations are current
- Denies taking any prescription drugs; admits using aspirin occasionally for aches and pains

Family History

- Father died at age 52 of heart attack.
- Mother, age 62, alive and well.
- Three siblings, all healthy.

Review of Systems

- **General Health Survey:** Usual state of health good
- **Integumentary:** No changes in skin, hair and nails; no lesions
- **HEENT:** No swollen glands/nodes; denies sore throat; no eye drainage
- **Respiratory:** No history of COPD
- **Cardiovascular:** No history of HTN or cardiovascular disease
- **Gastrointestinal:** No history of liver disease
- **Musculoskeletal:** Denies joint pain or swelling
- **Neurological:** No neurological problems, weakness or paralysis; denies personality changes or depression
- **Endocrine:** No history of thyroid disease or diabetes
- **Immune/Hematologic:** Has never been tested for HIV; no history of sickle cell anemia

Psychosocial Profile

- Cannot remember when he last had a physical or went to a doctor for illness. Does not perform testicular self-exam (TSE).
- Typical day: Awakens at 6:30 AM, has only coffee for breakfast, gets to work at 7:30 AM. Work is very physical and includes climbing up telephone poles and onto roofs of houses and crawling under houses. Usually arrives home by 5:30 PM. Spends evenings watching television or dating. Spends time with child every other weekend. Usually in bed about 10 PM on workdays.
- Skips breakfast, drinks 4 cups of coffee daily, eats out a lot, snacks on junk food, rarely has a nutritious meal.
- Besides work, hikes about every other weekend, plays tennis occasionally, does yard work.
- Sleeps about 7 hours a night on workdays, less on nights when he has dates. Naps on weekends to "catch up" on sleep.
- Has smoked a pack of cigarettes daily for the past 15 years. Drinks beer about 3 times per week and about 6 to 10 beers on weekends. Denies recreational drug use.
- Job is physically taxing and potentially dangerous because of climbing.
- Has good relationship with his one child and with his mother, who cleans, irons, and occasionally cooks for him.
- No community involvement, does not attend church.
- Lives alone since divorce 1 year ago, in single-family home with more space than he needs.
- Copes with stress by ignoring it.

Sexual History

- Currently sexually active
- Heterosexual
- Two sexual partners within past 6 months
- Inconsistent use of condoms
- Satisfied with sexual performance
- No problems achieving erection or ejaculation
- Does not perform testicular self-exam

Page 572: Critical Thinking Activity #1

- STDs
- Safe sex practices
- Nutritious diet
- Smoking and alcohol
- Health maintenance practices, such as TSE and yearly physicals.

Page 585: Key history findings

- Onset of dysuria 3 days ago. Clear urethral discharge occasionally at end of urine stream.
- Had two different sex partners within the past 6 months.
- Uses condoms "sometimes."
- Had chlamydia approximately a year ago and received antibiotics.
- Uses alcohol regularly.
- Has smoked one pack of cigarettes daily for 15 years.
- Does not perform TSE.

- Rarely has a nutritious meal.
- Cannot remember the last time he saw a doctor.

Page 585: Key physical examination findings

- Reddened urethral meatus
- Clear to white fluid discharge from penis
- Right inguinal lymphadenopathy

Page 585: Nursing diagnoses clustered supporting data

- States that he is concerned about STDs. Requests testing for all STDs including HIV.
- Is aware of effects of infections in reproductive system and of fact that some STDs are not curable. Verbalizes fears about being infected with an STD. States that he is concerned about telling sex partners. Scheduled for HIV antibody testing as well as tests for syphilis, gonorrhea, and chlamydia.
- Uses condoms only occasionally.
- Does not perform TSE. Uses tobacco and alcohol.

Page 585: Additional nursing diagnoses

- Role Performance, ineffective
- Self-Esteem, risk for situational low
- Sexual Dysfunction
- Sexuality Patterns, ineffective
- Infection, risk for

Page 585: Collaborative nursing diagnoses

Potential for altered reproductive health: sexually transmitted disease.

CHAPTER 18

Page 606: Case Study Evaluation

Biographical Data

- 68-year-old Caucasian female, widow
- Works as housekeeper for parish priest.
- Born and raised in United.States, Polish descent, Catholic religion
- Current health insurance: Medicare part A and B, supplemented with Medicaid.
- Source: Self, seems reliable.

Current Health Status

- "Several-year" history of aching joints in the evening after working all day.
- Discomfort first occurred in back and neck.
- Takes over-the-counter analgesic for pain with some relief.

Past Health History

- History of HTN
- Wrist fracture at age 65, caused by a fall on the ice. No pinning was performed.
- Cholestectomy at age 52, appendectomy at age 8, hysterectomy at age 35.
- Vaginal deliveries of 2 children with no complications.
- Denies allergies to food, drugs, or environmental factors.
- Medications include Zestril 10 mg OD for hypertension and Aleve once daily for arthritic pain.

Family History

- Mother had osteoporosis and HTN; died of cardiac problems at age 82.
- Father had HTN and died of heart attack at age 65.
- Sister, age 72, positive for osteoporosis and HTN.
- One daughter and one son, alive and well.
- All other known relatives alive and well.

Review of Systems

- **General Health Survey:** Describes usual state of health as "fair."
- **Integumentary:** Reports no changes in skin, hair, or nails.
- **HEENT:** Complains of pain and stiffness in neck; no swollen glands.
- **Respiratory:** No respiratory problems.
- **Cardiovascular:** Positive history of HTN, controlled with medication
- **Gastrointestinal:** No abdominal problems
- **Genitourinary:** No problems
- **Reproductive:** Postmenopausal since age 35
- **Neurological:** No changes in sensations
- **Immune/Hemotological:** No infections or bleeding
- **Endocrine:** No history of diabetes or thyroid disease

Psychosocial Profile

- Has a yearly exam because of HTN. Has not seen a gynecologist since her hysterectomy. Visits family physician every 3 months for HTN check.
- Arises at 6 AM. Does chores around own home and dresses for work. Workday is 9 AM to 5 PM. Typical day consists of daily chores around employer's home, including cooking, cleaning, and running errands. After work, she relaxes and watches the news and some television shows before going to bed at 9 PM.

- Admits she is a "tea and toast lady." Lives alone, so if she cooks, it is something quick, unless she goes out to eat with friends or family. Drinks 2 to 4 cups of caffeinated coffee/day. Has never been overweight.
- Activities include housecleaning and running errands uptown. No formal exercise program.
- Has no pets. Knits for a hobby while watching TV. Occasionally has dinner out or sees a movie with friends or family.
- Sleeps 4–5 hours uninterrupted, but often gets up at night to void.
- Denies smoking, alcohol use, or illicit drug use.
- Job requires some lifting (e.g., carrying vacuum cleaner upstairs) as well as bending.
- Says her self-esteem is "pretty good." Says she feels proud she can still earn a living. Admits she worries about living alone and developing health problems as she gets older, especially those that limit her mobility.
- Lives alone in a ranch home in suburbs; no steps. Is not afraid to be alone because of good neighbors.
- Has lunch or dinner once a week with daughter or son. Talks on phone to sister several times a week. Has friends in neighborhood, including younger neighbors who check on her.
- Copes with stress by talking with children or priest.

Page 606: Critical Thinking Activity #1

- **Musculoskeletal problem:** Osteoporosis
- **Risk factors:** Age, sex, race, family history, history of fracture, being postmenopausal, drinking 2 to 4 cups coffee a day, not exercising.

Page 635: Key history findings

- 68-year-old white female in for yearly routine examination.
- Concerned that she is "shrinking."
- Complains of back and neck discomfort at end of day for about past 5 years.
- Family history of osteoporosis in mother.
- Poor eating habits and sedentary lifestyle.
- Consumes 2 to 4 cups of coffee a day.
- History of hysterectomy because of dysfunctional bleeding at age 35. No use of estrogen replacement therapy.
- History of left wrist fracture age 65 caused by fall on ice.

Page 635: Key physical examination findings

- Height 5′5″; weight 125 lb (1 1/2 inch height loss since onset of menopause.)
- Gait steady, no support needed for ambulation.
- Mild muscle atrophy noted to quadriceps; all other muscles without atrophy. No involuntary movements.
- Shape and tone of muscles within normal limits.
- Contour smooth over joints. No tenderness, heat, redness, or pain palpated in any joint.
- Full ROM in all joints.
- Muscle strength 5/5.
- Limb length bilaterally: 80.5 cm leg; 40 cm thigh.
- Mild kyphosis noted when standing.

Page 635: Collaborative nursing diagnoses

- Complains of joint pain at end of day, back and neck pain
- Pain, atrophy of quadriceps
- Pain, atrophy of quadriceps
- Concerned about height loss; requesting information about osteoporosis

Page 635: Additional nursing diagnoses

- Activity Intolerance
- Body Image, disturbed
- Pain, chronic
- Self Care Deficit
- Sleep Pattern, disturbed

CHAPTER 19

Page 655: Critical Thinking Activity #1

- What does the pain feel like? How severe is it? Where does it hurt (point to spot)? Do you have any other symptoms, such as nausea or vision changes? Were you drinking or using drugs?

Pages 662–663: Case Study Evaluation

Biographical Data

- 21-year-old African-American male
- Baptist religion
- Senior in college; business major
- Insurance under family's plan while in college
- Lives on campus during school year; home is 1 hour from school
- Contact person: Janet Jones, mother
- Source: Self, seems reliable

Current Health Status

- Complains of headache and neck pain from hitting head in motor vehicle accident.
- Had a few beers earlier in night.
- Felt a little confused after accident and is not sure what happened. Does not know whether he lost consciousness.

Past Health History

- No hospitalizations or surgeries.
- Concussion in high school while playing football, otherwise negative for neurological problems.
- Fractured fibula freshman year in college while playing football; casted and healed without problem.
- Thinks immunizations are up to date but unsure of last tetanus shot.
- No known food, drug, or environmental allergies.
- No medications or other medical problems.

Family History

- Father, age 55, has HTN.
- Paternal uncle, age 60, has HTN.
- Paternal grandfather, died at 80 from CVA.
- Maternal aunt, age 50, has HTN.
- Maternal grandfather died at 75 from CVA.

Review of Systems

- **General Health Survey:** Usual state of health good until accident.
- **Integumentary:** No changes
- **HEENT:** Headache and neck pain; a little "dizzy."
- **Respiratory:** No problems
- **Cardiovascular:** No problems
- **Gastrointestinal:** Appetite usually good, but felt "a little sick after accident." No vomiting.
- **Genitourinary:** No problems
- **Reproductive:** Does not wish to discuss
- **Endocrine:** Negative
- **Lymphatic/Hematologic:** Negative

Psychosocial Profile

- Gets yearly physical exam for sports.
- Typical day consists of awakening at 9 AM, grabbing some breakfast, and heading to class. Goes to football practice from 3 PM to 6 PM 7 days a week, has dinner, relaxes, and does school work until about midnight. Usually goes to bed by 1 AM.
- Usually eats well; diet high in carbohydrates and protein.
- Practices football with team 3 hours a day, 7 days a week. Wears protective gear.
- Usually gets at least 8 hours of sleep a night.
- Denies use of drugs or nicotine. Admits to drinking alcohol on weekends; amount varies.
- Does well in school (GPA 3.0).
- Does not wish to discuss sexuality patterns.
- Friends and family are supports.
- Copes with stress by exercising, partying with friends on weekends.

Page 663: Critical Thinking Activity #2

- **Neurological problem:** Injury
- **Contributing factors:** Nutritional deficits; alcohol abuse; family history of HTN and CVA.

Page 669: Key history findings

- Drinks alcohol on weekends; had a few beers earlier in night.
- Felt a little confused after accident. Does not know whether he lost consciousness.
- Complains of headache, neck pain, and "a little dizziness."
- No vomiting after accident.
- Concussion in high school while playing football; otherwise, no neurological problems.
- Family history of HTN/CVA.
- Wears protective gear while playing football.

Page 669: Key physical examination findings

- Guarding and decreased ROM of neck
- 2-inch laceration on forehead
- Alcohol on breath

Page 669: Nursing diagnoses clustered supporting data

1. Reported head and neck injury from motor vehicle accident. Complains of headache and neck pain. Guarded movement of neck, increased neck ROM.
2. Reported head injury, headache, dizziness, recent memory loss.
3. Reported head injury, headache, dizziness, recent memory loss.

Page 669: Additional nursing diagnoses

Knowledge, deficient, related to substance abuse (alcohol)
Potential for increased ICP related to head injury

CHAPTER 20

Page 700: Critical Thinking Activity #1

- Nutrition: imbalanced, more than body requirements
- Sexuality patterns, ineffective
- Health-seeking behavior, re: osteoporosis
- Health maintenance, ineffective, related to diet
- Knowledge, deficient, of breast self-examination

Page 700: Critical Thinking Activity #2

- Breast exam
- Cardiovascular exam
- Musculoskeletal assessment for signs of osteoporosis such as loss in height

Page 700: Case Study Evaluation

Biographical Data

- 40-year-old Caucasian female
- Northern European extraction
- Protestant religion
- Married, with three children ages 12, 15, and 18
- Has a full-time, sedentary job as an accountant
- Source: Self; seems reliable

Current Health Status

- No current health problems
- Concerned about physiological changes of menopause and health care recommended for her age.
- Occasionally takes acetaminophen for tension headaches. No other medications.

Past Health History

- Had chickenpox, measles, mumps, and rubella as a child. Also had frequent bouts of strep throat as a child.
- Had an appendectomy at age 15. Was hospitalized for birth of her three children. Had a tubal ligation at age 35 for fertility control. Has never had a serious injury requiring hospitalization.
- No history of medical problems.
- No drug, environmental, or food allergies. Has taken penicillin without a reaction.
- Had all childhood immunizations. Last diphtheria-tetanus shot 10 years ago. Negative PPD skin test 5 years ago.
- Has not traveled in a foreign country within past year. Has never served in the armed services.

Family History

- Husband, age 45, alive and well
- Son, age 18, alive and well
- Daughter, age 15, alive and well
- Daughter, age 12, alive and well
- Mother, age 76, had breast cancer at age 54; osteoporosis and fractured hip at age 63.
- Father, age 78, has history of hypertension and had a myocardial infarction (MI) at age 68.
- Younger brother died in car accident at age 35.
- Two sisters, ages 42 and 50, alive and well.
- Maternal grandmother died of breast cancer at age 78.
- Maternal grandfather died of MI at age 81.
- Maternal uncle, age 80, has history of hypertension (HTN).
- Paternal grandmother died of cerebrovascular accident at age 82.
- Maternal aunt, age 78, has history of breast cancer and osteoporosis.
- Paternal grandfather died of MI at age 86.
- Paternal aunt, age 65, alive and well
- Paternal aunt, age 69, history of breast cancer
- Paternal uncle, age 71, history of HTN

Review of Systems

- **General Health Survey:** Client feels that her overall health is good. No fever, chills, fatigue, depression, or anxiety. She has occasional colds and has gained 10 lb in past year without a change in diet.
- **Integumentary:** No rashes, lesions, mole changes, or bruising. Skin is dry.
- **HEENT:** No headaches, frequent sore throats, hoarseness, or problems with vision, hearing, or sinuses.
- **Respiratory:** No shortness of breath, wheezing, or productive or nonproductive cough
- **Cardiovascular:** No history of HTN, heart problems or murmurs, blood clots/ phlebitis, chest pain, palpitations, edema, orthopnea, or claudication.
- **Breast:** Performs BSE occasionally, when she remembers. Has never had a mammogram. No breast pain, tenderness, lumps, discharge, or change in nipples. Breastfed all 3 children.
- **Gastrointestinal:** No nausea/vomiting, abdominal pain, dysphasia, heartburn, jaundice, hemorrhoids, or blood in stool. Has daily bowel movement, brown in color.
- **Genitourinary:** No dysuria, frequency or urgency, although reports occasional stress incontinence. Satisfied with sexual life except for increasing vaginal dryness. No breast masses or nipple discharge. Has breast pain 7 days before menstrual cycle. Occasionally does BSE.
- **Reproductive:** Last menstrual period 21 days ago. Menarche at age 14. Gravida 3, para 3. Menses are irregular, ranging from 23 to 45 days (cycle used to be 28 to 30 days). Menses last 5 days with moderate to heavy flow. Contraception method is tubal ligation.
- **Musculoskeletal:** No joint pains, swelling, or muscle weakness.
- **Neurological:** No dizziness, vertigo, syncope, head injuries, seizures, numbness, or tingling of extremities. Reports forgetfulness and difficulty concentrating. Has never been treated for mental disorders, depression, or anxiety, although she did visit a counselor about a family problem 3 years ago.

- **Endocrine:** No diabetes, thyroid disease, polyuria/polydipsia, or heat or cold intolerance. Weight gain of 10 lb last year.
- **Immune/Hematologic:** No current infections, allergies, cancer, bleeding, anemia, or blood transfusions. Blood type A+.

Psychosocial Profile

- Does not usually seek routine health care or screenings. Feels that she is healthy and does not need health care unless she is sick. Does not know her cholesterol level, has never had a mammogram, has not had a Pap smear or physical examination in 3 years.
- Typical day consists of arising at 6:00 AM, getting her children off to school and then going to work. She works from 8:00 AM to 5:00 PM 5 days a week. After work, she makes dinner for her family and reads or watches television. She goes to bed at 11:00 PM each night.
- Reports that she eats a balanced diet with foods from each of the major food groups each day, including three vegetables and two fruit servings. Admits to eating sweets and fried foods every day. Evaluation of daily calcium intake reveals that she usually ingests 500 mg a day. Has had an unexplained 10-lb weight gain in last year.
- 24-hour recall shows the following: Breakfast was two fried eggs, two slices of bacon, two slices of white toast with butter, one 4-oz. glass of orange juice, and a cinnamon bun with butter. Lunch was a chicken salad sandwich with mayonnaise on two slices of white toast, potato chips, two chocolate chip cookies, an 8-oz. cola, and a chocolate candy bar. Snack was one apple. Dinner was steak, baked potato with butter, string beans, tossed salad with Russian dressing, apple pie with ice cream, and 8 oz. of 2 percent lowfat milk.
- Admits that her only exercise is walking from her car to her office twice a day and walking up and down two flights of stairs several times a day. She walked on a daily basis in the past but stopped this year because of lack of time and inability to fit it into her schedule. For recreation she reads, does housework, and gardens on weekends.
- Hobbies include reading and gardening. Has a house cat.
- States that she usually sleeps well for 7 to 8 hours a night. Has occasional night sweats that awaken her.
- Has never smoked and is not exposed to smoke at home. Has smoke and carbon monoxide detectors at home. Drinks a glass of wine with dinner two to three times a week. Denies ever using illicit drugs.
- Identifies no occupational risks. Is not exposed to smoke at work. Drives 40 miles round trip to work each day. Wears seatbelt when driving.
- Attends church weekly with family. No religious or cultural influences that affect health practices.
- States that her marriage is supportive and comfortable. Describes good relationships with children, siblings, and parents.
- Uses prayer, friendships, and family support to deal with stress.

Page 701: Critical Thinking Activity #3

Strengths:

- Concerned about health and menopause
- No history of medical problems
- Supportive family
- Normal physical examination

Areas of concern:

- No regular exercise
- Sedentary job
- Weight gain of 10 lb
- Diet high in fat and sugar, low in calcium
- Infrequent BSE
- Family history of cancer, osteoporosis, and cardiiovascular disease
- Does not seek routine health care and screening

Page 708: List key history findings

- Concerned about menopause and health care recommended for her age group
- Sedentary job; no regular exercise routine
- Tubal ligation at age 35
- History of breast cancer in family: mother, grandmother, two aunts
- History of osteoporosis in family: mother and aunt
- 10-lb weight gain in past year
- Infrequent BSE; has never had mammogram
- Does not go for routine health screenings
- Has never had cholesterol checked
- Has high-fat, high-calorie diet with inadequate calcium intake

Page 708: List key physical examination findings

- Normal vital signs; height 5′5″, weight 145 lb
- No abnormalities noted in any body system

Page 709: Nursing diagnoses clustered supporting data

- Weight gain of 10 lb over past year and high-fat, high-calorie diet.
- Evidenced by inadequate health maintenance, infrequent BSE, no pelvic examination for 3 years.

Page 709: Collaborative nursing diagnoses

- Potential complication: CVD
- Potential complication: osteoporosis
- Potential complication: breast cancer

Page 709: Referrals

- Possible HRT: Perimenopausal
- Pelvic examination and Pap test: 3 years since last examination, hormonal changes
- Annual clinical breast examination: Infrequent BSE, family history of breast cancer, has never had a mammogram
- Mammogram: Same as above
- Cholesterol and thyroid screening: High-fat diet, family history of CVD, perimenopausal
- DEXA scan for bone density: Perimenopausal, family history of osteoporosis

CHAPTER 21

Page 723: Critical Thinking Activity #1

During the antepartal period, encourage exercise and reassure your Irish-American client that stretching and other activities that involve lifting her arms over her head will not cause the umbilical cord to become wrapped around the baby's neck. With Mexican-American clients, understand that because they view pregnancy as a "natural" and desirable condition, they may not seek early and ongoing prenatal care and instead rely on their family for advice and support. One approach to planning prenatal care would be to gain the support and acceptance of the family as you develop a timetable for the frequency of visits and discuss the goals of early and ongoing prenatal care.

In the intrapartum period, expect husbands of Arab-American and Egyptian-American clients to be voluntarily excluded from the birthing areas. For many cultures (Egyptian-American, Filipino-American, Greek-American) the client's mother will wish to be the primary labor support person.

Many cultures have certain beliefs regarding postpartum hygiene practices for the new mother. For example, your Egyptian-American client must avoid cold, which may result from bathing; your Filipino-American client may believe that showers can cause arthritis, so she will wish to take sponge baths only; and your Mexican-American client may wish to avoid showers altogether. Awareness of these different practices will be useful as you plan culturally appropriate care for your clients.

Page 723: Critical Thinking Activity #2

- **African-American:** Involve your client's grandmother and maternal relatives in the plan for prenatal, intrapartal, and postpartal care.
- **Amish:** Make certain that the prenatal classes are scheduled at a time when fathers can attend.
- **Arab-American:** Provide support, reassurance, and encouragement during labor, but do not emphasize relaxation and breathing techniques.
- **Chinese-American:** Consult with the dietary department to plan healthy meals for the postpartal mother that do not include fruits or vegetables.
- **Cuban-American, Egyptian-American, Filipino-American:** Involve the postpartal mother's family in the development of a plan of care for the new mother and her baby.
- **Greek-American:** Plan for alternatives to showering for postpartal mothers.
- **Iranian-American:** Soon after marriage, discuss preconception care and encourage healthy lifestyle practices to ensure a healthy pregnancy.
- **Irish-American, Mexican American:** Educate about the rhythm method of birth control.
- **Jewish-American:** Educate about birth control pills as one choice for contraception.
- **Navajo Native American:** Support and encourage the laboring woman who may wish to use special aids, such as a birthing necklace and a woven sash to facilitate the birth process.
- **Vietnamese-American:** Avoid touching the antepartal woman's head or the newborn's head.

Page 723: Critical Thinking Activity #3

- What do you and your family believe would be beneficial for you to do to remain healthy during your pregnancy?
- Can you identify some things that you could do, or not do, to improve your health and promote good health for your infant?
- Whom would you like to be present with you during labor?
- What activities would be important to you and to your family after your baby is born?
- What would you and your family like the nurses to do during your pregnancy, labor, and postpartal period?
- How would your family members like to participate in your birth experience?

Page 726: Critical Thinking Activity #4

Mrs. Ramirez reports that her last normal period was April 10 to 17. Using Naegele's rule, April 10 + 7 days = April 17. 3 months = January. Thus, her EDD is January 17.

Page 726: Critical Thinking Activity #5

- Fatigue
- Nausea and vomiting
- Breast enlargement, tingling, and tenderness

- Urinary frequency
- Amenorrhea

Page 730: Critical Thinking Activity #6

- Avoid an empty or overfull stomach.
- Eat dry carbohydrates on awakening and remain in bed until nausea subsides.
- Eat five to six small meals a day.
- Avoid fried, odorous, greasy, spicy, or gas-producing foods.
- Maintain good posture and do not lie down immediately after eating.

Page 732: Critical Thinking Activity #7

- Supportive and caring husband
- Enjoys her work
- Work is located near her home
- Works in a safe environment
- Obtains daily exercise
- Obtains adequate rest
- Maintains good nutrition
- Enjoys daily recreation
- Has yearly physical examination
- Does not smoke, use drugs, or drink alcoholic beverages
- Lives in a safe environment
- Has family support persons nearby
- Has a plan for infant care

Page 732: Case Study Evaluation

Biographical Data

- 24 years old, married, first pregnancy
- College graduate, full-time social worker
- Born and reared in the United States, Hispanic descent, Catholic religion
- Health insurance through own and husband's work plan.
- Referral: Routine prenatal care
- Source: Self, seems reliable

Current Health Status

- Fatigue
- Nausea and vomiting for 3 weeks
- Breast enlargement, tingling and tenderness
- Urinary frequency
- Amenorrhea

Past Health History

- Usual childhood illnesses
- No surgeries, hospitalizations, or allergies
- Immunizations current
- Takes one multivitamin with iron daily; no other medications
- Physical examinations yearly for 18 years; normal Pap smears
- Used oral contraceptives for 5 years without problems; discontinued them 8 months ago to attempt pregnancy
- No previous pregnancies

Family History

- Grandmother, age 64, takes medication to control high blood pressure.
- All other relatives alive and well; 2 older sisters married with children and experienced no complications during pregnancies; one younger sister is single.

Review of Systems

- **General Health Survey:** Very tired for past couple of months, needs to take a nap every day when she gets home from work. Body weight 125 lb, on the low end of her reported range of 126 to 128 lb. Has lost 2 lb since becoming pregnant.
- **Integumentary:** Noticed nipples getting darker and line on abdomen. Hair very oily.
- **HEENT:** No changes in head or neck. Has nasal stuffiness but no colds, allergies, or flu. Gums bleed with brushing; last dental exam 6 months ago. No eye changes.
- **Respiratory:** No changes.
- **Cardiovascular:** No history of MVP, palpitations, or edema.
- **Breasts:** Enlargement, tenderness, and tingling sensation.
- **Gastrointestinal:** Nausea and vomiting in the morning, usually subside by noon; says certain foods "just turn my stomach;" reports constipation.
- **Genitourinary:** Reports frequency of urination, no burning
- **Reproductive:** LMP 4/10/01.
- **Musculoskeletal:** No changes.
- **Neurological:** Occasional "lightheadedness;" no history of depression; excited at possibility of being pregnant.
- **Endocrine:** No history of gestational diabetes; reports heat intolerance.
- **Immune/Hematologic:** No history of anemia.

Psychosocial Profile

- Client is proactive regarding health care. Has yearly physical examination and Pap smear. Performs monthly BSE. Believes people are responsible for maintaining their own health.

- Typical day consists of arising at 6:30 AM and eating breakfast with husband. (Lately unable to enjoy usual breakfast of cold cereal and juice because of nausea.) Drives 4 miles to office 5 days a week and works from 8 PM to 5 PM at desk part of time and interviews clients in a clinic located on the ground floor of her office building for rest of time. Loves her work. In evenings she and husband prepare and eat supper, clean up dishes, take a walk in neighborhood, then relax watching television, playing cards,or reading. Client showers and goes to bed around 10 PM.
- Usually eats a healthy diet, but lately has been skipping breakfast because of nausea. As day progresses, is gradually able to eat bland food such as baked chicken, potatoes, and steamed vegetables.
- Walks daily for 45 minutes with husband.
- No pets. Recreation includes daily walk with husband, dinner at restaurant, or movie once a week, family get-togethers. Hobbies include reading and needlework.
- Sleeps around 8 1/2 hours normally, but lately gets very sleepy at work, especially in mid-afternoon. Combats sleepiness with a walk outside her office and an afternoon snack of fruit and yogurt or crackers. Takes a short nap after work. No problems falling asleep.
- Does not smoke, use drugs, or drink alcoholic beverages.
- No chemical exposure at work.
- Lives in a 1-story, 2-bedroom single family home in suburbs; has hot water, heating, and air conditioning; negative for radon gas. Will convert guest room into baby's room. No recent travel outside local community.
- Catholic religion, Hispanic nationality (third generation). No religious or cultural influences that affect health care, pregnancy, or delivery.
- Supportive, caring husband (nonsmoker) who is computer analyst for national company; married 5 years; attempted pregnancy for 6 months.
- Mother, mother-in-law, and three sisters live in same community and will assist with infant care. Client plans to breastfeed and stay at home for 6 weeks after birth and then return to job.

Page 742: Key history findings

- Well-developed, well-nourished 24-year-old Hispanic woman in no acute distress.
- Oriented to time, place, situation, person; affect pleasant and appropriate
- No complaints other than early pregnancy symptoms
- Vital Signs: Temperature 99.0°F; pulse 70 bpm, strong and regular; respirations 16/min, unlabored; BP 102/66
- Height: 5′ 5″; weight: 125 lb, prepregnancy weight 127 lb
- Normal cyclic menstruator, certain of date of last menstrual period; no contraception used during the past 8 months
- Desires pregnancy, excited and asking appropriate questions
- Taking multivitamins with iron and folic acid for past 8 months
- Supportive social situation: happily married, extended family nearby
- No medical conditions, current or past
- Exercises daily
- Nutritional status good except for 2-lb weight loss related to morning sickness; urine ketones negative today
- Desires to breastfeed
- Wishes to enroll in childbirth preparation and infant care classes

Page 742: Key physical examination findings

- Urine pregnancy test positive today
- Skin pink, warm, dry, good turgor, mucous membranes pink, moist
- No palpable cervical chain lymph nodes; slight thyroid enlargement, no nodularity or tenderness
- Lung sounds clear to auscultation bilaterally; heart: normal sinus rhythm
- Breasts: tenderness, venous congestion, prominence of Montgomery's tubercles, darkening of nipples and areolae, no nipple discharge
- Abdomen: linea nigra present, no masses, no enlargement, no FHTs auscultated with Doppler
- External genitalia: normal hair distribution, no varicosities, slight labial enlargement
- Extremities normal color, no edema, no varicosities, no tenderness, no increased warmth, DTRs 1+
- Pelvic examination:
  - Bartholin's and Skene's glands: nontender, no discharge
  - Cervix: positive Chadwick's sign, slight leukorrhea
  - Cervix long, thick, and closed. Cervical length: 3.0 cms; positive Hegar's sign
  - Uterus approximately orange-sized; no adnexal masses
  - Rectal mucosa pink, intact, no hemorrhoids

Page 743: Critical Thinking Activity #8

Strengths:

- Healthy
- No history of medical problems

- Planned pregnancy
- Supportive husband and family
- Preconception critical use of multivitamins with folate, lifestyle conducive to health

Areas of concern: None identified.

Page 743: Critical Thinking Activity #9

- An overview of the plan for prenatal care
- Self-care activities, including actions to prevent urinary tract infection (proper cleansing after urination, avoidance of bubble baths, adequate hydration and frequent bladder emptying)
- Routine practice of Kegel's exercises to strengthen and maintain pelvic floor muscle tone
- Maintaining adequate nutrition
- Getting adequate rest and exercise
- Involvement in childbirth preparation/parenthood education classes; development of a birth plan
- Maintaining intimacy and making necessary sexual adjustments as pregnancy progresses

Page 743: Critical Thinking Activity #10

Unless problems develop, she will probably need to return to the clinic every 4 weeks until her 28th week of pregnancy, then every 2 weeks until her 36th week of pregnancy, then every week from the 37th week until the time of birth.

Page 743: Critical Thinking Activity #11

The first prenatal visit is usually the most lengthy because you are obtaining the complete medical and obstetric history. On each subsequent visit, you should ask Mrs. Ramirez to describe any relevant events that have occurred since the last visit. Examples of questions you might ask are:

- How have you been doing since you were last here?
- Do you feel the baby move?
- Have you noticed any change in the baby's activity pattern?
- Have you experienced any pain?
- Have you experienced any nausea or vomiting?
- Have you experienced any bleeding?
- Have you noticed any unusual vaginal discharge, itching, or burning or experienced fluid leaking from your vagina?
- Have you experienced any severe back pain?
- Have you had any severe headaches or vision difficulties?
- Have you experienced a severe stomachache?
- Have you noticed any swelling in your hands, face, feet, or lower legs?
- Have you had any pain in your legs?
- Have you had any difficulty breathing?
- Have you had any abdominal pain or contractions?
- Do you have any problems when you urinate?
- Are you having regular bowel movements?
- Are you getting enough rest?
- Have you had any fever or chills?
- Are you getting daily exercise?
- How is your husband/significant other doing?
- Are you having any sexual difficulties?
- Have you made any changes to your birth plan?
- Have you enrolled in prenatal classes?
- Are you taking any medications?
- Is there anything you would like to share with me, or do you have concerns about something that I haven't covered?

Certainly this list of questions is not exhaustive, but it serves as a guide for the types of questions that you should ask at each prenatal visit.

Page 743: Nursing diagnoses clustered supporting data

- Pregnancy confirmed during this visit. Excited about this first pregnancy, asking about plan for prenatal care. Works full-time and wants to adjust work schedule to accommodate clinic visits.
- Weight loss of 2 lb since becoming pregnant. States that nausea and vomiting mostly occur in the morning on arising. Able to offset nausea and vomiting with diet modification. Urine negative for ketones today.
- States that she feels sleepy, especially in the mid-afternoon. Has begun going to bed earlier at night. Has a mid-afternoon snack and brief exercise in the mid-afternoon to offset fatigue.
- Has obtained a larger bra size; wears bra at all times when awake.
- Discontinued contraception 8 months ago to attempt conception. Began taking multivitamins with folic acid 8 months ago in anticipation of pregnancy. Maintains a healthy diet despite early morning nausea and occasional vomiting. Began prenatal care early in pregnancy. Exercises daily. Wishes to enroll in prenatal classes.

Page 743: Possible additional nursing diagnoses

- Body Image, disturbed
- Bowel Elimination, altered
- Sexuality Patterns, ineffective
- Adjustment, impaired
- Anxiety
- Infection, risk for
- Family Processes, interrupted
- Parenting, risk for impaired
- Comfort, altered
- Fear

- Coping, ineffective
- Self-Concept, altered

CHAPTER 22

Page 773: Critical Thinking Activity #1

During your physical examination, invite the parents to watch as you assess their baby. Take this opportunity to describe and explain findings. Include infant care such as handling, bathing, diapering, and safety precautions in your discussion.

Contact the hospital's patient education services regarding parenting and breastfeeding classes. Offer audiovisual tapes and printed matter. Refer parents to a lactation consultant.

Page 773: Critical Thinking Activity #2

Newborns should awaken and be alert for their feedings every 3 to 4 hours. Unarousable or lethargic behavior may indicate jaundice or infection, and medical advice should be sought.

Page 776: Case Study Evaluation

Health History

- Developmental
  - Sits
  - Bears weight on hands, stands with assistance
  - Rolls over
  - Controls head
  - Grasps objects
  - Is teething
  - Imitates sounds
  - Is attached to parents
  - Has separation anxiety
- Safety
  - Smoke and carbon monoxide detectors
  - Safety gates
  - Cabinet locks
  - Electrical outlet caps
  - Car seats
  - Medications and cleaning solutions out of reach
- Immunizations
  - Hepatitis B 1 and 2
  - DPT 1 and 2
  - Polio 1 and 2
  - HIB 1 and 2
  - PCV 1 and 2

Review of Systems

- **General Health Survey:** Very robust and active infant, healthy appearance.
- **Body Weight:** 16 lb, gained 2 lb since last month's visit for otitis media.
- **Integumentary:** No scaly skin.
- **Head and Neck:** Easily holds head upright and in alignment.
- **Eyes, Nose, and Throat:** Eyes: Normal response to visual stimuli, no drainage.
- **Ears:** Normal sound recognition and making sounds. No apparent abnormalities. Otoscope examination indicated because of recent otitis media.
- **Respiratory:** No breathing problems.
- **Cardiovascular:** No apparent distress. Active when awake.
- **Gastrointestinal:** Exclusively breastfed and nurses every 3 to 4 hours during the day, with daily bowel movements, yellow in color.
- **Genitourinary:** Normal urination pattern noted; 8 diapers a day.
- **Musculoskeletal:** Attempts to crawl; rolled over and sat up on her own (normal findings).
- **Neurological:** No abnormal movements, nurses well, no problems
- **Immunological:** No infection aside from otitis media.
- **Developmental:** Laughs easily with mother but is fearful of examiner. Normal age-related behavior observed.
- **Relationships:** Warm, caring responses noted toward baby from parents. Both parents say they enjoy parenthood very much.

Page 781: Critical Thinking Activity #3

Suggest that Mrs. Ramirez tap into other possible support systems, such as her other sisters, friends, neighbors, fellow workers, and members of her religious community. Community child-care resources that may be of assistance to the Ramirez family include:

- On-site job child-care center.
- Child-care centers connected with places of worship.
- Accredited child-care centers listed with the health department or local social service department.

Page 781: Key history findings

- Otitis media—one episode last month.
- Family members who cared for infant during mother's working hours have moved to another state, so mother has lost child-care/emotional supports.
- Mother concerned that infant is underweight.

Page 781: Key physical examination findings

- Diaper rash on labia and buttocks.
- Infant appears well nourished and is normal weight.
- Developmentally on target.

Page 781: Nursing diagnoses supporting data

- Irritating diaper rash noted on labia and buttocks. Mother eager to help condition.
- Otitis media—one episode last month.
- Mother's concern about Carmen's weight. Cultural interest toward large babies as healthy babies. Mother's lack of knowledge related to breastfeeding recommendation.
- Depended on family for emotional support and child care. Mother works full time. Husband supportive but works full time. No family or friends with children living locally.
- Mother eager to seek help and explore neighborhood resources for new friendships and child care.

Page 782: Additional nursing diagnoses

- Aspiration, risk for
- Infection, risk for
- Injury, risk for
- Poisoning, risk for
- Suffocation, risk for
- Trauma, risk for
- Pain
- Parenting, impaired

CHAPTER 23

Page 793: Critical Thinking Activity #1

The assessment is essentially the same as with other age groups except for the need to focus on growth and developmental changes that occur during the toddler/preschool years—for example, height and weight, body proportions (head), primary teeth, musculoskeletal and neurological development, and the struggle to develop a sense of autonomy.

Page 793: Critical Thinking Activity 2

- Answer questions honestly.
- Use concrete terms.
- Explain what you are doing.
- Involve the parent or caregiver.
- Use toys or games (e.g., puppets).

Page 793: Critical Thinking Activity #3

- Safety issues (injuries and poisonings)
- Nutrition
- Toilet training
- Sibling rivalry
- Temper tantrums
- Sleep problems
- Communicable diseases
- Abuse

Page 793: Critical Thinking Activity #4

For child:

- Anxiety, related to starting kindergarten.
- Anxiety, related to separation from parents
- Injury, risk for
- Nutrition: imbalanced, risk for
- Infection, risk for

For parents:

- Knowledge, deficient, related to dietary needs
- Knowledge, deficient, related to safety education

CHAPTER 24

Page 806: Critical Thinking Activity #1

The assessment is essentially the same as for other age groups, except for the need to focus on growth and developmental changes that occur during the school-age years—for example, height and weight, body proportions (head), secondary teeth, musculoskeletal and neurological development, and learning to work and play cooperatively.

Page 806: Critical Thinking Activity #2

- Answer questions honestly,
- Be concrete and explain what you are doing.

Page 806: Critical Thinking Activity #3

- Safety issues
- Nutrition
- Learning problems
- Alcohol and drug abuse
- Behavior problems (lying, cheating, and stealing)

Page 806: Critical Thinking Activity #4

- Anxiety, related to starting school
- Injury, risk for
- Nutrition: imbalanced, risk for
- Knowledge, deficient, related to dietary needs
- Knowledge, deficient, related to sex education
- Knowledge, deficient, related to substance abuse

Page 819: Critical Thinking Activity #5

The assessment is essentially the same as for other age groups, except for the need to focus on growth and developmental changes that occur during adolescence—for example, height and weight, sexual maturation, musculoskeletal development, and separating from parents and moving toward self-autonomy.

Page 819: Critical Thinking Activity #6

- Listen actively.
- Answer questions honestly.

- Be nonjudgmental.
- Avoid scare tactics.
- Maintain confidentiality.
- Explain what you are doing.

Page 819: Critical Thinking Activity #7

- Eating disorders
- Pregnancy
- STDs
- Emotional problems
- Substance abuse
- Violence
- Injuries and accidents

Page 819: Critical Thinking Activity #8

- Risk for identity conflict related to sexual maturation
- Nutrition: imbalanced, more or less than body requirements
- Sleep Pattern, disturbed, risk for
- Knowledge, deficient, related to safe sex practices
- Knowledge, deficient, related to sexual maturation

CHAPTER 25

Page 826: Critical Thinking Activity #1

In cultures in which older people are viewed with respect and as valued members of the family and society, health care is readily available. If the older person lives with his or her family, the family can be an important factor in the healthcare planning for the person. However, in cultures in which older people are perceived as a burden, health care for them may not be a priority.

Page 830: Critical Thinking Activity #2

- Liver: Decreased drug metabolism
- GI tract: Decreased absorption of medications
- Renal system: Decreased creatinine clearance may result in decreased drug clearance. Because of these changes, dosages of medications may need to be adjusted.

Page 838: Critical Thinking Activity #3

- Decreased GI tract motility
- Increased food intolerance
- Decreased dentin (may cause loss of teeth
- Decreased papillae on tongue(causes decreased taste)
- Delayed stomach emptying (causes decreased hunger sensation)

Page 843: Critical Thinking Activity #4

Strengths:

- Independent
- Supportive family
- Self-referral for health care
- Socially active
- Exercises routinely

Areas of concern:

- Fatigue
- Decreased appetite, activity tolerance, and muscle strength
- History of breast cancer, HTN, DJD
- Pain
- History of falls

Page 843: Case Study Evaluation

Biographical Data

- 80-year-old widow with four daughters
- Widowed for 15 years
- Resident of continuing care retirement community for 8 years
- Catholic religion, Slavic ancestry
- Not referred by doctor—came to outpatient office of her own accord

Current Health Status

- Complains of vague fatigue all day, decreased appetite, and inability to engage in usual activities such as walking group. Fatigue has been going on for several weeks and has gotten worse in the past week, despite going to bed around 9 PM and getting up at 8 AM. Is forcing herself to participate in social activities such as going to the dining room with friends for dinner. However, has no desire to eat.
- Takes Lasix 20 mg po qd for hypertension and Tamoxifen 20 mg bid to prevent recurrence of breast cancer

Past Health History

- Breast cancer 20 years ago
- Hypertension controlled by diuretics
- DJD, mostly in hips
- Cataract surgery 12 years ago (right eye) and 11 years ago (left eye)
- Lumpectomy, right breast, 23 years ago
- Elective left total hip replacement 17 years ago

Family History

- No known history of cognitive problems
- Believes that both of her parents died of heart disease in their 70s and 80s
- Does not know of any family history of cancer

Review of Systems

- **General Health Survey:** Complains of fatigue and "not feeling 'like myself.'" No changes in height or weight reported.
- **Integumentary:** Fair skin with no abnormal lesions. Complains of dry skin in winter.
- **HEENT:** No vision changes, dizziness, changes in smell or taste, or difficulty swallowing. Wears corrective lenses; has yearly eye exam. Reports being satisfied with quality of hearing.
- **Respiratory:** No cough or shortness of breath.
- **Cardiovascular:** No chest pain or shortness of breath during the day or at night. No shortness of breath while walking to the dining room. No leg cramping or pain either at rest or walking. Some swelling in ankles on arising, usually disappears in a few hours.
- **Gastrointestinal:** No indigestion or burning. Has a regular bowel movement daily and takes milk of magnesia rarely, only if she has not had a bowel movement in several days. Has not felt much like eating, but has not had stomach pain, nausea, or vomiting.
- **Genitourinary:** No discharge. Loses urine when she coughs, sneezes, or laughs, so wears a sanitary pad, which she changes two or three times a day. This problem has not gotten any worse recently. No vaginal discharge or bleeding. Menopause at age 51; was never on hormone replacement therapy. Last Pap test about 14 years ago; last mammogram 3 years ago.
- **Neurological:** No dizziness, change in cognition, problems with balance, tremor, seizure, or difficulty with concentration. Is very happy at continuing care retirement community and feels strongly that this was the best move for her because she could no longer manage her home independently. Enjoys living near friends, participating in activities, and having her daughters visit. Is glad they do not have to take care of her or worry about her being home alone. No previous history of depression.
- **Musculoskeletal:** Mild morning stiffness, usually gone by the time she has breakfast. Takes Tylenol when pain is bothersome. Had two falls since moving into the facility but no falls over past 6 months. No increase in joint pain or warmth or swelling of joints.
- **Immune/hematologic:** Reports feeling more tired than usual.
- **Endocrine:** No weight changes, increased thirst or urination. Heart does not flutter, race, or skip beats.

Psychosocial Profile

- Typical day starts around 8 AM. She fixes herself breakfast in her efficiency apartment, feeds her cat, then has coffee and watches television. Does laundry, light housecleaning, and "putters around" apartment. Midmorning usually goes to the activity room to socialize or play cards with other residents. Fixes own lunch. Until recently, walked 20 minutes three times a week with walking group in afternoon. Goes on planned outings with other residents. Sees daughters every weekend for lunch or dinner, shopping, and mass on Sunday. Previously went to bed at 11 PM but has been retiring at 9 PM for past few weeks because of fatigue.
- Does not smoke and rarely has a glass of wine socially.

Functional assessment

- Performs all personal care independently. Does own laundry, shopping, finances, and cleaning aside from the vacuuming, which is done by the facility every 2 weeks.
- Walks independently with a rolling walker. Has been participating in walking group and until recently was walking for 20 minutes three times per week.

Page 856: List key history findings

- Age 80, widow
- Lives in retirement community
- Supportive family
- Self-referral for health care
- Independent
- Fatigue for several weeks
- Decreased appetite
- Decreased activity tolerance
- History of HTN, breast cancer, DJD with total hip replacement
- Medications: Tylenol prn for joint pain, Lasix, Tamoxifen
- No bowel movement for several days
- No abdominal pain, nausea, or vomiting
- Increase in sleep from 9 hours to 12 hours
- Uses walker to ambulate
- Usually walks 20 minutes 3 times a week
- History of falls

Page 856: List key physical examination findings

- Well groomed, pleasant, appropriate behavior
- AAO × 3, memory intact
- VS WNL, afebrile
- Wears glasses
- Abdomen: positive tenderness RUQ, positive palpable liver edge
- Decreased muscle strength in lower extremities, decreased range of motion
- Gait steady with walker and wide base of support
- Kyphosis
- No evidence of depression

Page 856: Nursing diagnoses clustered supporting data

- Reports loss of appetite; does not feel like eating
- DJD; history of falls; uses assistive device (walker)
- Complains of fatigue; unable to participate in walking program
- Complains of having no energy; unable to participate in usual activities

Page 856: Additional nursing diagnoses

- Pain, Chronic, related to joint stiffness
- Incontinence, Stress Urinary, related to relaxed pelvic muscles
- Fluid Volume, Risk for Deficient, related to use of diuretics and loss of appetite
- Skin Integrity, Risk for Impaired, related to stress incontinence

APPENDIX B

Growth Charts

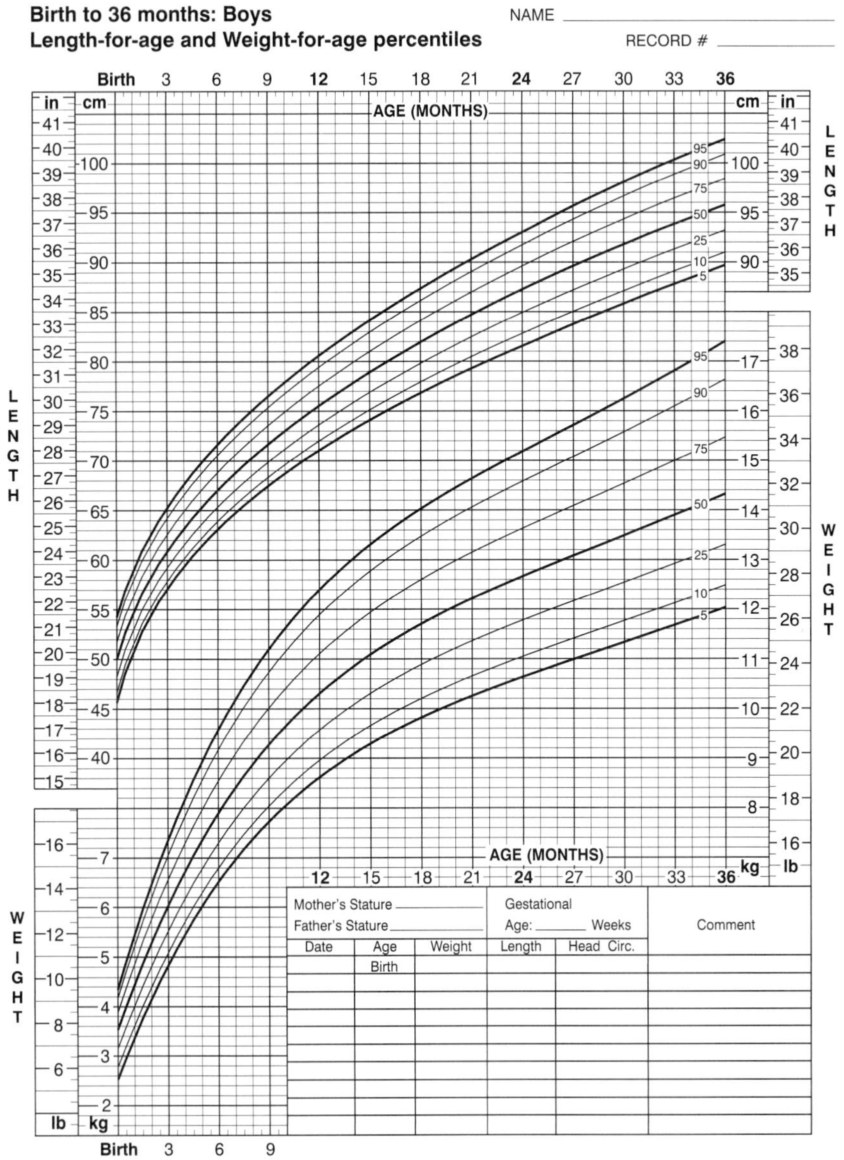

Pubished May 30, 2000 (modified 4/20/01).
SOURCE: Developed by the National Center for Health Statistics in collaboration with the National Center for Chronic Disease Prevention and Health Promotion (2000).
http://www.cdc.gov/growthcharts

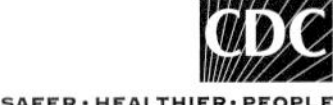

SAFER · HEALTHIER · PEOPLE™

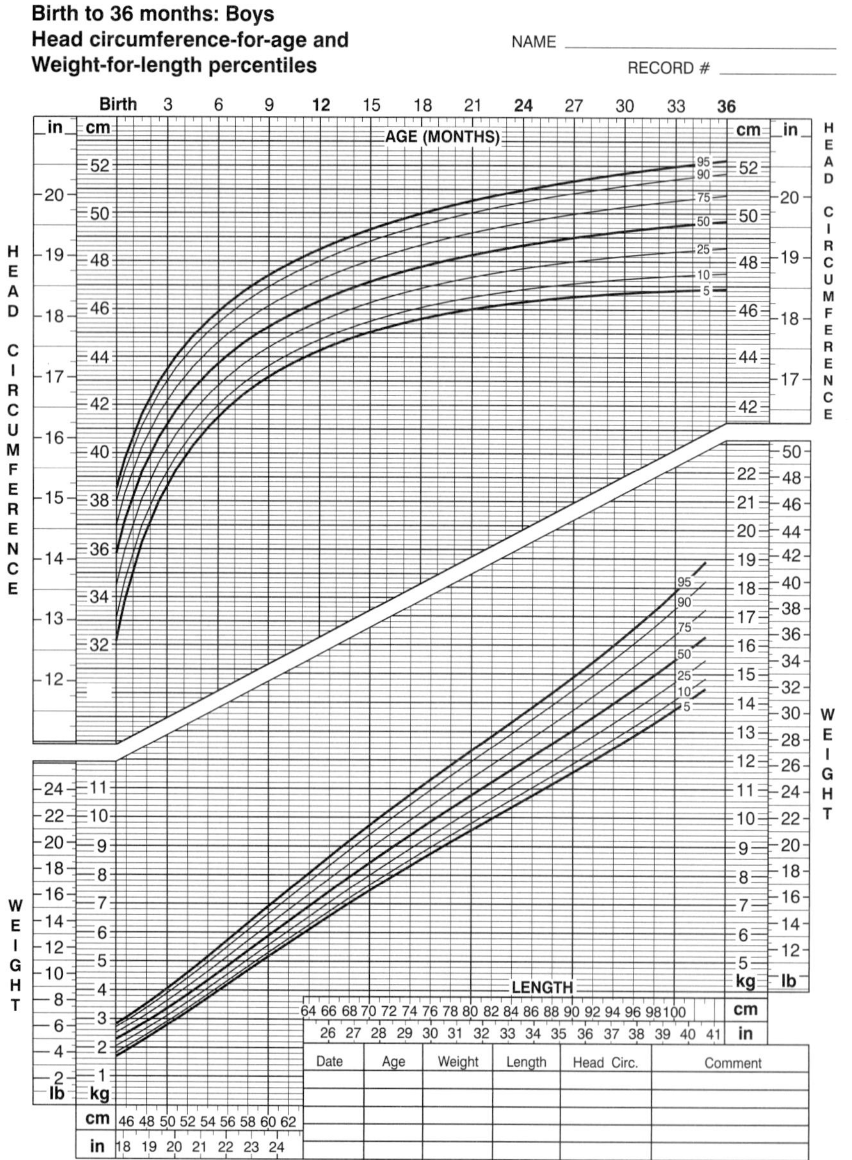

Published May 30, 2000 (modified 10/16/00).
SOURCE: Developed by the National Center for Health Statistics in collaboration with the National Center for Chronic Disease Prevention and Health Promotion (2000).
http://www.cdc.gov/growthcharts

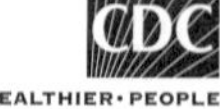

SAFER · HEALTHIER · PEOPLE™

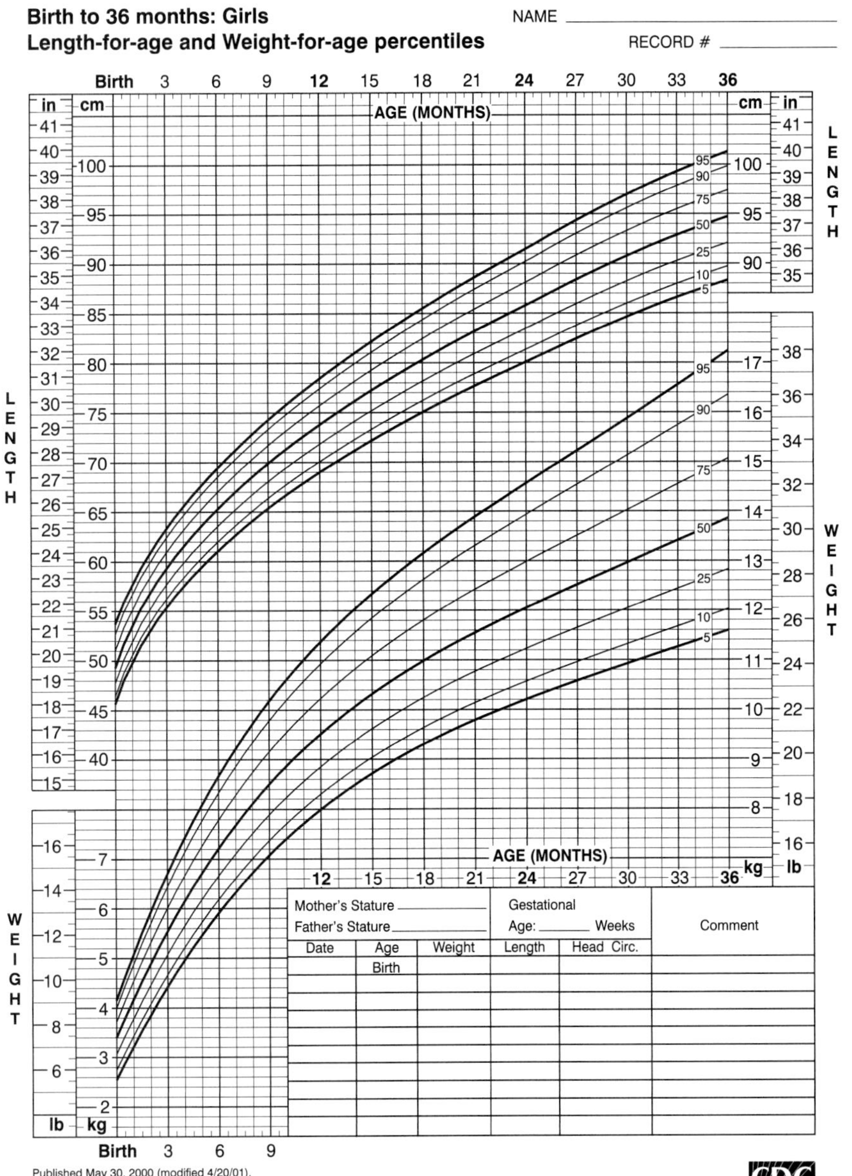

Published May 30, 2000 (modified 4/20/01).
SOURCE: Developed by the National Center for Health Statistics in collaboration with the National Center for Chronic Disease Prevention and Health Promotion (2000).
http://www.cdc.gov/growthcharts

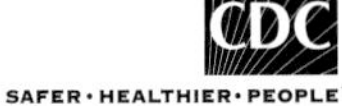

SAFER · HEALTHIER · PEOPLE™

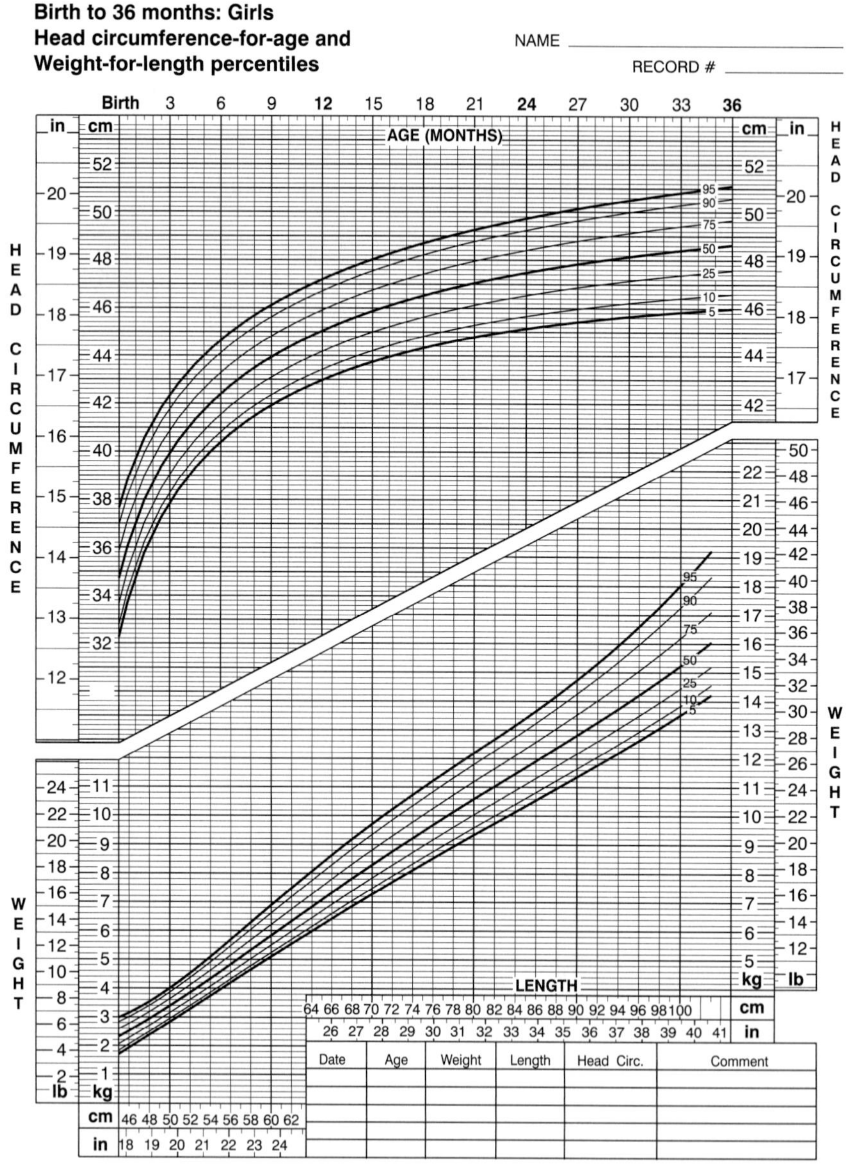
Birth to 36 months: Girls
Head circumference-for-age and
Weight-for-length percentiles
NAME
RECORD #
Birth 3 6 9 12 15 18 21 24 27 30 33 36
AGE (MONTHS)
HEAD CIRCUMFERENCE
WEIGHT
LENGTH
Date Age Weight Length Head Circ. Comment
Published May 30, 2000 (modified 10/16/00).
SOURCE: Developed by the National Center for Health Statistics in collaboration with
the National Center for Chronic Disease Prevention and Health Promotion (2000).
http://www.cdc.gov/growthcharts
SAFER · HEALTHIER · PEOPLE™

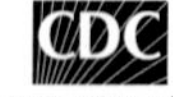
CDC

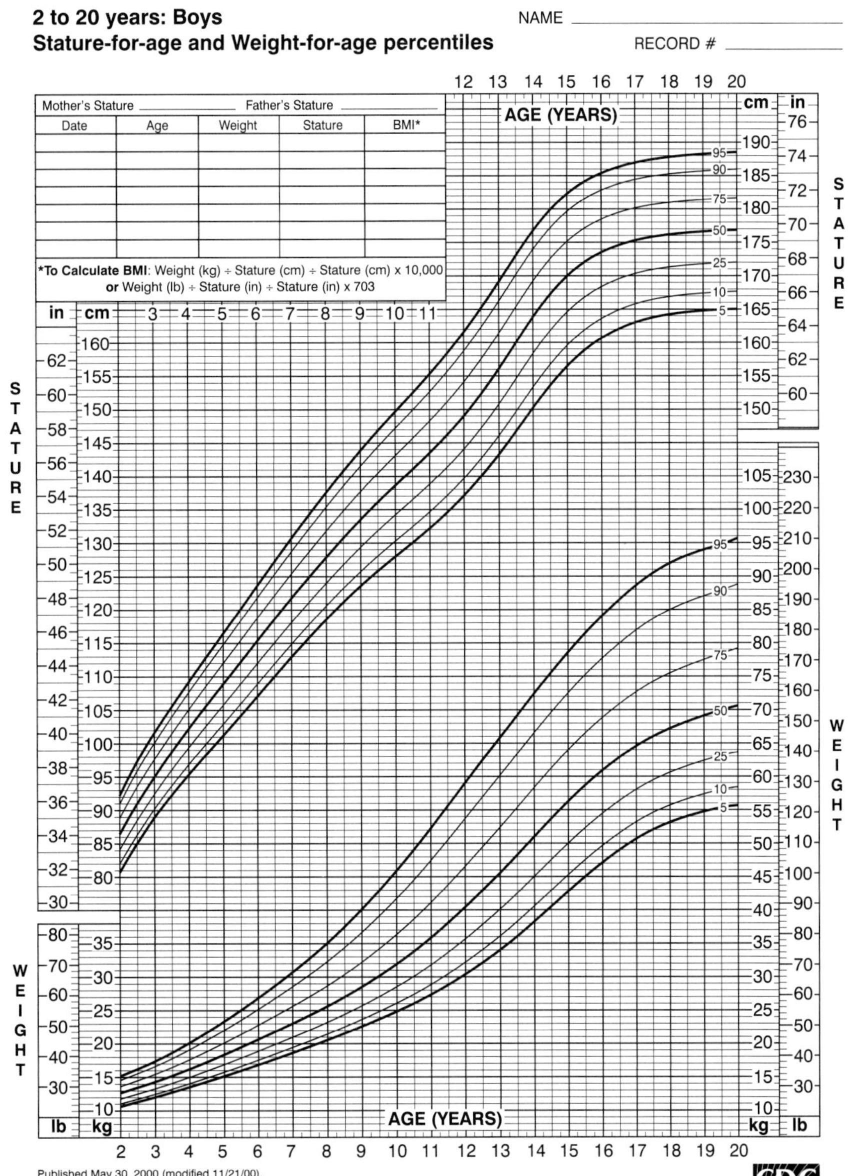
2 to 20 years: Boys
Stature-for-age and Weight-for-age percentiles
NAME
RECORD #
Mother's Stature
Father's Stature
Date
Age
Weight
Stature
BMI*
*To Calculate BMI: Weight (kg) ÷ Stature (cm) ÷ Stature (cm) x 10,000
or Weight (lb) ÷ Stature (in) ÷ Stature (in) x 703
AGE (YEARS)
STATURE
WEIGHT
in
cm
kg
lb
95
90
75
50
25
10
5
2 3 4 5 6 7 8 9 10 11 12 13 14 15 16 17 18 19 20
Published May 30, 2000 (modified 11/21/00).
SOURCE: Developed by the National Center for Health Statistics in collaboration with
the National Center for Chronic Disease Prevention and Health Promotion (2000).
http://www.cdc.gov/growthcharts

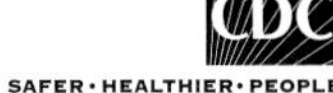
CDC
SAFER • HEALTHIER • PEOPLE™

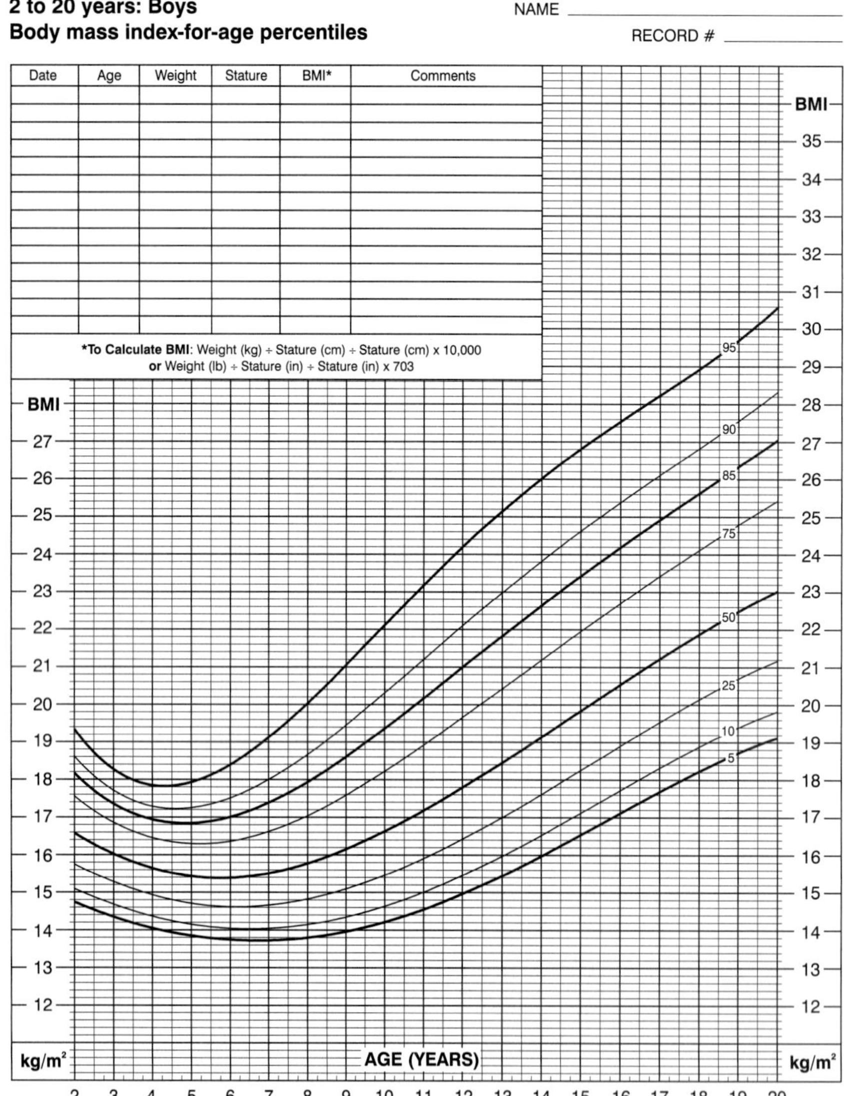

Published May 30, 2000 (modified 10/16/00).
SOURCE: Developed by the National Center for Health Statistics in collaboration with the National Center for Chronic Disease Prevention and Health Promotion (2000).
http://www.cdc.gov/growthcharts

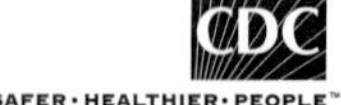

SAFER · HEALTHIER · PEOPLE™

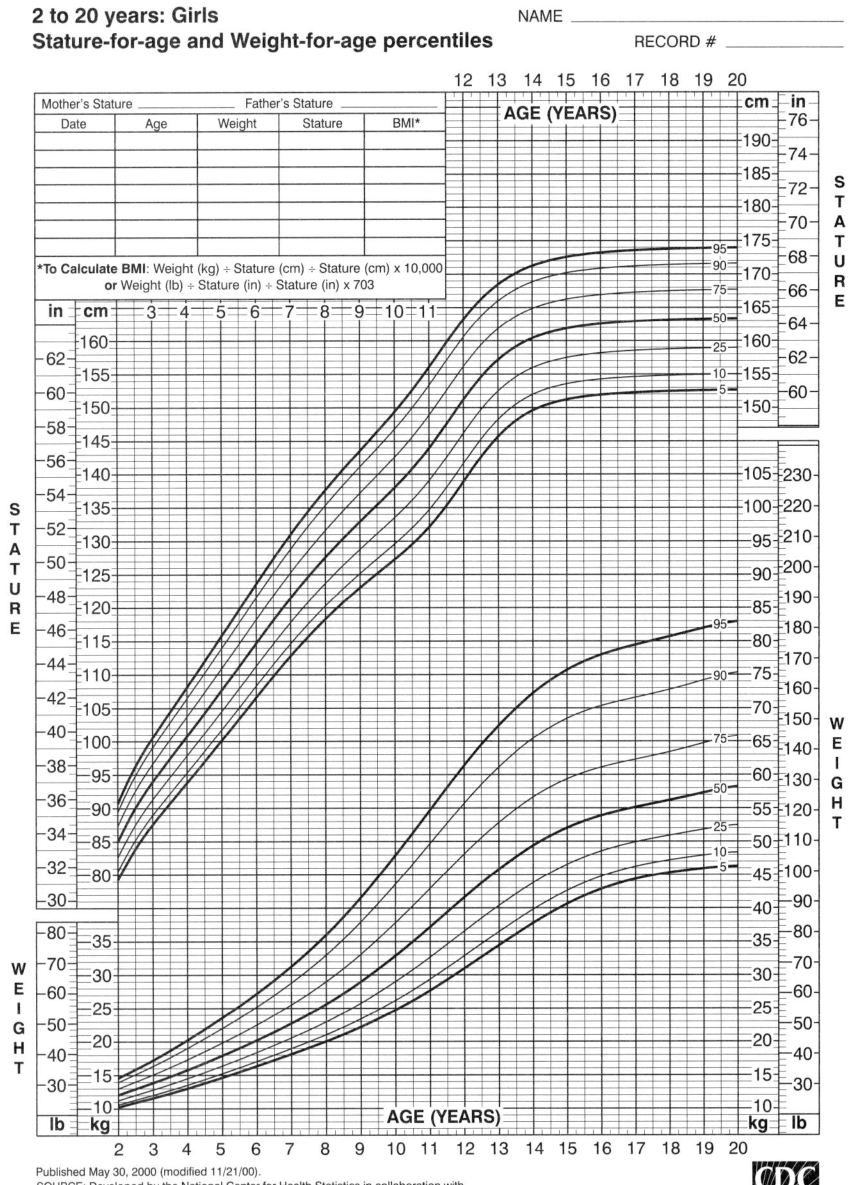
2 to 20 years: Girls
Stature-for-age and Weight-for-age percentiles
NAME
RECORD #
Mother's Stature
Father's Stature
Date
Age
Weight
Stature
BMI*
*To Calculate BMI: Weight (kg) ÷ Stature (cm) ÷ Stature (cm) x 10,000
or Weight (lb) ÷ Stature (in) ÷ Stature (in) x 703
AGE (YEARS)
STATURE
WEIGHT
in
cm
kg
lb
Published May 30, 2000 (modified 11/21/00).
SOURCE: Developed by the National Center for Health Statistics in collaboration with
the National Center for Chronic Disease Prevention and Health Promotion (2000).
http://www.cdc.gov/growthcharts
CDC
SAFER • HEALTHIER • PEOPLE™

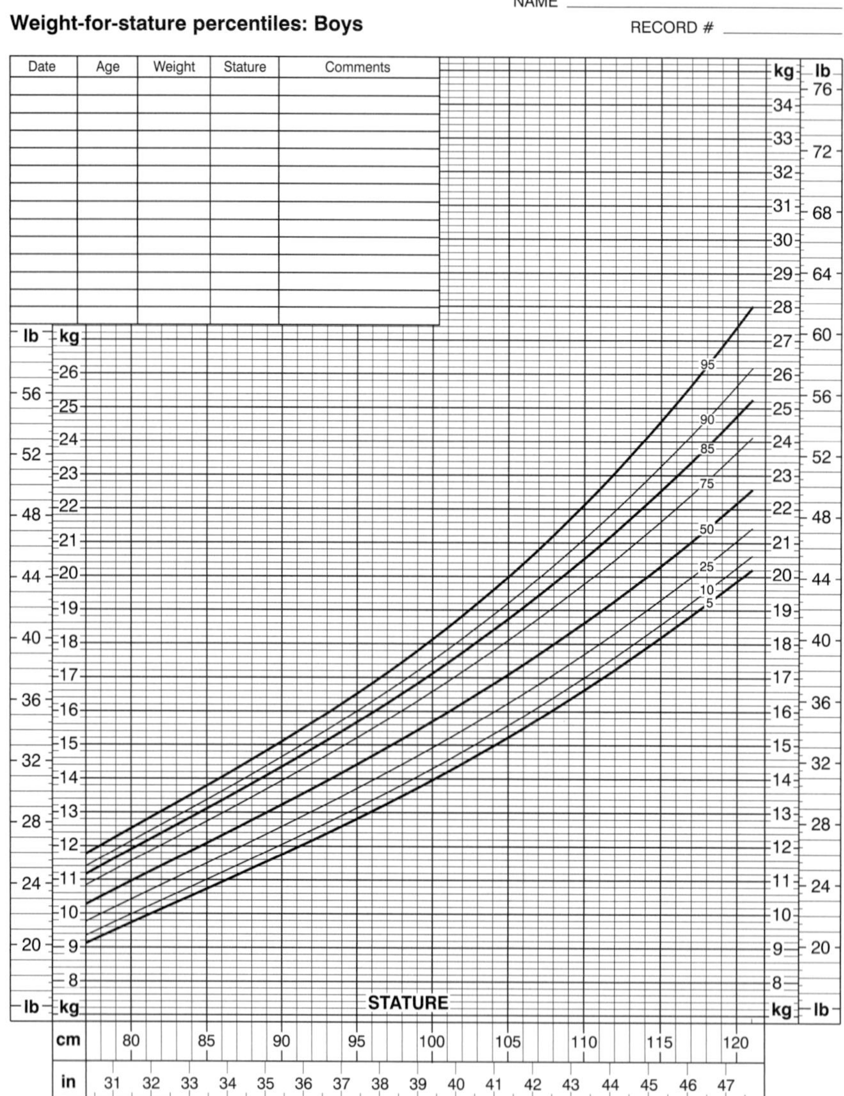

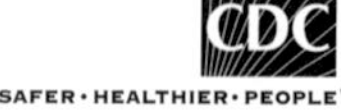

Published May 30, 2000 (modified 10/16/00).
SOURCE: Developed by the National Center for Health Statistics in collaboration with the National Center for Chronic Disease Prevention and Health Promotion (2000).
http://www.cdc.gov/growthcharts

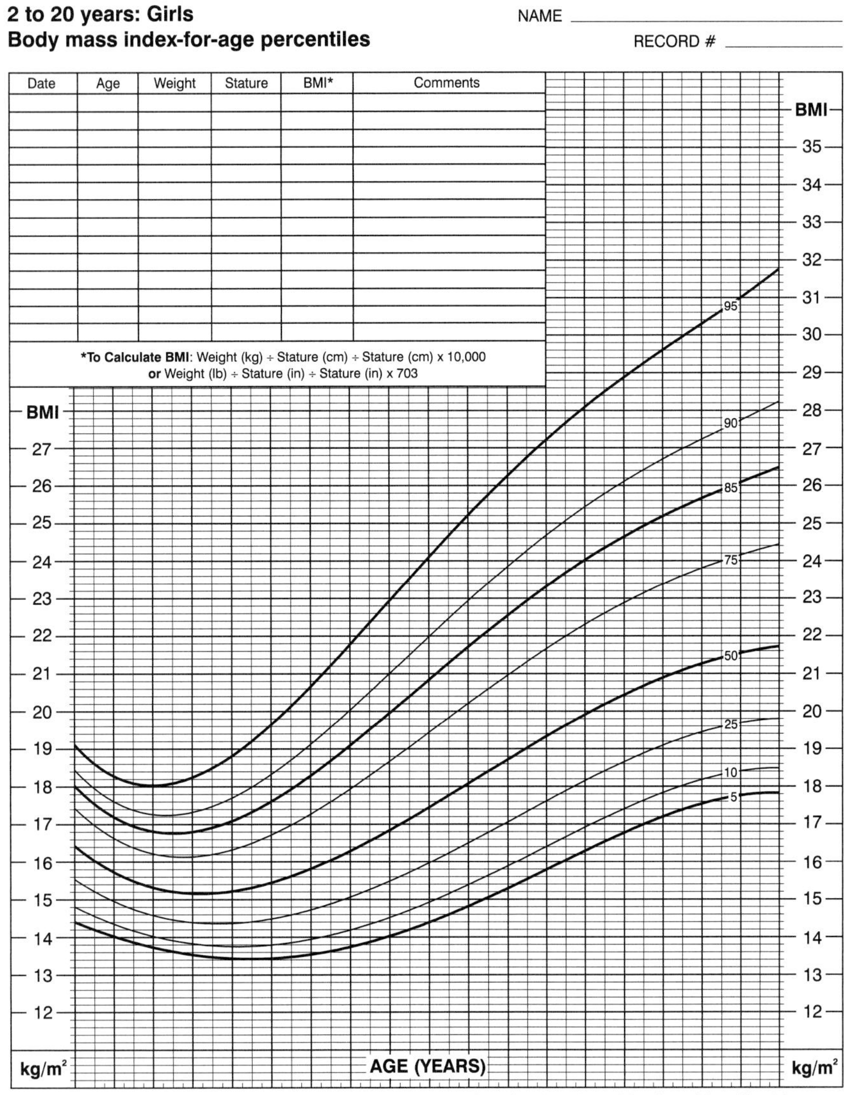

Published May 30, 2000 (modified 10/16/00).
SOURCE: Developed by the National Center for Health Statistics in collaboration with
the National Center for Chronic Disease Prevention and Health Promotion (2000).
http://www.cdc.gov/growthcharts

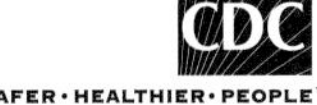

SAFER • HEALTHIER • PEOPLE™

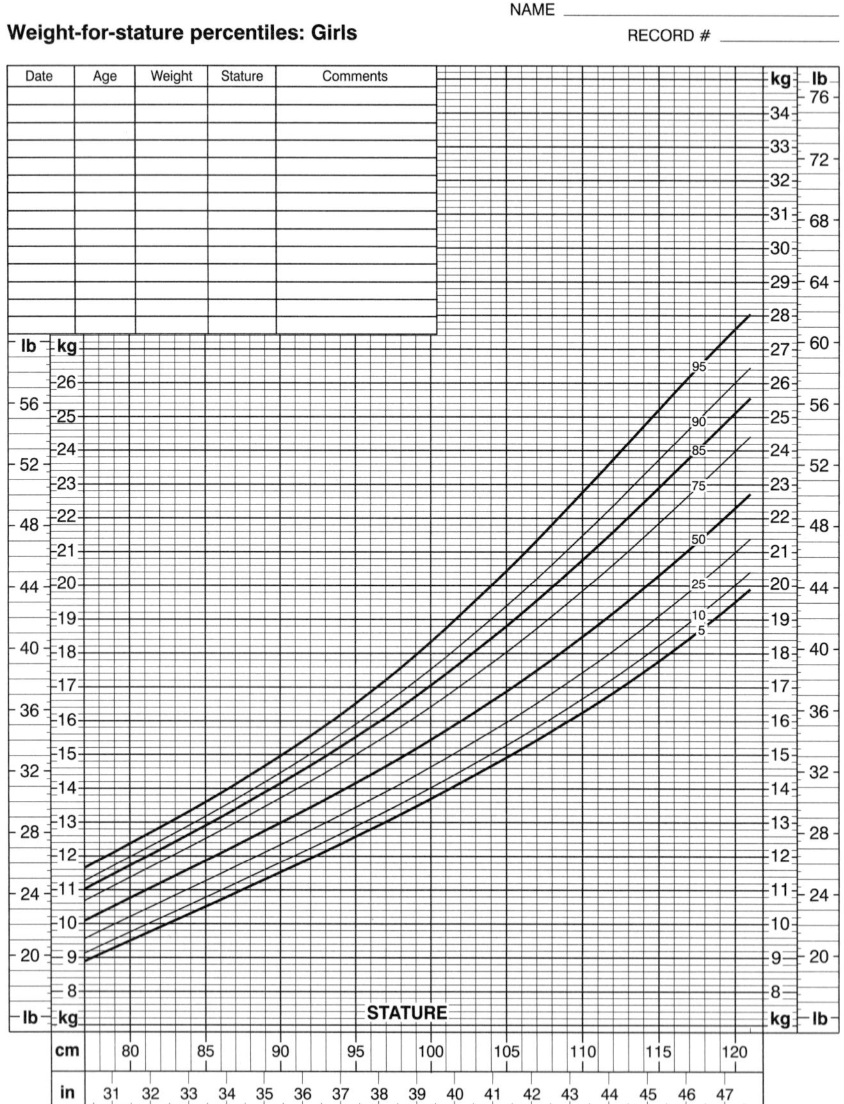

Published May 30, 2000 (modified 10/16/00).
SOURCE: Developed by the National Center for Health Statistics in collaboration with the National Center for Chronic Disease Prevention and Health Promotion (2000).
http://www.cdc.gov/growthcharts

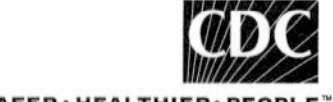

SAFER • HEALTHIER • PEOPLE™

APPENDIX C

Guidelines

Guidelines for Cultural Assessment*

According to Purnell and Paulanka (2003), culture is the "totality of socially transmitted behavioral patterns, arts, beliefs, values, customs, lifeways, and all other products of human work and thought characteristics of a population of people that guide their worldview and decision making."

Because cultural background encompasses every aspect of a person's life, you need to be aware of how it influences your client's health and wellness. Consider the following areas when determining the influence of culture on your client's health.

Overview

- Inhabited localities and topography
  - In what part of the world does this person's cultural or ethnic group originate?
  - What is the climate and topography there?
- Heritage and residence
  - Where does this person's cultural or ethnic group reside now?
  - What is the approximate population of the group here?
- Reason for migration and associated economic factors
  - What were the major factors that motivated this person's cultural/ethnic group to emigrate?
  - What were the economic or political factors that influenced this group's acculturation and professional development in America?
- Educational status and occupations
  - What value does the person's cultural group place on education?
  - What are the predominant occupations of the group's members?

Communication

- Dominant language and dialects
  - What is the dominant language of the group?
  - Does the person use that language or a dialect that may interfere with communication?
  - Are there specific contextual speech patterns for this group? If so, what are they?
  - What is the usual volume and tone of speech?
- Cultural communication patterns
  - Is the person willing to share thoughts, feelings, and ideas?
  - What is the practice and meaning of touch in the person's society? With family, friends, strangers, same sex, opposite sex, and healthcare providers?
  - What are the personal spatial and distancing characteristics when communicating one-to-one? With friends vs. strangers?
  - Does this group use eye contact? Does avoidance of eye contact have special meaning? Is eye contact influenced by socioeconomic status?
  - Do various facial expressions have specific meanings? Are facial expressions used to express emotions?
  - Are there acceptable ways of standing and greeting outsiders? If so, what are they?
- Temporal relationships
  - Are people primarily past, present, or future oriented? How do they see the context of past, present, and future?
  - Are there differences in interpretation of social time versus clock time? If so, what are they?
  - Are people expected to be punctual in terms of jobs, appointments, and social engagements?
- Format and names
  - What is the format for a person's name?
  - How does one expect to be greeted by strangers and healthcare practitioners?

Family Roles and Organization

- Head of household and gender roles
  - Who is the perceived head of household?
  - How does this role change during different developmental aspects of life?
  - What are the gender-related roles of men and women in the family system?
- Prescriptive, restrictive, and taboo behaviors
  - What are the prescriptive, restrictive, and taboo behaviors for children?
  - What are the prescriptive, restrictive, and taboo behaviors for adults?
- Family roles and priorities
  - What family goals and priorities are emphasized by this culture?
  - What are the developmental tasks of this group?
  - What is the status and role of older people in the family?
  - What are the roles and importance of extended family members?
  - How does one gain social status in this cultural system? Is there a caste system?
- Alternative lifestyles
  - How are alternative lifestyles and nontraditional families viewed by the society?

*Source: Adapted from Purnell & Paulanka, 2003.

Workforce Issues

- Culture in the workplace
  - Are workforce issues, such as education, affected by immigration? If so, how?
  - What are the specific multicultural considerations when working with this culturally diverse person or group?
  - What factors influence patterns of acculturation in this cultural group?
  - How do the person's or group's healthcare practices influence the workforce?
- Issues related to autonomy
  - What are the cultural issues related to professional autonomy, superior or subordinate control, religion, and gender in the workforce?
  - Are there language barriers? For example, do people sometimes misunderstand English expressions by interpreting them concretely?

Biocultural Ecology

- Skin color and biologic variations
  - Are there skin color and physical variations for this group? If so, what are they?
  - What special problems or concerns might the skin color pose for healthcare practitioners?
  - What are the biologic variations in body habitus or structure?
- Diseases and health conditions
  - What are the risk factors for people related to topography or climate?
  - Are there any hereditary or genetic diseases or conditions that are common with this group? If so, what are they?
  - Are there any endemic diseases specific to this cultural or ethnic group? If so, what are they?
  - Are there any diseases or health conditions for which this group has increased susceptibility? If so, what are they?
- Variations in drug metabolism
  - Does this group have any specific variations in drug metabolism, drug interactions, and related side effects? If so, what are they?

High-Risk Behaviors

- Are any high-risk behaviors common in this group? If so, what are they?
- What are the patterns of use of alcohol, tobacco, recreational drugs, and other substances in this group?

Healthcare Practices

- What are typical health-seeking behaviors for this group?
- What is this group's usual level of physical activity?
- Do people use safety measures, such as seat belts?

Nutrition

- Meaning of food
  - What does food mean to this group?
- Common foods and food rituals
  - What specific foods, preparation practices, and major ingredients are commonly used by this group?
  - Are there any specific food rituals for this group? If so, what are they?
- Dietary practices for health promotion
  - Are enzyme deficiencies or food intolerances commonly experienced by this group? If so, what are they?
  - Are large-scale or significant nutritional deficiencies experienced by this group? If so, what are they?
  - Are there native food limitations in America that may cause special health difficulties? If so what are they?

Pregnancy and Childbearing Practices

- Fertility practices and views regarding pregnancy
  - What are the cultural views and practices related to fertility control?
  - What are the cultural views and practices regarding pregnancy?
- Prescriptive, restrictive, and taboo practices in the childbearing family
  - What are the prescriptive, restrictive, and taboo practices related to pregnancy, such as food, exercise, intercourse, and avoidance of weather-related conditions?
  - What are the prescriptive, restrictive, and taboo practices related to the birthing process, such as reactions during labor, presence of men, position of mother for delivery, preferred types of health practitioners, or place of delivery?
  - What are the prescriptive, restrictive, and taboo practices related to the postpartum period, such as bathing, cord care, exercise, food, and roles of men?

Death Rituals

- Death rituals and expectations
  - Are there culturally specific death rituals and expectations? If so, what are they?

- What is the purpose of the death rituals and mourning practices?
- What specific practices (e.g., cremation) are used for disposal of the body?

- Responses to death and grief
  - How are people expected to show grief and respond to the death of a family member?
  - What is the meaning of death, dying, and afterlife?

Spirituality

- Religious practices and use of prayer
  - How does the dominant religion of this group influence healthcare practices?
  - Are there activities such as prayer, meditation, or symbols that help people reach fulfillment? If so, what are they?
- Meaning of life and individual sources of strength
- What gives meaning to people's lives?
- What is the person's source of strength?
- Spiritual beliefs and healthcare practices
  - What is the relationship between spiritual beliefs and healthcare practices?

Healthcare Practices

- Health-seeking beliefs and behaviors
  - What predominant beliefs influence healthcare practices?
  - What is the influence of health promotion and prevention practices?
- Responsibility for health care
  - Is the focus of acute-care practice curative or fatalistic?
  - Who assumes responsibility for health care in this culture?
  - What is the role of health insurance in this culture?
  - What are the behaviors associated with the use of over-the-counter medications?
- Folklore practices
  - How do magicoreligious beliefs, folklore, and traditional beliefs influence healthcare behaviors?
- Barriers to health care
  - Are there barriers to health care such as language, economics, and geography for this group? If so, what are they?
- Cultural responses to health and illness
  - Are there cultural beliefs and responses to pain that influence interventions? If so, what are they?
  - Does pain have special meaning?
  - What are the beliefs and views about mental and physical illness in this culture?
  - Does this culture view mental handicaps differently from physical handicaps?
  - What are the cultural beliefs and practices related to chronicity and rehabilitation?
  - Are there any restrictions to the acceptance of blood transfusions, organ donation, and organ transplantation for this group? If so, what are they?

Healthcare Practitioners

- Traditional versus biomedical care
  - What are the roles of traditional, folklore, and magicoreligious practitioners, and how do they influence health practitioners?
  - How does this culture feel about healthcare practitioners providing care to patients of the opposite sex?
  - Does the age of the practitioner make a difference? If so, what?
- Status of healthcare providers
  - How does this culture feel about healthcare providers?
  - What is the status of healthcare providers in this culture?
  - How do different healthcare practitioners in this culture view each other?

Example: Cuban-Americans

Overview

- Cubans are of Hispanic origin.
- Culture influenced by Spain, United States, and Soviet Union.
- 860,000 in the United States, mainly in New York and Florida
- Cuban climate tropical
- Political and economic reasons for immigration
- Educational attainment higher than other Hispanic groups.
- High proportion self-employed
- High proportion in industry, such as wholesale/retail trade, banking/credit, insurance, and real estate

Communication

- Dominant language is Spanish.
- Values *simpatico*—smooth interpersonal relationships, courtesy, respect without harsh criticism
- *Personalismo*—interpersonal relationships more important than bureaucratic relationships
- *Choteo*—light-hearted attitude with teasing and bantering
- Animated facial expressions, eye contact, hand gestures, speech loud and fast
- Touching in form of handshakes and hugs
- More present oriented, deal with current issues, use a flexible time frame, which may make appointment setting difficult

- Feel a sense of "specialness" about themselves and culture and convey this in communication
- Use both mother's and father's surnames. For example, Regina Morales Colon, in which Morales is the patriarchal surname and Colon the matriarchal. If Regina marries Mr. Ordonez, she would drop the matriarchal name and add her husband's name, becoming Regina Morales de Ordonez.

Family Roles and Organization

- Family is most important unit.
- Patriarchal, male dominant, and aggressive; female dependent.
- Double standard applied to male and female behavior.
- Children are pampered and protected.
- Children are expected to respect parents, follow *el buen camino*—the straight and narrow.
- Expectations for boys and girls are different.
- Families are tightly knit.
- Family is most important source of emotional and physical support
- *Compaadrazgo* (godparents) are considered part of family.
- High proportion of older persons live with family members.
- High proportion of women are divorced.
- Gay lifestyle is contradictory to prevailing machismo image.

Workforce Issues

- Have been economically successful in United States, with 57 percent employed in professional and technical jobs.
- Many own businesses.
- Tend to be lineal in relationships at work, rather than collegial.
- Carry concept of personalismo through to work.
- May speak Spanish when talking with Cuban friends and family and speak English professionally.

Biocultural Ecology

- Skin and hair vary from light to dark.
- Slightly higher incidence of obesity than other Hispanic groups.
- Lower incidence of hypertension than whites and blacks.
- High incidence of dental problems may be a result of diet high in sugars and starches.
- 42 percent of Cuban men smoke.
- Cuban-American women in 30s have higher incidence of smoking than national average.
- High mortality rates among adolescents and young adult because of violence.
- Suicide rates higher than white non-Hispanics.
- A little heaviness seen as attractive. Diets are high in calories, starches, and saturated fats.
- Have high levels of preventative health behaviors.

Nutrition

- Food has powerful social meaning—promotes sense of community, perpetuates customs and heritage.
- Root crops are staples, such as yams, yucca, malanga, boniato, plantains, and grains.
- Main course is meat, pork, or chicken.
- Diet high in calories, starches, and saturated fats.
- Leisurely noon meal and late dinner.
- Diet lacking in leafy green vegetables (fiber).

Pregnancy and Childbearing Practices

- Low rate of reproduction
- Many folk beliefs about pregnancy. For example, believe you need to eat for two, which leads to excessive weight gain during pregnancy.
- Childbirth is time of celebration.
- Traditionally, men do not participate in birthing.
- Family members and friends often care for the mother and baby for 4 weeks postpartum.
- Breastfeeding considered better than bottle. Child is weaned early at 3 months and introduced to solid foods.
- Believe that fat child is healthy child.
- Believe that breastfeeding can lead to deformity or asymmetry of breasts.

Death Rituals

- Large gathering of family at deathbed.
- Death rite may include animal sacrifice or *santería*.
- Candles used after death to light path to afterlife.
- Wake (*velorio*) lasts 2 to 3 days until funeral.
- Bereavement is expressed openly.
- Relatives light candles, pray, and visit gravesite on anniversary of death

Spirituality

- 85% Catholic
- Devoted to Blessed Virgin Mary, Jesus, and saints.
- Pictures of saints (*estampitas*) may be placed under pillow or beside bed of someone who is ill.
- Formal religious observance is an important source of support.
- Family is most important source of strength, identity, and emotional security.
- Take fatalistic view, feeling they have no control over circumstances influencing life.
- Practice folk remedies, most of which are harmless.

Healthcare Practices

- Family is primary source of health advice, usually older woman in the family.
- Poverty may be a barrier to health care.
- Herbal teas used to treat common ailments.
- Loneliness, depression, anger, anxiety may occur from losses caused by migrating from homeland.
- Dependency acceptable with sick role.
- Blood transfusions acceptable.
- Use both traditional and biomedical health care.
- Underrepresented in healthcare occupations.

Guidelines for Environmental Assessment*

Shorter stays in acute-care settings have increased the need for nursing care at home. Home care nursing can occur at both the primary and tertiary levels. At the primary care level, you will make postpartum visits to new mothers and babies. At the tertiary level, you will make follow-up visits to patients discharged from the hospital.

Assessing the Home

In the home, your assessment is based on the health history and physical examination findings. You need to assess your patient's response to the treatment plan and also identify any risk factors in his environment that may affect his or her health and well-being. Remember, the treatment plan established in the hospital will be effective only if your patient is able to follow it at home.

Begin by determining if your patient is able to perform activities of daily living (ADLs); then assess basic needs and environmental safety hazards. Also assess support systems and self-esteem or self-actualization. Keep in mind that financial status and religious and cultural beliefs will influence health beliefs and practices.

Assessing the Home

AREAS/QUESTIONS TO ASK	RATIONALE/SIGNIFICANCE
Physical Needs	
Food What does the patient eat and drink? Who prepares food? Who buys food? Is food being stored properly? Is kitchen accessible? Clean? Are appliances in good operating condition? If you detect a nutritional deficit, does patient's illness have an effect on appetite? Is there an unexplained weight loss or gain? Does the patient drink alcohol? Does he or she have a dental problem? Are financial hardships limiting purchase of foods? Is the patient taking multiple medicines? Does he or she eat alone? Does he or she need assistance in eating?	Identifies: • Need for referrals for assistance, such as financial support, Meals on Wheels, home health aides. • Self-care deficits • Teaching needs • Nutritional deficits or problems affecting nutritional status
Elimination Is the bathroom accessible? Does patient need a commode? Does he or she need a raised toilet seat? Grab bars?	Identifies: • Need for assistive devices • Self-care deficits • Risk for falls • Risk for incontinence problems
Bathing Does patient take baths, showers, or sponge baths? Does he or she care for his or her hair and teeth? Does he or she need assistance in bathing? Does he or she have a shower chair? Does the bathtub have grab bars? Rubber mats? Nonskid tiles?	Identifies: • Need for assistive devices • Self-care deficits • Risk for falls

*Compiled By Patricia M. Dillon, RN, MSN, DNSc

Assessing the Home

AREAS/QUESTIONS TO ASK	RATIONALE/SIGNIFICANCE
Dressing Does patient have clean clothes? Do clothes fit? Does he or she need assistance with dressing? Do shoes fit properly? Who does the laundry?	Identifies: • Self-care deficits • Risks for falls or skin breakdown • Need for home health aide
Sleep Where does the patient sleep? How much time does he or she spend in bed? Does the patient need a special mattress or bed? Are bedrails needed? How far is the bed from the bathroom? From other family members? Is there privacy for members in household?	Identifies • Risk for skin breakdown • Need for special equipment • Safety issues
Medications Is patient able to take own medications as prescribed? Is he or she taking any over-the-counter medications, vitamins, or herbal supplements? Does he or she need medications pre-poured? Does he or she have any impairments that would prevent him or her from self-administering medications safely (e.g., cognitive or visual impairments)? Are medications safely stored? Can patient open medication containers? If using syringes, how does patient dispose of them? Obtain supplies? What is the name of patient's pharmacy? His or her medication insurance plan? Does patient have the finances to pay for medications and treatment? Does patient understand what medications he or she is taking and their purpose?	Identifies: • Compliance with medical treatment plan and reasons for noncompliance • Problems associated with polypharmacy (e.g., side effects, drug interactions) • Safety issue surrounding medication preparation and administration • Need for assistive devices • Need for referral or visiting nurse • Teaching needs • Financial needs for obtaining prescriptions
Shelter Is home maintained and clean? Who is responsible for managing and cleaning it? Are plumbing and sewage systems working properly? What type of heating is there (gas, electric, oil, wood)? Central heating or space heating? Is heating system working properly? Is there air conditioning? Fans? Is ventilation adequate? Do windows open and close easily and completely? What type of insulation is there? Is home in need of repair (e.g., peeling paint or cracks in foundation or windows)? Is there evidence of insect or rodent infestation? Has home been tested for radon?	Identifies: • Safety issues • Need for referrals • Need for assistance with home management and maintenance
Assessing Environmental Safety	
Mobility/Fall Prevention Is patient able to walk? Is his or her gait steady? Does patient use assistive devices correctly? Do devices fit through pathways and doorways? Is house one level or more? Are there elevators or stairs?	Identifies: • Risk for fall/injury • Need for assistive devices • Need for referrals • Need for teaching

(Continued)

Assessing the Home *(Continued)*

AREAS/QUESTIONS TO ASK	RATIONALE/SIGNIFICANCE
Mobility/Fall Prevention (Continued) Can patient enter and exit home without difficulty? Are pathways and stairs clear? Are there throw rugs? Are there sturdy handrails on the stairs? Are first and last steps clearly marked? Are floors slippery or uneven? Is there adequate lighting in hallways, stairs, and path to bathroom? Is there need for restraints? If yes, what type and when? Are carpets in good repair without tears? Can patient walk on carpet? Does he or she have to hold onto furniture to maintain balance? If yes, is furniture sturdy and stable enough to provide support? Are chairs sturdy and stable? Are there any cords or wires that may present a tripping hazard?	
Fire/Burn Prevention Are there working smoke detectors on each floor? Carbon monoxide detectors? Fire extinguisher? Is there an escape plan in case of fire? Are wires, plugs, and electrical equipment in good working condition? Is client using a heating pad or portable heaters safely? Does he or she smoke? If yes, does he or she smoke safely? Are there signs of cigarette burns? Are there signs of burns in the kitchen? Is stove free of grease? Does patient use oxygen? If yes, is tank stored safely away from heat or flame?	Identifies: • Risk for injury • Safety issues • Teaching needs • Referrals (e.g., local fire company for free smoke detectors)
Crime/Injury Are there working locks on doors and windows? Is client able to make emergency calls? Are emergency numbers readily available? Is phone readily accessible? Are there firearms in home? If yes, are they safely secured with ammunition stored separately? Is there any evidence of criminal activity? Are poisonous or toxic substances properly stored?	Identifies safety issues • Need for referral to local police • Teaching needs
Assessing Support Systems, Self-Esteem, and Self-Actualization	
Roles What roles does person play because of illness? How has this affected other family members?	Identifies: • Source of stress, depression, and anxiety • Need for referrals
Caregivers Is there a caregiver? Is caregiver competent, willing, and supportive? Does caregiver need support? Can caregiver hear client? Is there a need for an intercom, "baby monitor," or bell?	Identifies • Supports • Need for referrals (e.g., caregiver may need support, respite care, or home health aide). • Need for assistive devices • Teaching needs
Communication Is phone in easy reach?	Identifies: • Emergency supports

Assessing the Home

AREAS/QUESTIONS TO ASK	RATIONALE/SIGNIFICANCE
Communication *(Continued)* Can client dial phone and see numbers? Does he or she need oversized numbers, audio enhancer, or a memory feature? Is there a daily safety check system? Should there be an alert system like Lifeline? Are emergency numbers for police, fire, ambulance, nurse, doctor, relative, or neighbor clearly marked? How does patient get mail?	Identifies: • Teaching needs • Need for assistive devices • Safety issues
Family/Friends/Pets Who visits patient? Family, friends, church members? Who can drive patient to doctor appointments, church, and other places? Are there any pets? Is patient able to take care of them properly? Are pets well behaved?	Identifies: • Supports • Need for referrals • Ability to maintain follow-up care • Teaching needs
Self-Esteem and Self-Actualization What does client like to do? Are there creative ways to enable him or her to do activities he or she enjoys? Are there meaningful solitary activities patient can do, such as reading or listening to music? Interactive activities?	Identifies: • Sources of meaning in patient's life • Need for referral to community resources (e.g., library, senior citizen groups).

Source: Adapted with permission from Narayan, M. (1997). Environmental assessment, *Home Healthcare Nurse, 15* (11): p. 798. Lippincott-Raven.

Assessing the Community

According to Smith and Maurer, a community is an "open social system characterized by people in a place over time who have common goals." Some examples of a community are a town, a school, or a nursing home. Assessment involves assessing the people within the community, the environment of the community, and the interaction between the two to identify any actual or potential health problems.

Assessing the Community

QUESTIONS TO ASK YOURSELF	RATIONALE/SIGNIFICANCE
Boundaries What is the geographic description of the community (e.g., a town) or the criteria for membership in the community (e.g., a school)?	Can be real, concrete or conceptual. Identify who and what is included in the community.
What are the neighboring areas (e.g., a city if the community is a suburb, or an archdiocese if the community is a private Catholic school)?	Allows you to focus assessment on the community.
Are boundaries open or closed?	Some boundaries may exclude certain groups (e.g., communities with only high-priced housing may exclude lower socioeconomic groups).
What is the purpose or goals of the community (e.g., a school's mission statement)?	Reflects purpose of community. For example, the goal of a Catholic school would be to educate children in Christian values.

(Continued)

Assessing the Community *(Continued)*

QUESTIONS TO ASK YOURSELF	RATIONALE/SIGNIFICANCE
Physical Characteristics	
How old is the community?	Older, well-established community may have more resources available than new, developing community. Or, older community's resources may be outdated, not meeting current needs.
What are community's demographics (e.g., age, race, sex, ethnicity, housing, density of population)?	Can identify health care needs of community by identifying health problems associated with age, gender, or race. For example: • Older adults have a higher incidence of health problems and need more services than younger adults. • Hypertension (HTN) screening services are greater for black males because they have a higher incidence of this problem. • Women need women's healthcare services such as breast self-exam teaching and mammography. • Ethnic groups may have specific health concerns. Cultural beliefs, values, and customs influence what and how health issues are addressed. • Type and condition of housing influences health (e.g., overcrowding increases incidence of communicable diseases). Also reflects how community values individual members.
What are community's physical features?	• Can influence community's behavior and health (e.g., exposure to toxic substances).
Psychosocial Characteristics	
What is the community's predominant religion, socioeconomic class, educational level, type of occupation, and marital status?	Religion influences what and how health issues are addressed (e.g., abortion/birth control contradicts Catholic beliefs). Socioeconomic class reflects affordability and accessibility of health care services. People in

Assessing the Community

QUESTIONS TO ASK YOURSELF	RATIONALE/SIGNIFICANCE
Psychosocial Characteristics *(Continued)*	low socioeconomic areas may not have financial resources for health care or be able to practice preventive health care. Limited financial access to health care raises community's morbidity and mortality rates.
	Educational level identifies health teaching needs and approaches. The higher their educational level, the more likely people are to practice preventative health behaviors.
	Occupation can identify specific health issues for the group (e.g., blue-collar workers may have a higher incidence of musculoskeletal problems, whereas white-collar workers may have a higher incidence of stress-related diseases).
	Marital status may identify stability and support sources within community.
External Influences	
Does the community receive any external funding?	Federal or state funding and grants may be available for health services.
Are there facilities outside community that are available to community members? Is there access/transportation to these facilities? Are adequate healthcare providers available to community?	Identifies healthcare facilities needed (e.g., rural areas may need to go outside community for health services).
Are volunteer groups available to the community?	Volunteer groups can be a valuable resource, especially if healthcare providers are limited.
How is health information communicated to community?	Determines if there is a need for further and better means of communication.
What laws affect the community?	Laws, such as zoning or pollution laws, can influence healthcare issues. Federal and state programs also can affect the health and well being of the community, such as senior citizens.
Are values of external influences consistent with those of community?	Inconsistent values can affect health care issues. For example, a rural community may depend on federal funding for free

(Continued)

Assessing the Community *(Continued)*

QUESTIONS TO ASK YOURSELF	RATIONALE/SIGNIFICANCE
External Influences *(Continued)*	mammograms, but the amount of funding fails to adequately cover the service. Or a community may feel that cleaning up a polluted stream is urgent, but external influences may disagree.
Internal Functions	
Human Services	
What human services are available within community? Nurses, doctors, volunteers? Is access to services adequate?	Determines if services meet community's needs.
What is community's budget? How much is allocated for healthcare services?	Identifies value of healthcare services and need for external funding sources.
What and how many healthcare facilities (hospitals, nursing homes, daycare) are available in community? Are there enough to meet people's needs? Are they well equipped? Accessible?	Determines availability and accessibility of health care facilities.
Does facility have goods and supplies to produce its goods? What is the product? What is the facility's contribution to the community?	Identifies both positive and negative effects to community (e.g., if facility is drug treatment center, drug dealers and abusers, as a community in itself, exert a negative effect on community at large).
Is education appropriate, accessible, and adequate for community? What types of schools are there? How much money is budgeted for education?	Identifies adequacy and availability of schools.
Politics	
What is the organizational structure of the community? Elected vs. appointed positions? Terms? Formal vs. informal leaders?	Helps identify how decisions are made and who has power.
How are decisions made? Majority rule or consensus? Is community independent or dependent?	Identifies approaches needed to bring about change. Identifies role of nurse within community (e.g., if community is dependent, nurse may need to take more active role).
What are rules and laws of community?	Identifies laws that regulate behaviors.
Formal and informal?	Identifies expectations, peer pressures.
Communication	
Nonverbal: What is personality of community? How do people respond to outsiders?	Identifies approaches toward community.
Verbal: Who communicates with whom? What are means of communication? Is communication vertical or horizontal?	
Values	
What does the community value? What is important?	Identifies what is important to community.
Does the community have any traditions?	Can influence healthcare practices.

Assessing the Community

QUESTIONS TO ASK YOURSELF	RATIONALE/SIGNIFICANCE
Values *(Continued)*	
Are there subgroups within the community?	Can have own values and norms that affect community and influence healthcare practices.
What is the condition of the physical environment? Clean, dirty, in disrepair?	Condition of environment reflects value place on it by community.
How is health defined by the community?	Identifies value community places on health.
How much does community value health?	
What type of health care facilities are there? How frequently are they used?	
Is the community homogeneous or heterogenous?	Identifies approaches toward community.
Health Behavior/Health Status	
People	
What is the growth rate of the community? Relationship between birth and death rates? Relationship between immigration and emigration? Is population young or old? Is it mobile?	Identifies health status and needs of community (e.g., health needs for retirement community are different from those of a community with mostly young couples). Indirectly identifies teaching needs. Identifies factors within community that affect health.
What are morbidity and mortality rates? The prevalence and incidence of disease?	Identifies focus and direction of health care needed by community. Identifies health teaching needs for community.
What types of risky behavior occur in the community? Are there at-risk groups?	Identifies at-risk groups (e.g., homeless, drug addicts). Identifies need for intervention and teaching (e.g., binge drinking on college campuses).
What is the incidence of presymptomatic illnesses, such as HIV, HTN, or high cholesterol?	Identifies need for screening programs. Determines effectiveness of existing screening programs. Identifies health teaching needs.
What is the level of functioning of community (e.g., dependent vs. independent)?	Identifies type and direction of intervention needed to maintain and promote health.
Are there people with disabilities? How many people and what types of disabilities?	Identifies resources required to meet need of community members with disabilities.
Environment	
What is the quality of the air?	Identifies possible exposure to pollutants.
What is the quality of the food supply?	Identifies possible contamination causing gastrointestinal (GI) diseases (e.g., salmonella).

(Continued)

Assessing the Community *(Continued)*

QUESTIONS TO ASK YOURSELF	RATIONALE/SIGNIFICANCE
What is the quality of the water supply? It the water public or well? Is it fluoridated?	Identifies possible contamination causing GI problems (e.g., ***Giardia lamblia,*** lead).
What is the quality of the soil?	Identifies possible contamination with radioactive material, human or animal excreta, ***Ascaris*** worm.
Is there adequate housing?	Identifies possible crowding, radon and lead exposure.
What is the quality of home and work site?	Identifies possible occupational health risks.
What is the quality of solid waste disposal?	Identifies possible source of contamination.
What is the quality of hazardous waste disposal?	Identifies possible contamination from toxic substances.
Is there infestation by insects, rodents, and animals? Use of pesticides?	Identifies disease carriers (e.g., mosquito carries malaria and West Nile virus; deer ticks carry Lyme disase; animals can transmit rabies). Pesticide use increases risk for exposure to toxic chemicals.
Are there natural disasters in the community? Incidences of violence or terrorism?	Identifies sources of stress (e.g., tornados, school shootings, terrorist attacks).

Source: Data from Smith, C. & Maurer, F. (2000). *Community health nursing theory and practice,* 2nd ed. Philadelphia: W. B. Saunders.

Guidelines for Assessing the Homeless Person*

Homelessness can be defined as a state in which a person has no permanent night-time residence or resides in a temporary shelter or a public or private place not intended for sleeping.

Homelessness affects men, women, and children of all ages, races, religions, and walks of life. An estimated 760,000 people in the Unites States are homeless, and this estimate is probably low. Of the homeless, about 46 percent are single men, 36.5 percent are families with children, and 14 percent are single women. Fifty-six percent of the homeless are black, 27 percent white, and 13 percent Hispanic. Approximately 20 percent of the urban homeless are veterans. In all, 40 percent of homeless men are veterans, 25 to 33 percent are mentally ill, and 45 percent suffer from substance abuse. Families with children (often single mothers) are the fastest-growing group among the homeless.

*Data collected by Ann Stewart, PhD, and Patricia Dillon, RN, MSN, DNSc

Stages of Homelessness

- *Stage 1:* Episodic—homeless from time to time
- *Stage 2:* Temporary—homeless, but continue to identify with the mainstream of society
- *Stage 3:* Chronic—homelessness becomes the norm.

Causes of Homelessness

Some causes of homelessness include unemployment, underemployment, poverty, domestic violence (50 percent of homeless women with children have experienced abuse), eviction, and deinstitutionalization.

Effects of Homelessness

- Lack of food, clothing, medical services, and social supports
- Vulnerability to crimes such as robbery, assault, and rape
- Impaired recovery from illness as a result of inadequate wound care, poor nutrition, and exposure

- Increased risk for episodic and chronic health problems
- Lack of follow-up care because there is no phone or address
- Feelings of low self-esteem, hopelessness, and powerlessness

Barriers to Health Care for Homeless

- No health insurance
- No primary care provider
- Noncompliance with treatment; no follow-up
- Negative attitudes of healthcare providers.

Performing the Assessment of the Homeless Person

The components of the health history and physical examination are the same as for other patients. However, when dealing with homeless clients, your approach and focus differ.

Approach and Focus

- Provide unconditional positive regard for the homeless client.
- Be accepting and nonjudgmental.
- Listen.
- Be sensitive to the reality of the homeless situation.
- Be direct in your communication with the client.
- Ask permission to touch the client. (Physical privacy may be one of the few prerogatives the client has left.)
- Focus more on addressing an immediate problem than on getting a complete history and physical examination.
- Use event markers for time periods; days, months, and years may not be meaningful to the homeless person.
- Schedule healthcare appointments early in the day because shelter management requires a person be present in the afternoon to secure a bed for the night. "Claiming a bed" may take priority over health care.
- Respond accurately and simply if the homeless person expresses concern about how his or her personal revelations are recorded and how the information will be used.
- Realize that the homeless person may be homeless by choice, be impatient, refuse to make eye contact, take a long time to respond, express minor complaints such as headache, have a mailing address or contact person, and see healthcare needs and priorities differently from you.

Health History

The table below outlines a thorough health history for a homeless client.

Taking the Health History

AREA/TYPES OF QUESTIONS	RATIONALE/SIGNIFICANCE
Biographical Data	
Ask where patient is staying.	Less threatening to ask than "What is your address?" Questions about family members, telephone numbers, or additional demographic data may not be appropriate and may be met with silence. May also be reluctant to identify government agencies.
Current Health Survey	
Ask about injuries first.	Client may synthesize life and environmental factors to explain symptoms in ways that may not have occurred to you. Begin with questions about injuries; this may be a marker for time in an unstructured life.
Ask about symptoms of communicable diseases that may not have been reported.	Increased risk for communicable diseases as a result of crowded living quarters.
Ask about respiratory diseases, such as tuberculosis (TB).	Risk is high for those who sleep in close quarters in shelters or crowded spaces.
Ask about dermatological problems such as lesions, infestation.	No change of socks, no clean clothes, exposure to extremes, poor hygiene, living in close quarters increase risk.
Past Health History	
Ask about past injuries, infections, communicable diseases, hospitalizations, substance abuse, psychiatric problems.	Determines compliance and/or completion of treatment and follow-up.

(Continued)

Taking the Health History *(Continued)*

AREA/TYPES OF QUESTIONS	RATIONALE/SIGNIFICANCE
Family History	May not want to discuss family.
Review of Systems	
Ask about problems in the following systems that you may have missed in the current health survey.	Homeless patients are at increased risk for:
Integumentary	Skin problems (see Current Health Status); scabies, lice.
HEENT	Ear and eye problems with children; dental problems with all ages.
Respiratory	Upper respiratory tract infections (URIs), TB.
Cardiovascular	Hypertension (HTN).
Gastrointestinal	Alcohol abuse increases risk for GI disorders and poor nutrition.
Genitourinary	*Women:* Pregnancy, lack of prenatal care. *All:* Poor nutrition, complications, sexually transmitted diseases (STDs).
Musculoskeletal/Neurological	Neurological and psychiatric disorders.
Hematologic/Immune/Endocrine	Anemia related to dietary deficiency, HIV/AIDS; diabetes.
Psychosocial Profile	
Ask about:	
Health Practices and Beliefs	Gives client opportunity to present positive aspects of life. Acknowledging positive behaviors may help establish bond between you and client. Barriers to health care and limited resources limit preventive behaviors. Client's healthcare practices are often crises/problem oriented and treated symptomatically. Follow-up is difficult.
Typical Day	May consist of being on feet all day, looking for food and a place to sleep.
Nutritional Patterns	Nutrition is a problem. Tell client about available resources (e.g., food stamps, soup kitchens).
Activity and Exercise Patterns	Center on survival and meeting basic needs.
Sleep/Rest Patterns	Finding a safe place to sleep is a problem.
Personal Habits	Substance abuse and associated health problems are common among homeless people, but do not assume this is the case with your patient. Ask, "Do you smoke, drink alcohol, or use drugs?" If the answer is yes, ask "How much?"
Occupational Health Patterns	Patient may be working, but income may not be sufficient to maintain housing.
Socioeconomic Status	Homelessness denotes low socioeconomic status, poverty. Ask if client is a veteran. Identify available resources and make appropriate referrals.
Environmental Health Patterns	Thermoregulatory problems (hypo/hyperthermia) resulting from exposure. Alcohol increases risk for hypothermia. Using fire to keep warm increases risk for burns. Because the homeless person often wears everything he or she owns, risk for heat exhaustion, heat stroke, and dehydration increases in warm weather. Increased risk for being a victim of crime, robbery, assault, and rape.
Roles/Relationships/Self-Concept	Low self-esteem, anxiety, and depression are common.
Cultural Influences	Can be seen in both legal and illegal immigrants. Many groups have high poverty rates (e.g., 30% of Hispanics live in poverty). In homeless, language barriers can also add to problem of accessing health care.
Religious Influences	Faith-based organizations are often major service providers for basic needs. Spiritual support may be integrated.
Sexuality Patterns	Homeless client may still be sexually active and in a committed relationship. Ask, "Are you sexually active? With men, women, or both? Do you have genital itching, burning, or other symptoms?" Ask if client is a victim of abuse—50% of homeless women with children have been victims of domestic abuse.

Physical Assessment

Conduct the physical assessment using tools and techniques appropriate for the age and gender of the client. Use gloves if risk for exposure to bodily fluids exists; otherwise, direct touch can convey trust. With the homeless client, the customary head-to-toe approach may not be practical. Close, face-to-face contact at the beginning of the exam may be seen as invasive or threatening by the client. Simply reverse the order, working from toe to head. This also minimizes the power position of the nurse standing over the client, giving directions while performing the exam.

Pay special attention to the client's feet. The homeless are at risk for foot problems because they are often on their feet most of the day, wearing poorly fitted shoes with no change of socks. Regardless of your findings, the act of touching and examining the feet demonstrates a thoroughness of approach and simple caring.

Also keep in mind that the homeless person may have all of his or her possessions on his or her person and may be reluctant to remove clothes. Assure the person that his or her clothing and belongings will be safe, and allow him or her to keep personal items.

The table below outlines a thorough physical assessment of a homeless client. Instead of performing a total assessment, you will usually focus on a specific area identified as a problem from the history data. Be as thorough as necessary to meet your client's health needs and as thorough as your client permits.

Performing the Physical Examination

AREA	RATIONALE/SIGNIFICANCE
General Health Survey	
Inspect general appearance, signs of injury, dress and grooming.	May have signs of injury—homeless people are more vulnerable to crime. Poor hygiene resulting from lack of resources may warrant referral.
Note any odors.	Body odors may be caused by poor hygiene or alcohol abuse.
Take vital signs: temperature, respirations, blood pressure (B/P)	Hypo/hyperthermia from exposure often present. Upper respiratory problems common. HTN is chronic health problem.
Integumentary	
Inspect skin for lesions, color changes; inspect hair for infestation.	Lice or scabies caused by crowded living conditions. High incidence of hepatitis related to I.V. drug use. Cirrhosis related to alcohol abuse. Minor skin problems common. Poor wound healing because of poor nutrition.
Inspect feet for lesions and edema.	Being on feet most of day increases risk for peripheral-vascular disease (PVD). Diabetes is also a chronic problem.
HEENT	
Inspect mouth and throat.	Dental problems and URI common among homeless.
Respiratory	
Auscultate lungs	Respiratory problems and TB common.
Cardiovascular	
Palpate peripheral pulses	PVD common.
Auscultate heart for normal and extra sounds	HTN common.
Gastrointestinal	
Auscultate bowel sounds.	GI problems common.
Palpate abdomen.	Cirrhosis, pancreatitis associated with alcohol abuse common.
Genitourinary	
Inspect genitalia.	Homeless people, especially women, are susceptible to rape, increasing risk for STDs and pregnancy.
Musculoskeletal	
Inspect and palpate muscles.	Homeless people are susceptible to trauma from beatings.

(Continued)

Performing the Physical Examination *(Continued)*

AREA	RATIONALE/SIGNIFICANCE
Neurological	
Assess mental status.	Head trauma may result from beatings. Substance abuse (drugs and alcohol) can affect neurological status. Seizures can result from trauma and substance abuse. Psychiatric problems common, including depression, schizophrenia, and organic brain syndrome.

Guidelines for Assessing Abuse*

Abuse can take many forms, can affect any age group, and knows no socioeconomic boundaries. It can be physical, sexual, emotional, or a combination of two or all of these. It may also be directed at property. As a nurse, you need to be alert for signs and symptoms of abuse at all levels of health care for all of your patients. This section covers child abuse, spousal or partner (domestic) abuse, and elder abuse.

Types of Abuse

- **Physical Abuse:** Physical contact with intent to harm, ranging from slapping, hitting, and biting to murder. Physical abuse includes **neglect**—depriving a person of basic needs such as food, water, or sleep.
- **Sexual Abuse:** Sexually oriented behavior without the consent of the other person or persons involved, ranging from sexually degrading remarks to rape.
- **Psychological (Emotional) Abuse:** Verbal abuse or actions that can be considered degrading, belittling, or threatening, used for control, often by evoking fear in the victim. This type of abuse is difficult to assess.
- **Property Abuse:** Deliberate destruction of a person's belongings.

Assessing Child Abuse

Child abuse and neglect are the leading cause of death in children under 3 years.

More than 2 million cases of are reported every year. Child abuse can take the following forms:

- **Physical Abuse:** Includes actual physical trauma, such as bruising, breaking bones, intentional burns, and shaken-baby syndrome. It also includes Munchausen syndrome by proxy (MSBP), in which the parent or caretaker intentionally causes a child to be ill to gain sympathy and recognition.
- **Neglect:** Failure to meet the child's basic needs.
- **Sexual Abuse:** Includes actual intercourse with either vaginal or anal penetration, genital fondling and other inappropriate touching, or pornographic photography of the child.
- **Psychological Abuse:** Includes emotional detachment from the child, constant belittling, fostering and enabling substance abuse and delinquency, and failing to provide adequate supervision.

Assessing for Physical Abuse

As you go through the assessment, ask yourself: Are the injuries inconsistent with the child's age or developmental stage (e.g., 1-month-old baby falling out of crib)? Is evidence of old fractures or trauma seen on current x rays?

Taking the Health History

Obtain separate statements from parents or caregivers. Be alert for inconsistencies (e.g., parent saying that hand-mark bruising on the child was inflicted by another child). Ask the following questions:

- Ask yourself: What is your perception of the child (e.g., difficult or quiet)?
- Ask the parent or caregiver:
  - Does the child have a history of past health problems? Where was the child treated? (Frequent emergency room visits signal abuse. Parents may use different healthcare centers to avoid suspicion.)
  - What is the child's feeding history? (Compare the history given to the child's physical growth and development.)
  - Ask the child (if old enough): What types of stress do you have in your life? Who are your supports?

Suspect MSBP if:

- Child does not respond to usual treatment.

*Information compiled by Patricia M. Dillon, RN, MSN, DNSc, Barbara Jones, MSN, DNSc, and Kathleen Killinger, MSN, CRNP, PhD.

- Laboratory results are inconsistent with history or physically impossible.
- Parent seems very knowledgeable about medical treatment.
- Signs and symptoms of illness do not occur when parent is not present.
- Similar findings or unexplained deaths have occurred in siblings.
- Parent craves adulation for his or her care of child.

Performing the Physical Examination

Obtain growth measurements and compare them with previous measurements. Nutritional neglect can cause failure to thrive.

- Look for distended abdomen, a sign of malnutrition.
- Observe child's grooming, dress, and hygiene.
- Examine all body surfaces for bruises, burns, and skin lesions, looking especially for the following signs of physical abuse:
  - Bruises that form the outline of a hand (from parent grabbing child)
  - Linear bruises (from belts)
  - Bruises on head, face, ears, buttocks, and lower back (consistent with abuse)
  - Obviously nonaccidental burns (e.g., burns on both lower legs)
  - Burn outline of an entire object, such as multiple cigarette burns on various parts of body
  - Detached retina and hemorrhages and subdural hematoma (shaken-baby syndrome)

Assessing for Sexual Abuse

Taking the Health History

Be nonjudgmental when questioning caregivers about possible sexual abuse. Obtain the following information from patients or their caregivers:

- Ask children over 2 1/2 years directly about being touched in "private parts." With older children, use an approach such as: "Sometimes people you know may touch or kiss you in a way that you feel is wrong. Has this ever happened to you?" With adolescents, use an approach such as: "Sometimes people touch you in ways you feel are wrong. This can be frightening, and it is wrong for people to do that to you. Has this ever happened to you?"
- Determine whether there has been a sudden onset of bedwetting in a child who was previously not a bedwetter.
- Determine whether the child masturbates or sexually acts out with other children.
- Determine whether the child has genitourinary symptoms, such as burning, itching, or vaginal discharge.
- Determine whether the child has a history of running away from home, especially to unsafe situations as opposed to a friend's home.

Performing the Physical Assessment

Look for genital and anal irritation, discharge, swelling, redness, and bruising. In girls, carefully evaluate the vaginal introitus for evidence of penetration. During the exam, observe the child's behavior:

- Is the child overly solicitous in a sexual manner?
- Does he or she dress or act provocatively?
- Is he or she overly fearful of the exam, especially the genital exam?

Assessing for Psychological Abuse

Taking the Health History

Ask the parent or caregiver the following questions:

- Was this child the result of a planned pregnancy? What were the birth and postpartum period like? Were there many stressors at home at the time of your child's birth?
- How would you describe your child now?
- How is this child compared to others in your family?
- Is there a history of physical or developmental problems? If so, what kinds of supports do you receive?
- Has the child had many illnesses? If so, what are they? How has this affected your life?
- What are your expectations of the child?
- What form of discipline works best for the child?

Performing the Psychological Assessment

During the exam, observe the following:

- Compare parental description of the child to what you actually observe.
- Observe child-parent interaction. Is it distant or engaging? How does the parent comfort the child?
- If other siblings are present, does the parent respond to them differently from the child in question?
- Does the parent openly and repeatedly belittle the child (e.g., saying: "You're so dumb")?
- Does the child have developmental delays, poor social skills, speech problems, or regression?

Assessing Spousal or Partner Abuse (Domestic Violence)

Domestic violence is the leading cause of injury to women. One in every three women has been abused by a spouse or partner at least one time during the relationship. Here are more facts about domestic violence:

- Fifty percent of homeless women and children have been victims of abuse.
- The battering cycle consists of the tension-building phase, the battering phase, and the apologetic phase.
- Abuse occurs in same-sex relationships as well as heterosexual relationships.
- Abusers are usually emotionally dependent and egocentric.
- The battered partner is usually unsure, economically and emotionally dependent, and exhibiting learned helplessness.
- Spousal or partner abuse can take the form of physical, sexual, or psychological abuse (or a combination of two or all of these), or property abuse.
- Emotional abuse is difficult to assess because the effects are not as visible as those of physical abuse.
- To gain power and control, the abuser may:
  - Use coercion and threats, such as threatening to leave the partner or commit suicide.
  - Use intimidation to evoke fear by destroying personal belongings or hurting pets.
  - Degrade and belittle, making the partner feel that it is his or her fault, make him or her feel guilty, or blame abuse on him or her.
  - Isolate the partner by limiting contacts with family and friends.
  - Control or limit finances.
  - Put children in the middle of the situation or threaten to take them away.
  - If male, use male privilege by enforcing dominant role.

Assessing for Physical Abuse

Taking the Health History

Ask the client:

- What is your chief complaint? Complaints are often vague and nonspecific; for example, headaches, GI complaints, asthma, fatigue, and chronic vague pain.
- Do you have trouble sleeping? Do you have nightmares?
- Have you ever been hospitalized? Frequent ER visits are common, with injuries becoming progressively more severe. Current x rays may reveal old fractures.
- How did the injury happen? Injury may not match the explanation (e.g., black eye from walking into door).
- Do you have a history of depression or attempted suicide? Abuse victim with a sense of hopelessness and powerlessness may be depressed and attempt suicide.
- Are you taking any prescribed or over-the-counter medications? Do you drink alcohol? If so, how much? Substance abuse may be used as an attempt to deal with physical abuse.
- Have you had any weight or appetite changes? Anorexia and bulimia are not uncommon.
- Have you ever been sexually assaulted? Are you satisfied with your sexual relationship with spouse or partner? Domestic violence can take the form of sexual abuse.

Performing the Physical Examination

Assess for injuries suggesting abuse, such as cigarette burns; black eyes; facial injuries, injuries to the chest, back, breast, or abdomen; bruising on genitalia; or bruises in the shape of a hand or belt.

During the exam, observe for the following:

- Patient's lethargic, passive behavior
- Patient's poor eye contact and anxious or fearful behavior
- Patient' s visible fear when partner is in room; looking to partner before responding to questions
- Partner answering for patient and being overly condescending

Assessing Elder Abuse and Neglect

More than 800,000 cases of elder mistreatment are reported annually. Elder abuse can be physical, sexual, or psychological. It can also take the form of neglect or financial or property abuse. During your assessment, be alert if the caregiver speaks for the patient, refuses to let the patient be examined alone, or underreacts when confronted with findings suggesting abuse.

Assessing for Physical Abuse

Taking the Health History

Ask the following questions of the patient and caregiver:

- How did the injury happen? Suspect abuse if injury does not match explanation (e.g., caregiver says injury is from fall, but patient has no difficulty with balance or walking).
- When did the injury occur? Lengthy interval between injury and treatment suggests abuse.
- Who is the primary healthcare provider? "Doctor shopping" (using different healthcare providers) suggests abuse.
- To patient: Do you feel safe in your home?
- To patient: Are there any situations in which you feel afraid?

- To patient or caregiver: Have you ever given/taken the wrong dose of medication? Repeated medication errors by caregiver (e.g., oversedating patient) suggest abuse.

Performing the Physical Examination

During the exam, observe for the following:

- Whiplash burns from rope or cord
- Cigarette burns on palms and soles of feet
- Injuries with a pattern, such as that of a belt buckle or electrical cord
- Oral ecchymosis or injury from forced oral sex
- Whiplash injuries from shaking
- Hyphema, subconjunctival hemorrhage, detached retina, ruptured tympanic membrane
- Bruises on trunk, breast, abdomen, genitalia, and buttocks (bathing suit zone)
- Bleeding or bruising of genitalia, poor sphincter tone, and bruises on inner thighs
- Bruising on wrists and ankles from being bound or restrained
- Immersion burns (may follow a stocking-glove pattern)
- Evidence of old injuries
- Anxiety and depression

Assessing for Neglect

The following are signs of neglect in a patient:

- Never changing clothes or wearing clothes that are dirty or inappropriate for the weather
- Poor hygiene or body odor
- Ingrown nails
- Decayed or missing teeth
- Untreated sores or pressure sores
- Matted hair
- Hypo/hyperthermia
- Untreated medical problems
- Dehydration
- Malnutrition, failure-to-thrive syndrome
- Weight loss
- Abnormal blood chemistry
- If you are making a home visit: Clutter, disconnected utilities, neglected pets, animal or human excrement, spoiled food

Assessing for Financial Abuse

The following are signs of financial abuse:

- Unusual activity in patient's bank account
- Bank statements diverted from patient's home
- Sudden disappearance of caregiver
- Patient asked to sign documents such as power of attorney
- Large withdrawals from patient's account
- Family that is reluctant to spend money on patient
- Disappearance of personal belongings
- Isolation of patient by caregiver
- Forged signatures on checks and documents
- Caregiver who is evasive about sources of income
- Lack of solid, legal financial arrangements in place for older person

Documentation

Physical, sexual, and financial abuse are crimes in all states. In most states, suspicion of abuse is grounds for reporting. Make sure that you document your findings clearly and objectively. Be specific and thorough because your assessment findings are crucial in early detection and prompt intervention.

APPENDIX D

Bibliography

Chapter 1

American Nurses' Association (1980). *Nursing: A social policy statement* (Publication Code: NP-63, 35M). Kansas City: ANA.

Benner, P. (1984). *From novice to expert: Excellence and power in clinical nursing practice.* Menlo Park, CA: Addison-Wesley.

Benner, P., Tanner, C., & Chesla, C. (1996). *Expertise in nursing practice, caring, clinical judgement and ethics.* New York: Springer Publishing.

Carpenito, L. (1997). *Nursing diagnosis application to clinical practice* (7th ed.). Philadelphia: Lippincott Williams & Wilkins.

Doenges, M., Moorhouse, M., & Geissler, A. (1997). *Nursing care plans: Guidelines for individualizing patient care* (5th ed.). Philadelphia: F. A. Davis.

Maslow, A. (1970). *Motivation and personality* (2nd ed.). New York: Harper & Row.

Morton, P. (1993). *Health assessment in nursing* (2nd ed.). Philadelphia: F. A. Davis.

Nightingale, F. (1859). *Notes on nursing: What it is, and what it is not.* Philadelphia: J. B. Lippincott.

Purnell, L. D., & Paulanka, B. J. (2003). *Transcultural healthcare: A culturally competent approach* (2nd ed.). Philadelphia: F. A. Davis.

Standards of Practice (1992). Kansas City, MO. American Nurses Association.

Stuart, G., & Laraia, M. (2001). *Principles and practice of psychiatric nursing* (7th ed.). Philadelphia: C. V. Mosby.

Taylor, C., Lillis, C., & LeMone, P. (2001). *Fundamentals of nursing: The art and science of nursing care* (4th ed.). Philadelphia: Lippincott Williams & Wilkins.

Weeks, C. (1891). *Textbook on nursing.* New York: Appleton.

Wilkenson, J. (1991). *Nursing process in action.* Redwood City: Addison-Wesley Nursing.

Chapter 2

Carpenito, L. (1997). *Nursing diagnosis application to clinical practice* (7th ed.). Philadelphia: Lippincott Williams & Wilkins.

Craven, R., & Hirnle, C. (2000). *Fundamentals of nursing human health and function* (3rd ed.). Philadelphia: Lippincott Williams & Wilkins.

Doenges, M., Moorehouse, M., & Geissler, A. (1997). *Nursing care plans: Guidelines for individualizing patient care* (4th ed.). Philadelphia: F. A. Davis.

Morton, P. (1993). *Health assessment in nursing* (2nd ed.). Philadelphia: F. A. Davis.

Purnell, L., & Paulanka, B. (2003). *Transcultural health care: A culturally competent approach* (2nd ed.). Philadelphia: F. A. Davis.

Stuart, G., & Laraia, M. (2001). *Principles and practice of psychiatric nursing* (7th ed.). Philadelphia: C. V. Mosby.

Taylor, C., Lillis, C., & LeMone, P. (2001). *Fundamentals of nursing: The art and science of nursing care* (4th ed.). Philadelphia: Lippincott Williams & Wilkins.

USDHHS (1998). *Put prevention into practice: Clinician's handbook of preventative services* (2nd ed.). Washington, DC: AHCPR.

Wong, D., & Hockenberry-Eaton, M. (2001). *Wong's essentials of pediatric nursing* (6th ed.).Philadelphia: C. V. Mosby.

Chapter 3

Lewis, S., Heitkemper, M., & Dirksen, S. (2000). *Medical surgical nursing assessment and management of clinical problems* (5th ed.). Philadelphia: C. V. Mosby.

Lowdermilk, D., Perry, S., & Bobak, I. (1999). *Maternity nursing* (5th ed.). Philadelphia: C. V. Mosby.

Morton, P. (1992). *Health assessment in nursing* (2nd ed.). Philadelphia: F. A. Davis.

Purnell, L., & Paulanka, B. (2003). *Transcultural healthcare: A culturally competent approach* (2nd ed.). Philadelphia: F. A. Davis.

Taylor, C., Lillis, C., & LeMone, P. (2001). *Fundamentals of nursing: The art and science of caring* (4th ed.). Philadelphia: Lippincott Williams & Wilkins.

Wong, D., & Hockenberry-Eaton, M. (2001). *Wong's essentials of pediatric nursing* (6th ed.). Philadelphia: C. V. Mosby

Chapter 4

American Red Cross (March 1997). *Health and safety services instructional system: Manual for the instructor trainer candidate.* American Red Cross.

Eiss, A. F., & Harbeck, M.B. (1969). *Behavioral objectives in the affective domain.* Washington, DC: National Education Association.

Felder, R. M., & Solomon, B. A. (retrieved 17 March 2002). *Learning styles and strategies.* Published online at ww2.ncsu.edu/unity/lockers/users/f/felder/public/ILSdir/styles.htm

Houle, C. O. (1974). *The design of education.* San Francisco: Jossey-Bass.

Martin, B. L. (1989). A checklist for designing instruction in the affective domain. *Educational technology, 29,* 7–15.

Taylor, Lillis, & LeMone (2001). *Fundamentals of nursing: The art and science of nursing care* (4th ed). Philadelphia: Lippincott Williams & Wilkins.

Chapter 5

American Academy of Family Physicians (1999). *Summary of policy recommendations for periodic health examination.* Washington, DC.

Burggraf, V., & Barry, R. J. (2000). Healthy People 2010—Protecting the health of older individuals. *Journal of Gerontological Nursing, 26*(12), 16–22.

Brazelton, T. (1990). Saving the bathwater. *Child Development, 61,* 1661–1671.

Child health guide (2000). Washington, DC: U.S. Department of Health and Human Services, Public Health Service, Agency for Healthcare Research and Quality.

Erikson, E. (1963). *Childhood and society* (2nd ed.). New York: Norton.

Lindberg, J. B., Hunter, M. L., & Kruszewski, A. Z. (1998). *Introduction to nursing: Concepts, issues, and opportunities* (3rd ed.). New York: Lippincott Williams & Wilkins.

Pender, N. J. (1996). *Health promotion in nursing practice* (3rd ed.). Stamford, CT: Appleton & Lange.

Richardson, G. E., & Berry, N. F. (1987). Strength intervention: An approach to lifestyle modification. *Health Education, 18*(3), 42–46.

Staying healthy at 50+ (2000). Washington, DC: U.S. Department of Health and Human Services, Public Health Service, Agency for Healthcare Research and Quality.

Stolte, K. M. (1996). *Wellness nursing diagnosis for health promotion.* New York: J. B. Lippincott Raven.

Chapter 6

American Diabetes Association (1993). *Medical management of pregnancy complicated by diabetes.* Alexandria, VA: American Diabetes Association.

American Diabetes Association (1994). *Maximizing the role of nutrition in diabetes management*. Alexandria, VA: American Diabetes Association.

American Heart Association (1999). *Heart and stroke guide*. www-medlib.med.utah.edu/infofair/slides/hile/tsld016.htm

Centers for Disease Control (1999). *Overweight prevalence among adults 20–74 years old, according to age, race, sex, and hispanic origin, selected periods, 1960–1994. http://webapp.cdc.gov/aging/obesez.html*

Dudek, S. (1997). *Nutrition handbook for nursing practice* (3rd ed.). Philadelphia: Lippincott Williams & Wilkins.

Estes, M. E. Z. (1998). *Health assessment and physical examination*. Albany, NY: Delmar Publishers.

Frisancho, A. R. (1981). New norms of upper limb fat and muscle areas for assessment of nutritional status. *American Journal of Clinical Nutrition Association, 30*:2540–2548.

Glenn, F. B., Glenn, W. D., & Duncan, R. C. Fluoride tablet supplementation during pregnancy for caries immunity: A study of the offspring produced. *American Journal of Obstetrics and Gynecology, 143*(5): 560–564.

Havala, S., & Dwyer, J. (1993). Position of the American Dietetic Association: Vegetarian diets. *Journal of the American Dietetic Association, 93*(11), 1317–1319.

Jarvis, C. (1996). *Physical examination and health assessment* (2nd ed). Philadelphia: W. B. Saunders.

Lee, R., & Nieman, D. (1996). *Nutritional assessment* (2nd ed.). St. Louis: C. V. Mosby.

Leitch, I. (1942). The evolution of dietary standards. *Nutrition Abstracts and Reviews,* 11, 109–117.

Looker, A. C., Dallman, P. R., Carroll, M. D., Gunter, E. W., & Johnson, C. L. (1997). Prevalence of iron deficiency in the United States. *Journal of the American Medical Association, 277*(12), 973–976.

Lutz, C., & Przytulski, K. (2001). *Nutrition and diet therapy* (3rd ed.). Philadelphia: F. A. Davis.

Messina, V. K., & Burke, K. I. (1997). Position of the American Dietetic Association: Vegetarian diets. *Journal of the* American Dietetic Association, *97*(11), 1317–1321.

Metropolitan Life Insurance Company (1999). *Height and weight tables (online): http://www.metlife.com/Lifeadvice/Tools/Heightnweight/Docs/frametable.html*

Mitchell, M. K. (1994). *Nutrition across the lifespan*. Philadelphia: W.B. Saunders.

National Center for Health Statistics (1976). *NCHS Growth Charts. Monthly Vital Statistics Report,* 25(3). Supplement (HRA)76–1120. Rockville, MD: Health Resources Administration

National Center for Health Statistics (1998). *Health, United States, 1998, with socioeconomic status and health chartbook*. Hyattsville, Maryland: U.S. Department of Health And Human Services, Centers for Disease Control and Prevention, National Center for Health Statistics. DHHS Publication number (PHS) 98–1232.

National Cholesterol Education Program (1993). *Second report of the expert panel on detection, evaluation, and treatment of high blood cholesterol in adults*. Bethesda, MD: U.S. Dept. of Health and Human Services, Public Health Service; National Institutes of Health; National Heart, Lung, and Blood Institute.

Pipes, P.L, & Trahms, C.M. (1993). *Nutrition in infancy and childhood*. St. Louis: C.V. Mosby.

Purnell, L., and Paulanka, B. (2003). *Transcultural health care: A culturally competent approach* (2nd ed.). F. A. Davis, Philadelphia, 1998.

Ritchey, A. K. (1987). Iron deficiency in children. Update on an old problem. *Postgraduate Medicine, 82*(2), 59–63, 67–69.

Rexrode, K. M., Carey, V. J., Hennekens, C. H., Walters, E. E., Colditz, G. A., Stampfer, M. J., Willett, W. C., & Manson, J. E. (1998). Abdominal adiposity and coronary heart disease in women. *Journal of the American Medical Association, 280*(21): 1843–1848.

Rose, E. A., Porcerelli, J.H., & Neale, A.V. (2000). Pica: Common but commonly missed. *Journal of the American Board of Family Practice, 13*(5), 353–358.

Rowland, M. L. (1989). A nomogram for computing body mass index; using the nomogram. *Dietetic Currents,* 16(2), 6–7. Columbus, OH: Ross Laboratories.

United States Department of Agriculture & Department of Health and Human Services: *Food guide pyramid. http://www.usda.gov/cnpp/pyramid.html*

United States Department of Agriculture (1995). *Nutrition and Your Health: Dietary Guidelines for Americans. http://www.hoptechno.com/dietary.htm*

United States Department of Agriculture & Department of Health and Human Services (1990). *Nutrition and your health: Dietary guidelines for Americans*. Home and Garden Bulletin No 232, Washington, DC: U. S. Government Printing Office.

Walker, S.P., Rimm, E.B., Ascherio, A., Kawachi, I., Stampfer, M.J., & Willett, W.C. (1996). Body size and fat distribution as predictors of stroke among U.S. men. *American Journal of Epidemiology, 144*(12):1143–1150.

Whaley, L. F., & Wong, D. L. (1991) *Nursing care of infants and children* (4th ed.), St. Louis: Mosby-Year Book.

Williams, C. L., Bollela, M., & Wynder, E. L. (1995). A new recommendation for dietary fiber in childhood. *Pediatrics, 96,* 985–988.

World Health Organization (2000). Nutrition: Aims and objectives. *http://www.who.int/nut/aim.htm*

Chapter 7

Berger, K.J., & Williams, M.B. (1999). *Fundamentals of nursing: Collaborating for optimal health* (2nd ed.). Stamford, CT: Appleton & Lange.

Burgess, W.A.(1997).*Psychiatric nursing*. Stamford, CT: Appleton & Lange.

Carson, V.B.(1989). *Spiritual dimensions of nursing practice*. Philadelphia: W. B. Saunders.

Carson, V.B., & Green, H. (1992). Spiritual well-being: A predictor of hardiness in persons with acquired immunodeficiency syndrome. *Journal of Professional Nursing, 8*(4), 209–220.

Dossey, B., & Dossey, L. (1998). Attending to holistic care. *American Journal of Nursing98*(8), 35–38.

Ellis, J.R., & Nowlin, E.A. (1994). *Nursing: A human needs approach*. (5th ed.). Philadelphia: Lippincott Raven.

Ellison, C., & Paloutzian, R.(1983). Spiritual well-being: Conceptualization and measurement. *Journal of Psychology and Theology, 11*(4), 330–340.

Fehring, R.J., Brennan, P.F., & Keller, M.L. (1987). Psychological and spiritual well-being in college students. *Research in Nursing and Health, 10,* 391–398.

Fehring, R.J., Miller, J.F., & Shaw, C. (1997). Spiritual well-being, religiosity, hope, depression, and other mood states in elderly people coping with cancer. *Oncology Nursing Forum, 24*(4), 663–671.

Highfield, M.F. (1997). Spiritual assessment across the cancer trajectory: Methods and reflections. *Seminars in Oncology Nursing, 13*(4) 237–241.

Hungelmann, J., Kenkel-Rossi, E. Klassen, L., & Stollenwerk, R. (1996). Focus on spiritual well-being: Harmonious interconnectedness of mind-body-spirit-use of the JAREL Spiritual Well-Being Scale. *Geriatric Nursing: American Journal of Care for the Aging, 17*(6), 262–266.

Hungelman, J., Kenkel-Rossi, E., Klassen, L., & Stollenwerk, R. (1987). Marquette University College of Nursing, Milwaukee, WI.

Kozier, B., Erb, G., Blais, K., & Wilkinson, J.M. (1998). *Fundamentals of nursing: Concepts, process, and practice* (5th ed.). NY: Addison-Wesley.

Mickley, J.R., Soeken, K., & Belcher, A. (1992). Spiritual well-being, religiousness and hope among women with breast cancer. *IMAGE: Journal of Nursing Scholarship, 24*(4) 267–272.

Moberg, D.O. (1984). Subjective measures of spiritual well-being. *Review of Religious Research, 25,* 351–364.

Nagai-Jacobson, M.G., & Burkhardt, M.A. (1989) Spirituality: Cornerstone of holistic nursing practice. *Holistic Nursing Practice, 3*(3), 18–26.

Potter, P.A. & Perry, A.G. (2001). *Fundamentals of nursing* (5th ed). St. Louis: C. V. Mosby.

Purnell, L.D., & Paulanka, B.J. (2003). *Transcultural health care: A culturally competent approach* (2nd ed.). Philadelphia: F. A. Davis.

Reed, P. (1986). Developmental resources and depression in the elderly. *Nursing Research, 35,* 368–374.

Ross, L. (1995). The spiritual dimension: Its importance to client's health, well-being and quality of life and its implications for nursing practice. *International Journal of Nursing Studies, 32*(5), 457–468.

Shelly, J.A., & Fish, S. (1988). *Spiritual care: The nurse's role.* (3rd ed.). Downers Grove, IL: Intervarsity.

Stoll, R. I. (1989). The essence of spirituality. In V.B. Carson (Ed.), *Spiritual dimensions of nursing practice.* Philadelphia: W. B. Saunders.

Chapter 8

Carpenter, D. (Ed.) (1998). Handbook of signs and symptoms. Springhouse, PA: Springhouse Corporation.

Epstein, O., Perkin, G., deBono, D., & Cookson, J. (1997). *Clinical examination* (2nd ed.). Philadelphia: C. V. Mosby.

Goldsmith, L., Lazarus, G., & Tharp, M. (1997). *Adult and pediatric dermatology: A color guide to diagnosis and treatment.* Philadelphia: F. A. Davis.

Goroll, A., & Mulley, A. (2000). *Primary care medicine* (4th ed.). Philadelphia: Lippincott Williams & Wilkins.

Lewis, S., Heitkemper, M., & Dirksen, S. (2000). *Medical-surgical nursing assessment and management of clinical problems* (5th ed.). Philadelphia: C. V. Mosby.

Mangione, S. (2000). *Physical diagnosis secrets.* Philadelphia: Hanley & Belfus, Inc.

McPhee, S., Lingappa, V., Ganong, W., & Lange, J. (1997). *Pathophysiology of disease: An introduction to clinical medicine.* Stamford, CT: Appleton & Lange.

Morton, P. (1993). *Health assessment in nursing* (2nd ed.). Philadelphia: F. A. Davis.

National Institutes of Health (NIH) (2000), Of mice and skin: Custom rodents. COX-1 show value against skin cancers. National Institute of Arthritis and Musculoskeletal and Skin Diseases. *www.nih gov/niams/news/spotlight/ofmice.htm*

NIH (2000). Scientists scrutinize sun and skin. National Institute of Arthritis and Musculoskeletal and Skin Diseases. *www.nih gov/niams/news/spotlight/ofmice.htm*

Purnell, L., and Paulanka, B. (2003). *Transcultural health care: A culturally competent approach* (2nd ed.). Philadelphia: F. A. Davis.

Ries, L., Eisner, M., Kosary, C., Hanbey, B., Miller, B., Clegg, L., & Edwards, B. (eds.). (2000). SEER cancer statistics review, 1973–1997. Bethesda, MD: National Cancer Institute.

Sellers, R. (1996). *Differential diagnosis of common complaints* (3rd ed.). Philadelphia: W. B. Saunders.

Sommers, M., & Johnson, S. (1997). *Davis's manual of nursing therapeutics for diseases and disorders.* Philadelphia: F. A. Davis.

Swartz, M. (1998). *Textbook of physical diagnosis: History and examination.* Philadelphia: W. B. Saunders.

Thompson, J., McFarland, G., Hirsch, J., & Tucker, S. (1997). *Mosby's clinical nursing.* St. Louis: C. V. Mosby.

Van Wynsberghe, Noback, C., & Carola, R. (1995). *Human anatomy and physiology* (3rd ed.). New York: McGraw-Hill.

Venes, D. (ed.). (2001). *Taber's cyclopedic medical dictionary* (19th ed.). Philadelphia: F. A. Davis.

Weber, J., & Kelley, J. (1998). *Health Assessment in Nursing.* New York: Lippincott Raven.

Chapter 9

Greenlee, R., Hill-Harmon, M. B., Murray, T.,& Then, M. (2001). Cancer statistics *CA: A Cancer Journal for Clinicians, 51*(1), 15–36.

Hurst, J. (1996). *Medicine for the practicing physician.* Stamford, CT: Appleton & Lange.

Mengel, M., & Schwieber, L. (1996). *Ambulatory medicine: The primary care of families.* Stamford, CT: Appleton & Lange.

NIH (2000). *CancerNet: Screening for oral cancer. http://www.meb.uni-bonn.de/cancernet/304725.html*

NIH (2000) *Oral cancer. http://webmd.lycos.com/encyclopedia/article/2730.308*

NIH (2000). *Cancer of the larynx. http://www.cancer.gov/cancerinfo/wyntk/larynx*

Pai, S., Ghezzi, E., & Ship, J. (2000). Development of a visual analogue scale questionnaire for subjective assessment of salivary function. *Oral Surgery, Oral Medicine, Oral Pathology, Oral Radiology, and Endodontics, 91*(3), 311–316.

Porth, C. (1998). *Pathophysiology: Concepts of altered health states.* Philadelphia: Lippincott Williams & Wilkins.

Springhouse (2000). *Professional guide to signs and symptoms.* Springhouse , PA: Springhouse Corporation.

Swartz, M. (1998). *Textbook of physical diagnosis: History and examination.* Philadelphia: W. B. Saunders.

Thompson, J., McFarland, G., Hirsch, J., & Tucker, S. (1997). *Mosby's clinical nursing.* St. Louis: C. V. Mosby.

Chapter 10: The Eye

Barkauskas, V., Stoltenberg-Allen, K., Baumann, L., & Darling-Fisher, C. (1998). *Health and physical assessment* (2nd ed.). St. Louis: C. V. Mosby.

Coleman, A. L. (1999). Glaucoma. *The Lancet, 354,* 1803–1810.

Committee on Practice and Ambulatory Medicine, Section on Ophthalmology (1996). Examination and vision screening in infants, children and young adults. *Pediatrics, 98*(1), 153–158.

Downey, D., & Leigh, J. (1998). Eye movements: Pathophysiology, examination, and clinical importance. *Journal of Neuroscience Nursing, 30*(1), 15–22.

Fong, D. S. (2000). Age-related macular degeneration: Update for primary care. *American Family Physician, 61,* 3035–3042.

Gilman, S., & Newman, S. (1996). *Essentials of clinical*

neuroanatomy and neurophysiology (9th ed.). Philadelphia: F. A. Davis.

Greenstein, B., & Greenstein, A. (2000). *Color atlas of neuroscience.* New York: Thieme.

Hoglund, T. (2000). *Food and drug administration approves photodynamic therapy in the treatment of wet AMD.* The Foundation Fighting Blindness, *http://www.blindness.org*

Jarvis, C. (2000). *Physical examination and health assessment* (3rd ed.). Philadelphia: W. B Saunders.

Knoop, K. J., Stack, L. B., & Storrow, A. B. (1997). *Atlas of emergency medicine.* New York: McGraw-Hill.

Mir, A. M. (1995) *Atlas of clinical diagnosis.* Philadelphia: W. B Saunders.

Morton, P.G. (ed.) (1993). *Health assessment in nursing* (2nd ed.). Springhouse Corporation, Springhouse, PA.

Shingleton, B., & O'Donoghue, M. (2000). Blurred vision. *New England Journal of Medicine, 343*(8), 556–562.

Snell, R., & Lemp, M. (1998). *Clinical anatomy of the eye* (2nd ed.). Malden, MS: Blackwell Science, Inc.

Skorin, L. (2000). Corneal and eyelid anomalies. *Consultant,* 265–272.

United States Department of Health and Human Services (1998). *Put prevention into practice: Clinician's handbook of preventative services* (2nd ed.). Washington, DC: U. S. Government Printing Office.

Weinstock, F. J., & Weinstock, M. B. (1996). Common eye disorders: Six clients to refer. *Postgraduate Medicine, 99*(4), 107–116.

Wong, D., Wilson, D., Hockenberry-Eaton, M., Winkelstein, M., & Schwartz, P. (2001). *Wong's essentials of pediatric nursing* (6th ed.) Philadelphia: C. V. Mosby.

Chapter 10: The Ear

Barkauskas, V., Stoltenberg-Allen, K., Baumann, L., & Darling-Fisher, C. (1998). *Health and physical assessment.* (2nd ed.). St. Louis: C. V. Mosby.

Gilman, S., & Newman, S. (1996). *Essentials of clinical neuroanatomy and neurophysiology* (9th ed.). Philadelphia: F. A. Davis.

Greenstein, B., & Greenstein, A. (2000). *Color atlas of neuroscience.* New York: Thieme.

Jarvis, C. (2000). *Physical examination and health assessment* (3rd ed.). Philadelphia: W. B Saunders.

Juhn, S., Li, W., Kim, J., Javel, E., Levine, S., & Odland, R. (1999). Effects of stress-related hormones on inner ear fluid homeostasis and function. *The American Journal of Otology, 20,* 800–806.

Knoop, K. J., Stack, L. B., & Storrow, A. B. (1997). *Atlas of emergency medicine.* New York: McGraw-Hill.

Lang, L. (1994). Environmental impact on hearing: Is anyone listening? *Environmental Health Perspectives Supplements, 102*(11) 924–930.

Meyer, C., Witte, J., Hildmann, A., Hennecke, K. H., Schunck, K. U., Maul, K., Franke, U., Fahnenstich, H., Rabe, H., Rossie, H., Hartmann, S., & Gortner, L. (1999). Neonatal screening for hearing disorders in infants at risk: Incidence, risk factors, and follow-up. *Pediatrics, 104*(4), 900–904.

Mir, A. M. (1995) *Atlas of clinical diagnosis.* Philadelphia: W. B Saunders.

Moore, K. L. , & Persaud, T. V. (1998). *The developing human: Clinically oriented embryology* (6th ed.). Philadelphia: W. B. Saunders.

Prasher, D. (1998). New strategies for prevention and treatment of noise-induced hearing loss. *The Lancet, 352,*1240–1242.

Schlauch, R., S., & Samuel, L. (1995). Evaluating hearing threshold differences between ears as a screen for acoustic neuroma. *Journal of Speech and Hearing Research, 38*(5),1168–1174.

Silverthorn, D. (1998). *Human physiology: An integrated approach.* Upper Saddle River, NJ: Prentice Hall.

United States Department of Health and Human Services (1998). *Put prevention into practice: Clinician's handbook of preventative services* (2nd ed.). Washington, DC: U. S. Government Printing Office.

Watts, R. L., & Koller, W., C. (1997). *Movement Disorders: Neurological Principles and Practice.* New York: McGraw-Hill.

Chapter 11

Ambrose, M. (1998). Chronic dyspnea. *Nursing98, 28*(5), 41–46.

Brooks-Brunn, J. (1995). Postoperative atelectasis and pneumonia. *Heart and Lung, 24*(2), 94–111.

Carpenter, D. (ed.) (1998). *Handbook of signs and symptoms.* Springhouse, PA: Springhouse Corp.

Carpenito, L. (1997). *Nursing diagnosis application to clinical practice* (7th ed.) Philadelphia: Lippincott Williams & Wilkins

DeGowin, R. L. (1994). *De Gowin and DeGowin's diagnostic examination* (6th ed.). New York: McGraw-Hill.

Desphpande, V., Pibeam, S., & Dixon, R. (1988). *A comprehensive review of respiratory care.* Norwalk, CN: Appelton & Lange.

Doenges, M.E., & Moorhouse, M.F. (1998). *Nurse's pocket guide: Diagnoses, interventions, and rationales.* Philadelphia: F. A. Davis.

Epstein, O., Perkin, G., deBono, D., & Cookson, J. (1997). *Clinical examination* (2nd ed.). Philadelphia: C. V. Mosby.

Goroll, A., May, L., & Mulley, A. (1995). *Primary care medicine office evaluation and management of the adult patient* (3rd ed.). Philadelphia: Lippincott-Raven.

Guyton, A. C. (1991). *Textbook of medical physiology* (8th ed.). Philadelphia: W. B. Saunders.

Hanson, C. (1996). *Instant nursing assessment: Gerontologic.* New York: Delmar.

Isselbacher, K., Braunwald, E., Wilson, J. Martin, J. Fauci., & Kasper, D. (Eds.) (1995). *Harrison's principles of internal medicine (13th ed.) companion handbook.* New York: McGraw-Hill.

Marieb, E. N. (1992). *Human anatomy and physiology* (2nd ed.). Menlo Park, CA: Benjamin/Cummings.

Mezey, M., Rauckhorst, L., & Stokes, S. (1993). *Health assessment of the older individual* (2nd ed.). New York: Springer.

Morton, P. (1993). *Health assessment in nursing* (2nd ed.) Springhouse, PA: Springhouse.

Polaski, A., & Tatro, S. (1996). *Luckmann's core principles and practice of medical-surgical nursing.* Philadelphia: W. B. Saunders.

Scanlon, V., & Sanders, T. (1995). *Essentials of anatomy and physiology* (2nd ed.). Philadelphia: F. A. Davis.

Sellers, R. (1996). *Differential diagnosis of common complaints* (3rd ed.). Philadelphia: W. B. Saunders.

Thomas, C.L. (ed.). (1997). *Taber's cyclopedic medical dictionary* (18th ed.). Philadelphia: F. A. Davis.

Wilkins, R., Hodgkins, J., & Lopez, B. (1996). *Lung sounds: A practical guide* (2nd ed.). Philadelphia: C. V. Mosby.

Chapter 12

Carpenter, D. (ed). (1998). *Handbook of signs and symptoms.* Springhouse, PA: Springhouse.

Cray, J., Kothare, V., & Weinstock, D. (eds.) (1999). *Auscultation skills: Breath and heart sounds*. Springhouse, PA: Springhouse.

Doenges, M., Moorehouse, M. & Geissler, A. (1997). *Nursing care plans: Guidelines for individualizing patient care* (4th ed.). Philadelphia: F. A. Davis.

Epstein, O., Perkin, G., de Bono, D., & Cookson, J. (1997). *Clinical examination* (2nd ed.). Philadelphia: C. V. Mosby.

Erickson, B., Littman, D., Liebson, P., Stovall, W. & Tavel, M. (1997). *3M education program cardiac auscultation—Heart Sounds Study Guide*. St. Paul: 3M.

Goroll, A., & Mulley, A. (2000). *Primary care medicine*. Philadelphia: Lippincott Williams & Wilkins.

Isselbacher, K., Braunwald, E., Wilson, J., Martin, J., Fauci, A., & Kasper, D. (1995). *Harrison's principles of internal medicine* (15th ed.). New York: McGraw-Hill.

Lewis, S., Heitkemper, M., & Dirksen, S. (2000). *Medical-surgical nursing assessment and management of clinical problems* (5th ed.) Philadelphia: C. V. Mosby.

Mangione, S. (2000). *Physical diagnosis secrets*. Philadelphia: Hanley & Belfus, Inc.

Mason, D. (2000). *Listening to the heart*. Philadelphia: F. A. Davis.

Morton, P. (1993). *Health assessment in nursing* (2nd ed.). Philadelphia: F. A. Davis.

Scanlon, V., & Sanders, T. (1995). *Essentials of anatomy and physiology* (2nd ed.). Philadelphia: F. A. Davis.

Sellers, R. (1996). *Differential diagnosis of common complaints* (3rd ed.). Philadelphia: W. B. Saunders.

Sommers, M., & Johnson, S. (1997). *Davis's manual of nursing therapeutics for diseases and disorders*. Philadelphia: F. A. Davis.

Stampfer, M., Hu, F., Manson, J., Rimm, E., & Willett, W. (2000). Primary prevention of coronary heart disease in women through diet and lifestyle. *The New England Journal of Medicine, 343*(1): 16–22.

Van Wynsberghe, Noback, C., & Carola, R. (1995). *Human anatomy and physiology* (3rd ed.). New York: McGraw-Hill.

Venes, D. (ed.). (2001). *Taber's cyclopedic medical dictionary* (19th ed). Philadelphia: F. A. Davis.

Chapter 13

Anand, S.S., et al. (1998). Does this patient have deep vein thrombosis? *Journal of the American Medical Association,* 279:1094.

Barkauskas, V. H., Stoltenberg-Allen, K., Bauman, L. C., & Darling-Fisher, C. (1994). *Health and Physical Assessment*. St. Louis: C.V. Mosby.

Bichler, L. M. (1999) Foot ulcers in diabetes: *Advance for Nurse Practitioners, 7,* 50.

Bickley, L. S., Hoekelman, R. A., & Bates, B. (1998). *Bates' guide to physical examination and history* taking. Philadelphia: Lippincott Williams & Wilkins.

Blank, C. A., & Irwin, G. H (1990). PV disorders—assessment and intervention *7:*777.

Carman, T. L., & Fernandez, B. B (1999). Issues and controversies in venous thromboembolism. *66:*113, 1999.

Carpenito, L .1997) *Nursing diagnosis application to clinical practice* (7th ed.) Philadelphia: Lippincott Williams & Wilkins.

Criqui, M. H., & Denenberg, J. O (1999). American Heart Association's hypertension primer. Council on high blood pressure research. Dallas: American Heart Association.

Dains, J. E., Baumann, L. C., & Scheibel, P (1998). *Advanced health assessment and clinical diagnosis in primary care*. St. Louis: C.V. Mosby.

Ginsberg, J. S. (1996) Management of venous thromboembolism. *New England Journal of Medicine, 335,*1816.

Guyton, A. C. (1991) *Textbook of medical physiology* (8th ed.) Philadelphia: W. B. Saunders.

Gray, B. H., & Sullivan, T. M. (1997). Vascular claudication: How to individualize treatment:
Cleveland Clinic Journal of Medicine, 64, 429.

Howes, P. S. (1998) Treating intermittent claudication: *RN, 98,*16A.

Lemone, P., & Burke, K. M (1996) *Medical surgical nursing—Critical thinking in client care*. Menlo Park, CA: Addison-Wesley.

Lymphoedema Foundation at Post Office Box 834, San Diego, CA 92014-0823 or Tollfree at 1-800-LYMPH-DX.

Morton, P.G. (1995). *Health assessment* (2nd ed.) Philadelphia: Springhouse.

Petrella, R. J. (1999). Exercise for older patients with chronic disease: *The Physician and Sportsmedicine, 27,* 79.

Powers, K.B., Vacek, J.L., & Lee, S. (1999). Noninvasive approaches to PV disease. *Postgraduate Medicine, 106,* 52.

Purnell, L., and Paulanka, B. (2003). *Transcultural health care: A culturally competent approach* (2nd ed.). Philadelphia: F. A. Davis.

Rice, K.L. (1998). Peripheral arterial occlusive disease, part 1: Navigating a bottleneck: *Nursing98, 28,* 33.

Ridkler, P.M. (1997). Age-specific incidence rates of venous thromboembolism among heterozygous carriers of factor V Leiden mutation. *Annals of Internal Medicine, 126,* 528.

Seidel, H. M., Ball, J. W., Dains, J. E., & Benedict, G. W. (1995) *Mosby's Guide to Physical Examination* (3rd ed.). St. Louis: C.V.Mosby.

Seller, R. H (1996) *Differential Diagnosis of Common Complaints*. Philadelphia: W. B. Saunders.

Taber's Cyclopedic Medical Dictionary, Philadelphia: F.A. Davis.

UKCC Professional Development Categories (1997). The assessment and treatment of patients with lyphoedema, *Nursing Standard, 11,* 49.

Zafar, M. U., & Farkouh, M. E. (1999). Diagnosing and managing lower extremity arterial disease. *Internal Medicine, 20,* 31.

Chapter 14

American Cancer Society (2002). *CA: A Cancer Journal for Clinicians Cancer Statistics 2002*. Volume 52, No 1. Atlanta, GA: American Cancer Society.

Lewis, S., Heitkemper, M., & Dirksen, S. (2000). *Medical-Surgical Nursing Assessment and Management of Clinical Problems* (5th ed.). Philadelphia: C. V. Mosby.

Molyneaux, D. (1995). *Predicting the practice and teaching of breast self-examination of student nurses*. Unpublished doctoral dissertation, Widener University, Chester.

Morton, P. (1993). *Health assessment in nursing* (2nd ed.). Philadelphia: F. A. Davis.

Tanner, J. (1962). *Growth at adolescence* (2nd ed.). Oxford: Blackwell Scientific.

Chapter 15

Alberts, D. S., Martinez, M. E., Roe, D. J., Guillen-Rodriguez, J. M., Marshall, J. R., Van Leeuwen, J. B., Reid, M. E., Ritenbaugh, C., Vargus, P. A., Battacharyya, A. B., Earnest, D. L., Sampliner, R. E., & the Phoenix Colon Cancer Prevention Physician's Network (2000). Lack of effect of a high-fiber cereal supplement on the recurrence of colorectal adenomas. *The New England Journal of Medicine, 342*(16), 1156–1162.

American Institute for Cancer Research (2000). Cancer researchers agree: New colon cancer studies send wrong message. Located on the internet at: *http://www.aicr.org/r042000.htm*

Anderson, K. (1996). *Mosby's medical, nursing and allied health dictionary* (4th ed.). St. Louis: C. V. Mosby.

Barkauskas, V. H., Stoltenberg-Allen, K., Baumann, L. C., & Darling-Fisher, C. (1998). *Health and physical assessment* (2nd ed.). St. Louis: Mosby-Year Book, Inc.

Bates, B., Bickley, L. S., & Hoekelman, R. A. (1995). *Physical examination and history taking* (6th ed.). Philadelphia: Lippincott-Raven.

Becker, K. L., & Stevens, S. A. (1988). Performing in-depth abdominal assessment. *Nursing88, 18*(6), 59–63.

Black, J. M., & Matassarin-Jacobs, E. (1993). *Luckmann and Sorenson's medical-surgical nursing: A psychophysiological approach* (4th ed.). Philadelphia: W.B. Saunders Company.

Burkhart, C. (1992). Guidelines for rapid assessment of abdominal pain indicative of acute surgical abdomen. *Nurse Practitioner: American Journal of Primary Healthcare, 17*(6), 39, 43–46.

L.J. (1997). *Nursing diagnosis: Application to clinical practice* (7th ed.). Philadelphia: Lippincott Williams & Wilkins.

Giger, J. N., & Davidhizar, R. E. (1995). *Transcultural nursing assessment and intervention* (3rd ed.). St. Louis: C. V. Mosby.

Harris, J. (1986). Pediatric abdominal assessment. *Pediatric Nursing, 12*(5), 355–362.

Holmgren, C. (1992). Perfecting the art of abdominal assessment. *RN, 53*(3), 28–34.

Ignatavicius, D. D., Workman, M. L., & Mishler, M. A.(1995). *Medical-surgical nursing: A nursing process approach* (2nd ed.). Philadelphia: W. B. Saunders.

Jarvis, C. (2000). *Physical examination and health assessment* (3rd ed.). Philadelphia: W.B. Saunders.

Langan, J. C. (1998). Abdominal assessment in the home: From A–Z. *Home Health-Care Nurse, 16*(1), 50–58.

Lawrence, D. M. (1993). Gastrointestinal trauma. *Critical Care Nursing Clinics of North America, 5*(1), 127–140.

Metheny, N. A., Stewart, B. J., Smith, L., Yan, H., Diebold, M., & Clouse, R. E. (1999). PH and concentration of bilirubin in feeding tube aspirates as predictors of tube placement. *Nursing Research, 48*(4), 189–197.

Munn, N. E. (1988). Diagnosis: Acute abdomen. *Nursing88, 18*(9), 34–42.

Niles, M. A., Bufffington, C., Cowan, G., & Hepworth, J. T. (1998). Comparison of lifestyles among obese and nonobese African American and European American women in the community. *Nursing Research, 47*(4), 251–257.

O'Hanlon-Nichols, T. (1998). Basic assessment series: Gastrointestinal System. *American Journal of Nursing, 98*(4), 48–53.

O'Toole, M. T. (1990). Advanced assessment of the abdomen and gastrointestinal problems. *Nursing Clinics of North America, 25*(4), 771–775.

Piscara, V.H. (1999). Recognizing the various presentations of appendicitis. *The Nurse Practitioner, 24*(8), 48–55.

Porth, C. M. (1994). *Pathophysiology concepts of altered health states* (4th ed.). Philadelphia: Lippincott-Raven.

Santilli, J, & Santilli, S.(1997). Diagnosis and treatment of abdominal aortic aneurysms. *American Family Physician [on line]*, *56*(4), 1–12.

Schatzin, A., Lanza, E., Corle, D., Lance, P., Iber, F., Caan, B., Shike, M., Weissfeld, J., Burt, R., Cooper, M. R., Kikendall, J. W., Cahill, J., & the Polyp Prevention Trial Study Group(2000). Lack of effect of a low-fat, high fiber diet on the recurrence of colorectal adenomas. *The New England Journal of Medicine, 342*(16), 1149–1155.

Seidel, H. M., Ball, J. W., Dains, J. E., & Benedict, G. W. (1999). *Mosby's guide to physical examination* (4th ed.). St. Louis: C. V. Mosby.

Shaw, B. (1995). Primary care for women: Comprehensive assessment of gastrointestinal disorders. *Journal of Nurse-Midwifery, 40*(2), 216–30, 59–64.

Shaw, B. (1996). Management and treatment of gastrointestinal disorders. *Journal of Nurse-Midwifery, 41*(2), 155–172.

Slota, M. (1982). Abdominal assessment. *Critical Care Nurse, 2,* 78–81.

Smith, C .E. (1988). Assessing bowel sounds: More than just listening. *Nursing88, 18*(2), 42–43.

Stone, R. (1996). Primary care diagnosis of acute abdominal pain. *The Nurse Practitioner, 21*(12), 19–41.

Thibodeau, G. A., & Patton, K. T. (1993). *Anatomy and physiology* (2nd ed.). St. Louis: Mosby-Year Book, Inc.

Thibodeau, G. A., & Patton, K. T. (1999). *Anthony's textbook of anatomy and physiology* (16th ed.). St. Louis: C. V. Mosby.

Thompson, J. M., & Wilson, S. F. (1996). *Health assessment for nursing practice*. St.Louis: Mosby-Year Book, Inc.

Town, J. (1997). Bringing acute abdomen into focus. *Nursing97, 27*(5), 52–58.

Wong, D. (1999). *Nursing care of infants and children* (6th ed.). St. Louis: Mosby.

Wright, J. (1997). Seven abdominal assessment signs every emergency nurse should know. *Journal of Emergency Nursing, 23, 446–450.*

Zator Estes, M. E. (1998). *Health assessment and physical examination*. Albany: Delmar Publishers.

American Cancer Society (2000). The colon and rectum cancer resource center. Available at: *www3.cancer.org/cancerinfo/load_cont.asp?st=ds&ct=10* and *www3.cancer.org/cancerinfo/load_cont.asp?st=pr&ct=10.*

Chapter 16

Allen, K., & Phillips, J. (1997). *Women's health across a lifespan*. Philadelphia: Lippincott Williams & Wilkins.

Barkauskas, V., Stoltenberg-Allen, K., Baumann, L., & Darling-Fisher, C. (1998). *Health and physical assessment* (2nd ed.). St. Louis: C. V. Mosby.

Bates, B. (1999). *A guide to physical examination* (7th ed.). Philadelphia: Lippincott Williams & Wilkins.

Centers for Disease Control and Prevention (1998). *Guidelines for treatment of sexually transmitted diseases. MMWR,* Rep 47 (RR-1), 1–118.

Harlan, L. C., Bernstein, A. M., & Kessler, L. F. (1991). Cervical cancer screening. *Journal of Public Health, 81*(7), 855–890.

Hawkins, J., & Roberto-Nichols, D. (1997). *Protocols for nurse practitioners in gynecologic settings*. Tiresias Press, Inc.

Morton, (1993). *Health assessment in nursing* (2nd ed.). Springhouse, PA: Springhouse.

Noble, J. (1996). *Textbook of primary care medicine*. St. Louis: C. V. Mosby.

Seidel, H., et al. (1999). *Mosby's guide to physical exam*. St. Louis: C. V. Mosby.

Chapter 17

American Academy of Pediatrics (1999). *Periodic survey of fellows #37, pediatrician attitudes, experiences mixed on circumcision counseling. HTTP://WWW.aap.org/research/p537a.htm>*

American Cancer Society, Inc. (1994). *Cancer facts and figures.* (On-line). *Internet Address:bcic/acsz/gifs/fact.map.*

Bates, B. (1999). *A guide to physical examination* (7th ed.). Philadelphia: Lippincott Williams & Wilkins.

Centers for Disease Control and Prevention (1998). Guidelines for the treatment of sexually transmitted diseases. *Morbidity and Mortality Weekly Report,* Rep 47 (RR-1), 1–118.

Holmes, K. K., March, P. A., & Sparling, P. F.(1990). *Sexually transmitted diseases* (2nd ed). New York: McGraw-Hill.

Jaffe, M., & McVan, B. (1997). *Davis's laboratory and diagnostic test handbook.* Philadelphia: F. A. Davis.

Lerman, S. E., & Liao, J. C.(2001). Neonatal Circumcision. *Pediatric Clinics of North America, 48*(6):1539–1557.

Lewis, S., McLean Heitkemper, M., & Ruff Dirksen, S. (2000). *Medical surgical nursing assessment and management of clinical problems* (5th ed.). Philadelphia: C. V. Mosby.

Morton, P. G. (1993). *Health assessment in nursing* (2nd ed.) Philadelphia: F. A. Davis.

Tanner, J. M. (1962). *Growth at adolescence* (2nd ed.). Oxford: Blackwell Scientific Publications.

Walsh, P. C., Retik, A. P., Stamey, T. A., & Vaughn, E. D. (1992). *Campbell's urology* (6th ed.). Philadelphia: W. B.Saunders.

Wynsberghe, D., Noback, C., & Carola, R. (1995). *Human anatomy and physiology* (3rd ed.). New York: McGraw-Hill, Inc.

Chapter 18

Alexander, M., & Kuo, K. N. (1997). Musculoskeletal assessment of the newborn. *Orthopaedic Nursing, 16*(1), 21–31.

Allison, M., & Keller, C. (1997). Physical activity in the elderly: Benefits and intervention strategies. *Nurse Practitioner, 22*(8), 53–69.

Behrman, R.E., & Vaughan, V. C.(eds). (1996). *Nelson textbook of pediatrics* (15th ed.). Philadelphia: W. B. Saunders.

Benetti, M. C., & Marchese, T. (1996). Management of common musculoskeletal disorders. *Journal of Nurse Midwifery, 41*(2), 173–187.

Birnbaum, J. S. (1976). *The musculoskeletal manual.* Orlando, FL: Grune & Stratton.

DeGowin, E., & DeGowin, R. (1987). *Bedside diagnostic examination* (5th ed.). New York: Macmillan.

Gordon, M. (1979). Assessing activity tolerance. *American Journal of Nursing, 76,* 72–75.

Hunt, A. H. (1996). The relationship between height change and bone mineral density. *Orthopaedic Nursing, 15*(3), 57–64.

Jones, A. K. (1997). Primary care management of acute low back pain. *Nurse Practitioner, 22*(7), 50–68.

Jones-Walton, P. (1990). Orthopaedic nursing assessment. *Advanced Clinical Care, 5*(3), 22.

Killam, P. (1989). Orthopaedics assessment of young children: Developmental variations. *Nurse Practitioner, 14*(7), 27–32.

Lewis, S., Heitkemper, M., & Dirksen, S. (*2001*). *Medical surgical nursing assessment and management of clinical problems* (5th ed.). Philadelphia: C. V. Mosby.

Maldonado, A. (1995). Comprehensive assessment of common musculoskeletal disorders. *Journal of Nurse Midwifery, 40*(2), 202–215.

Mason, K. (1989). Pediatric orthopaedics: Developmental norms. *Orthopedic Nursing, 8*(4), 45–50.

McIntosh, E. (1997). Low back pain in adults: Guidelines for the history and physical exam. *Advanced Nursing Practice, 5*(8), 16–25.

Milde, F. (1988). Impaired physical mobility. *Journal of Gerontological Nursing, 14*(3), 20–24, 38–40.

Muscari, M.E. (1998). Preventing sports injuries. *American Journal of Nursing, 98*(7), 58–60.

O'Hanlon-Nichols, T. (1998). A review of the adult musculoskeletal system. *American Journal of Nursing, 98*(6), 48–52.

Riggs, B., & Melton, L. (1995). The worldwide problem of osteoporosis: Insights afforded by epidemiology. *Bone, 17*(*Suppl.5*), 505S–511S.

Ross, C.A. (1997). A comparison of osteoarthritis and rheumatoid arthritis: Diagnosis and treatment. *Nurse Practitioner, 22*(9), 20–41.

Treml, L.A. (1996). Assessing patient mobility: Mobility screening a part of a community-based geriatric assessment. *Home Care Provider, 1*(1), 26–29.

Shaefer, K. M. (1997). Health patterns of women whith fibromyalgia. *Journal of Advanced Nursing, 26,* 565.

Spence, A., & Mason, E. (1987). *Human anatomy and physiology* (3rd ed.). Menlo Park, CA: Benjamin-Cummings.

Williams, M. A., Oberst, M. T., Bjoklund, B. C., & Hugher, S. H. (1996). Family caregiving in cases of hip fracture. Rehabilitation Nursing, *21*(3), 124–131, 138.

Wallace, M. (1994). Assessment and management of pain in the elderly. *MEDSURG Nursing, 3,* 293–298.

Woodhead, G. A. & Moss, N. M. (1998). Osteoporosis: Diagnosis and prevention. *Nurse Practitioner, 23*(11), 18–37.

Chapter 19

Carrozzella, J., & Jauch, E. (2002). Emergency stroke management: A new era. *Nursing Clinics of North America, 37*(1), 35–58.

Goroll, A., & Mulley, A. (2000). *Primary Care Medicine* (4th ed). Philadelphia: Lippincott Williams & Wilkins.

Hock, N. (1999). Brain attack: The stroke continuum. *Nursing Clinics of North America, 34*(3), 689–724.

Lewis, S., Heitkemper, M., & Dirksen, S. (2001). *Medical Surgical Nursing Assessment and management of clinical problems* (5th ed). Philadelphia: C. V. Mosby.

Lower, J. (2002). Facing neuro assessment fearlessly. *Nursing 2002, 32*(2), 58–64.

Morton, P. (1995). *Health assessment in nursing* (2nd ed.). Philadelphia: F. A. Davis.

Neatherlin, J. (1999). Foundation for practice: Neuroassessment for neuroscience nurse. *Nursing Clinics of North America, 34*(3), 573–592.

National Institute of Neurological Diseases, United States Department of Health and Human Services, National Institutes of Health: Stroke scales.

Purnell, L., & Paulanka, B. (2003). *Transcultural health care: A culturally comptent approach* (2nd ed.). Philadelphia: F. A. Davis.

Ringleb, P., Schellinger, P., Schranz, C., & Hacke, W. (2002). Thrombolytic therapy within 3 to 6 hours after the onset of ischemic stroke: Useful or harmful? *Stroke, 33*(5), 1437–1441.

Scanlon, V., & Sanders, T. (1995). *Essentials of anatomy and physiology* (2nd ed.). Philadelphia: F. A. Davis.

Thomas, C. (ed.) (1997). *Taber's cyclopedic medical dictionary* (18th ed.). Philadelphia: F. A. Davis.

USNIH, NINDS (1999–2000). *Brain basics: Preventing stroke.* Bethesda: NIH Neurological Institute.

Walley and Wong, 2001

Van Wynsberghe, D., Noback, C., & Carola, R. (1995). *Human anatomy and physiology* (3rd ed.). New York: McGraw-Hill, Inc.

Chapter 20

AWHONN 1999). *Monograph I: Postmenopausal health and the importance of prevention.* Chicago: Pragmation.

AWHONN (1999). *Monograph II: Disease prevention strategies among postmenopausal women*. Chicago: Pragmation.

Carpenito, L. (1997). *Nursing diagnosis: Application to clinical practice* (7th ed.). Philadelphia: Lippincott Williams & Wilkins.

DeGowin, R. L. (1994). *DeGowin and De Gowin's diagnostic examination* (6th ed.). New York: McGraw-Hill.

Doenges, M. E., Moorhouse, M. F., & Geissler, A. C. (1997). *Nursing care plans: Guidelines for individualizing patient care* (4th ed.). Philadelphia: F. A. Davis.

Goroll, A., May, L., & Mulley, A. (1995). *Primary care medicine: Office evaluation and management of the adult patient* (3rd ed.). Philadelphia: Lippincott-Raven.

Morton, P. (1993). *Health assessment in nursing* (2nd ed.). Springhouse, PA: Springhouse.

North American Nursing Diagnosis Association (2001). *NANDA nursing diagnoses: Definitions and classification, 2001–2002*. Philadelphia: NANDA.

Polanski, A., & Tatro, S. (1996). *Luckmann's core principles and practice of medical-surgical nursing*. Philadelphia: W.B. Saunders.

Report of the U.S. Preventive Services Task Force (1996). *Guide to clinical preventive services: An assessment of 169 interventions*. Baltimore: Williams &Wilkins.

Scanlon, V., & Saunders, T. (1999). *Essentials of anatomy and physiology* (3rd ed.). Philadelphia: F. A. Davis.

Taylor, C., Lillis, C.,& LeMone, P. (2001). *Fundamentals of nursing: The art and science of nursing care* (4th ed.). Philadelphia: Lippincott Williams & Wilkins.

Venes, D. (ed.) (2001). *Taber's cyclopedic medical dictionary* (19th ed.). Philadelphia: F. A. Davis.

Chapter 21

Carcio, H. A. (1999). *Advanced Health Assessment of Women*. Philadelphia: Lippincott Williams & Wilkins.

Cunningham, F. G., MacDonald, P. C., Gant, N. F., Leveno, K. J., Gilstrap III, L. C., Hankins, G. D. V., & Clark, S. L. (1997). *Williams' Obstetrics* (20th ed.). Stamford, CT: Appleton & Lange.

Darcus, J. V., Meyer, N. L., & Sibai, B. M. (1996). How preconception counseling improves pregnancy outcome. *Contemporary OB/GYN, 40*(6), 11–115.

Ferguson, H. W., & Hisley, S. M. (2000). *Nurse Test: Maternal-Newborn Nursing* (2nd ed.). Springhouse, PA: Springhouse.

Gorrie, T. M., McKinney, E. S., & Murray, S. S. (1998). *Foundations of Maternal-Newborn Nursing* (2nd ed.). Philadelphia: W. B. Saunders.

Hoebel, C. J. (1998). Routine antenatal laboratory tests and specific screening tests. *Contemporary OB/GYN, 56*(2), 25–34.

Jarvis, C. (1996). *Physical Examination and Health Assessment* (2nd ed.). Philadelphia: W. B. Saunders.

Lowdermilk, D. L., Perry, S. E.,& Bobak, I. M. (1997). *Maternity and Women's Health Care* (6th ed.). St. Louis: C. V. Mosby.

Niebyl, J. (1995). Folic acid supplementation to prevent birth defects. *Contemporary OB/GYN, 40*(6), 43–39.

O'Brien, B., & Zhou, Q. (1995). Variables related to nausea and vomiting during pregnancy. *Birth, 22*(2), 93–96.

Pillitteri, A. (1995). *Maternal & Child Health Nursing*. Philadelphia: Lippincott-Raven.

Purnell, L. D., & Paulanka, B. J. (2003). *Transcultural health care: A culturally competent approach* (2nd ed.). Philadelphia: F. A.Davis.

Rogers, J., & Davis, B. (1995). How risky are hot tubs and saunas for pregnant women? *MCN American Journal of Maternal Child Nursing, 20*(3), 137–139.

Simpson, K. R., & Creehan, P. A. (1996). *AWHONN Perinatal Nursing*. Philadelphia: Lippincott-Raven.

Spector, R. E. (1991). *Cultural diversity in health and illness* (3rd ed.). Norwalk, CT: Appleton & Lange.

Weber, J., & Kelley, J. (1998). *Health Assessment in Nursing*. Philadelphia: Lippincott Williams & Wilkins.

Wheeler, L. (1997). *Nurse mid-wifery handbook: A practical guide to prenatal and postpartum care*. Philadelphia: Lippincott-Raven.

Youngkin, E. Q., & Davis, M. S. (1998). *Women's Health: A Primary Care Clinical Guide* (2nd ed.). Stamford, CT: Appleton & Lange.

Chapter 22

Ballard, J., et al. (1991). New Ballard score, expanded to include extremely premature infants. *Journal of Pediatrics, 119*(3), 417–423.

Barkauskas, V., Stoltenberg-Allen, K., Baumann, L., & Darling-Fisher, C. (1998). *Health and physical assessment* (2nd ed.). St. Louis: C. V. Mosby.

Creehan, P. (2001/2002). Sending baby home safely. *Lifeline, 5*(6), 60–70.

Dickason, E., Lang Silverman, B, & Kaplan, J. (1998). *Maternal-infant nursing care* (3rd ed.). Philadelphia: C. V. Mosby.

Fuller, J., & Schaller-Ayers, J. (2000). *Health assessment: A nursing approach*. Philadelphia: Lippincott Williams & Wilkins.

Gardner, P., & Georges, P. (2001). Recommended schedules for routine immunization of children and adults. *Infectious Disease Clinics of North America, 15*(1), 1–8.

Lowdermilk, D. L., Perry, S. E., & Bobak, I. M. (2000). *Maternity and women's health* care (7th ed.). St. Louis: C. V. Mosby.

National Highway Traffic Safety Administration (2000). Traffic safety facts for 1999, Washington, DC: U.S. Department of Transportation. *http://www.nsc.org/lrs/statinfo/99report.htm*

Nichols, F. H., & Zwelling, E. (1997). *Maternal-newborn nursing: theory and practice*. Philadelphia: W. B. Saunders.

Olds, S. B., London, M. L., & Weiland Ladewig, P. A. (2000). *Maternal newborn nursing: A family and community-based approach* (6th ed.) Upper Saddle River: Prentice-Hall Health.

Purnell, L., & Paulanka, B. (2003). *Transcultural health care: A culturally competent approach* (2nd ed.). Philadelphia: F. A. Davis.

Weber, J.R. (2001). *Nurses' handbook of health assessment* (4th ed.). Philadelphia: Lippincott Williams & Wilkins.

Wilson, D. D. (1999). *Nurses' guide to understanding laboratory and diagnostic tests*. Philadelphia: Lippincott Williams & Wilkins.

Wilson, S. F., & Giddens, J. F. (2001). *Health assessment for nursing practice* (2nd ed.). St. Louis: C. V. Mosby.

Wong, D., & Hockenberry-Eaton, M. (2001). *Wong's essentials of pediatric nursing* (6th ed.). Philadelphia: C. V. Mosby.

Chapter 23

American Academy of Pediatrics (1991). *Caring for your adolescent: Ages 12–21*. New York:Bantam Books.

American Medical Association (1999). *Implementation guide for school-based health centers*. American Medical Association.

Berti, L., Zylbert, S., & Rolnitzky, L. (2001). Comparison of health status of children

Erikson, Erik (1968). *Identity youth and crisis*. New York: W.W. Norton & Company.

Green, Morris (Ed. (1994). *Bright futures: Gidelines for health su-*

pervision of infants, children, and adolescents. Arlington, VA: National Center for Education in Maternal and Child Health.

Mobley, C., & Evanshevski, J. (2000). Evaluating health and safety knowledge of preschoolers: Assessing their early start to begin health smart. *Journal of Pediatric Health Care, 4*(4), 160–165.

Morton, P. (1995). *Health assessment in nursing.* Philadelphia: F. A. Davis.

Seidel, H. M., Ball, J. W., Dains, J. E., & Benedict, G. W. (1999). *Mosby's guide to physical examination* (4th ed.). St. Louis: C. V. Mosby.

Thomas, C. (ed.). (1997). Taber's cyclopedic medical dictionary (18th ed.). Philadelphia: F. A. Davis.

United States Department of Health and Human Services (USDHHS) (1997). *Put prevention into Practice.* Wash. DC: USDHHS.

Using a school-based health center for comprehensive care. *Journal of Pediatric Health Care, 15*(5): 244–249.

Wong, D., Hockenberry-Eaton, M., Wilson, D., Winkelstein, M. & Schwartz, P. (2001). *Wong's Essentials of Pediatric Nursing* (6th ed.). Philadelphia: C. V. Mosby.

Chapter 24

American Academy of Pediatrics. (1991). *Caring for your adolescent: Ages 12–21.* New York: Bantam Books.

American Medical Association (1999). *Implementation guide for school-based health centers.* American Medical Association.

Berti, L., Zylbert, S., Rolnitzky, L. (2001). Comparison of health status of children

Erikson, Erik (1968). *Identity youth and crisis.* New York: W.W. Norton & Company.

Green, Morris (ed.) (1994). *Bright futures: guidelines for health supervision of infants, children, and adolescents.* Arlington, VA: National Center for Education in Maternal and Child Health.

Mobley, C., & Evanshevski, J. (2000). Evaluating health and safety knowledge of preschoolers: Assessing their early start to begin health smart. *Journal of Pediatric Health Care, 14*(4), 160–165.

Morton, P. (1995). *Health assessment in nursing.* Philadelphia: F. A. Davis.

Seidel, H. M., Ball, J. W., Dains, J. E., & Benedict, G. W. (1999). *Mosby's guide to physical examination* (4th ed.). St. Louis: C. V. Mosby.

Thomas, C. (ed.). (1997). *Taber's cyclopedic medical dictionary* (18th ed.). Philadelphia: F. A. Davis.

United States Department of Health and Human Services (USDHHS) (1997). *Put prevention into* Practice. Wash. DC: USDHHS.

Using a School-based Health Center for Comprehensive Care. Journal of Pediatric Health *care, 15*(5): 244–249.

Wong, D., Hockenberry-Eaton, M., Wilson, D., Winkelstein, M., & Schwartz, P. (2001). *Wong's Essentials of Pediatric Nursing* (6th ed.). Philadelphia: C. V. Mosby.

Chapter 25

Abdul, A., & Mourad, F. (1998). Constipation: Common-sense care of the older client. *Geriatrics, 51,* 28–36.

Advisory Committee on Immunization Practices, Centers for Disease Control and Prevention. *Http://www.americangeriatrics.org/immsched.html*

Agachan, F., Chen, T., Pfeifer, J., Reissman, P., & Wexner, S. (1996). A constipation scoring system to simplify evaluation and management of constipated clients. *Diseases of the Colon and Rectum, 39,* 681–685.

Alessi, C., Yoon, E., Schnelle, J., Al-Samarrai, N., & Cruise, P. (1999). A randomized trial of a combined physical activity and environmental intervention in nursing home residents: Do sleep and agitation improve? *Journal of the American Geriatric Society, 47,* 784–792.

American Cancer Society mammography guidelines. (1983). *California Cancer Journal Clinicals, 33,* 255–259.

American Medical Association, Council on Scientific Affairs (1997). Mammographic screening in asymptomatic women aged 40 years and older. *Journal of the American Medical Association, 261,* 2535–2542.

Bartkiw, T., & Pynn, B. (1994). Burning mouth syndrome: An overlooked condition in the geriatric population. *Geriatric Nursing, 15,* 241–245.

Benson, S. (1975). Simple chronic constipation: Pathophysiology and management. *Post-graduate Medicine, 5,* 55–60.

Bravo, G., Gauthier, P., Roy, P., Payette, H., Gaulin, P., Harvey, M. Peloquin, L, & Dubois, M. (1996). Impact of a 12-month exercise program on the physical and psychological health of osteopenic women. *Journal of the American Geriatrics Society, 44,* 756–762.

Buchner, D., Cress, M., Wagner, E., de Lateur, B., Price, R., and Abrass, I. (1993). The Seattle FICSIT/MoveIt study: the effect of exercise on gait and balance in older adults. *Journal of the American Geriatrics Society, 41,* 321–325.

Cassell, C., Cohen, H., Larson, E., Resnick, N., Rubenstein, L, & Sorensen, L. (1996). *Geriatric medicine.* New York: Springer.

Chandler, J. (1996). Understanding the relationship between strength and mobility in frail older persons: A review of the literature. *Topics of Geriatric Rehabilitation, 11,* 20–37.

Chaouloft, F. (1997). Effects of acute physical exercise on central serotonergic systems. *Medicine and Science in Sports and Exercise, 29,* 58–62.

Clark, D. (1999). Physical activity and its correlates among urban primary care clients aged 55 years or older. *The Journal of Gerontology, 54B,* S41–S48.

Costanza, M. (1992). Breast cancer screening in older women: Synopsis of a forum. *Cancer, 69,* 1925–1931.

Daly, M. Nutritional status and involuntary weight loss. In A. Adelman & M. Daly (2000). 20 common problems in geriatrics. New York: McGraw-Hill, pp. 337–367.

Dishman, R. (1994). Motivating older adults to exercise. *Southern Medical Journal, 87,* s79–s82.

Dobbs, R., Chalett, A. & Bowes, S. (1993). Is this walk normal? *Age and Ageing, 22,* 25–30.

Dungan, J., Brown, K., and Ramsey, B. (1996). Health maintenance for independent frail older adults: Can it improve physical and mental health? *Journal of Advanced Nursing, 23,* 1185–1193.

Dunlap, R. (1997). Teaching advance directives: The why, when and how. *Journal of Gerontological Nursing, 23,* 11–16.

Duke University Center for the Study of Aging and Human Development, The multidimensional Functional Assessment Questionnaire, ed. 2, pp. 169–170; 154–156; 157–162. Duke University, North Carolina.

Elliott, J. (1988). Swallowing disorders in the elderly: A guide to diagnosis and treatment. *Geriatrics, 43,* 95–99.

Emanuel, E., & Emanuel, L. (1992). Proxy decision making. *Journal of the American Medical Association, 267,* 2221–2226.

Elward, K., & Larson, E. (1992). Benefits of exercise of older adults. *Clinics of Geriatric Medicine, 8,* 35–50.

Erikson, E. (1982). The life cycle completed: A review. New York: Morton.

Ettinger, W. (1996). Physical activity and older people: A walk a day keeps the doctor away. *Journal of the American Geriatrics Society, 44,* 207–208.

Folstein, M., Folstein, S., & McHugh, P. (1975). Mini-mental state: A practical method for grading the cognitive state of clients for the clinician. *Journal of Psychiatric Research, 12,* 189–198.

Goldberg, T., & Chavin, S. (1997). Preventive medicine and screening in older adults. *Journal of the American Geriatrics Society, 45,* 341–354.

Goroll, A., & Mulley, A. (2000). *Primary care medicine* (4th ed.). Philadelphia: Lippincott Williams & Wilkins.

Gregg, E., Cauley, J., Seeley, D., Ensrud, K, & Bauer, D. (1998). Physical activity and osteoporotic fracture risk in older women. *Annals of Internal Medicine, 129,* 81–88.

Gruber, M., & Lance, P. (1998). Colorectal cancer detection and screening. *Lippincott's Primary Care Practice, 2,* 369–376.

Gudas, S. (1996). Implications of oncology in the aged. In Lewis, C. (ed.) *Aging The health care challenge.* Philadelphia: F. A. Davis, pp. 225–260.

Hanson, C. (1996). *Gerontologic instant nursing assessment.* New York: Delmar.

Heuvelen, M., Kemper, G., Orem, H. & Rispens, P. (1998). Physical fitness related to age and physical activity in older persons. *Medicine and Science in Sports and Exercise, 30,* 434–441.

Hogan, T. Geriatric emergencies. In C. Cassel et al. (eds.) *Geriatric medicine.* New York: Springer-Verlag, 1996.

Jacoby, S. (1999). Great sex: What's age got to do with it? *Modern Maturity, 9,* 43–45.

Johanson, J. F. (1998). Geographic distribution of constipation in the United States. *The American Journal of Gastroenterology, 93,* 188–191.

Katz, S., Ford, A, & Moskowitz, R. (1963). Studies of illness in the aged: The index of ADL. *Journal of the American Medical Association, 185,* 914–919.

Kane, R. (1996). The defeat of aging versus the importance of death. *Journal of the American Geriatrics Society, 44,* 321–325.

Kaplan, G., Strawbridge, W., Camacho, T., & Cohen, R. (1993). Factors associated with change in physical functioning in the elderly. *Journal of Aging and Health, 5,* 140–153.

King, A., Oman, R., Brassington, G., Bliwise, D., & Haskell, W. (1997). Moderate-intensity exercise and self-rated quality of sleep in older adults. *Journal of the American Medical Association, 257,* 32–37.

Lavker, R. (1995). Cutaneous aging: Chronologic versus photoaging. In B. Gilchrest (Ed.), *Photodamage.* Boston: Blackwell Sciences, pp. 125–133.

Lachs, M., Feinstein, A., & Cooney, L. A simple procedure for general screening of functional disability in elderly clients. *Annals of Internal Medicine, 112,* 699–702.

Lewis, S., Heitkemper, M., & Dirksen, S. (2000). *Medical surgical nursing assessment and management of clinical problems* (5th ed.). Philadelphia: C. V. Mosby.

Lichtenstein, M., Bess, F., & Logan, S. (1988). Validation of screening tools for identifying hearing-impaired elderly in primary care. *Journal of the American Medical Association, 259,* 2875–2878.

Mahoney, F., & Barthel, D. (1965). Functional evaluation: The Barthel Index. *Maryland State Medical Journal, 14*(2), 61–65.

Mahoney, J., Drinka, T., Abler, R., Gunter-Hunt, G., Matthews, C., Gravenstein, S., & Carnes, M. (1994). Screening for depression: Single question versus GDS. *Journal of The American Geriatrics Society, 42,* 1006–1007.

Maslow, A. (1954). *Motivation and personality.* New York: Harper & Row.

Mayfield, D., McLeod, G., & Hall, P. (1974). The CAGE questionnaire: Validation of a new alcoholism screening instrument. *American Journal of Psychology, 131,* 1121–1123.

Meador, J. (1995). Cerumen impaction in the elderly. *Journal of Gerontological Nursing, 25,* 43–45.

Metter, E., Lynch, N., Conwit, R., Lindle, R., Tobin, J., & Hurley, B. (1997). Muscle quality and age: Cross-sectional and longitudinal comparisons. *International Journal of Sports Medicine, 3,* S225–S231.

Mezey, M., Rauchhorst, L., & Stokes, S. (1993). *Health assessment of the older individual,* 2nd ed. New York: Springer.

Miller, C. (1990). *Geriatric Nursing, 11*(6), 301–302.

Morey, M., Pieper, C., & Cornoni-Huntley, J. (1998). Physical fitness and functional limitations in community-dwelling older adults. *Medicine & Science in Sports & Exercise, 30,* 715–723.

Morrell, C. H., Gordon-Salant, S, Pearson, J. D., Brant, L. J., Fozard, J. L. (1996). Age- and gender-specific reference ranges for hearing level and longitudinal changes in hearing level. *Journal of Acoustic Society of America, 100* (4 Pt 1), 1949–1967.

Morris, B., Van Niman, S., Perlin, T., Lucie, K., Vieth, J. Agricola, K., & McMurray, M. (1995). Healthcare professionals? Accuracy in predicting clients? Preferred code status. *The Journal of Family Practice, 40,* 41–44.

Nahm, E., & Resnick, B. (in press). End of life care preferences of older adults. *Nursing Ethics.*

National Institute of Health Consensus Development Conference statement (1995). Physical activity and cardiovascular health, pp 1–12.

Nesher, G., & Moore, T. (1994). Clinical presentation and treatment of arthritis in the elderly. *Clinics in Geriatric Medicine, 10,* 659–675.

Odenheimer, G., Funkenstein, H., & Beckett, L. (1994). Comparison of neurologic changes in successfully aging persons vs. the total aging population. *Archives of Neurology, 51,* 573–580.

Okumiya, K., Matsubayashi, K., Wada, T., Kimura, S., Doi, Y., and Ozawa, T. (1996). Effects of exercise on neurobehavioral function in community-dwelling older people more than 75 years of age. *Journal of the American Geriatrics Society, 44,* 569–572.

Parkatti, T., Deeg, D., Bosscher, R., & Launer, L. (1998). Physical activity and self-rated health among 55- to 89-year-old Dutch people. *Journal of Aging and Health, 10,* 311–326.

Pate, R., Pratt, M., & Blair, S. (1995). Physical activity and public health: A recommendation from the centers for Disease Control and Prevention and the American College of Sports Medicine. *Journal of the American Medical Association, 253,* 402–407.

Parker, J., Vukov, L., & Wollan, P. (1996). Abdominal pain in the elderly: Use of temperature and laboratory testing to screen for surgical disease. *Family Medicine, 28,* 193–197.

Pearson, J. D., Morrell, C.H., Gordon-Salant, S., Brant, L. J., Metter, E. J., Klein, L. L., & Fozard, J. L. (1995).Gender differences in a longitudinal study of age-associated hearing loss. *Journal of Acoustic Society of America, 97*(2), 1196–1205.

Pescatello, L., DiPietro, L., Fargo, A., Ostfeld, A., & Nadel, E. (1994). The impact of physical activity and physical fitness on health indicators among older adults. *Journal of Aging and Physical Activity, 2,* 2–13.

Potter, P., & Perry, A. (1999). *Basic nursing,* 4th ed. Philadelphia: C. V. Mosby.

Purnell, L., & Paulanka, B. (2003). *Transcultural health care: A culturally competent approach* (2nd ed.). Philadelphia: F. A. Davis.

Province, M., Hadley, E., Hornbrook, M., Lipsitz, L., Miller, J., Mulrow, C., Ory, M., Sattin, R., Tinetti, M., & Wolf, S. (1995).

The effects of exercise on falls in elderly clients. *Journal of the American Medical Association, 253,* 1341–1347.
Resnick, B. (1998). Health care practices of the old-old. *American Academy Journal of Nurse Practitioners, 10,* 147–155.
Resnick, B. (1998). Functional performance of older adults in a long term care setting. *Clinical Nursing Research, 7,* 230–246.
Resnick, B. (1999). Atrial fibrillation in the older adult: Presentation and Management. *Geriatric Nursing, 20,* 1–6.
Resnick, B. (2000). Health promotion practices of the older adult. *Public Health Nursing, 17*(3), 160–168.
Resnick, B. (2001). Geriatric health promotion. *Medscape Nursing, 1*(1)@ 2001 Medscape, Inc.
Rodeheffer, R, Gerstenblith, G., & Becker, L. (1994). Exercise cardiac output is maintained with advancing age in healthy subjects: Cardiac dilation and increased volume compensate for a diminished heart rate. *Circulation, 69,* 203–213.
Royall, D., Mulroy, A., Chiodo, L., & Polk, M. (1999). Clock drawing is sensitive to executive control: a comparison of six methods. *Journal of Gerontology, 54B,* P328–P333.
Saltzstein, S., Behling, C., & Baergen, R. (1998). Features of cancer in nonagenarians and centenarians. *Journal of the American Geriatrics Society, 46,* 994–998.
Schiffman, S. (1997). Taste and smell losses in normal aging and disease. *Journal of the American Medical Association, 256,* 1357–1360.
Seeman, T., Charpentier, P., Berkman, L., Tinetti, M., Guralnik, J., Albert, M., Blazer, D., & Rowe, J. (1993). Predicting changes in physical performance in a high-functioning elderly cohort: MacArthur studies of successful aging. *Journal of Gerontology, 49*(3), M97–M107.
Scanlon, V, .& Sanders, T. (1995). *Essentials of anatomy and physiology* (2nd ed.). Philadelphia: F. A. Davis.
Sherman, J., Abel, E., & Tavakoli, A. (1996). Demographic predictors of clinical breast examination, mammography, and Pap test screening among older women. *Journal of the American Academy of Nurse Practitioners, 8*(5), 231–236.
Ship, J. A., Pearson, J. D., Cruise, L. J., Brant, L. J., & Metter, E. J. (1996). Longitudinal changes in smell identification. *Journal of Gerontology, Series A, Biological Sciences and Medicine and Medical Sciences, 51*(2):M86–M91.
Sonnenberg, A, & Koch, T. (1989). Physician visits in the United States for constipation. *Digestive Diseases and Science, 34,* 606–611.
Talley, N., Flemin, K., Evans, J. O'Keefe, E., Weaver, A., Sinsmeister, A., & Melton, L. Constipation in an elderly community: A study of prevalence and potential risk factors. *The American Journal of Gastroenterology, 91,*19–25.
Teno, J., Branco, K., Mor, V., Phillips, C., Hawes, C., Morris, J., & Fries, B. (1997). Changes in advance care planning in nursing homes before and after the client self-determination act: Report of a 10-State survey. *Journal of the American Geriatrics Society, 45,* 939–944.
Tinetti, M., & Ginter, S. (1988). Identifying mobility dysfunctions in elderly clients: Standard neuormuscular examination or direct assessment? *Journal of the American Medical Association, 259,* 1190–1193.
Van Wynsberghe, D., Noback, C. & Carola, R. (1995). *Human anatomy and physiology* (3rd ed.). New York: McGraw-Hill.
Venes, D. (ed.). (2001). *Taber's cyclopedic medical dictionary,* (19th ed.). Philadelphia: F. A. Davis.
Watson, Y., Arfken, C., & Birge, S. (1993). Clock completion: An objective screening test for dementia. *Journal of the American Geriatrics Society, 41,* 1235–1240.
Weinberg, A., Pals, J., McGlinchey-Berroth, R., & Minaker, K. (1994). Indices of dehydration among frail nursing home clients: Highly variable but stable over time. *Journal of the American Geriatics Society, 42,* 1070–1073.
Weinstein, B. (1994). Age related hearing loss: How to screen for it and when to intervene. *Geriatrics, 49,* 40–46.
Whitehead, W., Drinkwater, W., & Cheskin, L. (1989). Constipation in the elderly living at home: Definition, prevalence, and relationship to lifestyle and health status. *Journal of the American Geriatrics Society, 37,* 423–429.
Whitehead, W., Chaussade, S., Corazziari, E., & Kumar, D. (1991). Report of an international workshop on management of constipation. *Gastroenterology International, 4,* 99–113.
Yesavage, J., Brink, T., Rose, T., Lum, O., Huang, V., Adey, M., & Leirer, O. (1983). Development and validation of a geriatric depression screening scale: A preliminary report. *Journal of Psychiatric Research,17,* 37–49.
Young, D., Appel, L., Jee, S. & Miller, E. (1999). The effects of aerobic exercise and tai chi on BP in older people: Results of a randomized trial. *Journal of the American Geriatrics Society, 47,* 257–284.

Appendix C Guidelines for Assessing the Homeless Person

Hitchcock, J., Schubert, P., & Thomas, S. (1999). *Community health nursing caring in action.* Albany: Delmar.
O'Connell, J. J., & Groth, J. (1991). *The manual of common communicable diseases in shelters.* Boston: Boston Health Care for the Homeless Program.
Smith, C., & Maurer, F. (2000). *Community health nursing theory and practice* (2nd ed.). Philadelphia: W. B. Saunders.
The Stewart B. McKinney Homeless Assistance Act, (1987). Public Law 100–107.
Web Sites:
Healthcare for the Homeless Information Resource Center: General information, research, reports, bibliographies, history, links
The National Coalition for the Homeless: information about the homeless condition, legislation and police, links

Illustration Credits

Chapter 1

Figure 1–1, p. 4: From Doenges, M., Moorhouse, M., & Geissler, A. (1997). *Nursing care plans: Guidelines for individualizing patient care* (5th ed.). Philadelphia: F. A. Davis, p. 7, with permission.

Chapter 8

Figure 8–4, p. 177: Courtesy of MCP-Hahnemann University Department of Dermatology, Philadelphia, PA.

Figure 8–5, p. 177: Goldsmith, L. A., Lazarus, G. S., & Tharp, M. D. (1997): *Adult and pediatric dermatology; A color guide to diagnosis and treatment,* Philadelphia: F. A. Davis, with permission.

Art for all figures depicting abnormal conditions, pp. 159–193: Courtesy of MCP-Hahnemann University Department of Dermatology, Philadelphia, PA; ©3M Health Care, used with permission; and Goldsmith, L. A., Lazarus, G. S., & Tharp, M. D. (1997): *Adult and pediatric dermatology: A color guide to diagnosis and treatment,* Philadelphia, F. A. Davis, with permission.

Chapter 9

Art for Inspection of the Head and Face, pp. 217–218: Acromegaly, Cushing's syndrome courtesy of MCP-Hahnemann University Department of Dermatology, Philadelphia, PA. Bell's palsy courtesy of Wills Eye Hospital, Philadelphia, PA.

Art for Inspection of the Nose, pp. 221–222: Polyps and Deviated septum courtesy of J. Barabe, CMSP Clearing House.

Art for Inspection of the Mouth and Throat, pp. 223–228: Cheilitis, Allergic response, Cancer on lip, Malocclusion, Tetracycline staining, Fluorosis, Leukemia, Early HIV peridontitis, Advanced HIV peridontitis, Lichen planus, Leukoplakia, Cancer on oral mucosa, Fordyce granules, Torus palatinus, Torus mandible, Cocaine use, Geographic tongue, Parotitis, Glossitis, Cancer of the tongue, Herpangioma courtesy of Tina S. Liang, DMD, Bala-Cynwyd, PA. Chancre, Aphthous ulcer from Goldsmith, L. A., Lazarus, G. S., & Tharp, M. D. (1997): *Adult and pediatric dermatology: A color guide to diagnosis and treatment,* Philadelphia, F. A. Davis, with permission. Dental caries, Gum hyperplasia, Gingival recession, Chronic gingivitis, HIV palatal candidiasis courtesy of Robert A. Levine, DDS, PC, Philadelphia, PA, and Sheryl Radin, DDS, Pediatric Dentistry. Red, "beefy" tongue courtesy of SPL, CMSP Clearing House. Black, hairy tongue courtesy of MCP-Hahnemann University Department of Dermatology, Philadelphia, PA. Enlarged tonsils with exudates courtesy of SIU BIOMED, CMSP Clearing House.

Art for Inspection of the Neck, p. 231: Cervical adenitis courtesy of MCP-Hahnemann University Department of Dermatology, Philadelphia, PA.

Art for Common Abnormalities, pp. 241–243: Acute cervical adenitis courtesy of MCP-Hahnemann University Department of Dermatology, Philadelphia, PA. Polyps courtesy of J. Barabe, CMSP Clearing House. Tonsillitis, Enlarged tonsils with exudates courtesy of SIU BIOMED, CMSP Clearing House.

Chapter 10

Art for Assessing the Extraocular Muscles, pp. 267–269: Exotropia, Congenital exotropia courtesy of Wills Eye Hospital, Philadelphia, PA.

Art for Inspecting the External Structures, pp. 269–277: Soft contact lenses, Hard contact lenses, Lice, Blepharoconjunctivitis, Entropion, Ectropion, Exophthalmos, Ptosis, Squamous cell carcinoma, Xanthelasma, Chalazion, Hordeolum, Dacryocystitis, Acute allergic conjunctivitis, Pterygium, Pinguecula, Subconjunctival hemorrhage, Nevus, Papilloma, Diffuse episcleritis, Arcus senilis, Corneal abrasion, Healing corneal ulcer, Mature cataract, Anisocoria, Adie's pupil, Hypopyon, Hyphema, Acute angle closure courtesy of Wills Eye Hospital, Philadelphia, PA.

Art for Performing an Ophthalmic Examination, pp. 280–282: Normal fundus, Acute papilledema, Chronic papilledema, Glaucomatous optic nerve, Optic neuritis, Optic nerve pallor, Hypertensive changes, Diabetic retinopathy, Malignant hypertension, Age-related macular degeneration, Advanced macular degeneration courtesy of Wills Eye Hospital, Philadelphia, PA.

Art for Common Abnormalities (eyes), pp. 285–287: All figures courtesy of Wills Eye Hospital, Philadelphia, PA.

Art for Focused Assessment of the External Ear: Congenital ear anomaly and low-set ears from *Variations and minor departures in infants,* Mead Johnson Nutritional Division, Evansville, IN, with permission.

Art for Performing an Otoscopic Examination, pp. 304–305: Exostosis, Foreign body, External otitis, Normal tympanic membrane, Serous otitis, Otitis media, Perforated TM, Hemotympanum, Adhesive otitis media, Cholesteatoma from *A guide to the use of diagnostic instruments in eye and ear examinations,* Welch Allyn, Inc., Skaneateles Falls, NY, with permission.

Art for Common Abnormalities (ears), pp. 311–312: All figures courtesy of Ann Marie Ramsey, RN, MSN, CPNP, Section of Pediatric Otolaryngology, University of Michigan Medical Center.

Chapter 13

Art for Inspecting the Veins and Lymph Nodes, pp. 426–428: Lymphedema courtesy of MCP-Hahnemann University Department of Dermatology, Philadelphia, PA. Venous stasis ulcer and Arterial insufficiency from: © 3M Health Care, used with permission.

Chapter 15

Boxes, Four-Quadrant Method and Nine Regions of the Abdomen, p. 490: From Thompson, J. M., & Wilson, S. F. (1996). *Health assessment for nursing practice.* St.Louis: Mosby-Year Book, pp. 448–449, adapted with permission.

Chapter 16

Art for Inspecting the External Genitalia, pp. 542–544: Pubic lice courtesy of Wills Eye Hospital, Philadelphia, PA. Herpes vulvovaginitis courtesy of MCP-Hahnemann University Department of Dermatology, Philadelphia, PA.

Art for Speculum Examination of the Internal Genitalia, pp. 546–547: Chadwick's sign courtesy of Women's Health Care Group, Philadelphia, PA.

Chapter 17

Art for Inspecting the Genitalia, pp. 576–578: Chancre, Genital herpes from Goldsmith, L., Lazarus, G., & Tharp, M. (1997). *Adult and pediatric dermatology: A color guide to diagnosis and treatment.* Philadelphia: F. A. Davis, p. 464. Chancroid, Genital warts on penis, Genital warts on scrotum, Tinea cruris courtesy of Hahnemann University Department of Dermatology, Philadelphia, PA.

Art for Common Abnormalities, pp. 586–588: Chancroid, Genital warts courtesy of Hahnemann University Department of Dermatology, Philadelphia, PA.Chancre, Genital herpes from Goldsmith, L., Lazarus, G., & Tharp, M. (1997). *Adult and pediatric dermatology: A color guide to diagnosis and treatment.* Philadelphia: F. A. Davis, p. 464.

Chapter 18

Art for Assessing Joints and Muscles, pp. 620–632: Rheumatoid arthritis, Heberden's nodes, Gouty arthritis, Callus courtesy of MCP-Hahnemann University Department of Dermatology, Philadelphia, PA.

Chapter 21

Art for Head-to-Toe Physical Assessment, pp. 733–742: Chadwick's sign, Circular cervical opening: nulliparous, Slit-like cervical opening: multiparous courtesy of Women's Health Care Group, Philadelphia, PA.

Chapter 22

Figure 22–1, p. 750: From Venes, D. (ed.): *Taber's cyclopedic medical dictionary* (19th ed.), F.A. Davis, 2001, p. 425.

Chapter 23

Art for Performing a Head-to-Toe Physical Assessment, pp. 789–793: Baby bottle caries courtesy of Robert A. Levine, DDS, PC, Philadelphia, PA, and Sheryl Radin, DDS, Pediatric Dentistry.

Chapter 25

Art for Head-to-Toe Physical Assessment, pp. 844–852: Acrocordon, Senile purpura, Heberden's nodes courtesy of MCP-Hahnemann University Department of Dermatology, Philadelphia, PA. Arcus senilis courtesy of Wills Eye Hospital, Philadelphia, PA.

Index

An "f" following a page number indicates a figure; a "b" following a page number indicates a box.